ZINSSER

MICROBIOLOGY

16th Edition

Zinsser
MICROBIOLOGY
16th Edition

Edited by

Wolfgang K. Joklik, D.Phil.

James B. Duke Distinguished Professor of Microbiology and Immunology
Chairman, Department of Microbiology and Immunology
Duke University School of Medicine

Hilda P. Willett, Ph.D.

Professor of Microbiology
Duke University School of Medicine

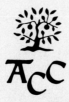

APPLETON-CENTURY-CROFTS/New York

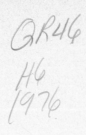

Library of Congress Catalog Card Number: 76-23518

Prentice-Hall International, Inc., London
Prentice-Hall of Australia, Pty. Ltd., Sydney
Prentice-Hall of India Private Limited, New Delhi
Prentice-Hall of Japan, Inc., Tokyo
Prentice-Hall of Southeast Asia (Pte.) Ltd., Singapore

PRINTED IN THE UNITED STATES OF AMERICA
0-8385-9976-1

To the memory of

PHILIP HANSON HISS, JR.,
HANS ZINSSER,
AND STANHOPE BAYNE-JONES

*whose labors over more than one third of a
century have made this textbook a favorite
with students of medicine and public health*

Contributors

Wolfgang K. Joklik, D. Phil.

James B. Duke Distinguished Professor of Microbiology and Immunology; Chairman, Department of Microbiology and Immunology, Duke University School of Medicine

Hilda P. Willett, Ph.D.

Professor of Microbiology, Duke University School of Medicine

D. Bernard Amos, M.D.

James B. Duke Distinguished Professor of Immunology and Professor of Experimental Surgery, Duke University School of Medicine

C. Edward Buckley III, M.D.

Associate Professor of Medicine and Associate Professor of Immunology, Duke University School of Medicine

Rebecca H. Buckley, M.D.

Associate Professor of Pediatrics and Associate Professor of Immunology, Duke University School of Medicine

Richard O. Burns, Ph.D.

Professor of Microbiology, Duke University School of Medicine

Thomas R. Cate, M.D.

Formerly Associate Professor of Medicine, Duke University School of Medicine; Presently Associate Professor of Medicine, Baylor College of Medicine

Norman F. Conant, Ph.D.

James B. Duke Distinguished Professor of Mycology Emeritus, Duke University School of Medicine

James J. Crawford, Ph.D.

Associate Professor of Oral Biology and Endodontics, University of North Carolina School of Dentistry

Peter Cresswell, Ph.D.

Assistant Professor of Immunology, Duke University School of Medicine

Jeffrey R. Dawson, Ph.D.

Assistant Professor of Immunology, Duke University School of Medicine

Thomas E. Frothingham, M.D.

Professor of Pediatrics and Professor of Community Health Sciences, Duke University School of Medicine

Harry A. Gallis, M.D.

Associate in Nephrology and Associate in Microbiology, Duke University School of Medicine

John F. Griffith, M.D.

Associate Professor of Pediatrics and Assistant Professor of Medicine, Duke University School of Medicine

Laura T. Gutman, M.D.

Assistant Professor of Pediatrics and Assistant Clinical Professor of Pharmacology, Duke University School of Medicine

Gale B. Hill, Ph.D.

Assistant Professor of Obstetrics and Gynecology; Assistant Professor of Microbiology, Duke University School of Medicine

Samuel L. Katz, M.D.

Wilburt C. Davison Professor of Pediatrics and Chairman, Department of Pediatrics, Duke University School of Medicine

David J. Lang, M.D.

Professor of Pediatrics and Associate Professor of Microbiology, Duke University School of Medicine

John E. Larsh, Jr., Sc.D.

Professor of Parasitology, School of Public Health and School of Medicine, University of North Carolina and Duke University School of Medicine

Nelson L. Levy, Ph.D.

Assistant Professor of Immunology, Duke University School of Medicine

Thomas G. Mitchell, Ph.D.
Assistant Professor of Microbiology, Duke University School of Medicine

Suydam Osterhout, M.D., Ph.D.
Professor of Microbiology and Professor of Medicine, Duke University School of Medicine

Emily G. Reisner, Ph.D.
Associate in Immunology, Duke University School of Medicine

Wendell F. Rosse, M.D.
Professor of Medicine and Professor of Immunology, Duke University School of Medicine

Hilliard F. Seigler, M.D.
Associate Professor of Surgery and Associate Professor of Immunology, Duke University School of Medicine

Daniel J. Sexton, M.D.
Formerly Fellow in Medicine, Duke University School of Medicine; Presently Resident in Medicine, University of Missouri Medical Center, Columbia, Missouri

David T. Smith, M.D.
James B. Duke Distinguished Professor of Microbiology Emeritus, Duke University School of Medicine

Ralph Snyderman, Ph.D.
Associate Professor of Medicine and Associate Professor of Immunology, Duke University School of Medicine

Robert W. Wheat, Ph.D.
Professor of Microbiology and Assistant Professor of Biochemistry, Duke University School of Medicine

John K. Whisnant, Jr., M.D.
Associate in Medicine, Duke University School of Medicine

Catherine M. Wilfert, M.D.
Associate Professor of Pediatrics and Associate Professor of Microbiology, Duke University School of Medicine

Peter Zwadyk, Ph.D.
Associate Professor of Pathology and Assoicate Professor of Microbiology, Duke University School of Medicine

Preface

With each passing year the term *microbiology* becomes a less satisfactory umbrella for the many disciplines that it attempts to cover. Bacteriology, immunology, virology, mycology, and parasitology have each long since become separate and independent disciplines in their own right, and they are together in a single text, not because they are in any way related, but simply because they deal with the agents of infectious disease in man and with the mechanisms employed by the host in his defense.

In spite of the undeniable triumphs of antibiotic chemotherapy, which has saved untold millions of lives during the past three decades and which very likely represents the greatest single triumph of biomedical science, "microbes" are by no means "conquered"; they continue to cause infections that demand a large amount of the physician's time. Discoveries in this field continue to be made at a breathtaking pace: New infectious agents, unsuspected properties of known agents, additional mechanisms for the genesis and persistence of infection, and advances in our understanding of the behavior of infectious agents at the molecular, cellular, and organismal levels are constantly reported. As a result, the scope and complexity of the material to be presented to students expand rapidly, and although the literature abounds with excellent papers and reviews, the compilation of a comprehensive textbook of manageable size becomes increasingly difficult.

This new edition of Zinsser Microbiology, the 16th, is designed to fulfill several clearly definable needs. First, it is intended for use by medical students experiencing their first exposure to medical microbiology. To that end, there is presented, in addition to a description of the pathogenic infectious agents and the diseases that they cause, a discussion of the biochemistry, molecular biology, and genetics of microorganisms, the purpose of which is not only to permit an understanding of the basic principles, for example, of

the mode of action of antimicrobial agents, the mechanisms of virus multiplication, and molecular and cellular immunology, but also to provide a firm basis for growth with the field during the remainder of the student's professional career. Second, the book is intended as a comprehensive text for advanced medical students, house officers, and practicing physicians, providing in a single volume information not only on the more common infectious diseases endemic in the United States, but also on diseases such as diphtheria, poliomyelitis, and smallpox, which are seen so rarely nowadays that they may not be recognized by the younger physicians. Finally, the book is designed as a reference source for instructors; to that end each chapter is supplemented with a selection of both reviews and important original papers that will permit a rapid entrée to any specialized topic that may require further study.

The 16th edition represents a very extensive revision of the 15th edition. The section on medical bacteriology, Section III, has been completely rewritten by a group of new contributors who bring to the subject a fresh approach and new viewpoints. The section has been carefully edited by a single author so as to ensure coverage of all important areas, a uniform format, and stylistic homogeneity. Emphasis is placed on correlating the basic and clinical aspects of each infectious agent so that the student may acquire an appreciation of how fundamental research may be used in unravelling the complexities of the host–parasite relationship. Each chapter consists of (1) an introduction to the important biologic properties of the organism, (2) a description of the clinical infection in man, including a discussion of mechanisms of pathogenicity, (3) a section on laboratory diagnosis that provides information on modern culture and immunologic procedures, and (4) a discussion of the currently recommended treatment.

Another section that has been completely rewritten

is that on immunology (Section II), where a group of authors has combined to provide a comprehensive account of both basic and clinical immunology. The section on bacterial physiology (Section I) has been extensively revised, particularly the chapters that deal with the molecular basis of genetics and gene transfer. Emphasis in this section continues to be placed on properties and mechanisms unique to bacterial cells, the mode of action of antibacterial agents, and the mechanisms of macromolecular biosynthesis. In the section on basic virology (Section IV) several chapters, such as those on viral genetics and tumor viruses, have been completely rewritten because of the multitude of recent advances, while the remainder have been extensively revised. The final three sections, those on clinical virology, mycology, and parasitology, have been brought up to date by their authors. However, here also there are several entirely new chapters, including those on arboviruses, progressive multifocal leukoencephalopathy, and general characteristics of fungi.

In reference to the bibliography, we have once again elected not to reference specific statements in the text but to append to each chapter a list of recent reviews and key original papers. The former will quickly guide the reader to any specific aspect of microbiology and immunology that he wishes to pursue; the latter makes available the detailed considerations and circumstances that have gone into the genesis of key discoveries, and many of the papers that are cited already are, or no doubt will soon become, "classics."

We have tried not to increase the size of the book—not an easy task in view of the enormous amount of new information that has accumulated since the publication of the last edition in 1972. Obviously, this has entailed the omission of a certain amount of older material; however, we are confident that there are no major gaps and that in our presentation of the newest advances we have not sacrificed careful and logical explanations of fundamental principles.

With two notable exceptions, all contributors to this edition are (or were) on the faculty of Duke University Medical Center, and most of them have an appointment in the Department of Microbiology and Immunology. The two contributors who are not at Duke are Dr. John E. Larsh, Jr., who, as in several previous editions, wrote the section on parasitology, and Dr. J. J. Crawford, who has once again contributed the chapter on the oral flora. Both are on the staff of the University of North Carolina at Chapel Hill; Dr. Larsh is also an Adjunct Professor of Microbiology at Duke University.

The list of individuals who have helped to produce this volume extends far beyond the circle of our colleagues who contributed textual material and to whom we are profoundly indebted. We would especially like to thank our many colleagues who permitted us to use illustrative material, and who almost invariably supplied us with original photographs, and the many publishers who allowed us to reproduce previously published material. We would also like to thank Lynda Frejlach, who did a superb job in drawing the innumerable charts and diagrams, and the many secretaries who have cheerfully typed and retyped the manuscript many times. Finally, we wish to express our appreciation to the staff of Appleton-Century-Crofts for their efficient cooperation in producing this new edition.

Wolfgang K. Joklik

Hilda P. Willett

Preface to the First Edition

The volume here presented is primarily a treatise on the fundamental laws and technic of bacteriology, as illustrated by their application to the study of pathogenic bacteria.

So ubiquitous are the bacteria and so manifold their activities that bacteriology, although one of the youngest of sciences, has already been divided into special fields—medical, sanitary, agricultural, and industrial—having little in common, except problems of general bacterial physiology and certain fundamental technical procedures.

From no other point of approach, however, is such a breadth of conception attainable, as through the study of bacteria in their relation to disease processes in man and animals. Through such a study one must become familiar not only with the growth characteristics and products of the bacteria apart from the animal body, thus gaining a knowledge of methods and procedures common to the study of pathogenic and nonpathogenic organisms, but also with those complicated reactions taking place between the bacteria and their products on the one hand and the cells and fluids of the animal body on the other—reactions which often manifest themselves as symptoms and lesions of disease or by visible changes in the test tube.

Through a study and comprehension of the processes underlying these reactions, our knowledge of cell physiology has been broadened, and facts of inestimable value have been discovered, which have thrown light upon some of the most obscure problems of infection and immunity and have led to hitherto unsuspected methods of treatment and diagnosis. Thus, through medical bacteriology—that highly specialized offshoot of general biology and pathology—have been given back to the parent sciences and to medicine in general methods and knowledge of the widest application.

It has been our endeavor, therefore, to present this phase of our subject in as broad and critical a manner as possible in the sections dealing with infection and immunity and with methods of biological diagnosis and treatment of disease, so that the student and practitioner of medicine, by becoming familiar with underlying laws and principles, may not only be in a position to realize the meaning and scope of some of these newer discoveries and methods, but may be in a better position to decide for themselves their proper application and limitation.

We have not hesitated, whenever necessary for a proper understanding of processes of bacterial nutrition or physiology, or for breadth of view in considering problems of the relation of bacteria to our food supply and environment, to make free use of illustrations from the more special fields of agricultural and sanitary bacteriology, and some special methods of the bacteriology of sanitation are given in the last division of the book, dealing with the bacteria in relation to our food and environment.

In conclusion it may be said that the scope and arrangement of subjects treated in this book are the direct outcome of many years of experience in the instruction of students in medical and in advanced university courses in bacteriology, and that it is our hope that this volume may not only meet the needs of such students but may prove of value to the practitioner of medicine for whom it has also been written.

It is a pleasure to acknowledge the courtesy of those who furnished us with illustrations for use in the text, and our indebtedness to Dr. Gardner Hopkins and Professor Francis Carter Wood for a number of the photomicrographs taken especially for this work.

P. H. Hiss, Jr.

H. Zinsser

Contents

SECTION THREE: MEDICAL BACTERIOLOGY

ZINSSER

MICROBIOLOGY

16th Edition

1

The Historical Development of Medical Microbiology

The history of many concepts now embodied in the doctrines of bacteriology is an account of attempts to solve the problems of the origin of life, the putrefaction of dead organic materials, and the nature of communicable changes in the bodies of living men and animals. The visible aspects of these phenomena were as apparent and as interesting to ancient observers as they are to modern biologists. In the past, notions of ultimate causes were derived from the available factual knowledge colored by the theologic and philosophic tenets of the time. The early history of what has become the science of microbiology is to be found, therefore, in the writings of the priests, philosophers, and scientists who studied and pondered these basic biologic problems.

Infection and Contagion Among ancient peoples epidemic and even endemic diseases were regarded as supernatural in origin and sent by the gods as punishment for the sins of man. The treatment and, more important, the prevention of these diseases were sought by sacrifices and lustrations to appease the anger of the gods. Since man is willful, wanton, and sinful by nature there was never any difficulty in finding a particular set of sins to justify a specific epidemic.

The concept of contagion and the practice of hygiene were, however, not entirely unknown to ancient man. The Old Testament is often quoted as indicating the belief that leprosy was contagious and could be transmitted by contact. The principle of contagion by invisible creatures was later recorded by Varro in the second century BC, and the concept was familiar to Greek, Roman, and Arabic writers. Roger Bacon, in the thirteenth century, more than a millennium later, postulated that invisible living creatures produced disease. The Venetian, Fracastorius, in 1546, wrote from a knowledge of syphilis that communicable disease was transmitted by living germs, "seminaria morbi," through direct contact or by intermediary inanimate fomites and through air "ad distans." Fracastorius expressed the opinion that the seeds of disease, passing from one infected individual to another, caused the same disease in the recipient as in the donor. This clear expression of the germ theory of disease was ahead of its time and awaited experimental observation and proof of the reality of these hypothetical living germs.

First Observation of Bacteria The direct observation of microorganisms awaited development of the microscope. The human eye cannot see objects smaller than 30 μ (1/1000 inch) in diameter, and although the knowledge of magnifying lenses reaches back to the time of Archimedes, the science of optics was not clarified until the fourteenth century by the Franciscan monk, Roger Bacon. The telescope was invented by Galileo in 1608, followed by the microscope in the same century. The first person known to have made glass lenses powerful enough to observe and describe bacteria was the amateur lens grinder, Anton van Leeuwenhoek (1632-1723), of Delft, Holland. In letters to the experimentalist group, The Royal Society of London, Leeuwenhoek described many "animalcules," including the three major morphologic forms of bacteria (rod, sphere, and spiral), various free-living and parasitic protozoa from human and animal feces, filamentous fungi, and globular bodies we now know as yeasts, and he discovered spermatozoa. In his lifetime he made some 250 single-lensed microscopes. He searched everywhere in this new microcosmic world he had discovered. In letters from 1676 to 1683, he described the sizes, shapes, and even the motility of bacteria (Fig. 1-1) using simple single biconvex lens microscopes, such as illustrated in Figure 1-2. There is no doubt that he saw the most

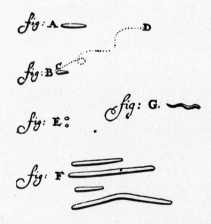

FIG. 1-1. Leeuwenhoek's picture of bacteria from the human mouth. Dobell's identifications are as follows: A. A motile *Bacillus*. B. *Selenomonas sputigena*. E. Micrococci. F. *Leptothrix buccans*. G. probably *Spirochaeta buccalis*. (From Dobel: Anton van Leeuwenhoek and His "Little Animals," 1932. Courtesy of Harcourt, Brace and Co.)

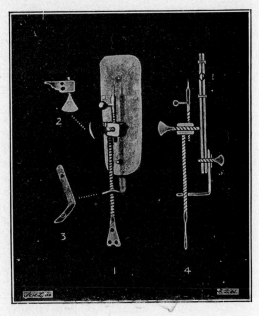

FIG. 1-2. Leeuwenhoek's "Microscope." (From Dobell: Anton van Leeuwenhoek and His "Little Animals," 1932. Courtesy of Harcourt, Brace and Co.)

usual forms of bacteria, the cocci, bacilli, and spirochetes. His observational reports were enthusiastic and accurate and developed some interest at the time, but unfortunately Leeuwenhoek did all this as a hobby and left no students to continue his work. However, in 1678, Robert Hooke, who developed the compound microscope, confirmed Leeuwenhoek's discoveries. Microorganisms were then occasionally studied by those primarily interested in classifying the various life forms observable with the microscope. These observations lay dormant and were not exploited by those interested in disease. The following 125 to 150 years witnessed the gradual development of knowledge and acceptance of the experimental method, which slowly disseminated throughout the expanding learned centers of the world. Improved microscopes became generally available only in the 1800s as a result of the Industrial Revolution which allowed rapid technologic advances. Even then, no notable advance in microbiology was accomplished until after the attention of the scientific world was focused on microbes and their role in the controversies of the doctrine of spontaneous generation and the associated phenomenon of fermentation.

Spontaneous Generation   The controversy over man's ability to create life carried over from Greek mythology. Even Aristotle (384-322 BC) thought animals could originate from the soil. Samson, in the Bible (Old Testament), and again Virgil, about 40 BC, described recipes for producing bees from honey, and for centuries it was believed that maggots could be produced by exposing meat to warmth in the air. This was not refuted until Francesco Redi (1626-1697) proved that gauze placed over a jar containing meat prevented maggots forming in the meat. Redi also observed that adult flies, attracted by the odor of meat through the gauze, laid eggs on the cloth, and maggots developed from the eggs. Recipes for producing mice and other similar life forms in litter and refuse were gradually disproved and discarded in similar fashion. However, the question was not settled in all minds. When microbes were discovered, their association with putrefaction and fermentations again raised the question of spontaneous generation. John Needham, in 1749, observed the appearance of microorganisms in putrefying meat and interpreted this as spontaneous generation. Spallanzani, however, boiled beef broth for an hour, sealed the flasks, and observed no formation of microbes. Needham, and 100 years later, Pouchet (1859), argued that access of air was necessary for the spontaneous generation of microscopic living beings. Disproof came from several lines of evidence. Franz Schulze (1815-1873) passed air through strong acids and then into boiled broth, while Theodor Schwann (1810-1882) passed air through red hot tubes and observed no growth. About 1850, Schroeder and von Dusch filtered air through cotton filters into broth and observed no growth. Pasteur was able to filter microorganisms from the air and concluded that this was the source of contamination. He developed an aseptic technique, using heat, in order to transfer and work with his microbes and, finally, in 1859, in public controversy with Pouchet, prepared boiled broths in flasks with long narrow gooseneck tubes which were open to the air. Air could pass but microorganisms settled in the gooseneck, and no growth developed in any of the flasks. Finally, a British physicist, John Tyndall (1820-1893), proved that dust carried the germs, and the story was complete. Tyndall also found that bacterial spores could be killed by successive heating, a process now known as tyndallization.

The Germ Theory of Disease EMPIRICAL OBSERVATIONS. A firm basis for the causal nature of infectious disease was established only in the latter half of the nineteenth century. One of the first proofs came from Agostino Bassi who, in the early 1800s, proved that a fungus, later named *Botrytis bassiana* in his honor, caused a disease of silkworms called "muscardine" in France and "mal segno" in Italy. In 1839, Schoenlein found the causative fungus in lesions of favus, and in 1846 Eichstedt noted the contagiousness of pityriasis versicolor and discovered a fungus in skin scrapings from patients.

In the 1840s, the American poet-physician, Oliver Wendell Holmes, wrote "The Contagiousness of Puerperal Fever," in which he suggested that disease was caused by germs carried from one new mother to another. In 1861, Ignaz Semmelweis, who had drastically decreased childbirth deaths by antiseptic techniques and practices, published his extremely important "The Cause, Concept and Prophylaxis of Childbed Fever." However, the importance of antiseptics in reducing contagious disease was not fully realized until the late 1870s, when Joseph Lister demonstrated the value of spraying operating rooms with aqueous phenol.

LESSONS LEARNED FROM FERMENTATIONS. Further emphasis on microbial activities came from the work of Louis Pasteur from the 1850s to the 1880s. In studies on the diseases of wine, Pasteur demonstrated that alcoholic fermentation of grapes, fruit, and grains was caused by microbes, then called "ferments." In good wine batches certain types of "ferments" existed in the vats, while in poor or bad fermentations other types of microbes were found, some of which Pasteur found to be capable of growing anaerobically. He suggested eliminating the bad types of "ferments" from fresh juices by heating at 63C for one half-hour, then cooling and reinoculating with a culture from the satisfactory vats. Pasteur's success with the problems of the wine industry led the French government to request that he study a disease, pébrine, which was ruining the silkworm industry in Southern France. Pasteur struggled with this problem for several years before he isolated the causative organism and showed that farmers could eliminate the problem by using healthy noninfected breeding stock.

OBSERVATIONS AND EXPERIMENTS WITH ANIMALS. In 1850 Rayer and Davaine observed rod-shaped microorganisms in the blood of animals which had died of anthrax. Rayer recalled the experiments in 1825 of Barthélemy who had shown that anthrax was transmissible by inoculation in series in sheep, and by 1863 Davaine had experimentally transmitted anthrax by blood containing these rods but not by normal blood from which rods were absent. In 1872 Obermeier discovered the relationship of a spirillum to relapsing fever and demonstrated for the first time the presence of a pathogenic microorganism in the blood of a human being.

IMPORTANCE OF PURE CULTURE TECHNIQUES. Through all this time, etiologic research was not based on pure culture work. Pure cultures were obtained largely by accident, and investigators had no way, except by crude morphologic microscopic examination, of knowing when contaminants were present. This resulted in much equivocal thinking and work that hindered progress.

The first pure or axenic culture technique was developed by Joseph Lister in 1878. Lister used a syringe to make serial dilutions in liquid media to obtain pure cultures of a simple type of organism which he named *Bacterium (Lactobacillus) lactis*. Meanwhile, Koch, as a student of Henle who insisted on proof that an organism caused disease, was also developing and refining techniques for the isolation of pure cultures. From the work of others, notably Ehrlich, Koch learned methods of staining bacteria on glass with aniline dyes for microscopic observation. In his early work on anthrax, Koch used sterile aqueous humor of the eyes of animals as a growth medium. But, having seen the advantages of older solid but opaque media such as potato, beets, starch, bread, egg white, and meat, Koch developed a transparent solid medium by mixing gelatin with Löffler's peptone solution. The gelatin mixture liquefied on warming, could be heat-sterilized and aseptically poured into plates, and upon cooling, it solidified. Microorganisms streaked upon it developed into macroscopic colonies where they were deposited as the result of the growth of a single invisible cell. However, gelatin liquefies at a relatively low temperature (26C), and Koch later switched to agar, the transparent red seaweed extract which solidifies below 43C.

ETIOLOGIC PROOF OF INFECTIOUS AGENTS.
Koch was able to isolate the anthrax organism in pure culture by streaking on his solid media and found that even after many transfers, the organism could still cause the same symptoms and disease when inoculated into animals. On the basis of his experiences, Koch formulated criteria which provided proof that a specific bacterium caused a disease. We now call these Koch's postulates.

1. The organism must always be found in the diseased animal, but not in healthy ones.
2. The organism must be isolated from diseased animals and grown in pure culture away from the animal.
3. The organism isolated in pure culture must initiate and reproduce the disease when reinoculated into susceptible animals.
4. The organism should be reisolated from the experimentally infected animals.

Koch's work thus provided impetus and means for proof of the germ theory of disease.°

The 20-year period following Koch's work was the Golden Age of Bacteriology. By 1900 almost all the major bacterial disease organisms had been described. The list included anthrax *(Bacillus anthracis)*, diphtheria *(Corynebacterium diphtheriae)*, typhoid fever *(Salmonella typhosa)*, gonorrhea *(Neisseria gonorrhoea)*, gas gangrene *(Clostridium perfringens)*, tetanus or lockjaw *(Clostridium tetani)*, dysentery *(Shigella dysenteriae)*, syphilis *(Treponema pallidum)*, and others.

Viruses Only with advances in technique and improvement in apparatus is it possible to make fundamental advances through new ideas and observations. The development of bacteriologic filters and the discovery of viruses is a case in point.

BACTERIOLOGIC FILTERS.
As an alternate to heat sterilization, unsuccessful efforts to re-

° *The leprosy organism has not been grown in vitro as yet, nor have all of Koch's postulates been fulfilled with some long-term viral diseases. Current thought suggests that in some viral diseases certain symptoms may occur long after the initial infection, while in others, fastidious or latent agents may not be directly demonstrable.*

move bacteria from solutions by filtration through paper and similar materials led Chamberland and Pasteur to test and develop unglazed porcelain as the first successful bacterial filter (1871-1884). The Berkefeld filter of Kieselguhr (diatomaceous earth) was developed shortly thereafter in 1891. Synthetic polymer filters of cellulose nitrate, cellulose acetate, polyester, and so forth, also introduced earlier, have come into common use only in the last two decades because of technical advances allowing quality control of pore size. It is of interest to note that these are essentially space-age products developed in part for the rapid removal of microorganisms from jet and rocket fuels.

DISCOVERY OF VIRUSES.
The tobacco mosaic disease agent was first discovered by Iwanowski in 1892 in bacteria-free filtrates of diseased plant leaf juices. This finding, confirmed by Beijerinck in 1899, marked the beginning of studies on the so-called filterable agents.

The filterable agent causing foot-and-mouth disease in cattle, the first described animal virus, was discovered by Löffler and Frosch in 1898. The yellow fever virus of humans was discovered in 1900 by Walter Reed and his coworkers. Bacterial viruses, or bacteriophages, were discovered in 1915 by Twort in England and d'Herelle in France.

Viruses could not be grown in artificial media, and Koch's criteria could not be specifically applied. Because these pathogens require a living host for propagation, rapid progress in their study developed only in recent years. Again, as in the Golden Age of Bacteriology, technology had to be developed. Outstanding were the development of the electron microscope, ultracentrifugation, tissue culture, and the application of sophisticated microchemical and biochemical techniques.

It is of interest to note that some filterable agents first thought to be viruses, such as *Mycoplasma*, *Rickettsia*, and *Chlamydia*, have been found instead to be bacteria. These organisms are fastidious in growth requirements: Almost all require living host cells. However, ultrastructure and chemical analyses have shown these infectious agents to be bacteria.

Immunity Ancient peoples immunized themselves against venomous snakes by introducing small amounts of venom into scratches in the skin. The Chinese used variolization with dried material from dermic smallpox lesions for 20 centuries. This practice spread through Asia by trade routes and was well accepted in the Middle East. Later, apparently quite independently, Edward Jenner (1749-1823) noticed that milkmaids who developed cowpox were immune to smallpox. He developed the concept of "vaccination" and was able to protect susceptible people by vaccinating them with cowpox. Pasteur developed a chicken cholera vaccine in 1877. He inoculated chickens with old attenuated cultures so that a mild disease rendered the chickens immune to virulent organisms. He called this "vaccination," after Jenner's procedure. Shortly afterward, in 1881, applying the same concept, Pasteur prepared temperature-attenuated anthrax grown at 42 to 43C and protected sheep by first injecting them with these bacteria before challenging them with virulent anthrax grown at lower temperatures. Salmon and Smith, in 1884-1886, used heat-killed cultures of hog cholera bacillus to develop resistance or immunity in swine against challenge by live virulent organisms. Pasteur developed rabies vaccine in 1886, again using the idea of injecting an attenuated living disease agent. In this case, Pasteur used dried animal spinal cords without, apparently, recognizing the viral form of the disease agent.

Two schools of thought arose in explanation of the increased resistance following vaccination. Metchnikoff developed, in the 1880s, the cellular theory of protection; Bordet and others proposed the humoral, or specific, antibody concept of immunity. There is now evidence that both theories are correct. The last two decades have resulted in the isolation and, in large measure, the structural description of the major humoral immune proteins, the immune gamma globulins. These are now commonly referred to as IgA, IgG, IgD, IgM, and IgE. The function of these various immunoglobulins are currently being intensively studied. For example, the correlation of the well-known immediate allergic response with the release of histamine from mast cells as a result of the reaction between humorally injected antigen and mast cell-bound IgE was elucidated in 1970. Much current work is also being devoted to the mechanisms of cellular interactions in immune reactions which occur not only in infectious disease caused by bacteria, viruses, and fungi but also in rejection reactions of tissue and organ transplants, and of cancer cells.

Antimetabolites Many antimetabolites, which were pioneered in concept by Ehrlich in the mid to late 1800s, are now accepted household words, eg, penicillin. The modern era of antibiotics developed only after Domagk reported in 1935 that Prontosil had a dramatic effect on streptococcal infections. It was soon discovered that Prontosil was converted in the body to sulfanilamide, the active chemical agent. The success of the sulfonamides catalyzed new interest in chemotherapeutic agents. In the 1940s, as the result of the stimulus of World War II, Florey and Chain and their associates reinvestigated Fleming's penicillin, isolated and characterized it, and demonstrated its practical clinical value. As a result of millions of tests with thousands of organisms, we now have numerous other antibiotics active against almost all types of bacteria.

With the recognition that metabolic and structural differences, at the molecular level, exist between pathogenic microorganisms and human or animal hosts, the rationale of developing new chemotherapeutic compounds is now often based on exploiting these differences. There is every reason to believe that newer, more specific and potent drugs will be discovered. However, chemotherapy has created new problems. Many previously susceptible organisms are now resistant to therapeutic levels of many widely used drugs. In addition, drug sensitization reactions or allergies occasionally develop, clinical syndromes are modified, and the normal ecologic flora of the body is disturbed.

Impact of Microbiology on Genetics and Biochemistry, and the Development of Molecular Biology The enormous advantages of homogeneous populations of cells for every conceivable type of investigation was soon realized. As a result, many of the epoch-making advances during the last century in cell physiology, biochemistry, and genetics have resulted from studies with microorganisms or materials isolated from them. Over the last two decades, these advances have led to a precise way of investigating the structure and function of nucleic acids and proteins, which has become known as "molecular biology." For example, the demonstration of the central role of DNA as the repository of genetic information resulted from the studies of Griffith in the 1920s that pneumococci could be transformed from one capsular type to the other, followed by the investigations of Avery and associates, who succeeded, during the 1940s, in isolating DNA from the pneumococci and in demonstrating that it was actually the transforming factor. Final proof beyond doubt was provided by the demonstration of Hershey and Chase in 1952 that viral nucleic acid itself contained all the information necessary for virus multiplication. At the same time, Watson and Crick developed the double-helix model of DNA, which led them to suggest that one of the complementary DNA strands could serve as a template for the synthesis of the other, thus providing a description of self-perpetuating gene replication and continuity.

Demonstration of the transcription from DNA of information in the form of messenger RNA synthesized in complementary sequence to DNA soon followed, again in a microbial system. Messenger RNA was then found to be translated into polypeptides on ribosomes. By the mid 1960s Nirenberg and others had worked out the nature of the triplet RNA base sequences corresponding to the codon signals for each amino acid.

More recently, attention has focused on the nature of the signals which specify initiation and termination of transcription and translation. Although the major portion of all of this research work was and is being carried out with microbial systems, evidence is constantly coming to hand which suggests that similar mechanisms operate in the cells of higher organisms and, more particularly, in mammalian cells. An important factor in this connection has been the development of the technique of tissue culture, which permits animal cells to be grown, cloned, and passaged like microorganisms. Tissue culture of animal cells provided the essential experimental tool for the development of animal virology, which is now being studied so intensively at the molecular level that it should be possible to develop a rational system of antiviral chemotherapy within the next one or two decades, thus enabling viral diseases to be brought under effective control. Finally, the application of the concepts concerning the regulation of gene expression which are being yielded by work with microbial systems to animal cells should, in the foreseeable future, provide insight into the fundamental control mechanisms operating in both normal and abnormal cell differentiation, including cancer.

FURTHER READING

Bulloch W: The History of Bacteriology. London, Oxford Univ Press, 1938

Dobell C: Anton van Leeuwenhoek and His "Little Animals." New York, Harcourt, Brace, 1932

Dubos RJ: Biochemical Determinants of Microbial Disease. Cambridge, Mass, Harvard Univ Press, 1954

Dubos RJ: Louis Pasteur, Free Lance of Science. Boston, Little, Brown, 1950

Florey HW: Antibiotics. London, Oxford Univ Press, 1949

Marquardt M: Paul Ehrlich. New York, Henry Schuman, 1951

Meleney FL: Treatise on Surgical Infections. London, Oxford Univ Press, 1948

Metchnikoff, E. Immunity in Infective Diseases. Binnie FG (trans). Cambridge, Mass, Harvard Univ Press, 1905

Tyndall J: Essays on the Floating-Matter of the Air in Relation to Putrefaction and Infection. New York, D Appleton and Co, 1882

SECTION 1
BACTERIAL PHYSIOLOGY

2
The Classification and Identification of Bacteria

PROTISTS

Protists include the bacteria, blue-green bacteria (algae), fungi, and protozoa, which were recognized by Haeckel in 1866 as a group of single-celled microorganisms which do not form highly differentiated tissue and organ systems. With the exception of some fungi and algae, protists are unicellular or coenocytic (many nuclei per cell), and each cell is capable of independent life. At most, some algae and fungi form tissuelike aggregates of primitively differentiated cells, such as the plantlike frond of seaweeds and the mushrooms of the Basidiomycetes. The general relationship of the relatively primitive bacteria and blue-green bacteria to other protists is indicated in Figure 2-1 on the basis of increasing intracellular and intercellular complexity, in analogy with an ancestral family tree. The level of cellular organization is emphasized, rather than phylogeny, because exact and fine details of the evolution of ancestral lines are difficult to establish. For example, the bacteria (the schizomycetes or fission fungi), like the blue-green bacteria and fungi (eumycetes, the true fungi), in the past have been traditionally and arbitrarily classified phylogenetically as primitive types of plants because they produce cell walls, as do plants, and because a few bacteria and all of the

blue-green bacteria are photosynthetic, as are the more highly developed eucaryotic algae and plants. Additionally, the bacteria and the blue-green bacteria have many related cell wall and cytoplasmic features. In contrast, the photosynthetic bacteria do not produce oxygen, as do the photo-oxygen-evolving blue-green bacteria and more highly developed eucaryotic algae and plants. The summation of all these features allows only the suggestion that the bacteria, the blue-green bacteria, and the higher algae may have shared at some time in evolution an ancestral relationship with plants.

The problem of defining ancestral (phyletic) relationships among the bacteria, algae, fungi, and protozoa becomes even more complex. Unfortunately, the fossil record does not indicate the order of appearance of these microorganisms. Here again, cellular organization and metabolic patterns must be used for comparisons. For example, only a few species of non-photosynthetic bacteria and only a few lower fungi, as well as the red and brown algae and higher plants, produce cellulose-containing cell walls. This would indicate the possibility of vague ancestral relationships, at a very early stage in evolution, among the bacteria, fungi, and even the predominantly xylan-producing (hemicelluloselike) and mannan-producing green algae *(Chlorophyceae)* on the one hand, and the cellulose-producing members of the plant kingdom on the other. However, it is also possible that the ability to synthesize cellulose was developed more than once at various points in time by various nonrelated organisms. It is therefore difficult to know whether similar characteristics are due to convergent, divergent, or parallel evolution. In this respect, some lower fungi, that is, some Phycomycetes, normally produce motile cells during their development, which are therefore animal cell-like and indistinguishable from protozoa. Also, it is possible to convert *Euglena gracilis*, by drug treatment in the laboratory, from a photosynthetic alga to a nonchloroplast-containing protozoonlike cell which resembles the protozoon *Astasia longa*. However, both of these organisms appear to obtain food by absorption through their plasma membranes, as do bacteria, algae, fungi, and plants. In contrast, true protozoa and other members of the animal kingdom engulf food within membrane-bound vacuoles.

Consideration of the variety and breadth of

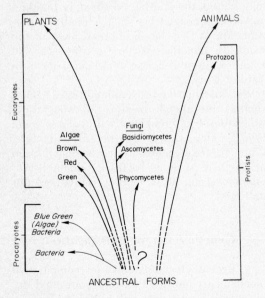

FIG. 2-1. Suggested relationship of procaryotic and eucaryotic protists, based on increasing levels of intracellular and intercellular complexity.

the above differences allows the suggestion that a multiplicity of life forms evolved simultaneously in several directions (that is, polyphyletic evolution) from a variety of primitive forms ancestral to the presently known procaryotes. For this reason, many taxonomists now believe that Kingdom status should be given to presently existing life types, such as the procaryotes, algae, fungi, and protozoa, along with the plants and animals. As a result, the procaryotes and their hypothetical ancestral forms are now grouped together in the Kingdom Procaryotae.

PROCARYOTES AND EUCARYOTES

Protists include two types of cells, the procaryotes (*pro-*, indicating a primitive nucleus) and the eucaryotes (from the Greek *eu-* true, and *-caryote-* nucleus), which are differentiated on the basis of nuclear structure and cellular organization. The bacteria and blue-green bacteria (algae) are procaryotic cells which divide amitotically by binary fission and are generally characterized as having naked, nonmembrane-bound nuclear deoxyribonucleic acid (DNA) without associated basic protein, and a semirigid cell wall of unique composition. In contrast, eucaryotic cells have a true, membrane-bound nucleus, usually containing multiple chromosomes, a mitotic apparatus, a well-defined endoplasmic reticulum, mitochondria, and a characteristic 9 + 2 fibrillar flagella structure. Eucaryotic protists include the fungi, the red, green, and brown algae, and protozoa. The higher plants and animals are, of course, also eucaryotes, which develop highly differentiated cells, tissues, and organ systems.

BACTERIAL CLASSIFICATION

According to the Linnaean scheme of classification used for higher plants and animals, bacteria may be classified as to Kingdom, Class (*-aceae*), Order (*-ales*), Family (*-aceae*), Tribe (*-ieae*), and a specific name comprised of a binomial for *Genus* and *species* designations. The specific name includes a latinized generic and a trivial species name. Concepts useful in

describing relatedness in higher eucaryotic life form have not been adequate for procaryotic cells, in that attempts to set up traditionally ordered schemes of relationships among diverse bacterial groups have failed for lack of information. Without an accurate fossil record to trace the development of the various branches of the evolutionary family tree, it is futile to construct arbitrarily phyletic classifications based on comparisons of the extremely diversified present-day bacterial life forms. For this reason, the current trend is to use a pragmatic approach in describing larger groups of bacteria without implying degrees of relatedness between them. This approach is used in the Eighth Edition of *Bergey's Manual of Determinative Bacteriology*, published in 1974, which is the classification and nomenclature system most widely followed in the United States. For example, the kingdom Procaryotae is recognized as containing two major Divisions, the Cyanobacteria or blue-green bacteria (algae), and the Bacteria. The latter division includes some 19 parts or bacterial groups which are given vernacular descriptions. Some 15 of these groups contain the three major classes of nonphotosynthetic bacteria which are of medical interest. These include (1) a diversity of cell-walled cocci, rods, and spiral bacteria, (2) the obligate intracellular eucaryotic parasitic rickettsia, and (3) the cell wall-less mycoplasmas, but not the gliding, sheathed, or budding and/or appendaged bacteria. A modified presentation of the classification of most of the medically important bacteria according to the Eighth Edition of *Bergey's Manual* is given in Table 2-1.

Well-known trivial or commonly used names, such as the tubercle bacillus (*Mycobacterium tuberculosis*) and typhoid bacillus (*Salmonella typhi*), often appear in medical literature. When a generic (genus) name is vernacularized in English, such as bacillus, salmonella, or pneumococcus, it is neither capitalized nor italicized.

Genetic Basis for Classification

Recent developments in comparative biochemistry indicate that gene-controlled stable metabolic patterns, cell polymers, and organelle structures have yielded information of possible evolutionary significance. An often

TABLE 2-1 GRAM-POSITIVE BACTERIA, NONPHOTOSYNTHETIC

Large Group of Similar Organisms Order (=ales) Family (=aceae) Genus	Important Species	Characteristic Features
Cocci (Order unassigned)		
Micrococcaceae		
Micrococcus	M. luteus M. roseus	Cocci single, in clusters or packets, metabolism strictly respiratory, aerobes
		Aerobic to facultatively anaerobic, nonmotile
Staphylococcus	S. aureus S. epidermidis	Cocci single, in chains or irregular masses, metabolism respiratory and fermentative, facultative anaerobes
Streptococcaceae		
Streptococcus	S. pyogenes S. pneumoniae S. species	Cocci, in pairs or chains, homofermenters, produce lactic acid, facultatively anaerobic, nonmotile, metabolism fermentative
Peptococcaceae		
Peptococcus	P. asaccharolyticus	Cocci single, in pairs, tetrads, or masses
		Anaerobic, nonmotile
Peptostreptococcus	P. anaerobius P. intermedius	Cocci in pairs or chains
Methane-producing Organisms (Order unassigned)		
Methanobacteriaceae		
Methanobacterium	M. ruminantium	Strict anaerobes, nonmotile, oval rods to cocci in pairs or chains, only methane producers in human gut
Endospore-forming Rods (Order unassigned)		
Bacillaceae		
Bacillus	B. anthracis	Aerobic rods
		Motile with peritrichous flagella or nonmotile
Clostridium	C. botulinum C. perfringens C. tetani	Anaerobic rods

13

TABLE 2-1 GRAM-POSITIVE BACTERIA, NONPHOTOSYNTHETIC (cont.)

Asporogenous Rod-shaped Organisms (Order unassigned)			
Lactobacillaceae			
Lactobacillus	*L. acidophilus* *L. casei*	Homofermenting rods, produce lactic acid, catalase and cytochromes absent, nonmotile	
Genera of uncertain affiliation			
Listeria	*L. monocytogenes*	Small coccoid rods, catalase-positive, motile	
Erysipelothrix	*E. rhusiopathiae*	Catalase-negative, non-motile rods, often produce filaments	Aerobic
Actinomycetes (and Related organisms)			
Coryneform bacteria (Corynebacteriaceae)			
Corynebacterium	*C. diphtheriae*	Generally aerobic, catalase positive rods, nonmotile	
Propionibacteriaceae			
Propionibacterium	*P. acnes*	Anaerobic to aerotolerant, nonmotile, heterofermenting rods, produce propionic, acetic acids	
Eubacterium	*E. lentum*	Obligate anaerobes, fermentative or nonfermentative	
Actinomycetales			
Actinomycetaceae			
Actinomyces	*A. israelii* *A. naeslundii* *A. propionica*	Anaerobic to facultatively anaerobic	Non-acid-fast, predominantly diphtheroid in shape, tend to form branching filaments, no spores
Arachnia			
Bifidobacterium	*B. eriksonii*	Anaerobic	
Bacterionema	*B. matruchotii*	Facultative anaerobe	
Rothia	*R. dentocariosa*	Aerobe	

Genus	Important Species	Characteristic Features
Mycobacteriaceae *Mycobacterium*	*M. tuberculosis*	Catalase-positive rods, acid-fast aerobes, nonmotile, no spores
Nocardiaceae *Nocardia*	*N. asteroides* *N. brasiliensis*	Aerobes, may form true mycelium, sometimes acid-fast, aerial spores usually absent
Streptomycetaceae *Streptomyces*	*S.* species	Aerobic soil organisms, antimetabolite producers, nonmotile, ray-forming rods, form true mycelia, buds or spores, most species are nonpathogens
Micromonosporaceae *Micropolyspora*	*M. faeni*	Aerobic, optimal growth at 50C, cause farmer's lung disease

TABLE 2-1   GRAM-NEGATIVE BACTERIA, NONPHOTOSYNTHETIC

	Important Species	Characteristic Features
Large Group of Similar Organisms **Class (=es)*** **Order (=ales)*** **Family (=aceae)** **Tribe (=ieae)*** **Genus**		
The Spirochetes (Class and Tribe unassigned) Spirochaetales Spirochaetaceae *Treponema* *Borrelia* *Leptospira*	*T. pallidum* *B.* species *L. interrogans*	Spiral cells, motile
Spiral and Curved Bacteria Spirillaceae *Spirillum*	*S. minor*	Aerobic, motile, causes rat-bite fever

TABLE 2-1 GRAM-NEGATIVE BACTERIA, NONPHOTOSYNTHETIC (cont.)

Campylobacter	C. fetus, C. sputorum	Oxidase-positive, microaerophilic to anaerobic, motile with polar flagella	
Aerobic Rods and Cocci (Class, Order, and Tribe unassigned) Pseudomonadaceae Pseudomonas	P. aeruginosa	Oxidize organic compounds, aerobic rods, motile with polar flagella	
Rhizobiaceae Rhizobium	R. species	Stimulate nitrogen-fixing root nodules on leguminous plants	
Halobacteriaceae Halobacterium	H. species	Generally require greater than 2 M NaCl for growth	
Genera of uncertain affiliation Brucella Bordetella Francisella	B. species, B. pertussis, F. tularensis	Coccoid rods, facultatively anaerobic, most species nonmotile	
Facultatively Anaerobic Rods (Class and Order unassigned) Enterobacteriaceae Escherichieae Escherichia Edwardsiella Citrobacter Salmonella Shigella	E. coli, E. tarda, C. species, S. typhi, S. dysenteriae	Mixed acid fermentation of sugars	Facultatively anaerobic rods, oxidase-negative, catalase-positive, motile with peritrichous flagella or nonmotile
Klebsiellieae Klebsiella Enterobacter Hafnia Serratia	K. pneumoniae, E. aerogenes, H. alvei, S. marcescens	Butylene glycol fermentation of sugars	
Proteae Proteus	P. vulgaris, P. mirabilis	Characteristically produce urease	

Yersinieae		
Yersinia	*Y. enterocolitica*	
	Y. pestis	
	Y. pseudotuberculosis	
Erwinieae		
Erwinia	*E. amylovora*	Plant pathogens
Vibrionaceae		
Vibrio	*V. cholerae*	Comma-shaped rods
Aeromonas	*A. hydrophila*	Straight rods
Pleisiomonas	*P. shigelloides*	Facultatively anaerobic, oxidase-positive, motile with polar flagella

Genera of uncertain affiliation

Chromobacterium	*C. violaceum*	
Flavobacterium	*F. meningosepticum*	
Haemophilus	*H. influenzae*	Require X and V factors from blood
Pasteurella	*P. multocida*	
Actinobacillus	*A. lignieresii*	
Cardiobacterium	*C. hominis*	
Streptobacillus	*S. moniliformis*	
Calymmatobacterium	*C. granulomatis*	

Anaerobic Bacteria (Class, Order, and Tribe unassigned)

Bacteroidaceae		
Bacteroides	*B. fragilis*	Obligate anaerobes, nonmotile, may be associated with anaerobic infections
Fusobacterium	*F. nucleatum*	
Leptotrichia	*L. buccalis*	

Cocci and Coccobacilli (Class, Order, and Tribe unassigned)

Neisseriaceae		
Neisseria	*N. meningitidis*	
	N. gonorrhoeae	Cocci in pairs, adjacent sides flattened
Branhamella	*B. catarrhalis*	Oxidase-positive aerobes, nonmotile
Moraxella	*M. lacunata*	
Acinetobacter	*A. calcoaceticus*	Short plump rods

17

TABLE 2-1 GRAM-NEGATIVE BACTERIA, NONPHOTOSYNTHETIC (cont.)

Veillonellaceae		
Veillonella	V. parvula	Anaerobic cocci, nonmotile
Acidaminococcus	A. fermentans	
The Rickettsias (Class unassigned)		
Rickettsiales		Majority are intracellular parasites
Rickettsiaceae		
Rickettsieae		
Rickettsia	R. species	Minute, coccobacilli, transmitted by arthropods
Rochalimaea	R. quintana	
Coxiella	C. burnetti	
Bartonellaceae		
Bartonella	B. bacilliformis	Nonmotile polymorphic coccobacilli, often occur in chains, causes Oroya fever
Chlamydiales		
Chlamydiaceae		
Chlamydia	C. trachomatis	Intracellular parasites, nonmotile
The Mycoplasmas		
Mollicutes		
Mycoplasmatales		
Mycoplasmataceae		
Mycoplasma	M. pneumoniae	Smallest free-living cells with complex growth cycle, pleomorphic, lack cell wall, nonmotile

*If assigned.
Modified from Buchanan and Gibbons (eds): *Bergey's Manual of Determinative Bacteriology,* 8th ed. 1974. Baltimore, Williams & Wilkins

quoted example is the observation that in a wide group of organisms, including bacteria, actinomycetes, blue-green bacteria, water molds, green algae, and vascular plants, the biosynthesis of the amino acid L-lysine occurs by decarboxylation of a common intermediate, α,ϵ-diaminopimelic acid.

$$
\begin{array}{ccc}
\text{COOH} & & \text{COOH} \\
| & & | \\
\text{H}_2\text{NCH} & & \text{H}_2\text{NCH} \\
| & & | \\
(\text{CH}_2)_3 & \longrightarrow & (\text{CH}_2)_3 + \text{CO}_2 \\
| & & | \\
\text{HCNH}_2 & & \text{H}_2\text{CNH}_2 \\
| & & \\
\text{COOH} & &
\end{array}
$$

D,L-diaminopimelic   L-lysine
acid (meso DAP)

By contrast, a different pathway, the aminoadipic acid pathway, is used for lysine biosynthesis by euglenoid algae, certain fungi including the Ascomycetes (for example, *Neurospora*), Basidiomycetes, and others. A second set of examples includes the observation that almost all bacteria, actinomycetes, and blue-green algae produce a semirigid cell wall structure of similar composition which is variously called murein, peptidoglycan, or mucopeptide (Chap. 6), and the fact that various microbial antigens including proteins, surface polymers including capsules, teichoic acids, and 0 antigens can be used for comparison of bacterial relatedness. Finally, comparison of homology, both of composition and of sequence, of deoxyribonucleic acids (DNA), ribonucleic acids (RNA), and proteins allows examination of organisms at the genetic level.

Because these developments are still in progress, a complete correlation with the present empirical classification in Table 2-1 cannot yet be made. However, the older empirically developed relationships based on recognition of phenotypic expression of various traits and features are, after all, a reflection of gene pool expression and correlate in general with the results obtained by newer approaches which aim at defining relatedness on a molecular basis. Such information may or may not be of phylogenetic significance. However, it is of use in assessing the similarity of present-day microorganisms.

Relatedness Based on Nucleic Acid Homology

Genetic information is encoded in DNA base sequence. As organisms drift apart by mutation, recombination, transduction, and selection in different environments (that is, evolution), their genomes change in size, nucleotide base composition, and nucleotide base sequence. The approximate sizes of the genomes of several bacteria are listed in Table 2-2. Analysis by both chemical and physicochemical methods shows that base composition is constant and characteristic for each organism. It is generally expressed in terms of the mole fraction of guanine plus cytosine (that is, G + C/G + C + A + T, expressed as a percentage); values of percent GC for different organisms vary from 25 to 75 (Table 2-3). At the level of descriptively defined species, it is to be noted that several genera exhibit similar DNA base composition. However, similarity of base composition does not necessarily signify DNA homology, that is, similarity in base sequence. For example, the genomes of all vertebrates, including man, contain approximately 44 mole percent GC, as do those of some microorganisms. Obviously, different organisms with similar DNA base compositions must have heterologous base sequences. Measurement of DNA homology has been quantified by several procedures which determine the extent of formation of molecular hybrids from two DNA strands of different origin. The generalized

TABLE 2-2 APPROXIMATE DNA CONTENT PER GENOME OF VARIOUS ORGANISMS

Species	Daltons
Mammalian sperm	18×10^{11}
Salmonella typhimurium	28×10^8
Escherichia coli	25×10^8
Bacillus subtilis	20×10^8
Haemophilus influenzae	16×10^8
Neisseria gonorrhoeae	9.8×10^8
Rickettsia rickettsii	9.8×10^8
Chlamydia trachomatis	6.6×10^8
Mycoplasma species	4×10^8
Coliphage T4	1.3×10^8

Modified from Kingsbury: J Bacteriol 98:1400, 1969; Muller and Klotz: Biochem Biophys Acta 378:171, 1975; Sober (ed): Handbook of Biochemistry, 1968. Courtesy of Chemical Rubber Co; Sorov and Becker: J Mol Biol 42:581, 1969

TABLE 2-3   NUCLEOTIDE BASE COMPOSITION OF THE DNA
OF VARIOUS BACTERIA

Organism	%GC
Clostridium perfringens, C. tetani	30–32
Staphylococcus aureus	32–34
Bacillus cereus, B. anthracis, B. thuringiensis, Mycoplasma gallisepticum, S. faecalis, Treponema pallidum, Veillonella parvula	34–36
Streptococcus (Diplococcus) pneumoniae, S. salivarius, S. pyogenes, Lactobacillus acidophilus, Listeria monocytogenes, Proteus vulgaris, P. mirabilis, Haemophilus influenzae	38–40
Moraxella bovis	40–42
Bacillus subtilis, Chlamydia trachomatis	42–44
Vibrio comma, Pasteurella pestis, Corynebacterium acnes	46–48
Neisseria gonorrhoeae	48–50
Neisseria meningitidis, Bacteroides fragilis, Escherichia coli, Citrobacter freundii, Shigella dysenteriae, Salmonella typhi, S. typhimurium, S. enteritidis, S. arizona, S. ballerup	50–52
Enterobacter aerogenes, Corynebacterium diphtheriae	52–54
Klebsiella pneumoniae, K. rhinoscleromatis, Brucella abortus	54–56
Lactobacillus bifidis	56–58
Serratia marcescens	58–60
Pseudomonas fluorescens	60–62
Pseudomonas aeruginosa, Mycobacterium tuberculosis	66–68
Micrococcus luteus (lysodeikticus), Nocardia sp.	70–80

Modified from Marmur, Falkow, and Mandel: Annu Rev Microbiol 17:329, 1963

procedure is illustrated in Figure 2-2. As indicated in Table 2-4, this approach has been useful in demonstrating the relative order and degree of DNA similarity of closely related groups of bacteria. In addition, the lack of DNA homology between dissimilar organisms is also clear, but this very specificity also limits the usefulness of this approach, since it cannot be used to study the relationship of dissimilar bacterial groups.

The Bacterial Species

According to present definitions, each kind of bacterium may be considered a species. A clearer definition is difficult until a genetic or phylogenetic description is available. For example, many bacterial groups are comprised of slightly different strains which form interrelated groups of dynamically evolving organisms (in analogy with closely related, continually subdividing branches from a growing ancestral tree). Within such a group, clusters of high-density areas (not necessarily at dead center) contain biotypes from which a strain may be chosen arbitrarily to best represent a species. Such a type strain, even if well chosen, may not exhibit all features expressed by the totality of the species cluster. Obviously the border-lines of such groups are not clear-cut, and many marginally interrelated strains are found

in the laboratory. An example of a group which forms a constellation of similar clusters is provided by the Enterobacteriaceae. Its members share a common gene pool, as evidenced by their ability to undergo intergeneric transformation, conjugation, or transduction (Chap. 8).

Species are therefore still arbitrarily defined by a descriptive array of features encompassing a spectrum of phenotypic expressions which describe a sampling of the potential of a particular gene pool. Features used include, more or less in sequence, the morphologic appearance of bacterial cell shape, size, flagellar pattern if motile, capsule occurrence, colonial morphology, and pigmentation; staining properties, including the gram, capsule, spore, acid-fast, and flagella visualizing stains; metabolic patterns, including growth requirements and conditions, ability to ferment sugars and produce or utilize unique chemicals, energy-yielding patterns, and characteristic metabolic products; macromolecular composition and structure, for example, the specific antigenic pattern of surface macromolecules, and the chemical composition and structure of the cell wall and DNA; the ecology of source and habitat; and the ability to parasitize or to be pathogenic.

The student will soon recognize that the lack of a definitive unifying criterion for species designation in bacteria has understandably

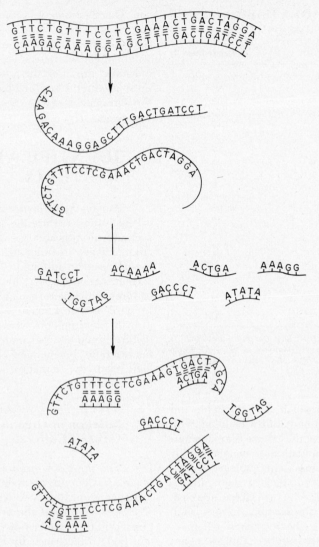

FIG. 2-2. DNA-DNA hybridization for comparison of the nucleotide base sequences of the DNAs of two bacterial species. DNA from one species is denatured by heating or treatment with alkali, so as to separate the two strands; these are then generally entrapped in some supporting matrix, so as to prevent their reassociation. To them small, broken, denatured (and therefore likewise single-stranded) DNA oligonucleotide strands derived from the second species are added, which are radioactively labeled. The mixture is then heated and allowed to cool slowly. During this annealing process, any oligonucleotide stretches able to base-pair will form double-stranded hybrid stretches which are resistant to solubilization by digestion with deoxyribonuclease, whereas unpaired single strands are susceptible. If, therefore, the two DNA samples are entirely homologous, all radioactively labeled DNA will hybridize and be converted to the DNase-resistant form; if they are completely dissimilar, all labeled DNA will remain enzyme sensitive.

resulted in variation in levels at which groups are divided, depending upon whether the describing investigator is a "splitter" or a "lumper." In the splitter category are those who have designated each *Salmonella* serotype a species with its own name; the lumpers, on the other hand, have designated individual serotypes as numbered types within a single species of, say, *Klebsiella, Streptococcus,* or *Pneumococcus*.

Type Cultures

The microbial taxonomist is continually faced with the practical problem of discerning

TABLE 2-4   DNA HOMOLOGIES AMONG SOME BACTERIA

DNA Source	% Relatedness
	(to *E. coli*)
Escherichia coli	100
Shigella dysenteriae	89
Salmonella typhimurium	45
Enterobacter aerogenes	35
Serratia marcescens	20
Proteus vulgaris	10
Pseudomonas aeruginosa	1
Bacillus subtilis	1
Brucella neotamae	0
	(to *N. meningitidis*)
Neisseria meningitidis	100
Neisseria gonorrhoeae	80
Neisseria perflava	55
Neisseria subflava	48
Neisseria catarrhalis	15
Neisseria caviae	10
Mima sp.	5
Herellea	5
Escherichia coli	3
Monkey kidney	0.1

Modified from Brenner: Int J Syst Bacteriol, 23:298, 1973; Brenner, Martin, and Hoyer: J Bacteriol 94:486, 1967; Kingsbury: J Bacteriol 94:870, 1967; McCarthy and Bolton: Proc Natl Acad Sci USA 50:156, 1963

identifying features which are both stable and characteristic. High mutability coupled with rapid growth rate generally cause the characteristics of bacterial populations to change rapidly in response to environmental selection pressures. For this reason, stock or type cultures are frequently stored in a viable, minimal, or nongrowth state (for example, freeze-dried) from which they can be recovered when required. Representative type cultures maintained in The American Type Culture Collection, Washington, D. C., are available for comparison.

Numerical Taxonomy

Because of the difficulties in constructing phylogenetic classifications which are based on only a few arbitrarily weighted characteristics, descriptive taxonomy has been revived for many strains in the form of computerized numerical comparisons of large numbers of diagnostic features. First devised by Michel Adanson in the eighteenth century, this system gives equal weight to all features chosen for compari-

son. Designations of groups are then made on the basis of the degree of similarity, quantitatively defined as the similarity coefficient (S value). Characteristics chosen for numerical taxonomy are often the arbitrary features presently used for describing bacterial species, and the agreement between the two systems is not surprising.

IDENTIFICATION OF BACTERIA

Among the primary concerns of the medical microbiologist are the isolation and rapid, accurate identification of disease-causing microorganisms, in order that adequate specific therapy can be initiated. This can be accomplished in most cases* by determinative procedures which, after isolation of the organism in pure culture,† make use of knowledge of growth requirements, visible (colony) growth features, microscopic morphology and staining reactions, biochemical characteristics, serologic reactivity, animal pathogenicity, and antibiotic sensitivity.

Isolation of Organisms in Pure (Axenic) Culture

The approach used for the isolation of organisms depends upon the source of the clinical specimen. Blood, spinal fluid, and closed abscesses may yield almost pure bacterial cultures, while specimens of sputum, stool, skin, and body orifices usually contain mixtures of organisms. The specimen is generally streaked onto solid agar-containing medium so as to separate the bacterial population into individual cells. Pathogens present in small numbers in mixtures of organisms may be missed, since they may be overgrown by other bacteria, or they may be killed by metabolic acids or other products resulting from growth of nonpathogens. Pathogens may also be missed if their growth requirements are not met. For this reason, selective culture techniques are employed

*Exceptions occur in the case of exotoxin-producing bacteria. Refer to discussions on botulism, tetanus, and staphylococcal food poisoning.
†Pure in the sense of axenic, that is, free of other organisms, rather than pure in the genetic sense.

in order to establish an environment in which the pathogen has a survival advantage: These include the use of selective media which are of specific pH, ionic strength, or chemical composition, or which contain inhibitors, or which lack nutrients for all but the organism in question. Control of gas phase and temperature of the growth environment must also be considered. Alternatively, for fastidious bacteria, enrichment media are used which contain nutrients ecologically favorable to the organism to be isolated. Such media include heated blood agar (chocolate agar), blood agar, and nutrient agar and sometimes inhibitors as discussed in later chapters under growth, nutrition, and specific organisms. The response of the unknown bacterium to such media is sometimes useful in identification. For example, *Haemophilus influenzae* requires for growth both pyridine

nucleotide and hemin, the iron porphyrin derived from hemoglobin, and therefore will grow on chocolate agar but not on blood agar. Unless the red cells are ruptured, the red cell pyridine nucleotide and hemin are not available to the bacterium.

Bacterial Colony Morphology

Bacteria multiply rapidly and form macroscopic, visible masses of growth when inoculated onto appropriate medium containing 2 percent agar and incubated 18 to 48 hours in a favorable atmosphere. For some species, such as the tubercle bacillus, *Mycobacterium tuberculosis*, a longer period of incubation is required. Ideally, a colony is composed of the descendents of a single cell, but it may of

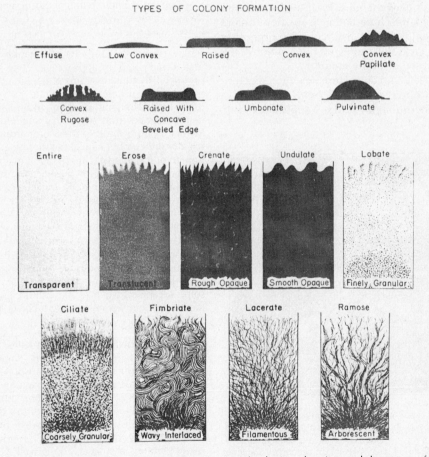

FIG. 2-3. Types of colony morphology, showing the structure of colonies, elevation, and the nature of the edges.

course also develop from two or more organisms or from a clump of cells. Such a colony may have the gross appearance characteristic of a certain type of bacterium although it may contain contaminating organisms. The gross characteristics of colonies of different species of organisms grown under standard conditions are of considerable aid in identification, since colonies differ in size, shape, color, odor, texture and degree of adherence to the medium. Colony morphology is related in part to motility or to postfission bacterial movements which depend on division planes formed by different species (Fig. 2-3). Colonies have been described as loop-forming (wavy edges characteristic of long filaments, such as those of *Bacillus anthracis*), folding and snapping (serrated or crenated edges such as those formed by *Yersinia pestis* and *Corynebacterium diphtheriae*), and slipping (smooth or lobate edges with spreading smooth growth films, characteristic of *Proteus vulgaris* or *Escherichia coli*). If the bacteria are first mixed into liquefied agar medium before pouring into a petri dish, colony morphology may also vary, depending on the location of the bacterium on or in the medium.

The serologic characteristics of a bacterium are often correlated with mucoid(M), smooth(S), or rough(R) colony appearance (Fig.

2-4). M or S colonies are characteristic of bacteria recently isolated from natural habitats and are sometimes referred to as wild-type.

THE MUCOID COLONY.   M colonies exhibit a waterlike glistening confluent appearance and are characteristic of organisms which form slime or well-developed capsules. Notable examples are *Klebsiella pneumoniae, Streptococcus (Diplococcus) pneumoniae, H. influenzae,* and the pathogenic yeast, *Cryptococcus neoformans.* The capsular polymers may be group-, species-, or stain-specific and are usually antigenic for mice and men. The capsule functions as a defense mechanism against phagocytosis, and among pathogenic bacteria encapsulated organisms usually, but not always, are more virulent than noncapsulated forms.

THE SMOOTH COLONY.   S colonies give the appearance of homogeneity and uniform texture without appearing as liquid as mucoid colonies. S-form bacteria produce a polymer, such as the somatic O-polysaccharide antigen of the gram-negative colityphoid-paratyphoid-dysentery group known as the enterobacteria, which is characteristic of the species.

THE ROUGH COLONY.   R colonies are granulated and rough in appearance. They are usually produced by mutant strains of bacteria which lack part of the specific carbohydrate polymer structures found in gram-positive and gram-negative cells obtained from smooth or mucoid colonies. Reversion from the R to the S prototrophic form is usually difficult but can sometimes be achieved by growth of rough organisms in medium containing R antisera, by growth in the presence of mutagens, or by passage through animals. In some encapsulated organisms, such as *Serratia marcescens,* the colony form may change from M↔S↔R. Virulence is commonly, but not always, associated with the M- or S-type colonies. Rough forms of enteric bacteria are usually nonpathogenic and are easily killed by phagocytes, in contrast to the more resistant parent or wild-type S colony bacteria. However, with some organisms, such as the anthrax bacillus and the human and bovine types of tubercle bacilli, the R forms are more virulent.

THE L COLONY.   L colonies were first associated with certain bacilli, notably *Streptobacillus moniliformis,* but have also been isolated from *H. influenzae* and various enteric bacteria. The rigid cell wall which is characteristic of bacteria is absent in L forms. Exposure to penicillin and other drugs and growth in osmotically supportive media facilitates L colony formation. Small coccoid and filamentous forms are observed, as well as large globoid forms which also contain the minute forms.

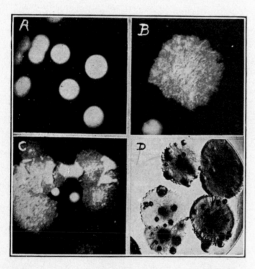

FIG. 2-4. Types of bacterial colonies. A. Smooth: B. Rough: C. Smooth developing from rough colonies. A, B, and C are from a culture of an acid-fast bacterium. D. Colonies of the cholera vibrio with secondary daughter colonies.

L forms normally resynthesize a cell wall once the penicillin or other drug is removed.

Microscopic Morphology and Staining Reactions

Light microscopic examination of gram-stained preparations is routinely used to determine the shape of bacteria. Common shapes are cocci (spherical), bacilli (rodlike), and spiral forms. The gram stain also allows a check on contamination by noting morphologic and staining homogeneity. Depending upon source and growth features, other differential stains may be used, as in the case of acid-fast staining of sputum smears or cultures. Special stains may also be used to detect capsules, flagella, spores, or intracellular inclusion bodies.

THE GRAM STAIN. A heat-fixed bacterial smear on a glass slide is treated with the basic dye, crystal violet. All organisms take up the dye. The smear is then covered with Gram's iodine solution (3 percent I_2-KI in water or a weak buffer, pH 8.0, in order to neutralize acidity formed from iodine on standing). After a water rinse and decolorization with acetone, the preparation is washed thoroughly in water and counterstained with a red dye, usually safranin. The stained preparation is then rinsed with water, dried, and examined under the light microscope.

Bacteria can be differentiated into two groups by this stain, devised in the early 1880s by the Danish bacteriologist, Christian Gram. Gram-positive organisms stain blue, while about one-third of the cocci, one-half the bacilli, and all spiral organisms stain red and are said to be gram-negative. Animal cells also stain gram-negative, and the gram-stain procedure can therefore be used to detect large gram-positive bacteria, such as *Nocardia asteroides*, in tissues.

The mechanism of the gram stain is related not only to the chemistry but also to the thickness of the cell wall, pore size, and permeability properties of the intact cell envelope. Gram-positive bacteria stain gram-negative if they lose osmotic integrity by rupture of the plasma membrane. Autolyzed, old, or dead gram-positive cells and isolated cell envelopes stain gram-negative. A unique bacterial cell-wall chemical composition does not appear to explain the gram stain, since thick-walled yeast cells, which also stain gram-positive, have a chemical composition and structure different from gram-positive bacteria.

THE ACID-FAST STAIN. The mycobacteria are lipophilic and difficult to stain, but once stained, they are resistant to destaining. Typically, a sputum or culture smear on a glass slide is stained with carbolfuchsin by steaming over a flame for several minutes. The phenol appears to aid penetration of the dye through the mycobacterial lipid. The slide is then rinsed with water, destained with acid alcohol, and counterstained briefly with methylene blue. When examined under the light microscope, mycobacteria appear as bright red bacilli against a light blue background.

Biochemical Characteristics

Various strains, species, and genera of organisms exhibit characteristic patterns of substrate utilization, metabolic product formation, and sugar fermentation. The latter are used routinely in the identification of enterobacteria: the salmonella characteristically ferment sugars with production of acid and gas, in contrast to the anaerogenic (nongas-producing) shigella.

Serologic Reactivity

The antigenic reactivity of an organism is often determined in order to identify the serogroup or serotype to which the organism belongs. These reactions are usually carried out on microscope slides by mixing a drop of antiserum containing specific antibody which reacts with a known cellular component. Visible reactions observed include flagellar clumping, cellular agglutination, and capsular reactions detected as an increase in the refractive index around the cell. Extracts of cells also may be used for the detection of antigenic reactivity, a precipitate being formed on addition of specific antiserum.

Bacteriophage Typing

Epidemiologists have found bacteriophage typing to be of use in tracing the development and source of outbreaks of certain bacterial diseases, including for example, those caused by *Staphylococcus aureus, S. typhi*, and *Pseudomonas aeruginosa*. This is possible because different strains of a serologically or otherwise identical species of bacteria are susceptible to one or more different strains or types of species-specific bacterial viruses known as bacteriophage, or phage. Suspensions of each bacteriophage type are deposited on an agar plate newly inoculated with the suspected pathogen. Susceptible bacteria are lysed by the phage, leaving clear areas known as plaques (Chap. 96).

Pathogenicity for Animals

Identification of certain organisms is aided by inoculation into animals. Some organisms, such as the spirochete which causes syphilis, *Treponema pallidum*, cannot be grown in vitro but can be isolated by testicular inoculation and transfer in rabbits. In other instances a pathogen which can be cultivated in vitro may be differentiated from similar pathogens by inoculation into susceptible animals which destroy the contaminant but yield to infection by the pathogen. For example, isolation of pneumococci present in only small numbers in contaminated sputum or in nasopharyngeal throat washings can be accomplished by inoculation into the mouse peritoneum where the encapsulated pneumococcus thrives and from which it can be recovered in pure culture. Similarly, subcutaneous inoculation into the groin of the guinea pig is used to differentiate pathogenic tubercle bacilli from similar, nonpathogenic mycobacteria.

Antibiotic Sensitivity

Antibiotics vary in their effect on different bacterial species and on strains of even the same species. Each pathogen must be tested for sensitivity to various concentrations of effective antimetabolites in order to determine the concentration level at which its growth is inhibited. The dosage necessary to give the blood level required for adequate therapy can then be established.

FURTHER READING

Books and Reviews

Barghoorn ES: The oldest fossils. Sci Am May 1971, p 30

Britten RJ, Kohne DE: Repeated sequences in DNA. Science 161:529, 1968

Buchanan RE, Gibbons NE (eds): Bergey's Manual of Determinative Bacteriology, 8th ed. Baltimore, Williams & Wilkins, 1974

Edwards PR, Ewing WH: Identification of Enterobacteriaceae, 2nd ed. Minneapolis, Burgess Pub Co, 1970

Jones D, Sneath PHA: Genetic transfer and bacterial taxonomy. Bacteriol Rev 34:40, 1970

Kennell DE: Principles and practices of nucleic acid hybridization. Prog Nucleic Acid Res Mol Biol 11:259, 1971

Mandel M: New approaches to bacterial taxonomy, perspective and prospects. Annu Rev Microbiol 23:329, 1969

Margulis L: Origin of Eukaryotic Cells. New Haven, Yale Univ Press, 1970

Marmur J, Falkow S, Mandel M: New approaches to bacterial taxonomy. Annu Rev Microbiol 17:239, 1963

Meynell GG, Meynell E: Theory and Practice in Experimental Bacteriology. New York, Cambridge Univ Press, 1970

Raff RA, Mahler HR: The non-symbiotic origin of mitochondria. Science 177:575, 1972

Stanier RY: Toward a definition of the bacteria. In Gunsalus IC, Stanier RY (eds): The Bacteria. New York, Academic Press, 1964, vol 5, pp 445-464

Stanier RY, Doudoroff M, Adelberg EA: The Microbial World, 3rd ed. Englewood Cliffs, NJ, Prentice-Hall, 1970

Selected Papers

Brenner DJ: Deoxyribonucleic acid divergence in Enterobacteriaceae. Developments Indust Microbiol 11:139, 1970

Cohen SS: Are/Were mitochondria and chloroplasts microorganisms? Am Sci 58:281, 1970

Gillis M, DeLey J, DeCleene M: The determination of molecular weight of bacterial genome DNA from renaturation rates. Eur J Biochem 12:143, 1970

Margulis L: Evolutionary criteria in thallophytes: a radical alternative. Science 161:1020, 1968

Raven PH: A multiple origin for plastids and mitochondria. Science 169:641, 1970

Whittaker RH: New concepts of kingdoms of organisms. Science 163:150, 1969

3
Bacterial Morphology and Ultrastructure

THE BACTERIAL CELL

Bacteria characteristically produce a cell envelope which includes a layered cell wall and external surface adherents known as capsules or slimes. The cell wall contains a rigid structure, known as the murein sacculus or peptidoglycan, which encloses and protects the protoplast from physical damage, such as by freezing and conditions of low osmotic pressure, and generally allows bacteria to tolerate a strikingly wide range of environmental conditions. The protoplast itself is defined as the naked cytoplasmic membrane and its contents. Appendages include flagella, which are organs of locomotion, and threadlike pili, which appear to serve adhesive functions. Internally, bacteria are relatively simple cells. Major cytoplasmic structures include mesosomes, which are derived from the membrane, and a central fibrillar chromatin network or nuclear body surrounded by an amorphous cytoplasm which contains ribosomes. A typical gram-negative bacterium is shown in schematic form in Figure 3-1. Inclusion bodies or storage granules vary in chemical nature according to species. Certain structures are limited to only a few bacteria. These include endospores, which are produced only by members of the family Bacillaceae, and thylakoids, which are the bacteriochlorophyll-containing, membrane-derived organelles of the photosynthetic bacteria. Bacteria do not produce intracellular organelles, such as mitochondria, nuclear membranes, a mitotic apparatus, an endoplasmic reticulum, or the complex 9 + 2 flagella characteristic of eucaryotic cells.

BACTERIAL SIZE AND FORM

Bacteria exhibit a wide range of sizes, as indicated in Figure 3-2, and appear under the light or electron microscope as spheres (cocci), rods (bacilli), and spirals (spirochetes) (Fig. 3-3). Free cocci appear perfectly spherical. They also occur in pairs as diplococci, in chains as streptococci, and in tetrads or in grapelike clusters depending on division planes. Bacilli vary considerably in length, from very short bacilli, sometimes called coccobacilli, to long rods which vary in length from 2 to 10 times their diameter. The ends of bacilli may be gently rounded, as in enteric organisms such as *Salmonella typhi*, or squared, as in *Bacillus anthracis*. Long threads of bacilli which have not separated into single cells are known as filaments. Fusiform bacilli, which occur in the oral and gut cavities, are tapered at both ends.

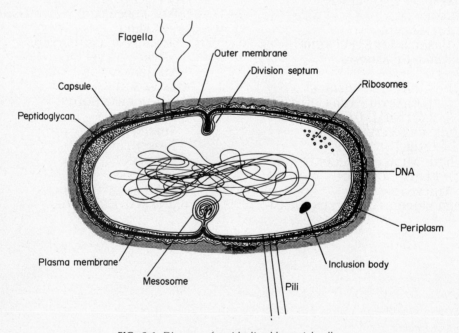

FIG. 3-1. Diagram of an idealized bacterial cell.

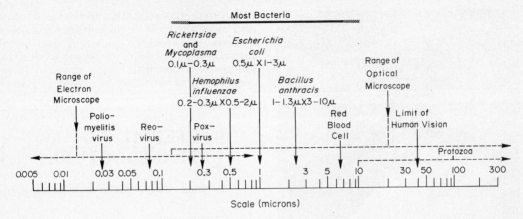

FIG. 3-2. Relative sizes of bacteria.

Curved bacterial rods, or spirilla, vary from small, comma-shaped or mildly helical-shaped organisms with only a single curve, such as *Vibrio cholera*, to the longer sinuous spirochete forms such as the *Borrelia, Treponema,* and *Leptospira*, which have from 4 to 20 coils.

Visualization

The Light Microscope The human eye cannot detect an object less than one-thousandth inch (30 μ) in diameter, and the light microscope, which has a resolving power of about 2,000 A or 0.2 μm, must be used to see bacteria.* Furthermore, because the refractive index of bacteria is similar to that of most aqueous suspending media, they are not easily seen unless they are suspended in glycerol or nonaqueous solutions, which enhance resolution, or if they are stained, which is almost always done in order to determine gross morphology. Capsules can be visualized in the light microscope as halos around cells suspended in India ink. Flagella, which are 0.01 to 0.02 μm in diameter, are below the limit of resolution of the light microscope and must be specially stained with dyes which adhere to flagellar protein and augment their size.

PHASE CONTRAST MICROSCOPY. Phase contrast light microscopes, which enhance refractive index differences of cell components, can be used to visualize live bacteria and to reveal some details of their internal structure. Capsules, endospores, and motility also can be observed.

Resolution, R, depends upon wavelength, λ, and the numerical aperture, NA, according to $R = \dfrac{0.6\lambda}{NA}$. The NA is usually about 1.5 and the wavelength 0.5 μ.

DARKFELD MICROSCOPY. This technique makes use of light redirected from the sample against a darkfield background and has been used to demonstrate the very thin spirochete which causes syphilis, *Treponema pallidum.*

The Electron Microscopes Bacterial ultrastructure was demonstrated only after the development of the electron microscope, which has a resolving power of about 0.001 μ, that is, some 200 times that of the light microscope. Preparations

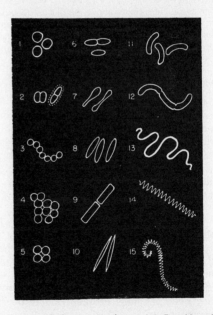

FIG. 3-3. Morphology. 1. Single cocci. 2. Cocci in pairs. 3. Cocci in chains. 4. Cocci in clusters. 5. Cocci in tetrads. 6. Coccobacilli. 7. Club-shaped bacilli. 8. Bacilli with rounded ends. 9. Bacilli with square ends. 10. Fusiform bacilli. 11. Vibrios. 12. *Spirillum.* 13. *Borrelia.* 14. *Treponema.* 15. *Leptospira.*

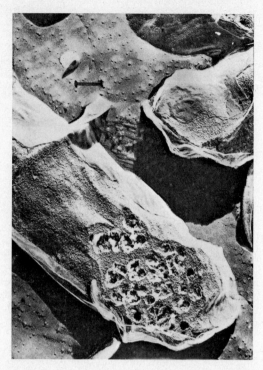

FIG. 3-4. Structure of *E. coli* after freeze etching. The lower cell is dividing, with division plane and intact cell surface on the left, exposed protoplasmic membrane in the center, and protoplasm on the right. Two distinct wall layers can be seen at the cut surfaces above the plasma membrane, which is studded with particles. The granular protoplasm contains open areas in which some fibrillar material can be seen. The bar equals 0.25 μ. (From Bayer and Remsen: J Bacteriol 101:304, 1970)

must be fixed, stained and dried. Improved techniques of fixation, embedding, and thin sectioning have gradually allowed better and better definition of structural components. The fine detail of flagella and pili as well as of the cell envelope, membrane, and of the internal cell fine structure can be visualized by either shadow casting or negative or specific staining procedures.

NEGATIVE STAINING. This technique, which is used for ultrafine structure work, involves the application of solutions of salts containing heavy metal atoms such as phosphotungstate, phosphosilicate, or ammonium molybdate. The electron-dense material deposits on the sample and forms a delicate, finely detailed outline of structural components.

THIN SECTIONS. Thin sections of 0.1 μ or less, as compared to the usual 2 to 7 μ sections used in light microscopy, allow resolution and study of structures by electron microscopy without background interference from other components.

FREEZE ETCHING. This technique involves freezing of specimens in situ with dry ice or liquid nitrogen. The specimen surface is then barely shaved or scratched with a microtome, followed by surface replication with carbon or metal. These preparations allow examination of surface layer and inner structures (Fig. 3-4).

BACTERIAL ULTRASTRUCTURE

Surface Adherents and Appendages

Capsules and Slimes Virulence of pathogens often correlates with capsule production. For example, virulent strains of such pathogens as the pneumococcus produce quantities of copious capsular polymers which protect the bacteria from phagocytosis. These bacteria form watery, mucoid, or smooth (S) colonies on solid media in contrast to non-capsule-forming rough (R) strains. Loss of capsule-forming ability by S→R mutation correlates with loss of virulence and increased ease of destruction of R cells by phagocytes.

Capsules and slimes are loosely differentiated on the basis that capsules tend to form gels which adhere to the cell, whereas slimes and extracellular polymers are more easily washed off. Capsules are easily visualized by negative staining; the capsule appears as a bordered halo of light surrounding the cell suspended in India ink (Fig. 3-5). Capsules may also be specially stained. If cells produce no visually demonstrable capsule and still react serologi-

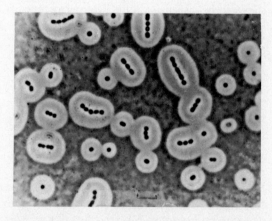

FIG. 3-5. Demonstration of capsules of *Acinetobacter calcoaceticus (Bacterium anitratum)* cells suspended in India ink and observed by phase contrast microscopy. (From Juni and Heym: J Bacteriol 87:461, 1964)

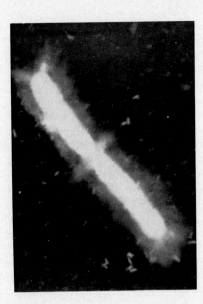

FIG. 3-6. Electron micrograph of *Bacillus megaterium*. Treatment with specific antipolysaccharide serum reveals microcapsulelike cell wall polysaccharide which is probably covalently linked to underlying murein sacculus. (From Baumann-Grace and Tomcsik: Schweiz Z Pathol Bakt 21:906, 1958)

cally with anticapsule sera, they are said to produce microcapsules (Fig. 3-6).

Capsules appear to be dispensable, since loss of the ability to produce capsules has no effect on growth rate or viability. In addition to genetic capability, environment and cultural conditions also markedly influence capsule production. In general, polysaccharide capsule production is enhanced by large amounts of carbohydrate and the restrictive growth conditions of low nitrogen, sulfur, or phosphorus, and low temperature or high salt concentration. In contrast, the *B. anthracis* polypeptide capsule, which is composed of D-glutamic acid linked through gamma carboxyl groups, is produced in large amounts only when the organism is grown in an environment containing a high CO_2 concentration. Other factors may also affect capsule production. For example, the hyaluronic acid capsule of groups A and C of *Streptococcus pyogenes* can be demonstrated only very early in the growth of hyaluronidase-producing strains.

Several different types of genetically determined capsular polysaccharides may be produced by subgroups of a single species. These can often be differentiated serologically, hence the term serogroup or serotype. For example, over 70 immunologically distinct capsular

polysaccharide serotypes of *Streptococcus (Diplococcus) pneumoniae* have been defined. Other organisms, such as *Klebsiella*, *Escherichia*, and *Haemophilus*, also produce several capsular-type polysaccharides. Differences in capsular types are detected by Neufeld's quellung reaction, in which cells are mixed with specific anticapsule serum. If the appropriate capsular substance is present, a swelling appears around the cell.

Flagella Motile bacteria can be detected in several ways. Movement can be observed microscopically in fluid (in a hanging drop or under a coverslip), by spread of bacterial growth as a film over agar, or as turbidity spreading through soft 0.3 to 0.5 percent (semisolid) agar. Motility is a characteristic of most vibrios, spirilla, and spirochetes, some bacilli, and a few nonpathogenic cocci. Motile bacteria produce one or more flagella which can be visualized directly by darkfield microscopy and in stained preparations by light and electron microscopy. Flagella can also be detected serologically: Flagellated cells react with specific antisera to give a typical loose, flocculent agglutination.

Flagella are long (3 to 20 μm), thin, wavy filaments of uniform diameter (0.01 to 0.013 μm) and terminate in a square tip. A helical structure is observed by negative staining at very high magnification under the electron microscope. The wave length and thickness of the helical filament are characteristic of each species, but some bacteria exhibit biplicity, that is, they have two flagella of different wave lengths (Fig. 3-7).

Flagellated bacteria are either peritrichously or polarly flagellated. Polar flagellated species of the Order *Pseudomonadales* have either one polar flagellum, when they are said to be monotrichous, a tuft of several polar flagella (lophotrichous), or flagella at both poles (amphitrichous). By contrast, members of the Order *Eubacteriales* have flagella distributed over the entire cell surface and are said to be peritrichous. The number of flagella in this case may vary from a few, as in some *Escherichia coli*, up to several hundred or thousand, as may sometimes be observed on *Proteus* species which swarm as a thin film or membrane on agar media surfaces. The term "H antigen" denoting flagellar antigen, derives from the German word *Hauch*, indicating a spreading film of growth, like breath condensing on a cold

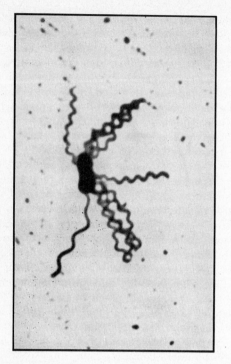

FIG. 3-7. Flagella of *Proteus*. Stained by Leifson's method. One normal and several curly forms. (From Leifson, Cahart, and Fulton: J Bacteriol 69:73, 1955)

cell wall is necessary for both flagellar growth and function, since removal of the rigid cell wall layer by lysozyme under appropriate conditions stops motility if flagella are present or prevents reflagellation if flagella were removed before lysozyme treatment. Reversible immotility results when cells are plasmolyzed. The mechanism by which flagella produce motility in bacteria is unknown, but both the wall and plasma membrane are obviously involved.

Filaments are composed of a protein monomer called "flagellin," which is characteristic of a particular bacterial species and which is similar in properties to contractile proteins such as myosin. In contrast to myosin, however, the bacterial filament has no ATPase activity. The isolated filaments can be dissociated into flagellin by heat, by treatment with mild acid below pH 4.0 and optimally near pH 3.0 to 3.4, or by 4 to 5 M urea. The monomer, flagellin, of molecular weight about 40,000, has the remarkable ability to reaggregate and form polymers: It reassociates to form single strands at pH values of 4.0 to 4.5 and re-forms flagellumlike helically intertwined filaments at pH values near 6.0.

In *Salmonella* organisms where phase varia-

glass surface, whereas the term "O or somatic O antigen" of nonflagellated forms was derived from the German term *ohne Hauch*, indicating a nonspreading type of growth.

The flagellum is composed of three distinct parts: the filament, the hook, and the basal body. The filament is external to the cell and connects to the hook at the cell surface. The hook-basal body structure is embedded in the cell envelope. Hook and filament can easily be differentiated, since the hook is curved and slightly larger in diameter than is the filament (0.017 vs 0.012 μm). The hook and basal body exhibit different antigens and are less soluble in acids and urea than is the filament.

The complete flagellum tripartite structure can be isolated as an intact unit from detergent-treated bacterial protoplast lysates. The isolated organelles, purified by differential and gradient centrifugation, retain the morphologic identity seen in intact cells (Fig. 3-8).

FILAMENTS.   Filaments, which are external to the cell, are easily removed by shaking bacteria with glass beads or by agitating them in a blender. The cells remain viable and regain motility as the flagella regrow. The intact

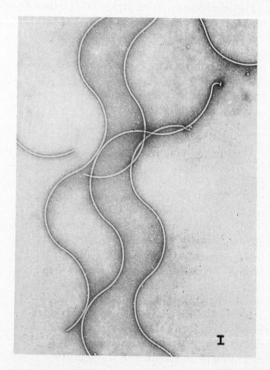

FIG. 3-8. Flagella of *Bacillus subtilis*. Bar equals 0.1 μ. (From Dimitt and Simon: J Bacteriol 105:369, 1971)

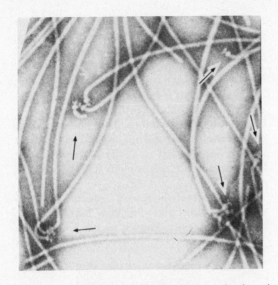

FIG. 3-9. Flagella of *E. coli,* showing filaments, hook, and basal body complex. × 66,000. (From DePamphlis and Adler: J Bacteriol 105:376, 1971)

tion has been described, two flagellar filament antigens which are specified by separate structural genes, the H genes, are alternately produced. Mutation in the H genes produces altered flagellins which can be recognized antigenically and functionally.

BASAL BODY STRUCTURE. The hook and basal body are distinct morphologically. The hook of *E. coli* is some 0.045 μm long, composed of five to six concentric helical coils, and connects to the basal body, 0.027 μm in length. The basal body has two pairs of 0.0225 μm diameter rings mounted on a rod, as shown in Figures 3-9 and 3-10. The outer pair of rings, contiguous with the outer membrane (O-antigen complex) of the gram-negative cell, is not found in flagella from gram-positive organisms, but both *E. coli* and *Bacillus subtilis* flagella exhibit a similar lower ring, or ring pair, which associates with the plasma membrane.

AXIAL FILAMENTS. The spirochetes, ie, the treponemes, leptospires, and borrelia, are

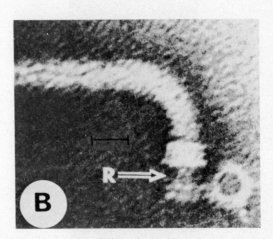

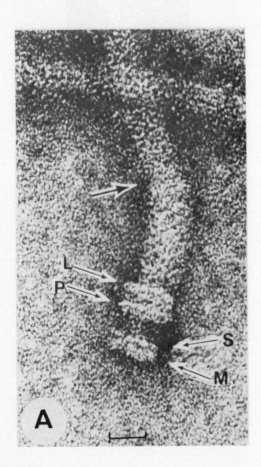

FIG. 3-10. Hook-basal body complex of flagella from *E. coli.* A. Basal end of intact flagellum. Unlabeled arrow marks the junction between the hook and the filament. The top pair of rings are connected near their periphery and resemble a closed cylinder. The individual rings are referred to as the L ring (for attachment to outer—lipopolysaccharide-O-antigen complex—membrane of the cell wall), the P ring (for its association with the peptidoglycan layer of the cell wall), the S ring (for supramembrane, which appears to be located just above the cytoplasmic membrane), and the M ring (for its attachment to the cytoplasmic membrane). Uranyl acetate. B. Note upper L-P ring cylinder. R marks rod connecting the top and bottom rings. A detached ring has associated with the bottom rings. Phosphotungstic acid. Bar equals 0.03 nm. (From DePamphlis and Adler: J Bacteriol 105:384, 1971)

motile cells which move by a traveling helical wave. Spirochetes produce flagellumlike sheathed axial filaments around which the cell is coiled. These filaments are located in the periplasmic space between the inner and outer membranes of the cell. *Treponema microdentium* produces two filaments per cell, *T. reiteri* produces six to eight, and some species produce more. The filaments do not run from one pole of the cell to the other; instead, they originate at opposite poles of the cell and overlap at the center. No obvious connection holds the two overlapping ends together (Fig. 3-11).

Treponeme axial filaments resemble flagella in length, diameter, and proximal hook at attachment sites. Highly purified axial filaments dissociate at low and high pH into a protein monomer with a molecular weight of 37,000. The axial filament is often surrounded by a sheath of unknown composition which is easily removed by distilled water.

Leptospira axial filaments are more complex than those of treponemes. They are composed of an inner case and an outer coat and are slightly larger, that is, 0.025 μm in diameter, than those of the treponemes (0.017 μm).

Pili Metal-shadowed electron micrographs of many gram-negative bacteria reveal hairlike filaments, known as pili or fimbriae,

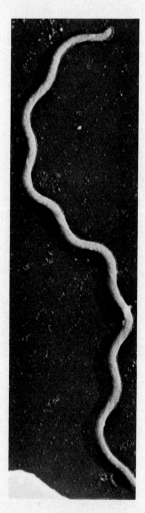
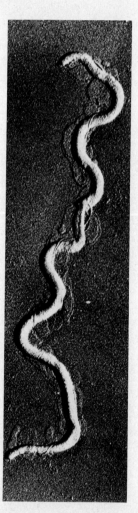

FIG. 3-11. Axial filaments of *Treponema zuelzerae*. Left. Intact cell shadowed with gold. Axial filament faintly visible under outer envelope. Right. After treatment with distilled water, shadowed with gold-palladium. A single axial filament originates at each pole. In the region of overlap, the two filaments have separated from each other and from the cell, the outer envelope of which has been disrupted. × 15,000. (From Bharrier, Eiserling, and Rittenberg: J Bacteriol 105:413, 1971)

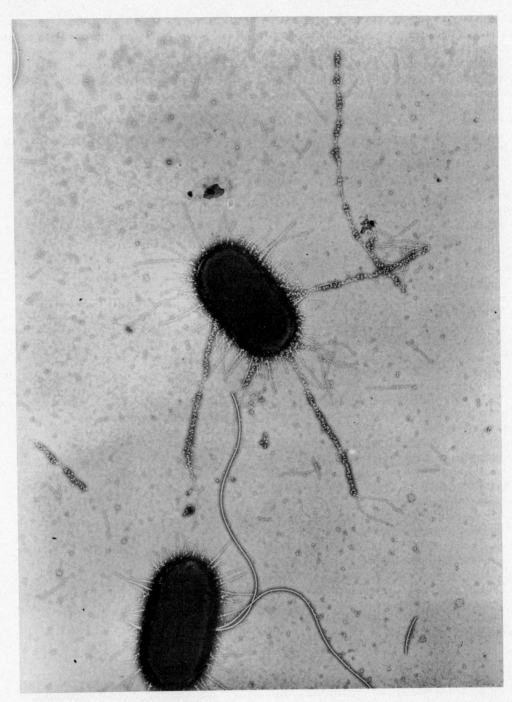

FIG. 3-12. Negatively stained *E. coli* K12 Hfr Cavalli. Note two long, large flagella; F type sex pili with round RNA bacteriophage absorbed to their sides and filamentous DNA bacteriophage absorbed to their tips; and phage-free short common pili. (Courtesy of Dr. Charles C. Brinton)

extending from the cell. These appendages do not confer motility on the cell and are straighter, thinner, and shorter than are flagella. Pili, which are composed of self-aggregating protein monomers (pilin) of 17,000 daltons, originate in the cell membrane. Pili vary from species to species in number, diameter, and length. One of the best sources of richly piliated bacteria is the infected human urinary tract. At least eight morphologic types of pili are known which may be classified as either common or sex pili on the basis of function; both may occur either independently or simultaneously on the same cell (Fig. 3-12). For example, some 100 to 200 ordinary or common pili of 7 μm diameter by 0.5 to 2 μm length may be evenly distributed over the entire cell surface (peripiliation) of *E. coli*, whereas only 1 to 4 sex pili 8.5 μm in diameter are usually found at random sites.

With the single exception of *Corynebacterium renale*, the occurrence of true pili on gram-positive bacteria has not been documented.

Pili appear to serve adhesive functions. Common pili adhere to latex, red blood cells, and glycoproteins of the gut. Piliated cells form pellicles on liquid media, and thereby gain the survival advantage of access to oxygen in dense growth suspensions. The production of pili can be tested by flooding bacterial colonies on an agar plate with a concentrated suspension of red blood cells. When these are rinsed off with saline, only pili-producing colonies retain red cells. Some degree of tissue specificity has been indicated. For example, the pili-mediated adhesion of *Shigella flexneri* to red cells and tissues is specifically inhibited by D-mannose and α-D-methyl-mannoside. And apparently only piliated gonocci (ie, Kellogg types 1 and 2) are infectious. It is not known, however, to what extent pili play a role in the ecology of host-parasite interactions by enabling specific bacterial colonization.

Sex pili, either type F or I, are necessary for the transfer of genetic material from donor to recipient cells during bacterial conjugation (Chap. 8). These pili are detected by the ability of cells to donate genes to recipients, by the presence of a specific sex pilus antigen, or by the ability of the suspected pilus-bearing bacteria to inactivate certain bacteriophages which attach specifically to sex pili (Chap. 70). The latter include both isometric RNA phages which attach to the side of sex pili and filamentous single-stranded DNA phages which attach to their tips. No conjugation or gene transfer occurs if sex pili are not produced or are removed by mechanical disruption or if the tip of the sex pilus is blocked by bacteriophage.

Topography and Visible Ultrastructure of the Bacterial Cell Envelope

Surface Patterns Examination by electron microscopy of different bacteria after negative staining reveals a surprisingly wide range of detailed surface patterns. The gram-positive staphylococcal, lactobacillal, and streptococcal cell surfaces appear smooth and devoid of regular patterns. The surfaces of *Clostridium botulinum* and *B. anthracis* (Sterne) reveal linear patterns of what are thought to be protein particles 6 to 8 nm in diameter. Tetragonal patterns are observed in *Bacillus polymyxa* and various other *Bacillus* species, and hexagonal patterns occur in still other bacilli and a few gram-negative organisms (Fig. 3-13). In contrast to the smooth or finely patterned surface of gram-positive bacteria, most gram-negative species exhibit a strikingly convoluted cell surface (Fig. 3-14).

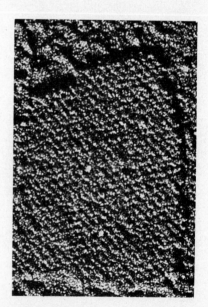

FIG. 3-13. Electron micrograph of a fragment of the envelope of *L. hyalina,* showing the surface pattern after tryptic digestion. $\times$ 160,000 (Courtesy of Drs. J. A. Chapman and M. R. J. Salton)

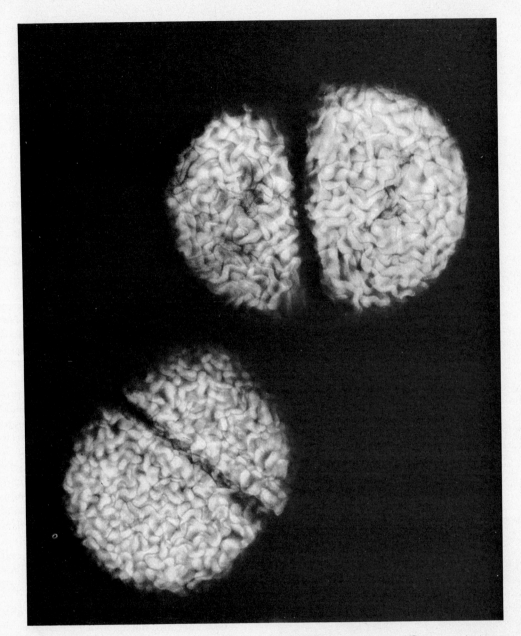

FIG. 3-14. Convoluted surface pattern of whole cells of *Veillonella parvula,* a gram-negative bacterium which is a common inhabitant of the human oral cavity. Negative stain, phosphotungstic acid. (From Bladen and Mergenhagen: J Bacteriol 88:1482, 1964)

The Cell Envelope The bacterial cell envelope serves functionally in several ways. It necessarily interacts with the environment and therefore influences host-parasite interactions. The cell surface contains receptor sites for bacterial viruses and bacteriocins (Chap. 70), is the site of antibody and complement reactions (Chap. 16), and often contains components toxic to the host.

The bacterial cell envelope includes the inner plasma membrane, the overlying semirigid murein sacculus or cell wall, and external specialized or adherent structures. This multilayered organelle of the procaryotic bacterial cell

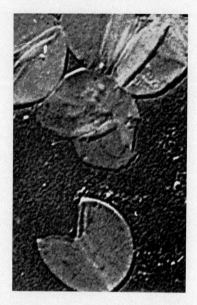

FIG. 3-15. Electron micrograph of cell wall of *Streptococcus faecalis*. (From Bibb and Straughn: J Bacteriol 1094, 1962)

comprises some 20 percent or more of the cell's dry weight. Envelope components are not visible in the darkfield or light microscope but can be observed after appropriate staining in both the light and electron microscopes.

THE MUREIN SACCULUS OR PEPTIDOGLYCAN.

The semirigid, cell-wall peptidoglycan layer or

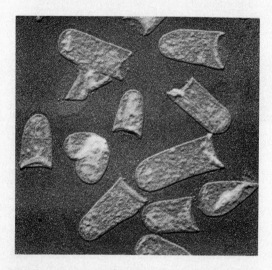

FIG. 3-16. Electron micrograph of cell envelopes of *Mycobacterium tuberculosis*. × 22,000. (From Larson et al: Bacteriol Rev 27:341, 1963)

murein sacculus (wall, from the Latin *murus*) is found in all bacteria except the cell wall-less mycoplasma and halobacteria. Although it is not yet known what determines cell shape, the peptidoglycan layer is responsible for the maintenance of a particular bacterial cell shape. This can be demonstrated by plasmolysis, by isolation of the particulate envelope after mechanical disruption of the bacterial cell, or by lysozyme digestion. In the first two instances the tough cell wall retains the morphologic identity of the cell. And further, the isolated cell walls or envelopes of cocci resemble grape hulls (Fig. 3-15), while isolated envelopes of bacilli appear as long deflated balloons (Fig. 3-16). If whole cells or isolated envelopes are treated with lysozyme, the particulate cell wall is characteristically dissolved.

THICKNESS.   Cell envelopes of various organisms usually range from 0.150 μm to 0.500 μm in thickness as measured in thin sections but reach up to 0.8 μm in some strains of *Lactobacillus acidophilus*. Walls of young, rapidly growing bacterial cells are thinner than those of cells in old cultures or cells limited in protein synthesis by lack of a required amino acid or by antimetabolites. *Staphylococcus aureus* cell walls, for example, may increase from 0.3 to 1.0 μm in thickness when protein synthesis is inhibited by chloramphenicol. The underlying plasma membrane remains approximately constant in thickness, about 8 nm, in both gram-positive and gram-negative bacteria and exhibits a typical trilaminar dark-light-dark unit-membrane structure. Pores of 1 to 10 nm diameter can be demonstrated in isolated cell walls by molecular sieving; membrane pores appear to be about 1 nm in diameter.

Differences Between Gram-positive and Gram-negative Bacterial Cell Envelopes

THE GRAM-POSITIVE CELL WALL. *Teichoic Acids, Specific Polysaccharides, and Proteins.*
Gram-positive bacteria characteristically produce a variety of specific polysaccharides and proteins which in most cases are covalently attached to the peptidoglycan. The better-known polysaccharides include teichoic acids, many of the pneumococcal capsular substances, and the streptococcal group polysaccharides. D-Polyglutamic acid polymers are produced by some bacillus species, and the M

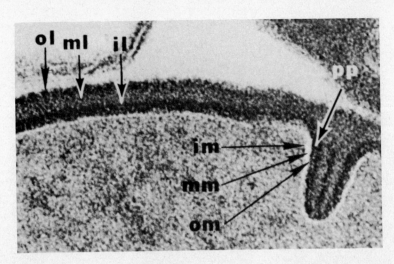

FIG. 3-17. Cell wall transverse thin section of *Staphylococcus aureus*. ol, outer dense layer; ml, middle layer; il, inner dense layer; pp, periplasm; om, outer layer of cytoplasmic membrane; mm, middle nondense layer of membrane; im, inner dense layer of membrane. × 230,000 (From Popkin, Theodore, and Cole: J Bacteriol 107:907, 1971)

protein of the group A streptococcus is a well-known virulence factor. The exact location and topographic arrangement of these substances is as yet unknown. Thin cross-sections of gram-positive cells reveal a relatively thick, contiguous cell wall layer overlying the plasma membrane. This layer can be dissolved by lysozyme in most instances, and can also be shown to be finely differentiated into as yet incompletely identified compact sublayers (Fig. 3-17). Although both protein and polysaccharide are thought to contribute to the layered wall substructure, only proteins have been definitely identified visually. These include the regular surface pattern proteins of various bacilli and other organisms (Fig. 3-13) and the serologic type-specific M protein of the group A streptococci. The M protein forms a diffuse, thick, externally fimbriate wall layer which can be removed by trypsin without destroying cell viability.

THE GRAM-NEGATIVE ENVELOPE. *The Outer Membrane and Lipoprotein.* In contrast to the generally compact appearance of gram-positive cell walls, gram-negative bacteria exhibit three distinct and more loosely arranged envelope layers (Fig. 3-18). These include the convoluted, wrinkled, creviced, or undulating outer membrane (OM) 6 to 20 nm thick, which contains the O antigen, a middle dense layer 1.5 to 3 nm thick, and the inner plasma membrane about 7.5 nm thick. Both the outer membrane

and the plasma membrane of the gram-negative bacterial cell exhibit typical trilaminar unit membrane structure. The middle dense layer can be removed by lysozyme; it corresponds to the rigid peptidoglycan and is much thinner than the corresponding layer in typical gram-positive cell walls. Lipoprotein globules, covalently linked to the outer surface of the murein layer, are found in *E. coli* and the salmonellae. The outer membrane, which is a complex of phospholipid, protein, and lipopolysaccharide, can be removed by various reagents, such as detergents (eg, 2 percent SDS) or 45 percent aqueous phenol, leaving behind the murein sacculus, which encompasses the protoplast.

The outer membrane appears to provide a permeability barrier which ordinarily protects gram-negative bacteria from a wide variety of antimetabolites (eg, actinomycin), detergents, drugs, and enzymes (eg, lysozyme). This has been shown largely in studies of the effect of ethylenediaminetetraacetate (EDTA) treatment, which removes some 30 to 60 percent of the outer membrane and increases permeability.

Protoplasts and Spheroplasts Bacteria ordinarily lyse when the rigid peptidoglycan layer of the cell envelope is dissolved by lysozyme or other agents. However, if stabilized by hypertonic solutions of sucrose or salts (eg, 0.3 to 0.5 M), a wall-less osmotically sensi-

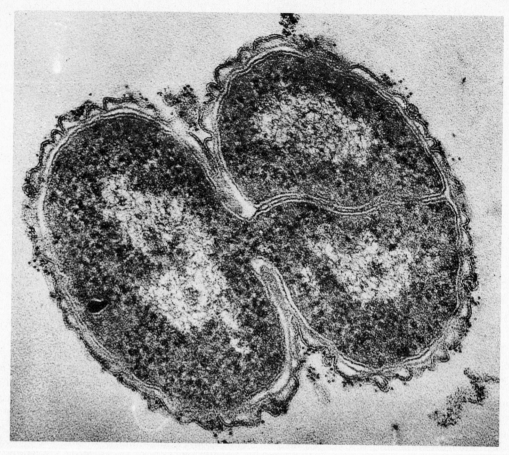

FIG. 3-18. Transverse thin section of *Veillonella parvula*. The layered structure of the gram-negative cell envelope includes a convoluted outer unit membrane, a middle dense layer, and the plasma unit membrane. Note formation of division septa and fibrillar chromatin network in the cell interior. Dark spots of ferritin-labeled O-specific antibody are found primarily on the outside surface of the outer membrane. (From Bladen and Mergenhagen: Ann NY Acad Sci 2:288, 1966)

tive spherical body called a "protoplast" is liberated. If there is doubt about retention of envelope components, the osmotically sensitive body is called a "spheroplast." Gram-positive bacteria treated in this fashion generally yield protoplasts, whereas gram-negative organisms yield spheroplasts, since some outer membrane components inevitably are retained. Spheroplasts can also be produced by growth in hypertonic environments in the presence of peptidoglycan-synthesis inhibitors, such as penicillin (Fig. 3-19), or by withholding a compound, such as diaminopimelic acid, which is required for the growth of a mutant organism.

Periplasm Periplasm, which occurs in the space between the plasma membrane and the outer membrane, may readily be observed

in gram-negative bacteria (Fig. 3-20) but only with difficulty in gram-positive bacteria (Fig. 3-17). The periplasmic space appears to vary with growth conditions and may also vary somewhat from one bacterium to another. In *E. coli*, the periplasmic space has been shown by cytochemical staining to contain various proteins, including alkaline phosphatase, acid hexosephosphatase, and cyclic phosphodiesterase. It is also thought to contain hydrolytic enzymes, such as phosphatase, DNase I, RNase I, and plasmid-controlled penicillinases, in addition to proteins which specifically bind sugars, amino acids, and inorganic ions (Chap. 5). These can be released from the cell by osmotic shock, ie, rapid dilution of hypertonic (0.5M sucrose) cell suspensions, after EDTA treatment. Other enzymes, such as the chromosomally con-

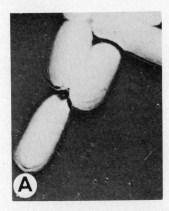

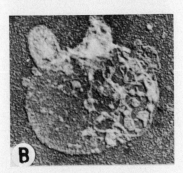

FIG. 3-19. Spheroplast of *E. coli* W 173-25. A. Untreated cells. B. Cell treated for 90 minutes with 500 units of penicillin. × 9,000. (From Schwarz, Asmus, and Frank: J Mol Biol 41:419, 1969)

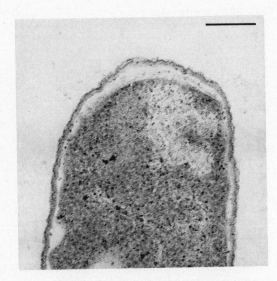

FIG. 3-20. Periplasmic space of *Citrobacter freundii* shown in thin section. Bar equals 0.2 μm. (Courtesy Dr. Sara Miller)

trolled penicillinases of *E. coli*, may be membrane associated, since they are released from the cell only during spheroplast formation (Chaps. 8 and 10).

Cytoplasmic Structures

The Plasma Membrane   Beneath the rigid cell wall layer and in close association with it is the delicate cytoplasmic membrane, vitally important to the cell. In thin sections the plasma membrane shows a typical unit-membrane or trilaminar sandwich structure of dark-light-dark layers of about 0.0025 μm each.

THE MEMBRANE AS AN OSMOTIC BARRIER.   Although bacteria are normally regarded as extremely tolerant to osmotic changes in their external environment, some species, especially gram-negative ones, readily undergo either plasmolysis or plasmoptysis when placed in media of varying salt concentrations. Placing cells in hypertonic solutions results in plasmolysis, that is, shrinkage of the membrane and cytoplasm from the cell wall, which may be observed with both the light and electron microscopes. Unless the cell is specially treated, a few points of connection between membrane and wall generally remain (Fig. 3-21). Gram-negative cells are more easily plasmolyzed than are gram-positive cells, which correlates with their relative internal osmotic pressures.

The presence of an osmotic barrier in bacteria is also indicated by their ability to concentrate certain amino acids against concentration gradients. In gram-positive bacteria a gradient of 300- to 400-fold may exist across the surface layers. Such substances as phosphates, phosphate esters, purines, pyrimidines, and other soluble materials may be present within the cell in a highly concentrated state, and contribute to the internal osmotic pressure. Osmotic activity is also indicated by the cells' selective permeability toward various compounds, especially organic acids.

MEMBRANE-ASSOCIATED STRUCTURES.   Membranes isolated after careful lysis account for some 30 percent or more, of the cell weight. The reason for this surprisingly high value is that numerous structures are attached to bacterial cell membranes; among these are DNA, ribosomes, messenger RNA, and multienzyme complexes. As an example, up to 90 percent of the ribosomes may be isolated as a membrane-polyribosome-DNA aggregate. Since, in thin sections, ribosomes are generally interspersed throughout the cytoplasm and since DNA is usually centrally located in the cell, it is probable that a delicate, and as yet unvisualized, interconnecting cytoplasmic reticulum exists.

MEMBRANE COMPONENTS. Cleanly isolated membranes are composed of approximately 60

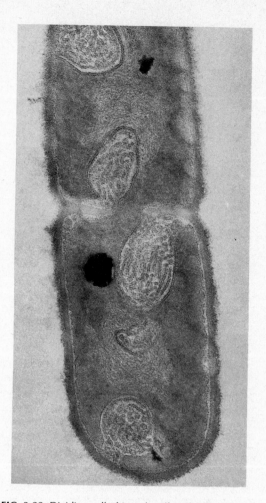

FIG. 3-22. Dividing cell of *Lactobacillus plantarum* showing prominent mesosomes associated with a newly forming crosswall. The immature type of mesosome seen at the bottom is not associated with nucleoplasm, in contrast to the upper mature mesosomes which are surrounded by a triple-layered boundary and are continuous with the nucleoplasm. The black bodies are inclusion granules. × 94,300. (From Kakefuda, Holden, and Utech: J Bacteriol 93:474, 1967)

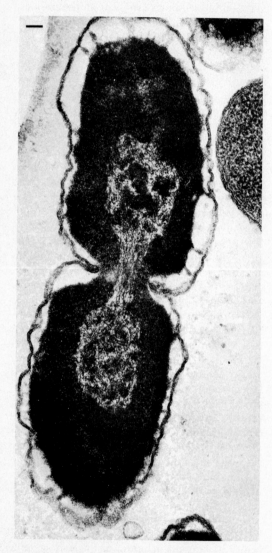

FIG. 3-21. Plasmolyzed dividing cell of *E. coli* B in an almost longitudinal section. Note associations between wall and cytoplasmic membrane and division of nuclear material in the central portion. (Bar equals 0.1 μm (From Bayer: J Gen Microbiol 53:395, 1968)

to 70 percent protein and 20 to 30 percent lipid and small amounts of carbohydrate. Phosphatidylethanolamines and glycolipids are found as major constituents, along with carotenoids and quinones (such as coenzyme Q). Choline and sphingolipids are absent; polyunsaturated fatty acids and steroids are rare. The mycoplasma, which do not make a rigid cell wall, incorporate steroids from the environment into their plasma membranes. Glycolipids found in most bacterial membranes include diglycosyldiglycerides which are found primarily in gram-

with division septa (Figs. 3-22 and 3-23). Attachment of mesosomes to both DNA chromatin and membrane has been demonstrated by
thin-section electron microscopy. Formation of
protoplasts (or spheroplasts) results in eversion
of tubular or vesicular mesosomal components
which remain attached at one end to the outside of the membrane, whereas the enclosing
mesosomal sacs disappear and are apparently
pulled into the membrane by the stretched
protoplast (Fig. 3-24).

The Nuclear Body Bacterial DNA can be
detected as nucleoids or chromatin bodies by
light microscopy using Feulgen staining. It is
difficult to demonstrate chromatin bodies by
direct staining because of the high concentration of ribonucleic acid. However, pretreatment with ribonuclease removes all or nearly
all of the RNA, and chromatin bodies can then
be seen at all stages of the growth cycle. No histones have been detected in bacteria.

Electron microscopy of stained thin sections
reveals nuclear material as an inrregular, thin
fibrillar DNA network which frequently runs
parallel to the axis of the cell. A direct attachment to the membrane is sometimes obvious.
Often the mesosome, itself a membrane-associated structure, serves as a DNA-membrane
attachment site. During multiplication, bacterial DNA remains as a diffuse chromatin network
and never aggregates to form a well-defined
chromosome during cell division, in contrast to
the eucaryotic chromosomes. When bacterial
cells are very gently lysed, the bacterial chromosome may be visualized by radioautography
as a circular molecule (Fig. 7-4). Although bacterial DNA represents only 2 to 3 percent of the
cell weight, it occupies about 10 percent of the
cell volume. This loose arrangement allows for
the ready diffusion of soluble materials to all
parts of the nuclear structure.

Ribosomes Negatively stained thin sections allow resolution by electron microscopy
of small cytoplasmic particles which correspond to the ribosomes present in pellets after
lysed protoplasts or disrupted bacterial cells
are centrifuged at 100,000 g. Ribosomes are
composed of approximately 30 percent protein
and 70 percent RNA and account for up to 40
percent of the protein and 90 percent of the
ribonucleic acid of the cell. Gentle lysis of
growing cells yields almost all ribosomes as

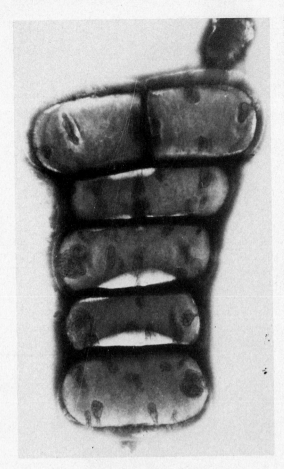

FIG. 3-23. Mesosomes of *Bacillus subtilis* shown by nega-
tive staining. × 30,000. (From Fitz-James: In Guze (ed):
Microbial Protoplasts, Spheroplasts and L-forms, 1968.
Courtesy of Williams and Wilkins)

positive bacterial membranes, which also contain lipoteichoic acids. Polyisoprenoid alchols
are found in small amounts.

Various enzymic activities have been found
associated with membrane proteins. These include the energy-producing bacterial cytochrome and oxidative phosphorylation system,
the membrane permeability systems discussed
in later chapters, and various polymer-synthe-
sizing systems. An ATPase has been isolated
from knoblike membrane structures.

Mesosomes These membrane-associated
organelles are more easily demonstrated in
gram-positive than in gram-negative bacteria.
Mesosomes are usually seen as cytoplasmic
sacs which contain whorled lamellar, tubular,
or vesicular structures and are often associated

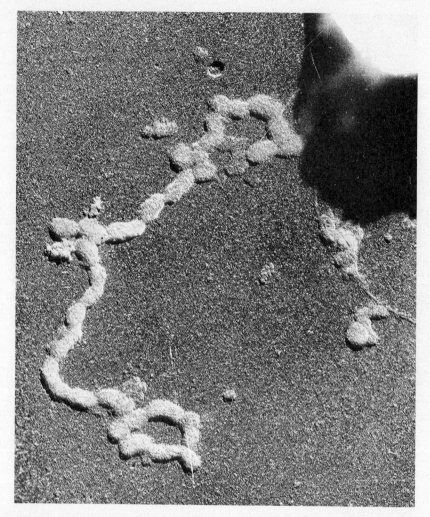

FIG. 3-24. Shadowed preparation of a protoplast of *Bacillus megaterium* showing everted mesosomal tubule in the form of a pearl string. × 22,000. (From Ryter: Bacteriol Rev 32:39, 1968)

polyribosome-membrane aggregates which contain all components of the protein-synthesizing mechanism; polyribosomes are chains of 70S ribosomes (monomers) attached to messenger RNA (Fig. 3-25). Ribosome numbers in the cell vary according to growth conditions; rapid-growing cells in rich medium contain many more ribosomes than do slow-growing cells in poor medium.

SUBUNITS. The stability of ribosomes depends on the presence of Mg^{++}. In low concentrations of magnesium (less than 10^{-4}M Mg^{++}), 70S ribosomal monomers dissociate into 50S and 30S subunits. The 30S subunit measures approximately 0.007 by 0.016 μm and weighs

about 800,000 daltons. It is composed of a single 16S RNA molecule with a molecular weight of about 500,000 daltons and some 20 protein molecules. The 50S subunit measures about 0.014 by 0.016 μm and weighs 1.64 times 10^6 daltons. It is composed of one 23 S RNA molecule with a molecular weight of 1.1 times 10^6 daltons, a 5S RNA molecule (40,000 daltons), and some 30 protein molecules.

BIOSYNTHESIS. Several intermediates in ribosome synthesis have been isolated. For example, 16S ribosomal RNA can be found in the form of a complex with protein which sediments with 26S and is a precursor of the 30S subunit. Similarly, one of the precursors of the

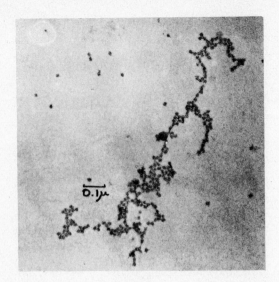

FIG. 3-25. Polyribosomes from *E. coli*. Note the membrane fragment in the center. Negative staining with uranyl acetate. (Courtesy of Dr. A. Rich)

50S subunit is a 32S particle which contains only about two-thirds of the protein complement of the complete 50S subunit. Stages in the genesis of ribosomal subunits are also revealed by measuring the degree of methylation of ribosomal RNA. For example, the RNA molecule present in the 32S precursor complex contains no methyl groups, and the RNA molecule in a 43S precursor particle is less methylated than the 23S RNA molecule present in intact 50S subunits. The 5S RNA component is found only in mature 50S subunits.

PROTEINS.   Most, if not all, of the protein molecules which comprise the ribosomal subunits are different; in other words, the protein complement of the smaller subunit consists of about 20 different molecules, that of the larger of about 30. All these proteins have been separated and partially characterized. Ribosomal proteins range in molecular weight from 10,000 to 65,000.

Ribosomal subunits are more or less completely dissociated into their components by concentrated salt solutions, with the actual degree of dissociation depending on the nature of the ions and their concentration. The more easily dissociated proteins, in particular those liberated by 2 to 3 M cesium chloride, are known as "split" proteins, while those that remain associated with the RNA under these

conditions are the "core" proteins. Ribosomal subunit cores and split proteins are nonfunctional in protein synthesis on their own, but if incubated together in vitro, they reconstitute to yield subunits indistinguishable from native particles in all respects, including ability to synthesize protein.

Polyamines Bacteria do not synthesize histones, but they do produce polyamines, which are required for the growth of some *Haemophilus* species and are found associated in general with bacterial DNA, ribosomes, and membranes. The three principal ones are:

Putrescine: $H_2N(CH_2)_4NH_2$
Spermidine: $H_2N(CH_2)_4NH(CH_2)_3NH_2$
Spermine:
$H_2N(CH_2)_3NH(CH_2)_4NH(CH_2)_3NH_2$

The precise function of polyamines is not known, but they seem to exert most of their effects by more or less completely replacing or substituting for Mg^{++}, which is itself essential for the stability of DNA, ribosomes, and membranes. In support of this view, polyamines are known to exert an antimutagenic effect, they prevent dissociation of 70S ribosomes to 30S and 50S components, and they increase the resistance of protoplasts to osmotic lysis. Furthermore, it is found that the amount of spermidine varies inversely with the amount of Mg^{++} in ribosomes, and that 30S and 50S ribosomal subunits remain associated in the absence of Mg^{++} if spermidine is present. From this, it would appear that charge neutralization of polyanionic polymers such as nucleic acid may be at least partly nonspecific.

Cytoplasmic Granules The cytoplasm of growing cells generally appears remarkably homogeneous. However, granules which can be identified by appropriate staining procedures tend to appear in older cells. Usually they represent accumulation of food reserves, such as polysaccharides, lipids, and polyphosphate complexes, and they vary in amount with the type of medium and the functional state of the cells. Glycogen is the major storage material of enteric bacteria and may account for as much as 40 percent of the weight of some bacterial species. Similarly some *Bacillus* and *Pseudomonas* species accumulate as much as 7 to 30 percent of their weight as poly-β-hydroxybutyrate. Another type of inclusion granule is

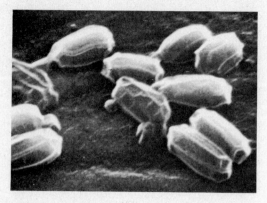

FIG. 3-26. *Bacillus polymyxa* endospores examined in a scanning electron microscope. Both parallel ribbing and random reticulation of the surface structure are exhibited. × 4,800. (From Murphy and Campbell: J Bacteriol 98:727, 1969)

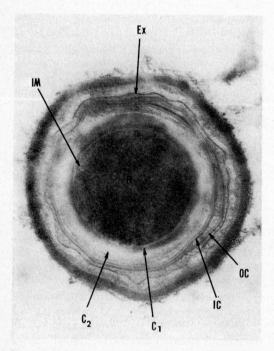

FIG. 3-27. Cross-section of a *Bacillus cereus* endospore before release from parent cell, showing various spore coats and layers. Ex, exosporium; IM, inner membrane; R, ribosomal aggregates; OC, outer coat; IC, inner coat; C_1, inner dense cortical layer; C_2, less dense cortical layer. Note that parent cell still surrounds the exosporium. ×75,000 (From Ellar and Lundgren: J Bacteriol 92: 1748, 1966)

the metachromatically staining Babes-Ernst or volutin granule, which is thought to consist chiefly of polyphosphate and which is found in abundance in diphtheria and plague bacilli, mycobacteria, and some other bacteria; they stain red with toluidine blue and methylene blue.

Bacterial Endospores   Endospore formation is a distinguishing feature of organisms of the family Bacillaceae, which includes members of the aerobic genus, *Bacillus*, and the anaerobic genus, *Clostridium*. Endospores resist adverse environmental conditions of dryness, heat, and poor nutrient supply. If present in inadequately heat-sterilized canned foods, spores of the anaerobic *Clostridium* germinate, grow, and cause spoilage. In the case of *C. botulinum*, this is especially dangerous because spoilage may not be obvious even though accompanied by the production of deadly exotoxin. Other spore formers, such as the gas-gangrene bacillus, *C. perfringens*, or the tetanus bacillus, *C. tetani*, produce their toxic effects only when a medium of dead or injured tissue affords the spore a nidus for growth in the animal body.

The true endospore is a highly refractile body formed within the vegetative bacterial cell at a certain stage of growth. The size, shape, and position of the spore are relatively constant characteristics of a given species and are therefore of some value in distinguishing one kind of bacillus from another (Fig. 3-26). The position of the spore in the cell may be central, subterminal, or terminal. It may be the same diameter as the cell, smaller, or larger, causing a swelling of the cell. Various protective spore coats are formed within the vegetative cell before death and dissolution of the parent cell (Fig. 3-27). These include a rigid peptidoglycan layer which, in the case of *Bacillus pumilis*, differs in composition from that of the parent vegetative cell. Spore surface antigens are usually different from those of the parent vegetative bacilli.

FURTHER READING

Books and Reviews

Archibald AR, Baddiley J, Blumson NL: The teichoic acids. Adv Enzymol 30:223, 1968

Bayer ME: Ultrastructure and organization of the bacterial envelope. Ann NY Acad Sci 235:6, 1974

Driel DV, Wicken AJ, Dickson MR, Knox KW: Cellular location of the lipoteichoic acids of *Lactobacillus fermenti* NCTC 6991 and *Lactobacillus casei* NCTC 6375. J Ultrastruct Res 43:483, 1973

Glauert AM, Thornley MJ: The topography of the bacterial cell wall. Annu Rev Microbiol 23:159, 1969

Higgins ML, Shockman GD: Procaryotic cell division with respect to wall and membranes. CRC Crit Rev Microbiol 1:29, 1971

Ino T: Genetics and chemistry of bacterial flagella. Bacteriol Rev 33:454, 1969

Kalckar HM: The periplasmic galactose binding protein of *Escherichia coli*. Science 174:557, 1971

Knox KW, Wicken AJ: Immunologic properties of teichoic acids. Bacteriol Rev 37:215, 1973

Meynell E, Meynell GG, Datta N: Phylogenetic relationships of drug-resistance factors and other transmissible bacterial plasmids. Bacteriol Rev 32:55, 1968

Neidhart FC: Effects of environment on the composition of bacterial cells. Annu Rev Microbiol 17:61, 1963

Nomura M: Bacterial ribosomes. Bacteriol Rev 34:228, 1970

Rogers HJ: Bacterial growth and the cell envelope. Bacteriol Rev 34:194, 1970

Ryter A: Association of the nucleus and the membrane of bacteria: a morphological study. Bacteriol Rev 32:39, 1968

Salton MRJ: The Bacterial Cell Wall. Amsterdam, Elsevier Publ Co, 1964

Salton MRJ: Bacterial membranes. CRC Crit Rev Microbiol 1:161, 1971

Wannamaker LW, Matsen JM (eds): Streptococci and Streptococcal Diseases. New York, Academic Press, 1972

Selected Papers

Boman HG Nordstrom K, Normark S: Penicillin resistance in *Escherichia coli* K 12: synergism between penicillinases and a barrier in the outer part of the envelope. Ann NY Acad Sci 235:569, 1974

Brinton CC Jr: Contributions of pili to the specificity of the bacterial surface, and a unitary hypothesis of conjugal infectious heredity. In Davis B, Warren L (eds): The Specificity of Cell Surfaces. Englewood Cliffs, NJ, Prentice-Hall, 1967, pp. 37-70

Davies JE, Benveniste RE: Enzymes that inactivate antibiotics in transit to their targets. Ann NY Acad Sci 235:130, 1974

Flessel CP, Ralph P, Rich A: Polyribosomes of growing bacteria. Science 158:658, 1967

Kurland CG: Ribosome structure and function emergent. Science 169:1171, 1970

Lieve L: The barrier function of the gram-negative envelope. Ann NY Acad Sci 235:109, 1974

Wetzel BK, Spicer BK, Dvorak HF, Heppel LA: Cytochemical localization of certain phosphatases in *Escherichia coli*. J Bacteriol, 104:529, 1970

4
Energy Metabolism

Bacterial cells, like the cells of all living organisms, accomplish work. For this they require a source of energy. Although the wide variety of compounds that serve as a source of energy for microorganisms is almost limitless, there is a remarkable simplicity in the basic metabolic patterns utilized to transform this energy into a useful form. Many of these systems are fundamentally similar to those found in the higher forms of life, but superimposed on these basic mechanisms are examples of differentiation unique to the bacterial world.

The systems in bacteria that transform chemical and radiant energy into a biologically useful form include respiration, fermentation, and photosynthesis. In respiration, molecular oxygen is the ultimate electron acceptor, while in fermentation, the foodstuff molecule is usually broken down into two fragments, one of which is then oxidized by the other. In photosynthesis, light energy is converted into chemical energy. In all types of cells, however, and regardless of the mechanism used to extract useful energy, the reaction is accompanied by the formation of adenosine triphosphate (ATP). ATP is a common intermediate of both energy-mobilizing and energy-requiring reactions, and its formation provides a mechanism by which the available energy may be channeled into the energy-requiring biosynthetic reactions of the cell. The study of energy metabolism is the study of ATP production.

The metabolic activity of bacteria is very high. This is manifested both in a very rapid rate of cell division and in a high rate of catabolism. Associated with these processes is a very noticeable evolution of heat, much greater than for other organisms. Since the heat produced during metabolism represents that fraction of the total free-energy change which is unavailable to the organisms for the performance of work, bacteria in general are less efficient as converters of free energy than are organisms with a slower metabolic rate.

BIOENERGETICS

Fundamentally, the bacterial cell is a physical-chemical system whose activities occur in large part by the flow of chemical energy. The same laws of thermodynamics that deal with energy and its transformations also hold in the biologic world.

In the cell where work is performed under

TABLE 4-1   RELATIONSHIP BETWEEN THE EQUILIBRIUM CONSTANT AND THE STANDARD FREE ENERGY CHANGE AT 25C

k_{eq}	$\Delta F'$ cal/mole
0.001	+4,089
0.01	+2,726
0.1	+1,363
1.0	0
10.0	−1,363
100.0	−2,726
1,000.0	−4,089

isothermal conditions, that fraction of the system's energy that tends to carry out the work process is referred to as the free energy, ΔF. In such systems, however, there is a large energy fraction that cannot be made to perform in the manner required of work, and this energy is regarded as unavailable or "lost to entropy." The driving force of all processes is the tendency to seek the position of maximum entropy, and heat is either given up or absorbed by the system from the surroundings to reach this state.

The fundamental equation relating these changes is

$$\Delta F = \Delta H - T\Delta S$$

where ΔH is the total energy of the system and $T\Delta S$ the increase in entropy.

The free energy change of chemical reactions can in principle be quite accurately measured. Since the equilibrium reached in a chemical reaction is a function of the drive toward minimum free energy of the reaction components, the equilibrium constant is a mathematical function of the free energy change of the components of the reaction (Table 4-1). When the equilibrium constant is high, the reaction tends to go to completion, and the standard free energy change is negative. Such a reaction is an exergonic or downhill reaction and proceeds with a decline of free energy. When the equilibrium constant is low, the reaction does not go far in the direction of completion, the free energy change is positive, and energy must be put into the system. Such processes are endergonic or uphill reactions.

Energy from Organic Compounds   The heterotrophic bacterial cell ultimately derives its energy from the chemical energy stored in the molecules of its carbon substrate. This is accomplished by a sequence of oxidative reactions during which utilizable energy is released. In biologic oxidations as well as in chemical ones, the essential characteristic is the removal of electrons from the substance being oxidized. Since the majority of biologic oxidations involve a dehydrogenation, biologic oxidations may be expressed more simply in terms of the transfer of hydrogen. In the transfer of hydrogen from the substrate to a final hydrogen acceptor, reducing equivalents are removed, two at a time, and passed via a graded series of oxidation-reduction systems such that the derivatives en route are alternately reduced and oxidized. The occurrence of several reversible oxidation-reduction reactions between the initial substrate and final oxidant makes for a smoother release of energy, providing a system whereby oxidations involving large amounts of energy resulting from the complete oxidation of a carbohydrate are split up into several integrated partial reactions, and the energy is stored or liberated in smaller packets.

The calculation of free energy changes for oxidation-reduction reactions is based on the oxidation-reduction potential, a quantitative measure of the ability of the system to accept or donate electrons reversibly with reference to the standard hydrogen electrode. In biologic systems the normal potential at a given pH is referred to by the symbol E'_0. A knowledge of the potential of any two oxidation-reduction systems enables one to predict the direction of interaction. A system with a more positive normal oxidation-reduction potential than another system has a greater tendency to take up electrons, ie, it is a stronger oxidizing agent. The standard free energy change of oxidative reactions in calories per mole may be calculated from equilibrium data.

Key Position of Adenosine Triphosphate   In both aerobic and anaerobic cells all of the utilizable energy released by oxidation is transformed to ATP for use in driving the various energy-requiring reactions involved in the biosynthesis of cell material. The amount of ATP available from a particular substrate depends on whether the organism employs a fermentative type of metabolism or whether the compound is completely oxidized to CO_2 and H_2O.

ATP occurs in all types of cells: animal, plant, and microbial. Its free energy of hydrol-

TABLE 4-2   Standard Free Energy of Hydrolysis of Phosphorylated Compounds

	$\Delta F^{o'}$ kcal	Direction of Phosphate Group Transfer
Phosphoenolpyruvate	−14.8	
1,3-Diphosphoglycerate	−11.8	
Acetyl phosphate	−10.1	
ATP	− 7.3	
Glucose-1-phosphate	− 5.0	
Fructose-6-phosphate	− 3.8	
Glucose-6-phosphate	− 3.3	↓

ysis is significantly higher than that of simple esters, glycosides, and many phosphorylated compounds. Molecules such as ATP, which are characterized by a free energy of hydrolysis at pH 7 more negative than 7 kcal per mole, are classified as high-energy compounds. These energy-rich compounds include a number of other important molecules: acetyl phosphate, aminoacyl adenylates, phosphoenolpyruvate, and the esters of coenzyme A and lipoic acid, all of which serve as a driving force for the various endergonic reactions of the cell.

The standard free energies of hydrolysis of various phosphate compounds are shown in Table 4-2. Compounds with the more negative values have a higher equilibrium constant than those lower in the scale. This scale is thus a quantitative measure of the affinity of the compound for its phosphoryl group. Those high in the scale tend to lose their phosphate groups, and those lower in the scale tend to hold on to their phosphate groups. ATP is unique because its free energy of hydrolysis occupies the midpoint of a thermodynamic scale of phosphorylated compounds.

The ATP-ADP system functions as an intermediate carrier of phosphate groups. ADP (adenosine diphosphate) serves as a specific acceptor of phosphate groups from cellular phosphate compounds of very high potential formed during the oxidation of substrate by the cell. The ATP so formed then donates its terminal phosphate group enzymatically to phosphate acceptor molecules, such as glucose, transforming them to phosphate derivatives with a higher energy content. The direction of enzymatic phosphate group transfer is specified by this thermodynamic scale. Phosphate groups are transferred only from compounds of high potential to acceptors of low potential, ie, down the scale.

GENERATION OF ATP. There are five known types of metabolic reaction that eventually lead to the production of ATP: (1) substrate level oxidative phosphorylation, (2) phosphorolysis of C—C, C—N, or C—S bonds, (3) dehydration of 2-phosphoglycerate, (4) oxidative phosphorylation linked to electron transport, and (5) photosynthetic phosphorylation.

In the first group, substrate-level oxidative phosphorylation, the oxidation of aldehydes or keto acids is accompanied by esterification of P_i, resulting in the formation of acyl-P, followed by a transfer of its phosphate to ADP. The oxidative step of the glycolytic pathway catalyzed by glyceraldehyde-3-phosphate dehydrogenase is an example of this type of reaction. The second group contains reactions leading to ATP formation by the cleavage of C—C, C—N, or C—S bonds. Microorganisms, particularly anaerobic bacteria, use such reactions to obtain energy for growth by the breakdown of citrulline, purines, and glycine. The cleavage of xylulose-5-P and of fructose-6-P are energy-yielding reactions also belonging to this group. The third type of reaction represents a mechanism of dehydration linked to the production of a compound with a high-energy group potential. The only well-established representative in this group is the dehydration of 2-P-glycerate to P-enolpyruvate during glycolysis. The last two groups contain the electron transport-linked reactions of oxidative phosphorylation and of photosynthesis that give rise to ATP formation.

ENERGY-YIELDING METABOLISM

There is among bacteria a remarkable diversity and individuality of metabolites consumed via the various catabolic routes. In spite of individual variations, however, there is a conspicuous degree of order and simplicity in metabolic patterns and a central area of metabolism that provides a direct link between catabolic and biosynthetic pathways.

Glucose occupies an important position in the metabolism of most biologic forms, and its dissimilation provides a metabolic pathway common to most forms of life. The ability to utilize a sugar or related compound of a configuration different from glucose is the result of the organism's ability to convert the substrate to intermediates common to the pathways for glucose fermentation.

Glycolytic Pathway The major route of glucose catabolism in most cells is that of glycolysis, in which the glucose molecule is degraded to two molecules of lactic acid without the intervention of molecular oxygen. The basic concepts of glycolysis are incorporated in the Embden-Meyerhof-Parnas scheme, shown in Figure 4-1. The sequence consists of 11 enzymatic reactions. Although the basic pathway is the same for all cell types, the properties of certain of the enzymes in the pathway are not uniform in all species or cell types. Such variations apparently are introduced for purposes of cellular differentiation and control of specific steps in the pathway.

Glycolysis consists basically of two major phases. In the first, glucose is phosphorylated and cleaved to form glyceraldehyde-3-PO_4. In the second phase this 3-carbon intermediate is converted to lactic acid in a series of oxidoreduction reactions that are coupled to the phosphorylation of ADP. A mechanism is thus provided for the conservation of the energy originally present in the glucose molecule.

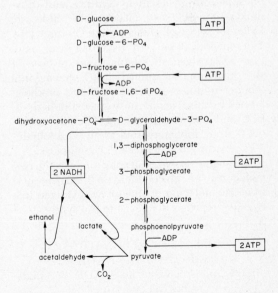

FIG. 4-1. The Embden-Meyerhof-Parnas glycolytic scheme.

The conversion of glucose to glyceraldehyde-3-PO_4 proceeds as follows:

(1) glucose + ATP → glucose-6-PO_4 + ADP
(2) glucose-6-PO_4 ⇌ fructose-6-PO_4
(3) fructose-6-PO_4 + ATP ⇌ fructose-1,6-diPO_4 + ADP
(4) fructose-1,6-diPO_4 ⇌ glyceraldehyde-3-PO_4 + dihydroxyacetone-PO_4

Reaction 3, the phosphorylation of D-fructose to fructose-1,6-diphosphate, occupies a very strategic position in the glycolytic pathway. Alternate pathways of hexose metabolism diverge from the other hexose phosphates in the earlier part of the pathway. This reaction may be regarded as the first one characteristic of the glycolytic sequence proper and thus constitutes a very important branch and control point, subject to strong metabolic regulation. Phosphofructokinase, the enzyme catalyzing this pathway, is an allosteric enzyme responding to fluctuations in adenine nucleotide levels. Control at this point ensures that when an abundant supply of ATP is available as occurs when lactate and pyruvate are oxidized to CO_2 via the citric acid cycle, glycolysis will be essentially blocked, and glucose synthesis will be favored. The reverse is also true. When glycolysis is absolutely required for energy generation, glycolysis will be favored and carbohydrate synthesis turned off.

Reaction 4, the cleavage of fructose-1,6-diphosphate to glyceraldehyde-3-PO_4 and dihydroxyacetone-PO_4, is catalyzed by aldolase. Different types of aldolases are produced by different cell types. In bacteria, fungi, and blue-green algae, the aldolases are of class II and differ from the animal class I enzyme in a number of their properties. Of the products formed by this reaction, only glyceraldehyde-3-PO_4 can be directly degraded. The other product is reversibly converted to glyceraldehyde-3-PO_4 by the enzyme triose-PO_4-isomerase.

During the second stage of glycolysis the two molecules of glyceraldehyde-3-PO_4 formed from one molecule of glucose are oxidized in a two-step reaction that leads to the synthesis of ATP.

(5) glyceraldehyde-3-PO_4 + NAD^+ + P_i ⇌ 1,3-diphosphoglycerate + NADH + H^+
(6) 1,3-diphosphoglycerate + ADP ⇌ 3-phosphoglycerate + ATP

In the first of these reactions, the aldehyde group of glyceraldehyde-3-phosphate is oxidized to the oxidation level of a carboxyl group. The other important component of the reaction is the oxidizing agent, nicotinamide adenine dinucleotide (NAD), that accepts electrons from the aldehyde group of glyceraldehyde-3-PO_4. The electrons are then carried to pyruvate that is formed later in the glycolytic pathway.

In the next reaction the 1,3-diphosphoglycerate that was formed in reaction 5 transfers a phosphate group to ADP, with the resultant formation of 3-phosphoglycerate. As a result of these two reactions the energy derived from the oxidation of an aldehyde group to a carboxylate group has been conserved as the phosphate bond energy of ATP.

These two reactions are a prototype example of substrate-level oxidative phosphorylation. In these reactions the phosphorylation of ADP is coupled to the NAD-linked oxidation of glyceraldehyde -3-PO_4, as shown in Figure 4-2. In this type of coupling, hydrogen is transferred from an initial donor to a final acceptor via transitional intermediates and via intermediate carrier compounds. The common covalent intermediate 1,3-diphosphoglycerate is the common covalent intermediate in the above reactions.

The dehydration of 2-phosphoglycerate to phosphoenolpyruvate, as shown in Figure 4-1, is the second reaction of the glycolytic sequence in which a high-energy phosphate bond is generated. The formation of this bond involves an internal rearrangement of a phosphorylated molecule leading to the conversion of a phosphoryl group of low energy into one of high energy. In the subsequent reaction the phosphate group from phosphoenolpyruvate is transferred to ADP, yielding ATP and pyruvate.

In the glycolytic pathway a total of 4 moles of ATP are formed per mole of glucose used. Since 2 moles of ATP are used in the initial

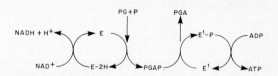

FIG. 4-2. Primary chemical coupling between the phosphorylation of ADP and the NAD-linked oxidation of 3-phosphoglyceraldehyde (PG) to 3-phosphoglycerate (PGA) via 1,3-diphosphoglycerate (PGAP). E/E-2H and E′/E′-P stand for 3-phosphoglyceraldehyde dehydrogenase and 3-phosphoglycerate kinase, respectively.

steps, the net ATP yield is 2 moles per mole of glucose fermented.

The stoichiometry observed in the production of pyruvate from hexoses is:

$$C_6H_{12}O_6 + 2\ NAD^+ + 2\ ADP + 2\ P_i \rightleftharpoons$$
$$2CH_3COCOO^- + 2\ NADH + 2\ ATP$$
$$\Delta F^{\circ\prime} = 15\ kcal/mole$$

Only a very small proportion of the total free energy potentially derivable from the breakdown of a hexose molecule is actually made available via this pathway. This is because of the inherent inefficiency of the system, as well as the fact that the reaction products are compounds in which carbon is still at a relatively reduced level. The ultimate fate of the key metabolite pyruvate depends upon the means employed for the regeneration of NAD^+ from NADH. For this purpose microorganisms have evolved a variety of pathways.

Pentose Phosphate Pathway Whereas the EMP scheme is the major pathway in many microorganisms, as well as in animal and plant tissues, it does not represent the only available pathway for carbohydrate metabolism. The pentose phosphate pathway or hexose monophosphate shunt functions in the fermentation of hexoses, pentoses, and several other carbohydrates in a number of microorganisms. The point of departure of this route from the EMP system is the oxidation of glucose-6-phosphate to 6-phosphogluconate, which in turn is converted to pentose phosphates. The oxidation of glucose-6-phosphate is catalyzed by glucose-6-P dehydrogenase, an important enzyme of wide distribution. NADP is the specific coenzyme for most of these enzymes. In each oxidation one molecule of NADP is converted to NADPH, a supply of which is required by the cell for reductive biosynthetic reactions.

When glucose is fermented through the pentose phosphate pathway, the net yield of ATP is half of that characteristic of the EMP pathway. This lower energy yield is characteristic of a pathway of dehydrogenation before cleavage. There are several variations of the pentose

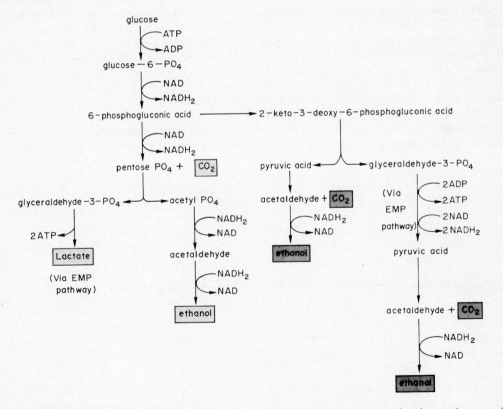

FIG. 4-3. Alternate pathways of glucose fermentation in certain bacteria. The pentose phosphate pathway used in heterolactic fermentation is shown on the left. A variation of this pathway, the Entner-Doudoroff pathway on the right, results in the alcoholic fermentation of glucose.

phosphate pathway. One major fermentation pattern, the heterolactic, follows this route and provides an explanation for the source of ethanol in those organisms that lack aldolase and triose-PO_4 isomerase (Fig. 4-3).

ENTNER-DOUDOROFF PATHWAY. Although this pathway has been established as a functional system for only *Pseudomonas lindneri*, enzymes characteristic of the pathway have been detected in other species. The pathway diverges at 6-P-gluconate from the pentose phosphate pathway. In this sequence, 6-P-gluconate is dehydrated and then cleaved to yield one molecule of glyceraldehyde-3-P and one molecule of pyruvate, from which ethanol and CO_2 are formed via the same series of reactions as in alcoholic fermentation by yeast.

FATE OF PYRUVATE UNDER ANAEROBIC CONDITIONS

The fermentation of glucose is always initiated by a phosphorylation at the expense of ATP, to yield glucose-6-P. The pyruvic acid to which glucose-6-P is converted is a key intermediate in the fermentative metabolism of all carbohydrates. In its formation, NAD is reduced, and must be reoxidized in order to achieve a final oxidation-reduction balance. This reoxidation characteristically occurs in the terminal step reactions and is accompanied by

the reduction of a product derived from pyruvic acid.

Bacteria differ markedly from animal tissues in the manner in which they dispose of the pyruvic acid. In mammalian physiology the main course of respiration is such that substrates are oxidized to CO_2 and H_2O, oxygen being the ultimate hydrogen acceptor. Among the bacteria, however, incomplete oxidation is the rule rather than the exception, and the products of fermentation may accumulate to an extraordinary degree. The final product in certain organisms is either alcohol or lactic acid; in others the pyruvic acid is further metabolized to such products as butyric acid, butyl alcohol, acetone, and propionic acid. Bacterial fermentations are of practical importance because they provide products of industrial value and are useful in the identification of bacterial species (Fig. 4-4).

ALCOHOLIC FERMENTATION. The oldest known type of fermentation is the production of ethanol from glucose. In yeasts that carry out an almost pure alcoholic fermentation, the alcohol arises from the decarboxylation of pyruvic acid with the formation of acetaldehyde and carbon dioxide. The acetaldehyde is then reduced to ethanol by alcohol dehydrogenase, and the NADH is reoxidized. Although a number of bacteria produce alcohol, it is produced via other pathways.

HOMOLACTIC FERMENTATION. All members of the genera *Streptococcus* and *Pediococcus*

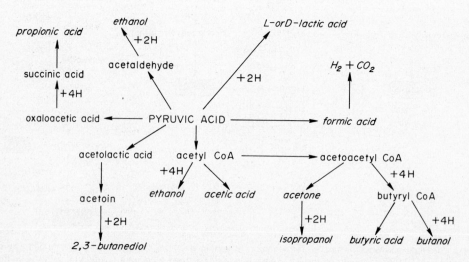

FIG. 4-4. Fate of pyruvate in major fermentations by microorganisms.

and many species of *Lactobacillus* ferment glucose predominantly to lactic acid with no more than a trace accumulation of other products. In the dissimilation of glucose by the homofermenters, pyruvate is reduced to lactic acid by the enzyme lactic dehydrogenase, with NADH acting as the hydrogen donor. The homofermentative mechanism owes its characteristically high yields of lactic acid to the action of aldolase, which cleaves the hexose diphosphate into two equal parts, both of which form pyruvate, and hence lactate. The same fermentation occurs in animal muscle.

HETEROLACTIC FERMENTATION. In addition to the production of lactic acid, some members of the lactic group, *Leuconostoc* and certain *Lactobacillus* species, produce a mixed fermentation in which only about one-half of the sugar is converted to lactic acid, the remainder appearing as CO_2, alcohol, formic acid, or acetic acid. The heterolactic fermentation differs fundamentally from the homolactic type in that the pentose phosphate pathway is employed rather than the EMP scheme. The release of carbon 1 of glucose as CO_2 is characteristic of glucose fermentations by all heterolactic organisms. Also of significance is the finding that the energy yield as measured by growth is one-third lower per mole of glucose fermented than observed for homolactic organisms.

PROPIONIC ACID FERMENTATION. Propionic acid bacteria are gram-positive, nonspore-forming rods closely related to the lactobacilli. The propionic acid that they produce from glucose or from lactic acid contributes to the characteristic taste and smell of Swiss cheese. The ability of these organisms to ferment lactate is significant in that it allows the organism to net an additional ATP.

The early stages in hexose fermentation,

3 $CH_3CHOHCOOH$

↓ −6H

3 $CH_3COCOOH$

ADP + P_i ⌉
                +6H
ATP ⌋

2 CH_3CH_2COOH + CH_3COOH + CO_2

in these organisms, are those of the EMP scheme. The latter stages, either from pyruvate or lactic acid, are highly complex and are cyclic in nature.

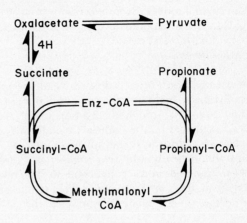

MIXED ACID FERMENTATION. This type of fermentation is characteristic of most of the *Enterobacteriaceae*. In it the metabolism of pyruvate leads to a number of different products, whose nature and quantitative relationships vary with the organism. All of the enterobacteria produce formate, which either accumulates or which under acid conditions is converted by formic hydrogenlyase to molecular hydrogen and carbon dioxide. The formic acid produced in this fermentation is derived from pyruvate in a cleavage involving CoA to yield acetyl-CoA and formate. The acetyl-CoA is rapidly converted to acetyl phosphate. The combined reaction whereby formate and acetate are produced from pyruvate is known as the phosphoroclastic split.

$$CH_3COCOOH + HSCoA \rightleftharpoons CH_3CO \cdot SCoA + HCOOH$$
$$CH_3CO \cdot SCoA + P_i \rightleftharpoons HSCoA + CH_3COOP$$

The conversion of formate to CO_2 and H_2 is the result of hydrogenlyase activity. Hydrogenlyase is an inducible enzyme whose formation is prevented by aerobiosis. Fermentations by *Escherichia coli* and most *Salmonella* are characterized by CO_2 and H_2 production, but in *Shigella* and *Salmonella typhi* no CO_2 and H_2 are produced, and an equivalent amount of formic acid accumulates. The inability of *S. typhi* and *Shigella* to cleave formate is useful in the diagnostic bacteriology laboratory.

$$HCOOH \rightarrow H_2 + CO_2$$

The overall fermentation by *E. coli* is as follows:

$$2 \text{ glucose} + H_2O \rightarrow 2 \text{ lactate} + \text{acetate} + \text{ethanol} + 2 CO_2 + H_2$$

The ethanol formed by *E. coli* comes from acetyl-CoA via acetaldehyde and its subsequent reduction; the lactic acid is produced via the EMP scheme.

BUTANEDIOL FERMENTATION. Several groups of organisms, including *Enterobacter, Bacillus*, and *Serratia*, produce 2,3-butanediol in fermentations which are otherwise of the mixed acid type. Pyruvate is the precursor of acetoin (acetylmethylcarbinol), two molecules being decarboxylated in its conversion to one molecule of the neutral acetoin. The reduction of acetoin then produces 2,3-butanediol.

$$2 CH_3COCOOH \rightarrow CH_3\overset{|}{C}OHCOOH + CO_2$$

pyruvic acid $\qquad$ $\underset{\text{acetolactic acid}}{COCH_3}$

$$\downarrow$$

$$(2H)$$

$$\underset{\text{2,3-butanediol}}{CH_3CHOHCHOHCH_3} \leftarrow \underset{\text{acetoin} + CO_2}{CH_3CHOHCOCH_3}$$

This reduction is slowly reversible in air and, when made strongly alkaline, is the basis for the Voges-Proskauer reaction, a test for acetoin.

The diversion of part of the pyruvate to 2,3-butanediol greatly reduces the amount of acid produced relative to the mixed acid fermentation and is responsible for the positive methyl red reaction often used in the differentiation of *E. coli* and *Enterobacter*.

BUTYRIC ACID FERMENTATION. Among the primary characteristic products of carbohydrate fermentation by many organisms in the genus *Clostridium* are butyric acid, acetic acid, CO_2, and H_2. The key reaction in this type of fermentation is the formation of acetoacetyl-CoA by the condensation of two molecules of acetyl-CoA derived from acetate or from pyruvate.

$$2 CH_3CO \cdot SCoA \rightleftharpoons CH_3COCH_2CO \cdot SCoA + HSCoA$$

This C_4 compound is the key to all of the C_4-forming reactions of the clostridia. Subsequent reduction of the primary acidic products of the butyric acid fermentation results in the accumulation of neutral end products: butanol, acetone, isopropanol, and ethanol. The end products of clostridial fermentations can thus be very numerous.

FERMENTATION OF NITROGENOUS ORGANIC COMPOUNDS. Some of the clostridia, including some of medical importance, *Clostridium sporogenes*, *C. histolyticum*, and *C. tetani*, are not primarily butyric acid fermenters. Among these organisms the most characteristic type of amino acid fermentation is the Stickland reaction, a coupled oxidation-reduction involving a pair of amino acids, one of which serves as the electron donor and the other as the electron acceptor. An example of this type of reaction is the fermentation of alanine and glycine.

$$\text{alanine} + 2 \text{ glycine} + 2 H_2O \rightarrow 3 \text{ acetic acid} + 3 NH_3 + CO_2$$

Single amino acids also are fermented by certain clostridia, as are a variety of nitrogen-containing ring compounds.

AEROBIC RESPIRATION

In aerobic cells, energy is obtained from the complete oxidation of the substrate, with molecular oxygen serving as the ultimate hydrogen acceptor. In respiration the large amount of energy set free in the formation of water is made available to the process. The pathways of aerobic dissimilation are exceedingly complex. They consist of many enzymes and a large number of biochemical reactions. The most important respiratory mechanism for terminal oxidation is the tricarboxylic acid cycle of Krebs, which together with the known reactions of glycolysis, can account for the complete oxidation of glucose. This cycle is unique in that it provides the cell not only with an energy source but also with carbon skeletons for the synthesis of cellular material.

Tricarboxylic Acid Cycle In aerobic cells, the pyruvate formed from the glycolytic pathway is enzymatically oxidized by pyruvate dehydrogenase to a two-carbon compound, acetyl-CoA.

$$CH_3COCOOH + NAD + CoA\text{-}SH \rightarrow CH_3CO\text{-}S\text{-}CoA + CO_2 + NADH$$

The electrons accepted from pyruvate by NAD

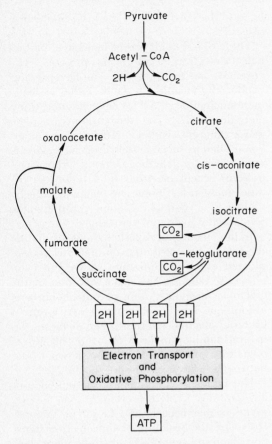

FIG. 4-5. The tricarboxylic acid cycle. The four pairs of H atoms liberated are fed into the respiratory chain.

enzymatic mechanisms for replenishing the TCA intermediates as they are diverted to biosynthetic pathways. The most important of these anaplerotic (filling-up) reactions is the enzymatic carboxylation of pyruvate to oxaloacetate.

$$\text{pyr} + CO_2 + \text{ATP} \rightleftharpoons \text{oxaloacetate} + \text{ADP} + P_i$$

The reaction is catalyzed by pyruvate carboxylase, an allosteric enzyme containing biotin. The rate of the forward reaction is very low unless acetyl-CoA, the fuel of the TCA cycle, is present in excess.

GLYOXYLATE CYCLE. In aerobic microorganisms there is no mechanism for synthesizing pyruvic acid directly from acetic acid. Therefore, during the oxidation of acetic acid or of other substrates such as the higher fatty acids, which are converted to acetyl-S-CoA without the intermediate formation of pyruvic acid, a modification of the TCA cycle, the glyoxylate cycle, comes into play. This modification constitutes a bypass of some of the reactions of the TCA cycle. It does not result in the conversion of acetate to CO_2 but in the net conversion of two acetyl residues to oxaloacetic acid. The need for a net input of oxaloacetate arises from the diversion of several of the intermediates of the TCA cycle into biosynthetic pathways (Fig. 4-6).

are carried in the form of NADH to the respiratory chain.

In the first reaction of the cycle, the acetyl group of acetyl-CoA is condensed with oxaloacetate to form citric acid (Fig. 4-5). In one turn of the cycle this 6-carbon molecule is then decarboxylated and oxidized to regenerate the 4-carbon oxaloacetate and liberate two carbon atoms as CO_2. In so doing four pairs of electrons are enzymatically extracted from the intermediates of the cycle. Anything capable of generating acetyl-CoA can be oxidized via the cycle. Also, important synthetic mechanisms utilize reactants of the cycle to provide a common meeting ground for carbohydrate, lipid, and protein metabolism.

ANAPLEROTIC REACTIONS. Under normal conditions the reactions by which the TCA cycle intermediates are formed and drained away remain in balance. This is made possible by

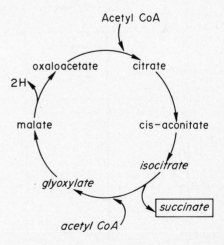

FIG. 4-6. The glyoxylate cycle. This cycle provides both energy and four-carbon intermediates for biosynthetic purposes. In each turn of the cycle two molecules of acetyl-CoA enter, and one molecule of succinate is formed. The reactions in the pathway between isocitrate and malate are catalyzed by auxiliary enzymes; all of the others are reactions of the TCA cycle.

Electron Transport In each revolution of the TCA cycle there are four dehydrogenations. In three of these, NAD serves as the electron acceptor; in the fourth the electron acceptor is flavin adenine dinucleotide. The reoxidation of these reduced coenzymes is accomplished by passing of the electrons through a series of intermediate carriers, capable of undergoing freely reversible oxidation and reduction. The last carrier in the series reacts with oxygen in a reaction mediated by a terminal oxidase. The series of carriers that link the dehydrogenation of an oxidizable substrate with the reduction of molecular oxygen to water is termed the "electron transport chain." The carriers participate in a series of reactions of gradually increasing E'_0 values. Thus, electrons will tend to pass from the more negative carrier NAD in Figure 4-7 to the more positive carrier above it on the scale. A decline in free energy is associated with each electron transfer and is directly related to the magnitude of the drop in electron pressure.

Three different classes of molecules participate in electron transport: flavoproteins, cytochromes, and the quinones. The flavoproteins contain the vitamin riboflavin, either as flavin mononucleotide (FMN) or flavin adenine dinucleotide (FAD). The flavoproteins mediate many different oxidation-reduction reactions. Some, such as succinic dehydrogenase, are active in primary dehydrogenations. Other flavoproteins accept electrons from reduced pyridine nucleotides. Some are autoxidizable by molecular oxygen in a reaction resulting in the formation of hydrogen peroxide.

In the electron transport chain of respiration the reoxidation of the flavoproteins is accomplished either by quinones or by the cytochromes. Whereas the major quinone of the electron transport system of mitochondria is ubiquinone, additional quinones play a role in bacterial electron transport. One of these, the natural napthoquinone K_9H, occurs in *Mycobacterium phlei* and has been shown to act between the flavoprotein and cytochrome b.

The typical electron transport sequence of flavoprotein → cyto b→ cyto c → cyto a → O_2 found in mammals is also found in bacteria. However, the structure of the electron transport chain in bacteria appears to be more complex in that a number of transport chain systems may exist. The flavoprotein dehydrogenases may be inputs to a number of the chain systems, and the chains may be more branched in structure than is found in mammalian systems. A bacterial respiratory chain should be conceptualized as a three-dimensional model, with each member having possibly more than one input and output, rather than as a two-dimensional linear and almost unbranched chain as is often done in representations of the mammalian respiratory chain.

BACTERIAL CYTOCHROMES. The cytochromes are heme-containing protein components of the electron transport chain. Although basically similar to the mammalian cytochromes, the bacterial cytochromes possess properties not encountered in mammalian systems. In bacteria the classes of cytochromes, their structure, functions, location, and conditions for existence exhibit greater variability. The wide variety of bacterial cytochromes has been grouped into four broad classes that may be

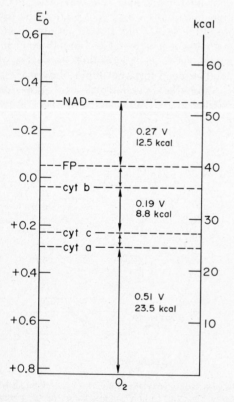

FIG. 4-7. Release of free energy as a pair of electrons passes down the respiratory chain to oxygen. Sufficient energy is generated in three of the segments for the formation of a molecule of ATP: between NAD and FP, between cyt b and cyt c, and between cyt a and O_2.

identified by their characteristic absorption spectra. The conditions under which a bacterium is grown markedly affects both the total and relative amounts of the cytochrome components in the organism. Whereas mammalian cytochromes function primarily as members of a respiratory electron transport chain, bacterial cytochromes also transport electrons to nonoxygen acceptors; in *E. coli*, for example, cytochromes function as part of the nitrate reductase system. They also play a role in photosynthesis (p. 61).

Location of Bacterial Cytochromes. In eucaryotic cells the cytochromes are located within mitochondria; in procaryotic cells they are associated with the membrane fraction. The isolation procedure for extracting cytochromes from bacteria usually involves protoplast or spheroplast formation followed by osmotic shock to produce a membranous ghost. The cytochromes may then be released from their membrane environment by sonication.

Oxidative Phosphorylation The movement of electrons down the respiratory chain of carriers is coupled with the production of energy-rich phosphate bonds as a result of oxidative phosphorylation. The multiplicity of catalysts in the chain provides a device for bleeding off the energy in convenient packets. Oxidative phosphorylation is, thus, the process whereby the large amount of free energy liberated during the complete oxidation of metabolites via the citric acid cycle can be utilized to drive the synthesis of ATP.

Although many bacteria can carry out oxidative phosphorylation, bacterial systems differ from intact mammalian systems in a number of ways. They have lower P:O ratios, fail to exhibit respiratory control, and are quite variable in their properties even within a particular group of bacteria.

In mitochondrial systems the number of moles of ATP formed relative to the gram atoms of oxygen consumed, ie, the P:O ratio, approaches integral values for different substrates undergoing one-step oxidation. When a single pair of electrons travels from NADH to oxygen along the respiratory chain in mitochondria, three molecules of ATP are formed from ADP and phosphate. Since the formation of three moles of ATP requires the input of at least 3 times 7,000 cal, and the oxidation of NADH

delivers 52,000 cal (Fig. 4-7), the oxidative phosphorylation of three moles of ADP conserves 3 (7,000/52,000) or about 40 percent of the total energy yield when one mole of NADH is oxidized by oxygen. In the respiratory chain of mammalian systems there are three segments in which there is a relatively large free-energy drop: from NAD to flavoprotein, from cytochrome b to cytochrome c, and from cytochrome a to oxygen. It is at these points in the respiratory chain that high-energy intermediates are generated during electron transfer. In many bacteria it appears that there are only one or two of these oxidation-phosphorylation coupling points. Loss of these sites and the presence of nonphosphorylative electron transport bypass reactions, both of which have been demonstrated, may account for the lower P:O ratios observed in most bacteria.

In certain bacteria, however, such as *M. phlei*, 3 moles of ATP are synthesized per mole of oxidized substrate by three distinct respiratory chains. A comparison of the effect of uncoupling agents in this organism with their effect in mitochondrial systems has revealed both similarities and striking differences. The differences are of fundamental importance, emphasizing the existence in the bacterial system of an exquisitely sensitive site not present in mammalian systems.

Mitochondrial systems are characterized by a tight coupling of oxidation to phosphorylation, thus providing a means by which the rate of oxidation of foodstuffs is regulated by the requirements of the cell for useful energy. The utilization of ATP to drive the various energy-requiring processes of the cell automatically increases the available supply of ADP and inorganic phosphate. This in turn becomes available to react in the coupling mechanism and to permit respiration to proceed. Respiratory control has not been demonstrated in fractionated bacterial systems or even in intact bacterial cells. For example, when biosynthesis is stopped for some reason and ATP consumption ceases, respiration continues at the same rate.

Although mitochondria of different animal species and of different organs have in general the same or similar properties, this is not true of preparations from bacteria. In bacteria, oxidative phosphorylation not only differs from that in higher organisms but is quite variable even within a particular group of bacteria. Especially variable are such properties as the requirement of cofactors and sensitivity to various inhibitors.

Flavin-mediated Reactions In some anaerobic microorganisms flavins are active both in the primary dehydrogenation of organic substrates and in the oxidation of reduced pyridine nucleotides. Some of these flavoproteins are autoxidizable by molecular oxygen, a reaction that is accompanied by the formation of hydrogen peroxide, which is highly toxic.

$$FPH_2 + O_2 \rightarrow FP + H_2O_2$$

Aerobic organisms produce catalase, an enzyme that breaks down the hydrogen peroxide to water and oxygen. This is a very useful laboratory test for distinguishing the catalase-producing staphylococcus from the streptococcus, which is catalase negative.

$$2 H_2O_2 \rightarrow 2 H_2O + O_2$$

The combined action of two enzymes, a flavoprotein NADH oxidase and a peroxidase, provides another mechanism for the destruction of hydrogen peroxide.

$$NADH + H^+ + O_2 \xrightarrow{\text{NADH oxidase}} NAD^+ + H_2O_2$$

$$NADH + H + H_2O_2 \xrightarrow{\text{peroxidase}} NAD^+ + 2 H_2O$$

$$\text{Sum: } 2 NADH + 2H^+ + O_2 \longrightarrow$$
$$2 NAD^+ + 2 H_2O$$

Most anaerobic organisms lack both catalase and peroxidase.

AUTOTROPHIC METABOLISM

There is in nature a large and widely distributed group of microorganisms that play an important role in the maintenance of the nitrogen, carbon, and sulfur cycles. These are the autotrophic bacteria, which differ from the heterotrophs in their ability to utilize CO_2 as a major source of carbon. They obtain their energy either from the respiration of inorganic electron donors (chemoautotrophy) or from the absorption of visible light (photosynthesis).

Chemoautotrophy A number of special physiologic groups of bacteria can use inorganic compounds such as H_2, NH_3, NO_2^-, Fe^{++}, S,

and H_2S. The organisms that can use H_2 as an energy source are aerobic organisms that also can utilize organic compounds. These organisms possess the enzyme hydrogenase which activates molecular hydrogen.

$$H_2 \rightleftharpoons 2 H^+ + 2 e$$

The acceptors that function subsequent to the primary step vary with the kinds of coupling reactions that exist between hydrogenase and the ultimate oxidant. A coupling with pyridine nucleotides and the electron-transport system occurs in a number of organisms, with oxygen serving as the ultimate oxidant.

$$H_2 \rightarrow NAD \rightarrow FP \rightarrow cyt\ c \rightarrow cyt\ a$$

In the nitrifying bacteria *Nitrosomonas* and *Nitrobacter*, and the sulfur-oxidizing chemoautotrophs the E'_0 values for the oxidations involved do not permit a coupling with the reduction of NAD. In some of these organisms the electrons enter the transport chain at the level of cytochrome c.

$$2 NH_3 + 3 O_2 \rightarrow 2 NO_2^- + 2 H + 2 H_2O$$
$$2 NO_2^- + O_2 \rightarrow 2 NO_3^-$$
$$2 H_2S + O \rightarrow 2 S + 2 H_2O$$
$$2 S + 2 H_2O + 3 O_2 \rightarrow 2 SO_4^{-2} + 4 H^+$$

Most of the organisms in this group are obligate autotrophs, incapable of using organic substrates as an energy source.

ANAEROBIC RESPIRATIONS. Among bacteria there also exists another unique variation in energy metabolism. A number of bacteria are capable of respiring under completely anaerobic conditions by utilizing nitrate, sulfate, or carbonate as a terminal inorganic electron acceptor. The reaction $NO_3^- + 2 e + H^+ \rightarrow NO_2^- + H_2O$ is mediated by nitrate reductases. The nitrite formed is very toxic, and growth is limited except in organisms such as *Bacillus* and *Pseudomonas*, which can by a process of denitrification reduce nitrate beyond the level of nitrite to molecular nitrogen.

$$2 NO_3^- + 10 e^- + 12 H^+ \rightarrow N_2 + 6 H_2O$$

For these organisms nitrate can be a physiologically useful electron acceptor. The enzymes involved in denitrification are linked to the normal aerobic respiratory chain, making possible the transfer of electrons to nitrate and its partial reduction products. Denitrification is an alternative mode of respiration used by these organisms for growth in the absence of oxygen. Oxygen represses synthesis of the enzymes essential for nitrification, and in its presence respiration proceeds through the aerobic electron transport chain.

Other examples of anaerobic respiration include the use by a small number of obligate anaerobes of sulfate or of carbonate as an electron acceptor, yielding sulfide and methane as end products.

$$SO_4^{-2} + 8\,e^- + 8\,H^+ \rightarrow S^{-2} + 4\,H_2O$$
$$4H_2 + CO_2 \rightarrow CH_4 + 2\,H_2O$$

PHOTOSYNTHESIS. The reactions whereby light energy is converted into chemical energy are known as photosynthesis. Mechanistically this is the most complex mode of energy-yielding metabolism. Although the overall reaction is basically the same in all photosynthetic organisms, bacteria possess an evolutionarily more primitive mechanism.

Photosynthesis consists of an oxidation-reduction sequence in which carbon dioxide is reduced to the level of carbohydrate at the expense of a variety of hydrogen donors activated by light reactions.

$$2\,H_2A + CO_2 \rightarrow (CH_2O) + H_2O + 2\,A$$

The nature of the compound H_2A varies with the organism, and it is this property that distinguishes bacterial photosynthesis from that present in evolutionarily higher forms. In plants and algae that can grow aerobically in the light, H_2A can be water, and oxygen is liberated in the reaction, but in photosynthetic bacteria that are obligate anaerobes, H_2A must be supplied as reduced sulfur or organic compounds. The photosynthetic bacteria are typically aquatic species and include the green and purple sulfur bacteria and the purple nonsulfur bacteria.

Photosynthetic Apparatus. Photosynthesis occurs in a membrane system containing pigments, electron carriers, lipids, and proteins. In bacteria this apparatus is much simpler than the chloroplasts of plants. The basic membranous unit is an enclosed sac or thylakoid which contains the chlorophyll and carotenoid pigments that function in the absorption of light energy.

Photosynthetic Electron Transport. Whereas plants have two distinct photochemical re-

action centers, bacteria have only one. The primary photochemical event is initiated when a molecule of chlorophyll in this center absorbs a quantum of light. The chlorophyll serves in some manner to effect a photochemical separation of oxidizing and reducing power, resulting in a flow along two transport systems. One of these systems accepts the electron delivered to the acceptor; the other replaces it. In a photosynthetic bacterium such as *Rhodospirillum rubrum*, ferredoxin serves as the immediate electron acceptor and a cytochrome c-like protein as the electron donor to the activated chlorophyll (Fig. 4-8). The flow of electrons is accompanied by the generation of ATP.

The fixation of the CO_2 into carbohydrate requires a supply of both NADPH and ATP. This relationship may be summarized in the following general statement.

$$H_2A + NAD(P)^+ + yADP + yP_i \xrightarrow{mh\nu}$$
$$A + NAD(P)H + H^+ + yATP$$

For photosynthetic bacteria the H_2A may be an inorganic substance, such as H_2S, or an organic compound, such as succinate. The energy of absorbed photons drives this reaction. In this event the flow of electrons is open or noncyclic. In the absence of oxidizable substrate, however, light-induced electron flow occurs along a circular path (Fig. 4-8). The electrons that come from the excited chlorophyll molecule may quite simply return to it again after they have traveled a circular route around the closed chain of electron carriers. This circuitous flow of electrons is a device to conserve some of the energy of the high-energy electrons that leave

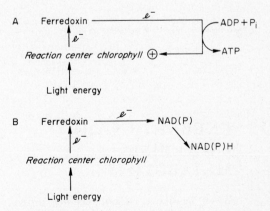

FIG. 4-8. Cyclic (A) and noncyclic (B) photophosphorylation. In the cyclic pathway the photosynthetic electron transport system is shown in italics.

the excited chlorophyll. In cyclic photophosphorylation the formation of ATP proceeds by a coupling mechanism that is similar in principle to the coupling mechanisms involved in respiratory chain phosphorylation in the mitochondria. Cyclic photophosphorylation may represent the most primitive form of photosynthesis, useful to organisms in an environment rich in organic compounds and requiring only ATP.

Dark Phase of Photosynthesis. The formation of glucose in photosynthesis is a dark process which begins with the reduced NADP and ATP generated by light. The mechanism by which CO_2 fixation occurs in all photosynthesizing organisms is cyclic in nature and occurs in both eucaryotic and procaryotic organisms. This complex series of reactions in known as the Calvin cycle, the initial reaction of which is the synthesis of ribulose-1,5-diphosphate from ribulose-5-phosphate.

ribulose-5-PO$_4$ + ATP → ribulose-1,5-PO$_4$ + ADP

ribulose-1,5-PO$_4$ + CO_2 → 2 3-phosphoglyceric acid

These two reactions are specific for organisms that use CO_2 as a sole carbon source and are not found in organisms that have a heterotrophic metabolism. The reduction of the two molecules of 3-phosphoglycerate occurs at the expense of NADPH and ATP formed in the light reaction. The two molecules of 3-phosphoglyceraldehyde thus formed are then converted into glucose, essentially by reversal of the reactions of glycolysis.

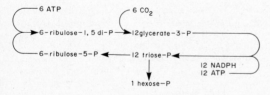

ENERGETICS OF BACTERIAL METABOLISM

When facultative organisms are grown under aerobic conditions, growth is always more vigorous than that obtained under anaerobic conditions. This is because of the greater amount of phosphate-bond energy made available by respiration.

The anaerobic breakdown of the glucose molecule to lactate is accompanied by the phosphorylation of 2 moles of ADP and proceeds with a free energy decline of −38,000 calories per mole. This is 16,000 calories less than the calculated −56,000 calorie free energy change, which would be expected from the simple breakdown of glucose to lactate. In the intact cell a significantly large part of this free energy loss is conserved in the form of ATP. In the breakdown of 1 mole of glucose to the level of lactate, 16/56 or approximately 28 percent of the energy is thus conserved in the two moles of ATP formed.

In growth under aerobic conditions the combined processes of glycolysis and oxidative phosphorylation provide a total of 38 moles of ATP. Since the calculated $\Delta F'$ for the complete combustion of glucose is −686,000 cal/mole, and since an approximate input of 8,000 cal/mole of ATP is required, the efficiency of energy conservation under aerobic conditions is (38 times 8,000)/686,000, or approximately 45 percent (Table 4-3).

This energy that is conserved in the form of ATP is used by the cell to perform its various activities. The most important forms of work carried out by the bacterial cell at the expense of ATP are active transport and the biosynthesis of cellular components from small precursor molecules. Almost all of the energy of bacterial cells is put into biosynthetic work. Their sole mission is to multiply. Since bacteria normally live in natural environments over which they have no control and from which they cannot escape, the ability to multiply rapidly fits them to survive. For this task a large amount of energy is required.

GROWTH YIELD.   Many studies have been made attempting to evaluate the energetic efficiency of bacterial growth. When growth is limited by the energy source, the total growth obtained in a culture is proportional to the amount of carbohydrate added. When anaerobic organisms employing a fermentative metabolism are grown in a complex medium, the substrate is used almost exclusively for the generation of ATP. Since the amount of ATP produced by various fermentations can be calculated, the growth yield as a function of ATP (Y_{ATP}) provides a means of determining the efficiency

TABLE 4-3 ENERGETICS OF GLUCOSE METABOLISM

	ATP Yield	$\Delta F'$ (calories)
Glucose → 2 lactic acid	2	56,000
Glucose + 6 O_2 → 6 CO_2 + H_2O	38	686,000
Sequence		
Glucose → fructose-1, 6-diP	−2	
2 Triose P → 2,3-phosphoglyceric acid	+2	
2 NAD^+ → 2 NADH → 2 NAD^+	+6	
2 Phosphoenolpyruvic acid → 2 pyruvic acid	+2	
2 Pyruvic acid → 2 acetyl CoA + 2 CO_2		
2 NAD^+ → 2 NADH → 2 NAD^+	+6	
2 Acetyl CoA → 4 CO_2	+24	
Net: $C_6H_{12}O_6$ + 6 O_2 + 6 H_2O	+38	

with which ATP is used by different organisms. The growth yields for different organisms utilizing a wide variety of substrates and employing different pathways are constant; values of approximately 10 g of cell material per g-mole of ATP have been obtained. This value is considerably less than would be expected if all the ATP used in cellular growth was coupled to biosyntheses. It would thus appear, on the basis of these and thermodynamic considerations, that bacteria are inefficient as converters of free energy and that there is a large outflow of entropy from the cell.

CONTROL OF ENERGY METABOLISM

If a microorganism is to function efficiently, the rate of metabolism along the various metabolic pathways must be controlled in such a way that optimal use is made of the available substrates. For this purpose the microbial cell has evolved a number of mechanisms, some of which control its energy-supplying processes. In its natural habitat the cell is confronted with a variety of carbon-containing materials as potential energy sources. The survival of a particular species in its highly competitive environment has resulted from the ability of that species to adapt to new experiences in its environment. In so doing the enzymatic machinery for the degradation of a wide variety of organic compounds is produced. Although the potential for the dissimilation of different substrates is great, the enzymes for such activities are produced only when need-

ed. How this is accomplished, ie, what are the determinants that control how much of a specific protein is to be synthesized at any one moment in an organism's history, is discussed in detail in Chapter 9. Controls of this type are exceedingly common in microorganisms and are referred to as "induction" and "repression." In general, induction exerts effective control of catabolic sequences involving carbon and energy sources, where the synthesis of enzymes catalyzing a particular sequence is turned on or off, depending on the demands for that specific sequence. The study of the utilization of the disaccharide lactose by *E. coli* has provided knowledge of the fundamental principles involved in this type of control, much of which can probably be extended to other systems and organic substrates.

Catabolite Repression This type of control is frequently observed when organisms are grown on glucose or some other rapidly metabolizable energy source. Often referred to as the "glucose effect," catabolite repression results in a repression of synthesis of enzymes that would metabolize the added substrate less rapidly than glucose. When the lac system is induced, the rate of synthesis of β-galactosidase is considerably reduced in cultures growing upon glucose, compared with cells for which some other metabolite is provided as the carbon source. Glucose elicits catabolite repression by depressing the level of 3'-5' cyclic AMP in the cell. The addition of cyclic AMP to cultures overcomes glucose repression by stimulating the production of the inducible enzyme, β-galactosidase. The level of cAMP in the cell reflects its energetic needs. The level is low when the available energy exceeds the biosynthetic requirement for energy; the level of cAMP rises when the organism's carbon supply is depleted. The molecular aspects of catabolite repression are presented in Chapter 9.

Pasteur Effect   In facultative organisms the fermentative capacity of the cell is blocked in the presence of sufficient oxygen, and the energy is supplied almost exclusively by respiration. As a result, less glucose is consumed, and lactate does not accumulate. This phenomenon, first recognized by Pasteur in fermenting yeast, is known as the Pasteur effect. The benefits of this effect are obvious in terms of the energy gain realized in switching from an anaerobic metabolism to an aerobic one. Anaerobic glycolysis releases only about 8 percent of the energy that is obtained from the complete breakdown of glucose. Therefore, if oxygen is available, and the glucose is oxidized to CO_2 and water without the accumulation of lactic acid, the energy needs of the cell can be met by the utilization of less glucose.

Several factors may be responsible for the Pasteur effect, but the most important probably relates to altered levels of ADP and ATP. Both inorganic phosphate and ADP are required in glycolysis for substrate-level phosphorylation. In the generation of ATP via the respiratory pathways, however, the supply of phosphate and ADP available for glycolysis is diminished, thus altering the ADP/ATP ratio. Increased levels of ATP inhibit phosphofructokinase activity, thereby decreasing the flow of glucose into the glycolytic pathway.

The inhibition of phosphofructokinase activity by ATP is illustrative of regulation of an allosteric enzyme by a negative effector. The reaction catalyzed by phosphofructokinase, the formation of fructose-1,6-diphosphate from fructose-6-phosphate, is a critical control point subject to strong metabolic regulation. It is susceptible to strong inhibition by high concentrations of ATP and is activated by ADP or AMP. Such controls ensure that whenever a plentiful supply of ATP is available, as when pyruvate is metabolized aerobically to CO_2 via the TCA cycle, glycolysis will be essentially blocked. The reverse is also true. When glycolysis is absolutely required for the generation of energy, ie, when the ATP drops to low levels and ADP or AMP accumulate, glycolysis will be favored.

LOCALIZATION OF ENZYMIC ACTIVITIES

In eucaryotic organisms, the mitochondrion and the chloroplast contain the units which transform oxidative energy into the bond energy of ATP. No mitochondria are found in bacteria, but a functional equivalent is present. In such cells either the cell membrane itself or extensions of the membrane contain the subunits that carry out energy transductions. Although bacteria have essentially one membrane system, this system is a composite of almost all the membrane systems found in the more complex forms of life.

The main components of the respiratory chain — succinic dehydrogenase, NADH dehydrogenase, cytochromes of groups A, B, and C, ubiquinones, and naphthoquinones — are found in membranes or in particles obtained by homogenization and subsequent differential centrifugation. The membranes and their fragments also contain several enzymes of the TCA cycle and firmly bound dehydrogenases.

Owing to the small size of the bacterial cell and the nature of the open membrane system of which the respiratory apparatus is an integral part, there is in bacteria direct interaction between the membranes carrying the respiratory chain and the cytoplasm which is the source of coenzymes, substrates, and ADP. The metabolites that accumulate in the cytoplasm as a result of glycolysis are rapidly oxidized by the enzymes in the membranes.

FURTHER READING

Asano A, Cohen NS, Baker RF, Brodie AF: Orientation of the cell membrane in ghosts and electron transport particles of *Mycobacterium phlei*. J Biol Chem 248: 3386, 1973

Forrest WW, Walker DJ: The generation and utilization of energy during growth. In Rose AH, Wilkinson JF (eds): Advances in Microbial Physiology. New York, Academic Press, 1971, vol 5, pp 213-274

Gel'man NS, Lukoyanova MA, Ostrovskii DN: Respiration and Phosphorylation of Bacteria. New York, Plenum Press, 1967

Gunsalus IC, Stanier RY (eds): The Bacteria. New York, Academic Press, 1961, vol 2

Lehninger AL: Bioenergetics. New York, Benjamin, 1965

Lehninger AL: Biochemistry. New York, Worth Publishers, 1970

Mahler HR, Cordes EH: Biological Chemistry. New York, Harper, 1966

Mitchell P: Reversible coupling between transport and chemical reactions. In Bittar EE (ed): Membranes and

Ion Transport. London, Wiley-Interscience, 1970, chap 7, pp 192-256

Ramaiah A: Pasteur effect and phosphofructokinase. In Horecker BL, Stadtman ER (eds): Current Topics in Cellular Regulation. New York, Academic Press, 1974, vol 8, pp 297-308

Rickenberg HV: Cyclic AMP in prokaryotes. Annu Rev Microbiol 8:353, 1974

San Pietro A: Ferredoxin and photosynthetic pyridine nucleotide reductase in biological oxidations. In Singer TP (ed): Biological Oxidations. New York, Interscience, 1968, pp 515-523

Sanwal BD: Allosteric controls of amphibolic pathways in bacteria. Bacteriol Rev 34:20, 1970

Smith L: The respiratory chain system of bacteria. In Singer TP (ed): Biological Oxidations. New York, Interscience, 1968, pp 55-122

Stanier RY, Doudoroff M, Adelberg EA: The Microbial World, 3rd ed. Englewood Cliffs, NJ, Prentice-Hall, 1970

Thimann KV: The Life of Bacteria, 2nd ed. New York, Macmillan, 1963

Vernon LP: Photochemical and electron transport reactions of bacterial photosynthesis. Bacteriol Rev 32:243, 1968

White DC, Sinclair PR: Branched electron-transport systems in bacteria. In Rose AH, Wilkinson JF (eds): Advances in Microbial Physiology. New York, Academic Press, 1971, vol 5, pp 173-211

5
Physiology of Bacterial Growth

The growth of bacteria consists of the specific balanced synthesis of the components of protoplasm from the nutrients present in the immediate environment. It is a process that shows continuous change with time and is one of the prime characteristics of living matter.

As a group bacteria are extremely omnivorous organisms. They are able to support their metabolic processes by utilizing quite diverse food sources, ranging from completely inorganic substrates to very complex organic materials. In fact, there is probably not a single naturally occurring organic compound that cannot be utilized by one or more kinds of bacteria. This ability is indeed proof of the tremendous adaptability of bacteria and reflects their capacity to respond successfully to a stimulus that is completely foreign to their past history.

NUTRITIONAL REQUIREMENTS

Sources of Energy and Carbon Two basic patterns characterize the nutritional requirements of bacteria and reflect the metabolic potentialities of the organism (Table 5-1). At one end of the spectrum are the autotrophic bacteria, or lithotrophs, that require only water, inorganic salts, and CO_2 for growth. These organisms synthesize a major portion of their essential organic metabolites from CO_2. Their energy requirements are derived either from light or from the oxidation of one or more inorganic

materials. Photosynthetic autotrophs (photolithotrophs) obtain energy for their synthetic activities by the utilization of radiant energy. These are anaerobic organisms containing a magnesium porphyrin pigment closely related to chlorophyll a of green plants. Chemosynthetic autotrophs (chemolithotrophs) obtain their energy by the oxidation of an inorganic substrate, such as iron, sulfur, ammonia, or nitrite, the nature of which is specific for that particular organism. The nitrification of ammonia in the soil is brought about by certain of these organisms.

At the other end of the spectrum are the heterotrophic bacteria (organotrophs) that are unable to grow with CO_2 as the sole source of carbon but require that it be supplied in an organic form. This group contains all of those bacteria pathogenic for man. For the heterotrophic bacteria a portion of the organic compound that serves the organism as an energy source invariably is used for the synthesis of many or all of the organic compounds required by the organism. Although glucose is used quite widely in routine laboratory practice as the organic source of carbon, a variety of other substances also can be used as an exclusive or partial source of carbon by different strains of bacteria.

Growth Factor Requirements Many of the bacteria in the heterotrophic group are unable to grow unless supplied with growth factors. These substances, usually provided in the medium in the form of yeast extract or whole blood, include the B-complex vitamins, amino

TABLE 5-1   CLASSIFICATION OF BACTERIA ACCORDING TO SOURCE
OF CARBON AND ENERGY

Type	Carbon Sources	Energy Sources	Electron Donors	Example
Photolithotrophs	CO_2	Light	Inorganic compounds (H_2S, S)	Green and purple sulfur bacteria
Photoorganotrophs	Organic compounds (in addition to CO_2)	Light	Organic compounds	Purple non-sulfur bacteria
Chemolithotrophs	CO_2	Oxidation-reduction reactions	Inorganic compounds (H_2, S, H_2S, Fe, NH_3)	Hydrogen, sulfur, iron and denitrifying bacteria
Chemoorganotrophs	Organic compounds	Oxidation-reduction reactions	Organic compounds (glucose)	Most bacteria

acids, purines, and pyrimidines. The B-complex vitamins play a catalytic role within the cell either as components of coenzymes or as prosthetic groups of enzymes. Organisms that do not require an exogenous source of a given growth factor are capable of synthesizing their own.

Oxygen Requirements The oxygen requirement of a particular bacterium reflects the mechanism employed for satisfying its energy needs. On the basis of their oxygen requirements bacteria may be divided into four groups: the obligate anaerobes, which will grow only under conditions of high reducing intensity; facultative anaerobes, which are capable of growth under both aerobic and anaerobic conditions; obligate aerobes, which require oxygen for growth; and microaerophilic organisms, which grow best at low oxygen tensions, high tensions being inhibitory. Catalase, peroxidase, and a functional cytochrome system, which are present in aerobic bacteria, are lacking in the anaerobic organisms. The absence of catalase and the resulting accumulation of hydrogen peroxide may be responsible in some anaerobic bacteria, such as *Clostridium*, for the toxic effect of oxygen (p. 646).

Lack of catalase, however, is an insufficient explanation for the toxicity of oxygen. Anaerobes also lack superoxide dismutase, an enzyme in aerobic and aerotolerant organisms that is essential for the organism's defense against oxygen and superoxide radical (O_2^-) toxicity. A number of biochemical reactions generate O_2^-. Among these are the autoxidations of hydroquinones, leucoflavins, and tetrahydropteridines. The catalytic actions of several enzymes also evolve O_2^-. The reaction, catalyzed by superoxide dismutase,

$$O_2^- + O_2^- + 2\,H^+ \rightarrow O_2 + H_2O_2$$

is induced by oxygen. The presence in cells of induced high levels of the enzyme renders them resistant to hyperbaric oxygen.

Oxidation-Reduction Potential The oxidation-reduction potential (Eh) of the culture medium is a critical factor determining whether growth of an inoculum will occur when transferred to fresh medium. The Eh of most media in contact with air is about +0.2 to 0.4 volt at pH 7. The strict anaerobes are unable to grow unless the Eh of the medium is at least as

low as −0.2 volt. The establishment of anaerobic conditions in culture may be accomplished by the exclusion of oxygen or by the incorporation in the medium of sulfhydryl-containing compounds, such as sodium thioglycollate (mercaptoacetate). The growth of both aerobic and anaerobic bacteria also lowers the oxidation-reduction potential of the environment. This observation is of extreme clinical importance in wound infections where a mixed population of aerobic and anaerobic organisms is capable of setting up an infection in an initially aerobic setting (Chap. 49).

Temperature For each bacterium there is an optimal temperature at which the organism grows most rapidly and a range of temperatures over which growth can occur. Cellular division is especially sensitive to the damaging effects of high temperature; very large and bizarre forms are often observed in cultures grown at a temperature higher than that supporting the most rapid division rate.

Bacteria are divided into three groups on the basis of the temperature ranges through which they grow: psychrophilic, −5 to 30C, optimum at 10 to 20C; mesophilic, 10 to 45C, optimum at 20 to 40C; and thermophilic, 25 to 80C, optimum at 50 to 60C. The optimum temperature is usually a reflection of the normal environment of the organism. Thus, bacteria pathogenic for man usually grow best at 37C. One very practical example of the importance of temperature on the growth of microorganisms in vivo is found in studies with *Mycobacterium leprae*. Growth of this organism is temperature dependent, as reflected by the distribution of lesions in clinical cases of leprosy. The skin usually shows the most obvious lesions; the internal organs are not infected. This correlation led, after many years of failure, to the successful passage of the organism in mice by inoculation of the foot pads, a site with a reduced body temperature.

pH The pH of the culture medium also affects the growth rate, and here also there is an optimal pH with a wider range over which growth can occur. For most pathogenic bacteria the optimal pH is 7.2 to 7.6. Although a given medium may be initially suitable for growth, subsequent growth may be severely limited by products of the metabolism of the organisms themselves. This is especially pronounced in bacteria exhibiting a fermentative type of metabolism where large amounts of inhibitory organic acids accumulate.

THE UPTAKE OF NUTRIENTS

Exoenzymes

Bacteria, in common with all living organisms, are surrounded by a semipermeable membrane that restricts the entry of both small molecules and high-molecular-weight compounds into the cell. Highly specialized systems have been evolved for transport of small molecules across the membrane barrier. However, large molecules found in the organism's natural environment cannot be utilized unless the organism possesses exoenzymes that are liberated outside the cell. The development of such systems has permitted certain bacteria to occupy specific ecologic niches and has played an important role in the conservation and recycling of carbon, nitrogen, and other elements.

ENRICHMENT CULTURE. If one looks in the right place and in the proper way, one will always find some organism that can break down any selected naturally occurring substance. This hypothesis is the basis for the enrichment culture technique used in isolating organisms capable of breaking down substances of high molecular weight. In attempting to find an organism that can degrade a particular substrate, the substrate is added to a medium containing essential inorganic salts, which is then inoculated with a mixture of organisms derived from a source in which it is probable that destruction of that substrate has been occurring. Soils and muds are the most useful sources of inoculum, and it was from such a source that organisms were isolated capable of degrading the polysaccharide capsule of the pneumococcus, thus facilitating biochemical analysis.

Many of the exoenzymes elaborated by bacteria are extracellular, appearing free in the medium. Others are cell bound, being found on the surface of the cell outside the cytoplasmic membrane. The surface enzymes are either bound to the membrane or are found in the periplasmic space between the wall and membrane. Distinction between the latter two types may be made by determining whether the cell-bound enzyme is extracted by procedures that remove the cell wall and retain the intact cytoplasmic membrane of the protoplast.

Among the substances attacked by exoenzymes are such polysaccharides as cellulose, starch, and pectins; mucopolysaccharides, including chitin, hyaluronic acid, and chondroitin sulfate; proteins; lipids; and nucleic acids. A number of the more invasive pathogenic bacteria, including *Streptococcus pyogenes*, *Staphylococcus aureus*, and members of the *Clostridium* group, elaborate a variety of exoenzymes that destroy various components of the body tissues and thus contribute to the overall pathogenesis of infection.

There is little definitive information on the site of formation of exoenzymes and the mechanism by which they are liberated from the cell. Also, no universal statement can be made concerning the stage of the growth cycle during which they are produced. Although many of the exoenzymes such as the lecithinase of *C. perfringens* and the hyaluronidase of *S. aureus*, are formed toward the end of the logarithmic phase of growth, others, including the nicotinamide adenine dinucleotidase of *S. pyogenes* and the proteinase of *C. botulinum,* are formed in approximately equivalent proportions during most of the growth cycle. Regardless of the mechanism of formation and secretion of the exoenzymes, however, their production by various microbial species in their natural habitat is of tremendous evolutionary, medical, and economic importance.

Membrane Transport

In order for growth of the bacterial cell to occur the plasma membrane must permit the entry of essential nutrients and the exit of cell wastes and must prevent essential metabolites from diffusing out. The properties of the plasma membrane that enable it to regulate the entry and exit of materials are of prime importance to life itself. The movement of water and various solutes through the plasma membrane is a dynamic process. The living cell is never in equilibrium with its environment in terms of the concentration of materials on either side of the membrane. When complete equilibrium with the solutes in the environment does occur, the cell is dead.

Movement of substances through the cell membrane is not determined solely by the concentration gradient. Few substances move as freely as water. Usually the molecules that enter the cell most readily are those with the highest partition coefficients (ratio of solubility of the compound in a nonpolar and polar solvent). This can be attributed to the molecular arrangement of the lipids and protein in the cell membrane. Bacterial membranes, as those of animal and plant cells, are visualized as consisting of two layers of lipid molecules arranged with their hydrocarbon chains oriented inward toward each other to form a continuous hydrocarbon phase and with their respective hydrophilic groups arranged outwardly, the entire double layer of lipid molecules being sandwiched between two layers of protein. The layers and pores in the plasma membrane are dynamic in nature, and at times a lipid chain appears to make contact with the exterior of the membrane. For the biochemist, however, concerned with the metabolic roles and dynamic aspects of membranes, the bimolecular leaflet model is inadequate. Alternate views have developed that consider membranes as aggregates of lipoprotein subunits, which in themselves are the fundamental units of both structure and function. This model shifts the emphasis from the lipids to the proteins, which are the usual biologic mechanism for specificity and versatility. It also regards the functional and structural components of the membrane as different properties of the same lipoprotein molecules. With the available data it is quite consistent that different membranes may have different structures, that different portions of the same membrane may have different structures, or that the same section of membrane may exist in different states at different times. Although a number of additional factors other than lipoidal solubility of the molecule affect the rate of entry of a substance into the bacterial cell, none of these factors can account for the high degree of selectivity exhibited by the membrane. To accomplish this, stereospecific transport systems are built into the cytoplasmic membrane in such a manner as to provide for selective permeability and the facilitated diffusion of solutes. In other cases the substance is moved through the cell membrane against a concentration gradient. This movement, referred to as active transport, occurs at the expense of metabolic energy. Since the cytoplasmic membrane of bacteria is poorly permeable to hydrophilic organic compounds, the entry of most organic nutrilites is mediated by transport systems.

Properties of Transport Systems   Extensive studies of rates of entry and exit in uninhibited and inhibited cells have established certain properties of transport systems. (1) Transport systems, like enzymes, are quite specific. A single transport system can catalyze the translocation of a limited number of substrates with similar chemical structures. Proteins of the membrane constitute the recognition sites because they are the only molecules which have the observed degrees of specificity to discriminate between possible substrates. (2) The initial rate of entry of a substrate depends on its concentration, as if there were a limited number of independent absorption sites. (3) The flow of one substrate can stimulate the flow in the opposite direction of a second similar substrate, as though the two processes shared a component of the system. Such a component could be a carrier molecule in the membrane that cycles between the inward and outward states. (4) Active transport which occurs at the expense of metabolic energy is inhibited when the cell's energy production is inhibited by compounds, such as iodoacetate or azide, as would be expected for a process that expends energy in moving the substrate through the cell membrane against a concentration gradient.

Progress in the understanding of transport phenomena has been slow because of the technical difficulties associated with biochemical studies on fragile membranes. Primarily, however, progress has been slowed by the difficulties involved in making an intellectual transition from the classical concept of metabolic enzymology in which a cell was regarded as a bag of enzymes to the concept of vectorial metabolism in which the directional aspect of the diffusion of substrates and group transfers through the catalytic carrier systems in the lipid membranes must also be explained.

Analysis of kinetic data has resulted in a model dividing transport into three steps (Fig. 5-1). In the first step, recognition, the substrate combines with a specific molecule on the outer membrane surface. The second step, transloca-

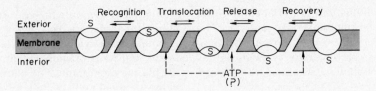

FIG. 5-1. Model of transport system showing binding and translocation substrate (S) across the membrane. Energy is required at one of these steps. (After Pardee: Science 162:632, 1968)

tion, moves the substrate across the membrane. During the final step, the recovery step, the substrate is released inside the cell, and the system returns to its original state. In active transport systems, energy is supplied at one of these steps.

β-Galactoside Transport System One of the most extensively studied bacterial transport systems is the β-galactoside transport system of *Escherichia coli.* Lactose does not enter the cells of this organism by a process of free diffusion but rather by a highly specific, genetically controlled transport system. The existence of transport systems for sugars was first inferred during analyses of enzyme induction in both wild-type and mutant cells of *E. coli.* Some mutants are unable to form the enzyme β-galactosidase but are able to concentrate lactose by a factor of several hundred times. By contrast, other mutants have been found that contain β-galactosidase but which cannot grow when lactose is the only carbon source supplied. Chemical analysis shows that these mutant cells are cryptic, ie, their β-galactosidase activity remains hidden and undetectable unless the cells are disrupted. Such cells are unable to take up lactose from the medium. The transport factor which is present in the first mutant and absent in the second exhibits high stereospecificity, and its formation is blocked by inhibitors of protein synthesis.

Cohen and Monod provided the decisive genetic and kinetic evidence for such transport systems in bacteria and coined the term "permease" for the stereospecific protein involved in the transport of lactose into the cell. A membrane-associated protein, M protein, has been isolated from spheroplast membranes of *E. coli.* It is the product of the y gene of the lactose operon and has all of the functional characteristics expected of β-galactoside permease. It is localized in the membrane fraction of *E.*

coli, is absent in y⁻ mutants and in uninduced cells, and has a high affinity for thiodigalactosides.

Kennedy proposed a working model of the β-galactoside transport system in which the M protein operates as a membrane carrier. This membrane carrier exists in two conformational states. When it is external it is in the M form, but when internal it is in the M_i conformational state. The carrier in its M form combines with lactose at the outer membrane surface, forming a complex of the Michaelis-Menten type. The sugar then passes through the membrane as the β-galactoside M complex. In the presence of an energy source, the protein is postulated to undergo transformation to the form M_i, which has little affinity for the sugar, thus leading to accumulation of the sugar within the cell. An interesting feature of this model is that it requires no energy to carry lactose into the cell, but in order to accumulate lactose against a gradient, the same system requires a source of metabolic energy.

Other Transport Proteins Proteins with affinities for a variety of molecules, such as inorganic sulfate, glucose, galactose, and various amino acids, have now been isolated and identified with specific transport systems. The transport proteins isolated to date are similar but not identical in composition and are all of approximately the same size with a molecular weight of 30,000. In contrast to the M protein of the β-galactoside transport system, these binding proteins have been isolated from the fluid obtained by subjecting bacteria to osmotic shock.

Energy-coupling Proteins Two mechanisms have been discovered for providing the energy required by transport systems in which uptake takes place against a concentration gradient. The first involves the transport of a variety of carbohydrates into bacterial cells by the action of a phosphotransferase system. The transfer of phosphate from phosphoenolpyruvate to various carbohydrates is catalyzed according to the following reactions.

(1) Phosphoenolpyruvate + HPr $\xrightleftharpoons{\text{Enz I, Mg}^{++}}$ pyruvate + phospho-HPr

(2) Phospho-HPr + sugar $\xrightarrow{\text{Enz II, Mg}^{++}}$ sugar-P + HPr

Sum: Phosphoenolpyruvate + sugar → pyruvate + sugar-P

The system is composed of two enzymes, I and II, and a heat-stable, low-molecular-weight protein, HPr, which functions as a phosphate carrier in the overall reaction. Enzyme II, the membrane-bound component of the system, is responsible for the specificity of various systems with respect to the various sugars studied. The phosphotransferase system can be adapted to many of the models offered to explain the processes of active transport and facilitated diffusion. In general, these models explain facilitated diffusion by the action of a specific carrier or permease molecule. Active transport results when facilitated diffusion is coupled with an energy-yielding process. In the phosphotransferase system, Enzyme II, known to be associated with the cell membrane fraction and to be specific for certain sugars, may be regarded as the carrier or permease proteins that transport the sugars across the membrane. By coupling Enzyme II with Enzyme I, HPr, and phosphoenolpyruvate, the sugar would be removed from Enzyme II, and active transport would result. There is very little if any passive transport, suggesting that the energy donor is required for the translocation step. There is really no clear evidence as to how translocation, the central process of transport, operates. Enzyme II, the membrane-bound component of the phosphotransferase system, may be capable of undergoing conformational changes within the membrane matrix. By the use of a variety of techniques which alter the phospholipids of the membrane without affecting the activity of the phosphotransferase system, the transport (vectorial phosphorylation) properties of the membrane can be functionally separated from the barrier properties of the membrane.

Another system in which the energy requirements for transport have been studied is the membrane adenosine triphosphatase involved in the transport of monovalent cations across the plasma membrane. The plasma membranes of most animal cells contain a Na^+- and K^+-dependent ATPase which is believed to be involved in the linked active transport of these cations. There is substantial evidence that the mechanism of these animal ATPases involves a Na^+-dependent phosphorylation and a K^+-dependent dephosphorylation of the enzyme. In bacteria the membrane ATPase is also thought to be involved in the active transport of monovalent cations across the plasma membrane. In the bacterial systems studied, however, the reaction mechanism appears to be different from that described in animal cells. The mechanism of the Na^+- and K^+-dependent ATPases of animal cells involves the formation of a phosphorylated enzyme intermediate. Studies with a purified membrane adenosine triphosphatase from *Streptococcus faecalis* failed to demonstrate a phosphorylated intermediate or to exhibit an exchange reaction. Competitive inhibition was observed by the products P_i and ADP. These findings have suggested a reaction mechanism in which all possible enzyme-substrate and enzyme-product complexes dissociate rapidly and reversibly, and the only slow step is the interconversion of the enzyme-substrate to the enzyme-product complex.

GROWTH OF BACTERIAL POPULATIONS

Bacteria, unlike the higher forms of life, do not have an obligatory life cycle. When bacterial cells are placed in a nutritionally complete medium, the cells grow larger and eventually divide to form two cells. This continues with the production of a population of vegetative, undifferentiated cells. In a bacterial culture, however, growth is a phenomenon of the individual cell whose ability to grow and reproduce itself depends upon its ability to form new protoplasm from the nutrients available.

Growth of bacteria involves two closely related problems, the growth of the individual bacterium and the growth of populations or cultures. For obvious practical reasons bacteria are usually studied not as individuals but as aggregates of very large numbers of cells.

In the development of a bacterial culture there is an increase both in cell mass and in number of organisms, but there is no constant relationship between the two parameters. In quantitative studies dealing with cell growth it is therefore necessary to distinguish between cell concentration, or the number of cells per unit volume of culture, and bacterial density, defined as total protoplasm per unit volume. In most problems dealing with the biochemistry and physiology of bacteria, the significant variable is bacterial density. Knowledge concerning the actual cell concentration is more pertinent in problems concerned with cell division, genetics, or infection.

Determination of Bacterial Mass Various techniques are in general use for estimating bacterial densities and cell concentrations. Unfortunately, no single method determines mass and number in a single operation. Cell mass can be determined directly in terms of dry weight. Although this method is time consuming, it is especially useful for reference in isolation and purification work and in the basic calibration of other methods.

The most widely used method for estimating total microbiologic material in suspension is the measurement of turbidity or optical density of a broth culture in a spectrophotometer. Turbidimetric techniques are especially useful in determining mass of cells while they are growing, as in the evaluation of drug action on bacteria. Other methods that have been employed include nitrogen determination and measurement of cell volume after centrifugation. These methods are useful when difficulty is encountered with clumping of cells and light adsorption by colored materials in the turbidimetric assay. In addition, data on packed cell volume have proved useful for permeability studies on microorganisms.

Determination of Cell Number In studies where information is needed on the number of organisms in a culture, enumerations are performed either by total direct counts or by indirect viable counts. Total counts of both living and dead organisms may be made by means of a counting chamber, such as the Petroff-Hauser counter, which is similar in principle to the hemacytometer but more reliable for bacterial counts. More convenient than the counting-chamber technique, however, is the Coulter counter, an electronic particle counter that measures both the distribution of sizes and the numbers in bacterial suspensions.

For determination of viable numbers it is necessary to plate out a sample of the culture. The microbial population is diluted in a nontoxic diluent, and an aliquot of the diluted population is dispersed in or on a suitable solid medium, such that each viable unit forms, after incubation, a colony. The number of viable individuals or clusters originally present is determined from the colony count and the dilution. Samples containing fewer than 100 microorganisms per milliliter, such as urine or clear natural water, often require concentration rather than dilution before counting. This is done by filtering a known volume of sample through a sterile membrane of pore size capable of retaining all the bacteria, then transferring the membrane to an absorbent pad saturated with a broth medium.

BACTERIAL CULTURE SYSTEMS

Properties of a Closed System As bacteria are usually grown in the laboratory in batch culture the conditions approximate that of a closed system. If a suitable medium is inoculated with bacteria and small samples are taken out at regular intervals, a plotting of the data will yield a characteristic growth curve (Fig. 5-2). The changes of slope on such a graph indicate the transition from one phase of development to another. Usually logarithmic values of the number of cells are plotted rather than

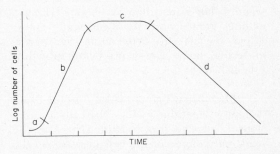

FIG. 5-2. Bacterial growth curve showing the four phases of growth. a. The lag phase. b. The exponential phase. c. The stationary phase. d. The phase of decline.

arithmetic values. Logarithms to the base 2 are the most useful of the plots, since each unit on the ordinate represents a doubling of population.

The period initiated immediately on planting the inoculum is a period of stationary population, the lag phase. During a considerable part of this phase the growth rate continuously increases up to its maximum value, which is reached in the logarithmic or exponential phase of the growth curve. Growth will continue in an unhindered manner at this maximum rate, which is characteristic of the particular strain and of the particular culture medium, until the population reaches a certain level. A period of decreasing multiplication rate leads to the final period of stable population, the stationary phase, where the number of newly formed cells is balanced by the number of dying cells.

LAG PHASE.   The course of the growth curve which is based on the number of bacteria does not express accurately all changes occurring in such a culture. During the early hours of growth the cells increase considerably in size at a time when little or no cell division is occurring. There is an increase in total protein, ribonucleic acid, and cell phosphorus, a marked increase in metabolic activity, and an increased susceptibility to many harmful physical and chemical agents. Often referred to as a phase of rejuvenescence or physiologic youth, it is a phase of adjustment necessary for the replenishing of the internal supply of intermediate metabolites and corresponds to the time required for the metabolism of the culture to build up to a steady state, which is necessary if cell synthesis is to occur at a maximum rate. Under suitable conditions the lag phase may be so shortened as to be imperceptible, as occurs when a large inoculum is obtained from a culture growing in its logarithmic phase. When inocula are taken from the period of decline, hours may elapse before growth is established.

EXPONENTIAL GROWTH PHASE.   In the exponential or logarithmic phase the cells are in a state of balanced growth. During this state the mass and volume of the cell increase by the same factor in such a manner that the average composition of cells and the relative concentrations of metabolites remain constant for a certain period of time. During the period of balanced growth the rate of increase can be expressed by a natural exponential function.

The cells are dividing at a constant rate determined by both the nature of the organism and the environmental conditions. There is a wide diversity in the rate of growth of the various microorganisms. In *E. coli* grown in broth at 37C, the doubling time is approximately 20 minutes. This compares with a minimum doubling time for mammalian cells at the same temperature of approximately 10 hours.

STATIONARY PHASE.   With the ordinary methods of cultivation, the accumulation of waste products, exhaustion of nutrients, change in pH, and other obscure factors exert a deleterious effect on the culture, resulting in a decreased growth rate. During the stationary phase the viable count remains constant for a variable period depending upon the organism, but eventually this gives way to a stage of decreasing population. In some cases the cells in dying cultures become quite elongated, abnormally swollen, or distorted, a manifestation of unbalanced growth.

Growth Rate and Doubling Time   Knowledge of the growth rate is important in determing the state of the culture as a whole. If one assumes the doubling of the initial mass M_1 in time g, the final concentration of microorganisms M is

$$(1) \qquad M = M_1 2^n$$

where n is the number of cell divisions in time t. The equation

$$(2) \qquad g = \frac{t}{n}$$

expresses the doubling time or mean generation time and is the reciprocal of the growth-rate constant ρ, which is usually expressed as the number of doublings per hour. The term "doubling time" represents the average generation time of the culture as a whole, usually determined by doubling of the microbial mass in the culture. The doubling time g is best determined by calculation. To accomplish this the increase of cell mass is determined in a known time interval, and the generation time is calculated from the values obtained. Rearranging equation (2) to the form $n = \frac{t}{g}$ which is substituted into equation (1) we have

$$(3) \qquad M = M_1 2^{\frac{t}{g}}$$

By conversion to the logarithmic form and rearranging we obtain

$$(4) \qquad g = \frac{\ln2 \, t}{\ln M - \ln M_1} = \frac{0.69 \, t}{\ln M - \ln M_1}$$

Equation (4) is the formula for calculating the doubling time from two measurements that give the increase of the mass in time t. Measurements must be performed under constant conditions, and the amount of microorganisms is best determined as dry weight. From equation (4) may be derived the growth rate, ρ.

$$\rho = \frac{\ln M - \ln M_1}{0.69 t}$$

For calculating the specific growth rate or exponential growth rate of an organism the logarithmic form of equation (3) is used.

$$(5) \qquad \ln M = t \frac{\ln2}{g} + \ln M_1$$

For the logarithmic phase of growth, the expression $\frac{\ln2}{g}$ is a constant. Therefore, in equation (5) we can substitute μ. The resulting equation expressing the increase of mass within a certain time, is the equation of a straight line.

$$(6) \qquad \ln M = \mu t + \ln M_1$$

When the values of t are plotted on the abscissa and the values of $\ln M$ on the ordinate, a straight line is obtained, and the constant μ is the slope of this straight line. It determines the growth rate of the bacterial mass as a function of time. It is therefore called the "specific growth rate" or "instantaneous growth rate constant." Its value can be determined either graphically, by calculation,

$$(7) \qquad \mu = \frac{\ln2}{g} = \frac{0.69}{g}$$

or it can be calculated directly from equation (6)

$$\mu = \frac{\ln M - \ln M_1}{t}$$

where the time t is the interval $t_1 - t_2$ during which the bacterial mass M_1 increased to the value of M.

The instantaneous growth rate μ is specific for every organism and culture medium. It is governed primarily by such factors as the growth capacity of the organism, but it also is affected by the environment. In order to express the real maximum value, the value corresponding to the logarithmic phase of the growth curve, the culture must grow in an unrestricted medium with substrate and growth factors in excess so that the growth rate is independent of these.

Continuous Culture In many physiologic studies it is desirable that the cells be examined in the exponential or steady state of growth. It is impossible, however, to provide such conditions over a long period of time in an intensively metabolizing batch culture. Continuous culture techniques circumvent this problem. These are open systems in which advantage is taken of the relation existing between the growth rate and the concentration of a limiting factor.

The chemostat is a continuous system cultivator in which the medium is thoroughly mixed to obtain maximum homogeneity (Fig. 5-3). The fresh nutrient medium flows into the cultivator at a defined and constant rate. The volume is kept constant by a device that allows culture medium together with part of the grown organisms to leave the culture vessel at the same rate. The ratio of the inflowing amount of nutrient medium per hour to the volume of the culture is the dilution rate, D. If the dilution rate is kept constant, the concentration of all the components becomes constant, and a steady state is established that may be maintained for a long period of time.

The key to an understanding of the mode of action of the chemostat lies in the way in which the growth rate depends on the concentration of a limiting growth factor in the culture medium. In a batch culture, substrate is consumed as the organisms grow. As a result the substrate

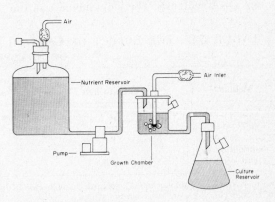

FIG. 5-3. Simplified diagram of a chemostat.

concentration continually decreases, and the growth rate decreases. In a chemostat, however, the continued addition of fresh medium fixes the substrate concentration and the growth rate at some predetermined value. The chemostat is useful in the study of population genetics and in the study of regulatory mechanisms that control the flow of material into the major classes of macromolecules.

EFFECT OF GROWTH RATE ON STRUCTURE AND COMPOSITION OF BACTERIA. The structure and chemical composition of bacteria vary with the growth rate. These changes are shown in Table 5-2 in which the growth rate was controlled by providing different carbon and nitrogen sources. The size of the cell is directly related to their growth rate, and the average number of nuclear bodies per bacterium is greater at the faster growth rates. The greatest change, however, is the concentration of RNA, especially ribosomal RNA. Such findings emphasize the importance of the number of ribosomal particles present in the cell in limiting bacterial cell growth.

The response of RNA to changes in growth rate has been demonstrated in a number of shift experiments, either a shift-up if the change of medium leads to an increase in growth rate, or a shift-down if there is a decrease (Fig. 5-4). In both types of experiments it has been shown that the first process to respond to the change in environment is the synthesis of RNA. When bacteria growing at 37C under conditions of balanced growth in one medium are transferred to another medium that will support a higher growth rate, the transition is characterized by a sudden increase in the rate of RNA synthesis, followed more slowly by corresponding changes in the rates of protein and DNA synthesis. The slow increase in the

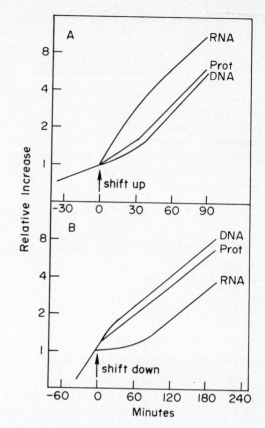

FIG. 5-4. Relative rate of RNA, DNA, and protein synthesis in *E. coli* following a shift in medium. A. Cells were shifted up from a glucose salts medium to a nutrient broth. B. Cells growing in nutrient broth are shifted down to a glucose salts medium. The value of each component is normalized to 1.0 at 0-time.

rate of protein synthesis after a shift to a richer medium is closely correlated with the increase in total RNA per cell. Observations such as these contribute to our understanding of factors controlling the rate of growth of bacteria and provide a basis for studies designed to answer

TABLE 5-2   THE EFFECT OF GROWTH RATE ON CELL SIZE AND COMPOSITION OF *S.* TYPHIMURIUM

Medium	Growth Rate	Dry Weight per Cell	Nuclei per Cell	RNA per Nucleus
	$\mu°$	g $\times 10^{-15}$		g $\times 10^{-15}$
Lysine salts	0.6	240	1.1	22
Glucose salts	1.2	360	1.5	31
Nutrient broth	2.4	840	2.4	65
Heart infusion	2.8	1090	2.9	84

From Schaechter, Maaløe, and Kjeldgaard: J Gen Microbiol 19:603, 1958
°Growth rate expressed as generations/hour

the question of why a bacterium can replicate in 20 minutes whereas it takes the most rapidly dividing mammalian cell 10 hours.

Synchronous Growth As bacteria are usually grown, cell division occurs at random, giving a mixture of cells representing all phases of the division cycle. Studies on such cultures yield average values only. There are techniques, however, that synchronize division and induce all of the cells in a bacterial culture to divide simultaneously. By withdrawing cells representing a single age class, a sample is obtained large enough for analysis by standard biochemical techniques. Among the problems that can be studied by this technique are the rate of synthesis of a macromolecule, the initial rate of induced enzyme synthesis or mutation induction, the quantity of a macromolecule, or the effect of inhibitors. Two fundamentally different experimental approaches have been employed. In the first approach the cells are sorted out according to age or size. In methods of the second type a culture is treated to yield a synchronously dividing population. The former procedures are preferable, since they are less likely to introduce distortions in the physiologic state of the cells.

SELECTION BY SIZE AND AGE. One useful technique for synchronization of bacteria is based on size selection by filtration. This method takes advantage of the cyclic changes in size that accompany the division cycle. A culture is filtered through a stack of filter papers that retains the larger cells near the top of the pile and allows the small cells to pass through and to be collected in the filtrate. The cells in the filtrate, or those obtained by eluting selected papers, grow synchronously during subsequent incubation.

In another technique for obtaining synchrony, cells of uniform age are selected from a growing population. A population of cells is passed through a membrane filter of pore size small enough so that the bacteria remain irreversibly bound on the surface of the membrane. When the filter is then inverted and medium passed through, the only cells appearing in the eluted medium are the unbound sister cells which would be the youngest cells in a log phase culture. Under the proper conditions, new daughter cells can be removed for extended periods of time from the population growing

on the surface, and these cells would grow synchronously (Fig. 5-5). This technique has been very useful in studies on the biochemical events accompanying the bacterial division cycle.

SELECTION BY INDUCTION TECHNIQUES. Most of the earlier techniques for obtaining synchronized cells have used shock treatments, such as variations in temperature, starvation, and illumination. Although synchronized growth is induced by these techniques and the degree of synchrony is usually as good as or better than that achieved by selection techniques, induction techniques introduce physiologic abnormalities.

One of the earliest techniques utilized temperature and was based on the assumption that the processes that occur during the division cycle are differentially sensitive to temperature. If the temperature of an exponentially growing culture is reduced from 37C to 25C for 15 minutes and then returned to 37C, cell division of most of the cells is synchronized. The most successful methods of synchronizing bacterial growth with temperature shifts have involved repeated changes in temperature at intervals of a generation time.

Starvation treatments of various forms have also been used extensively. A phasing of cell division was observed in cultures of a thymine-requiring mutant following withdrawal and readdition of thymine to the cultures. Starva-

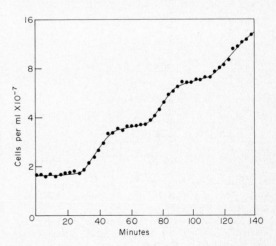

FIG. 5-5. Cells of *E. coli* synchronized by the selection of newly formed cells eluted from membrane filter. (After Helmstetter: Methods in Microbiology, vol 1. Courtesy of Academic Press)

tion for glucose, either alone or in conjunction with a cold shock, also phases cell division.

THE GROWTH OF SINGLE CELLS

Cells that are growing are destined to divide. Cell division takes place at different intervals depending on the species and environmental conditions. Within a short period, often as short as 20 minutes, a bacterium can create a complete duplicate of itself, which in turn is capable of duplicating. This process requires the synthesis of the millions of parts of the parent cell and their organization into the various homo- and heteropolymers which are the functional units of the cell.

In order to understand bacterial growth it is necessary to have some knowledge of the temporal sequence of events during a single cell cycle and an understanding of how these biochemical events are interrelated. Bacteria do not exhibit the characteristic cell-division cycle observed in eucaryotic organisms. Whereas in eucaryotic organisms DNA synthesis is confined to a single phase of the cell cycle, the S

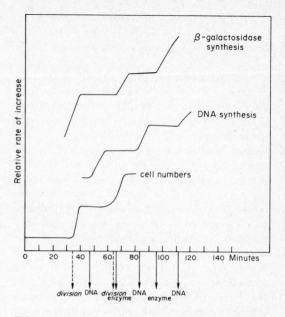

FIG. 5-7. Use of a synchronized population of *E. coli* to study temporal control of gene expression. (After Donachie and Masters: The Cell Cycle. Courtesy of Academic Press)

phase, in bacteria that are growing exponentially DNA synthesis occurs virtually throughout the entire division cycle. Also, in bacteria the duplication sequences do not necessarily follow one after the other, but instead they overlap, the amount of overlapping depending on the growth medium. Bacterial duplication begins with the initiation of DNA replication, followed by the complete duplication and separation of the DNA replicas, and formation of a septum near the equatorial plane so that two cells, each one containing half the DNA content of the mother, are formed (Fig. 5-6).

Techniques that achieve synchrony in a dividing population in a metabolically undisturbed state have proved invaluable in studies of the bacterial division cycle (Fig. 5-7). Autoradiography and marker-frequency analysis have been used for the study of particular aspects of the division cycle in asynchronous cultures. Morphologic details related to the division process have been provided by examination of serial ultrathin sections with the electron microscope.

Bacterial Cell Division   Genetic information necessary for duplication of the bacterial cell is contained within the bacterial chromo-

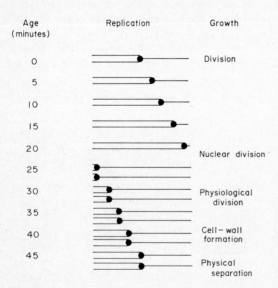

FIG. 5-6. DNA replication in *E. coli* growing with a doubling time of 45 minutes. Newborn cells at 0-time possess half-replicated chromosomes. The end of a round occurs at 20 to 25 minutes. Nuclear division occurs, and a new round of replication begins. At the time of division, cells contain two half-replicated chromosomes. (After Clark: J Bacteriol 96:1223, 1968)

somes. The number of chromosomes in a cell and the extent of their replication are determined by the physiologic state and age of the cell. Chromosomes of cells in very slowly growing cultures appear to have but a single replication point. Observations of gaps in DNA synthesis in these cells indicate that chromosome replication occupies only part of the cycle. Cells in rapidly growing cultures, however, contain multiple replication points. Because replication occurs simultaneously at several points along these chromosomes, the entire chromosome can be replicated in a fraction of the time that would be required if there were but a single replication fork. Genetic material can thus be duplicated at rates that otherwise could not be attained.

Initiation of Chromosome Replication During division, in order to insure the segregation of equal portions of the genetic material among the progeny, chromosome replication and cell division are coordinated in such a manner that the frequency of initiation of replication determines the rate of cell division. In *E. coli* replication of the DNA requires approximately 40 minutes from time of initiation to completion. Cell division takes place about 20 minutes after the completion of each round of chromosome replication.

As presently conceptualized, a duplication sequence begins with the initiation of chromosome synthesis at a unique site, the replicator site of the chromosome. Initiation of chromosome replication requires protein synthesis and depends on the achievement of a critical cell mass:DNA ratio. Chromosome replication begins when a fixed amount of protein initiator substances has accumulated regardless of the position of other replication points on the chromosome. Thus, in a given culture medium the rate of cell division is determined by the time required for accumulation of the initiator. Initiation is not influenced by the presence, absence, position, or rate of movement of replication points on the chromosome.

At least three classes of protein synthesis are essential for cell division. The first is required for the initiation of chromosome replication itself, the second is a 40-minute period that takes place concurrently with chromosome replication, and the third is a short period of RNA and protein synthesis that must take place at, or subsequent to, the time of completion of chro-

mosome duplication. In cells growing under conditions in which the time for formation of initiator is longer than the time required for a replication point to traverse the chromosome, a new round of replication is not initiated until after the previous replication point has reached the chromosome terminus. In this case, there is a period devoid of DNA synthesis between rounds of chromosome replication. Conversely, in cells growing in media in which the inter-initiation time is shorter than that required for a round of replication, new rounds are initiated before the previous replication point has reached the terminus. In this situation, cells contain chromosomes with three or more rep-

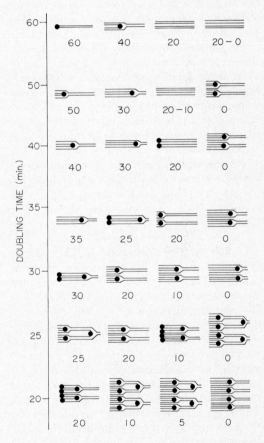

FIG. 5-8. Relationship between chromosome replication and the division cycle in *E. coli* B/r growing at different rates. The time required for a replication point to proceed from the origin to the terminus of the genome is 40 minutes; the time between the end of a round of chromosome replication and cell division is 20 minutes. The black dot indicates a replication point, and the numbers indicate the time in minutes prior to cell division. (After Cooper and Helmstetter: J Mol Biol 31:521, 1968)

lication points, as have been observed in rapidly growing cells (Fig. 5-8). Helmstetter's model of DNA replication is based on the constancy at all growth rates of two periods: (1) the interval between the end of a round of DNA replication and cell division and (2) the time required for a replication point to traverse the genome. The first of these periods could be considered analogous to the G_2 period in eucaryotic cells; the second period, analogous to the S period, is the time required for the synthesis of DNA.

Chromosome Duplication The replication of bacterial DNA begins by the gradual separation of the two strands at the replicator site to form a Y-shaped locus, the replication fork, which represents a growing point. The replicating enzyme system attaches to the DNA at this site and moves along the entire chromosome replicating the parent DNA as the double helix slowly rotates and unwinds. After a replication point reaches the terminus of a chromosome, the two newly replicated sister chromosomes separate from each other. Although the process has been referred to as "nuclear division," it is not strictly analogous to nuclear division in eucaryotic organisms, since the chromosomes separate gradually throughout the entire period of replication. The enzymatic mechanisms of DNA replication are discussed in Chapter 7.

Role of Cell Membrane in Chromosome Separation Electron microscopy has failed to show any bacterial structure equivalent to the mitotic apparatus of higher cells. It is evident, however, that there must be some mechanism that ensures equitable separation of chromosomes after each replication. The replicon method proposed by Jacob and his associates provides an explanation of how this might be achieved. The model suggests that the cellular DNA is attached to the bacterial membrane where replication occurs by passage of the DNA through an enzyme complex in the membrane. Separation and equipartition of the DNA copies results from the synthesis of new cell membrane in an annular region between attachment points.

This model is supported by both biochemical and morphologic criteria. Biochemical analyses have demonstrated that in gently lysed prepa-

rations of bacteria, the actively replicating portion of the DNA is associated with a membrane fraction. Electron microscopic studies have provided a morphologic basis and have shown that in gram-positive organisms extensions of the cytoplasmic membrane, the mesosomes, are in contact with the bacterial chromosome (Fig. 5-9). Serial sections through dividing cells have indicated that in the course of replication the mesosomes with thin attached chromosomes split in two and move apart, each carrying with it one of the two sister chromosomes. Evidence that the separation of the mesosomes is achieved by the synthesis of new membrane in the region between them was obtained by following the distribution of a specific marker, potassium tellurite, in the membrane during growth. Potassium tellurite is deposited selectively in the reduced form at the oxidation-reduction sites of the membrane as crystals that are visible in the electron microscope. The observed distribution of crystals supports the hypothesis that new membrane is generated in the region of the point of attachment of the chromosome to the membrane.

In gram-negative bacteria where mesosomal formation is minimal, the chromosome is either

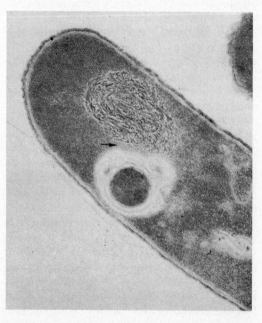

FIG. 5-9. Section of *E. coli* showing the physical association of DNA with a mesosome. (From Altenberg: J Bacteriol 103:231, 1970)

attached to the membrane without the mediation of mesosomes, or it is attached to their base. There appears to be no unique membrane attachment site on the *E. coli* genome; either the genome is attached to the membrane at random or to a number of fixed or changing attachment points.

Terminal Steps in Cell Division Following the separation of the two daughter chromosomes the cell initiates synthesis of a transverse septum. The temporal relationship between replication of the chromosome and synthesis of the transverse septum is closely regulated. The completion of a round of replication and a period of protein synthesis that normally occurs concurrent with chromosome replication are both required for cell division. Cell division occurs at a fixed time after the termination of a round of DNA replication. This time period represents the time required for the expression of the many special reactions involved in septum formation, membrane growth, and wall synthesis.

The importance of the coupling between DNA replication and cell division has been emphasized by the finding of a number of mutants in which the regulation of cell division is disrupted. Many of these are conditional lethal mutants that grow normally at 30C but are unable to form colonies at 41C. In some of these mutants specific differences in membrane proteins have been observed, some of which correlate well with an interference of septum formation and inhibition of cell division.

SEPTUM FORMATION. Compartmentalization of physiologic division of the cell occurs prior to the actual physical separation of the daughter cells. This is the time at which the cytoplasmic events at one end of the cell become independent of cytoplasmic events occurring at the opposite end. The end of a round of replication occurs well in advance of this compartmentalization.

This stage of growth is characterized by the development of a weak septum followed by the formation of a strong crosswall. As emphasized previously, the position and timing of septum formation are crucial if each daughter cell is to receive a full complement of the parental material. The process of septum formation is poorly understood, and little is known of the

physiologic events that periodically initiate it. Although it is generally agreed that the completion of chromosome replication triggers cell division, perhaps by transcription of genes located at the chromosome terminus, other factors such as the presence of polyamines and heat-labile proteins also play an important role.

CELL WALL GROWTH. During balanced growth a greater surface area is normally required to cover a greater volume. In several gram-positive species, cell wall growth appears to be limited to discrete areas at the equator. These areas have been located in a number of gram-positive organisms by staining the cell surface with fluorescent antibodies and observing the location of the label during subsequent growth (Fig. 5-10). In gram-negative organisms, however, although zonal growth of the murein component also occurs, the lipopolysaccharide of the cell envelope probably is added by diffuse intercalation during cell elongation.

The nascent crosswall of the growing cell originates within the area enclosed by a mesosome (Fig. 5-11). Subsequent inward growth of the wall is preceded by a corresponding inward proliferation of the mesosome, which is formed by a concentric infolding of the plasma membrane. As the mesosome, followed by the grow-

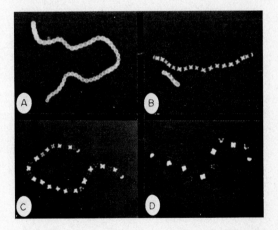

FIG. 5-10. Growth of the wall of *Streptococcus pyogenes,* followed by ultraviolet photomicrography of growing chains of cells after initial labeling with fluorescent antibody. A. Immediately after antibody treatment, showing even fluorescence of cells. B. Cells after 15 minutes of growth. C. After 30 minutes. D. After 60 minutes. New (nonfluorescent) wall material is formed around the equator of each cell. (From Cole: Bacteriol Rev 29:326, 1965)

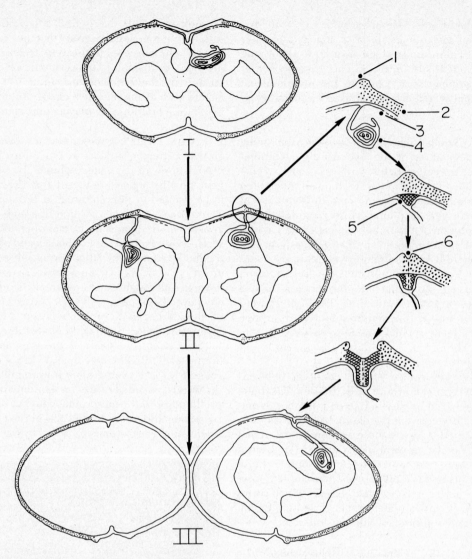

FIG. 5-11. Diagrammatic representation of cell-wall division model for *Streptococcus faecalis*. This simulated time-lapse sequence was reconstructed from a large number of electron micrographs. 1. Wall band. 2. Cell wall. 3. Cell membrane. 4. Mesosome. 5. New wall synthesis. 6. Wall notch. (Adapted from Higgins and Shockman: Crit Rev Microbiol 1:29, 1971)

ing transverse septum, moves toward the center of the cell, the membranes at its base continue to form around the newly synthesized cell wall.

Both peripheral wall elongation and centripetal crosswall extension apparently result from biosynthetic activity in the vicinity of the leading edge of the crosswall. An interplay of murein-hydrolyzing and murein-synthesizing enzymes has been invoked to explain the sequence of interrelated events associated with the enlargement of the cell wall. A closed mole-

cule like the structural component of the cell wall, the murein sacculus, can only be modified when covalent bonds are split. The hydrolases would provide both space and acceptor sites for incoming subunits, which in a second step would be condensed into the preexistent murein. The sites at which murein hydrolases are active correspond to the zones where murein is synthesized.

SEPARATION OF BACTERIA.   Separation of the two daughter cells takes place some time after the completion of the transverse septum. The separation begins with the appearance of a constriction between the subsequent daughter cells and a thickening of the cell wall in the constriction region. Further thickening of the cell wall accompanies constriction between the cells until the pole of the cell assumes its characteristic rounded shape. The normal thickness of the cell wall, however, is achieved only after constriction is complete and the two daughter cells have separated completely. Separation of the daughter cells is mediated by murein hydrolases that are localized at the site of septum formation and which are latent in nondividing cells.

Asymmetrical Cell Division Regulation of the site at which cell division occurs along the length of rod-shaped bacteria is under genetic control. In rod-shaped bacterial cells, division sites arise normally in an equatorial position, partitioning the daughter genomes into cells of approximately the same length. A number of bacterial mutants have been described, however, in which the division site location is abnormal. The most extensively studied of these are the minicells of *E. coli*. These are tiny, spherical cells produced from the ends of the parent rod-shaped cells. *E. coli* minicells lack host chromosomes although they may contain episomal DNA if the parent cell contains an episome. Minicells lacking DNA are unable to synthesize any polymer whose synthesis is DNA-dependent. Minicell formation also occurs in mutants of *Bacillus subtilis* as a result of abnormal division site location. Motility is retained in *B. subtilis* minicells, an indication of functional energy metabolism. Such cells are produced by a structurally normal division mechanism and contain a normal cell surface. Minicells have been very useful in many areas of experimentation, although the mechanism responsible for abnormal division site location is unknown.

A series of temperature-sensitive mutants of *E. coli* K 12 also has been isolated which grow normally at 30C but cease DNA synthesis at 40C after a small portion of the chromosome has been replicated. Most of these mutants are unable to form a septum, so that the cells continue to elongate and to produce long filamentous cells without septa. However, a small number of these thermosensitive mutants can still form septa and undergo cell division. In these mutants the septa are not formed near the equatorial plane as in the wild-type parent but to one side of the DNA, so that of the two daughter cells formed, one contains all of the DNA of the mother bacterium and the other contains none. This type of anucleate cell, however, differs from the minicell in that it is about the same size as a normal wild-type cell.

DIFFERENTIATION IN BACTERIAL CELLS

Sporulation and Germination One of the most unusual properties of certain bacteria is the ability to form endospores. At some point in the vegetative cell cycle of spore-forming organisms, growth is arrested, and the cell undergoes progressive physiologic and morphologic changes that result in the formation of an endospore. A spore is a dormant structure capable of surviving for prolonged periods and endowed with the capacity to reestablish the vegetative stage of growth under appropriate environmental conditions. The process involved in sporulation, as well as the breaking of the spore's dormancy and subsequent emergence of a vegetative cell, represents a primitive example of unicellular differentiation. Studies of these phenomena provide model systems for understanding the mechanisms by which sequential morphologic and biochemical events are ordered and controlled in a differentiating system.

Properties of Endospores Endospores are formed by organisms of the genera *Bacillus*, *Clostridium*, and *Sporosarcina* during the stationary phase of growth after certain essential nutrients in the medium have been exhausted. A single spore is produced within a vegetative cell and differs from it in its morphology and composition, increased resistance to adverse environments, and absence of metabolic activity. Although the thermoresistance of spores has been the major concern of medical microbiologists because of the problems associated with the control of infections caused by spore-forming organisms, spores also have an increased resistance to the lethal effects of desiccation, freezing, radiation, and deleterious chemicals. The primary selective value of the spore, however, lies in its longevity in the soil coupled with its ability to germinate under the proper environmental conditions.

CHEMICAL BASIS OF SPORE RESISTANCE. Resistance to various chemical and physical agents appear at different stages during sporulation, concomitant with changes in the physicochemical composition of the sporulating cell. The resistance to radiation, drying, and chemical agents appears after the cell becomes refractile and depends at least in part upon the properties of the cystine-rich spore coat proteins. Thermal resistance is probably due to the very low content of water, which renders the proteins and nucleic acids more resistant to denaturation. This dehydration occurs late in sporulation at the time of cortex formation and at the time that the spore first appears as a refractile object. The massive synthesis of dipicolinic acid during this stage may be responsible for the dehydration. Dipicolinic acid, a chelating agent, is a spore-specific component present in high concentrations in all bacterial endospores (Fig. 5-12). It is present in the cortex of the mature spore as the calcium salt and accounts for 5 to 15 percent of its dry weight. Both calcium and dipicolinic acid are required for heat resistance.

Metabolic Differences Between Vegetative Cells and Spores As a bacterial cell passes from the vegetative state to the sporulating state, it undergoes dramatic changes in its morphology and physiology. During sporulation certain compounds such as poly-β-hydroxybutyrate, accumulate and are later utilized. Extensive turnover of macromolecules occurs, and some enzyme levels change drastically. New and characteristic spore structures are synthesized, while previously existing structures are degraded.

The pools of small molecules found in spores are distinctly different from those of vegetative cells. There is an accumulation of dipicolinic acid, divalent cations, and high levels of L-glutamic acid. The predominant component of the

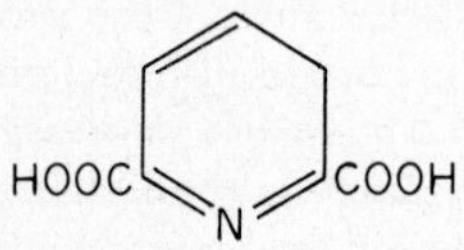

FIG. 5-12. Dipicolinic acid (pyridine-2,6-dicarboxylic acid).

drastically reduced acid-soluble phosphate pool is 3-phosphoglyceric acid, which constitutes as much as 75 percent of the acid-soluble phosphate in the spore but no more than 5 percent of the acid-soluble phosphate of the vegetative cell. Spores contain very low levels of ATP, whereas ATP is a major component of vegetative cells.

During sporulation many differences occur both qualitatively and quantitatively in the pattern of enzyme activities. Some of these differences are associated with mechanisms related to spore formation; some with components of the spore itself. The heat-stable catalase of spores is immunologically distinct from the vegetative cell enzyme; glucose dehydrogenase, a ribonuclease, and spore lytic enzymes are present only in the spore and absent from the vegetative cells. These enzymes as well as the spore coat proteins represent spore-specific gene products.

Initiation of Sporulation Sporulation is a response to nutritional deprivation. Although limitation of any one of a variety of nutrients can initiate sporulation, the most pronounced effect is exerted by the carbon and nitrogen sources available. The regulation of spore formation in the bacterial cell is negative; the cell makes an inhibitor or repressor from some ingredient in the medium that prevents the initiation of sporulation. When this ingredient is exhausted, inhibition is released, and the cells sporulate. A metabolizable supply of both carbon and nitrogen are required to inhibit sporulation. If there is a deficiency in the supply of either of these, inhibition will be relieved and sporulation initiated.

The Biochemistry of Sporulation At some period in the development of a cell, the metabolism is irreversibly channeled in the direction of sporulation. There is no single point of commitment for the sporulation process as a whole but a separate point of commitment for each new specific macromolecule. An examination of thin sections of sporulating cells in the electron microscope has shown that an ordered series of cytologic and structural changes accompanies the physiologic changes associated with sporulation. The morphologic changes observed in *B. subtilis* have been presented in Figure 5-13 as a time scale divided into seven sequentially appearing stages. The process is

STAGE	MORPHOLOGIC EVENT	BIOCHEMICAL EVENT
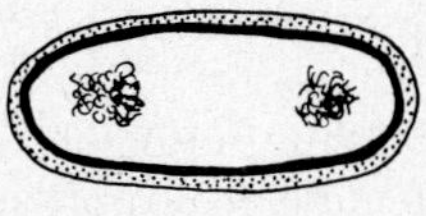	Vegetative cell	
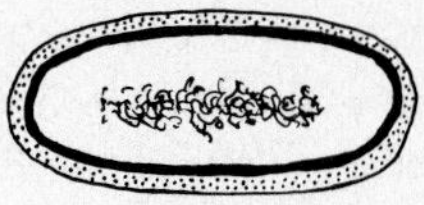	Chromatin filament	Exoenzymes Antibiotic
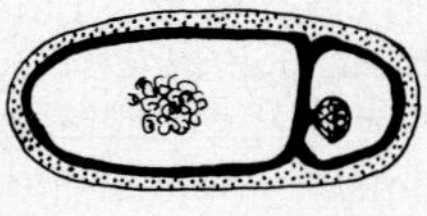	Spore septum	Alanine dehydrogenase
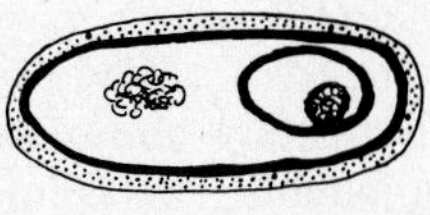	Spore protoplast	Alkaline phosphatase Glucose dehydrogenase Aconitase Heat−resistant catalase
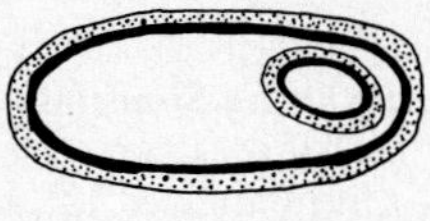	Cortex formation (refractility)	Ribosidase Adenosine deaminase Dipicolinic acid
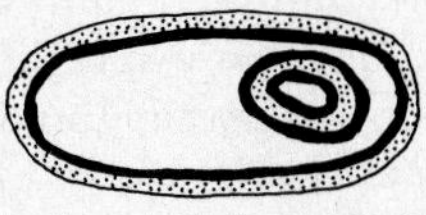	Coat formation	Cysteine incorporation Chemical resistance
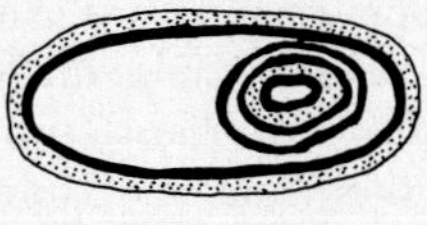	Maturation	Alanine racemase Heat resistance

FIG. 5-13. Morphologic and biochemical events associated with sporulation. A composite diagram of data obtained with different species of *Bacillus*. (After Mandelstam: Microbial Growth. Nineteenth Symp Soc Gen Microbiol. Courtesy of Cambridge University Press)

timed from the end of exponential growth at t_0 and at hourly periods after this.

STAGE 0.   This represents the state of the cell at the end of exponential growth at a time when each vegetative cell contains two chromosomes.

STAGE I.   This stage is characterized by the formation from the more disperse nuclear bodies of a broad axial chromatin filament, which occupies the center of the cell. During this stage the most characteristic events are the production and excretion into the medium of antibiotics and various exoenzymes. The importance of antibiotic and protease production in the formation of spores is emphasized by the finding that mutants unable to produce these substances are almost invariably also asporogenous. Proteases probably play a role in the intracellular turnover of protein, but the correlation between sporulation and antibiotic production is more difficult to explain.

STAGE II.   This stage is characterized by the formation of a forespore septum near one pole of the cell. Septum formation follows the separation of the two discrete chromatin bodies in the axial filament and movement of one of them to the end of the cell, resulting in the segregation of the nuclear material into two compartments, the mother cell and the forespore units. The forespore septum is formed de novo and does not result from the rearrangement of preexisting membrane. During this period there is a marked increase of alanine dehydrogenase, a component important in germination.

STAGE III.   During this stage the spore protoplast is formed as a consequence of the unidirectional growth of the cytoplasmic membrane of the sporangium. Among the enzymes whose activity is increased markedly during this stage are glucose dehydrogenase and aconitase. Aconitase is an example of an enzyme appearing during the early stages of sporogenesis that is, like sporulation itself, subject to catabolite repression. With the exhaustion of glucose and glutamate at the end of vegetative growth, repression is relieved, aconitase is formed, and functional tricarboxylic acid and glyoxylic acid cycles produced. Heat-resistant catalase and alkaline phosphatase also appear during Stage III.

STAGE IV.   Cortex formation occurs during this stage at a time when the spore appears for the first time as refractile objects. Metabolic activity of the forespore at the end of Stage IV is considerably less than that of vegetative cells; beyond this stage the forespore probably contributes little to its own development. The activity of both ribosidase and adenosine deaminase increases during Stage IV, and the synthesis of dipicolinic acid begins.

STAGE V.   This is the period of coat formation. Deposition of spore coat protein and the incorporation of cystine lead to a completed coat structure.

STAGE VI.   Spore maturation occurs during this stage. Changes occur in the fine structure of the cytoplasm of the spore protoplast which make it more homogeneous and electron-dense. There is continued synthesis of or modification of cortical peptidoglycan and uptake of dipicolinic acid and calcium. Alanine racemase, an enzyme important in spore germination, is formed, and a number of ill-defined changes occur which make the spores resistant to organic solvents and to heat.

STAGE VII.   The mature endospore is liberated from the mother cell. This is initiated by a lytic enzyme synthesized or activated subsequent to maturation of the endospore.

Protein Synthesis during Sporulation   With the appearance of the forespore the cell becomes a compartmentalized structure. In the compartment developing into the forespore, DNA replication is inhibited and the substances synthesized are spore-specific. In the second compartment, the sporangium, synthesis of vegetative DNA continues, and products of the vegetative cell continue to be produced. Thus, in the sporulating cell both the vegetative and spore genomes are transcribed. The mRNA contains some of the same mRNA molecules as derepressed cells transferred from a rich medium to a poor one and, in addition, molecules specific to sporulation. There is no evidence that the mRNA produced late in sporulation is stable and retained in the spore for protein synthesis during outgrowth.

ROLE OF RNA POLYMERASE.   The changes that occur during sporulation result from the turnoff of certain vegetative genes and the expression of new classes of genes. Ribosomal RNA genes are not transcribed in sporulating cells. The turnoff, however, of ribosomal RNA genes during sporulation is brought about by a mechanism different from that responsible for stringent control of ribosomal RNA synthesis. The most attractive model that has been proposed suggests that early in passing from the vegetative to the sporulating state, the template specificity of the RNA polymerase is altered. The vegetative sigma factor does not function in sporulating cells, while the core enzyme, the machinery for polymerizing RNA, is conserved. The reason for failure of the sigma factor to function may be explained by differences observed between the β subunits in vegetative and sporulation RNA polymerase cores. The two β polypeptides of vegetative RNA polymerase have a molecular weight of 155,000 daltons. In sporulation RNA polymerase, one of these β subunits, has a molecular weight of only 110,000 daltons. Although this modification of vegetative RNA polymerase is critical to sporulation and may be the event responsible for the turnoff of some vegetative genes during sporulation, a more precise explanation is still needed for the mechanism by which the transcription of new genes is directed. The spore genome is present in vegetative cells but is repressed under conditions of rapid growth. At the end of exponential growth the level of intracellular catabolites is altered, and the gene governing the synthesis of a sporulation initiation factor is derepressed. The nature of this sporulation initiation factor, however, remains to be clarified.

Germination and Outgrowth Simultaneous structural and physiologic changes also are manifested during the transformation of a dormant spore into a vegetative cell. The process of spore germination consists of three sequential phases: (1) an activation state that conditions the spore to germinate in a suitable environment, (2) a germination stage, during which the characteristic properties of the dormant spore are lost, and (3) an outgrowth stage during which the spore is converted into a new vegetative cell.

Activation is a reversible process that conditions the spore for germination. Spores do not germinate or germinate very slowly unless activated either by heat or various chemical treatments. Activation probably involves a reversible denaturation of a specific macromolecule.

Germination is an irreversible process triggered by the exposure of activated spores to specific stimulants, such as amino acids, nucleosides, and glucose. This is the stage during which the dormant stage is ended. During the early stages of germination there is a loss of refractility, swelling of the cortex, and appearance of fine nuclear fibrils. Accompanying these changes is a loss of resistance to deleterious physical and chemical agents, increase in the sulfhydryl level of the spore, a release of spore components, and an increase in metabolic activity. The germination of spores is not inhibited by antibiotics that perturb protein and nucleic acid synthesis, indicating that the enzymes responsible for germination are already present in the spore.

During outgrowth there is de novo synthesis of proteins and structural components that are characteristic of vegetative cells. During this stage the spore core membrane develops into the cell wall of the vegetative cell. Outgrowth is a period of active biosynthetic activity and is markedly inhibited by interference with the energy supply or by antibiotics that inhibit cell wall, protein, or nucleic acid synthesis.

If heat-activated spores are germinated under suitable conditions a high degree of synchrony is obtained. Such a synchronous population provides a model system for the study of the initiation of transcriptional and translational events occurring during differentiation. Since the dormant spore is devoid of functional mRNA the conversion of the spore to a vegetative cell during outgrowth requires transcription and de novo synthesis of gene products. The appearance of these gene products is ordered, determined by the time of transcription of particular genes. Ribosome synthesis starts early, vegetative cell wall synthesis later, and DNA synthesis begins just before division of the cell. During a stepwise doubling of cell members for several generations, the initiation of certain enzymes occurs at a specific time during each division cycle and results in a doubling of each enzyme during only a fraction of the total cycle.

FURTHER READING

Books and Reviews

Abrams A, Smith JB: Bacterial membrane ATPase. In Boyer PD (ed.): The Enzymes. New York, Academic Press, 1974, Vol 10, pp 395-429

Adler J: Chemotaxis in bacteria. Annu. Rev Biochem 44: 341, 1975

Coleman R: Membrane-bound enzymes and membrane ultrastructure. Biochim Biophys Acta 300:1, 1973

Doi RH: Role of proteases in sporulation. Curr Top Cell Reg 6:1, 1972

Donachie WD, Masters M: Temporal control of gene expression in bacteria. In Padilla EM, Whitson GL, Cameron IL (eds): The Cell Cycle. New York, Academic Press, 1969, pp 37-76

Fridovich I: Superoxide dismutases. Annu Rev Biochem 44:147, 1975

Guirard BM, Snell EE: Nutritional requirements of microorganisms. In Gunsalus IC, Stanier RY (eds): The Bacteria. New York, Academic Press, 1962, vol 4, pp 33-93

Harold FM: Conservation and transformation of energy by bacterial membranes. Bacteriol Rev 36:172, 1972

Helmstetter CE: Methods for studying the microbial division cycle. In Norris JR, Ribbons DW (eds): Methods in Microbiology. London, Academic Press, 1969, vol 1, pp 327-363

Helmstetter CE: Regulation of chromosome replication and cell division in Escherichia coli. In Padilla EM, Whitson GL, Cameron IL (eds): The Cell Cycle. New York, Academic Press, 1969, pp 15-35

Kaback HR: Transport across isolated bacterial cytoplasmic membranes. Biochim Biophys. Acta 265:367, 1972

Kepes A: Galactoside permease of Escherichia coli. In Bronner F, Kleinzeller A (eds): Current Topics in Membranes and Transport. New York, Academic Press, 1970, vol 1, 101-133.

Maaløe O, Kjeldgaard NO: Control of Macromolecular Synthesis. New York, Benjamin, 1966

Malek I, Fenel Z: Theoretical and Methodological Basis of Continuous Culture of Microorganisms. New York, Academic Press, 1966

Mallette MF: Evaluation of growth by physical and chemical means. In Norris JR, Ribbons DW (eds): Methods in Microbiology. London, Academic Press, 1969, vol 1, pp 521-566

Mandelstam J: Regulation of bacterial spore formation. Microbial Growth. Nineteenth Symp Soc Gen Microbiol. London, Cambridge Univ Press, 1969, pp 377-402

Oxender DL: Amino acid transport in microorganisms. In Hokin LE, (ed): Metabolic Pathways; Metabolic Transport. New York, Academic Press, 1972, vol 6, pp 133-185

Reusch VM Jr, Burger MM: The bacterial mesosome. Biochim Biophys Acta 300:79, 1973

Roseman S: Carbohydrate transport in bacterial cells. In Hokin LE (ed): Metabolic Pathways: Metabolic Transport. New York, Academic Press, 1972, vol 6, pp 41-89

Simoni RD, Postma PW: The energetics of bacterial active transport. Annu Rev Biochem 44:523, 1975

Slepecky RA: Synchrony and the formation and germination of bacterial spores. In Padilla EM, Whitson GL, Cameron IL (eds): The Cell Cycle. New York, Academic Press, 1969, pp 77-100

Stanier RY, Doudoroff M, Adelberg EA: The Microbial World, 3rd ed. Englewood Cliffs, NJ, Prentice-Hall, 1970

Tosteson DC (ed): The Molecular Basis of Membrane Function. Englewood Cliffs, NJ, Prentice-Hall, 1969

Selected Papers

Asghar SS, Levin E, Harold FM: Accumulation of neutral amino acids by Streptococcus faecalis. Energy coupling by a proton-motive force. J Biol Chem 248:5225, 1973

Clark DJ: Regulation of deoxyribonucleic acid replication and cell division in Esherichia coli B/r. J Bacteriol, 96: 1214, 1968

Cooper S, Helmstetter CE: Chromosome replication and the division cycle of Escherichia coli B/r. J Molec Biol 31:519, 1968

Dix DD, Helmstetter CE: Coupling between chromosome completion and cell division in Escherichia coli. J Bacteriol 115:786, 1973

Ellar DJ, Lundgren DG, Slepecky RA: Fine structure of Bacillus megaterium during synchronous growth. J Bacteriol, 94:1189, 1967

Esser AF, Souza KA: Correlation between thermal death and membrane fluidity in Bacillus stearothermophilus. Proc Natl Acad Sci USA 71:4111, 1974

Greenleaf AL, Linn TG, Losick R: Isolation of a new RNA polymerase-binding protein from sporulating Bacillus subtilis. Proc Natl Acad Sci USA 70:490, 1973

Higgins ML, Daneo-Moore L, Boothby D, Shockman GD: Effect of inhibition of deoxyribonucleic acid and protein synthesis on the direction of cell wall growth in Streptococcus faecalis. J Bacteriol 118:681, 1974

Jacob F, Brenner S, Cuzin F: On the regulation of DNA replication in bacteria. Cold Spring Harbor Symp Quant Biol 28:329, 1963

Jones NC, Donachie WD: Chromosome replication, transcription and control of cell division in Escherichia coli. Nature [New Biol] 243:100, 1973

Jones THD, Kennedy EP: Characterization of the membrane protein component of the lactose transport system of Escherichia coli. J Biol Chem 244:5981, 1969

Leighton TJ: An RNA polymerase mutation causing temperature-sensitive sporulation in Bacillus subtilis. Proc Natl Acad Sci USA 70:1179, 1973

Losick R, Shorenstein RG, Sonenshein AL: Structural alteration of RNA polymerase during sporulation. Nature 227:910, 1970

Norris TE, Koch AL: Effect of growth rate on the relative rates of synthesis of messenger, ribosomal and transfer RNA in Escherichia coli. J Mol Biol 64:633, 1972

Pardee AB: Membrane transport proteins. Science 162: 632, 1968

Rogers HJ: Bacterial growth and the cell envelope. Bacteriol Rev 34:194, 1970

Ryter A: Association of the nucleus and the membrane of bacteria: a morphological study. Bacteriol Rev 32:39, 1968

Schaeffer P: Sporulation and the production of antibiotics, exoenzymes, and exotoxins. Bacteriol Rev 33:48, 1969

Setlow P, Kornberg A: Biochemical studies of bacterial sporulation and germination. J Biol Chem 245: 3637, 1970

Van Golde LMG, Schulman H, Kennedy EP: Metabolism of membrane phospholipids and its relation to a novel class of oligosaccharides in Escherichia coli. Proc Natl Acad Sci USA 70:1368, 1973

6

Composition, Structure, and Biosynthesis of the Bacterial Cell Envelope and Energy Storage Polymers

LIPOPOLYSACCHARIDE BIOSYNTHESIS
LIPID A BIOSYNTHESIS (REGION
  III)
CORE POLYSACCHARIDE
  BIOSYNTHESIS (REGION II)
O ANTIGEN BIOSYNTHESIS
  (REGION I)

The bacterial cell surface and envelope components are of medical interest for many reasons. There was early recognition that cell surface antigens may play a role in the virulence of pathogens and that these antigens were useful for serologic identification and vaccine prophylaxis. The biosynthesis of the cell wall structure unique to bacteria later was found to be inhibited by various antibiotics, a fact which established a strong rationale for the study of the cell envelope as an approach to selective chemotherapy.

Envelope components provide survival value to microorganisms by serving one or more of many functions. Acidic polymers act as water and divalent metal (eg, Mg^{++} and Ca^{++}) sequestering agents, whereas the lipophilic integument of the acid-fast and gram-negative bacteria provides barriers to the entrance of various noxious chemicals and perhaps prevents loss of needed metabolites. The outer membrane of gram-negative bacteria may also serve to position periplasmic nutrient gathering and protective hydrolases outside the cytoplasmic membrane where they are most needed. In addition, the chemical and structural diversity of bacterial surface components is overwhelming. This is important, since, in host-parasite interactions,

the production of parasite-specific antibody aids in phagocytosis (Chaps. 16, 18). It follows that bacterial pathogens which produce copious amounts of different capsular polysaccharides and other envelope polymers (ie, virulence factors) will be difficult to phagocytose early in infection, until antibody production becomes sufficient. And though little specific information is yet available, it would appear that human and animal systems have difficulty in destroying enzymatically some of the more unusual components of bacterial integuments.

GROSS COMPOSITION OF THE BACTERIAL ENVELOPE

The structure and chemical nature of bacterial envelopes fall into three categories which correlate with whether a bacterium stains gram-positive, gram-negative, or acid-fast (Chap. 2). Other than in cell wall peptidoglycans, which are of remarkably similar general structure, the three groups of organisms differ considerably in the types of envelope lipids, polysaccharides, and proteins produced and in their ultrastructural arrangement. These differences are most notable in the occurrence of an outer membrane on gram-negative bacteria that is not found on gram-positive and acid-fast bacteria and the presence in both gram-positive and acid-fast bacteria of polysaccharides linked to peptidoglycan, a pattern not found in gram-negative cells. In addition, acid-fast and related organisms produce a variety of complex lipids not found in gram-positive or gram-negative organisms. The different types of envelope components produced by the three groups of organisms are summarized in Table 6-1. The

TABLE 6-1 COMPARISON OF CHARACTERISTIC TYPES OF BACTERIAL ENVELOPE COMPONENTS

Gram-positive Bacteria	Acid-fast Bacteria	Gram-negative Bacteria
Peptidoglycan 0.02 to 0.06 μ (multilayer)	Peptidoglycan 0.01 μ (monolayer ?)	Peptidoglycan 0.01 μ (monolayer ?)
Proteins	(Lipoproteins ?)	Lipoproteins
(Lipoteichoic acids)	Mycolic acid-glycolipids	Outer membrane
Teichoic acids	Arabinogalactans	Lipopolysaccharide
Teichuronic acids	Wax D	Lipoprotein
Polysaccharides	Cord factor	Phospholipid
	Sulfolipids	Polysaccharides
	Mycosides	

chemical composition, structure, biosynthesis, and, as indicated, the general location of many of these components within the various layers of the cell envelope can be described. However, the exact topologic, three-dimensional orientation, physical interrelationships, and function of many of these polymers as yet can only be inferred.

THE CELL WALL SACCULUS

Peptidoglycan (Murein or Mucopeptide)

The cell wall is a single, giant bag-shaped macromolecule composed of a network of cross-linked peptidoglycan. This supermolecule and associated components may account for 10 to 40 percent of the cell dry weight. The glycan component is invariably constituted of the two amino sugars, glucosamine and muramic acid. These occur as alternating β-1,4-linked N-acetyl-D-glucosamine (GlcNAc) and N-acetylmuramic acid [3-0-(1'-D-carboxyethyl)-N-acetyl-D-glucosamine] (ie, MurNAc) residues (Fig. 6-1). Chains vary from < 10 to > 170 disaccharide units. The glycan and peptide units are linked through the lactic acid carboxyl group of MurNAc to the amino terminus of a tetrapeptide. These glycotetrapeptides are cross-linked through the tetrapeptide units, forming a continuous sheet which is the cell wall peptidoglycan bag-shaped sacculus. The invariant feature

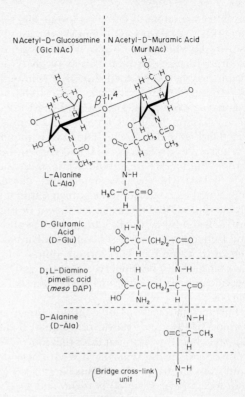

FIG. 6-1. Structure of the peptidoglycan repeating unit.

of the tetrapeptide component is the presence of D-alanine, which is always the linkage unit between peptidoglycan chains.

Peptide Structure and Variations As shown in Figure 6-1, the muramic acid-linked

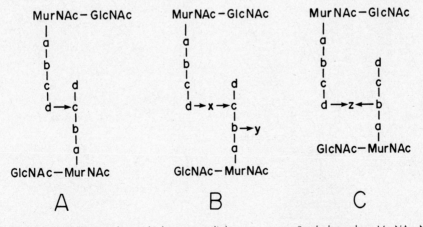

FIG. 6-2. General patterns of bacterial peptidoglycan cross-linkage structures. Symbols used are MurNAc, N-acetylmuramic acid; GlcNAc, N-acetylglucosamine; a,b,c,d are peptide units; y, amide substituent linked to α-carboxyl of D-isoglutamic or 3-hydroxyglutamic acid; x and z are bridge peptide amino acids. Type C bridge units, z, contain two —NH— termini, ie, —NH—R—NH—.

peptide component of many bacteria is the tetrapeptide, -L-Ala-D-isoGlu-mesoDAP (or L-Lys)-D-Ala, which may be generalized as a-b-c-d. Cross-linkage between two peptidoglycan chains may be established directly or through an interposed peptide bridge, as illustrated in Figure 6-2. The peptidoglycans of most organisms conform to the two types, A and B, illustrated in Figure 6-2, type C being rarely found. For example, *Escherichia coli* and *Corynebacterium diphtheriae* are of type A (Fig. 6-2A and Fig. 6-3A), whereas *Staphylococcus aureus* accomplishes interchain cross-linkage through an interposed peptide bridge as shown in Figure 6-2B and Figure 6-3B. Variations in peptide and bridge structures of several organisms are shown in Table 6-2. The various amino acids thus far found in peptidoglycans at the various peptide and bridge positions are shown in Table 6-3.

Further modifications of peptide structures include the in vivo removal of terminal D-alanine residues from tetrapeptides (eg, Fig. 6-3A) as in *E. coli*, or the removal of whole peptide units from the glycan chain. This happens in *E. coli*, which loses some 30 percent, and in *Micrococcus luteus*, where half or more of the glycan chains are free of tetrapeptide units. In contrast, *S. aureus* glycan appears to retain all of its tetrapeptide units which are highly cross-linked (Fig. 6-3B). In addition, peptidoglycan-bound proteins occur in both gram-positive and gram-negative species and perhaps also in acid-fast organisms. For example, in *E. coli*, a lipoprotein is attached covalently to the ε-amino group of diaminopimelic acid (Figs. 6-3A and 6-4).

STRENGTH AND SHAPE.   The alternating L- and D-amino acid sequence of the peptidoglycan tetrapeptide adds structural strength (D-, L-heteropolymers are known to be stronger than L- or D-homopolymers) and allows amino acid R-groups to align on one side of the peptide chains: intrapeptidoglycan hydrogen bonding (as shown with models) can occur between juxtaposed chains aligned in this way. Further, the equatorial or planar β-1, 6 linkage and the pyranose ring forms of the MurNAc-GlcNAc components of the glycan chains in peptidoglycan conform to the most thermodynamically stable of polysaccharide structures. The same type structure is also found in chitin and cellulose.

Cell shape is not determined by peptidoglycan chemical structure, since rod-shaped and spherical *E. coli* yield chemically similar peptidoglycan. The three-dimensional or spatial organization of the peptidoglycan chains is unknown. X-ray crystallography indicates an amorphous (ie, noncrystalline) arrangement of peptidoglycan. For *E. coli*, which contains approximately 10^6 repeating units, the amount of peptidoglycan allows only one to three layers of peptidoglycan. In a gram-positive cell, which may contain 20 times as much or more peptidoglycan, there could be as many as 40 layers.

Glycan Variations   These include (1) the occurrence of N-glycoyl-muramic acid in *Myco-*

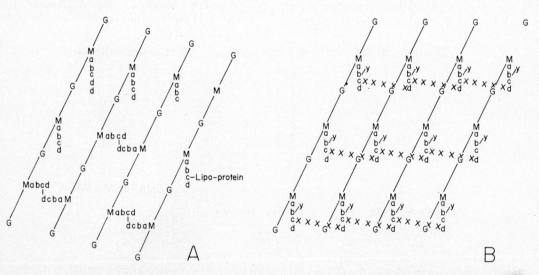

FIG. 6-3. A. Schematic generalization of *E. coli* peptidoglycan structure. B. Schematic generalization of *Staphylococcus aureus* H peptidoglycan structure. M (N-acetylmuramic acid), G (N-acetylglucosamine), a (L-alanine), b (D-glutamic acid), c (either meso-diaminopimelic acid (in A) or L-lysine (in B), d (D-alanine), X (pentaglycine bridge), y (−NH₂).

TABLE 6-2 VARIATIONS IN PEPTIDOGLYCAN STRUCTURE

Organism	Peptide Components	Bridge Units	Bridge Linked to	Structure Type*
Escherichia coli	—L-Ala-D-Glu-mesoDAP-D-Ala—	None	—mesoDAP—	A
Bacillus megaterium	—L-Ala-D-Glu-D-mesoDAP-D-Ala—	None	—mesoDAP—	
Bacillus subtilis	—L-Ala-D-Glu-mesoDAP · NH$_2$-D-Ala—	None	—mesoDAP—	
Corynebacterium diphtheriae	—L-Ala-D-isoGlu · NH$_2$-mesoDAP · NH$_2$-D-Ala—	None	—mesoDAP—	
Mycobacterium tuberculosis	—L-Ala-D-isoGlu · NH$_2$-mesoDAP · NH$_2$-D-Ala—	None, and mesoDAP(2:1)	—mesoDAP—	A,B
Streptococcus pyogenes (beta hemolytic group)	—L-Ala-D-isoGlu · NH$_2$-L-Lys-D-Ala—	—(L-Ala)$_2$—	—L-Lys—	B
Streptococcus (viridans group)	—L-Ala-D-isoGlo · NH$_2$-L-Lys-D-Ala—	—(L-Ala)$_3$—	—L-Lys—	
Streptococcus faecalis (enterococci)	—L-Ala-D-isoGlu · NH$_2$-L-Lys-D-Ala—	—(L-Ala)$_3$—	—L-Lys—	
Streptococcus cremoris (lactic group)	—L-Ala-D-isoGlu · NH$_2$-L-Lys-D-Ala—	—(L-Ala-L-Thr)—	—L-Lys—	
Lactobacillus casei	—L-Ala-D-isoGlu · NH$_2$-L-Lys-D-Ala—	—(isoAsp · NH$_2$)—	—L-Lys—	
Lactobacillus acidophilus	—L-Ala-D-isoGlu · NH$_2$-L-Lys-D-Ala—	—(isoAsp · NH$_2$)—	—L-Lys—	
Staphylococcus aureus H	—L-Ala-D-isoGlu · NH$_2$-L-Lys · D-Ala—	—(Gly)$_5$—	—L-Lys—	
Staphylococcus epidermidis	—L-Ala-D-isoGlu · NH$_2$-L-Lys-D-Ala—	—(Gly$_m$-Ser)$_n$—	—L-Lys—	
Micrococcus (lysodeikticus) *luteus*	—L-Ala-(D-Glu—Gly)-L-Lys-D-Ala—	—(L-Ala-D-Glu-L-Lys-D-Ala)—	—L-Lys—	B
Butyribacterium rettgeri	—L-Ser-(D-Glu—D-Lys)-L-Orn-D-Ala—	—(D-Orn and L-Lys)—	—D-isoGlu—	C

Adapted from Ghuysen: *Bacteriol Rev* 32:425, 1968; Wietzerbin et al: *Biochemistry* 13:3471, 1974

Abbreviations: Ala, alanine; DAP, diaminopimelic acid; DAP · NH$_2$, diaminopimelic acid-ϵ-amide; Glu, glutamic acid; iso Glu · NH$_2$, glutamic acid-α-amide; Lys, lysine; Thr, threonine; isoAsp · NH$_2$, aspartic acid-α-amide; Gly, glycine; Ser, serine; Orn, ornithine.
*Structure Type: refer to Figure 6-2

TABLE 6-3   Amino Acids Found in Peptidoglycans

Position	Amino Acids Identified
a	L-**Ala**, Gly, L-Ser
b	D-**iso-Glu**, 3-Hyg
c	L-**Lys, meso-DAP,** DD-DAP, L-DAB, L-Hse, DD-DAP, L-Ala, L-Glu, L-Orn, *meso*-HyDAP, L-Hyl, Nγ-acetyl-L-DAB
d	D-**Ala**
x	**Gly, L-Ala, L-Thr, L-Ser, D-Asp,** D-Ser, D-Glu, D-Gly(NH$_2$), D-Asp(NH$_2$, L-Lys, *meso*-DAP
y	Gly, Gly(NH$_2$), D-Ala(NH$_2$)
z	D-Lys, L-Lys, D-Orn, Gly, D-DAB

Modified from Schleifer and Kandler: Bacteriol Rev 36:407, 1972; Wietzerbin et al: Biochemistry 13:3471, 1974

Positions shown are as indicated in Figure 6-2. Amino acids shown in heavy type have been found frequently in many different bacteria. The muramic acid-linked tetrapeptide residues are shown as a, b, c, d, bridge peptide units as x and z, and y is the second peptide (glutamic acid) residue α-carboxyl substituent. The cross-linking bridge unit in a given organism usually consists of one or two amino acids: for example, the amino acids D-Asp, D-Asp-(NH$_2$), D-Glu-(NH$_2$), and meso-DAP occur as single residue bridges, whereas in the case of some micrococci such as M. luteus, the cross-link bridge unit consists of a tetrapeptide unit (see Table 6-2). Symbols used are as follows: 3-Hyg, threo-3-hydroxyglutamic acid; DAP, diaminopimelic acid; DAB, 2,4-diaminobutyric acid; HyDAP, meso-2,6-diamino-3-hydroxy-β-pimelic acid; L-Hse, homo-serine; L-Hgl, hydroxylysine.

bacterium and *Nocardia kirovani*, (2) the partial substitution of muramic acid lactam in spore peptidoglycan, (3) the occurrence of small amounts of the D-mannosamine muramic acid derivative (2 percent of total muramic acid) in *M. luteus*, (4) the occurrence of free amino groups on the glucosamine and muramic acid groups of peptidoglycans, and (5) the occurrence of 0-acetyl groups on muramic acid. In addition, phosphodiester groups, which often are substituted on the C-6 hydroxyl groups of muramic acid, may serve as links to such polymers as teichoic acid, teichuronic acids, and other polysaccharides, whereas glycosyl substituents attached at the C-6 hydroxyl

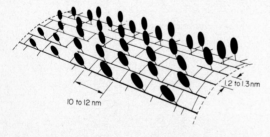

FIG. 6-4. Postulated structure of the lipoprotein-peptidoglycan structure of gram-negative bacteria. The longitudinal lines represent glycan chains cross-linked by peptide units spaced 1.2 to 1.3 nm apart. The actual orientation of peptidoglycan chains in the cell is unknown, and the glycan chains could be oriented in any direction. (After Braun: J Infect Dis 128 [Suppl]:1S, 1973)

of muramic acid may serve as links for neutral polymers. One example of the latter is the rhamnosyl-muramic acid linked C-polysaccharides of the streptococci.

Cell Wall Lytic Enzymes   Because of their D-amino acid content and lack of aromatic amino acids, peptidoglycans are not susceptible to L-proteases, such as trypsin and chymotrypsin, which often are used to remove nonpeptidoglycan proteins from cell wall preparations. However, bacteriolytic enzymes which act on peptidoglycans occur widely and have been very useful in elucidating peptidoglycan structures. These enzymes fall into three major groups: (1) endo-β-1,4-N-acetylhexosaminidases which cleave the glycan strands either between N-acetylmuramic acid and N-acetylglucosamine (for example, the muramidases or lysozymes of egg white, tears, and white blood cells) or between the alternative acetylglucosamine-muramic acid glycoside linkages (for example, the β-N-acetylhexosaminidases), (2) endopeptidases, many of which attack D-alanine at bridge peptide cross-linkages, whereas others may specifically hydrolyze the interpeptide bridge linkages, as in the case of lysostaphin, which splits glycylglycine bonds in the pentaglycine bridge of *S. aureus* (Fig. 6-3B), and (3) amidases which cleave the glycan-peptide junction between N-acetylmuramic acid and L-alanine, thereby separating the glycan strands from the interlocking peptides.

Many of the lytic enzymes described above are found as bacterial autolysins. One of the most notable autolysins is the N-acetylmuramyl-L-alanine amidase found in *Streptococcus (Diplococcus) pneumoniae* which is activated by low pH or bile salts.

LYSOZYME RESISTANCE. Lysozyme is apparently a very important first line of host resistance to bacterial infection (6 to 15 μg/ml human serum). Susceptibility to lysozyme varies from one bacterium to another, but gram-positive organisms are generally more sensitive than gram-negative cells, due to the outer membrane barrier of the latter. In either case, organisms usually are more sensitive in log phase of growth (minimal peptidoglycan) than at the stationary phase of growth (eg, continuance of peptidoglycan synthesis, after protein synthesis stops, yields thicker cell walls). Also, lysozyme resistance of some organisms can be attributed to modification of peptidoglycan structure through O-acetylation of N-acetylmuramic acid residues (eg, *S. aureus*), or by removal of N-acetyl groups from N-acetylglucosamine, which leaves lysozyme-resistant free amino groups on the peptidoglycan chain glucosamine residues (eg, *Bacillus* species).

NONPEPTIDOGLYCAN COMPONENTS

Envelope Proteins

Both gram-positive and gram-negative cells produce envelope proteins which may influence host-parasite interaction. These proteins include the cell wall-bound virulence factor, or M proteins, of the group A streptococci, the *S. aureus* A protein (SpA), which reacts with the Fc fragment of IgG (Chaps. 2 and 6), and the lipoprotein of *E. coli*.

Envelope Polysaccharides

Capsular Polysaccharides A variety of chemically diverse capsule and surface polymers are produced by both gram-positive and gram-negative bacteria. Among the best known capsular polymers are the soluble specific substances (SSS) or acidic polysaccharides produced by the pneumonia-causing organisms, *S. (D.) pneumoniae* and *Klebsiella pneumoniae*

(Friedländer's bacillus), and hyaluronic acid, which is produced by group A *Streptococcus pyogenes*. These polymers are composed of repeating oligosaccharide units of two to four monsaccharides, one of which is usually a uronic acid. The *Klebsiella* polymers often contain acetic and pyruvic acids and sometimes the methyl ethers of hexoses. Examples of medically interesting types of capsules are listed in Table 6-4.

Although capsular polysaccharides may be washed off bacterial cells, small amounts often remain cell bound and are detectable by sensitive serologic procedures. In the case of the pneumococci, many of the capsular polysaccharides have the chemical structure of teichoic acidlike polymers which are thought to be cell wall bound. However, because of the ease with which the pneumococci autolyze, it is difficult to know whether the easily removed capsular materials are in fact excreted as extracellular polysaccharides, as opposed to cell wall-bound, autolytically released teichoic acids, or whether they may be lipoteichoic acids pulled from the cell by the long water-soluble polymer chains after or before loss of a lipophilic cytoplasmic membrane anchor. In the case of gram-negative cells, covalent linkage of polysaccharides to peptidoglycan is unknown. However, capsularlike acid polymer chains linked to outer membrane lipopolysaccharides are found in various gram-negative bacteria.

Capsular polysaccharides have in some cases been shown to be bacteriophage (ie, bacterial viruses) receptors. These bacteriophages produce specific depolymerases, which apparently serve to dissolve the capsule at the site of attachment in order to allow the virus access to the cell below the capsule.

The Integument of Gram-positive Bacteria Cell wall polysaccharides of gram-positive bacteria contribute 10 to 50 percent of the mass of the cell wall, and, in many instances, these polymers appear to be covalently linked to peptidoglycan. Cell surface polysaccharides produced include lipoteichoic, teichoic, teichoic-like and teichuronic acids on the one hand, and nonteichoic-acidic and neutral polysaccharides on the other.

TEICHOIC ACIDS. Teichoic acids (wall, from the Greek *teichos*) are polymers of phosphodiester-linked polyols (Fig. 6-5), which in several cases have been shown to be linked to the cell wall through muramic acid-6-phosphate. Up to 50 percent of the peptidoglycan

TABLE 6-4 VARIOUS KINDS OF BACTERIAL SURFACE POLYMERS

Bacterium	Surface Polymer	Components
1. *Bacillus anthracis*	Polypeptide capsule	$[-\alpha\text{-}D\text{-}(-)\text{-glutamic acid}]_n$
	Teichoic acid	Polyolphosphate, glucose
2. *Yersinia (Pasteurella) pestis*	Protein	Protein
3. *Streptococcus pyogenes*	Hyaluronic acid capsule	$[-\text{N-Acetyl-}D\text{-glucosamine-}\beta\text{-}$ $1,4D\text{-glucuronic acid-}\beta\text{-}1,3\text{-}]\ 1_n$
	M (virulence) antigens	Proteins
	Group A polysaccharide	Polyrhamnan, N-acetyl-D-glucosamine
4. *Staphylococcus aureus*		
Smith strain	Polysaccharide	$[2\text{-N-}(\text{-N-acetyl-alanyl)-}D\text{-}$ glucosamine uronic acid$]_n$
Copenhagen strain H	Teichoic acid	Ribitol-1,5-phosphodiester, N-acetylglucosamine, D-alanine
	Protein A	Protein
5. *Staphylococcus epidermidis*	Teichoic acid	Glycerol-1,3-phosphodiester, D-glucose
6. *Streptococcus (Diplococcus) pneumoniae*	Type II	D-Glucose, L-rhamnose, D-glucuronic acid
	Type III	D-Glucose, D-glucuronic acid
	Type V	D-Glucose, D-glucuronic acid, N-acetyl-L-pneumosamine (2-acetamido-2,6-dideoxy-L-talose), N-acetyl-L-fucosamine (2-acetamido-2,6-dideoxy-L-galactose)
	Type VI (teichoic acid)	[Galactose, glucose, L-rhamnose, ribitol-PO$_4$]$_n$
	Type XVIII (teichoic acid)	[D-Glucose, D-galactose, L-rhamnose, glycerol-PO$_4$, O-acetyl]$_n$
7. *Escherichia coli*	Vi antigen capsule	[N-Acetyl-D-galactosamine uronic acid]$_n$
	Colominic acid	[N-Acetylneuraminic acid]$_n$
	Polysaccharides	Acidic polymers of various uronic acids, hexoses, and amino sugars
	K 88 (protein)	Protein
	Mucus antigen (colanic acid)	Glucuronic acid, galactose, fucose
8. *Haemophilus influenzae*	Type a capsules	Glucose, phosphate
	b	Polyribose-ribitol phosphate
	c	Hexose, phosphate
	d	N-Acetyl-D-glucosamine uronic acid
	e	Hexose, N-acetyl-D-glucosamine
	f	Galactosamine, phosphate
9. *Klebsiella pneumoniae*	Type 1 capsule	D-Glucose, fucose, glucuronic acid, pyruvic acid
10. *Neisseria meningitidis*	Capsular polysaccharides	
	Serogroup A	[N-Acetyl-,O-acetyl-mannosamine]$_n$ phosphate
	Serogroup B	[N-Acetylneuraminic acid]$_n$
	Serogroup C	[N-Acetyl, O-acetylneuraminic acid]$_n$
11. *Pseudomonas aeruginosa*	Capsules	Alginic acidlike polymer (mannuronic and guluronic acids) DNA, various other polysaccharides

may be combined with teichoic acids in the bacilli and staphylococci. Cell wall teichoic acids usually contain ribitol, or occasionally glycerol, and appear to be covalently linked to peptidoglycan through substituted phosphodiester groups on the C-6-hydroxyl of N-acetylmuramic acid residues. Membrane or lipoteichoic acids (LTA) which are not cell wall-bound are glycerophosphate polymers which terminate in glycolipid (Fig. 6-6). Lipoteichoic acid, which remains membrane associated in protoplasts, appears to be anchored in the cytoplasmic membrane.

Teichoic acids are specifically modified in different bacteria by addition to the polyol units of ester-linked D-alanine, D-lysine, or O-

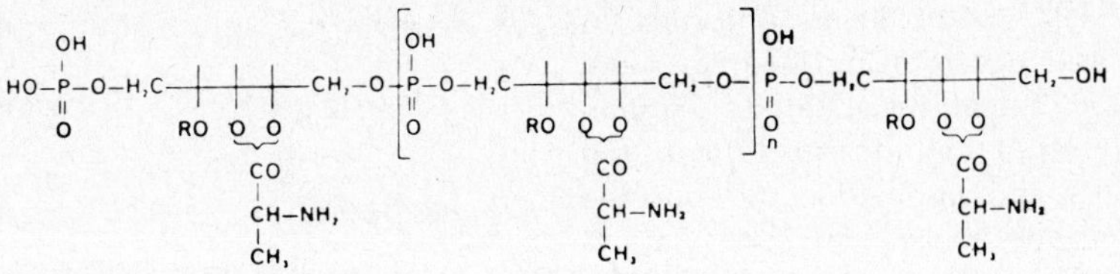

FIG. 6-5. Ribitol teichoic acids. *Bacillus subtilis:* R = β-glucosyl; n = 7; *Staphylococcus aureus* H: R = α- and β = N-acetylglucosaminyl; n = 6; *Lactobacillus; is arabinosus* 17-5: R = α'glucosyl; alternate ribitol residues also have α-glucosyl at the 3-position; n = .4-5. (From Baddiley: Endeavour 23:33, 1964)

glycoside-linked glucose, galactose, or N-acetylhexosamines. The substituted teichoic acids are important as specific cell surface antigens of *Staphylococcus, Streptococcus, Lactobacillus,* and *Bacillus* species. For example, almost all (96 percent human strains of *S. aureus* produce glucosamine-substituted ribitol cell wall teichoic acids, whereas *Staphylococcus epidermidis* appears to produce glucose-substituted glycerol teichoic acids.

Many teichoic acidlike polymers also occur in a variety of bacteria. These polymers are composed of phosphodiester-linked sugar repeating units, repeating units built of oligosaccharide-phosphate only, or oligosaccharides linked to a polyolphosphate. A notable example is the teichoic acidlike C polysaccharide of *S. (D.) pneumoniae,* which contains choline. This polymer is composed of phosphate, N-acetyl-D-galactosamine, D-glucose, N-acetyl-2, 4-diamino-2, 4, 6-trideoxyhexose, ribitol, and choline, and functions in cell wall division. If cells are grown on ethanolamine instead of choline, the C polysaccharide contains ethanolamine, and the cells do not divide.

TEICHURONIC ACID. This polymer is produced by various *Bacillus* species and is composed of N-acetylgalactosamine (GalNAc) and glucuronic acid (GlcUA), linked as the disaccharide repeating unit (GlcUA $\xrightarrow{1,3}$ GalNAc)$_n$, but contains no phosphate. Teichuronic acid may be found in the same cell together with teichoic acid. Teichuronic acid is apparently also covalently linked to cell wall and is synthesized in large amounts by cells deprived of phosphate and which cannot therefore make teichoic acids.

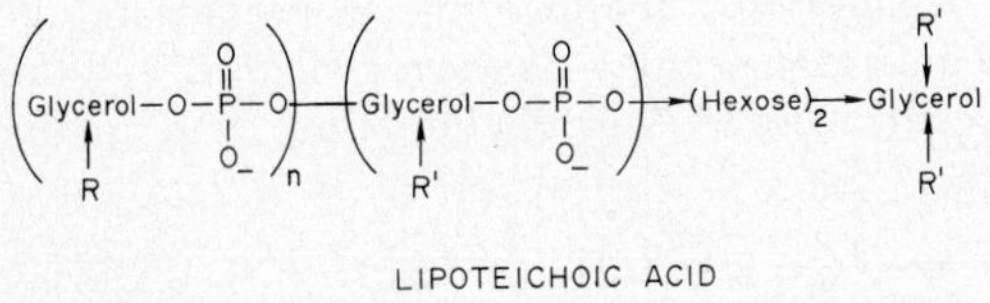

ACIDIC AND NEUTRAL CELL WALL POLYSACCHARIDES. Acidic or neutral polysaccharides which do not contain phosphate are also found in the cell walls of many bacteria. The significance of small amounts of cell wall-bound hexose polymers in various organisms is as yet unknown. One example of an acidic polysaccharide is the antitumorigenic polysaccharide of *Propionibacterium (Corynebacterium parvum) acnes.* Another example is a characteristic highly branched, group-specific, and cell wall-bound L-rhamnose polymer which occurs in the group B and group G streptococci and which is substituted with N-acetyl-D-glucosamine in group A streptococci and with N-acetyl-D-galactosamine in group C organisms. Rhamnose-containing polymers also are found in cell walls of some corynebacteria (primarily plant and animal pathogens).

The Integument of Acid-fast and Related Bacteria Members of the genus *Mycobacterium* and some *Nocardia* species, which characteristically stain red with carbolfuchsin and resist decolorization with acid-alcohol, are said to be "acid-fast." This staining property appears to correlate with the presence of cell wall-bound mycolic acids in the intact bacterium. Mycolic acids occur principally as esters bound to cell wall polysaccharides and as components of extractable (ie, free) glycolipids known as

LIPOTEICHOIC ACID

FIG 6-6. Postulated structure of lipoteichoic (membrane teichoic) acid includes possibility of fatty acid (R') substituted glycerophosphate interposed between glycerol teichoic acid chain and glycolipid. R-H or glycosyl; R'-H, or esterified fatty acid residue; hexose disaccharide may be either α-1,2 or β-1,6 glucosylglucose, or α-1,2 galactosylglucose; n > 28. (After Knox, Wicken: Bacteriol Rev 37:215, 1973)

"cord factors." The latter occur uniformly in mycobacteria and nocardia and also in some members of the non-acid-fast genus *Coryne-bacterium* (the latter include the human and animal parasites and pathogens but not the plant-associated corynebacteria). The corynebacteria, nocardia, and mycobacteria (ie, the CNM group of bacteria) also share a similar cell wall peptidoglycan structure and cross-linkage pattern, in addition to sharing a common antigen which is probably peptidoglycan-bound arabinogalactan. Arabinomannans and galactosamine-containing polymers also occur, but the relationship of these to the arabinogalactans is obscure. Only the nocardia and mycobacteria produce cell wall-bound mycolic acids. The CNM group of organisms is considered to be gram-positive but is not reported to produce teichoic acid.

MYCOLIC ACIDS.   The general structure of mycolic acids as α-substituted, β-hydroxy fatty acids is shown in Figure 6-7. The biosynthesis of the complex, branched-chain fatty acids is thought to proceed by condensation of the carboxyl groups of one long-chain fatty acid to the α-position of another:

$$(1) \qquad R'—COOH + \underset{\underset{R}{|}}{CH_2}—COOH \rightarrow$$

$$R'—\underset{\underset{OH}{|}}{CH}—\underset{\underset{R}{|}}{CH}—COOH$$

The corynebacteria, nocardia, and mycobacteria each produce characteristic types of mycolic acids, which are presumably synthesized by similar mechanisms from similar precursors. As might be expected, the chain lengths and complexity of mycolic acids increase from the corynemycolic acid (about $C_{32\text{-}36}$) through the nocardic acids (about C_{50}) and mycolic acids (up to C_{90}) (Figs. 6-8 – 6-10). The synthesis of mycolic acid in *Mycobacterium tuberculosis* is re-

A $C_{32}H_{62}O_3$

$$CH_3(CH_2)_5 CH{=}CH—(CH_2)_7\underset{\underset{C_{14}H_{29}}{\overset{\overset{OH}{|}}{\underset{|}{C}}}}{\underset{H}{C}}—CH—COOH$$

B $C_{32}H_{64}O_3$

$$CH_3(CH_2)_{14}\underset{\underset{H}{\overset{\overset{OH}{|}}{\underset{|}{C}}}}{C}—\underset{\underset{C_{14}H_{29}}{|}}{CH}—COOH$$

C $C_{36}H_{68}O_3$

$$CH_3(CH_2)_7 CH{=}CH(CH_2)_7\underset{\underset{H}{\overset{\overset{OH}{|}}{\underset{|}{C}}}}{C}—\underset{\underset{\underset{\underset{HC(CH_2)_7CH_3}{\|}}{HC}}{\overset{}{(CH_2)_6}}}{CH}COOH$$

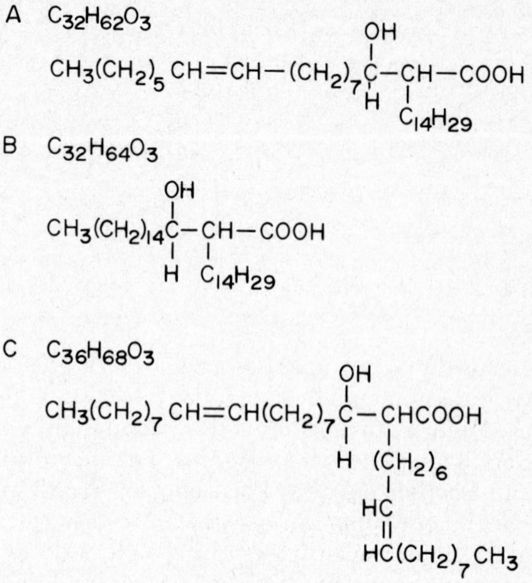

FIG. 6-8. Corynemycolic acids. A. Corynemycolenic acid. B. Corynemycolic acid. C. Corynemycoladienoic acid. (After Lederer: Pure Appl Chem 25:135, 1971)

ported to be inhibited by isoniazid (Chap. 10) by an unknown mechanism.

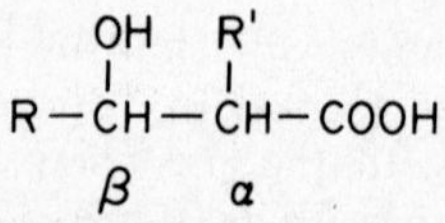

PEPTIDOGLYCAN.   The cell wall of *M. tuberculosis* contains approximately equal amounts of peptidoglycan, arabinogalactan, and lipid. Greater than 50 percent of the lipid components are esterified mycolic acids, whereas some 25 percent appear to be normal fatty acids. The presence of nonpeptidoglycan amino acids has led to the postulation of possible cell wall-bound lipoproteins similar to those found in gram-negative bacteria, but this possibility has not been documented. The common peptidoglycan structure of *C. diphtheriae*, *Nocardia*, and *M. tuberculosis* was presented in Figure 6-2A and Table 6-2. Notable features are the presence of an alternative *meso*-diaminopimelic acid-peptide bridge which may occur in the mycobacteria, and the occurrence of N-glycoylmuramic acid in the

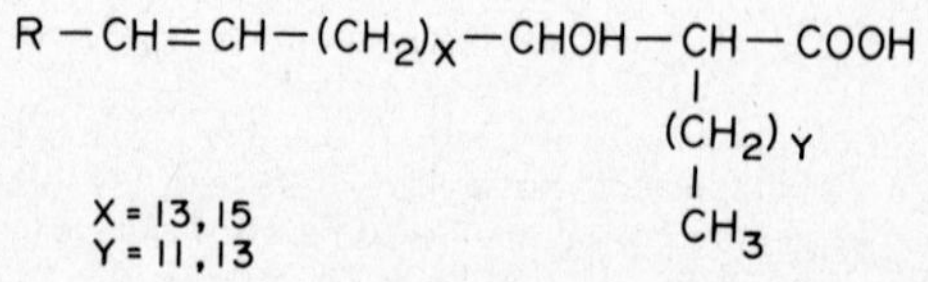

$$R—\underset{\underset{\underset{\underset{CH_3}{|}}{(CH_2)_Y}}{|}}{CH}{=}CH—(CH_2)_x—CHOH—CH—COOH$$

$$X = 13,15$$
$$Y = 11,13$$

$$\underset{\beta \qquad \alpha}{R—\underset{\underset{}{|}}{\overset{\overset{OH}{|}}{CH}}—\underset{\underset{}{|}}{\overset{\overset{R'}{|}}{CH}}—COOH}$$

FIG. 6-7. Mycolic acids, showing general structure as α-substituted, β-hydroxy fatty acids.

FIG. 6-9. Nocardic acids.

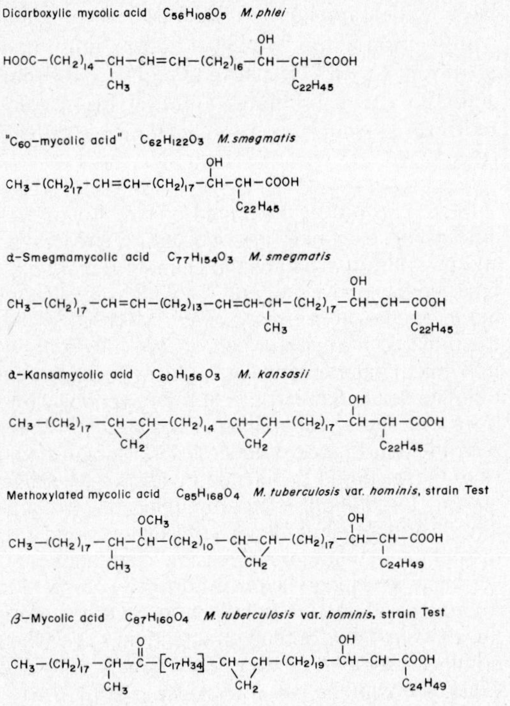

Dicarboxylic mycolic acid $C_{56}H_{108}O_5$ *M. phlei*

$$HOOC-(CH_2)_{14}-CH-CH=CH-(CH_2)_{16}-\underset{\overset{|}{OH}}{CH}-CH-COOH$$
$$\quad\quad\quad\quad\quad\underset{CH_3}{|}\quad\quad\quad\quad\quad\quad\underset{C_{22}H_{45}}{|}$$

"C_{60}-mycolic acid" $C_{62}H_{122}O_3$ *M. smegmatis*

$$CH_3-(CH_2)_{17}-CH=CH-(CH_2)_{17}-\underset{\overset{|}{OH}}{CH}-CH-COOH$$
$$\quad\quad\quad\quad\quad\quad\quad\quad\quad\quad\quad\quad\underset{C_{22}H_{45}}{|}$$

α-Smegmamycolic acid $C_{77}H_{154}O_3$ *M. smegmatis*

$$CH_3-(CH_2)_{17}-CH=CH-(CH_2)_{13}-CH=CH-CH-\underset{\overset{|}{OH}}{(CH_2)_{17}}-CH-CH-COOH$$
$$\quad\quad\quad\quad\quad\quad\quad\quad\quad\quad\quad\quad\underset{CH_3}{|}\quad\quad\quad\quad\quad\underset{C_{22}H_{45}}{|}$$

α-Kansamycolic acid $C_{80}H_{156}O_3$ *M. kansasii*

$$CH_3-(CH_2)_{17}-\underset{\overset{|}{CH_2}}{CH}-CH-(CH_2)_{14}-\underset{\overset{|}{CH_2}}{CH}-CH-(CH_2)_{17}-\underset{\overset{|}{OH}}{CH}-CH-COOH$$
$$\quad\quad\quad\quad\quad\quad\quad\quad\quad\quad\quad\quad\quad\quad\quad\quad\quad\quad\quad\underset{C_{22}H_{45}}{|}$$

Methoxylated mycolic acid $C_{85}H_{168}O_4$ *M. tuberculosis* var. *hominis*, strain Test

$$CH_3-(CH_2)_{17}-\underset{\overset{|}{CH_3}}{\underset{|}{CH}-\overset{OCH_3}{CH}}-(CH_2)_{10}-\underset{\overset{|}{CH_2}}{CH}-CH-(CH_2)_{17}-\underset{\overset{|}{OH}}{CH}-CH-COOH$$
$$\quad\quad\quad\quad\quad\quad\quad\quad\quad\quad\quad\quad\quad\quad\quad\quad\quad\quad\quad\underset{C_{24}H_{49}}{|}$$

β-Mycolic acid $C_{87}H_{160}O_4$ *M. tuberculosis* var. *hominis*, strain Test

$$CH_3-(CH_2)_{17}-\underset{\overset{|}{CH_3}}{\underset{|}{CH}-\overset{O}{\overset{||}{C}}}-[C_{17}H_{34}]-CH-CH-(CH_2)_{19}-\underset{\overset{|}{OH}}{CH}-CH-COOH$$
$$\quad\quad\quad\quad\quad\quad\quad\quad\quad\quad\quad\quad\underset{CH_2}{|}\quad\quad\quad\quad\quad\quad\underset{C_{24}H_{49}}{|}$$

FIG. 6-10. Mycolic acids. (After Lederer: Pure Appl Chem 25:135, 1971)

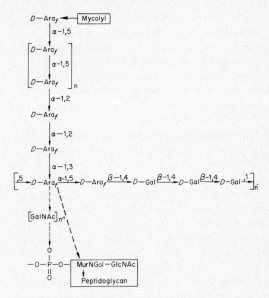

FIG. 6-11. Postulated mycolyl-arabinogalactan-peptidoglycan structure of mycobacterial cell wall equivalent to a monomer of Wax-D. Linkages shown between mycolic acid and arabinogalactan and arabinogalactan components are known. Both phosphodiester and glycoside linkages between arabinogalactan and peptidoglycan have been postulated, and postulated inclusion of galactosamine as part of Wax-D structure is tentative. Note substitution of muramic acid with N-glycoyl (ie, N-Gol) groups. See Table 6-2 for peptidoglycan structure. (After Asselineau, Lederer: In Bloch (ed): Lipid Metabolism, 1960 Courtesy of John Wiley; Lederer: Pure Appl Chem 25:135, 1971; Goren: Bacteriol Rev 36:33, 1972, Misaki; Seto, Azume: J Biochem 76:15, 1974)

peptidoglycans of the mycobacteria and at least some nocardia but not in the corynebacteria, and the occurrence of muramic acid phosphate. The latter is thought to serve as a linkage between cell wall-bound arabinogalactans and peptidoglycan, although glycosidic linkage of arabinogalactan may occur, possibly through N-acetylgalactosamine. The exact structure and linkages between mycolyl-arabinogalactan, N-acetylgalactosamine, and peptidoglycan are unknown. A possible structure for cell wall-linked mycolyl-polysaccharide-peptidoglycan is shown in Figure 6-11. As indicated in Figure 6-11, mycolic acids are bound to cell wall uniformly through the C-5-hydroxyl of D-arabinose residues of the arabinogalactan. In the mycobacteria, cell wall esterified mycolic acids vary between 76 to 90 carbons, whereas in nocardia, esters of C_{56} to C_{60} nocardic acids are found.

WAX-D AND IMMUNOADJUVANT ACTIVITY. Fractionation of chloroform-soluble extracts of mycobacteria and nocardia yield ether-soluble and acetone-insoluble fractions called "Wax-

D." These fractions, with molecular weights up to 30,000, are split by saponification into equal amounts of mycolic acid and water-soluble peptidoglycan-arabinogalactan. Similar material can be prepared from isolated defatted cell walls by treatment with lysozyme and other lytic enzymes. Wax-D therefore equates to the general structure shown in Figure 6-11. This structure, ie, the cell wall skeleton of BCG (Bacillus of Calmette-Guérin, an attenuated *M. tuberculosis* strain used for human immunization against tuberculosis), has been found to exhibit antitumor activity in mice.

Originally, interest in Wax-D developed because this fraction retained much of the immunoadjuvant activity of the whole mycobacterial cell (Chap. 13). Although at first it was thought that mycolic acids were the components necessary for adjuvant activity, it gradually became obvious that only the Wax-D fractions which contained peptidoglycan were active. Reasonably homogeneous, mycolic acid-free, water-soluble arabinogalactan-peptidoglycans of 20,000 MW have now been obtained which retain full immunoadjuvant activity, indicating that mycolic acid is unnecessary. In addition, water-soluble peptidoglycan subunits of a variety of bacteria have been found to have immunoadjuvant activity, the minimal structure being N-acetylmuramyl-L-alanyl-D−*iso*-glutamine.

GLYCOLIPIDS.   Several unusual glycolipids occur in the acid-fast and related bacteria which are not cell wall bound. These include cord factors, sulfolipids, mycosides, and lipopolysaccharides.

TREHALOSE MYCOLATES.   Toxic petroleum ether-soluble glycolipids were first discovered in virulent *M. tuberculosis* which grew in culture as serpentine cords. Cord factors have been shown to be 6, 6'-dimycolyl esters of the α, α'-1, 1'-linked glucose disaccharide, trehalose (Fig. 6-12A). These glycolipids are found throughout the corynebacteria, nocardia, and mycobacteria. *C. diphtheriae* produces trehalose esterified with the C_{32} acids, corynemycolic acid, and corynemycolenic acid, whereas the *Corynebacterium hofmani* analog contains the C_{36} corynemycoladienoic acid (Fig. 6-8). In some *Nocardia* species, only nocardic acids are found, but in *N. asteroides*, cord factors contain a mixture of C_{28} to C_{36} corynemycolic acids, whereas the cell wall is esterified with C_{50} to C_{56} nocardic acids. The cord factor of *M. tuberculosis* contains a series of myco-

lates, which appears to reflect the mycolic acid composition of the whole bacterium, ranging in size from C_{78} to C_{90}. These mycolic acids characteristically contain one methyl group, one methoxyl group, and a cyclopropane ring (Fig. 6-10).

Interest in cord factors centers on their toxic properties. For example, mycobacteria increase the susceptibility of experimental animals to gram-negative endotoxin, a property for which cord factor alone appears to be responsible. More generally, the multiple injection of cord factor, mixed in oil, into mice intraperitoneally, induces wasting and ultimate death. Similar injection intravenously into mice can cause granulomatous responses in lungs with the appearance of tubercles indistinguishable from those caused by infection with live *M. tuberculosis*. In addition, some immunity may be conferred. At the cellular level, cord factors appear to disrupt mitochondria, decreasing respiration and oxidative phosphorylation. And finally, a specific "cord factor" fraction isolated from *M. tuberculosis* (ie, BCG) exhibits antitumor activity in mice when administered in a mixture (cf, Freund's adjuvant, Chap. 13) with the cell wall skeleton of BCG.

Sulfolipids appear to be periphally located within the envelope and appear to be responsible for the neutral-red staining properties of cord-forming mycobacteria. Sulfolipids appear to be nontoxic but potentiate the toxicity of cord factor. The principal sulfatide of *M. tuberculosis* has been identifed as 2,3,6,6'-tetraacyltrehalose-2-sulfate (Fig. 6-12B).

MYCOSIDES.   These nonimmunogenic and apparently nontoxic compounds are presumed to be peripherally located, since the production

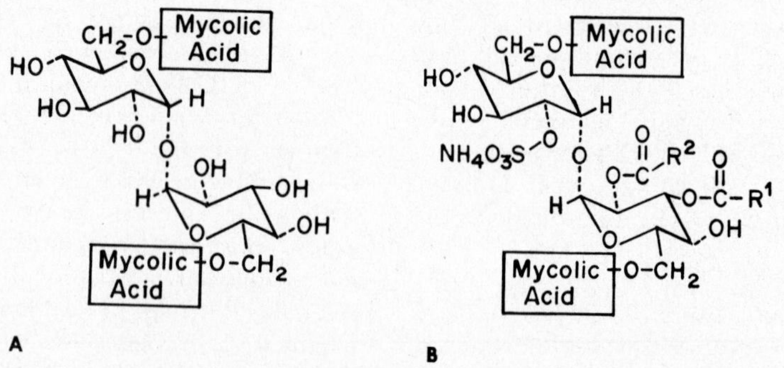

A   **B**

FIG. 6-12 A. Cord factors, 6, 6'-dimycolyl-trehalose. B. Sulfolipids, 2, 3, 6, 6'-tretracyl-trehalose-2-sulfate, where R groups are different fatty acids. (After Goren: Bacteriol Rev. 36:33, 1972)

of specific mycosides often correlates with type of colonial growth and sometimes corresponds to susceptibility to specific bacteriophages. Chemically, the mycosides are of interest because they contain 6-deoxytalose and o-methyl ether derivatives of deoxytalose, fucose, and rhamnose. The mycosides A and B are phenolic glycolipids (Fig. 6-13), whereas mycosides C are a group of peptidoglycolipids (Fig. 6-14). Whether the type C mycolipids relate to postulated cell wall-bound lipoproteins is unknown. Mycosides C appear in some instances to be strain-specific phage sites.

PHOSPHOLIPIDS AND LIPOPOLYSACCHARIDES. These components are probably membrane associated, although their exact location within the cell is unknown. Mycobacterial phospholipids include diphosphatidylglycerol (cardiolipin) and phosphatidylethanolamine, which are found in common with other bacteria. In addition, the mycobacteria produce phosphatidylinositol mono- and oligosaccharides, such as tetracylated phosphatidylinositol pentamannosides.

Lipoglycans or lipopolysaccharides have also been described in the mycobacteria. *M. tuberculosis* and *M. phlei* produce a branched-chain polymer composed of eleven 6-0-methyl-D-glucose and seven D-glucose residues in α-1,4 linkage. The reducing terminus is linked to acylated glycerol. The polymer occurs acylated with 0 to 3 succinyl ester groups, 3 acetyl, and 1 each propionate, isobutyrate, and octanoate. An unusual α-1,4 linked 3-0-methyl-D-mannose polymer has also been described which is reported to stimulate the fatty acid synthetase of *M. phlei*.

The Integument of Gram-negative Bacteria

THE OUTER MEMBRANE. Gram-negative bacteria produce a unique three-layered envelope. This structure consists of an outer membrane overlying a thin peptidoglycan or murein layer, which may be separated by a periplasmic

$$R'O-\bigcirc-(CH_2)_n-\underset{\underset{OR}{|}}{CH}-CH_2-\underset{\underset{OR}{|}}{CH}-(CH_2)_4-\underset{\underset{CH_3}{|}}{CH}-\underset{\underset{CH_3}{|}}{CH}-CH_2-CH_3$$

Mycoside A R' = trisaccharide
2-O-methylfucose; 2-O-methylrhamnose; 2,4-di-O-methylrhamnose
n = 16, 17, 18, 19, 20

Mycoside B R' = 2-O-methylrhamnose
n = 14, 15, 16, 17, 18

R = palmitic acid
mycocerosic acid $C_{22}H_{45}-\underset{\underset{CH_3}{|}}{CH}-CH_2-\underset{\underset{CH_3}{|}}{CH}-CH_2-\underset{\underset{CH_3}{|}}{CH}-COOH$

FIG. 6-13. Mycosides A and B. (After Goren: Bacteriol Rev 36:33, 1972)

FIG. 6-14. Mycoside C. Sugar 1, diacetyl-6-deoxytalose; sugar 2, mono-O-methyl to tri-O-methyl-rhamnose. (After Goren: Bacteriol Rev 36:33, 1972)

space from the inner cytoplasmic membrane (Fig. 6-15; see also Figs. 3-18, 3-20).

The outer membrane, which contains the characteristic lipopolysaccharide (LPS) of gram-negative bacteria, also serves as a barrier which confers resistance to many antimetabolites, chemicals, and detergents. This barrier may be related to LPS, since removal of some 30 to 50 percent of the total LPS by EDTA treatment or mutational alteration of LPS structure results in decreased resistance to antibiotics and detergents.

Outer Membrane Composition. Outer and inner membranes can be separated by density-gradient centrifugation. The outer membrane is composed of LPS, phospholipids, and protein, which together comprise about 80 percent of the envelope. The phospholipids of the outer membrane appear to be qualitatively similar to those of the cytoplasmic membrane, whereas the outer-membrane proteins appear to be very different from the proteins of the cytoplasmic membrane. Outer-membrane proteins include phospholipase activities, small amounts

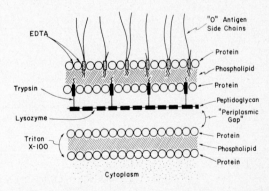

FIG. 6-15. Simplified diagram of the cell envelope of *E. coli.* Envelope components are listed on right and probable sites of attack of envelope disruption agents are indicated on the left. (From Schnaitman: J Bacteriol 108:553, 1971)

(approximately 10 percent) of at least two of the enzymes which serve in the synthesis of the LPS core structure, free murein-lipoprotein, and other proteins of unknown function.

OUTER MEMBRANE ATTACHMENT TO PEPTIDOG-LYCAN.   The mode of linkage between the outer membrane components and peptidoglycan is not completely known. Outer membrane is released from some cells during growth, indicating a transitional or loose linkage to the cell. Current evidence indicates that divalent metal ligands and lipophilic binding are involved in the attachment of the outer membrane to the murein (ie, peptidoglycan) layer. This view is based on the observations that EDTA treatment removes some 30 percent or more of the LPS from the cell wall, whereas detergents such as sodium dodecylsulfate (SDS) remove the entire outer membrane. The lipophilic attachment is thought to occur through interac-

tion of outer-membrane phospholipid, free lipoprotein, and the peptidoglycan-bound lipoprotein. There is also evidence for covalent linkage between LPS and lipoprotein.

LIPOPROTEIN AND PEPTIDOGLYCAN.   Lipoprotein contributes 40 percent or more of the mass of the isolated 4 percent SDS-insoluble cell wall sacculus of enterobacteria. It is probable that lipoprotein occurs in all gram-negative bacteria. The peptidoglycan structure of all gram-negative bacteria so far examined appears to be identical to the type A structure illustrated in Figure 6-2 and Table 6-2. The insoluble peptidoglycan, after trypsin digestion, which removes lipoprotein, seldom accounts for more than a small percentage of the cell dry weight. The lipoprotein is covalently linked to peptidoglycan through the trypsin-sensitive peptidoglycan sequence—Tyr-Arg-Lys—to *meso*-diaminopimelic acid (DAP) units

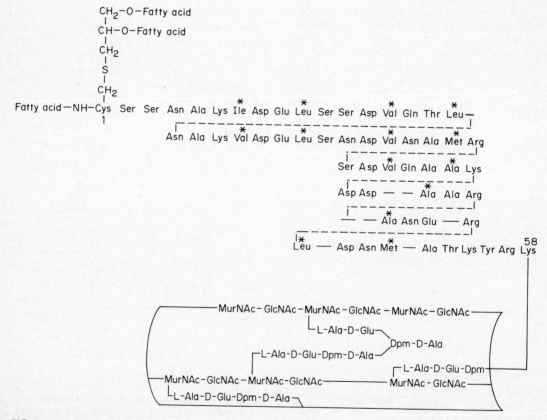

FIG. 6-16. Murein-lipoprotein structure. Sequence of amino acids is spaced to indicate possible evolution from a gene which originally coded for 15 amino acids and which was duplicated and then lengthened by addition of only the carboxy terminus four times. Presumed deletions of amino acids during evolution are indicated by dashes. (After Braun and Hantke: Annu Rev Biochem 43:89, 1974)

of the peptidoglycan (Fig. 6-16). The lipoprotein molecules appear by electron microscopy to be spaced every 10 to 12 nm on the outer surface of the peptidoglycan structure (Fig. 6-4). This corresponds to one lipoprotein for every 10 to 12 peptidoglycan disaccharide units 1.03 nm long, or some 10^5 bound lipoprotein molecules per cell.

A free form of the lipoprotein of molecular weight approximately 7,500 occurs in the outer membrane in twice the concentration of the bound form. The lipoprotein, which self-aggregates and is strongly lipophilic, appears to exist in 70 percent helix form. Because it binds avidly to lipid and protein, it is thought to aid in anchoring the outer membrane complex to the cell wall (Fig. 6-15). This view is supported by the fact that over 90 percent of the lipoprotein may be isolated with the outer membrane after lysozyme digestion of the peptidoglycan sacculus.

The lipoprotein contains no histidine, glycine, proline, phenylalanine, or tryptophan. The lipoprotein appears to be composed of repetitive sequences with nonpolar amino acids every 3.5 residues* (Fig. 6-16). The latter arrangement would allow the alignment of the nonpolar amino acid side-chain groups on one side of the helical structure. Such a structure could be of importance in binding with outer membrane phospholipid-free lipoprotein and lipopolysaccharide. The lipoprotein N-terminal amide fatty acids include palmitic acid (65 percent), palmitoleic acid (11 percent), and *cis*-vaccenic acid (11 percent). Ester-bound fatty acids include palmitic acid (45 percent), palmitoleic acid (11 percent), and *cis*-vaccenic acid (24 percent).

LIPOPOLYSACCHARIDE (LPS). Lipopolysaccharides are responsible for many of the biologic properties of gram-negative bacteria. Serologic specificity resides primarily in the variable polysaccharide portion of LPS, which corresponds to the somatic O antigen of gram-negative organisms. O antigens also act as specific receptor sites for certain bacteriophages. Heat-stable endotoxic properties (endotoxins, in contrast to extracellular or excreted protein exotoxins) of LPS are due to the glycolipid portion called "lipid A." Endotoxic properties include fever production (pyrogenicity), lethality, tissue necrosis activity, complement reactivity, B-cell mitogenicity, immunoadjuvant activity, and antitumor activity. It is not surprising, therefore, that endotoxins

have been subject to intensive investigation. However, the mechanisms of endotoxic action at the cellular and molecular levels remains unknown.

LIPOPOLYSACCHARIDE ISOLATION. The smooth (wild-type or complete) LPS may be extracted by a variety of procedures. Trichloroacetic acid, ethylene glycol, or cold aqueous phenol extraction yields a lipopolysaccharide-protein-phospholipid complex, whereas hot aqueous 45 percent phenol (68C) removes the protein, leaving the lipopolysaccharide complexed with phospholipid. This complex self-aggregates to form micelles of large molecular weight which can be separated from RNA and soluble polysaccharides by sedimentation. The phospholipid, sometimes referred to as phospholipid-B, can be removed by lipid solvent extraction procedures. A lipopolysaccharide-protein complex, reported to be covalently linked, can be prepared by 1 percent SDS extraction.

LPS which contains no side-chain and only minimal core units, ie, KDO-lipid A, can be obtained from cells by lipid solvent extraction procedures (chloroform-methanol, 4:1) and subsequent extraction with aqueous solvent systems (aqueous phenol).

LIPOLYSACCHARIDE STRUCTURE. The LPS is composed of three regions: Serologic specificity resides in region I, toxicity in region III.

O-specific Polysaccharide Region I	Core Polysaccharide Region II	Lipid A Region III

For serologic and biochemical studies, regions I and II can be separated from the water-insoluble region III by mild acid hydrolysis (pH 3). The complete structure of the lipopolysaccharide of *Salmonella typhimurium* is indicated in Figure 6-17.

O-Specific Polysaccharide (Region I). The O antigen polymer is composed of repeating oligosaccharide units of three to four monosaccharides. A variety of monosaccharides, including various pentoses, a 4-aminopentose, hexoses, 2-aminohexoses, 6-deoxy- and 3,6-dideoxyhexoses, 6-deoxyamino sugars with amino groups at the C-2, C-3, and C-4 position on the hexose carbon skeleton, and aminohexose uronic acids have been isolated from the region I polymers of various bacteria.

The LPS of *Salmonella, Escherichia, Shigella, Citrobacter,* and related genera often contain similar O antigen monosaccharides and can be grouped into a limited number of similar

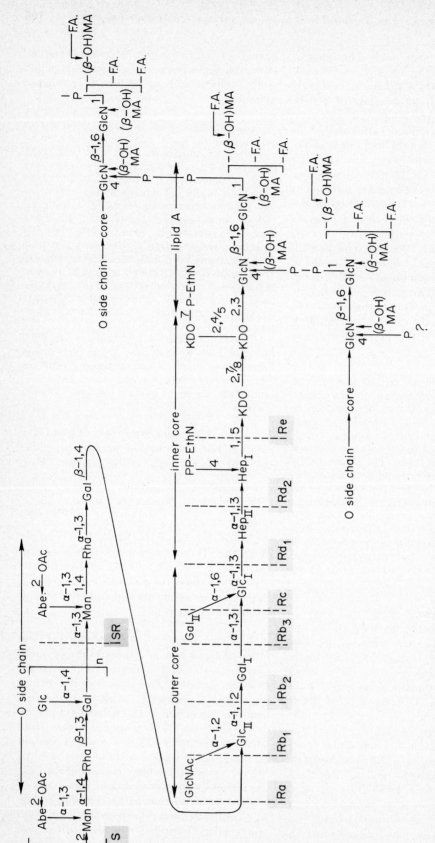

FIG. 6-17. Diagram of tentative lipopolysaccharide structure of *Salmonella typhimurium*. Note three regions indicated as O side-chain, core (outer and inner), and lipid A, the latter composed of phosphate-linked disaccharide units. Vertical dashed lines indicate limits of structures produced by mutants of S-form organisms (serologic smooth or wildtype), starting with SR (semirough) mutants, which produce LPS with only one repeating side-chain unit and continuing through R_a to R_e. Roman numerals indicate presumed order of addition of core sugars during biosynthesis, and glycosidic bonds are indicated where known. Abbreviations used: Abe, abequose (3,6-dideoxy-D-galactose); Ac, acetyl; EthN, ethanolamine; F.A., fatty acid; Gal, galactose; Glc, glucose; GlcN, glucosamine; Hep, L-glycero-D-mannoheptose; (β-OH)MA, β-hydroxymyristic acid; KDO, 2-keto-3-deoxymannooctulosonic acid; Man, mannose; Rha, rhamnose. (After Luderitz, Westphal, Staub, Nikaido: In Weinbaum, Ajl (eds): Microbial Toxins, 1971, vol 4. Courtesy of Academic Press; Rietschel, Gottert, Luderitz, Westphal: Eur J Biochem 28:166, 1972)

chemotypes on the basis of O antigen sugar composition. Sugar composition, sequence, linkage groups, and additional substituents (eg, acetyl group) determine the antigenic or serologic and bacteriophage specificity of the particular O antigen chain. Bacteriophage susceptibility and serologic specificity may not always coincide exactly with the chemical composition (Table 6-5). Bacteriophage attachment to these O antigens is determined by the specificity of phage depolymerases. Over a thousand different serologic combinations have been found in *Salmonella*.

Core Polysaccharide (Region II). This region is arbitrarily separated into inner and outer core areas. Inner core contains 2-keto-3-deoxyoctonic acid (KDO) and heptose, both of which are unique to bacteria, as well as phosphate and pyrophosphate-bound ethanolamine. The KDO is bound to the glucosamine of lipid A by an acid-labile (pH 3) ketoside linkage. The outer core is composed of the hexoses glu-

cose, galactose, and N-acetylglucosamine. All *Salmonella* are believed to share a common core polysaccharide which differs from that of *Shigella* or *Escherichia* species (Fig. 6-18). *Escherichia coli*, however, may produce three different core structures.

Lipid A (Region III). Lipid A is obtained from LPS by mild acid hydrolysis which cleaves the ketosidic KDO-lipid A linkage. Because of its high fatty acid content, lipid A behaves as a difficultly water-soluble phosphoglycolipid, which is separable from the water-soluble side-chain-core-KDO product. Lipid A contains 10 to 20 percent glucosamine-4-phosphate, ethanolamine, and 60 to 70 percent fatty acids. Because of its composition and solubility characteristics, lipid A is often called a glycolipid. The lipid A subunit is composed of a glucosamine disaccharide which is linked β-1,6 in *Salmonella* and *Serratia* (Fig. 6-19) and β-1,4 in *E. coli* and *Shigella*. The disaccharide units are thought to be linked through phos-

TABLE 6-5 SOME SALMONELLA LIPOPOLYSACCHARIDE O-SPECIFIC POLYSACCHARIDE REPEATING OLIGOSACCHARIDE UNITS

Serogroup	Salmonella species	Antigens	LPS Repeating Unit
A	*S. paratyphi A*	1,2,12	Par $\xrightarrow{\alpha\text{-}1,3}$ $\xrightarrow{,2}$ Man $\xrightarrow{\alpha\text{-}1,4}$ Rha $\xrightarrow{\alpha\text{-}1,3}$ Gal (Glc $\xrightarrow{\alpha\text{-}1,4}$), Ac $\xrightarrow{\alpha\text{-}1,}$
B	*S. typhimurium*	1,4,4,12	Abe-2-0-Ac $\xrightarrow{\alpha\text{-}1,3}$ $\xrightarrow{,2}$ Man $\xrightarrow{\alpha\text{-}1,4}$ Rha $\xrightarrow{\beta\text{-}1,3}$ Gal (Glc $\xrightarrow{\alpha\text{-}1,4}$) $\xrightarrow{\alpha\text{-}1,}$
D_2	*S. strasbourg*	(9),46	Tyv $\xrightarrow{\alpha\text{-}1,3}$ $\xrightarrow{,6}$ Man $\xrightarrow{\beta\text{-}1,4}$ Rha $\xrightarrow{\alpha\text{-}1,3}$ Gal (Glc $\xrightarrow{\alpha\text{-}1,4}$) $\xrightarrow{\alpha\text{-}1,}$
E_1	*S. anatum*	3,10	$\xrightarrow{,6}$ Man $\xrightarrow{\beta\text{-}1,4}$ Rha $\xrightarrow{1,3}$ Gal (Ac $\xrightarrow{}$) $\xrightarrow{\alpha\text{-}1,}$
E_2	*S. newington*	3,15	$\xrightarrow{,6}$ Man $\xrightarrow{\beta\text{-}1,4}$ Rha $\xrightarrow{\alpha\text{-}1,3}$ Gal $\xrightarrow{\beta\text{-}1,}$
E_3	*S. minneapolis*	3,(15),34	$\xrightarrow{,6}$ Man $\xrightarrow{\beta\text{-}1,4}$ Rha $\xrightarrow{\alpha\text{-}1,3}$ Gal (Glc $\xrightarrow{\alpha\text{-}1,4}$) $\xrightarrow{\beta\text{-}1,}$
E_4	*S. senftenberg*	1,3,19	$\xrightarrow{,6}$ Man $\xrightarrow{\beta\text{-}1,4}$ Rha $\xrightarrow{\alpha\text{-}1,3}$ Gal (Glc $\xrightarrow{\alpha\text{-}1,6}$) $\xrightarrow{\alpha\text{-}1,}$

Adapted from Lüderitz, Staub, Westphal; Bacteriol Rev 30:192, 1966; Lüderitz; Angew Chem 9:649, 1970: Lüderitz, West-phal, Staub, Nikaido: Bact Endotoxins 4:145, 1971.

Abbreviations: Ac, acetyl; Abe, abequose; Gal, galactose; Glc, glucose; Man, mannose; Par, paratose; Rha, rhamnose; Tyv, tyvulose.

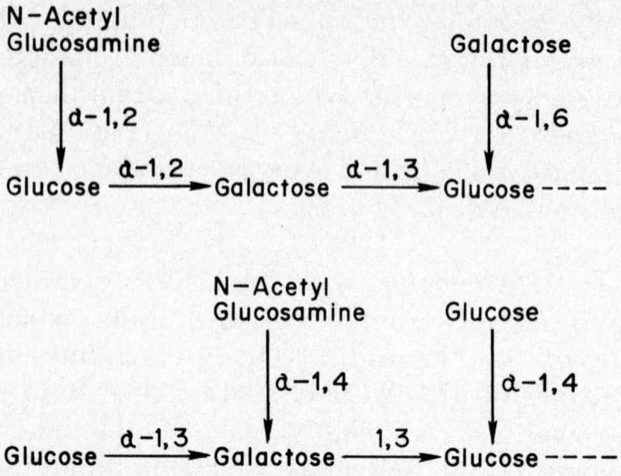

FIG. 6-18. Variation in lipopolysaccharide outer-core structure comparing similar structures of salmonella and shigella. (After Luderitz: Angew Chem 9:649, 1970)

phodiester or pyrophosphate groups. The glucosamine amino groups are acylated with β-hydroxy-fatty acids 10 to 17 carbons long, which appear to be characteristic of each bacterial family: for example, the 14-carbon β-hydroxymyristic acid (Fig. 6-19) is found in enterobacterial lipid A, while C-13 and C15 β-hydroxy-fatty acids are present in *Veillonella* species, and β-hydroxydecanoic acid occurs in *Pseudomonas* species. Saturated fatty acids found in enterobacterial lipid A include lauric, myristic, and palmitic acids.

BIOSYNTHESIS OF EXTRACELLULAR POLYSACCHARIDES AND INTRACELLULAR STORAGE POLYMERS

Extracellular Polymers   The extracellular slimes of some microorganisms, such as the lactic acid bacteria, are produced by a single transglycosylating enzyme from a single substrate in such quantity that viscous solutions result. As an example, *Leuconostoc mesenteroides* produces a predominantly α-1,6-linked polyglucan slime, or dextran, which is sometimes used as a blood plasma substitute. It is produced only when the proper substrate, sucrose (glucose-1,2-fructose), is supplied in the growth medium. The reaction requires a specific transglucosidase and proceeds by utilization of the energy inherent in the sucrose-glycoside bond (Fig. 6-20).

Glycogen   Bacterial glycogen, an intracellular α-1,4-linked polyglucan with α-1,6 branch points, is synthesized from adenosinediphosphateglucose by a variety of organisms, including *E. coli, Enterobacter aerogenes, M. luteus, Rhodopseudomonas* species, and the

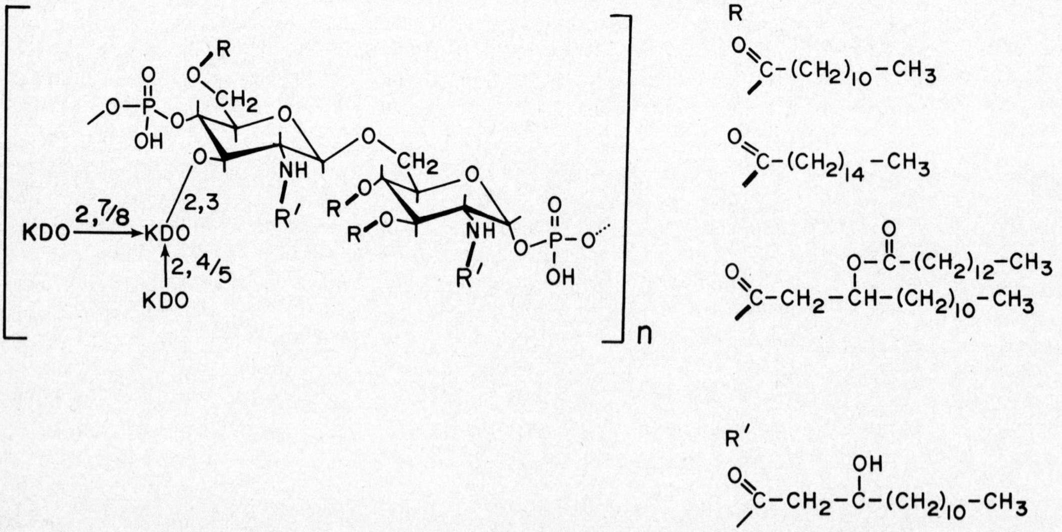

FIG. 6-19. Tentative structure of a KDO-lipid A unit of *Salmonella minnesota* R595 glycolipid. Fatty acid residues, myristic and palmitic acids, and β-hydroxymyristyl-β-hydroxymyristic acids occur at positions indicated by R. R′ indicates amide-linked β-hydroxymyristic acid. (After Rietschel, Gottert, Luderitz, Westphal: Eur J Biochem 28:166, 1972)

$$n \text{ Sucrose} \rightleftharpoons (- \text{Glucose} \xrightarrow{\beta-1,6})_n + n \text{ fructose}$$

FIG. 6-20. Dextran biosynthesis.

mycobacteria. It is produced at a rate that varies inversely with the growth rate and accumulates most readily in media rich in carbohydrate and poor in nitrogen or sulfur, which restrict growth but not metabolism. Glycogen synthesis occurs by transfer of glucose from ADP-glucose to the terminal nonreducing end groups of the glycogen polymer (Fig. 6-21). As in the animal system, branching is achieved by the action of an amylo-α-1,4 to α-1,6-transglucosylase.

$$\text{ADP}-\text{Glucose} + (\text{Glycogen})_n \longrightarrow$$

$$(\text{Glycogen})_{n+1} + \text{ADP}$$

FIG. 6-21. Glycogen synthesis in bacteria.

Poly-β-hydroxybutyric Acid (PHB) Some *Bacillus* species are capable of producing this chloroform-soluble polymer in amounts ranging from 7 to 40 percent of the dry cell weight. The polymer appears to be encased in a thin layer of protein which is assumed to contain the enzymes involved in its metabolism. Biosynthesis and degradation of PHB

$$\left[-\text{O}-\underset{\underset{\text{CH}_3}{|}}{\text{CH}}-\text{CH}_2-\underset{\underset{\text{O}}{||}}{\text{C}}- \right]_n$$

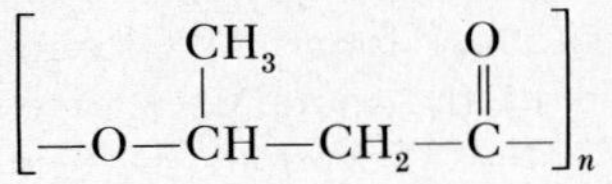

1. $2 \text{ Acetyl}\sim\text{SCoA} \rightleftharpoons$

$$\text{Acetoacetyl}\sim\text{SCoA} + \text{HSCoA}$$

2. $\text{Acetoacetyl}\sim\text{SCoA} + \text{NADH} \rightleftharpoons$

$$\beta-\text{OH}-\text{butyryl}\sim\text{SCoA} + \text{NAD}^+$$

3. $(\text{PHB})_n + \text{CoA}-\text{S}-\overset{\overset{\text{O}}{||}}{\text{C}}-\text{CH}_2-\text{CHOH}-\text{CH}_3 \rightleftharpoons$

$$(\text{PHB})_{n+1} + \text{HSCoA}$$

FIG. 6-22. Poly-β-hydroxybutyric acid biosynthesis.

$$^-\text{O}-\overset{\overset{\text{O}}{||}}{\underset{\underset{\text{O}_-}{|}}{\text{P}}}-\text{O}-\left(\overset{\overset{\text{O}}{||}}{\underset{\underset{\text{O}_-}{|}}{\text{P}}}-\text{O}\right)_n +\text{ATP} \xrightarrow{\text{Mg}^{2e}} \text{ADP} + {}^-\text{O}-\overset{\overset{\text{O}}{||}}{\underset{\underset{\text{O}_-}{|}}{\text{P}}}-\text{O}-\left(\overset{\overset{\text{O}}{||}}{\underset{\underset{\text{O}_-}{|}}{\text{P}}}-\text{O}\right)_{n+1}$$

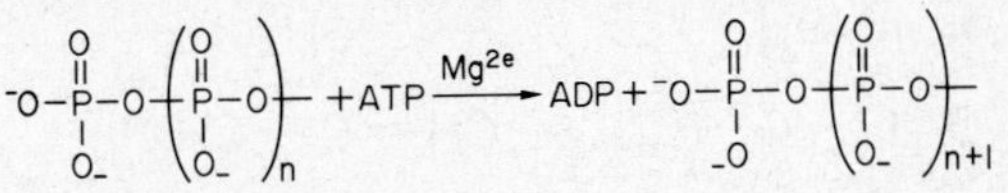

FIG. 6-23. Polyphosphate biosynthesis.

are apparently carried out by the same enzymes (Fig. 6-22). The polymer is depleted during growth and again accumulates during the stationary phase or restrictive conditions of growth.

Polyphosphate Babes-Ernst or volutin granules, thought to be polymetaphosphates, have been identified in various organisms, including *E. coli, E. aerogenes, C. diphtheriae,* mycobacteria, and the yeast, *Saccharomyces cerevisiae.* During active growth, only minute amounts of polyphosphates are detectable, whereas amounts equivalent to 1 to 2 percent of dry cell weight accumulate under conditions of restrictive growth in media poor in N or S. Synthesis of polyphosphate in *E. coli* proceeds as shown in Figure 6-23.

BIOSYNTHESIS OF CELL-ENVELOPE POLYMERS

Bacterial envelope polymers are synthesized by membrane-bound enzymes from nucleotide-sugar precursors which are synthesized in the cytoplasm. A membrane-bound cofactor, generally known as glycosylphosphate lipid carrier, is involved in the biosynthesis of peptidoglycan and the O-specific polysaccharide chain of lipopolysaccharides. The carrier lipid has been identified as the phosphomonoester of C_{55}-polyisoprenoid alcohol, undecaprenol (Fig. 6-24). This substance was first named "bactoprenol" before it was known that analogous lipid cofactors are also found in eucaryotic cells, including those of mammalian systems. The membrane-bound carrier forms glycosyl-pyrophospholipid oligosaccharide intermediates which are then transferred to form polymers. Similar membrane lipid-linked oligosaccharide derivatives are involved in the biosynthesis of membrane-bound mannan in *M. luteus (lysodeikticus)* and capsular polysaccharides in *E. aerogenes.*

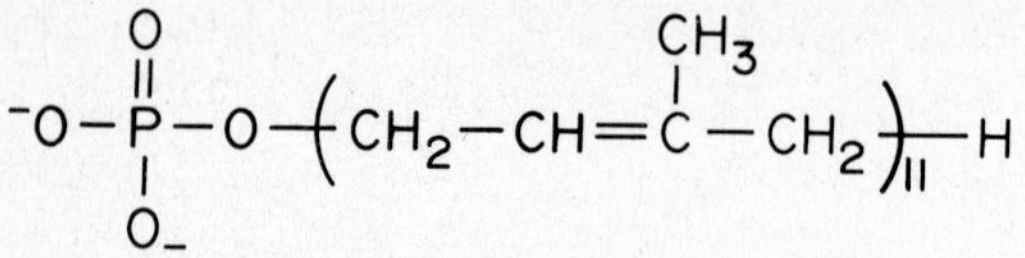

$$^-O-\overset{\overset{\displaystyle O}{\parallel}}{\underset{\underset{\displaystyle O_-}{|}}{P}}-O-\left(CH_2-CH=\overset{\overset{\displaystyle CH_3}{|}}{C}-CH_2\right)_{11}-H$$

FIG. 6-24. Phosphoundecaprenol.

Teichoic Acid and Teichuronic Acid Biosynthesis Polyolphosphodiester polymers, or teichoic acids, are formed by particulate enzyme systems from CDP-glycerol or CDP-ribitol (Fig. 6-25). The newly made teichoic acid chains are not transferred to preexisting peptidoglycan. The polyolphosphate chains appear to be added to nascent peptidoglycan chains during the synthesis of both polymer units in the membrane. The teichoic acid-bound peptidoglycan unit is then transferred as a unit to the growing cell wall peptidoglycan. The nature of the membrane-associated teichoic acid carrier is unknown, but it appears not to be undecaprenol. The synthesis of teichuronic acid appears to occur by a similar mechanism.

Peptidoglycan Biosynthesis There are five stages in the biosynthesis of bacterial peptidoglycan: (1) the biosynthesis of soluble precursors in the cytoplasm, (2) transfer of precursors to membrane-bound carrier lipid (phospholipolyisoprenol) and the formation of disaccharide pentapeptide units, (3) transfer of the disaccharide-pentapeptide to the cell wall, thereby extending the peptidoglycan backbone

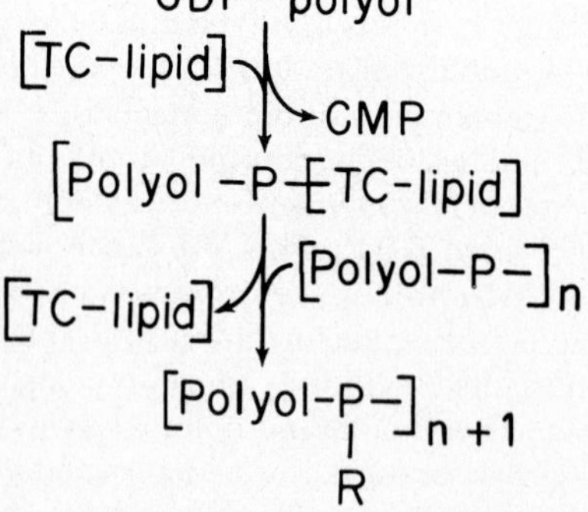

polymer, (4) formation of cross-links between peptidoglycan polymers, and (5) regeneration of monophosphocarrier lipid.

(1) The first stage of peptidoglycan synthesis involves formation of uridinediphospho-N-acetylmuramic acid (UDP-MurNAc) from uridinediphospho-N-acetylglucosamine (UDP-GlcNAc) by soluble cytoplasmic enzymes. First, the enolpyruvic acid group is transferred from phosphoenolpyruvic acid to the acetylglucosamine carbon-3-hydroxyl group, which is followed by its enzymic reduction by means of NADPH to a 3-0-lactic acid group. The amino acids of the pentapeptide are then added to the lactyl carboxyl group of UDP-MurNAc in stepwise fashion (Fig. 6-26), each addition except the last being catalyzed by a separate soluble enzyme and requiring ATP and a divalent cation, either Mg++ or Mn++. The last two amino acids are added to the MurNAc-tripeptide as the dipeptide, D-alanyl-D-alanine, by a reaction which also requires ATP and divalent cation. The D-alanine is produced from L-alanine by a racemase.

(2) A series of steps then occurs in the particulate membrane fraction (Fig. 6-27). First, the phosphoacetylmuramyl-pentapeptide group is transferred to the membrane-bound carrier lipid with formation of a pyrophosphate bridge and release of UMP (Fig. 6-27, step 1); then β-1,4-linked disaccharide-pentapeptide-pyrophospho-carrier lipid is formed by addition of acetylglucosamine from UDPGlcNAc to the C-4 hydroxyl of the muramic acid component (Fig. 6-27, step 2). Various modication steps may follow, depending upon the species; for example, *S. aureus* amidates the alpha-carboxyl

$$\begin{array}{c} \text{CDP-polyol} \\ [\text{TC-lipid}]\diagdown \\ \diagdown \text{CMP} \\ [\text{Polyol}-P-\text{TC-lipid}] \\ [\text{TC-lipid}]\diagup\diagdown[\text{Polyol}-P-]_n \\ [\text{Polyol}-P-]_{n+1} \\ | \\ R \end{array}$$

FIG. 6-25. Postulated sequence of polyolphosphate (teichoic acid) biosynthesis in gram-positive bacteria. Abbreviations used: CDP-polyol, cytidine diphosphate polyol; CMP, cytidine monophosphate; TC-lipid, teichoic acid carrier lipid; R, peptidoglycan biosynthetic intermediate. (After Fiedler, Mauck, Glaser: Ann NY Acad Sci 235:198, 1974)

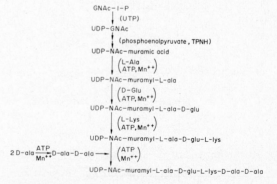

FIG. 6-26. Biosynthesis of the UDP-N-acetylglucosamine-N-acetylmuramic acid-pentapeptide precursor of cell-wall peptidoglycan.

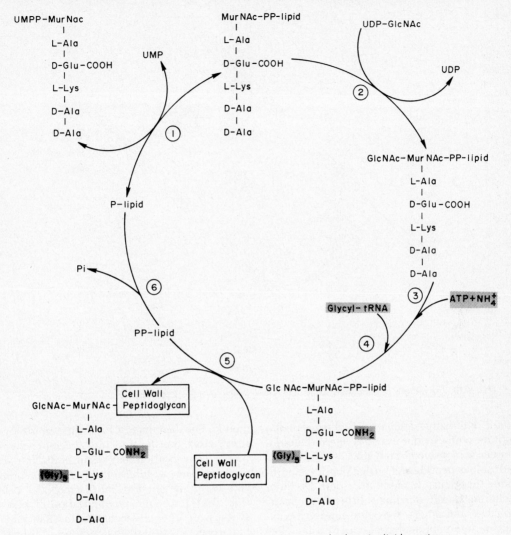

FIG. 6-27. Biosynthesis of peptidoglycan: membrane-involved carrier lipid reactions.

group of glutamic acid and also forms a penta-glycine bridge peptide by stepwise addition of glycine to the epsilon-amino group of the muro-peptide L-lysine residues by mediation of a special 4-thio-uridine-containing tRNA which differs from the glycine-tRNA involved in protein biosynthesis (Fig. 6-27, steps 3 and 4).

(3) The third stage, elongation of the peptidoglycan backbone, occurs by transglycosylation (translocation) of the disaccharide-penta-peptide unit from the carrier lipid to the cell wall acceptor peptidoglycan backbone (Fig. 6-27, step 5), thereby releasing the pyrophospho-carrier lipid, from which phosphatase regenerates the monophospho-carrier lipid by removal of phosphate (Fig. 6-27, step 6).

(4) The cell wall polymer formed at this stage is a noncross-linked peptidoglycan with pentapeptide units terminating in D-Ala-D-Ala·COOH. Closure of the peptide bridges linkages by transpeptidation to form the cross-linked murein polymer finishes the biosynthetic sequence. In *S. aureus*, this is accomplished by a reaction (Fig. 6-28) in which the penultimate D-alanine carboxyl group is linked to the free amino group of the pentaglycine bridge peptide of a neighboring peptidoglycan chain with concomitant release of the terminal D alanine.

This sequence of reactions is essentially similar in all bacteria studied so far. Differences known include the species-specific substitu-

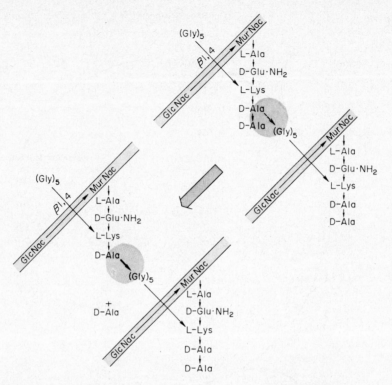

FIG. 6-28. Biosynthesis of peptidoglycan: bridge cross-linkage by transpeptidation and release of D-alanine.

tion of alternative amino acids during penta-peptide synthesis (for example, *meso*-diamino-pimelic acid instead of L-lysine, see Table 6-3) and various peptide and bridge peptide modification reactions. In addition, some bacteria, including *E. coli, Bacillus subtilis, Lactobacillus casei,* and others, appear to control the extent of interpeptidoglycan cross-linkage. Removal of whole peptides may occur by action of the autolysin, MurNAc-L-Ala amidase, as in the case of *E. coli* and *M. luteus,* in which 30 to 50 percent of the glycan chains occur free and uncross-linked. One or both D-alanines may be removed from soluble UDP-MurNAc-penta-peptide precursors and noncross-linked penta-peptidoglycan by carboxypeptidase. This is thought to explain the occurrence of tri- and tetrapeptides, as in *E. coli* (Fig. 6-3).

Lipopolysaccharide Biosynthesis The mechanism of lipid A synthesis is unknown. However, LPS core and side-chain are synthesized in the membrane in several stages. Lipid A (region III) serves as an acceptor for the stepwise addition of core polysaccharide units (region II), followed by the addition of preassambled O-specific polysaccharide units (re-

gion I). The completed LPS is then rapidly and irreversibly translocated into the outer membrane. Translocation may occur at discrete export sites, seen as adhesion sites between inner and outer membranes in plasmolyzed cells (Fig. 3-21), although randomization of newly synthesized lipopolysaccharide in outer membrane occurs within several minutes of growth.

Lipid A biosynthesis (Region III). The mechanism of lipid A biosynthesis is unknown. However, lipid A components serve as an acceptor for CMP-KDO, forming KDO-lipid A. KDO-lipid A appears to be necessary for growth. Mutant organisms which require arabinose-5-phosphate (Ara-5-P) for synthesis of KDO-8-phosphate cease growing after one generation of Ara-5-P starvation but remain viable.

Core Polysaccharide Biosynthesis (Region II). The basic mechanism of core polysaccharide synthesis involves membrane-associated enzymes which catalyze the stepwise addition of monosaccharides from nucleotide sugar intermediates to the nonreducing terminus of the growing core polymer (Table 6-6). Inner

TABLE 6-6 STRUCTURE AND BIOSYNTHETIC SEQUENCE OF LIPOPOLYSACCHARIDES OF CORE AND O POLYSACCHARIDE-DEFECTIVE SALMONELLA R MUTANTS

Source	O Antigen Polymer	Core Polysaccharide Components ←—Outer Core—→ ←— Inner Core —→	Lipid A	Mutant Chemotype
Rough (R-form) mutants	None	$(KDO)_3 \rightarrow$ Lipid A ↑ PP-EthN		Re
		$Hep \rightarrow (KDO)_3 \rightarrow$ Lipid A ↑ PP-EthN		Rd_2
		$Glc \rightarrow (Hep)_2 \rightarrow (KDO)_3 \rightarrow$ Lipid A ↑ PP-EthN		Rd_1P^-
		$Glc \rightarrow (Hep)_2 \rightarrow (KDO)_3 \rightarrow$ Lipid A ↑ ↑ P PP-EthN		RcP^+
		$Gal \rightarrow Glc \rightarrow (Hep)_2 \rightarrow (KDO)_3 \rightarrow$ Lipid A ↑ ↑ ↑ Gal PP-EthN PP-EthN		Rb
		$Glc \rightarrow Gal \rightarrow Glc \rightarrow (Hep)_2 \rightarrow (KDO)_3 \rightarrow$ Lipid A ↑ ↑ ↑ ↑ GlcNAc Gal PP-EthN PP-EthN		Ra
Semi-rough mutants	[Single repeating unit]₁	$\rightarrow Glc \rightarrow Gal \rightarrow Glc \rightarrow (Hep)_2 \rightarrow (KDO)_3 \rightarrow$ Lipid A ↑ ↑ ↑ ↑ GlcNAc Gal PP-EthN PP-EthN		SR
Smooth or S-form (parent wild-type)	[Multiple repeating units]ₙ	$\rightarrow Glc \rightarrow Gal \rightarrow Glc \rightarrow (Hep)_2 \rightarrow (KDO)_3 \rightarrow$ Lipid A ↑ ↑ ↑ ↑ GlcNAc Gal PP-EthN PP-EthN		

Adapted from Lüderitz: *Angew Chem* 9:20, 1970; Muhlradt; *Eur J Biochem* 18:20, 1971; Nikaido: *In Leive (ed): Bacterial Membranes and Walls*, 1973, vol 1. Courtesy of Marcel Dekker

Smooth and rough refer to serologic reactivity of polysaccharides. Addition of core monosaccharides is by single, stepwise addition. Addition of O antigen repeating units occurs in two steps: a single oligosaccharide repeating unit is attached to the core and serves as acceptor for the remainder of the preformed O antigen polysaccharide. Abbreviations: KDO, 2-keto-2-deoxyoctonic acid; Hep, heptose; Glc, glucose; Gal, galactose; GlcNAc, N-acetylglucosamine; P, phosphate; PP-EthN, pyrophosphorylethanolamine.

core units (KDO, heptose, phosphate, and ethanolamine) are added stepwise, followed by the outer core hexose units (glucose, galactose, and N-acetyl-D-glucosamine). The sequence of addition is ordered by specific enzyme recognition of both acceptor and activated nucleotide-sugar donor.

Much of the knowledge of core polymer structure and biosynthesis has been made possible by the availability of a series of *Salmonella* R or rough-form mutants which are defective in LPS biosynthesis (Table 6-6, Fig. 6-17). Such mutants are defective in their ability to synthesize nucleotide sugar precursors, such as UDP-galactose, or they lack one or more of the necessary nucleotide sugar transferases or O polymer transferases. By using cell envelope preparations from appropriate mutant organisms, the stepwise addition of each core component in sequence can be demonstrated. Phospholipid-free core polymers are inactive as acceptors of glucose or galactose; phosphatidylethanolamine is a physical cofactor which is necessary for binding of the appropriate UDP-glycosyl transferase to the acceptor molecule.

O ANTIGEN BIOSYNTHESIS (REGION I). The synthesis of the O antigen polysaccharide hapten is formally similar to that of peptidoglycan, in that soluble nucleotide sugars are utilized by membrane enzymes to synthesize carrier lipid-O antigen repeating oligosaccharide unit intermediates, which are then polymerized. The biosynthetic sequence in particulate cell envelope membrane preparations occurs in four stages: (1) preassembly of O antigen repeating units as oligosaccharide-pyrophosphate carrier lipid intermediates, (2) polymerization of the preassembled repeating units, (3) transfer of the O-chain polymer to LPS core polysaccharide, and (4) regeneration of monophospho-carrier lipid.

(1) The first step in synthesis of the oligosaccharide repeating unit of *S. typhimurium*, for example, involves the transfer of galactose-1-phosphate from UDP-galactose (UDPGal) to membrane-bound phospho-carrier lipid to form galactosyl-pyrophospho-carrier lipid with release of UMP. Transfer of L-rhamnose from thymidine diphosphorhamnose (TDPRha), mannose from guanosine-diphosphomannose (GDPMan) and abequose from cytidine diphosphoabequose (CDPAbe) follow to complete the tetrasaccharide repeating unit intermediate.

(2) This step involves the transfer of the proximal ends of growing chains from membrane-attached PP lipid to single newly formed oligosaccharide repeating units, which are themselves linked to membrane-bound PP lipid (Fig. 6-29). This is exactly the opposite of the mechanisms of intracellular biosynthesis of cytoplasmic polymers, such as glycogen, in which each new repeating unit is added to the distal ends of growing polymer chains.

(3) Transfer of O antigen oligosaccharide repeating units to the core polysaccharide involves two steps. First, a single repeating unit is transferred, and then a different enzyme transfers the polymerized O antigen polysaccharide.

(4) Monophosphopolyisoprenol, the P lipid carrier, is regenerated from the corresponding pyrophosphate by phosphatase action as described above for peptidoglycan synthesis.

Of interest is the ability of bacteriophage to change the composition and structure of the O antigen side-chain repeating units (Chap. 70).

FURTHER READING

Books and Reviews

Ashwell G, Hickman J: The chemistry of the unique carbohydrates of bacterial lipopolysaccharides. In Weinbaum G, Kadis S, Ajl SJ (eds): Microbial Toxins. New York, Academic Press, 1971, vol 4, pp 235-266

Barksdale L: *Corynebacterium diphtheriae* and its relatives. Bacteriol Rev 34:378, 1970

Blumberg PM, Strominger JL: Interaction of penicillin with the bacterial cell: penicillin-binding proteins and penicillin-sensitive enzymes. Bacteriol Rev 38:291, 1974

Braun V, Hantke K: Biochemistry of bacterial cell envelopes. Annu Rev Biochem 73:89, 1974

Braun V, Bosch V, Hantke K, Schaller K: Structure and biosynthesis of functionally defined areas of the *Escherichia coli* outer membrane. Ann NY Acad Sci 235:66, 1974

Galanos C: Physical state and biological activity of lipopolysaccharides. Toxicity and immunogenicity of the lipid A component. Z Immunitaetsforsch 149:214, 1975

Ghuysen JM: Use of bacteriolytic enzymes in determination of wall structure and their role in cell metabolism. Bacteriol Rev 32:425, 1968

Goren MB: Mycobacterial lipids. Bacteriol Rev 36:33, 1972

Heymer B: Biological properties of the peptidoglycan. Z Immunitaetsforsch 149:214, 1975

Kaplan MH: Nature of the streptococcal and myocardial antigens involved in the immunologic cross-reaction between group A streptococcus and heart. In Nowotny A (ed.): Cellular Antigens. New York, Springer-Verlag, 1972, p 70

Lederer E: The mycobacterial cell wall. Pure Appl Chem 25:135, 1971

Leive L: The barrier function of the gram-negative envelope Ann NY Acad Sci 235:109, 1974

Lüderitz O, Jann K, Wheat R: Somatic and capsular antigens of gram-negative bacteria. In Florkin M, Stotz EH (eds): Comprehensive Biochemistry. Amsterdam, Elsevier Publishing Company, 1968, vol 26A, pp 105-228

Lüderitz O, Staub AM, Westphal O: Immunochemistry of O and R antigens of *Salmonella* and related *Enterobacteriaceae*. Bacteriol Rev 30:192, 1966

Lüderitz O, Westphal O, Staub HM, Nikaido H: Isolation and chemical and immunological characterization of bacterial lipopolysaccharides. In Weinbaum G, Kadis S, Ajl SJ (eds): Microbial Toxins, New York, Academic Press, 1971 vol 4, p 145

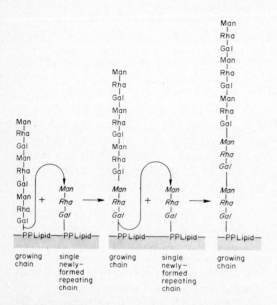

FIG. 6-29. Polymerization of preassembled repeating units during the biosynthesis of O antigen. Mechanism allows extension of growing polysaccharide side-chain into external environment without requiring movement of biosynthesis machinery.

Lüderitz O, Galanos C, Lehmann V, et al: Lipid A: chemical structure and biological activity. J Infect Dis 128 [Suppl]:9, 1972

Osborn MJ: Structure and biosynthesis of the bacteria cell wall. Annu Rev Biochem 38:501, 1969

Osborn MJ, Rick PD, Lehmann V, Rupprecht E, Singh M: Structure and biogenesis of the cell envelope of gram-negative bacteria. Ann NY Acad Sci 235:52, 1974

Preiss J: The regulation of the biosynthesis of α-1,4 glucans in bacteria and plants. In Horecker BL, Stadtman ER (eds): Current Topics in Cellular Regulation. New York, Academic Press, vol 1, p 125, 1969

Rietschel ET, Lüderitz O: Chemical structure of lipopolysaccharides and endotoxin immunity. Z. Immunitaetsforsch 149:201, 1975

Rogers HJ: Peptidoglycans (mucopeptides): structure, function, and variations. Ann NY Acad Sci 235:29, 1974

Rothfield L, Romero D: Role of lipids in the biosynthesis of the bacterial cell envelope. Bacteriol Rev 35:14, 1971

Schleifer KH, Kandler O: Peptidoglycan types of bacterial cell walls and their taxonomic implications. Bacteriol Rev 36:407, 1972

Schwab JH: Suppression of the immune response by microorganisms. Bacteriol Rev 39:121, 1975

Yotis, WW (ed): Recent advances in staphylococcal research. Ann NY Acad Sci: 236:520, 1974

Selected Papers

Adam A, Ellouz F, Ciorbaru R, Petit JF, Lederer E: Peptidoglycan adjuvants: minimal structure required for activity. Z Immunitaetsforsch 149:341, 1975

Antoine A, Tepper BS: Characterization of glycogens from mycobacteria. Arch Biochem 134:207, 1969

Fosgren A, Nordstrom K: Protein A from *Staphylococcus aureus:* the biological significance of its reaction with IgG. Ann NY Acad Sci 236:252, 1974

Heptinstall S, Archibald AR, Baddiley J: Teichoic acids and membrane functions in bacteria. Nature 225:519, 1970

Inouye M, Hirashima A, Lee N: Biosynthesis and assembly of a structural lipoprotein in the envelope of *Escherichia coli*. Ann NY Acad Sci 235:83, 1974

Kaletti J, Lüderitz O, Mlynarcik, Sedlak J: Immunochemical studies on Citrobacter O antigens (lipopolysaccharides). Europ J Biochem 20:237, 1971

Leloir LF: Two decades of research on the biosynthesis of saccharides. Science 172:1299, 1971

Misaki A, Seto N, Azuma I: Structure and immunological properties of D-arabino-D-galactans isolated from cell walls of *Mycobacterium* species. J Biochem 76:15, 1974

Movitz J: Study on the biosynthesis of protein A in *Staphylococcus aureus*. Eur J Biochem 48:131, 1974

Orskov F, Orskov I, Jann B, et al: Immunochemistry of *Escherichia coli* O antigens. Acta Pathol Microbiol Scand 71:339, 1967

Rick PD, Osborn MJ: Isolation of a mutant of *Salmonella typhimurium* dependent on D-arabinose-5-phosphate for growth and synthesis of 3-deoxy-D-mannooctulosonate (ketodeoxyoctonate). Proc Natl Acad Sci USA 69:3756, 1972

Scherrer R, Gerhardt P: Molecular sieving by the *Bacillus megaterium* cell wall and protoplast. J Bacteriol 107:718, 1971

Schnaitman CA: Effect of ethylendiaminetetraacetic acid, triton X-100, and lysozyme on the morphology and chemical composition of isolated cell walls of *Escherichia coli*. J Bacteriol 108:553, 1971

Sjoquist J, Movitz J, Johansson I, Hjelm H: Localization of protein A in the bacteria. Europ J Biochem 30:190, 1972

Stalenheim G, Gotze O, Cooper NR, Sjoquist J, Muller-Eberhard HJ: Consumption of human complement components by complexes of IgG with protein A of *Staphylococcus aureus*. Immunochemistry 10:501, 1973

Takayama K: Selective action of isoniazid on its synthesis of cell wall mycolates in mycobacteria. Ann NY Acad Sci 235:426, 1974

Wu MC, Heath EC: Isolation and characterization of lipopolysaccharide protein from *Escherichia coli*. Proc Natl Acad Sci USA 70:2572, 1973

7
Molecular Basis of Genetics

Heredity in bacteria, as in other organisms, is based on the chromosome. Unlike that of higher, differentiated organisms, the genetic apparatus of bacteria is not organized into discrete, morphologically identifiable structures, nor does it go through the gross morphologic changes of mitosis during the division cycle of the cell. The bacterial genome, ie, the total complement of hereditary units or genes, is usually contained in a single DNA molecule, although, as will be discussed in Chapter 8, extrachromosomal genetic elements, known as plasmids, also are widely distributed among bacteria. Bacteria are haploid, and in this respect they are analogous to gametes generated by the reduction of meiosis rather than to diploid somatic cells. However, the transmission of genetic information from generation to generation is linear, and in this respect bacteria are analogous to somatic cells. Although mitosis does not occur in bacteria, it is known that the daughter cells generated at each division cycle receive their proper apportionment of genetic information (Chap. 5).

Because of the difference between the chromosome structure of nucleated (eucaryotic) organisms and nonnucleated (procaryotic) bacteria and because of the sexual versus asexual modes of reproduction, one might expect that the rules and mechanisms governing gene expression in bacteria differ from those that operate in higher organisms. However, no contradictions have yet been found between the tenets of transmission genetics (ie, how the units of heredity behave from generation to generation) and the more recent formulations of biochemical and molecular genetics primarily derived from the study of bacteria and their viruses. In fact, genetic studies of bacterial systems continue to provide a unitary view of the molecular basis of heredity.

THE BACTERIAL CHROMOSOME

The bacterial chromosome is composed of DNA and, in contrast to the chromosome of eucaryotic organisms, contains no histones. The DNA of bacteria accounts for about 2 to 3 percent of the dry weight of the cell. Electron micrographs of appropriately fixed thin sections of bacteria reveal that the DNA exists as a fibrillar structure which appears to occupy a large portion of the cell's volume. Many of the DNA molecules extracted from bacterial cells are circular; the implication of this circularity will be discussed later.

The Structure of DNA DNA is extracted from bacteria as a high-molecular-weight heteropolymer of the deoxyribonucleotides of the purines, adenine and guanine, and the pyrimidines, cytosine and thymine. The linear integrity of the polymer is maintained by phosphodiester bonds involving the 3'-hydroxyl group of one deoxyribose molecule and the 5'-hydroxyl group of another deoxyribose molecule. Attached to the 1'-hydroxy group of each sugar is one of the four bases mentioned above. Analysis of the base composition of DNA shows that the amount of 6-amino bases (adenine and cytosine) equals the amount of 6-keto bases (thymine and guanine). The gross anatomy of the DNA molecule was first visualized by x-ray diffraction patterns which showed that it most probably was a multiple-stranded fiber about 22 angstroms in diameter, with a linear spacing of groups 3.4 Å apart along the fiber, and a repeating unit every 34 Å (Fig. 7-1).

Aided by x-ray measurements, Watson and Crick described the double helix structure of DNA in which two polyribonucleotide strands are aligned in an antiparallel fashion in a helical arrangement stabilized by hydrogen bonding between purine on one strand and pyrimidine on the other (Fig. 7-1). The resulting structure, with the appropriate restriction placed on it by the x-ray data, can be likened to a right-handed, circular stairway with the sugar-phosphate backbone as the railing and each planar, hydrogen-bonded adenine-thymine and cytosine-guanine base pair as a step. The description of the structure of DNA, which must be considered one of the most significant accomplishments of modern biology, provides a structure capable of fulfilling the general requirements for genetic material deduced from the results of transmission genetics, ie, (1) that it must achieve its own faithful replication and transmission from one generation to the next and (2) that it must preside over all of the physiologic processes of the cell. Studies in bacterial genetics have been directed toward describing the mechanisms whereby these events are fulfilled.

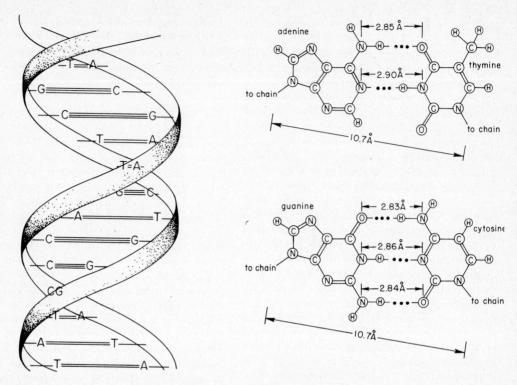

FIG. 7-1. The double helix. Two polydeoxyribonucleotides are wound around one another to form a double-stranded, right-handed helix, in which the two strands are oriented antiparallel to one another. X-ray studies indicate that each base is separated by 3.4 Å, and each turn of the helix is 34 Å—therefore 10 base pairs are required for each turn. The dimensions of the base pair formed by the hydrogen bonding between a purine and pyrimidine are depicted at the right.

DNA REPLICATION

The structure of DNA provides a clue to how new DNA molecules can be generated as precise copies of the old molecules. The possibility for replicating a linear molecule composed of two noncovalently associated strands whose nucleotide sequence is governed by the rather strict rules of base pairing is enzymatic polymerization, with each strand serving as template upon which to build the complementary strand. The polymerization can be viewed as proceeding with or without strand separation. Strand separation would result in a semi-conservative retention of one of the parent strands in each of the daughter DNA molecules. Polymerization without concomitant strand separation would result in one daughter molecule derived entirely from the parent and another totally new molecule.

That the replication of DNA occurs in a semi-conservative fashion was proved by use of a technique able to distinguish newly synthesized from parental DNA. The DNA of bacteria cultured in a medium containing a heavy isotope of nitrogen (^{15}N) is more dense than DNA containing the relatively abundant isotope, ^{14}N. These DNAs can be separated by isopycnic centrifugation. When an appropriate concentration of a heavy salt, such as cesium chloride, is centrifuged a concentration gradient is formed with the highest concentration located at a position in the centrifuge cell which is farthest from the axis of rotation. If DNA is added to the solution prior to centrifugation it will redistribute itself and come to rest in a narrow band at the position in the gradient where it displaces its own weight of the cesium chloride solution; in other words, the DNA will float at that position because the density of the cesium chloride solution which it displaces matches its own density. Owing to the gradient in the centrifuge cell, DNAs of different densities come to equilibrium at different positions—^{15}N DNA being more dense than ^{14}N DNA bands farther from the axis of rotation. Employing this procedure, cells which had grown for several generations in a medium containing the heavy isotope were transferred to medium containing ^{14}N, and the distribution of the isotopes was monitored after subsequent generations. Following one generation in the light medium the DNA was found to be of intermediate density, ie, between that of light and heavy DNA. After two generations the light and intermediate density DNAs were found in approximately equal amounts (Fig. 7-2). These results are consistent with a semiconservative mechanism for DNA replication. The intermediate density DNA represents a hybrid containing one strand of parental heavy DNA and one strand of newly synthesized light DNA. The experimental results cited above illustrate another very significant aspect of DNA replication, namely, that it occurs in a continuous and sequential fashion (evidenced by the fact that all of the heavy DNA becomes hybrid prior to the appearance of light DNA). Several experimental results are now available which not only substantiate this conclusion but which also indicate that the direction of chromosomal replication is constant and that

the initiation site is heritable, ie, each round of DNA replication is initiated at the same position on the chromosome.

The Replicon The concept that the replication of DNA molecules begins at one point on the chromosome and proceeds to the end of the chromosome is the basis for the replicon model of replication. Some bacterial cells may contain, in addition to their chromosomes, other autonomously replicating DNA molecules, known as plasmids (Chap. 8). These plasmids (as well as the chromosome per se) are replicons and constitute distinct genetic linkage groups which replicate and usually segregate independently. Each replicon possesses a unique site for replication initiation; these sites are termed replicators. Initiation of replication requires interaction of the replicator with protein initiator substances which are distinct from the DNA polymerase involved in the polymerization process. These initiator substances are specified by the replicon and are specifically involved in the initiation of the replication of the homologous replicon, although in the case of some of the smaller bacteriophages, DNA replication is dependent upon the host replication apparatus (Chap. 70). The initiator protein

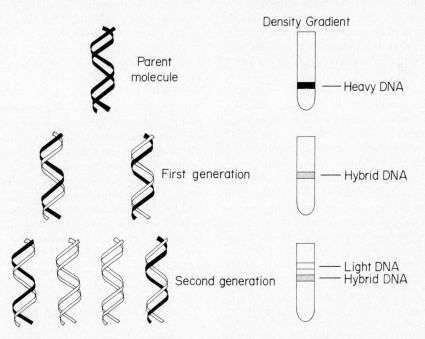

Density Gradient

Parent molecule — Heavy DNA

First generation — Hybrid DNA

Second generation — Light DNA / — Hybrid DNA

FIG. 7-2. The semiconservative replication of the bacterial chromosome. The left side of the figure depicts the distribution of uniformly labeled heavy (^{15}N) DNA following 0, 1, and 2 generations, respectively, in light (^{14}N) medium. The right side of the figure depicts the location at equilibrium in a cesium chloride gradient of heavy, hybrid, and light DNA.

substances are unstable or consumed in the initiation process, since if protein synthesis is prevented after initiation, replication will continue, but a new round of replication will not begin until protein synthesis is restored. Additional support for the presence of initiator proteins comes from the observation that mutant replicons which are unable to replicate at elevated temperatures can be caused to replicate at the nonpermissive temperature if present with a nonmutated replicon of the same type. In other words, the initiator substance produced by the nonmutated replicon is able to rescue the mutated replicon.

The Origin and Direction of Replication

The replicator, which is composed of a unique nucleotide sequence, is the heritable site of initiation of replication. The heritable nature of the replicator can be demonstrated in certain temperature-sensitive mutants *(dnaA)* of *Escherichia coli* deficient in initiation of chromosome replication. The inability of these mutants to initiate replication at 42C can be reversed if the chromosome acquires a new replicator. For example, integration of a fertility (F) factor, which itself is a replicon (Chap. 8), into the chromosome will restore chromosome replication at the nonpermissive temperature. This integrative suppression is caused by utilization of the DNA synthesis initiation site of the F factor.

Direct studies of chromosome replication employing synchronously growing cultures of *E. coli* show that the replicator is located near the *ilv* region on the chromosome. The results of these studies also show that replication of the *E. coli* chromosome is bidirectional, diverging from the point of initiation and terminating at a point that is 180 degrees away on the circular chromosome. The elegant experiments which permitted these conslusions involved the use of several strains of *E. coli*, each of

which has the Mu-1 prophage integrated at a known and unique position on the chromosome.[*] The DNA of each of these strains was labeled with ^{3}H-thymidine, and the cultures were then subjected to amino acid starvation. This procedure allows ongoing rounds of replication to be completed in the absence of reinitiation of new rounds of replication. Restoration of protein synthesis following amino acid starvation results in the synchronous reinitiation of chromosome replication. If DNA synthesis is reinitiated in the presence of the density label, 5-bromouracil, the rate at which the integrated Mu-1 DNA becomes copied during the course of chromosome replication can be followed because its DNA will be of hybrid density—if the Mu-1 prophage is located near the initiator region it will appear early in DNA of hybrid density; if it is located some distance from the initiator region it will appear as hybrid DNA later in the course of replication. Portions of the culture are removed following reinitiation of DNA synthesis, and the DNA is extracted, sheared, and subjected to isopycnic centrifugation so that bands of DNA of hybrid and light density form in the gradient. The amount of specific Mu-1 DNA in each band can be quantified by hybridization to purified Mu-1 DNA. Quantification is accomplished by measurement of the amount of radioactivity present in the previously labeled, conserved strand of the newly synthesized hybrid as well as in the unreplicated portion of the molecule. Figure 7-3 illustrates these results and compares the relative rate of appearance of the Mu-1 DNA with the known position of the integrated prophage in the strains employed for this analysis. This analysis shows that newly replicated prophage appears earliest in those strains where it is integrated close to, and on either side of, the *ilv* region, and latest when it is integrated 180 degrees away from the *ilv* region. Alternative techniques have been employed to show that several other replicons replicate in a bidirectional manner (eg, the chromosome of *Bacillus subtilis*, the genomes of coliphages λ and T4, and the genome of simian virus 40).

The Genetics of DNA Replication

The results of the amino acid starvation technique mentioned above suggest that the initiation and polymerization events in bacterial chromosome replication occur as distinct and

[*] *Mu-1 prophage, unlike most lysogenic phages (Chap. 70), is able to integrate into virtually any position on the chromosome. Specific integration can be directed by selecting for inactivation of genes within which the prophage integrate. Accordingly, for the purposes of the experiments described here, strains with Mu-1 prophage integrated at a specific site are obtained by using Mu-1 as a mutagen and selecting for specific amino acid auxotrophy or, in the case of the mal-organism, by selecting for an organism unable to grow on maltose as carbon source.*

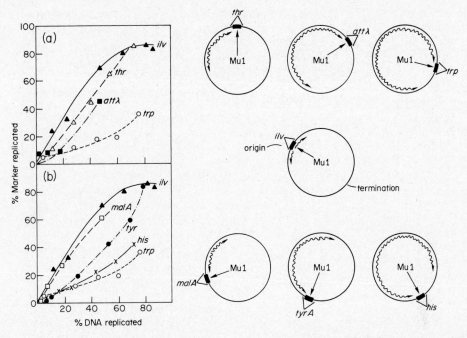

FIG. 7-3. The origin and direction of DNA replication in *E. coli*. The position of integration of Mu-1 prophage in the chromosome of the various strains used in this analysis is shown on the left. The details of the experiment are described in the text. (Left figure from Bird et al: J Mol Biol 70:549, 1972)

separable processes, and mutant methodology has verified this view. Mutant strains of *E. coli* have been isolated in which DNA replication occurs at 30C but not at 42C. The mutations thus far described as causing DNA synthesis to be temperature sensitive lie at six distinct loci on the *E. coli* chromosome; these genes are designated dnaA, B, C-D, E, F, and G. (The *dna C-D* designation stems from the original description of *dnaC* and *dnaD* mutations as being different, but these are now thought to affect the same gene.) It has been shown both by in vivo analysis and by use of in vitro DNA synthesizing systems that the *dnaA* and *dnaC-D* gene products are involved in initiation, whereas *dnaB, E,* and *G* are involved in the elongation process, and *dnaF* is the structural gene for nucleoside diphosphate reductase, which is not directly involved in DNA replication but which converts nucleosides to deoxynucleosides, which are subsequently used to synthesize DNA. The gene products of *dna A, B, C-D, E,* and *G* have been at least partially purified, but with the exception of the *dnaE* gene product, which is DNA polymerase III (see below), their precise roles are unknown. (It is known, however, that a DNA-dependent ribonucleoside triphosphatase activity is associated with the *dnaB* gene product.) The complexity of DNA replication is further amplified by the results of in vitro analysis which indicate that, in addition to gene products described above, several other proteins are involved.

Enzymology of DNA Replication

DNA Polymerase Enzymes capable of catalyzing the polymerization of deoxyribonucleotides have been extensively characterized, and much effort has been expended to identify the polymerase which functions in in vivo DNA replication. *Escherichia coli* contains three DNA polymerases, polymerase I, II, and III, each of which carries out a primer-dependent, template-directed polymerization of deoxyribonucleotide monophosphates in a 5'-OH to 3'-OH direction, ie, the nucleotide monophosphates are transferred from nucleotide triphosphates to the 3-OH group of the growing nucleotide chains. The polymerization is polarized so that the product strand is aligned antiparallel to the template molecule. Also, the product strand is complementary to the template strand, obeying the rules of pairing in that adenine, thymine, cytosine, and guanine on the

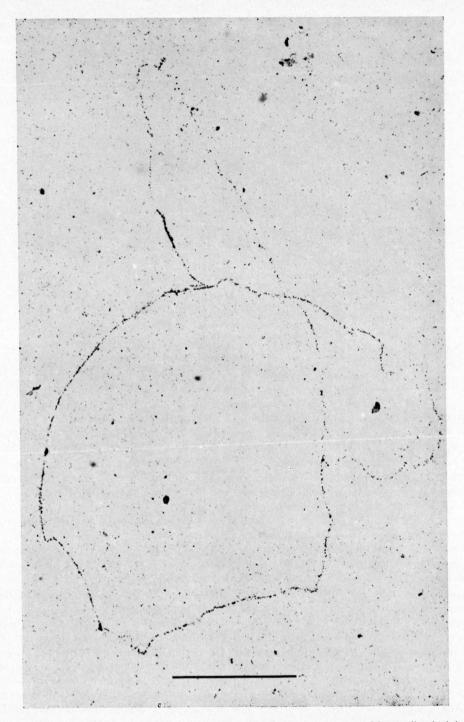

FIG. 7-4. Radioautograph of the chromosome of *E. coli* K12 Hfr. The DNA was extracted from cells which had been labeled with ³H-thymidine for two generations, and spread on a photographic emulsion. The outline of the DNA molecule is produced by the exposure of the silver grains in the emulsion to the β particles emitted by the isotope. The scale shows 0.1 mm. The molecule shown is thought to be undergoing replication; the loops are the daughter molecules. (From Cairns: Cold Spring Harbor Symp Quant Biol 28:43, 1963)

product strand are opposite thymine, adenine, quanine, and cytosine, respectively, on the template strand. The stoichiometry of these polymerase reactions is as follows:

$$
\begin{array}{l}
n1\ dATP \\
\quad + \\
n2\ dGTP \\
\quad + \\
n3\ dCTP \\
\quad + \\
n4\ dTTP
\end{array}
\;
\begin{array}{c}
\text{primer DNA} \\
\text{template DNA} \\
\xrightarrow{\hspace{1.2cm}} \\
Mg^{++}
\end{array}
\quad
\begin{array}{c}
\text{5'-primer DNA-3'} \\[4pt]
\left[
\begin{array}{c}
dAMPn_1 \\
dGMPn_2 \\
dCMPn_3 \\
dTMPn_4
\end{array}
\right]
\end{array}
+ (\Sigma n)\ PPi
$$

Much of the early enzymology of DNA polymerization was described by Kornberg and his collaborators using polymerase I, and it was thought that this enzyme, which represents the largest fraction of polymerase in *E. coli,* was the enzyme involved in in vivo chromosome replication. However, the isolation of mutants *(polA⁻)* which lack polymerase I activity, but which are able to grow in a normal way, prompted a search for other polymerases. These investigations led to the discovery of polymerases II and III, and it is now known that polymerase III is involved in chromosome replication. This conclusion stems from the observation that mutants *(dnaE)* in which chromosomal DNA synthesis is temperature sensitive contain a temperature-sensitive polymerase III but normal polymerases I and II. Significant roles for polymerase I and II are maintained, however, owing to their participation in the process of genetic recombination and in the repair of aberrant DNA. These processes are described in Chapter 8.

Two major problems are evident when considering the specificity of DNA polymerase: (1) in a continuous, semiconservative replication mechanism, how are antiparallel strands of DNA copied by an enzyme which effects elongation in a 5' → 3' direction when one of the strands requires growth in a 3' → 5' direction and (2) how is the absolute requirement for a primer satisfied? The first of these problems was solved when it was discovered, upon examination of DNA gently prepared from cells which had been briefly pulsed with ³H-thymidine, that most of the label was located in short (1,000 to 2,000 nucleotides) pieces (termed Okazaki fragments, after their discoverer), but if the radioactive thymidine was chased with nonradioactive thymidine most of the radioactivity was located in large molecular weight DNA. These data, together with other results of

studies of in vivo DNA replication, reveal that DNA synthesis occurs in a discontinuous manner. The rapidly labeled Okazaki fragments are located at the growing point of the DNA and are subsequently joined to form the characteristic, large DNA molecules (thus explaining the appearance of the chased label in the larger DNA). The second problem, a requirement for a primer in DNA replication, is solved by RNA. It has been shown in some systems, notably DNA viruses, that RNA synthesis is required for the initiation of DNA replication. Also, the short DNA replication intermediates (Okazaki fragments) described above contain RNA at their 5'-OH ends, showing that these fragments are formed by the addition of deoxyribonucleotides to 3'-OH ends of primer RNA. The specificity of known RNA polymerases is consistent with their role in primer synthesis, because they are capable of initiating a template-directed polymerization of ribonucleotides in the absence of a primer.

Ribonuclease H and Polynucleotide Ligase

Owing to the fact that chromosomes are uninterrupted polymers of deoxyribonucleotides, other enzymatic activities are required for the removal of the RNA which serves as primer, for filling the remaining gaps, and for sealing the single-stranded breaks in the incipient daughter strands of DNA. Bacterial cells contain a nuclease which specifically hydrolyzes RNA present in a RNA-DNA hybrid. This enzyme, which is known as ribonuclease H, is thought to serve in removing the RNA used for priming DNA synthesis. The gaps which remain after removal of the polyribonucleotides are filled by the action of DNA polymerase, and the remaining single-stranded break is sealed by the action of polynucleotide ligase. Polynucleotide ligase is specifically involved in sealing single-stranded breaks in DNA molecules, whether in chromosome replication or in the process of genetic recombination (Chap. 8). This enzyme reacts with single-stranded breaks having 5'-phosphoryl and 3'-OH termini in hydrogen-bonded juxtaposition, ie, the damaged strand must be paired with an undamaged, complementary strand at the point of the break. Ligase from *E. coli* requires nicotinamide adenine dinucleotide (NAD) for activity. The reaction proceeds via the adenylylation of the ligase by the AMP moiety of the NAD and the concomitant release of nicotinamide mononucleotide (NMN). The adenylated ligase reacts with the

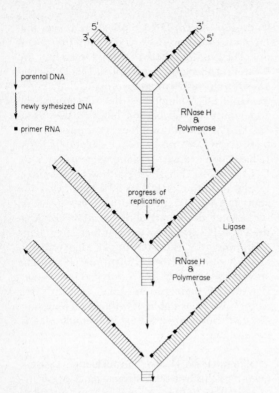

FIG. 7-5. Symmetrical replication of DNA. The sequential synthesis and joining of short pieces of DNA result in the continuous elongation of strands of daughter DNA.

single-stranded break to yield a repaired phosphodiester bond, free enzyme, and AMP. The reaction is represented as follows:

Ligase + NAD → LigaseAMP + NMN
Ligase-AMP + DNA (single-stranded breaks) →
DNA (repaired) + Ligase + AMP

Polynucleotide ligase is indispensable for the viability of *E. coli.* Mutants possessing temperature-sensitive ligase are killed when exposed to a temperature (40C) at which the altered enzyme is inactive. Other polynucleotide ligases have been described which use ATP rather than NAD in the adenylylation reaction; among these are the ligase specified by coliphage T4 and the ligase of animal cells. Figure 7-5 represents the current view of certain aspects of chromosome replication.

Other Aspects of DNA Replication

Double-stranded, helical DNA as a covalently closed circle exists as a supercoil. This conformation introduces additional complexities into consideration of DNA replication and segregation. Superhelicity can be relieved by nucleases which cause single-stranded nicks in the DNA. The action of such a nuclease at the growing point in DNA replication has been invoked to account for unwinding the double helix at its replication point and thereby relieving the torque that would otherwise be imparted to the remaining sections of the DNA molecule during replication. Other proteins which are capable of binding to DNA and facilitating unfolding of DNA have been described. The prototype of such proteins is the gene 32 protein of coliphage T4. The precise manner in which these proteins participate in DNA replication is unknown, and the unwinding problem in DNA replication remains largely unanswered.

Concatameric DNA Structures which contain sequentially joined copies of DNA molecules frequently are produced during the replication of small replicons, such as viral genomes and plasmids. It is thought that these intermediates are produced by an asymmetrical type of DNA replication which is envisioned to occur by the rolling-circle mechanism depicted in Figure 7-6. This model for the production of oligomeric (concatenated) DNA utilizes most of the elements involved in the symmetrical replication described above. Several of the consequences of this mode of DNA replication are described in Chapter 70.

The Membrane and the Replication and Segregation of DNA As was previously mentioned, bacteria do not possess a mitotic apparatus and therefore must have an alternative mechanism to insure the synchronization of daughter chromosome separation and cell division. The solution to this problem is inherent in the observation that the DNA is anchored to the bacterial membrane (Chap. 3). It is also known that DNA synthesis is associated with the membrane. Pulse-labeling experiments employing tritiated thymine have shown that the earliest labeled fraction of DNA is associated with the membrane, and DNA polymerase activity can be recovered from membrane preparations by the use of detergents. The current view of segregation holds that replication of the membrane-attached DNA is followed by separation of the replicas by membrane growth and

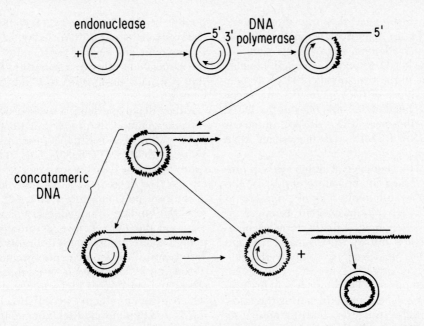

FIG. 7-6. Asymmetrical replication of DNA by the rolling-circle mechanism. One strand of a circular DNA duplex is cleaved by an endonuclease. The 3'-OH border of the single-stranded nick is used as a primer for DNA synthesis which uses the intact strand as template. Processive elongation of the DNA results in the continuous displacement of the plus strand. Initiation of DNA synthesis on the free plus strand (presumably preceded by the action of RNA polymerase to provide a primer) results in the formation of concatenated DNA molecules. This model explains the presence of concatameric DNA as intermediates in the replication of certain viral genomes and plasmids.

that septum formation then occurs near the equatorial plane of the cell, so that each daughter cell receives one-half of the DNA content of the mother cell. The fact that DNA is associated with the cell membrane, together with the rather plausible model for segregation outlined above, requires that with the separation of the newly formed DNA molecule (the chromatids), a new attachment point must be formed on the membrane. There is evidence that at least some replicons specify a membrane protein which forms part of the attachment complex and that synthesis of this protein is required for each round of replication.

DECODING THE CHROMOSOME

The information contained in the chromosome of procaryotic organisms resides in the order of the four nucleotides along its length. Linear arrays of a finite number of nucleotides with discrete beginnings and endings correspond to the hereditary units, the genes. That

the genetic determinants act as discontinuities (particulate) is known from the results of Mendel (segregation and independent assortment). Also, this linear arrangement (linkage) was inferred from the results of *Drosophila* breeding experiments conducted by T. H. Morgan and his students. It should be pointed out, however, that the linearity deduced by the early geneticists may not be topologically related to the simple arrangement of genes along the procaryotic chromosome. Procaryotic chromosomes consist of a single linear DNA molecule, but the eucaryotic chromosome may be a suprastructured composite of many molecules similar to a single procaryotic chromosome.

It is now known that discrete nucleotide sequences on the DNA molecule specify either a complementary molecule of RNA or regions which serve as elements to control the rate at which these molecules are produced. Unlike the DNA of the chromosome, RNA is single-stranded and contains ribose instead of deoxyribose. Also, whereas DNA contains thymine, RNA contains a different pyrimidine, namely uracil. In the process of transcribing DNA sequences into RNA sequences, the adenine, guanine, cytosine, and thymine of one strand of the DNA are paired with uracil, cytosine, guanine, and adenine, respectively, with the result that the RNA formed is complementary to only one of the two strands of DNA. In general, three types of RNA molecules are specified by the nucleotide sequences of the DNA; these are ribosomal RNA (rRNA), aminoacyl transfer RNA (tRNA), and messenger RNA (mRNA).

The primary sequence of amino acids in proteins is governed by the nature of mRNA, and because many different types of proteins, including a variety of enzymes, are required for cellular function, most of the bacterial chromosome specifies mRNA. Ribosomal RNA and tRNA, on the other hand, are employed mechanistically in protein synthesis, and fewer species are required. Therefore, less of the bacterial chromosome is used for storing the information for these structures. The predominating species of RNA in the bacterial cytoplasm is rRNA, because of its rapid rate of synthesis and relative stability. Whereas mRNA is rapidly hydrolyzed, rRNA as well as tRNA are conserved through many generations. The benefits derived from mRNA turnover are underscored upon considering the mechanisms whereby the bacterial cell regulates the synthesis of specific proteins (Chap. 9).

Transcription

The synthesis of the three types of RNA mentioned previously requires the enzyme RNA polymerase, the ribonucleoside triphosphates of adenine, uracil, cytosine, and guanine, and an appropriate DNA template. The polymerization of RNA occurs from the 5'-OH direction, ie, the ribonucleotides are linked by 3'-5'-phosphodiester bonds. The products of the polymerase reaction are polyribonucleotides, which are complementary to a strand of the DNA template, and inorganic pyrophosphate. If a completed RNA molecule is aligned on its DNA template the strands of the resulting duplex will be antiparallel to one another with the 5'-OH end of the RNA at the 3'-OH end of the DNA and vice versa.

RNA polymerase from *E. coli*, as well as from several other organisms, is a complex oligomeric protein consisting of three types of polypeptide chains designated β (MW 155,000), β' (MW 165,000), and α (MW 39,000). In the native enzyme one each of the β and β' subunits are associated with two α subunits; this structure is usually designated as $\beta\beta'\alpha2$ (core polymerase).

Although polymerizing activity resides in the core polymerase, its proper function requires participation of an additional protein known as sigma (σ) factor (MW 86,000). This factor, when combined with the core polymerase, has two effects: (1) it decreases the nonspecific binding of the core polymerase to DNA, and (2) it directs the binding of polymerase to specific regions on the DNA known as promoters (see below) where proper transcription is initiated. Two types of RNA polymerase-promoter complexes can be identified in vitro, those formed at low temperature or high-ionic strength and which are nonproductive in initiating RNA synthesis, and those formed at higher temperatures (25 to 30C) or low-ionic strength and which are productive in initiating RNA synthesis. The latter complex is thought to involve a separation of 6 to 8 nucleotide pairs of the helical DNA within the promoter; it is within this complex that the RNA molecule is initiated with a purine ribonucleotide triphosphate. The addition of the purine ribonucleotide is followed by the release of the sigma factor, which is then free to participate in another initiation event.

The functions of the various subunits of RNA polymerase are not completely understood. It is known, however, that the β' subunit is involved in the binding of RNA polymerase to DNA and that the β subunit is required for interaction with sigma factor. The role of the α subunit is unknown. Although several RNA polymerases have substructures similar to the one from *E. coli*, this structure is not a sine qua non for template-directed RNA synthesis. For example, a DNA-dependent RNA polymerase specified by coliphage T7 consists of a single polypeptide chain (MW 100,000), and the mitochondria of *Neurospora* contain one of MW 86,000.

An additional protein, the rho (ρ) factor, also has been implicated in faithful synthesis of RNA molecules. This factor is involved in termination of RNA synthesis. In vitro studies have shown that the ρ factor causes RNA synthesis to stop at specific sites of the DNA template.

Promoters The rate of elongation of the ribonucleotide chains encoded within the various productive regions of the bacterial chromosome is relatively constant, but the relative abundance of the transcripts varies over a wide range. This apparent discrepancy is explained by the fact that initiation rather than elongation of ribonucleotide chains is the rate-limiting step in RNA synthesis. This means that the sites of initiation, the promoters, vary in their efficiency in directing initiation. For example, in *E. coli*, it is estimated that the rate of initiation of ribosomal RNA is of an order of magnitude greater than that of messenger RNA. Also, mutant strains of bacteria can be selected in which mutations in a promoter region greatly decrease or enhance the rate of initiation of specific mRNA. The nucleotide sequences of several promoter regions have been determined, and certain aspects of their structure are discussed in Chapter 9.

Bipolarity of Information Transfer As was pointed out above, transcript RNA is complementary to one strand of the duplex DNA. One strand of the duplex chromosome does not serve as an exclusive template. In other words, the mRNA corresponding to a given gene may be transcribed from one of the DNA strands, while the mRNA of another gene may be transcribed from the other strand. The DNA is always read in a 3' to 5' direction, and the circular chromosome can therefore be viewed as being transcribed in a clockwise direction for some regions and in a counterclockwise direction for others. When both strands of a genome serve to specify RNA, transcription is said to be "symmetrical;" when RNA is produced exclusively from one strand of the duplex DNA the transcription is termed "asymmetrical." It should be emphasized that regardless of the direction of transcription, the RNA transcribed from a specific region is complementary to only one of the DNA strands of that region.

Polygenic Messenger RNA Bacterial mRNA molecules may contain the information for one or several genes. The genes encoded by polygenic mRNA molecules generally specify functionally related proteins, for example, the enzymes comprising a biosynthetic pathway. The physiologic significance of polygenic mRNA is the unit control of enzyme synthesis provided by this arrangement (Chap. 9).

Processing of RNA

Ribosomal and transfer RNA are derived from larger RNA molecules which represent the primary transcription products. These precursor RNA transcripts are processed by specific ribonucleases to produce the biologically active species which predominate in the bacterial cell.

The nucleotide sequences for 5S, 16S, and 23S ribosomal RNA are contained within a 30S precursor molecule. The 30S precursor apparently is processed very rapidly in vivo because it is undetectable in normal cells. This feature contrasts with the situation in animal cells, where precursor ribosomal RNA is readily detected by pulse-labeling techniques. However, 30S RNA is detectable in mutant strains of *E. coli* deficient in ribonuclease III (RNase III). The in vitro ability of purified RNase III to convert 30S precursor RNA to species of RNA which are similar to 5S, 16S, and 23S RNA supports a role for this nuclease in rRNA maturation. The nuclease activity of RNase III is specific for double-stranded RNA, suggesting that RNase III is an endonuclease which recognizes specific double-stranded regions of RNA. The processing of 30S precursor can be viewed as resulting from hydrolytic cleavage at a specific position caused by secondary structure within the single-stranded RNA. Secondary structure appears to be a common feature of RNA and occurs by hydrogen bonding between complementary regions within the molecule.

Transfer RNA also is processed from large precursor molecules. There are two general classes of precursor molecules, one which contains a single type of tRNA and another in which two or more types of tRNAs may be present. The first class requires removal of extraneous nucleotides from the 3'-OH and 5'-triphosphate ends. The second class, represented by the tRNA^ser-tRNA^thr precursor shown in Figure 7-7, requires an endonucleolytic cleavage to separate the two tRNAs and subsequent processing to remove extraneous nucleotides. Figure 7-7 illustrates the processing of the tandem transcript containing tRNA^ser and tRNA^thr. In the cases of tRNA^ser and tRNA^thr, the structure resulting from nucleolytic cleavage of the precursor contains the 3'-OH terminal sequence-CCA. This sequence is required for the subsequent participation of all tRNA molecules in protein synthesis, since it is this

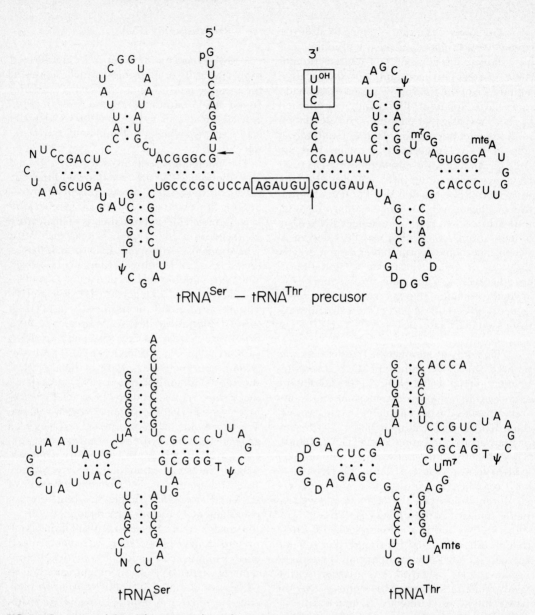

FIG. 7-7. Processing of tRNA. The arrows indicate the points at which RNase P or RNase P$_2$ act to initiate the processing of tRNA from precursor molecules. Subsequent trimming of the molecule is effected by the action of RNase II and possibly other nucleases. Processing of tRNA frequently results in the production of molecules which lack the essential-CCA 3' terminus. This trinucleotide sequence is added by the action of nucleotidyl transferase.

structure that is required for aminoacylation of tRNA. In some cases processing results in the formation of tRNA which does not contain the -CCA terminus. This problem is solved by the action of nucleotidyl transferase which specifically adds the -CCA trinucleotidyl terminus in a stepwise fashion. This enzyme also is involved in repairing damaged tRNA molecules.

Maturation of tRNA molecules involves additional modifications, as described on page 129.

The Genetic Code

The information contained in messenger RNA molecules is translated into the primary structure of proteins, that is, a given nucleotide sequence in mRNA provides a polypeptide chain with a definite sequence of amino acids. Since there are 20 different types of amino acids in proteins and 4 types of nucleotides in mRNA, it is clear that the number of nucleotides required to specify an amino acid must be greater than one. A coding sequence of two nucleotides would produce only 16 (4^2) possible coding combinations, and some of these combinations, or codons, would have to specify more than 1 amino acid. A doublet code would be ambiguous, which contradicts the observation that the amino acid sequence of proteins is stringently controlled. A triplet code, on the other hand, provides for 64 (4^3) combinations of the 4 nucleotides. That codons are, in fact, composed of sequences of 3 nucleotides was first deduced from the following types of experimentation using acridine mutagens. Acridine dyes, such as acridine orange and proflavin, are planar molecules which are capable of intercalating between the stacked bases of the DNA helix. Insertion of these agents in the DNA molecule causes distortions of the helical structure. It is thought that these distortions prevent precise pairing of homologous DNA molecules, so that during the process of genetic recombination (Chap. 8) additions or deletions of bases occur—either of these latter events causes inactivation of the gene product. Bacteriophages are particularly sensitive to mutagenesis by acridines because they undergo extensive recombination during their vegetative growth. In a series of bacteriophage mutants derived through mutagenesis with acridines some will contain deletions and others additions of bases. It has been shown, using the rII region (see complementation, p. 136) of coliphage T4, that some acridine-induced mutations will suppress others (ie, negate their effect) when present in the same gene. In other words two classes of acridine-induced mutations can be identified, designated plus and minus. All plus mutations suppress all minus mutations, but a plus mutation will not suppress another plus mutation, nor will a minus mutation suppress another minus mutation. These results are interpreted to mean that the plus mutations are insertions and the minus mutations deletions; a deletion can negate the effect of an insertion and vice versa. More significant, however, is the observation that two additional deletions can negate a deletion, and two additional

insertions can negate an insertion, but that a − + + or a + − − configuration remains mutant (Fig. 7-8).

The original (and current) interpretation of these results was based on the assumption that the translation of messenger RNA occurs in a polarized fashion and is phased with codon following upon codon. This notion was initially supported by the observation that the growth of polypeptide chains is from the amino terminal to the carboxyl terminal end and that the amino acids are added in a stepwise fashion. Also, the observation that many mutant proteins possess single amino acid replacements suggests that the code is nonoverlapping, since in a completely overlapping triplet code a change in any of the bases would result in a replacement of more than one amino acid (with the exception of the alteration of the first base of an initiating triplet, in which case only one amino acid would be altered). The experimental results described above suggest that the reading of the mRNA at positions following an insertion or a deletion is out of phase because of the change in triplet sequences. The reading phase is restored by introducing additional alterations which restore a meaningful sequence of triplets (Fig. 7-8).

tRNA and Codon Recognition Translation of mRNA into protein requires specific and faithful recognition of the triplet code and expenditure of energy for peptide bond formation. These requirements are fulfilled by tRNA and aminoacyl-tRNA synthetases. The essential role of aminoacyl-tRNA synthetase is twofold: (1) to raise the carboxyl group of the amino acid to an energy level sufficient for peptide bond formation and (2) the esterification of the activated amino acid to its cognate tRNA molecule. The synthesis of aminoacyl-tRNA occurs in a two-step process. First, an adenylate of the amino acid is produced by reaction with ATP, in which enzyme-bound aminoacyl-AMP and free pyrophosphate are formed. The amino acid is then transferred to the ribose moiety of the adenylribonucleotide at the 3′-OH end of the tRNA molecule. The ribose of the terminal nucleotide contains two unsubstituted hydroxyl groups, at the 2′ and at the 3′ position. Analyses of the specificities of aminoacyl-tRNA synthetases using tRNA molecules in which either the 3′OH or 2′OH is blocked by chemical modifica-

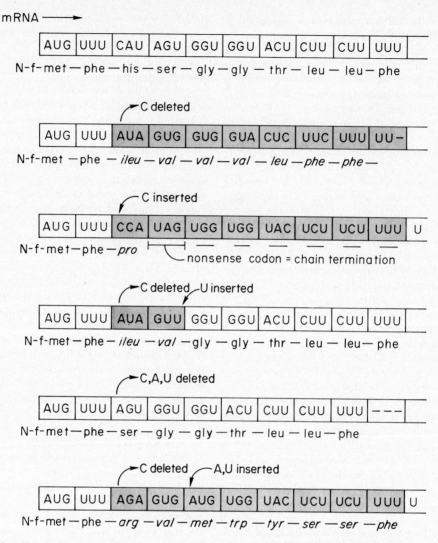

mRNA ——→

AUG | UUU | CAU | AGU | GGU | GGU | ACU | CUU | CUU | UUU

N-f-met — phe — his — ser — gly — gly — thr — leu — leu — phe

C deleted

AUG | UUU | AUA | GUG | GUG | GUA | CUC | UUC | UUU | UU–

N-f-met — phe — *ileu* — *val* — *val* — *val* — *leu* — *phe* — *phe* —

C inserted

AUG | UUU | CCA | UAG | UGG | UGG | UAC | UCU | UCU | UUU | U

N-f-met — phe — *pro* ——— nonsense codon = chain termination

C deleted, U inserted

AUG | UUU | AUA | GUU | GGU | GGU | ACU | CUU | CUU | UUU

N-f-met — phe — *ileu* — *val* — gly — gly — thr — leu — leu — phe

C,A,U deleted

AUG | UUU | AGU | GGU | GGU | ACU | CUU | CUU | UUU | – – –

N-f-met — phe — ser — gly — gly — thr — leu — leu — phe

C deleted   A,U inserted

AUG | UUU | AGA | GUG | AUG | UGG | UAC | UCU | UCU | UUU | U

N-f-met — phe — *arg* — *val* — *met* — *trp* — *tyr* — *ser* — *ser* — *phe*

FIG. 7-8. The effect of deletion and addition on the reading frame of mRNA. The change in reading frame resulting from additions or deletions of bases is illustrated by the shaded areas; the change in the amino acid sequence is depicted below each RNA molecule. The reading frame is restored by further additions or deletions. The meaning of the message is maintained only when the total number of bases deleted or inserted is equal to three. These results indicate that three bases are required to specify each amino acid. Note in the third example that the insertion of a single base generates a nonsense codon which causes polypeptide chain termination (p. 135).

tion reveal that some synthetases esterify amino acid to tRNA using the 3'OH, whereas others use the 2'OH. This discrimination is inconsequential for subsequent mRNA-directed, ribosome-mediated peptide bond formation, because this process requires tautomerization of the ester between the 3'OH and 2'OH positions. The significant property of aminoacyl-tRNA synthetases is that their specificity ensures the proper union of amino acid and tRNA.

Once the amino acid is attached to its adaptor tRNA molecule, it acts passively, and the specificity of the translation process resides only in the tRNA. An early observation to support this view is that if, in an in vitro protein-synthesizing system, cysteinyl-tRNA is catalytically reduced so as to remove the -SH group but leaving the amino acid alanine attached to the tRNA, alanine is incorporated into polypeptide chains where cysteine normally is found. This type of experiment conclusively illustrates the adaptor role for tRNA in protein synthesis.

The Structure of tRNA Transfer RNA molecules range from 73 to 93 nucleotides in length. Their small size and relative ease of purification have made possible a description of the nucleotide sequence of many of these important molecules. The results of sequence analysis reveal that the linear structure can be folded by virtue of hydrogen bonding to provide secondary structure. Analysis of the base composition of tRNAs reveals the existence of rare nucleotides, and it is now known that these represent posttranscriptional modifications of either the bases or the ribose portions of the usual four nucleosides found in RNA. A list of modified nucleosides is presented in Table 7-1.

Nucleotide composition and sequence data led to the conceptualization of tRNA molecules as shown in Figure 7-9A. Five domains (cloverleaf structure) which are common to all tRNA molecules are evident. The aminoacyl arm contains the -CCA-3'OH terminal sequence common to all tRNA molecules. The T arm contains the sequence thymidine-pseudouridine-cytosine, which is common to all tRNAs and probably represents the 50S ribosome-binding site, owing to its interaction with ribosomal 5S RNA. The anticodon arm contains the trinucleotide sequence which is complementary to mRNA-contained codons.

The D arm contains dihydrouracil, which is common to all tRNAs. The composition of the V or variable arm differs among tRNA molecules.

The cloverleaf representation of tRNA has been modified following x-ray crystallographic studies. These studies, which revealed a tertiary structure in the tRNA molecule, resulted in the representation depicted in Figure 7-9B. This picture, which represents a more precise orientation of the domains within the tRNA molecule, will aid further exploration of how these molecules interact with aminoacyl-tRNA synthetases and how they participate in protein synthesis.

Codon Assignments As previously pointed out, a triplet code of the 4 nucleotides provides for 64 possible combinations. Two approaches have been used to determine which codons correspond to each amino acid. One approach utilizes a cell-free protein-synthesizing system consisting of ribosomes, radioactively labeled amino acids, transfer RNA, an energy source, the necessary enzymes, and synthetic polyribonucleotides. The first code word was deciphered by Nirenberg and Matthei, who demonstrated that polyuridylic acid, when added to such a system, directed the synthesis of polyphenylalanine. The conclusion from this observation was that the code for phenylalanine is UUU. It was subsequently shown that polyadenylic acid and polycytidylic

TABLE 7-1 MODIFIED NUCLEOSIDES*

I	Inosine	s^2m^5U	2-thio-5-methyl uridine
m^1I	1-methyl inosine	V	5-oxyacetic acid uridine
m^1A	1-methyl adenosine	s^2am^5U	2-thio-5-acetic acid methyl ester uridine
m^2A	2-methyl adenosine	s^2cm^5U	2-thio-5-carboxymethyl uridine
m^6A	N^6-methyl adenosine	cmm^5U	5-carboxymethyl uridine methyl ester
i^6A	N^6-isopentenyl adenosine	cm^5U	5-carboxymethyluridine
ms^2i^6A	2-methylthio-N^6-isopentenyl adenosine	Um	2'-O-methyl uridine
t^6A	N^6-(N-threonylcarbonyl) adenosine	ψm	2'-O-methyl pseudouridine
m^1G	1-methyl guanosine	mam^5s^2U	5-methylaminomethyl-2-thiouridine
		X	3-(3-amino-3-carboxypropyl) uridine
m^2G	N^2-methyl guanosine	s^2m^5C	2-thio-5-methyl cytidine
m^2_2G	N^2-dimethyl guanosine	s^2C	2-thiocytidine
m^7G	N^7-methyl guanosine	Cm	2'-O-methyl cytidine
Gm	2'-O-methyl guanosine	ac^4C	N^4-acetyl cytidine
T	(ribo) Thymidine	m^3C	N^3-methyl cytidine
Ψ	Pseudouridine (5-ribofuranosyl uracil)	m^5C	5-methyl cytidine
D or hU	5,6-dihydrouridine		
s^4U	4-thiouridine		

After Kim: Prog Nucleic Acid Res Mol Biol 17:181, 1976
Modified nucleosides found as minor components in tRNA molecules. The biologic role of most of these modification is unknown.

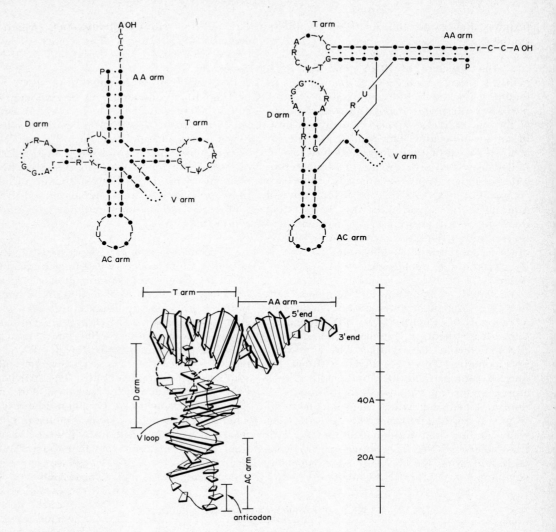

FIG. 7-9. The structure of transfer RNA. Sequence analysis of tRNA shows that the molecule can possess secondary structure maintained by intramolecular hydrogen bonding; the cloverleaf configuration is depicted above. The solid circles in the figure represent nucleotides which are generally variable among various tRNA molecules, the letters r and y indicate positions which are usually occupied, respectively, by purine and pyrimidine, R and Y indicate positions invariably occupied, respectively, by purine and pyrimidine, H indicates the position usually occupied by a modified nucleoside. X-ray crystallographic studies reveal additional structure and suggest the rearrangement of the relative position of the domains as depicted at the upper left. A three-dimensional representation of the tRNA molecule is shown on the left. (Courtesy of Dr. S. H. Kim)

acid specify polylysine and polyproline, respectively. (Polyguanidylic acid was inactive in the system; it forms multistranded helices because of hydrogen bonding and consequently will not bind to ribosomes.)

Similar approaches led to the tentative assignment of other codons and their amino acids. By using varying proportions of any two bases and the enzyme polyribonucleotide phosphorylase, polymer products with varying

degrees of enrichment for the bases can be synthesized and tested for directing polymerization of the various amino acids. The results of these experiments led to the tentative identification of many of the triplet codons. A more precise assignment of codons, based upon a technique developed by Nirenberg and Leder, involves the immobilization of aminoacyl-tRNA-triplet-ribosome complexes on nitrocellulose membranes. This technique is based on

TABLE 7-2   NUCLEOSIDE SEQUENCES OF RNA CODONS AND CORRESPONDING AMINO ACIDS

1st Base	2nd Base				3rd Base
	U	C	A	G	
U	Phe	Ser	Tyr	Cys	U
	Phe	Ser	Tyr	Cys	C
	Leu	Ser	Ochre*	*	A
	Leu	Ser	Amber*	Trp	G
C	Leu	Pro	His	Arg	U
	Leu	Pro	His	Arg	C
	Leu	Pro	Gln	Arg	A
	Leu	Pro	Gln	Arg	G
A	Ileu	Thr	Asn	Ser	U
	Ileu	Thr	Asn	Ser	C
	Ileu	Thr	Lys	Arg	A
	Met	Thr	Lys	Arg	G
G	Val	Ala	Asp	Gly	U
	Val	Ala	Asp	Gly	C
	Val	Ala	Glu	Gly	A
	Val	Ala	Glu	Gly	G

From Crick: Cold Spring Harbor Symp Quant Biol 31:1, 1966
*Nonsense codon

the observation that codon-anticodon recognition (association) is stabilized in the presence of ribosomes. This procedure employs triplets of known sequence, the syntheses of which were pioneered by Khorana and his co-workers, in a cell-free system containing ribosomes and different tRNA molecules bearing radioactively labeled amino acids. Using such a system it was demonstrated that UUU binds only phenylalanyl-tRNA, UUA binds only leucyl-tRNA, and so forth. The codon assignments of the 64 triplets, using this technique, are shown in Table 7-2.

These results show that the genetic code is degenerate in that each amino acid (with the exception of tryptophan) has more than one codon. It should be pointed out that if the cell contains the 61 different tRNA molecules, each one able to accept the amino acid which is cognate to its anticodon, mechanistically no degeneracy exists in the code, and although many more than 20 tRNA molecules have been separated by various techniques, it remains to be seen if any cell contains all 61 tRNAs. An alternate explanation of the apparent degeneracy is that proposed by Crick (the wobble hypothesis), which supposes that the first two positions of the triplet codon on messenger RNA pair precisely with the anticodon on tRNA, but pairing of the third position may be ambiguous accord-

ing to the nucleotide present at this position. For example, G at the third position of the anticodon may pair with U or C, U may pair with A or G, and so forth. The principle of the third position ambiguity also provides a mechanism that would protect the organism from certain mutational alterations in this position.

Three codons, UAG, UAA, and UGA* do not code for amino acids because tRNA molecules with corresponding anticodons normally do not exist. When these codons exist in a mRNA molecule, polypeptide chain growth terminates as described on page 135. These codons serve as translation termination signals.

Colinearity of the Gene and Its Products

Consideration of the colinearity of the gene, the mRNA which it specifies, and the sequence of amino acids in the ensuing polypeptide chain is an important prelude to a dis-

*The codons UAG, UAA, and UGA frequently are termed amber, ochre, and opal, respectively. The reason for this nomenclature is trivial but humanistic and is related on page 167 of Cairns J, Stent G S, Watson J D (eds): Phage and the Origin of Molecular Biology. Cold Spring Harbor Laboratory of Quantitative Biology, 1966.

cussion of the translation of mRNA into protein. Several lines of evidence now exist which prove that colinearity follows from the nucleotide sequence of the gene. The homology which exists between the DNA template and its product mRNA has been discussed above and is proved by the experimental demonstration that mRNA hybridizes only to the DNA which serves as template for its synthesis. The colinearity of the gene and its protein product was first inferred from the combined data of genetics and protein chemistry. For example, Yanofsky and his co-workers have carefully mapped the positions of a number of mutations in the structural gene for the A polypeptide chain of the tryptophan synthetase enzyme of *E. coli* and have correlated these map positions with the position of amino acid replacements in the polypeptide chain. Figure 7-10 illustrates how the original genetic data correlate with the sequence analysis. These assignments have been verified by the use of more recent RNA-sequencing techniques which show that amino acid substitutions in mutated proteins correspond precisely to nucleotide replacements in mRNA.

Translation of mRNA

The translation of mRNA is effected by a number of highly integrated reactions which insure that the genetic code is read with fidelity. It is known that mRNA translation requires, in addition to ribosomes and tRNA molecules, a number of protein factors and the nucleotide triphosphate, GTP. The role played by these various elements in protein synthesis is known in some detail, but the precise molecular mechanism of their action remains obscure.

All proteins are synthesized by a common mechanism, and the nature of the product is stringently specified by mRNA. It is this principle which separates the synthesis of protein from that of the relatively small polypeptides, such as certain antibiotics. In this latter case, amino acid sequences are governed by enzymes which are able to recognize amino acids and relatively small peptides as specific substrates for the formation of peptide bonds, ie, the short amino acid sequences of these peptides are not template directed but are the products of enzyme specificity. It should be clear, even with genetic considerations aside, that a large protein molecule is not synthesized by this mechanism because the number of enzymes involved would be prohibitive. The process by which ribosomes, aminoacyl-tRNA, and the various protein factors participate in mRNA-directed protein synthesis, although complex, nonetheless provides an efficient machinery relative to the task accomplished.

Messenger RNA is translated in a $5'-OH$ to $3'$-OH direction, and amino acids are added one at a time so that the polypeptide chain

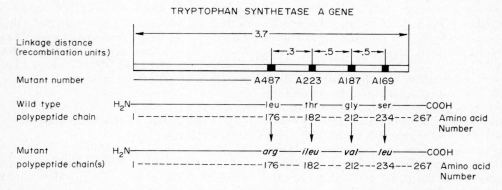

FIG. 7-10. Colinearity of a gene and its polypeptide product. In order to establish the colinearity of a gene and its polypeptide product a number of mutations are carefully mapped by recombination analysis. The positions of the mutations are then correlated with the positions of the amino acid replacements in the pertinent polypeptide chain. The gene on the *E. coli* chromosome which specifies the primary structure of the typtophan synthetase A protein is 3.7 recombinational units in length; the A protein contains 267 amino acids. The figure depicts the relative locations of a series of mutations in the A gene and the position of the amino acid replacement in the A protein. The genetic measurement which represents the frequency of recombination between the various mutants correlates well with the position of the ensuing amino acid replacement. Results with this system have been expanded to include over 20 such substitutions, many of which have been correlated with base changes in mutant mRNA.

grows from the amino terminal to carboxyl terminal residue. Protein synthesis proceeds in three consecutive phases, namely, initiation, elongation, and termination (Fig. 7-11).

Initiation Knowledge of the sequential growth of polypeptide chains, coupled with the observation that a large fraction of the total protein of bacterial cells contains methionine as the amino terminal amino acid, suggested that the initiation of protein synthesis occurs by a unique reaction. The discovery of N-formylmethionine (fMet) and its implication in the initiation of protein synthesis subsequently led to a clarification of this process, and it is now

thought that all proteins in procaryotic organisms are initiated with N-formylmethionine. The lack of formyl groups on some amino terminal methionyl residues and the observation that amino terminal acids other than methionine are found on some proteins of procaryotes reflect the activity of deformylases and aminopeptidases which act on these proteins after they are synthesized.

The initial step in protein synthesis in procaryotic cells is the formation of a complex consisting of mRNA, 30S ribosomes, and fMet-tRNA. At least three protein initiation factors and the codon AUG or GUG are required in this process. The initiation factors, known as

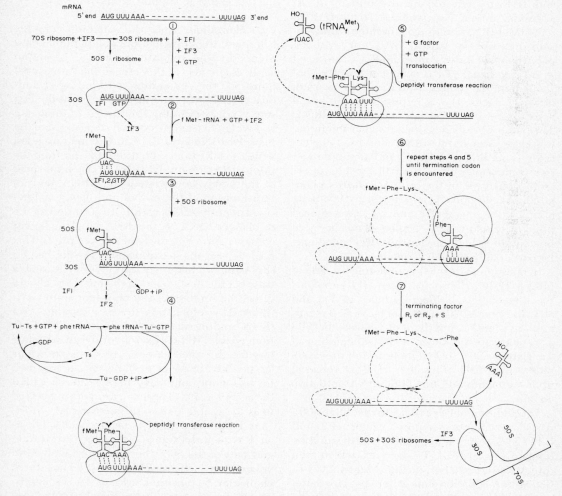

FIG. 7-11. Messenger RNA-directed protein synthesis. The details of the steps depicted are presented in the text. Steps 1 through 3 represent formation of the initiation complex, steps 4 and 5 represent elongation, and steps 6 and 7 represent termination.

IF1, IF2, and IF3, have been highly purified and characterized. IF1 is a small (MW 9,000), basic protein, IF2 is an acidic protein (MW 65,000), and IF3 is a basic protein (MW 29,000). All of these factors apparently are composed of single polypeptide chains and can be eluted from ribosomes with high ionic strength buffers.

The precise role of the initiation factors is not known. However, in vitro studies with natural and synthetic mRNAs have permitted a partial description of their function. The formation of the mRNA-30S-ribosome-fMET-tRNA complex occurs in two steps: (1) the binding of mRNA to a 30S ribosome, followed by (2) the binding of fMet-tRNA. It appears as if factors IF1 and IF3 are required for the initial mRNA-ribosome interaction, whereas factor IF2 directs fMet-tRNA binding. When the trinucleoside diphosphate ApUpG (AUG) or synthetic polyribonucleotides containing AUG are used as mRNA, factor IF1 is sufficient for 30S ribosome binding. When natural mRNA is used, however, factor IF3 is required for the initial reaction between 30S ribosomes and mRNA. This latter observation suggests that the initiation region of natural mRNA consists of nucleotides in addition to AUG. Added support for this contention comes from the results of sequence analysis of the mRNA from RNA-containing bacteriophages, where at least 90 nucleotides from the 5′-OH end are encountered prior to the first AUG triplet. Some of these nucleotides which border the AUG codon may be part of an initiation sequence.

In addition to its role in promoting binding of mRNA to 30S ribosomes, factor IF3 promotes the dissociation of 70S ribosomes to 50S and 30S ribosomes. This ability of factor IF3 is particularly significant in light of the facts that 70S ribosomes are produced at the completion of translation and that initiation requires 30S rather than 70S ribosomes. IF3 is released upon formation of the 30S-mRNA initiation complex.

The addition of fMet-tRNA to the mRNA-30S ribosome complex requires factor IF2 and GTP. This reaction apparently is preceded by formation of an IF2-GTP complex, which then directs the association of the fMet-tRNA with the mRNA-30S ribosome complex. This latter reaction does not require the hydrolysis of GTP, since complex formation also occurs in the presence of 5′-guanylylmethylenediphos-phonate, a GTP analog which is unable to undergo enzymatic hydrolysis. The terminal step in the initiation process is the addition of the 50S ribosome subunit to the mRNA-30S-ribosome-fMet-tRNA complex. This final step is accompanied by the release of factors IF1 and IF2 and the hydrolysis of GTP to GDP and iP by a GTPase activity which is associated with the IF2 factor. The hydrolysis of GTP at this point is presumably accompanied by a conformational change in the initiation complex which prepares it for participation in the elongation process. This view is supported by the observation that if 5′-guanylylmethylenediphosphonate is used in place of GTP in forming the initiation complex, the resulting complex is unable to support elongation.

Elongation   Once the initiation complex is formed, the growth of the polypeptide chain occurs by the repetitive addition of amino acids. Each step in this elongation process requires (1) the codon-directed binding of aminoacyl-tRNA to a binding site, which at the first step is adjacent to the fMet-tRNA binding site and which in each successive step is next to the peptidyl-tRNA site, (2) peptide bond formation which results from a peptidyl transfer from the fMet-tRNA or peptidyl-tRNA to the amino acid of the newly bound aminoacyl-tRNA, and (3) translocation of the mRNA and newly synthesized peptidyl-tRNA to the site occupied by the discharged tRNA (ie, the tRNA which no longer contains formylmethionine or peptide). This final step results in expulsion of the discharged tRNA and orientation of the ribosome in such a way that the next codon in the mRNA is able to direct the binding of the pertinent aminoacyl-tRNA. This elongation process identifies two tRNA-binding sites on the ribosome: The site from which fMet-tRNA or peptidyl-tRNA transfers the esterified carboxyl group is known as the peptidyl or donor site, and the site to which the incoming aminocyl-tRNA binds is called the acceptor site. (These are frequently referred to as the P and A sites, respectively.)

At least three protein factors and GTP, as well as peptidyl transferase, which is an integral part of the 50S ribosome, are involved in polypeptide chain elongation. The three elongation factors are known as Tu, Ts, and G. The T designation derives from the role these factors play in transferring aminoacyl-tRNA from the cytoplasm to the mRNA-ribosome complex. The Tu and Ts designations derive from the heat stability of the factors (unstable and stable, respectively). The G designation stems from a GTPase activity of the G factor. The Tu (MW 40,000) and Ts (MW 19,000) factors associate avidly; they purify and crystallize as a unit. In vitro studies have shown that the Tu-Ts complex reacts with GTP and aminoacyl-tRNA to form a Tu-aminoacyl-tRNA-GTP complex, which in turn reacts with either the initiation complex or a complex undergoing chain elongation. At this point the aminoacyl-tRNA binds to the acceptor site on the mRNA-ribosome complex, resulting in the release of Tu-GDP and iP. The Tu-Ts complex is regenerated by the displacement of GDP by Ts (Fig. 7-11, step 4). The role of GTP in this process is obscure. However, it is known that 5'-guanylylmethylenediphosphonate can replace GTP and promote transfer of aminoacyl-tRNA to the protein-synthesizing complex. In this latter case, the analog and Tu remain bound to the complex and subsequent peptide bond formation is prevented.

Addition of the aminoacyl-tRNA to the acceptor site is immediately followed by peptide bond formation between the esterified carboxyl group of the formylmethionine or the growing peptide chain of the tRNA at the donor site and the amino group of the amino acid bound by the tRNA at the acceptor site. This process results in occupancy of the donor site by a discharged tRNA and peptidyl-tRNA at the acceptor site. As mentioned above, the enzyme (peptidyl transferase) that effects peptide bond formation is part of the 50S ribosome. It should be emphasized that peptide bond formation, at this stage, does not require the expenditure of energy, since the esterified carboxyl group at the donor site is at a sufficiently high energy level to participate in group transfer. This is verified by the observation that isolated 50S ribosomes in the presence of 33 percent ethanol will catalyze peptide bond formation between aminoacyl-tRNAs in the absence of mRNA, 30S ribosomes, and GTP. The role of the ethanol is thought to expose or orient the peptidyl transferase so that it is active in the absence of the other components.

Following peptide bond formation and prior to the addition of the next aminoacyl-tRNA to the protein-synthesizing complex, the aminoacyl-tRNA acceptor site must be vacated and properly oriented with respect to the next co-don in the mRNA. These events are carried out by a simultaneous translocation of both the mRNA and the peptidyl-tRNA by a process which requires G factor and GTP. G factor possesses a potent GTPase activity which is manifested only in the presence of ribosomes, and it is thought that the presence of G factor as well as the hydrolysis of GTP are necessary for translocation. The G factor-GDP complex is released from the translation apparatus following translocation. Experiments with both synthetic and natural mRNA have shown that G factor and GTP hydrolysis are required for the recognition of the third and subsequent codons. In other words, the synthesis of mRNA-encoded peptides ceases at the dipeptide level in the absence of G factor and GTP.

Termination The process of polypeptide chain elongation described above results in a constant association of tRNA-attached growing polypeptide chain with the mRNA-ribosome complex. This process demands a mechanism for termination which results in the cessation of polypeptide chain growth, as well as in release of the tRNA from the carboxyl terminus of the polypeptide chain. It is known that termination is caused by information encoded in the mRNA and by protein release factors. Three codons, UAA, UAG, and UGA, for which there normally are no tRNA species with corresponding anticodons and which consequently do not serve to specify amino acids in polypeptide chains, serve as efficient termination signals. Two release factors (R1 and R2) act in conjunction with nonsense codons to effect release of the polypeptide chain. R1 acts in conjunction with either UAA or UAG, and R2 with UAA or UGA. Employing a system consisting of the triplet AUG, fMet-tRNA, and ribosomes it can be demonstrated that the triplets UAA, UAG, or UGA, in the presence of the appropriate release factor R1 or R2, cause the release of free formylmethionine from ribosomes. An additional factor, S, acts in conjunction with R1 and R2 to facilitate release. This factor has no release activity by itself but increases the affinity of the terminating codons in the release process.

Evidence exists which suggests that peptidyl transferase may be involved in the release process. For example, antibiotics that inhibit peptidyl transferase also inhibit the release reaction, and in the presence of 20 percent ethanol, formylmethionine is released from fMet-tRNA-AUG-ribosome complex in the presence of only R factor, ie, the termination codons are not required. Furthermore, it has been shown that the codon immediately preceding a terminating codon must be translated prior to release. This latter observation suggests that the peptide to be released must be esterified to tRNA which is at the peptidyl donor site, precisely the place where it acts as substrate for peptidyl transferase, and that the terminating codon must be in register at the acceptor site on the ribosome. One view of the role of peptidyl transferase in termination is that R factor converts peptidyl transferase into a hydrolase, which then transfers the peptidyl group of peptidyl-tRNA to water instead of to the amino group of the adjacent aminoacyl-tRNA.

Specificity Initiating of Codons As described above, the codons AUG and GUG are able to promote the formation of fMet-tRNA initiation complexes. In other words, AUG and GUG, when at initiating positions of the mRNA, code for fMet-tRNA. It is known that when these codons (AUG and GUG) are located at internal positions in an mRNA molecule, they code for methionine and valine, respectively, and the question arises as to how ambivalence in the specificity of these codons at initiating and internal positions is avoided. This problem is solved by the specificity of the T factors involved in the elongation process. Two types of methionine-accepting tRNA molecules are present in the cell, and the methionine of one of these tRNA molecules is able to be formylated whereas the methionine of the other is not, ie, the formylating enzyme recognizes only one type of methionyl-tRNA molecule. Conversely, the T factors of elongation will not form a complex with the fMet-tRNA but will with the Met-tRNA which is unable to be formylated. This lack of recognition by T factor insures that only the nonformylated Met-tRNA binds to the ribosome mRNA acceptor site when an internal AUG is encountered. The same situation applies to the internal GUG codon and valyl-tRNA.

An additional question that arises is: Why doesn't spurious initiation occur at internally positioned AUG or GUG codons? This question is answered by the extraneous nucleotides which precede the initiating triplet in mRNA. It is known that this untranslated region represents ribosome-binding sites; internal AUG and GUG codons lack this neighboring structure.

The Ribosome Cycle As pointed out above, protein synthesis involves an initial interaction of mRNA and 30S ribosomes followed by the production of mRNA-associated 70S ribosomes as a consequence of the addition of 50S ribosomes. In the course of the translation of an mRNA molecule, new initiation complexes are formed before the first 70S ribosome traverses the entire length of the mRNA molecule. This process of repetitive initiation results in the formation of polysomes, ie, mRNA molecules to which several 70S ribosomes are attached. Ribosomes are released from mRNA as 70S particles. The dissociation of 70S ribosomes to 30S and 50S ribosomal subunits occurs by the ribosome-dissociating activity of IF3; this process maintains an adequate pool of the particles which are reused for additional rounds of translation (Fig. 7-11).

Posttranslational Events and Complementation

It is evident from the foregoing discussion that the order of trinucleotides in mRNA governs the primary structure of proteins. However, the physiologic properties of these proteins, whether enzymatic or structural, always depend upon a secondary (folding of peptide chains governed by noncovalent interactions such as hydrophobic and coulombic forces) and frequently tertiary (covalent bonds other than peptide bonds, eg, disulfide bonds) and quaternary (subunit association) structure.

The folding of polypeptide chains, which imparts the proper conformation to biologically active proteins, occurs, for the most part, as a spontaneous process. In other words, the primary structure or sequence of amino acids directs the folding of the polypeptide chain. In vitro studies have shown that enzymes which are completely unfolded by chaotropic agents, such as guanidine hydrochloride plus reducing agents, upon removal of the denaturant will spontaneously refold with a high degree of fidelity to yield the native protein. Also, experiments have been performed which show that oligomeric proteins will faithfully form from subunits even when present with an excess of heterologous subunits.

Polypeptide chains frequently are folded in such a way that portions of the resulting structure possess discrete functions; these regions within polypeptide chains are known as domains. One of the premiere examples of a protein which possesses functionally discrete sections is immunoglobulin, in which portions of the molecule which contain antigen-binding sites are functionally distinct from that section of the antibody involved in other reactions, such as binding to cell surfaces and fixation of complement (Fig. 13-11).

The foregoing observations suggest that once the polypeptide chain is synthesized, it is removed from further genetic influence. This contention is, for the most part, true, although epigenetic modification of proteins can alter their physiologic function (Chap. 9). This relative separation of activity and genetic determination forms the basis for one of the most significant genetic tools, namely, complementation. Genetic complementation is frequently employed to determine whether or not mutants with the same phenotype lack the same function. For example, two bacterial mutants may be unable to synthesize a certain end product, and since the specific biosynthetic pathway may be composed of several different enzymes, the question arises as to whether or not the same enzyme is lacking in each mutant strain. Complementation analysis readily answers this question. If the genetic information from one of the organisms is introduced into the other organism (by use of the methods of gene transfer described in Chap 8) and the resulting diploid organism regains the ability to synthesize the end product, it may be concluded that the two mutations are located in regions of distinct genetic function. On the other hand, if inability to synthesize the end product persists in the diploid, it may be concluded that the two mutations affect the same unit of genetic function. In the first case cited above, it is obvious that the genetic information of the two organisms is complementary, each supplying the function which the other lacks.

In a case such as the biosynthetic pathway mentioned above, the complementation pattern can usually be verified by enzymatic analysis. However, in other situations, where the number and nature of elements participating in a given function are unknown, complementa-

tion analysis can reveal at least the number of genes involved in the process. The *rII* region of coliphage T4 is an excellent and classical exemplar of the latter case. Mutants bearing lesions in the *rII* locus are able to infect but are unable to grow in *E. coli* K12; however, they can grow in *E. coli* B. Benzer, who made what is considered one of the most refined genetic analyses of a single genetic region using this system, showed that simultaneous infection with certain pairs of phage mutants permitted growth of the virus, whereas infection with other pairs did not. Furthermore, he showed that this complementation occurred only when the two mutations resided on different phage genomes (ie, in the *trans* position). The same mutations, when located on a single genome (ie, in the *cis* position) did not show complementation (Fig. 7-12). This *cis-trans* test shows that the rII region is composed of two distinct regions of function. These two complementation groups are designated A and B. Therefore, *rIIA* and *rIIB* each code for a polypeptide, both of which are required for growth of phage T4 in E. coli K12.

The two examples cited above represent cases of interallelic complementation which results from the replacement of aberrant gene products with functionally active gene products. It should be pointed out that whereas complementation analysis can be used to determine the number of genes which participate in a given phenotypic expression, conclusions employing this principle must be tempered by the fact that, in certain cases, two different mutations affecting the same gene, when in the *trans* position, can restore the activity of the gene product. This phenomenon is known as intraallelic complementation and usually occurs where the active gene product is oligomeric. For example, an enzyme may be active only when the subunit specified by the gene is associated with others of its kind. A mutation may occur which causes a change to a conformation which is incompatible with enzyme activity. However, upon associating with another mutationally altered subunit with a different incompatible conformation, the respective restraints may be cancelled to produce an active enzyme. This type of complementation is depicted in Figure 7-13.

The genetic complementation tests described above are known as *cis-trans* analyses. Genetic regions which show complementation

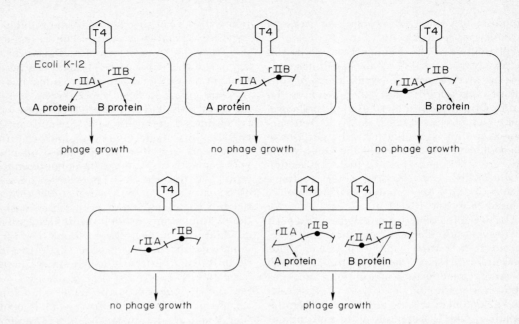

FIG. 7-12. Interallelic complementation. This figure depicts the results of a typical cis-trans analysis using the *rll* region of coliphage T4. In this test *E. coli* K12 is simultaneously infected with pairs of mutant strains of T4 bearing mutations in the rll region. Growth of the phage occurs only when the two mutations are located in regions of different genetic function. Two transcomplementing mutations when in the cis position (on the same chromosome) do not complement one another, thus illustrating that it is not the two mutations per se which permit growth of the phage but rather the presence of nonmutated alleles.

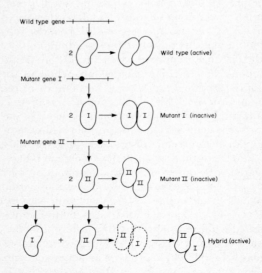

FIG. 7-13. Intraallelic complementation. The protein shown is active only in the dimeric state. The mutant protomers alone are unable to produce functional dimers. The hybrid dimers are active because the two types of mutant protomers mutually correct each other.

when aberrations are oriented in the trans position (ie, on different DNA molecules) are known as cistrons. The terms cistron and gene are not synonymous, and it is evident from the above discussion that cistrons can be genes or parts of genes.

Protein Synthesis in Eucaryotic Cells

Consideration of protein synthesis in eucaryotic cells, as the features of this process differ from that in procaryotic cells, is useful for the strategic development of antimicrobial agents, as well as for understanding possible mechanisms of pathogenesis. The basic features of protein synthesis are similar in the two classes of organisms, but differences do exist among the various elements involved. The cytoplasmic ribosomes of eucaryotic cells are different from those of procaryotes. They are typically larger, the monosome having a sedimentation coefficient of 80S and being composed of a 60S and a 40S ribosome. The 60S and 40S ribosomes of eucaryotes are analogous to the 50S and 30S ribosomes of procaryotic cells. Initiation of protein synthesis in eucaryotic cells requires the codons AUG or GUG. In contrast to procaryotic cells, however, methionine rather than N-formylmethionine is the initiating amino acid. Eucaryotic cells contain two types of methionine-accepting tRNA molecules; one is analogous to the fMet-tRNA of procaryotes in that it is used for initiation, whereas the other is used for reading internal AUG triplets. The functional analogy between the fMet-tRNA of procaryotic cells and the initiating Met-tRNA of eucaryotic cells is amplified by the observation that extracts of *E. coli* can formylate the initiating tRNA of certain eucaryotes which themselves lack the pertinent formylase activity. Also, when formylated, the initiating Met-tRNA of eucaryotic cells is active in bacterial initiation. Formation of the initiation complex in eucaryotes requires three protein factors which appear to function in a manner similar to the IF1, IF2, and IF3 of procaryotes.

Polypeptide chain elongation in eucaryotes proceeds in a manner similar to that in procaryotes. Peptidyl transferase is an integral part of the 60S ribosome, and two elongation factors, T1 and T2, and GTP are required. The T1 factor is analogous to the T factor of procaryotic cells, and it forms a complex with GTP and aminoacyl-tRNA to direct aminoacyl-tRNA binding to ribosomes. Unlike the T factor of procaryotes, T1 has not been resolved into two different proteins (viz, Tu and Ts). T factor can substitute for T1 in directing the binding of aminoacyl-tRNA to eucaryotic ribosomes, but T1 cannot substitute for T in a procaryotic system. The T2, or translocation, factor is functionally analogous to the procaryotic G factor; T2 appears to be functional only with 80S ribosomes and G only with 70S ribosomes. The termination of polypeptide chain synthesis in eucaryotes is thought to occur by a mechanism which is similar to that in procaryotes.

The foregoing outline of protein synthesis in eucaryotes pertains to this process as it occurs in the cytoplasm. It is known that the elements of protein synthesis in plastids such as mitochondria are more similar to the bacterial system than to the eucaryotic cytoplasmic system. For example, mitochondrial ribosomes are 70 S, initiation occurs with fMet-tRNA, and T factor can be separated into components similar to Tu and Ts.

The contrasts that exist between protein synthesis in procaryotic and eucaryotic cells suggest that agents ought to exist which selectively perturb this process in either type of cell. That selective toxicity does exist is illustrated in Chapter 10, where many antibiotics are described which act preferentially at some specific point in procaryotic protein synthesis. The selective inhibition of protein synthesis ought to occur in the opposite direction, ie, agents should exist which inhibit eucaryotic protein synthesis but which have little or no effect on procaryotes. One well-described protein which is elicited by a bacterium and which selectively blocks protein synthesis in eucaryotic cells is the toxin produced by *Corynebacterium diphtheriae;* the mode of action of this toxin is described in Chapter 33.

FURTHER READING

Books and Reviews

Altman S: Biosynthesis of transfer RNA in *Escherichia coli.* Cell 4:21, 1975

Chamberlin MJ: The selectivity of transcription. Annu Rev Biochem 43:721, 1974

Davis BD: Role of subunits in the ribosome cycle. Nature 231:153, 1971

Gefter ML: DNA replication. Annu Rev Biochem 44:45, 1975

The Genetic Code. Cold Spring Harbor Symp Quant Biol 31:1, 1966

Haselkorn R, Rothman-Denes LB: Protein synthesis. Annu Rev Biochem 42:397, 1973

Kim SH: Three-dimensional structure of transfer RNA. Prog Nucleic Acid Res Mol Biol 17:181, 1976

Kornberg A: DNA Synthesis. San Francisco, W. H. Freeman and Co, 1974

Watson JD: Molecular Biology of the Gene, 2nd ed New York, Benjamin, 1970

Selected Papers

Adams JM, Capecchi MR: N-formylmethioninyl-sRNA as the initiator of protein synthesis. Proc Natl Acad Sci USA 55:147, 1966

Anfinsen CB, Haber E: Studies on the reduction and reformation of protein disulfide bonds. J Biol Chem 236: 1361, 1961

Benzer S: The elementary units of heredity. In McElroy WD, Glass B (eds): The Chemical Basis of Heredity. Baltimore, Md, Johns Hopkins Press, 1957, p 70

Bird RE, Louarn J, Mortascelli J, Caro L: Origin and sequence of chromosome replication in *Escherichia coli.* J Mol Biol 70:549, 1972

Burgess RR, Travers AA, Dunn JJ, Bautz EKF: Factor stimulating transcription by RNA polymerase. Nature 221: 43, 1969

Caskey CT, Tomkins R, Scolnick E, Caryk T, Nirenberg M: Sequential translation of trinucleotide codons for the initiation and termination of protein synthesis. Science 162:135, 1968

Crick FHC: Codon-anti-codon paring: the wobble hypothesis. J Mol Biol 19:548, 1966

Crick FHC, Barnett L, Brenner S, Watts-Tobin RJ: General nature of the genetic code for proteins. Nature 192:1227, 1961

Dintzis HM: Assembly of the peptide chains of hemoglobin. Proc Natl Acad Sci USA 47:247, 1961

Ehrenstein G von, Weisblum B, Benzer S: The function of sRNA as amino acid adapter in the synthesis of hemoglobin. Proc Natl Acad Sci USA 49:669, 1963

Ginsberg D, Steitz JA: The 30S ribosomal precursor RNA from *Escherichia coli*. J Biol Chem 250:5647, 1975

Jacob F, Brenner S, Cuzin F: On the regulation of DNA replication in bacteria. Cold Spring Harbor Symp Quant Biol 28:329, 1963

Kim SH, Suddath FL, Quigley GJ, et al: Three-dimensional tertiary structure of yeast phenylalanine transfer RNA. Science 185:435, 1974

Meselson M, Stahl FW: The replication of DNA in *Escherichia coli*. Proc Natl Acad Sci USA 44:671, 1958

Nichols JL: Nucleotide sequence from the polypeptide chain termination region of the coat protein cistron in bacteriophage R17 RNA. Nature 225:147, 1970

Nirenberg MW, Matthei JH: The dependence of cell-free protein synthesis in *E. coli* upon naturally occurring or synthetic polyribonucleotides. Proc Natl Acad Sci USA 47:1588, 1961

Nirenberg MW, Leder P: RNA and protein synthesis: the effect of trinucleotides upon the binding of sRNA to ribosomes. Science 145:1399, 1964

Roberts JW: Termination factor for RNA synthesis. Nature 224:1168, 1969

Watson JD, Crick FHC: A structure for deoxyribose nucleic acid. Nature 171:737, 1953

Yanofsky C, Carlton BC, Guest JR, Helinski DR, Henning U: On the colinearity of gene structure and protein structure. Proc Natl Acad Sci USA 51:266, 1964

8

Genetic Variation and Gene Transfer

Although the hydrogen-bonded, helical structure of DNA imparts an extraordinary degree of stability to such a large molecule, this structure can be altered. Alterations, regardless of how subtle they may be, are passed, by virtue of the semiconservative mode of DNA replication, from generation to generation. Alterations or mutations in the DNA, if they persist, are usually reflected in a concomitant change in some property of the cell. Common types of mutations encountered in microbiology affect easily recognizable properties, such as nutritional requirements, morphology, and susceptibility to antibiotics and bacteriophage. Mutation in bacteria is not necessarily a dead-end process. Many well-described systems exist which provide for gene transfer among bacteria; these systems allow the assortment of mutationally derived characters.

MUTATION AND VARIATION

Recognition of mutant properties often depends upon the environment. For example, an auxotrophic mutant (ie, one with a nutritional requirement different from the parent) with a particular amino acid requirement is not recognized as such when growing in a medium containing the pertinent amino acid. However, a nutritional requirement is evident by the inability of such a mutant to grow in a medium lacking the amino acid. A prototrophic revertant (ie, an organism with the same nutritional requirements as the parent) would be recognized by its ability to grow in the absence of the amino acid. In other words, although the mutant genotype may be present in the cell, its phenotypic expression may not always be evident. This example serves to illustrate the genetic axiom that genotypes rather than phenotypes are inherited.

Mutations may occur spontaneously, or they may be induced by agents (mutagens) which directly or indirectly cause alterations in the structure of DNA. Spontaneous mutation frequencies are generally low, and occur with a probability of from 10^{-7} to 10^{-12} per organism. Events leading to potential mutations occur at a somewhat higher frequency, but many of these alterations do not persist because of repair mechanisms present in the organism; these mutation-mitigating mechanisms will be discussed later.

Organisms with altered characteristics, because of the low frequency of their occurrence, are difficult to detect in the absence of environments which allow them to multiply in preference to the overwhelming number of nonmutated cells. Conditions which favor the multiplication of a member of a heterogeneous population provide selective pressures that may be relatively strong or subtle. For example, if the amino acid auxotroph mentioned previously is inoculated into a medium which does not contain the pertinent amino acid, this medium would be selective for growth of prototrophic revertants. These conditions obviously provide very strong selective pressure for the appearance of prototrophs. In a different situation, an organism could mutate so that in a given environment it requires slightly less time to divide. When both the wild-type organism and the mutant can multiply, the population will be enriched for the faster growing organism, with the result that the original population will eventually be displaced by the progency of the more fit organism. In this latter case, the conversion of the population will not occur as rapidly as in the former, because the selective pressure is not as strong. Nonetheless, because of the usually short bacterial generation time, a relatively short period will allow the mutation-imparted growth advantage to be compounded through many generations with the result that the progeny of the mutated cell will prevail. This population conversion represents an example of Darwinism, ie, the appearance of a different organism by mutation and selection or genetic adaptation.

Mutagenesis   As was mentioned above, mutation frequencies can generally be increased by a variety of agents. It may not always be clear, however, whether a given agent is acting as a mutagen or providing an environmental background against which a mutant phenotype is preferentially expressed (selection). In order to answer this question the fluctuation test of Luria and Delbrück may be used. This test was originally used to determine whether the origin of bacteriophage-resistance in E. coli was Darwinian or Lamarckian, that is by spontaneous mutation and selection or by acquired immunity. This procedure was designed to determine whether bacteriophage-resistant organisms appeared prior to or following exposure to phage. A typical fluctuation test works as follows: When a series of petri plates seeded with bacteriophage are spread with approximately 10^9 cells from a single culture, a narrow fluctuation occurs in the number of resistant colonies per petri plate. However, when the original culture is used as the source of a small inoculum (approximately 1,000 cells) for a series of cultures (100) and allowed to grow, subsequent plating of 10^9 cells from the individual cultures shows a wide fluctuation in the number of resistant colonies per plate. These results are explained by the occurrence of random mutations in the individual cultures, the resistant mutants in some arising early and producing large clones within the cultures, and others arising late and therefore forming smaller clones. This experiment is depicted in Figure 8-1.

In general, there are four types of alterations which occur in the nucleotide sequence of DNA: (1) deletions, the loss of one or more nucleotides, (2) additions, the acquisition of one or more nucleotides, (3) transversions, the substitution of a purine for a pyrimidine and vice versa, and (4) transitions, purine/purine or pyrimidine/pyrimidine substitutions.

The effects of mutation are potentially unlimited. They may affect the properties of DNA with respect to its replicative function as well as information transfer. Most of the DNA is involved in specifying the primary structure of proteins, and therefore the probability is high that alterations in the nucleotide sequence will be expressed as alterations in proteins. It is now clear that aberrations produced by mutation can have multiple effects on the process of protein synthesis. Consider, for example, a deletion of nucleotides within a gene which, in addition to inactivating the gene product, may cause premature polypeptide chain termination by generating a nonsense codon. The fusion of the internal 3'-OH and 5'-OH ends created by the deletion may result in the production of a nonsense codon or in alteration of the reading frame which ultimately generates nonsense codons (Fig. 7, Chap. 7). Nonsense codons, when located in polygenic mRNA molecules, have a pleiotropic* effect on the expression of cistrons which are located distal to the nonsense codon and the initiating codon, ie, in the downstream direction of translation. These effects are polar, in that they cause decreased expression of distal genes. The reason for this perturbed expression is at least partially explained in terms of chain termination and ribosome dissociation, which cause a decrease in the rate of the initiation of translation of the next gene in the polygenic mRNA. Additions of nucleotides have similar effects. The most commonly encountered consequence of additions is alteration of the reading frame. It should be noted that additions and deletions can also correct previously generated frameshift mutations. This is the basis of the experiments which determined that the genetic code consisted of trinucleotides (Chap. 7).

Transversions and transitions also may cause nonsense mutations, but the probability of creating missense mutations is greater. A missense mutation is one in which the triplet code is altered so as to specify an amino acid different from that normally located at a particular position in a protein. The potential consequences of missense mutations are many. For example, the alterations can range from total inactivation of an enzyme to more subtle changes in cata-

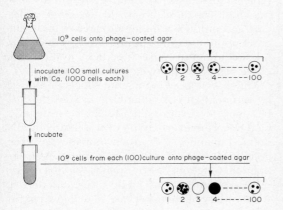

FIG. 8-1. A fluctuation test. The results of this experiment show that phage-resistant mutants appear spontaneously, prior to exposure to phage. The number of resistant mutants in each sample from a single culture is relatively constant. When several cultures are sampled, however, the number of mutants varies over a wide range, indicating that the mutants arise at different times in the course of the growth of the individual cultures. The time between the appearance of the mutant and sampling governs the number of resistant organism per culture.

*A pleiotropic mutation is one which affects more than one phenotype. In the case stated above the nonsense mutation causes (1) inactivation of the gene in which it is located and (2) decreased expression of genes located between it and the 3'-OH end of the polycistronic mRNA.

lytic ability expressed in such parameters as enzyme-substrate apparent dissociation constants (km) or maximum catalytic ability (V_{max}). However, even in cases where enzyme activity is altered, gross topologic changes do not occur, and these inactive enzymes are detectable with antibodies prepared against the native enzyme. Because of their serologic cross-reactivity these enzymatically inactive proteins have been termed CRM (cross-reactive material).

Missense, or partial missense, mutations also may give rise to temperature-sensitive gene products. A missense mutation may, for example, alter the internal bonding of a protein in such a way that its secondary or tertiary structure is compatible with biologic function at low, but not high, temperatures. The elevated temperature induces conformational changes which are incompatible with biologic function, and these mutations are termed "conditional." Many types of conditional mutants exist in which the function of a gene is normal or sufficient for survival under one set of circumstances but nonfunctional under different circumstances.

Mutagens Many physical and chemical agents are mutagenic, and although their modes of action may differ, they possess in common the ability to alter the nucleotide sequence of DNA. The foremost physical mutagenic agents are ultraviolet light and high-energy ionizing radiation. The primary effect of ultraviolet light on DNA is the production of pyrimidine dimers caused by linking the 5,6 unsaturated bonds of adjacent pyrimidines to form a cyclobutane ring (Fig. 8-2). Pyrimidine dimers are stable and can be quantified following irradiation of a bacterial culture and extraction of the DNA. The relative abundance of the three possible pyrimidine dimers is 50 percent thymine-thymine, 40 percent thymine-cytosine, and 10 percent cytosine-cytosine. The production of pyrimidine dimers within a DNA strand is by far greatest, although dimers formed between pyrimidines on adjacent strands occur at a frequency of about 10 percent.

The primary mutagenic effect produced by ultraviolet light is thought to be a consequence of the replication errors caused by the pyrimidine dimer-induced distortion of the DNA helix. Although pyrimidine dimerization proba-

FIG. 8-2. Pyrimidine dimers.

bly is the primary cause of mutation, secondary effects of ultraviolet irradiation also contribute to mutagenesis. Mutation frequencies are increased if culture medium is irradiated shortly before nonirradiated bacteria are placed upon it, suggesting that photoproducts, including free radicals, produced in the medium are mutagenic.

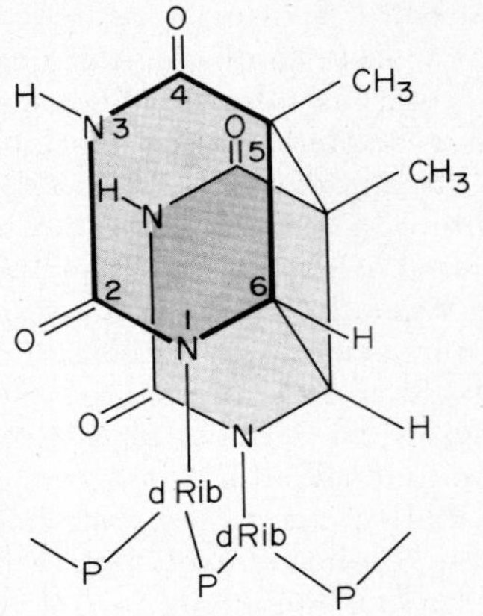

Ionizing radiations have greater penetrance than does untraviolet radiation and are effective by virtue of their ability to produce free radicals which tend to labilize molecules. This type of radiation is particularly efficient in causing single-stranded breaks in the DNA molecule and produce a high incidence of multisite or deletion mutations. Ionizations produced in the medium also cause alterations in the DNA of the organisms growing in the medium.

The discovery of mutagenic effects produced by various types of radiation provided the initial tool for experimentally altering genetic material. However, owing to the relatively ill-defined manner by which radiation causes genetic aberration, agents with more precisely defined functions were sought so that more precise modifications could be promoted. A wide variety of chemicals are now known to be mutagenic, and a great deal of experimental evidence has accumulated to provide insight into their mode of action.

The chemical mutagens can be classified according to the manner in which they alter nucleotide sequences. A general classification of chemical mutagens is as follows: (1) agents which alter the pyrimidines or purines so as to cause errors in base pairing, or which labilize the bases to spontaneous chemical modification, (2) agents which interact with the DNA and its secondary structure, producing local distortions in the helix and therefore promoting replication and recombination errors, and (3) base analogs which are incorporated into the DNA and cause replication errors. Examples of the first class are nitrous acid and alkylating agents. Nitrous acid deaminates adenine to form hypoxanthine. Adenine pairs with thymine during replication, but hypoxanthine pairs with cytosine, therefore causing a transition from an AT to a GC pair. Agents such as ethylethane sulfate or nitrogen and sulfur mustards cause alkylation at the 1 and 7 position of guanine. The alkylation may cause pairing errors or induce the slow hydrolysis of the purine, which results in depurination and gap formation in the DNA.

The foremost representatives of the second class of chemical mutagens are the acridine dyes, such as proflavine and acridine orange. These as well as other planar-type compounds are able to intercalate between the stacked bases which form the DNA helix and distort this structure in such a way that recombination between homologous chromosomes is attended by occasional insertion or deletions of bases. Additions and deletions cause a shift in the reading frame and therefore have profound effects on the gene product.

An example of a widely used mutagenic base analog is 5-bromouracil, which, when in the keto form, functions as an analog of thymine and pairs with adenine. However, rare tautomerization to the enol form occurs, and the analog is then more apt to pair with guanine. This copy error results in a transition from an AT pair to a GC pair (Fig. 8-3).

Mutations can also be caused intrinsically by aberrant DNA polymerase and possibly faulty repair and recombination mechanisms. Intrinsic mutagenesis is controlled by so-called mutator genes. For example, the gene specifying DNA polymerase in coliphage T4 becomes a mutator gene by mutations which alter its catalytic properties so that transversions of the GC→TA are produced by its activity. The *mut T* gene in *Escherichia coli* possesses an unknown function which causes AT→CG transversions. An additional mechanism for bringing about the loss of gene function is replicon inte-

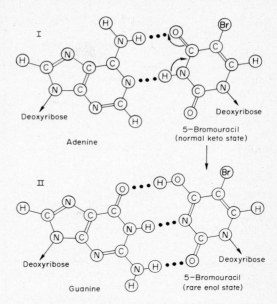

FIG. 8-3. Proper and spurious base pairing with the tautomers of 5-bromouracil. 5-Bromouracil is a thymine analog, which, when in its normal keto state, pairs with adenine but, when in its rarer enol state, pairs with guanine. Replication of 5-bromouracil-containing DNA is occasionally accompanied by the mispairing of the analog with guanine with the result that mutant daughter DNA molecules are produced.

gration (Chap. 7 and p. 155). In these cases an episome can integrate within a gene and inactivate it by gene splitting. This property of episomes has been extremely useful in genetic engineering experiments because the position in the chromosome for integration can be directed by selecting for the property caused by gene inactivation. Table 8-1 lists the actions of several mutagens that are widely used in studying bacteria and their viruses.

Bacteria as Indicators of Mutagenic/Carcinogenic Compounds The ease and economy with which bacterial systems serve as experimental tools have made them ideal for use as indicators of the mutagenic activity of various chemicals. Bacterial systems have been used to demonstrate the mutagenic effect of a number of known carcinogens. Ames and his collaborators, employing a series of well-defined histidine auxotrophs of *Salmonella typhimurium*, have shown that a number of carcinogenic compounds are capable of increasing the frequency of reversion to histidine sufficiency.

TABLE 8-1   MUTAGENS USED FOR BACTERIA

Mutagen	Apparent in vivo Specificity	Additional Advantages	Disadvantages
2-AP (2-aminopurine)	Transitions AT $\leftrightarrows$ GC	—	In some cases a weak mutagen
5-BU (5-bromouracil)	Transitions AT $\leftrightarrows$ GC	—	Must depress normal thymine incorporation; weak mutagen
NH₂OH (hydroxylamine)	Transitions AT $\leftrightarrows$ GC	—	In some cases a weak mutagen
Sodium bisulfite	Specific transition GC → AT	—	Weak mutagen
Mutator gene (*mutT*)	Specific transversion AT → CG	No treatment required	Genetic construction required
EMS (ethylmethane sulfonate)	Transitions and transversions	Powerful mutagen	Dangerous to handle
NG (nitrosoguanidine)	Transitions and transversions; induces small deletions at low rates	Very powerful mutagen	Dangerous to handle; frequent secondary mutations
ICR 191	Frameshifts; small insertions and deletions	Powerful mutagen	Compound difficult to obtain
Nitrous acid	Transitions and probably transversions; deletions	—	High amount of killing required for good mutagenesis
UV (ultraviolet radiation)	Transitions and probably transversions; deletions; possibly stimulates insertions and chromosomal rearrangements	—	High amount of killing required for good mutagenesis; certain strains too sensitive
Mu-1 phage	Insertions; some deletions	Random induction of nonleaky, polar, nonreverting mutations	—
Spontaneous (no mutagen)	Transitions; transversions; insertions; deletions (frameshifts)	Wide spectrum of mutants; no complications due to secondary mutations	Low level of mutants; many siblings in each culture

After Miller: Experiments in Molecular Genetics, 1972. Courtesy of Spring Harbor Laboratories

In practice, these tests are performed simply by spreading an auxotrophic strain of the bacterium on an agar plate containing minimal medium to which the suspected mutagen has been added. An increase in the spontaneous reversion rate is assessed by counting the revertant colonies which subsequently appear on the plate. A pharmacologic aspect can be introduced into this system by incorporating into the medium sterile microsomal preparations derived from various tissues. For example, it has been shown that cigarette smoke condensates display powerful mutagenic activity only if lung or liver microsomes are present in the test medium. The results of this approach to testing the mutagenic effects of carcinogens, together with other results, lend support to the theory that cancer can be caused by somatic mutations.

REPAIR OF GENETIC DAMAGE

The bacterial cell is not totally defenseless toward genetic damage. It is known that enzymes are present which are able to repair at least certain types of aberrant gene structure. The type of DNA repair which has received the most attention is reversal of damage induced by ultraviolet irradiation or, more specifically, reversal of pyrimidine dimer-imparted distortions.

Pyrimidine dimers can be removed by either of two processes. One process occurs only in the present of light and is known as photoreactivation or light repair, and the other, which does not require light, is known as dark repair. Photoreactivation occurs by separation of pyrimidine dimers by an enzyme (photolyase) which splits the cyclobutane ring joining the bases and regenerates the original pyrimidines. The enzyme performing this function is active only in the presence of long ultraviolet or short visible light (320 to 370 nm). Photoreactivation contributes to a large degree but is not totally effective in revitalizing cells following ultraviolet irradiation.

The mechanism of dark repair is not simple as that involved in photoreactivation and requires two distinct processes: (1) removal of the pyrimidine dimer and (2) reestablishment of the continuity of the DNA molecule. Removal of pyrimidine dimers occurs in two phases, the first of which is an incision by an endonuclease to produce a single-stranded nick bordered by a 3'-OH nucleotide and the 5'-phorphoryl pyrimidine dimer. The enzyme which effects incision is specified by the *uvrA* and *uvrB* loci. Inactivation of these functions by mutation prevents ultimate excision of pyrimidine dimers and renders the cell extrasensitive to UV irradiation. The initial single-strand scission exposes the pyrimidine dimer to an exonucleolytic activity which ultimately removes the dimer along with other nucleotides. This single-stranded nick also is a substrate for polynucleotide ligase and may be sealed prior to removal of the dimer. However, another protein, which is the product of the *uvrC* locus, is conjectured to function in repair by specifically impeding ligase-mediated repair of the original scission and therefore allowing the competing exonucleolytic activity to function. Mutations in *uvrC* also cause increased sensitivity to UV irradiation. Several exonucleolytic activities have been described which are potentially capable of removing the phosphoryl pyrimidine dimer exposed by the incision process described above. Some of these enzymes which hydrolyze phosphodiester bonds in the vicinity of pyrimidine dimers are exonuclease VII, so-called UV exonuclease, and the 5'-3' exonucleolytic activity associated with DNA polymerases I and II. These enzymes have been implicated in removal of pyrimidine dimers accompanied by formation of single-strand gaps

in the DNA. These gaps subsequently are filled by the action of DNA polymerase, which uses the free 3'-OH group of the nucleotide bordering the gap as primer and the intact strand as template. Once the gap is filled, the remaining single-strand nick is sealed by the action of polynucleotide ligase, completing the second phase of the repair process. A generalized view of this repair process is presented in Figure 8-4.

Analysis of DNA which has undergone pyrimidine dimer excision and repair reveals that the patched regions of the chromosome may contain either short (10 to 30 nucleotides) or long (1,000 to 3,000 nucleotides) single-stranded stretches of newly synthesized DNA. Investigation of the enzymes required for synthesis of these short and long patches reveals two pathways of repair. Both of these pathways require *uvr A, B,* and *C* gene products and are distinguished by the extent of gap formation which accompanies the postincision release of the 5'-phosphoryl-pyrimidine dimer. The short patch pathway of repair is thought to involve, in addition to the *uvr A, B,* and *C* products, polymerase I and ligase. Polymerase I, unlike polymerases II and III, specifically binds to DNA which contains single-stranded nicks. The binding of polymerase I is followed by a concerted 5'→3' exonucleolytic digestion and a polymerization by addition to the exposed 3'-OH termini border of the gap. These concerted activities result in nick translocation, a well-documented property of polymerase I. The exonuclease of polymerase I is ideally suited for removal of pyrimidine dimers because it is capable of exonucleolytically cleaving dinucleotides and oligonucleotides from 5' termini. The concerted polymerase and nuclease activities proceed until 10 to 30 nucleotides, including the pyrimidine dimer, are replaced, at which point the ligase restores the integrity of the repaired strand of DNA. This repair mechanism is consistent with the increased UV sensitivity of *polA*⁻(PolI⁻) strains.

The long patch pathway of repair is more complex and, in addition to the *uvr* gene products, requires an exonuclease activity specified by the *rec BC* genes (p. 171), DNA unwinding protein, exonuclease VII or UV exonuclease, and polymerases II and/or III. In this case, initial removal of pyrimidine dimers is probably accomplished by exonuclease VII or UV exonuclease followed by extensive gap widening by combined activities including a single-strand

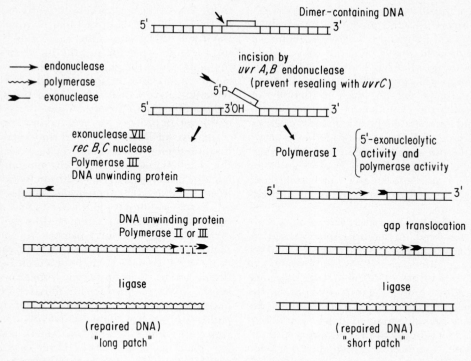

FIG. 8-4. The enzymatic repair of pyrimidine dimer-containing DNA. The pathway on the left represents short patch repair. The pathway on the right represents long patch repair.

nuclease activity of the *rec BC* exonuclease, and the 5′-3′ exonucleolytic activity associated with polymerase III. This widespread gap is then filled by the action of either polymerase II or polymerase III which, unlike polymerase I, initiates DNA synthesis within gaps (ie, they bind poorly if at all to nicks). The role of the unwinding protein in the long patch pathway of repair is thought to be twofold: it is required for processive° polymerization over long stretches of template, and it is able to block a single-strand endonucleolytic activity present in the *rec BC* nuclease (p. 171). This latter function allows the *recBC* nuclease to function in gap extension (by its exonucleolytic function) without destroying (by its endonucleolytic activity) the intact single strand of DNA which is to be used as template in subsequent gap filling by the polymerases.

Excision repair of pyrimidine dimers is not exclusively found in microorganisms, and many of the enzymes described above are found in eucaryotic organisms, including man. It is noteworthy that patients with xeroderma pigmentosum, a heritable disease which imparts extreme ultraviolet sensitivity to the skin, are defective in their ability to repair pyrimidine dimer-containing DNA.

Although the above discussion of repair mechanisms dealt with reversal of damage to DNA caused by ultraviolet irradiation, other types of damage can similarly be reversed. It is known, for example, that other classes of excision enzymes are capable of initiating removal of nucleotides containing monoadducts, such as alkylated bases. The repair of these lesions apparently involves the postincision mechanisms described above for pyrimidine dimers.

Repair of DNA damage also occurs by processes of genetic recombination. This type of repair is frequently referred to as postreplication repair and requires the *recA, B,* and *C* system. The role of these in recombination is described on page 171. Unlike the direct repair

°*A processive polymerase is one which effects continuous elongation of the polymer without being released from its primer-template complex. A processive nuclease is one which effects sequential hydrolysis of phosphodiester bonds without dissociating from its polymeric substrate.*

processes described above, postreplication repair results in the dilution of the aberrant structures by replication and concomitant recombination. The role of recombination mechanisms in repair processes is underscored by the increased sensitivity of *recA, B,* and *C* mutants to ultraviolet irradiation.

GENETIC SUPPRESSION

The previously described repair mechanisms reverse genetic aberration and restore the original phenotypic expression of the affected gene. Other mechanisms are available which do not correct the original mutation per se but which are capable of restoring the original phenotype. This occurs by the action of suppressor mutations. Suppression is defined as the reversal of a mutant phenotype by another mutation at a position on the DNA distinct from that of the original mutation. The presence of suppressor mutations is ascertained by demonstrating, with appropriate genetic analysis, that the original mutation can be recovered independently of the suppressor mutation, and vice versa.

Suppression is a generic term in that its molecular basis may be varied. Suppressor mutations may be categorized as follows: (1) The suppressor mutation may open an alternate pathway for the production of a product the synthesis of which is prevented by the primary mutation. A corollary to this type of suppression is that in which the second mutation augments a low residual activity caused by the primary mutation. (2) The suppressor mutation may be located in a gene whose mutated product may replace that of the affected gene. (3) The suppressor mutation may alter the internal environment of the cell so that the structure of the product of the mutated gene is restored to normal. (4) The suppressor mutation may introduce an additional alteration which completely or partially negates the effect of the primary mutation. This latter case includes not only interactions between missense mutations but also corrections of frameshift mutations by subsequent additions or deletions. (5) The suppressor mutations may alter the properties of one of the factors which participate in the transfer of information from DNA to protein. The first three mechanisms represent indirect suppression in which the consequence of the primary mutation is circumvented rather than corrected. The last two mechanisms provide for a correction within the product of the mutated gene. This is direct suppression.

Indirect Suppression Several examples of indirect suppression exist. Examples of (1), (2), and (3) listed above are as follows: (1) A *Neurospora* mutant with an effective decrease in synthesis of carbamylphosphate requires pyrimidines for growth. Carbamylphosphate is also used for arginine biosynthesis. If a mutation which lowers the activity of ornithine transcarbamylase, the enzyme utilizing carbamylphosphate for arginine biosynthesis, is introduced into the former mutant, the pyrimidine requirement is suppressed. Apparently the second mutation introduces a sparing effect on carbamylphosphate which allows this compound to be diverted from arginine to pyrimidine biosynthesis. (2) A mutation in one of two genes which code for the two polypeptide chains which form isopropylmalate isomerase, an enzyme specifically involved in leucine biosynthesis in *S. typhimurium*, can be suppressed by mutations far removed from the leucine locus. It is thought that this suppressor mutation allows a surrogate polypeptide chain to replace the mutated, nonfunctional polypeptide chain in the isomerase. (3) A mutation in *Neurospora* produces a tryptophan synthetase which is extremely sensitive to zinc and is therefore inactive. (All culture media contain traces of zinc as an impurity.) This mutation is suppressed by a mutation which prevents the organism from accumulating the toxic metal, thus providing an environment in which the zinc-sensitive enzyme is active.

Direct Suppression As pointed out above, direct suppression results in an alteration of the mutated gene product so that it is again functional. Direct suppression may be intragenic or intergenic. Both types have been extensively investigated.

Intragenic Suppression. Intragenic suppression requires two distinct mutations within a single gene, and the effect of one mutation cancels the other. An example of this type of suppression is a mutation in the tryptophan synthetase A protein of *E. coli*, which causes a substitution of a glycine with a glutamic acid residue in position of 120 of the polypeptide chain and inaction of the protein. Another mu-

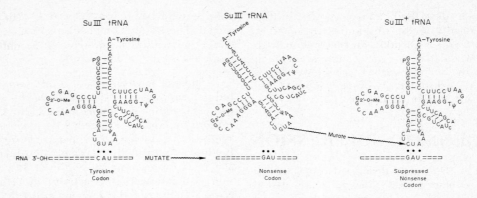

FIG. 8-5. Reading of a nonsense codon by a suppressor tRNA. The product of the *suIII* gene of *E. coli* is a tyrosin-accepting tRNA. A mutation affecting the anticodon region of this tRNA allows it to read the nonsense codon UAG.

tation causes a replacement of a tyrosine with a cysteine residue in position 175 of the polypeptide chain. This second mutation cancels the effect of the first mutation and restores activity. In this particular case the amino acid substitutions have reciprocal effects, ie, the glutamic acid or cysteine substitution alone produces an inactive protein.

INTERGENIC SUPPRESSION.   The most extensively studied case of intergenic suppression is that involving the nonsense codons UAA, UAG, and UGA. These triplets, when present in mRNA, cause termination of polypeptide chain extension. This characteristic is suppressible by mutations which alter elements which participate in the translation process. The molecular basis of this suppression is relatively well understood and involves mutational alteration of tRNA.

The most straightforward way of suppressing nonsense codons would be by altering the anticodon of a tRNA molecule so as to cause reading of the otherwise undecipherable triplet. This mechanism would seem to require that the cell contain duplicate tRNA molecules, each of which reads the same triplet. Otherwise any benefit derived by an anticodon alteration allowing nonsense codon translation would be negated by inability to read the normal, cognate codon. The *suIII* gene is an example of how this problem is solved. A mutation in the *suIII* gene, which is one of two tandem genes for a minor species of tRNA^{tyr}, causes suppression of UAG (amber) nonsense codons. Tyrosine-accepting tRNA from *suIII*$^-$ and *suIII*$^+$

strains have been sequenced.[*] The results of these analyses reveal that the only alteration in the *suIII* product is in the anticodon loop of the molecule where AUG in the wild type is changed to AUC in the mutant. The anticodon AUC reads the nonsense codon UAG. (Note that, by convention, nucleotide sequences are expressed in a 5′ to 3′ sequence, and therefore one of the triplets must be reversed in order to display the proper base pairing.) The result of the recognition of the UAG codon by the mutated tyrosine-accepting tRNA is the insertion of tyrosine into the polypeptide chains at the position of the nonsense codon-mediated chain termination.

Suppression of nonsense codons does not always require alterations in the anticodon of suppressor tRNA molecules. The nonsense codon UGA is suppressed by mutations in the gene which specifies tryptophan-accepting tRNA. This suppressor mutation results in an A to G substitution in the dihydrouracil arm, far removed from the anticodon. It is thought that this alteration in tRNA^{trp} increases wobble (p. 131) and allows C to pair with A while also maintaining normal C-G pairing. This type of change in the tRNA^{trp} molecule probably is the only one which is acceptable for viability of the organism, because there is a single gene for

[*]*Note that the suppressor allele designation is the reverse of genetic convention. Classically, wild-type alleles are designated with a (+) and mutated alleles with a (−). Suppressor alleles are designated as su$^+$ when active in suppression and su$^-$ when inactive. This is so regardless of their wild type or mutated character.*

tRNA[trp]. This situation provides an interesting contrast with the case of the tRNA[tyr] described above.

Figure 8-5 shows how the nonsense codons arising from sense codons are suppressed by mutant tRNAs. It is evident that suppression by this pathway results either in complete restoration of the amino acid sequence of the polypeptide or in substitution of an amino acid which is compatible with the biologic function of the protein. Similar suppression mechanisms exist for the remaining nonsense codon, UAA, as well as for missense mutations. Mechanisms for suppressing frameshift mutations also are available. One of these involves an additional nucleotide in the anticodon for phenylalanine tRNA in which case the anticodon reads UUUC rather than UUU as the codon for phenylalanine. This results in restoration of the reading frame which was shifted by the insertion of an extra base.

PHENOTYPIC SUPPRESSION

Mutations may also be suppressed by nonmutational alteration of the components of information transfer. For example, sublethal concentrations of streptomycin and other related antibiotics which cause misreading of the genetic code may allow missense or nonsense codons to be translated as sense codons. This phenomenon is described in detail in Chapter 10.

An additional type of phenotypic suppression is caused by incorporating base analogs into mRNA. For example, 5-fluorouracil, which is similar in structure to uracil, is incorporated into RNA. This analog causes ambiguity of translation, probably because it is recognized as C rather than U. Therefore, in transitions involving a change from C to U the mutant codon will be translated as sense instead of nonsense or missense.

Most agents capable of causing phenotypic suppression are effective at low concentrations. Higher concentrations are bactericidal or bacteriostatic. The ambiguities introduced by suppressing compounds, while being sufficient to return the function of a mutated gene, do not seriously detract from the transfer of information from normal genes. Bacterial systems, in most cases, possess supernumerary quantities of gene products, and a low level of ambiguity is sufficient to produce an effective quantity of functional gene product without effectively lowering the level of the functional product produced from a nonmutated gene.

GENE TRANSFER

Zygote formation, in eucaryotic cells, results from the fusion of the gametes of sexually compatible members of the same species. This sexual union contributes to invigoration of the species and speciation by allowing reassortment of traits acquired by mutation. Zygotes are formed in bacteria by more primitive means of gene transfer. Three general mechanisms are known whereby the genetic information of one bacterial cell can be introduced into a recipient bacterial cell. These are characterized by the vectors of transfer. The most primitive mode of transfer occurs by the process of transformation, in which naked DNA derived from one cell is taken up by another cell. Another type of relatively primitive transfer is accomplished by viral infection; this process is termed transduction. A third mode of transfer, which is probably most analogous to the fusion of gametes, is conjugation, where genetic transfer is preceded by cell-to-cell contact. It should be emphasized that this latter process does not involve cell fusion. Incomplete, rather than full, diploids result from gene transfer in bacteria. These partial diploids are known as merozygotes and consist of the entire genome (endogenote) derived from the recipient cell and the incomplete genome (exogenote) derived from the donor cell. Regardless of the mode of gene transfer, merozygotes support genetic recombination in which portions of the DNA of the exogenote effectively replace segments of the DNA of the endogenote.

Transformation

Historically, identification of the active transforming principle permitted the equating of genetic material with DNA. Avery, MacLeod, and McCarty showed that DNA purified from an encapsulated strain of pneumococcus was capable of imparting onto a nonencapsulated strain the ability to form capsules and that the resulting strain was genetically stable.

Bacterial transformation is presently the basis for several experimental determinations relative to the properties of DNA. The property of gene transfer by soluble DNA provides a test for the biologic activity of DNA which has been subjected to various in vitro treatments (such as with mutagens). Also, transformation may be used to assay the gene dosage in a given DNA solution, since the number of transformants (cells which have participated in recombination with externally added DNA) is directly proportional to the concentration of the pertinent genetic regions. In addition, transformation provides the only available test for the biologic activity of DNA that has been enzymatically synthesized in vitro.

The process of transformation has been extensively studied using pneumococcus, *Haemophilus influenzae, Bacillus subtilis,* and streptococci. *Escherichia coli* also can be transformed if it is first treated with $CaCl_2$ to render it permeable to DNA and if it lacks certain nucleases which would otherwise destroy the incoming DNA. In brief, transformation requires that DNA be adsorbed by the cell, gain entrance to the cytoplasm, and undergo recombination with the recipient genome. This phenomenon has been investigated with regard to the physical state of the donor DNA, the state of the recipient cell which allows competency (ie, ability to take up DNA), and the fate of the DNA upon entering the cell. Double-stranded DNA is more effective in transformation than is single-stranded DNA. However, under special circumstances single-stranded DNA is effective in infecting spheroplasts. The size of the DNA molecule is related to its transforming ability. Using a pneumococcal transforming system, it has been shown that DNA loses its ability to transform when the molecular weight falls below 0.3 million daltons.

Physiologic and genetic data suggest that the competent state requires the expression of a number of specific cellular properties which are needed for cells to adsorb DNA. In general, these properties appear to be related to the surface properties of the recipient cell. A competence factor can be eluted from the surface of competent cells, and this molecule, which is inactivated by trypsin, is able to restore competency to the cells. Another protein of unknown function also appears to be involved in the competent state, as is the appearance of new antigenic determinants and rearrangement of cell wall components.

Adsorption of transforming DNA by competent cells involves a reversible followed by an irreversible binding. Irreversibly bound DNA is resistant to deoxyribonuclease but is probably not inside the cell, since antibody prepared against single-stranded DNA is capable of halting subsequent transformation. At this stage the DNA is probably located in the periplasmic space. Irreversible binding of DNA requires energy, but not DNA, RNA, or protein synthesis. Shortly after DNA becomes irreversibly fixed to recipient cells, a brief eclipse period is encountered during which the transforming ability of the donor DNA cannot be recovered. However, isotopes from radioactively labeled donor DNA can be recovered, one-half being in the form of 5'-mononucleotides and the other half in high-molecular-weight form. These and other observations suggest that transforming DNA traverses the bacterial membrane, with a concomitant hydrolysis of one of the strands resulting in a single-stranded molecule gaining entrance to the cell. The fate of the DNA single strand is to synapse with homologous regions of the endogenote and to participate in recombination, ie, a portion of the recipient genome is replaced by the transforming DNA. The precise structure defining the synapse of the transforming single strand and the recipient DNA is not known. However, it is known that physical heterozygosis (the presence of alternate, allelic forms of a gene) of the hybrid recombinant DNA is paralleled by a genetic heterozygosis. Physical heterozygosis is demonstrated by the covalent association of exogenote DNA with that of the recipient cell. Genetic heterozygosis is shown by the observation that following transformation a DNA replication-dependent segregation of donor-type and recipient-type alleles occurs. Heterozygosity would be expected if transformation involves single-strand replacement, since the new duplex region would contain strands derived from two different alleles. Semiconservative replication of this region (with the genome) would result in a heterozygous cell until the two types of DNA molecules are separated by cell division-mediated segregation.

Conjugation

Bacterial cells frequently harbor extra-chromosomal, autonomously replicating DNA molecules known as plasmids. Two classes of plasmids exist: (1) those which replicate autonomously and (2) those which replicate autonomously but also can integrate into the chromosome and replicate as any other chromosomal character. The latter type of plasmid is usually referred to as an episome. Some types of episomes are capable of promoting gene transfer to compatible cells and therefore confer sexual fertility to cells which harbor them. This episome-imparted fertility is the basis for bacterial conjugation. Although the most extensively studied conjugal system is that found in *E. coli*, it is known that interchange of genetic material by conjugation can occur in other types of gram-negative cells as well.

The episome (fertility, or F, factor) which confers fertility to the *E. coli* cell is a double-stranded, circular DNA molecule with a molecular weight equivalent to 45 times 10^6 daltons. Although a DNA molecule of this size potentially codes for 40 to 60 proteins, very few of these have been identified. It is known that the fertility factor specifies a diffusable product which is necessary for its own replication. This episome also specifies the structural proteins of a surface structure, F pili, which are responsible for promoting the union of male cells (the F factor-bearing and F pili-bearing cell) and female cells (those not possessing F factor). The fertility factor (F) is able to exist in three states: (1) as an autonomously replicating episome, (2) as an integral part of the chromosome, and (3) as an autonomously replicating episome containing relatively small segments of material derived from the chromosome. The terminology applied to cells bearing the sex or fertility factor in these states are F+, Hfr, and F' respectively; cells not containing the fertility factor are termed F−. The types of male cells are characterized by the manner in which they effect gene transfer. The F+ cell is able to transfer only the genetic information contained in the fertility factor. The only genetic alteration effected by introduction of the fertility factor into an F− cell is conversion of the F− cell to an F+ cell. This transfer does not necessarily involve loss of maleness of the F+ cell; the reason for this will become obvious when the mechanism

of transfer is considered. Hfr cells are capable of transferring the entire chromosome of the cell, and although this occurs rarely, relatively large portions of the genome are transferred at a high frequency. However, an Hfr times F− cross rarely results in the acquisition of maleness by the F− cell. This is one of the original observations that led to an understanding of some of the characteristics of Hfr-mediated gene transfer.

It is known that the position of integration of the fertility factor in the chromosome specifies a breaking point which creates, at least operationally, a linear structure from the original circular one. This breaking point is within the fertility factor, so that each end of the chromosome is composed of part of the nucleotide sequence of the F factor. The chromosome is transferred in a polarized fashion, and upon passing into an F− cell, part of the fertility factor enters first and the remainder enters last. This relationship of the fertility factor and the mobilized chromosome, together with the susceptibility to shearing of DNA in the course of transfer, means that the complete F factor is rarely transferred. It can be demonstrated experimentally that genetic markers nearer the origin enter earlier and at a higher frequency than do markers located at more distal positions on the chromosome.

Fertility factor-mediated replicon transfer involves curtailment of initiation of DNA replication at the normal replicator site and initiation of a new round of replication presumably at the site of the origin of transfer. In a normal transfer, DNA replication occurs in the male cell, and a newly synthesized, semiconserved DNA molecule remains in the male. (This feature explains why the male cell does not lose maleness in a F+ times F− cross.) The remaining strand of the DNA undergoing transfer is passed to the female cell in a polarized, linear manner. This method of transfer, which involves a new round of DNA replication in the male cell, ensures postmating viability of the male cell. Although the normal transfer of DNA results in semiconserved DNA in both the male and female, it is of interest that DNA replication is not an absolute requirement for transfer of DNA. This can be demonstrated by blocking DNA synthesis in a male cell during conjugation and observing loss of viability of the male cell and the formation of recombinants in the female population. Apparently, in this case, conjugation results in suicide of male cell as a consequence of the accumulation of single-stranded, nuclease-sensitive DNA. A similar experiment can be performed in which DNA synthesis is prevented in the female, in which case single-stranded DNA derived from the male cell accumulates in the female cell. These observations suggest that the mechanism and energy for transfer of the DNA involves something other than DNA polymerization per se and may be related to those processes normally involved in unwinding the double helix at the growing point.

Hfr-mediated gene transfer provides a convenient method for locating the relative position of various genes on the chromosome. This is accomplished by performing crosses between appropriate genetically marked strains and interrupting transfer of the chromosome at various times by subjecting the conjugates to moderate shear forces and plating the male/female mixture on a medium which will kill the male cells but which is selective for the desired re-

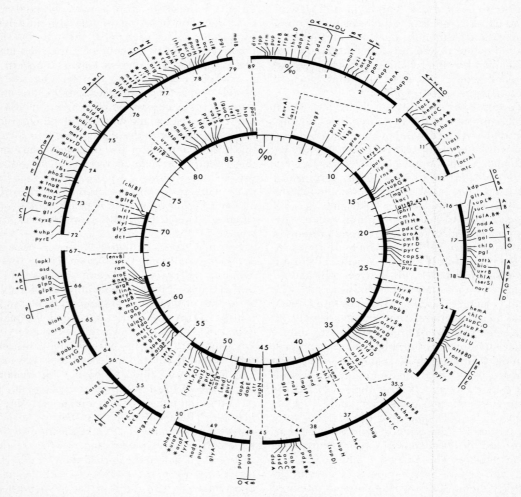

FIG. 8-6. Map of the *E. coli* chromosome. The inner circle bears the time scale 0 to 90 minutes, or the time required for transfer of the entire chromosome from a male to female cell. The positioning of 0-time is arbitrary, since different Hfr strains possess different origins of transfer. The meaning of the gene symbols may be found in the article credited below. The contour length of the *E. coli* chromosome is 1,000 μm, or about 3 times 10⁶ nucleotide pairs. Assuming that the average gene contains 1,000 nucleotide pairs, then the *E. coli* chromosome contains enough information for 3,000 genes. It is possible, therefore, that the map depicted above is only 10 percent saturated with respect to gene content (310 genes are shown). (From Taylor: Bacteriol Rev 34:155, 1970),

combinant cells. Viability of the zygote but death of the male cell is usually accomplished by using phage-resistant or antibiotic-resistant female cells and sensitive male cells. Application of this technique with a series of Hfr strains with the origin of transfer at different positions on the chromosome facilitated construction of the rather extensive genetic map of *E. coli* shown in Figure 8-6. The results of a typical interrupted mating experiment are shown in Fig. 8-7.

The Formation of Hfr Cells from F+ Cells
Hfr cells arise from F+ cells. The molecular event involved in this conversion is the integration of the fertility factor into the chromosome. This integration is not a particularly rare event and occurs normally in cultures of F+ cells. This fact accounts for the originally observed fertility of a mating between F+ and F− cells (fertility is defined here as the ability of markers from the chromosome of the F+ cell to recombine with those of the chromosome of F− cells) and provided for the discovery of bacterial sexuali-

ty. The introduction of alleles into F− cells from an F+ population occurs with a frequency of approximately 10^{-4} to 10^{-5} and virtually any chromosomal marker can be introduced. However, if a petri plate is spread with an F+ culture so as to give confluent growth and is then replica plated* to another plate freshly seeded with a related organism with a mutationally derived auxotrophic requirement, the pattern of restricted growth on the F− plate indicates that only organisms from discrete areas of the F+ plate are capable of introducing the wild-type allele into the F− cells. These areas represent clones containing the progeny of cells in which the fertility factor has integrated into the chromosome. From these areas of the plate organisms can be obtained which are able to transfer the pertinent marker with a much higher frequency than could the F+ strain. This quality of high-frequency transfer is the basis for the Hfr designation for this type of cell. Using the above procedure, Hfr strains can be isolated which have the fertility factor integrated at various points on the chromosome and which, consequently, will have origins of chromosomal transfer at defined points.

Formation of F′ Cells Disintegration of fertility factors from the chromosome can occur in two ways: The fertility factor itself can be regenerated, in which case it has all the properties of the original factor, or it may be released together with a portion of the chromosome. As previously mentioned, cells containing fertility factors bearing chromosome-derived genes are termed F-prime (F′). Like F factors, F′ factors also are circular and cells bearing them are capable not only of transferring the conjoined genes at a high frequency but also, in contrast to Hfr cells, of conferring maleness to female

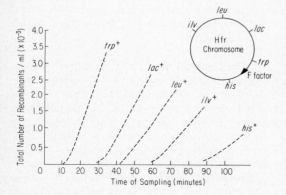

FIG. 8-7. Interrupted mating experiment. Hfr strain of *E. coli* with the fertility factor integrated at the position shown is mixed with an F-strain which is auxotrophic for the indicated amino acids. Samples are removed from the mating mixture at the times shown, subjected to moderate shear forces, and plated on medium which is selective for the desired recombinants and which prevents growth of the Hfr. The rate of appearance of recombinants equals the time of entry of the competent region of the Hfr chromosome and therefore represent the position of the various loci relative to the fertility factor. The decrease in the slopes of the lines representing the frequency of recombinants for late entering loci is because of the smaller number of zygotes formed which contain the relevant genetic loci. This decrease is because of accidental separation of mating pairs during the course of the linear, polarized transfer of the Hfr chromosome.

Replica plating is a technique which is widely used in the practice of bacterial genetics. It is a simple method whereby the properties of individual bacterial clones growing on a petri dish can be demonstrated by transferring a representative sample of each clone onto different selective media. In practice, a petri dish containing either confluent growth or well-defined bacterial colonies is brought into contact with a layer of sterile velveteen. The velveteen, which at this point holds an inoculum with a pattern equal to that of the original (master) plate, is then pressed onto sterile selective media contained in petri plates. The absence or presence of response of the various clones to the selective media permits identification of the desired variants.

cells at an equally high frequency. In other words, the shorter distance between the point of entry and the distally located portion of the fertility factor decreases the probability that the DNA will be sheared during transfer. Genetic transfer mediated by F′ cells is also known as sexduction. F′ cells have been particularly useful in genetic and biochemical analysis, because virtually entire populations of recipient cells can be converted to a homogeneous merodiploid state.

The three modes of existence of F factors (Fig. 8-8) described above are explained in terms of the circular nature of both the chromosome and the autonomously replicating episome (whether F or F′). Campbell proposed a model to explain episome integration which assumed circularity of both chromosome and episome and which involved a reciprocal crossing over between these circular structures. This model, which essentially has been proven, is the same as that for the integration of λ prophage (Fig. 70-15). Subsequent to the formulation of this model both the chromosome and the episome have been visualized by electron microscopy and shown to be circular. Also,

subsequent analysis of F′s strongly suggest that their release from the chromosome occurs by a similar, but reversed, process, also like the release of λ prophage. As with λ prophage, F′s have been described which contain both distally and proximally transferred segments of the original Hfr chromosome, ie, they contain chromosomal information from regions on both sides of the integrated F factor. Other F′s have been described which only contain the information on one side of the integrated fertility factor. Release also may occur in such a way as to leave a small portion of the F factor integrated in the chromosome. This results in the production of a sex factor affinity (sfa) locus which retains some homology with sex factors and therefore directs or favors their subsequent integration at that position on the chromosome. It is also known that the production of F′s results in a deletion in the chromosome including the F factor as well as conjoined DNA. All of these observations support a model for release which is the reverse of the process shown in Figure 70-15. The local looping of the chromosome governs the position of the reciprocal crossover event, which in turn governs the nature of F factor derivative which is produced. In other words, the size of the loop governs the amount of DNA released.

The Conjugal Act   Fertility factor-mediated gene transfer requires cell-to-cell contact. The affinity of male and female cells resides in the male-borne F pilus (Chap. 3). It is not clear whether the pilus serves as a conduit through which the male genome passes or whether it is simply a sensing device to recognize the female cell. F pili not only promote the male-female union but also retard union between male cells. This, however, is not an absolute impediment, and gene transfer can occur, although at a low frequency, between the different types of male cells. F pili can be removed from male cells by shearing or by allowing growth into the late stationary phase. Cells bearing fertility factors and which have had their pili removed are known as F⁻ phenocopies. Concomitant with effective male-female pair formation, the circular DNA bearing the fertility factor, whether the Hfr chromosome, F′, or F⁺, is converted to a form able to be transferred to the female cell in a sequential manner.

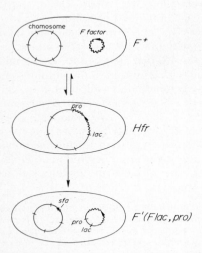

FIG. 8-8. The formation of Hfr and F′ cells. The random integration of the fertility factor occurs by a reciprocal recombination event between the circular factor and the circular chromosome. Disintegration of the fertility factor also occurs by reciprocal recombination. The site of recombination governs the chromosome-derived material which will be present in the F′. A portion of the fertility factor occasionally will remain in the chromosome, thus creating a sex factor affinity locus.

Transduction

The type of gene transfer in which the DNA of one bacterial cell is introduced into another bacterial cell by viral infection is known as transduction. The transfer of genetic material by bacteriophage can be classified according to the scope of potential transfer. Some types of bacteriophage are able to transfer genes derived from their previous host cells in a relatively indiscriminate manner, so that virtually any chromosomal marker can be transferred; this process is termed generalized transduction. However, other types of bacteriophage are capable of transferring only certain genes from the previously infected host; this process is termed specialized transduction.

The ability of a phage to mediate specialized or generalized gene transfer depends upon its relationship not only with the organism which is to serve as the source of genetic information to be transferred but also with the recipient organism. An understanding of the events which permit phage to mediate gene transfer depends upon a knowledge of the physiology and molecular biology of phage infection; this background information is presented in Chapter 70. An abbreviated and generalized outline of the infectious process is as follows: Adsorption of the bacteriophage to stereospecific receptor sites on the bacterial surface is followed by injection into the cell of the DNA contained within the phage particle. If the phage is of the virulent type, the genetic program of the DNA will be expressed, in which case an abundance of new phage particles will be produced and released by subsequent cell lysis. However, if the infecting phage is of the temperate type, alternative pathways are available following injection of the DNA. The vegetative program of the DNA may be expressed, in which case the lytic response ensues, or the vegetative program may be prevented by the production of a phage-specified repressor, in which case the phage DNA may enter into a benign relationship with the host cell. The presence of the phage repressor establishes a lysogenic state, in which the DNA of the phage may be incorporated into the host chromosome in such a way that the two genomes are linearly contiguous. The phage genome in this state is known as prophage. The cell acquires a significant new property as a consequence of lysogeny,

namely, that it is immune to infection by homologous phage. This immunity is important in demonstrating transduction.

Generalized Transducing Particles If, during phage maturation, host DNA rather than phage DNA is packaged into the phage capsid, a generalized transducing particle will be formed. This aberrant packaging occurs randomly with respect to the piece of host DNA which is occluded in the phage particle. Also it occurs at a relatively low frequency, and only a minor fraction of the population of a phage lysate contains host rather than viral DNA. The size of the host DNA contained in generalized transducing particles is similar to the size of the genome which is normally carried by the phage. This is reflected in the amount of genetic information that the particle subsequently is able to transfer. For example, the DNA molecular weight of coliphage P1 and *Salmonella* phage PLT 22 is 60 times 10^6 and 26 times 10^6, respectively, and genetic analysis has revealed that transducing fragments introduced into recipient cells by P1 are twice the size of those introduced by PLT 22. As pointed out in Chapter 70, progeny genomes appear to be derived from concatenates which are composed of multiple complements of the total phage genome. The scission of concatenate DNA by some phage, such as coliphage λ, occurs in reproducibly defined positions, so that the order of the genes in each phage particle is the same. However, in other phages, such as coliphage T4, the scission occurs at random. In the latter case, each phage particle will contain approximately equal lengths of DNA, but the terminal position of the DNA molecules in various particles will represent different genes. As will be seen in the following sections, the events by which DNA is packaged into the phage particle may be related to the ability of phage to carry DNA other than its own.

Specialized Transducing Particles The production of specialized transducing particles resides in the ability of certain phage genomes to integrate reversibly into the genome of the cells which they infect. As alluded to above, integration of the phage genome into the host chromosome occurs by a process similar to that described for fertility factor integration (p. 155). It is thought that production of specialized transducing DNA occurs by a process similar to that which produces F's, ie, when prophages are released from the chromosome, they frequently carry a portion of host DNA. There are significant quantitative and qualitative differences between the host DNA carried by F's and released prophage. For example, relatively long F's can be produced by the reciprocal crossover mechanism and still be recovered, owing to their mode of transfer. Only a limited amount of host DNA can be detected in the released prophage because of the limited size of DNA that can be packaged into the phage capsid. Also, the F factor-Hfr-F' route potentially produces episomes carrying a variety of host markers, but the release of prophage results in episomes containing but a few host determinants. The reason for this latter limitation is that prophage integrates at one or, at best, a few positions on the host chromosome (recall that F integration is not so restricted). The basis for specialized transduction is, therefore, the location of the prophage on the host chromosome (ie, which bacterial genes are contiguous with it) and the manner in which the prophage is released. It also should be pointed out that specialized transducing lysates are usually produced by induction of the release of the prophage by ultraviolet irradiation or by other treatment which destroys the lysogenic (immune) state.

The process just described for the formation of specialized transducing DNA results in exclusion of a portion of phage DNA from the transducing particle. The extent of the exclusion will depend upon how much of the host DNA is included in the excised prophage – the greater the amount of host DNA, the greater the exclusion of phage DNA. This principle has obvious consequences with respect to the viability of the particle which is subsequently released from the cell. For example, in the case of coliphage λ, which integrates on the host chromosome between the galactose and biotin loci, λgal transducing particles may be formed which are still capable of growing vegetatively. These particles are termed λpgal (p for plaque-forming) and they lack nonessential portions of the λ genome. However, other λ transducing particles which also carry galactose genes may be formed which are incapable of vegetative growth because they lack essential λ genes. These defective particles are termed λdgal (defective λ carrying galactose genes), and they

require helper phage if they are to grow. (The role of the helper phage is to provide the function lacking in the defective particle.) The question arises as to how defective phages which are released from the lysogenic state ever manage to undergo the vegetative cycle in the cell in which they originally are produced. This problem is solved by the abundance of normal phage particles that are produced upon induction. When released from one cell, they infect the cell carying the defective genome and serve as helper phage.

It should be emphasized that, whereas generalized transducing particles are produced during vegetative growth and maturation of the phage, specialized transducing particles arise only from cells which have been previously lysogenized. The aberrant maturation which gives rise to a generalized transducing particle occurs with a frequency of 10^{-5} to 10^{-6}. Specialized transducing particles arise with a similar frequency when lysogenic cells are induced to lyse (by ultraviolet irradiation or some other treatment), ie, most of the phages produced are normal.

Transmission of Genetic Information by Transducing Particles Specialized transducing particles are formed because of the special relationship which exists between the viral and the host genomes, and it is therefore obvious that only temperate phages demonstrate this ability. The reason why generalized transduction also requires a temperate phage vector is not quite so obvious and is probably more directly related to the events which occur at the time of DNA transfer to the recipient organism rather than to the manner in which generalized transducing particles are formed. Because of the low relative abundance of transducing particles, a high multiplicity of infection must be used to demonstrate transduction. Therefore, the probability is high that a cell receiving a transducing particle also will be infected by normal phage. If the nontransducing particles are of a virulent nature, death of the cell ensues, thus preventing recovery of recombinant cells. However, with temperate phage, the immunity which attends lysogeny is able to prevent lysis, and the DNA introduced by the phage is able to participate in recombination with the host chromosome. It is of interest to note that transduction with the virulent coliphage T1 can be demonstrated by employing genetic variants with reduced virulence. When T1 phage containing an amber mutation is grown in a strain of *E. coli* containing an amber suppressor mutation, a productive lysis ensues. If this lysate is then used to infect another strain of *E. coli* which does not contain the amber suppressor, the phage cannot grow and transduction can be demonstrated. Virulence is but one aspect of this question, however, since similar experiments with another virulent coliphage, T4, have failed to show transduction. Furthermore, T4 particles containing host-derived DNA cannot be demonstrated. Apparently the DNA packaging mechanism of some phages is able to distinguish between phage and host DNA, or perhaps, in some cases, host DNA is damaged too extensively following infection (see Chap. 70). The first contention is borne out by the inability to demonstrate generalized transduction with λ, which, because of its temperate nature, should allow it. However, recall that the concatenate-mediated packaging of λ DNA requires specific cleavage of the DNA, suggesting that the nuclease effecting this cleavage may be able to recognize specific regions on the λ genome. These regions may not be present on other DNA molecules.

The DNA contained in generalized transducing particles, upon injection into the host cell, is apparently available for recombination by the usual mechanisms, but the fate of the DNA of a specialized transducing particle is somewhat different. For example, when transducing a galactose-negative strain to galactose-positive, all of the *gal+* bacteria will be lysogenic for λ, either able to produce λ upon induction or at least immune to subsequent infection by λ. In other words, introduction of the galactose genes requires lysogenization. In the case of transduction by λd*gal*, galactose-positive cells will be produced only in the presence of helper phage. Also, phage can be recovered from the gal+ cells only if the induction (for example, by ultraviolet irradiation) is followed by the addition of a λ helper phage. This phage supplies the function lacking in the λd*gal* and allows it to mature and be released from the cell. The ability of this secondary lysate to effect transduction of the galactose genes will be much greater than that of the original lysate because approximately 50 percent of the phage released will be of the λd*gal* variety. Such preparations are known as Hft (high-frequency transducing) lysates. High-frequency trans-

ducing lysates provide a valuable source of DNA enriched for specific chromosomal genes and have been used extensively to study in vitro protein synthesis.

Abortive Transduction If the DNA from either type of transducing particle does not integrate into the chromosome, abortive transduction occurs, ie, the exogenote DNA does not replicate, and cell division is accompanied by the segregation of the transducing DNA to only one of the daughter cells. This phenomenon can be recognized by the appearance of microcolonies on the medium used for the expression of the transductants and owes its expression to the genetic complementation which occurs in the one cell which contains the transducing fragment. (The microcolony arises as a consequence of linear rather than exponential growth.) The phenomenon of abortive transduction has been used as an effective test for genetic complementation.

Episomes and Plasmids

As was pointed out above, episomes are extrachromosomal genetic units which are capable of replicating either autonomously or as integral parts of the host chromosome. Both the fertility factor and the DNA of temperate phage fit this definition. Other types of extrachromosomal genetic units, known as plasmids, are unable to integrate into the bacterial chromosome and are not transferred by an infectious process (although they can be transferred by transduction by generalized transducing phage).

Bacteriocinogenic Factors A variety of bacteria harbor extrachromosomal elements (bacteriocinogenic factors) which produce bactericidal proteins known as bacteriocins. Bacteriocins may be relatively low molecular weight, heat-stable, nonsedimentable proteins, or they may be large, sedimentable material which in electron micrographs appear as phage components. Bacteriocins bind to stereospecific sites on the bacterial surface, and either manifest their activity while bound or gain entrance to the cell. A single surface-bound molecule of bacteriocin frequently is bactericidal. The metabolic perturbation wrought differs among the various types of bacteriocins. Some of these effects are cessation of DNA, RNA, and protein synthesis, cessation of respiration, cellular leakage, and impairment of general metabolism.

The bacteriocins which have received the most attention are the colicins (those produced by *E. coli*), of which a large number exist. The mode of action of some of the colicins is known in some detail. Colicin E1 causes an impairment of ATP formation which is reflected in a cessation of protein synthesis, a perturbation of DNA and RNA synthesis, and an inability to accumulate certain compounds from the medium. Colicin E2 causes single-stranded nicks in DNA and therefore interferes with DNA synthesis. Colicin E3 inactivates 30S ribosomes by removing 50 terminal nucleotides from 16S RNA.

The presence of bacteriocinogenic factors in bacterial cells frequently is cryptic, owing to repression of bacteriocin production. However, as in the case of lysogenic phage, the repression can be destroyed by irradiation with ultraviolet light as well as by other treatments. Unlike induction of prophage, the derepression of bacteriocins does not always result in death of the cell. The bacteriocins consequently are analogous to defective prophage in this respect, although the basis for lack of killing may be different. It is known, for example, that the colicinogenic factor (Col E3) which contains the structural gene for colicin E3 also contains a structural gene for a colicin E3 immunity factor. This immunity factor, which is a protein of 10,000 MW, reacts stoichiometrically with the colicin E3 molecule to prevent its activity. It is highly probable that other bacteriocinogenic factors specify immunity substances which prevent self-destruction of the cells which harbor them.

Some colicinogenic factors appear to be analogous to F factors, whereas others act more like nonintegrating prophages. Colicinogenic factor E1, for example, specifies I-pilus formation and consequently promotes its own transfer by cell-to-cell contact. It has also been reported that other colicinogenic factors can promote host gene transfer. The responsible factor, like the fertility factor, may integrate into the host chromosome. Other types of colicinogenic factors which are incapable of autonomous transfer are able to be transferred with a helper F factor. Regardless of the episomal versus plasmid existence of bacteriocinogenic factors, most are inducible, as explained above, by treatment

with ultraviolet irradiation or mitomycin C. The bacteriocinogenic state in this respect appears analogous to the lysogenic state. As release from lysogeny results in expression of vegetative phage functions, so release from bacteriocinogeny results in expression of the bacteriocin gene. The reason for the existence of bacteriocinogenic factors is not entirely clear: Some may provide survival value by preventing colonization of ecologic niches by intruding organisms (such as in the case of *Col* E1, E2, and E3), and others may represent evolutionary intermediates between prophage and sexual fertility factors (granting the obvious advantages of sexuality).

Transmissible Drug Resistance   The practical aspects of infectious gene transfer are underscored by the existence among members of the Enterobacteriaceae of a genetic capability which allows the passage of antibiotic resistance from one organism to another. The potential hazard of this transfer lies in the fact that resistance to multiple antibiotics is involved. This phenomenon of transmissible drug resistance was discovered in Japan in 1959 when a strain of *Shigella flexneri* resistant to four drugs, chloramphenicol, tetracycline, streptomycin, and sulfonamides, was isolated from a case of dysentery. The occurrence of multiple-resistant strains of shigellae, salmonellae, *E. coli, Enterobacter, Proteus,* and related inhabitants of the animal or human intestine, as well as of other gram-negative cells, is now common throughout the world. The scope of resistance has expanded to include such drugs as ampicillin, kanamycin, neomycin, chloramphenicol, streptomycin, tetracycline, sulfonamides, and penicillin.

Multiple antibiotic resistance occurs by acquisition of an extrachromosomal element known as a resistance (R) factor, which is structurally similar to the F′ factor described above. The transfer of drug resistance occurs by a mechanism similar to F′ sexduction. The R factor is composed of two functionally distinct regions: one is a sex factor unit (frequently termed resistance transfer factor or RTF) which contains the information for conjugal transfer, and the other is a unit specifying drug resistance (frequently termed the r-determinant). These two elements may exist as separate, autonomously replicating elements, or they may be associated to form a unit similar to an F′.

The r-determinant may contain, as a single linkage group, information for more than one type of antibiotic resistance, in which case resistances will be transferred *en bloc*. As is the case with the F factor, RTFs specify characteristic sex pili; some RTFs produce F pili, others I pili (ie, similar to the type produced by colicinogenic factor E1), and still others produce unique N pili. Strains bearing the RTF and r-determinant as autonomous units may transfer the RTF, the determinant, or both. If only the RTF is transferred, the exconjugant recipient will not be drug resistant but will gain the ability to transfer the RTF. If only the r-determinant is transferred, the recipient will be drug resistant but will not be able to transfer the determinant.

However, if an RTF is subsequently acquired by an r-determinant-containing strain, transmissibility of the r-determinant will be restored. The degree of association-dissociation of RTF and r-determinant is a property of the individual R factor, as well as of the host in which it resides. For example the R1 plasmid, which contains determinants for resistance to ampicillin, chloramphenicol, streptomycin, sulfonamides, and kanamycin exists in *E. coli* as a single covalently closed circular molecule of 65 times 10^6MW, but when transferred to *Proteus mirabilis*, it exists as what appears to be an equilibrium mixture of the 65 times 10^6 MW species and two covalently closed circular molecules of 54 times 10^6 MW and 12 times 10^6 MW, representing the composite RTF and the r-determinant, respectively. R factors share an additional property with the F factor; they are episomal in nature and can effect chromosomal transfer. R factors apparently integrate into the chromosome by the reciprocal recombination characteristic of the F factor and λ prophage.

Resistance transfer factors are usually characterized according to the effect that they have on the fertility of F-bearing strains. Some inhibit fertility and are designated fi$^+$, whereas others do not and are designated fi$^-$. The ability of the fi$^+$ type to decrease the activity of the F factor is simply a reflection of the similarity between these two types of factors in that the repressor produced by the fi$^+$ RTF recognizes the F factor and represses its gene expression.

The mechanism of antibiotic resistance imparted by r-determinants is usually specific for each antibiotic. Examples of the antibiotic-inactivating enzymes as well as other resistance

principles elicited by r-determinants are presented in Chapter 10. It should be noted here, however, that even for a single mode of resistance, variations may exist depending upon the R factor involved. An excellent example of this is the R factor-determined penicillinases. Penicillinase (β-lactamase) hydrolyzes the β-lactam ring of penicillin to form penicilloic acid. The β-lactam ring is the functional group for inhibition of cell wall biosynthesis (Chap. 10) and its hydrolysis destroys the bactericidal action of penicillin. The β-lactamases specified by R factors can be grouped into at least four main types based upon their substrate specificities (ie, against the β-lactam type antibiotics, benzylpenicillin, ampicillin, cephaloridine, cephalexin, carbenicillin, and cloxacillin), immunologic cross-activity, and electrophoretic mobility.

It should be emphasized that chromosomal mutation also leads to antibiotic resistance in the Enterobacteriaceae, which is again exemplified by penicillinase production (viz, the *ampA* locus of the *E. coli* chromosome codes for a type I β-lactamase). The significant difference between chromosomally mediated and R factor-mediated resistance is that the latter imparts multiple resistance, whereas the former imparts resistance to a single class of drug. Episome-specified multiple resistance is brought about by a single event, namely, acquisition of the R factor. The development of multiple resistance based in the chromosome requires several mutational events, so that accumulation of multiple antibiotic resistance of the chromosomal type within a given strain requires sequential selection in the presence of a series of antibiotics. This fact forms one of the bases for using a combination of unrelated antibiotics in treatment of infectious disease.

The potential hazard of transmissible antibiotic resistance is amplified by the observation that transfer can occur among the various members of the Enterobacteriaceae. A strain of *E. coli* inhabiting the intestine of a healthy individual could possess an R factor. A shigella or other pathogen entering this setting could acquire multiple antibiotic resistance by transfer from the *E. coli*, with obvious repercussions upon attempting to clear the newly acquired pathogen from this site.

Penicillinase Plasmids Plasmids have been identified in *Staphylococcus aureus* as well as in other gram-positive bacteria which are of particular significance in antibiotic therapy because cells which harbor these extrachromosomal elements are resistant to certain antibiotics. The most extensively studied of this group of plasmids are the so-called penicillinase plasmids, which contain the determinants for the enzyme β-lactamase.

In general, the β-lactamases of plasmid-containing, gram-positive organisms are produced at a maximal rate only in the presence of penicillin (ie, induced), and the enzyme is found both associated with the cell and in the surrounding medium. These features are in contrast to the regulation and localization of the β-lactamases produced by gram-negative cells, where this enzyme is usually produced constitutively and remains cell associated.

At least three types of β-lactamases are produced by the plasmids of *S. aureus*. These have been designated types A, B, and C and are distinguished from one another on the basis of turnover number, immunologic cross-reactivity, substrate specificity, and amino acid sequence. The types of penicillinase produced by plasmid-containing *S. aureus* correlate with the typing of the particular strain on the basis of bacteriophage sensitivity (Chap. 26, p. 416). Penicillinase types A and C are produced by members of phage group I or III, but never II, and type B is produced by members of group II. This correlation may have its basis in the mechanism by which penicillinase plasmids are transferred among organisms.

Unlike the resistance transfer factor of the gram-negative cells, the plasmids of gram-positive cells do not promote conjugal transfer but must rely upon a virus vector (transduction) for their transfer. Many plasmid-containing strains of *S. aureus* found in nature are lysogenic, which raises the possibility that occasional release from the lysogenic state results in the production of transducing particles containing penicillinase-producing plasmids. Cohabitation of a resistant and a sensitive strain of *S. aureus* could result in acquisition of the penicillinase plasmid by the sensitive strain by generalized transduction. Since successful transduction requires compatibility between the surface of the bacterium and the attachment structure of the phage, the acquisition of the plasmid DNA would be restricted to a host able to receive the virus. The host range of the transducing phage could coincide with the host range of typing phage and consequently establish the above-mentioned correlations. Also, since lysogeny frequently accompanies gene transfer, this relationship could be perpetuated. However, because of the degree of genetic recombination which occurs in bacterial cells and because of the constant selective pressure provided by use of penicillin, this epidemiologic relationship would be expected to break down. This contention is supported by the description of a relatively rare type of plasmid which produces a noninducible penicillinase (type D) which is immunologically different from types A, B, and C and which is found in *S. aureus* cells of phage groups I, II, and III.

Penicillinase plasmids frequently contain other characteristics, such as resistance to erythromycin (or, in the case of the rare plasmid mentioned above, resistance to fusidic acid) and resistance to the inorganic ions, mercury, arsenate, cadmium, lead, and bismuth. Plasmids bearing determinants for resistance to other antibiotics may be present in *S. aureus* and in other gram-positive organisms. For example, resistance to streptomycin, tetracycline, neomycin, and fusidic acid are plasmid-borne is *S. aureus*.

Antibiotic resistance in *S. aureus* can also occur by mutation of the chromosome. Table 8-2 presents the relative frequency of the location of resistant determinants for a number of anti-

TABLE 8-2 GENETIC LOCI OF RESISTANCE TO VARIOUS ANTIBIOTICS IN S. AUREUS

Antibiotic Resistance in Clinical Strains	Genetic Locus
Penicillinase	Plasmid in > 95% of strains
Streptomycin	Probably plasmid in 30% of strains, chromosomal in 70%
Tetracycline	Generally plasmid
Erythromycin	Generally plasmid
Neomycin	Plasmid
Fusidic acid	Plasmid in 70% of strains, chromosomal in about 30%
Trimethoprim	Probably chromosomal in a few strains
Novobiocin	Probably chromosomal in one strain
Methicillin	Conflicting (see text)

Modified from Lacey and Richmond: In Yotis (ed): Recent Advances in Staphylococcal Research. Ann NY Acad Sci 236:395, 1974.

biotics. The appearance of methicillin resistance on this list is noteworthy, because this drug was primarily developed for its property of resistance to hydrolysis by β-lactamase. Methicillin resistance also exemplifies the apparent genetic complexities which accrue as a consequence of the selective pressures introduced by antibiotics. In methicillin resistance, it is uncertain whether the responsible genetic determinant is chromosomal or plasmidal or both because most of the strains isolated as methicillin resistant are nonetheless bearers of plasmids which produce a methicillin-inactive β-lactamase.

Plasmid Incompatibility Groups The various plasmids and episomes discussed above can be classified according to their ability to cohabitate. Plasmids which are distinguishable and which cannot coexist stably in the same cell belong to the same incompatibility group. Conversely, plasmids within one incompatibility group can coexist with those of another group.

The episomes of the Enterobacteriaceae have been placed into several incompatibility groups (group FI, FII, Iα, Iϵ, N, C, O, T, W, P, L, x). The relatedness of various functionally distinct episomes is underscored by the members of these incompatibility groups. For example, the fertility factor F, the colicinogenic factors Col v2 and Col v3, as well as resistance factor R 386, are members of the same group. Also, DNA hybridization studies indicate extensive homology among the DNA of plasmids within incompatibility groups and little homology between groups.

Incompatibility grouping potentially could be of epidemiologic value, for it provides a method of partially identifying R factors. For example, both of the resistance factors R 444 and R 390 carry resistant determinants for ampicillin, streptomycin, tetracycline, chloramphenicol, and sulfonamides, but R 444 belongs to incompatibility group FII, whereas R 390 belongs to group N. The epidemiologic sleuth finding these R factors in a case of dysentery might conclude that they arose from different origins, and he would be right, for R 444 was originally identified in *Proteus morganii*, and R 390 in *Proteus rettgeri*.

Plasmids found in other organisms can also be classified according to incompatibility groups. There are, for example, at least two incompatibility groups of penicillinase plasmids in *S. aureus*.

The molecular basis for incompatibility is obscure but may be related to the replicon properties of plasmids. It is known that plasmid replication is at least partially self-regulated and, therefore, a cytoplasmic, plasmid-specified repressor could possess ambivalent recognition of an incoming plasmid to prevent its replication. Maintenance of the plasmid at a membrane site may also be involved, since it is known that replication and segregation involves DNA-membrane association, and competition for membrane sites may cause incompatibility. The number and types of membrane sites may also explain why cells contain one or two copies of one type but ten or more copies of a different type of plasmid.

RESTRICTION AND MODIFICATION OF DNA

The foregoing outline of gene transfer suggests that the genotypes of bacteria are susceptible to alteration by the genophores with which they coexist in nature. This appears especially true with members of the Enterobacteriaceae, owing to shared mechanisms of gene transfer as well as to common ecology. However, a mechanism exists which tempers this potentially promiscuous interchange of genetic material. It is known that in many bacteria, endonucleases are present which protect the cell from invasion by DNA derived from other strains of bacteria, and these endonucleases are the basis for the phenomenon of restriction. These restricting endonucleases can be active against all types of foreign DNA, and the restriction is manifest regardless of the mode of infection with the foreign DNA, ie, by phage infection, conjugation (including sexduction), or transformation. Restriction systems are highly specific and are accompanied by equally specific modification systems. Modification resides in an enzyme which acts on the same site of the DNA that is recognized by the restriction system and alters it in such a way as to prevent subsequent cleaving of the DNA by restricting endonucleases. Restriction and modification enzymes exist as companions and constitute highly specific epigenetic systems. The genetic information for restriction-modification systems may be located on the chromosome or on plasmids, such as prophage, R factors, or bacteriocinogenic factors. It is tempting to speculate that the presence of restriction systems on plasmids adds a new dimension to the parasitism of this type of element, since it endows them with a mechanism for excluding other extraneous DNA.

The phenomenon of modification and restriction has been most extensively studied using DNA-containing bacteriophages as indicators for the presence of modifying and restricting activities. The degree of modification and restriction can be assessed by determining plating efficiency of the phage on a given host. (Plating efficiency equals the number of infective centers produced per phage particle.)

The specificity of modification and restriction can be exemplified by phage λ replicating in two different hosts, E. coli strains K12 and B. If a lysate of λ is prepared from E. coli K12 and then used to infect E. coli B, the plating efficiency is about 1×10^{-4}. However, the plating efficiency on strain K12 is 1. Conversely, if strain B is the original host, the plating efficiency on strain K12 is about 4×10^{-4}, and the efficiency of plating on strain B is 1. These results, explained in terms of modification and restriction, show that by growing in one strain, the phage acquires a strain-specific modification so that upon infecting the same strain it is protected from restriction. However, when grown on another strain with a different modification-restriction specificity, the phage is restricted. That the restriction is not absolute is shown by the fact that although the plating efficiency on a restricting host is decreased, some of the phage escapes the restriction. This fact reflects the epigenetic nature of modification in that it proceeds without DNA synthesis and is in fact a modification of existing DNA structure. Similarly, restriction does not require DNA synthesis. This is evident from the observation that a host which is lysogenically homoimmune for λ (ie, carrying a λ prophage), and which therefore does not allow replication of λ DNA, will restrict incoming, unmodified λ. The degree of restriction is reflected in the number of restriction sites present on the DNA molecule, ie, the number of sites subject to the endonucleolytic activity of the restriction enzyme. This can be demonstrated by determining the extent of restriction when a single DNA molecule is acted on by two restriction systems with different

specificities. For example, if E. coli K12 is lysogenized with phage P1 which carries its own restriction system, the restriction of E. coli B-grown λ is greater (plating efficiency equals 10^{-7}) on the lysogen (KP1) than it is on Strain K (plating efficiency equals 4 times 10^{-4}) itself.

The first description of a molecular basis for modification was glucosylation of the DNA of the T-even coliphages. When T-even coliphages are grown through one cycle in a mutant of E. coli that is unable to synthesize uridinediphosphoglucose, an intermediate in the phage DNA glucosylation reaction (Chap. 70), phages are produced which lack glucose on their DNA. These phages are unable to grow in E. coli containing a membrane-associated nuclease which is active on the nonglucosylated phage DNA; the phages are restricted. These phages will grow in Shigella which lacks the nuclease, and because Shigella possesses the glucosylating system, unrestricted phage will be produced, ie, the Shigella modifies the DNA. The Shigella-derived phage can now grow on the previously restrictive strain of E. coli because the phage DNA is once again glucosylated.

It is evident from the description of restriction and modification systems that their specificity resides in the host. It is for this reason that the term "host-controlled modification and restriction" is frequently applied to this phenomenon.

The quantitatively important modification mechanism now appears to involve methylation of specific sites on the DNA, which result in protection against the activity of restricting endonuclease. Two types of restriction-modification systems involving methylation have been described. Type I systems, represented by those of E. coli B and E. coli K12, are complex and require a number of participating factors for both the restricting and modifying activities. Restriction requires a divalent metal, S-adenosylmethionine, ATP, and double-stranded DNA as substrate for nucleolytic cleavage. The modification activity requires a divalent metal and S-adenosylmethionine, which serves as a methyl donor. Modification of the DNA involves transfer of the methyl group from S-adenosylmethionine to produce either 5-methylcytosine or N-6-methyladenine in the DNA, depending upon the specificity of the methylase. Genetic analysis has revealed that three loci are involved in type I restriction-modification systems, *hss, hsr,* and *hsm.* (*hs* stands for host specific, *s, r,* and *m* stand for specificity, restriction, and modification, respectively.)

Mutant strains have been selected which are phenotypically restrictionless (R⁻), and 50 percent of these are also modificationless (M⁻). Strains which are solely M⁻ for obvious reasons have not been obtained; this would be a lethal situation, since the presence of active restriction in the absence of modification would result in destruction of the cellular DNA. The frequency of the phenotypically R⁻M⁺ and R⁻M⁻ (50/50) strains show that the restriction and modification enzymes contain a common protein subunit. This view is supported by the results of biochemical analysis, which show that restriction and modification activities exist as a single functional unit (nuclease-methylase). This common subunit, which governs recognition of a common site on the DNA for the nuclease-methylase, is the product of the *hss* locus. The *hsr* and *hsm* loci produce subunits which are specifically involved in restriction and modification, respectively. Accordingly, R⁻M⁺ strains are mutant in *hsr,* and R⁻M⁻ strains are mutant in *hss.* Biochemical analyses of purified type I restriction and modification activities support this view.

The DNA specificity site for type I modification is the substrate for the methylation reaction, but it is not the substrate site for the endonuclease, ie, the enzyme must bind to the specificity site and then by some unknown mechanism migrate to other sites where endonucleolytic cleavage occurs. The modifying enzyme methylates both strands of DNA at the recognition site, although methylation of a single strand is sufficient to prevent restriction. Restricting type I endonucleases cause successive single-stranded breaks in the duplex DNA, but the enzymes are peculiar in that they do not turn over but remain bound to the DNA. This means that two molecules of the endonuclease are required to make a double-stranded scission at the restriction site. It also is of interest that the endonuclease catalyzes excessive DNA-dependent hydrolysis of ATP during restriction; the reason for this is unknown.

In vitro studies have shown that restriction of unmodified DNA at sites where both strands are unmethylated requires minutes, whereas methylation requires hours. This difference in kinetics suggests difficulties for operation of these phenomena in vivo, because the unmodified DNA produced by the rapid rate of DNA replication would be subject to hydrolytic destruction by the endogenous restricting endonuclease. This apparent difficulty is obviated by an important property of the purified endonucleases, namely, that they possess modifying activity, ie, the nuclease and methylase activities are properties of a single functional unit within the cell. Furthermore, the modifying activity of these endonucleases causes methylation at a very rapid rate at recognition sites in which one of the DNA strands is methylated. This is precisely the type of modification substrate which would be produced by the semiconservative replication of modified DNA—composed of one methylated parental strand and one unmethylated daughter strand. Purified type I endonuclease contains three types of protein subunits, two of which are found also in a corresponding modifying methylase which can be purified. These three proteins are the products of the *hss, hsr,* and *hsm* loci. These observations suggest that the dual functioning endonuclease-methylase enzyme is the element responsible for restriction and modification in vivo. The relative rates of nuclease and methylase activity on DNA with unmodified versus hemimodified restriction sites provide the organism with appropriate protection against incoming foreign DNA which lacks the specific methylation, while protecting its own DNA where potential restriction sites are fully or hemimethylated. The ability to isolate a nuclease-free methylase may simply be fortuitous in that it represents a derivative of the endonuclease-methylase.

The type II restriction and modification systems are also composed of endonucleases and methylases, but they are different in many respects from the type I systems. The type II endonucleases and methylases do not contain a common protein subunit, nor do the endonucleases contain methylase activity. The sole requirement for the restricting nucleolytic activity is Mg⁺⁺. Like type I methylases, the corresponding type II activity also uses S-adenosylmethionine as the methyl group donor. The most significant property of the type II systems is that the recognition site on the DNA is the substrate not only for the methylase but also for the endonuclease, ie, the cleavage occurs at the unmodified recognition site.

Because the nucleotide sequence at the recognition site governs the specificity of the re-striction-modification system and also is the site of action of the restricting nuclease, all the fragments produced from an unmethylated DNA molecule by a type II endonuclease contain the same termini. This has permitted sequence analysis of these recognition sites. The sequences of the recognition sites for many of the type II restriction enzymes have been determined. Table 8-3 lists several of these sequences together with the positions at which the double-stranded break occurs in the unmodified DNA and the positions of methylation in the modified DNA. An interesting common feature of all these sequences is the presence of dyad symmetry. This type of symmetrical structure appears to be prevalent in regions of DNA which are designed specifically to bind

proteins. Two types of scissions are made by type II restriction endonucleases: some cleave the double-stranded DNA to produce nonoverlapping ends, while others cleave on a bias to produce fragments with single-stranded complementary ends. These enzymes have been extensively used to analyze DNA molecules in much the same way as specific proteases are used to analyze proteins. Also, those restricting endonucleases which produce single-stranded, complementary termini have been used in genetic engineering experiments for constructing hybrid DNA molecules. This latter feat has been limited to small DNA molecules, such as bacterial plasmids or the amplified genes of eucaryotic cells, such as the ribosomal genes of the toad *Xenopus leavis*.

TABLE 8-3   TYPE II RESTRICTION–MODIFICATION RECOGNITION SITES*

Specificity Designation	Enzyme	Substrate ↓ = hydolysis • = methyl
Eco RI	Endonuclease	↓ GAATTC CTTAAG
	Methylase	• GAATTC CTTAAG •
Eco RII	Endonuclease	↓ NCCAGGN NGGTCCN ↑
	Methylase	• NCCAGGN NGGTCCN •
Hind II	Endonuclease	↓ NAAGCTTN NTTCGAAN
	Methylase	• NAAGCTTN NTTCGAAN •
Hind II	Endonuclease	↓ NGTPyPuACN NCAPuPyTGN ↑
	Methylase	• • NGTpyPuACN NCAPuPyTGN

*The nomenclature for restriction-modification systems uses the first letter of the genus designation, the first two letters of the species designation, a strain or type designation (if appropriate), and the identification of the genophore which codes for the system, if other than the chromosome. EcoRI signifies the restriction-modification system of Escherichia coli antibiotic resistance factor RI. A suggested nomenclature for restriction-modification systems is given in Smith and Nathans: J Mol Biol 81:419, 1973.

RECOMBINATION

The primary significance of the various types of gene transfer previously described is the formation of zygotes within which genetic recombination may occur. Recombination, simply defined, is the acquisition by one genetic linkage group (eg, the chromosome) of information from another linkage group. Recombination is recognized by the redistribution of traits in progeny organisms and may appear to be reciprocal or nonreciprocal. Mating experiments in eucaryotic organisms in which the redistribution of genetically linked (on the same chromosome) characters in progeny cells is scored represents reciprocal recombination and is detected because the recombinant chromosomes are recovered in the progeny. On the other hand, apparent nonreciprocal recombination is often noted in procaryotic organisms because one of the participating genophores frequently is not recovered.

Three classes of recombination can be recognized in bacteria and bacteriophage systems: (1) general recombination which involves exchanges between homologous regions of genophores, (2) site-specific recombination which occurs at unique nucleotide sequences (integration of a prophage, such as λ, at a specific site on the chromosome is an example of this type of recombination), and (3) illegitimate recombination or interaction of genophores where neither site specificity nor extensive homology is involved. Examples of illegitimate recombination include production of F′ episomes, formation of specialized transducing particles, and random integration of prophages into chromosomes from which the specific integration site has been deleted.

The types of interaction between the DNA molecules participating in a recombinational event are the basis for the above categories. It is clear that the initial interaction in general recombination is hydrogen bonding governed by complementary base sequences. The propinquity in site-specific recombination, however, is governed by specific nucleotide sequences and more or less specific recombination proteins. For example, integration of prophage λ into its specific site on the *E. coli* chromosome is brought about by a protein-mediated interaction of specific sites on the prophage and on the chromosome. In this case a specific recombination protein is specified by the *int* gene of the prophage (Chap. 70). The structural principle which underlies illegitimate recombination is obscure.

Mechanisms of Recombination Plausible models of genetic recombination have been fostered by description of the action of DNA of several enzymes, by mutant methodology, and by knowledge of the structural and mechanical properties of DNA.

Two early models of genetic recombination, which because of more recent findings, have been rejected but which nonetheless were of heuristic value, are embodied in the paradigms of copy choice and breakage reunion. The copy choice model was based on cytologic observations of chiasma formation, on genetic data of the transmission of traits in eucaryotic systems, and on the template-directed nature of DNA replication. Recombination by copy choice was envisioned to result from a conservative type of DNA replication which could switch between parental chromosomes as templates so as to form recombinant chromosomes containing regions homologous to one parental chromosome contiguous with regions homologous to the other parental chromosome. The essential feature of the copy choice mechanism is ruled out by the semiconservative nature of DNA replication and by the demonstration that incipient recombinant DNA molecules are composed of DNA derived from both parents and that this redistribution of DNA does not require vegetative replication of DNA.

The breakage and reunion model for genetic recombination largely derived from results of studies on the genetics of bacteriophage. The nature and the replication of bacteriophages make these relatively simple elements ideal material for the study of several molecular biologic problems including genetic recombination. The large number of progeny phage particles produced by a single bacterial cell, together with powerful selective techniques for scoring variants, permits recombinational analysis within very short segments of the phage genome. In fact, it was recombinational analysis of bacteriophage which resulted in the identification of a single base pair as the smallest unit of recombination (ie, crossing over occurs virtually anywhere along the length of the chromosome, intergenic or intragenic), thus dispelling the notion that recombination only occurred between genes. An additional advantage of the use of bacteriophages is their small chromosomes, which can be isolated intact. A typical genetic cross employing bacteriophage and the results of this cross are as follows. *Escherichia coli* simultaneously infected with appropriate genetically marked strains of coliphage T4, *AC*, and *ac* will issue four types of progeny: Two will be parental, *AC* and *ac*, and two will be recombinant, *Ac* and *aC*. However, about 1 percent of the recombinant phage will be heterozygous, ie, upon subsequent infection they will produce approximately equal numbers of particles which are homozygous with respect to the genotypes of the original, parental phage. Heterozygosity is generally considered a property of the diploid state and in classical genetic terms is defined as the presence of allelic forms of the same gene. Heterozygosity in phages, which are strictly haploid, was very revealing and is now known to represent heteroduplex DNA, ie, a region within the double-stranded DNA molecule composed of single strands from each parent. The distribution of heterozygous regions in recombinant phage chromosomes involving several markers is even more revealing. If, in a three-factor cross (*ABC* and *abc*), heterozygosity is noted in one region of a particle, it is usually absent from the remaining regions. Also, if heterozygosity occurs for the middle marker, the two outside flanking markers will be recombinant, each derived from one of the parents. Observations of this type, together with the description of putative recombinant intermediates of T4 which can be isolated from a polymerase I, ligase-negative strain of *E. coli*, fostered a breakage and reunion model for phage recombination. The recombinant intermediates alluded to above are joint molecules of T4 DNA, in which parental contributions are linked by noncovalently bound, presumably hydrogen-bounded heteroduplex regions. The use of the *polA⁻lig⁻* mutant prevents completion of the recombinant molecule and permits detection of these joint molecules. The simplest picture of recombination to emerge from these results with coliphage T4 is that, during phage growth, fragmented DNA molecules containing single-stranded ends are produced. The random reannealing of these single-stranded regions during a mixed infection, followed by the filling of any remaining gaps and sealing with ligase, results in the formation of recombinant molecules. This picture of recombination, which represents the antipode of the copy choice mechanism, is now thought to be oversimplified. The most significant contribution to our understanding of recombination which comes from these types of analyses is the demonstration that recombinant DNA molecules, at least in their incipient form, are composed of material derived from the participating chromosomes. This view is further supported by studies of bacterial transformation, where it has been shown by both genetic and physical means that heterozygous regions of recombinant bacterial chromosomes are composed of a single strand of input, transforming DNA and a strand of DNA of the recipient chromosome.

Current efforts to explain recombination are aimed at defining the molecular events involved in the formation of heteroduplex (heterozygous) DNA flanked by recombinant markers (ie, derived from each parent). Models of genetic recombination hold that heteroduplex DNA is formed by the assimilation of a single strand of DNA from one chromosome by another chromosome. The essential propinquity for this assimilation is complementarity of the bases within the participating regions of the chromosomes and therefore may be restricted in application to the process of generalized recombination. Some of the processes described below, however, should also apply to site-specific and illegitimate genetic recombination.

Single-strand assimilation is most probably initiated by a nuclease which produces a single-stranded nick in the donor duplex DNA

molecule. This initial scission is followed by displacement of the 5′ terminal bordering strand by the action of DNA polymerase which initiates DNA synthesis at the 3′-OH border of the scission. (This polymerization may, in fact, be preceded by gap formation.) The single strand which is locally freed from the duplex structure is then available for displacing a like strand from a homologous region of a recipient DNA molecule (Fig. 8-9). Although the precise mechanism of assimilation is obscure, results are available which show that superhelical, but not relaxed circular, phage DNA is capable of assimilating homologous, single-stranded DNA fragments in vitro and that the tripartite structure formed is relatively stable. These observations as applied to genetic recombination are consistent with the view that in the assimilation process the resident strand of the recipient DNA is removed by the action of nuclease following formation of a tripartite structure. Strand assimilation could be propagated by the simultaneous action of polymerase on the donor molecule and nuclease activity on the recipient molecule. This model, which is depicted in Figure 8-9, adequately explains heteroduplex formation but does not reveal how the rearrangement of the flanking arms of the participating chromosomes occurs so as to produce the recombinant configuration.

Two extremes can be visualized to explain the formation of recombinant molecules. One involves continued interaction of the type of structure shown in Figure 8-9 with recombination enzymes, and the other involves an isomerization of this putative recombinant intermediate. In the first process, the stepwise, or concerted, interaction of the initial recombinant intermediate with recombination enzymes results in a symmetrical cross-strand exchange (Fig. 8-9), which unlike the asymmetrical assimilations described above results in the formation of heteroduplex DNA in each of the participating molecules. The formation of recombinant molecules is completed by an additional symmetrical assimilation involving the DNA strands of the participating molecules which did not undergo the first cross-strand exchange. This process, depicted in Figure 8-10, requires participation of all four strands of DNA and would require a high degree of synchrony of the participating enzymes. An alternative mechanism for generating recombinant molecules following the asymmetrical strand

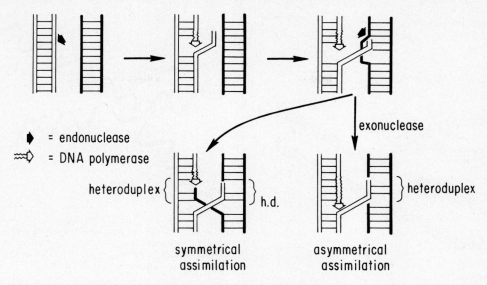

= endonuclease
= DNA polymerase

FIG. 8-9. Initiation of recombination by asymmetrical and symmetrical strand assimilation. Asymmetrical strand assimilation results in the formation of heteroduplex DNA in one of the participating molecules, whereas symmetrical exchange results in formation of heteroduplex DNA on both molecules. The arms of the chromosomes which flank the heteroduplex region are not recombinant in either case.

assimilation (Fig. 8-9) is by an isomerization brought about by rotating one pair of homologous arms 180 degrees about an axis between and parallel to them. The interconversion of recombinant and nonrecombinant forms is depicted in Figure 8-11. The recombinational event is terminated by nucleolytic cleavage of the cross strands as depicted in the figure. The isomerization model results in the formation of heteroduplex DNA in only one of the chromatids. This would seem to rule out its operation in vivo as a significant mechanism for genetic recombination, because genetic segregation data suggest that heteroduplex DNA frequently forms on both chromatids. This problem is read-

ily solved, and plausibility of the model is maintained by the process of rotary diffusion. Rotary diffusion of the cross strand occurs by rotating the individual DNA duplexes in the same sense. This results in migration of the cross strand and formation of heteroduplex DNA on both strands (Fig. 8-12).

It should be emphasized that the foregoing models for genetic recombination are purely speculative. The first model is based on extensive interaction of the participating molecules with various enzymes, whereas the second model requires a minimal interaction with these same enzymes, followed by molecular gymnastics which may appear restricted by the

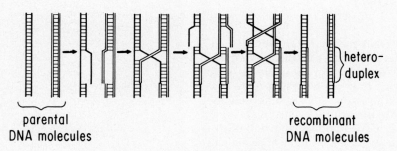

FIG. 8-10. The formation of recombinant DNA molecules. Recombinant DNA molecules can be formed by the participation of all four strands of DNA in single-strand assimilation reactions. The enzymes involved are described in the text. (Modified from Holliday: Genet Res 5:282, 1964)

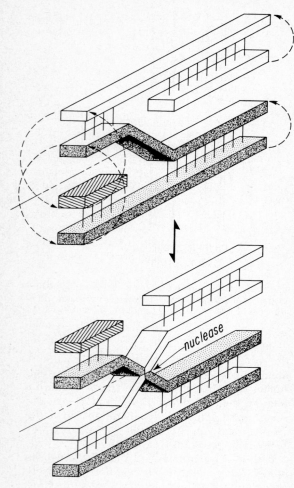

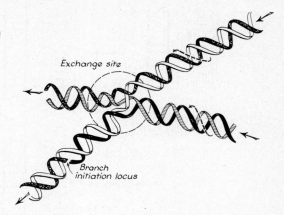

FIG. 8-12. Migration of a cross-strand exchange by rotary diffusion. Heteroduplex DNA can be formed on both DNA molecules by rotating each participating duplex in the same sense. (Courtesy of Dr. T. Broker)

FIG. 8-11. The formation of recombinant·DNA molecules by isomerization of an asymmetrical recombination intermediate. Recombinant molecules are formed by rotating one set of arms 180 degrees around an axis parallel to them. Heteroduplex regions on both of the participating molecules are generated by rotary diffusion of the cross strand (Fig. 8-12). The molecules are separated by the action of nuclease as shown.

tions for initiation of recombination exist and failure to observe these forms when these conditions are absent (Fig. 8-13). Also, space-filling models of the unions specified by the models show a remarkable preservation of base stacking and bond angles at cross-strand regions (Fig. 8-14).

The Genetics and Enzymology of Genetic Recombination   Several genetic loci thought to be involved in genetic recombination in *E. coli* have been identified, and the effect of mutation of these loci have been extensively investigated. Mutations in the *recA* locus cause almost total cessation of general recombination and

nature of the DNA molecule. However, theoretical calculations suggest that isomerizations of the type invoked above are possible, as is the rotary diffusion. It is of interest to note that complexities of structure, such as superhelicity, rather than impeding these events, may in fact facilitate them. The models above, both of which involve an intimate union of participating molecules, are supported by the isolation of branched DNA molecules of coliphage T4 extracted from cells in which permissive condi-

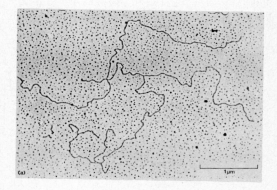

FIG. 8-13. Joint molecules of coliphage T4 DNA Radioautographs of DNA molecules isolated from T4-infected *E. coli*. (Courtesy of Dr. T. Broker)

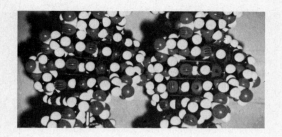

FIG. 8-14. Space-filling model of a cross-strand exchange between two molecules of DNA. The cross-strand exchange resulting from the symmetrical assimilation of single strands of DNA does not involve gross distortion of the participating molecules. Base stacking and bond angles are preserved (Courtesy of Dr. B. Alberts)

have wide-ranging pleiotropic effects, including increased sensitivity to UV and x-irradiation, as well as extensive hydrolysis of DNA following irradiation. Also, *recA* mutations have been described which are suppressible by amber suppressor mutations, suggesting that this genetic region specifies a protein. The nature of the *recA* gene product is unknown, but suggestions have been made to implicate it in the structure of DNA, so that *recA⁻* strains possess DNA which is less rigidly held in its supercoiled conformation (recall that superhelicity has been implicated in the isomerization described above). Still other suggestions have been made to implicate the *recA* gene product in the regulation of other proteins involved in genetic recombination.

The *recB* and *recC* genes are known to code for the two polypeptide chains of an ATP-dependent nuclease known as exonuclease V. Mutations in *recB* or *recC* decrease recombination frequencies, but not to the same extent as do *recA* mutations. *Escherichia coli* cells bearing mutations in *recB* or *recC* display a general decrease in viability, but unlike in *recA* mutants, DNA degradation is limited following UV irradiation. The *recB,C* endonuclease possesses activities which are compatible with its role in recombination as well as in its previously described role in repair mechanisms. It is an ATP-dependent double-stranded and single-stranded exonuclease, an ATP-stimulated single-stranded endonuclease, and also a DNA-dependent ATPase. The apparent importance of exonuclease V type activity is underscored by its presence in virtually all types of cells. Although its precise role in recombination is not known, the decrease in viability of cells

lacking this activity suggests that it might be involved in termination of recombination and/or separation of joint molecules.

Mutant methology has revealed more than one pathway for recombination in *E. coli*. The decreased recombination and viability of *recB⁻, C⁻ E. coli* can be suppressed by mutations in the *sbcB* locus which bring about a lack of exonuclease I. Although the basis of this suppression is obscure, *recB⁻ recC⁻ sbcB⁻* cells are recombination competent. However, recombination in *recB⁻ recC⁻ sbcB⁻* strains can be decreased to 0.05 to 0.5 percent of normal by mutation in the so-called *recF* or *recL* loci. These observations suggest that two recombination pathways normally are operative, a major one, the *RecBC* pathway and a minor one, the *RecF* pathway, and both of these pathways require an intact *recA* gene.

Several other proteins, in addition to those mentioned above, have also been implicated in genetic recombination. For example, the DNA polymerases I, II, and III and their associated nucleolytic activities might participate in the strand assimilation reactions depicted in Figures 8-9 and 8-10, and polynucleotide ligase would be required for sealing the nicks which are generated during recombination. It is known that at least some other proteins which participate in DNA replication are also involved in recombination. Notable among these are the DNA binding proteins which facilitate the melting as well as the reannealing of DNA by preventing it from assuming secondary structure. This latter type of protein is indispensable for the displacements and assimilations depicted in Figures 8-9 and 8-10.

Gene Conversion Heteroduplex DNA contains mispaired nucleotides owing to the allelic origin of the single strands of DNA which constitute these regions. These mismatches can be removed by either of two processes: (1) homozygous daughter duplexes can be generated by the subsequent replication of heteroduplex DNA or (2) the repair mechanisms which were previously described may correct the local distortions caused by imperfect base pairing. Repair results in gene conversion, ie, the loss of one of the input alleles in subsequent progeny cells. This phenomenon forms the basis for aberrant segregation which is frequently noted in the study of transmission genetics.

FURTHER READING

Books and Reviews

Anderson ES: The ecology of transferable drug resistance in the enterobacteria. Annu Rev Microbiol 10:131, 1968

Boyer HW: DNA restriction and modification mechanisms in bacteria. Annu Rev Microbiol 25:153, 1971

Boyer HW: Restriction and modification of DNA: enzymes and substrates. Fed Proc 33:1125, 1974

Broher TA, Doermann M: Molecular and Genetic Recombination of Bacteriophage T4. Annu Rev Genet 9:213, 1975

Cambell A: Episomes. New York, Harper, 1969

Clark AJ: Recombination deficient mutants of E. coli and other bacteria. Annu Rev Genet 7:67, 1973

Drake JW: The Molecular Basis of Mutation. San Francisco, Holden Day, 1970

Gorini L: Informational suppression. Annu Rev Genet 4:107, 1970

Gorini L, Beckwith JR: Suppression. Annu Rev Microbiol 20:401, 1966

Grossman L, Braun A, Feldberg, R, Mahler I: Enzymatic repair of DNA. Annu Rev Biochem 44:14, 1975

Hayes W: The Genetics of Bacteria and their Viruses, 2nd ed. New York, Wiley, 1968

Helinski DR: Plasmid determined resistance to antibiotics: molecular properties of R factors. Annu Rev Microbiol 27:437, 1973

Linn S, Lautenberger JA, Barnet E, Lackey D: Host controlled restriction and modification enzymes of Escherichia coli B. Fed Proc 33:1128, 1974

Miller JH: Experiment in Molecular Genetics. Cold Spring Harbor, NY, Cold Spring Harbor Laboratory, 1972

Radding CM: Molecular mechanics of genetic recombination. Annu Rev Genet 7:87, 1973

Strickberger MW: Genetics. New York, Macmillan, 1968

Watson JD: Molecular Biology of the Gene, 2nd ed. New York, Benjamin, 1970

Willetts N: The genetics of transmissible plasmids. Annu Rev Genet 6:257, 1972

Selected Papers

Alberts BM, Frey L: T4 bacteriophage gene 32: a structural protein in the replication and recombination of DNA. Nature 227:1313, 1970

Avery OT, MacLeod CM, McCarty M: Induction of transformation by a deoxyribonucleic acid fraction isolated from pneumococcus type III. J Exp Med 71:137, 1944

Broker TR, Lehman IR: Branched DNA molecules: Intermediates in T4 recombination. J Mol Biol 60:131, 1971

Cavalli S, Sforza LL, Lederberg J, Lederberg EM: An infective factor controlling sex compatibility in Bacterium coli. J Gen Microbiol 8:89, 1953

Goodman HM, Abelson J, Landy A, Brenner S, Smith JD: Amber suppression: a nucleotide change in the anticodon of tyrosin transfer RNA. Nature 217:1019, 1968

Gottesman S, Beckwith JR: Directed transposition of the arabinose operon: a technique for the isolation of specialized transducing bacteriophages for any Escherichia coli gene. J Mol Biol 44:117, 1969

Hedges RW, Datta N, Kontomichalou P, Smith JT: Molecular specificities of R factor-determined β-lactamases: correlation with plasmid compatibility. J Bacteriol 117: 56, 1974

Hirsh D: Tryptophan transfer RNA as the UGA suppressor. J Mol Biol 58:439, 1971

Holloman WK, Wiegand R, Hoessli C, Radding CM: Uptake of homologous single-stranded fragments by superhelical DNA: a possible mechanism for initiation of genetic recombination. Proc Nat Acad Sci USA 72: 2394, 1975

Horiuchi K, Zinder ND: Cleavage of bacteriophage f1 DNA by the restriction enzyme of Escherichia coli B. Proc Natl Acad Sci USA 69:3220, 1972

Jakes KS, Zinder ND: Highly purfied colicin E3 contains immunity protein. Proc Natl Acad Sci USA 71:3380, 1974

Kier LD, Yamasaki E, Ames BN: Detection of mutagenic activity in cigarette smoke condensates. Proc Natl Acad Sci USA 71:4159, 1974

Lacey RW, Richmond MH: The genetic basis of antibiotic resistance in S. aureus: the importance of gene transfer in the evolution of this organism in the hospital environment. In Yotis WW (ed): Recent Advances in Staphylococcal Research. Ann NY Acad Sci 236:395, 1974

Luria S, Delbrück M: Mutation of bacteria from virus sensitivity to virus resistance. Genetics 28:491, 1943

Meselson MS: Formation of hybrid DNA by rotary diffusion during genetic recombination. J Mol Biol 71:795, 1971

Meselson MS, Radding CM: A general model for genetic recombination. Proc Natl Acad Sci USA 72:358, 1975

Meselson MS, Yuan R: DNA restriction enzyme from E. coli. Nature 217:110, 1968

Morrow JS, Cohen S, Chang A, et al: Replication and transcription of eukaryotic DNA in Escherichia coli. Proc Natl Acad Sci USA 71:1743, 1974

Novick RP, Brodsky R: Studies on plasmid replication. I. Plasmid in compatibility and establishment in Staphylococcus aureus. J Mol Biol 68:285, 1972

Sarathy PV, Siddiqui O: DNA synthesis during bacterial conjugation. I. Effect of mating on DNA replication in Escherichia coli Hfr. J Mol Biol 78:427, 1973

Sarathy PV, Siddiqui O: DNA synthesis during bacterial conjugation: Is DNA replication in the Hfr obligatory or chromosome transfer? J Mol Biol 78:443, 1973

Setlow RB, Carrier WL: The disappearance of thymine dimers from DNA: an error correcting mechanisms. Proc Natl Acad Sci USA 51:226, 1964

Sigal N, Alberts B: Genetic recombination: The nature of a crossed strand-exchange between two homologous DNA molecules. J Mol Biol 71:789, 1972

Vovis GF, Horiuchi K, Zinder ND: Kinetics of methylation of DNA by a restriction endonuclease from Escherichia coli B. Proc Natl Acad Sci USA 71:3810, 1974

Zinder ND, Lederberg J: Genetic exchange in Salmonella. J Bacteriol 64:679, 1952

9

Regulatory Mechanisms

The unicellular nature of bacteria precludes any division of metabolic labor. Even within individual bacterial cells the lack of organelles, such as mitochondria and nuclei, requires that the various metabolic activities form an integrated biochemical microcosm. The expression of this integration in the remarkably ordered growth which is exhibited by relatively simple cells like *Escherichia coli* is based in the various regulatory mechanisms which the individual organisms have retained during the continuing evolutionary flux.

Regulatory mechanisms are usually categorized according to the level at which they act. Genetic regulatory mechanisms modulate the synthesis of the informational and catalytic macromolecules of the cell, and metabolic regulatory mechanisms modulate the activities of preformed macromolecules, such as enzymes. Bacteria have served as fruitful model systems both for the recognition of regulatory phenomena and for the study of the molecular mechanisms underlying these phenomena. Results of studies on the control of the synthesis and activity of bacterial enzymes have been particularly rewarding and have permitted the description of regulatory processes of general biologic significance.

REGULATION OF ENZYME SYNTHESIS

Chromosome Structure and Genetic Regulation As was pointed out in preceding chapters, the bacterial chromosome is a simple structure when compared to its counterpart in eucaryotic organisms. This simplicity, which is reflected in the lack of differentiation, means that the various functions contained within the bacterial chromosome are potentially capable of immediate expression. As the result of extensive biochemical, physiologic, and genetic studies, it is now known that gene expression in bacteria is rather stringently regulated. This regulation is of a type which allows the bacterial cell to alter its macromolecular constitution to best fit the prevailing environmental conditions. It is the limit of this response which contributes to the survival of a particular bacterial species within a given ecology.

The signals which govern genetic regulatory responses are immediately related to the growth and survival of a single cell and are in the form of energy and carbon cources and physical factors, such as temperature, oxygen pressure, hydrogen ion concentration, and other factors discussed in Chapter 5. The bacterial chromosome is in intimate contact with the remaining cytoplasm of the cell and is therefore able to respond in an immediate way to these signals. The regulation of gene expression in bacteria is equivalent to a modulation of the rate of initiation of transcription into RNA of specific regions of the chromosome. This dictum applies to transfer RNA and ribosomal RNA, as well as to the more variegated messenger RNA. The qualitatively important genetic regulation in bacterial cells, therefore, is at the level of transcription. This is not to say that regulation of translation, the other important level of information transfer, does not occur. Translational control may well be a fine adjustment in the rate of protein synthesis, and, in fact, we know that mechanisms for translational controls do exist in bacterial systems. For example, in RNA-containing bacteriophage, where the genome also is a messenger RNA, rather stringent translational controls operate. Many of the features of this type of control are described in Chapter 70.

Transcriptional controls reside in specific regulatory nucleotide sequences conjoined to other nucleotide sequences which are translated into RNA. These regulatory sequences interact with specific proteins which serve to enhance or retard transcription, and the positive or negative action of these regulatory proteins is effected by the physiologic signals alluded to above.

The foregoing brief outline of regulation of gene expression, which will be expanded below, raises the question as to whether or not other mechanisms are available for modulating the relative level of gene products in bacterial cells. A well-known phenomenon, which is usually thought of as operating in eucaryotic cells and which provides for additional gene products, is gene amplification, where multiple copies of particular genes greatly augment the level of products which result from the maximum intrinsic rate of transcription from a single gene. (Oocytes, which contain hundreds of copies of ribosomal RNA genes, are an example of gene amplification.) Gene amplification caused by multiple copies of genes within the bacterial chromosome occurs to a limited extent. In *E. coli,* for example, there are six copies of the ribosomal RNA gene, and some tRNA genes are duplicated. The question arises, however, whether the orientation of genes on the bacterial chromosome and the manner in which chromosome replication occurs, taken together, constitute a type of primitive gene amplification. It was pointed out in Chapter 8 that the replication of the *E. coli* chromosome is bidirectional, proceeding from a heritable origin located at 73 minutes on the standard map and terminating at a point of 180 degrees away. Also, it was pointed out in Chapter 5 that rapidly growing cells of *E. coli* inherit partially replicated chromosomes (thus reconciling a requirement of 40 minutes for a single round of chromosome replication and a 20-minute generation time). These facts mean that those genes which occupy positions on the chromosome within 45 degrees of either side of the origin will always be in the greatest abundance in rapidly growing cells. It may be significant that several genes whose products are found in high levels are located within this region, eg, ribosomal proteins, catabolite activator protein, adenyl cyclase, polymerase I, stringent factor, the isoleucine-valine-leucine biosynthetic enzymes (these amino acids account for 20 percent of the residues in *E. coli* protein), and many others. On the other hand, the genes for the biosynthetic enzymes of the amino acids histidine and tryptophan, which are present in low levels in *E. coli* proteins, as well as many other low-dosage genes are located on the chromosome at positions away from the origin of replication. Although the gene arrangement cited above may be fortuitous, it may reflect a subtle selective advantage by way of a primitive type of gene amplification.

Regulatory Elements

Genetic regulatory regions are of two types: They may be nucleotide sequences that provide specific recognition sites for regulatory proteins which enhance or retard transcription, or they may be nucleotide sequences that specify the primary structure of these regulatory proteins. These two types of regulatory loci are usually distinguished on the basis of their orientation relative to the genes they control. The regions that are targets for regulatory proteins are conjoined to the genes

whose activity they modulate and therefore are active in a *cis* configuration. The genes specifying the proteins which stereospecifically recognize *cis*-active regions need not be conjoined to the regions that they regulate and therefore are active in *trans* orientation, ie, regardless of where these proteins are produced on the chromosome, they ultimately diffuse through the cytoplasm to collide with their targets.

Operons   One of the most striking features of genetic organization in bacterial cells is the frequent clustering of genes which participate in related functions. These gene clusters may be expressed as a unit, so that a single RNA transcript contains the information for more than one product. Discrete, functional molecules are produced from these polygenic transcripts by processing, as in the case of ribosomal RNA and certain species of tRNA (Chap. 7, p. 125), or by translation, as in the case of polygenic mRNA. It should be emphasized, however, that not all RNA transcripts are polyfunctional. Proteins and tRNA molecules also are produced from primary transcripts which contain information for a single product. The response of both polygenic and monogenic systems to genetic regulatory signals is attributable to the *cis*-active regulatory sequences which precede the structural genes in question. These regions on the chromosome, ie, regulatory sequences, together with their conjoined structural gene(s) are known as operons, although as explained below, the original definition of this term was more restrictive.

Conjoined (cis) Regulatory Regions

Three general types of *cis*-active regulatory regions have been described: promoters, operators, and attenuators. Other more specialized types of *cis*-active regulatory elements have been described which bear some functional relationship to the three regions mentioned above but which also display basic differences. One of these, the initiator region of the arabinose operon, subsequently will be described.

Promoters   As pointed out in Chapter 7, the specificity of initiation of translation requires a signal to insure that template-directed RNA synthesis occurs in a meaningful way.

This is accomplished by the interaction of sigma factor-associated RNA polymerase with specific nucleotide sequences which are coupled to structural genes. The role of sigma factor is an essentially regulatory one in that it allows RNA polymerase to select initiation sequences from among all other nucleotide sequences on the chromosome. Initiation sequences, or promoters, are an integral part of all regions of transcription. Promoters are generally considered as positive regulatory regions in that they facilitate transcription. Accordingly, the sigma subunit of RNA polymerase also is positive in its action, because it endows the polymerase with this specific recognition property. Promoters may vary in their ability to initiate transcription and therefore can possess an intrinsic regulatory property. The presence of low and high efficiency promoters is evident by the different levels of various gene products in the absence of overriding regulatory signals. Also, promoter regions can be mutated to higher or lower levels of efficiency.

At least two general types of promoters have been identified in bacteria: catabolite-sensitive and catabolite-insensitive promoters. Catabolite-sensitive promoters require, in addition to holo-RNA polymerase (ie, containing sigma factor), a catabolite activator protein liganded with cyclic adenosine 3'5'-monophosphate (cyclic AMP) in order to initiate RNA synthesis. This requirement forms the basis for the mechanism of catabolite repression which will be described below. Catabolite-insensitive promoters require only sigma factor-associated RNA polymerase for initiation of RNA synthesis. The requirement of catabolite-sensitive promoters for a protein in addition to holo-RNA polymerase raises the possibility that other promoters may exist which require specific proteins for activation. It would seem that this latter situation would constitute an efficient and specific regulatory mechanism. However, systems which respond to specific metabolic regulatory signals possess other types of cis-active regulatory regions in addition to promoters.

Operators   Operator regions are nucleotide sequences which modulate the expression of conjoined genes by binding repressor proteins. Repressor-operator interactions constitute negative regulatory systems in that occupancy of the operator by a repressor molecule prevents transcription of structural genes into RNA. Repressor-operator interactions are more discriminating than are RNA polymerase-promoter interactions. Whereas holo-RNA polymerase binds to several types of promoter regions, repressors only bind to a limited number of stereospecific sites on the DNA. In fact, if a repressor binds to more than one operator, it does so because the functions which it regulates are related. Repressor binding is itself regulated by low-molecular-weight metabolic regulatory signals. The binding of these regulatory effector ligands to repressor proteins can have two types of effects: (1) in inducible systems, low-molecular-weight compounds specifically bind to repressor proteins and change their conformation so that they no longer bind to the operator, and (2) in repressible systems, specific low-molecular-weight compounds bind to repressor proteins and alter their conformation so that they bind to cognate operator regions. The two effects are able to account, respectively, for the physiologic phenomena of induction and repression, ie, inducing metabolites cause an increase in the differential rate of synthesis of specific enzymes by neutralizing the DNA-binding capacity of repressor, and repressing metabolites cause a decrease in the differential rate of synthesis of enzymes by activating the DNA-binding capacity of repressors. It should be pointed out, however, that in the case of many repressible systems, specific repressor proteins have not been identified and other elements are involved.

Operator regions are usually located between the promoter region and the structural gene whose expression they modulate. This orientation, together with other experimental results, promoted a paradigm for the regulation of transcription by operator-repressor interaction, the principal feature of which was steric hindrance by the operator-bound repressor of the migration of RNA polymerase from the promoter into the structural gene. This type of model visualized the promoter and operator as being functionally separate. However, it is now known, at least for some systems, that promoter and operator functions overlap. This will be clarified below.

Attenuator Regions   Messenger RNA molecules contain many extraneous nucleotides at their 5'-end which are not translated into protein. One of the roles invoked for the presence of these nucleotide sequences is ribosome binding and translation initiation complex formation. The presence of these nucleotides means that transcription of messenger RNA is initiated well before the first translation initiation AUG triplet. It has been shown, for some systems, that an additional *cis*-active regulatory region is encoded in the DNA which specifies this leader region of the mRNA. This regulatory region apparently modulates mRNA synthesis by causing termination of transcription. These regions, which are termed "attenuators," have been described in certain biosynthetic systems and are thought to abort productive transcriptional events in response to the same physiologic signal which prevents initiation of transcription. The nature of the element in the cells which conveys the signal of physiologic excess to the attenuator region is obscure but may be related to the potential regulatory elements discussed below (p. 183).

The Structure of CIS-Active Regulatory Regions

The nucleotide sequences of promoter, operator, and attenuator regions have been determined. This feat is usually accomplished by transcribing the DNA into RNA using RNA polymerase and then employing what have become routine procedures to determine the nucleotide sequence of the RNA. Figure 9-1 presents some of these sequences written in the form of double-stranded DNA. The most striking features of these structures is the presence of dyad symmetry. This symmetry is undoubtedly related to the ability of these regions to bind specifically the proteins which perform at these sites, for example, RNA polymerase in the case of promoters, and repressor proteins in the case of operators. This type of symmetry appears to be a common feature of nucleotide sequences designed to recognize proteins (Chap. 8). Many of the proteins which specifically bind to DNA contain subunits, which raises the possibility that the avidness of binding is attributable to the interaction of equivalent regions of these oligomeric proteins with the individual regions of the DNA which constitute the symmetry.

The foregoing description of regulatory regions is by no means complete but is based on what is known from some of the best-described genetic regulatory systems in bacteria. Illustrations of how these elements operate in specific systems are presented below.

The Lactose Operon

The lactose operon of *E. coli* is the prime example of a mechanism of genetic regulation expressed in molecular terms. The operon is composed of a promoter, an operator, and the structural genes for β-galactosidase, galactoside permease, and galactoside transacetylase. The gene for a repressor protein which specifically recognizes the operator region is located near, but is not contiguous with, the operon. Operator-repressor interaction is modulated by the level of inducer present. Although it was thought originally that lactose, the substrate for β-galactosidase, was the normal inducer for this system, it is now known that allolactose, produced by the activity of low uninduced levels of β-galactosidase, is the compound which binds to the repressor to inactivate its operator binding capability. Figure 9-2 depicts the original conceptualization of the lactose operon and the repressor-operator interaction which prevents formation of *lac* mRNA.

The observations which allowed Jacob and Monod to formulate the operon model for gene regulation followed upon the realization that the variation in the enzyme content of bacterial cells, which had been vaguely considered as an adaptive response to the environment, was, in fact, brought about by the ability of low-molecular-weight metabolites to induce formation of

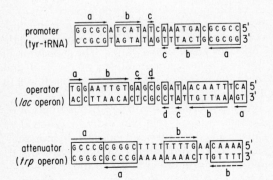

FIG. 9-1. The nucleotide sequence of *cis*-active regulatory regions. The sequence of promoters, operators, and attentuators displays dyad symmetry. Regions of symmetry are indicated by the letters and arrows.

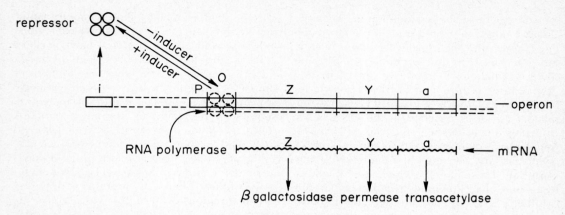

FIG. 9-2. The lactose operon. The structural genes for β-galactosidase, galactoside permease, and galactoside acetylase are Z, Y, and a, respectively. P is the promoter, the binding site for RNA polymerase. O is the operator region, the binding site for the repressor which is specified by the i gene. The repressor-bound operator prevents the formation of *lac* polycistronic mRNA. The equilibrium between operator-bound and free repressor is displaced toward the free repressor in the presence of inducer, thus allowing expression of the operon.

enzymes required for their own subsequent metabolism. For example, β-galactosidase is present at high levels in cells obtained from a medium containing lactose as the sole source of carbon but is present in very low levels in cells grown in a medium containing carbon source other than lactose. The mechanistic concept of induction as opposed to the physiologic concept of adaptation was amplified by the demonstration that β-galactosidase is synthesized de novo in response to induction and that compounds structurally related to lactose, but which are nonmetabolizable, are also able to cause formation of β-galactosidase. These gratuitous inducers proved particularly useful in studying the induction of β-galactosidase, because they showed that compounds need not be altered in order to induce, and their use did away with secondary effects which accrue as a consequence of metabolizing the inducer molecule (p. 181). Mutant methodology revealed that the structural gene for β-galactosidase is separate from the gene controlling inducibility. Mutant strains of *E. coli* were selected which lacked β-galactosidase activity but which contained immunologic cross-reactive material (CRM), whose level in the cell responded to the presence of inducers. The mutations responsible for lack of activity were shown to lie in the *lacZ* gene. Other mutant strains were isolated in which the formation of β-galactosidase was constitutive, that is, formed at a rapid differential rate in the absence of inducer. These mutations were reasoned to lie in a gene

controlling inducibility, and this gene, which is now known to specify the *lac* repressor protein, was termed the *lacI* gene (*I* for inducibility). The classical experiment which first demonstrated the behavior of the *lacI* gene product is described in Figure 9-3. Another type of mutation leading to constitutive synthesis of β-galactosidase also was described. This regulatory mutant was shown to behave in a strikingly different fashion from the *lacI* gene mutation. Whereas the *lacI⁺* gene was shown to be trans-dominant in merozygotes containing *lacI⁻Z⁺* on an endogenote and *lacI⁺Z⁻* on an exogenote, the second type of regulatory mutation was shown to affect the expression of the *lacZ* gene only when it was conjoined with it (ie, on the same genote). In other words, the second type of regulatory region is *cis*-dominant. This *cis*-dominant regulatory locus was termed the "operator (*lacO*)" locus and its constitutive allele "operator-constitutive (*Oᶜ*)." The behavior of the wild-type mutant alleles of the *lacI* and *lacO* genes in various merozygotes is shown in Table 9-1.

Another striking feature of the regulation of β-galactosidase is that two additional enzymes, galactoside permease and galactoside transacetylase, are coordinately synthesized with it, that is, the rate of synthesis of these three enzymes changes by a common factor when induced with various gratuitous inducers. Also, *lacI* and *lacO* mutations are pleiotropic in that they affect the rates of synthesis of all three enzymes coordinately. (A pleiotropic mutation

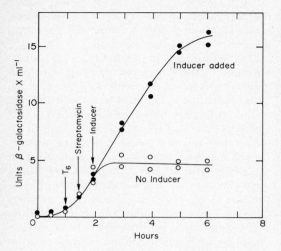

FIG. 9-3. The delayed expression of inducibility of β-galactosidase synthesis in merozygotes formed by conjugation between inducible β-galactosidase-positive males ($Hfr\ i^+\ z^+\ T_6{}^s\ Sm^r$) and constitutive β-galactosidase-negative females ($F^-\ i^-\ z^-\ T_6{}^r\ Sm^r$). The abscissa represents time after formation of the merozygote. Coliphage T6 and streptomycin are added to kill the male cells; the female cells and the zygotes are resistant. The female cell contains neither β-galactosidase (z^-) nor repressor (i^-). Introduction of the i^+, z^+ alleles from the male cell allows immediate and constitutive expression of the z gene. However, at later times the i^+ gene product, the repressor, accumulates to a level sufficient to repress the operon, and the synthesis of β-galactosidase then requires the presence of inducer. (From Pardee et al: J Mol Biol 1:165, 1959)

is one which affects more than a single phenotype.) The coordinate synthesis of these enzymes was correctly explained by Jacob and Monod in terms of a polygenic RNA molecule containing the information for the enzymes in question and under control of the *lacI* and *lacO* genes.

IN VITRO ANALYSIS OF THE LAC OPERON. The model presented above for regulation of the *lac* operon has been verified by in vitro analysis. The *lac* repressor has been isolated and characterized to the extent that its amino acid sequence is known, and x-ray crytallographic studies to determine its three-dimensional structure are presently underway. The affinity of various gratuitous inducers for the purified *lac* repressor corresponds to the in vivo inducing ability of these compounds. In fact, the binding of radioactive isopropylthiogalactoside (IPTG) was used to follow the repressor through the course of its purification. The *lac* repressor specifically binds to *lac* operator DNA contained in the DNA obtained from specialized transducing phages which carry the *lac* operon (Chap. 8), and this binding is reversed by inducing compounds. Direct verification of *lac* repressor action was obtained in an in vitro transcription system employing *lac* operon-containing phage DNA and purified *lac* repressor. In these experiments the presence of repressor specifically blocked formation of *lac* mRNA.

Additional aspects of the action of *lac* repressor were also revealed by in vitro analysis. It was found that repressor binding is extremely tight, with a dissociation constant of 10^{-12} moles per liter (ie, the rate of dissociation of the operator-repressor complex is much lower than the rate of its formation), and the role of inducer is to drive the repressor from the operator. The *lac* repressor prevents transcription by blocking the migration of RNA polymerase from the promoter into the structural genes. This action was demonstrated by preparing phage DNA which contains a *lac* operon, lacking its promoter, fused with the typtophan operon. In this case, initiation of RNA synthesis occurs at the *trp* operon promoter, and *lac* mRNA is formed by readthrough from this point. Using this type of DNA it was shown that *lac* repressor blocked the formation of *lac* mRNA but not *trp* mRNA.

TABLE 9–1 **SYNTHESIS OF β-GALACTOSIDASE IN MEROZYGOTES OF E. COLI**

Diploid Condition*		Synthesis of β-galactosidase
$I^+O^+Z^+/$	(*lac* region is haploid)	Inducible
$I^+O^+Z^-/$	(*lac* region is haploid)	Negative
$I^+O^+Z^-/I^+O^cZ^+$	(O^c is *cis* to Z^+)	Constitutive
$I^+O^cZ^-/I^+O^+Z^+$	(O^c is *trans* to Z^+)	Inducible
$I^-O^+Z^+/$	(*lac* region is haploid)	Constitutive
$I^-O^+Z^+/I^+O^+Z^-$	(I^+ is *trans* to Z^+)	Inducible

The various alleles are explained in the text.

Positive Regulation of Enzyme Synthesis

The regulation of the lactose operon described above represents an example of negative control, where a diffusible repressor protein causes gene inaction. Other systems are known in which induction requires activation of a regulatory protein by the inducing compound. In other words, these regulatory proteins bear a positive relationship with respect to the systems they regulate, and inactivation of these proteins, unlike the case of the *lac* repressor, results in absence of expression of the pertinent structural genes. Positive regulation is found in both catabolic and biosynthetic systems. For example, the genes responsible for rhamnose and maltose utilization are under positive control in *E. coli,* and several of the structural genes involved in cysteine biosynthesis are positively controlled by the *cysB* region in *E. coli* and *Salmonella typhimurium.*

The L-arabinose operon of *E. coli,* which is depicted in Figure 9-4, appears to be controlled in both a positive and a negative fashion. This operon, the expression of which is induced by L-arabinose, contains the structural genes for an isomerase, a kinase, and an epimerase. Linked to these genes is an initiator (*araI*) region and an operator (*araO*) region, as well as a region (*araC*) which specifies a protein that specifically interacts with L-arabinose to modulate expression of the operon. The *araC* gene product exists in two forms, one of which binds the operator to repress gene expression, while the other binds the initiator to promote gene expression. The initiator (*araI*) region of the operon may, in fact, represent a specialized promotor which requires *araC* protein interaction for RNA polymerase binding. The inducer, L-arabinose, has reciprocal effects on the two forms of the *araC* gene product, inactivating the repressor function and activating the positive regulatory function.

The positive role of the *araC* protein is demonstrated by the expression of the *ara* operon in merozygotes containing mutant alleles of *araC.* Two allelic forms, in addition to the wild type, of the *araC* gene have been identified, *araC*c and *araC*⁻, and they, respectively, result in pleiotropic constitutive and negative expression of the operon. Merozygotes containing an exogenote with an *araC*⁻ mutation and an endogenote with an *araC*c mutation exhibit constitutive synthesis of the L-arabinose enzymes encoded in the exogenote. The same condition, but with an *araC* (wild-type) allele on the endogenote, results in inducible expression of the exogenote. These results show that both the *araC*c and *araC* alleles are dominant to the *araC*⁻ allele, and this is true regardless of their *trans* or *cis* position, thus indicating that the *araC* gene specifies a diffusible product which is necessary for expression of the operon. The positive action of the *araC* protein is further demonstrated by the observation that strains bearing deletions of the *araC* gene also are pleiotropic-negative in *ara* operon expression.

In order to demonstrate the repressor character of the *araC* protein it is first necessary to select a mutant of *E. coli* in which the positive action of this product is no longer required. Such mutants can be selected from strains bearing a deletion of the *araC* gene, which can no longer grow on arabinose as the sole source of carbon. Mutation in the initiator region (*araI*c) restores the ability to synthesize the arabinose enzymes and therefore allows growth on arabinose as the sole source of carbon. When the *ara* Ic allele is present with the *araC* deletion, constitutive expression of the *ara* operon occurs. If, however, merozygotes are constructed which

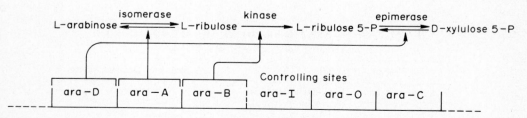

FIG. 9-4. The L-arabinose operon. The genes *D, A,* and *B* specify the structures of the enzymes indicated. The *C* gene specifies a protein which in one form acts as a repressor and binds to the operator (o) region and which in another form acts as a positive regulatory element and binds to the initiator (I) region. The initiator (I) region may be analogous to a promoter. (From Englesberg et al: J Mol Biol 43:281, 1969)

TABLE 9–2 EXPRESSION OF ARABINOSE OPERON IN MEROZYGOTES OF E. COLI

Diploid Condition*		Synthesis of L-arabinose Isomerase (A gene)
$A^+I^+O^+C^+/$	(ara region is haploid)	Inducible
$A^-I^+O^+C^+/$	(ara region is haploid)	Negative
$A^+I^+O^+C^-/$	(ara region is haploid)	Negative
$A^+I^+O^+C^c/$	(ara region is haploid)	Constitutive
$A^+I^+O^+C^-/A^-I^+O^+C^+$	(C^+ is trans to C^- and A^+)	Inducible
$A^+I^+O^+\triangle C/$	(ara region is haploid, $\triangle C$ is a deletion of C gene)	Negative
$A^+I^cO^+\triangle C/$	(ara region is haploid, lacks C gene but I^c mutated)	Constitutive
$A^+I^cO^+\triangle C/A^-I^+O^+C^+$	(C^+ is trans to the O^+ which is conjoined to functional A gene)	Inducible
$A^+I^c\triangle OC/A^-I^+O^+C^+$	(C^+ is trans to I^c and $\triangle OC$; $\triangle OC$ is a deletion of C gene and part of O gene)	Constitutive

*The various alleles are explained in the text.

contain a functional *araC* gene, the operon is repressed, and its expression requires the presence of L-arabinose. In this latter case, the regulation of the *ara* operon is similar to that of the lactose operon, with the *araC* protein acting in a manner analogous to the *lacI*-specified repressor. Added support for the repressor nature of the *araC* protein is the observation that *araC* is dominant to *araCᶜ*, ie, the constitutive expression of the arabinose operon as a consequence of an *araCᶜ* mutation can be restored to arabinose-inducible by the presence of a functional *araC* protein. This latter relationship between the *araC* and *araCᶜ* alleles is to be expected if the *araC* protein acts as a repressor. The operator, or site of action of the *araC* protein, is defined by mutation. Strains of *E. coli*

bearing a deletion which includes all of *araC* and which terminates somewhere between *ara C* and *araI* synthesize the arabinose enzymes in a constitutive manner. The expression of the genes which are located *cis* in relation to the deletion remain constitutive in merozygotes containing a *trans*-oriented *araC* gene. The expression of the L-arabinose operon in various types of merozygotes is shown in Table 9-2.

The observations outlined above are consistent with the ambivalent function of the *araC* protein and show that this regulatory element must exist in two forms, a repressor and a positive regulatory element. The site of action of the repressor is the operator, and the site of action of the positive element is the initiator (promoter). This view has been verified at least partially by in vitro studies which have shown that purified *araC* protein binds to DNA prepared from specialized transducing phage which carry the *ara* operon but not to comparable DNA which contains an *ara* operon with a deleted operator region. A model for regulation of the L-arabinose operon is depicted in Figure 9-5.

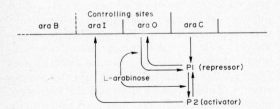

FIG. 9-5. A model for ambivalent function of the *araC* gene product. P1 is the repressor form of the C gene product and binds to the operator. In the presence of the inducer, L-arabinose, the affinity of P1 for the operator is decreased. P2 is the activator form of the C gene product and is in equilibrium with $P_2 1$. Binding of L-arabinose to P2 is required for its positive function in promoting operon expression. (From Englesberg et al: J Mol Biol 43:281, 1969)

Catabolite-sensitive Promoters and Catabolite Repression

The promoters of the *lac* and *ara* operons, as well as those of virtually all bacterial genetic systems which specify enzymes of a purely catabolic nature (ie, those enzymes whose function it is to metabolize compounds to substrates for subsequent use in amphibolic or anabolic pathways), contain catabolite-sensitive promoters, as do certain other regions as the bacterial chromosome. Operons which contain catabolite-sensitive promoters are subject to a general type of regulation which overrides their specific regulatory systems. The basis for this regulation is a requirement for the participation of a catabolite gene-activating protein (CAP) and adenosine 3′, 5′-cyclic monophosphate (cAMP) in the binding of RNA polymerase to catabolite-sensitive promoters. The CAP protein from *E. coli* is a dimer composed of 22,500 MW subunits which must bind cAMP in order to exert its transcription-enhancing activity. Conditions, whether physiologic or genetic, which decrease the intracellular level of cAMP retard transcription from catabolite-sensitive promoters. The most prominent physiologic condition which results in decreased intracellular levels of cAMP is provided by a growth medium containing a rapidly metabolizable carbohydrate; these are the conditions under which the phenomenon of catabolite repression is observed. Catabolite repression is among the earliest observations related to the regulation of enzyme synthesis and is simply defined as the ability of rapidly metabolizable substrates to depress the synthesis of specific proteins. Classically, the protein synthesis which was affected in this manner involved enzymes whose synthesis was induced by their respective substrates. However, it is now known that the synthesis of other types of proteins is also controlled by catabolite-sensitive promoters and is subject to catabolite repression.

A classic observation of the expression of catabolite repression is the diauxie growth curve which results from the growth of *E. coli* on a mixture of glucose and lactose as carbon sources. Figure 9-6 depicts the increase in cell numbers, the disappearance of glucose, and the rate of appearance of β-galactosidase in the course of growth and shows that the cells deplete the supply of glucose prior to the formation of β-galactosidase, which is necessary for the subsequent utilization of lactose for growth. The conservative nature of this type of regulatory mechanism is evident when the fate of the products, glucose and galactose, of the action of β-galactosidase on lactose is considered — glucose is metabolized by enzymes already present in the cell. The repressive effect of glucose

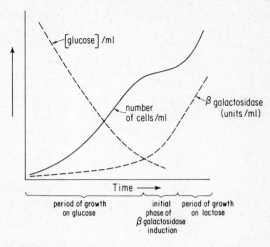

FIG. 9-6. The diauxie phenomenon. *E. coli* growing in a medium containing a mixture of glucose and lactose as sources of carbon will not utilize the lactose until the glucose is depleted. The catabolite repression of β-galactosidase formation exerted by the glucose is reflected in the growth of the cells. A growth lag which follows depletion of the glucose represents the time required for the synthesis of the β-galactosidase necessary for lactose utilization.

can be viewed as conserving the energy required to synthesize β-galactosidase, the activity of which would serve only to produce more glucose. A similar rationale is applicable to other catabolite-repressible systems. Because of this effect of glucose, this phenomenon originally was named "the glucose effect." However, this term was subsequently replaced with "catabolite repression" when it was realized that virtually any carbon source which was metabolized at a rate which exceeded the growth demands of the cell caused this repressive effect on sensitive systems. Cells which are cultivated under catabolite-repressing conditions contain low levels of cAMP. This observation has drawn attention to the enzymes responsible for maintaining the intracellular pool levels of this cyclic nucleotide. All cells contain adenyl cyclase, which catalyzes the formation of cAMP from ATP, and many cells also contain a cAMP phosphodiesterase, which converts cAMP to AMP. The regulated activity of these enzymes could be the basis of a homeostatic mechanism for regulating cAMP levels, a contention that has some support from the observation that glucose inhibits the activity of adenyl cyclase in *E. coli*. If this inhibition by glucose is specific and in fact is the basis for catabolite repression, it must be concluded that the ability of compounds other than glucose to exert catabolite repression is explained in terms of the rate of gluconeogenesis supported by these metabolites.

The important role that CAP and cAMP play in the versatility of catabolic processes of bacterial cells is demonstrated by the effect of mutations which inactivate either CAP or adenyl cyclase. Strains of bacteria in which the cyclase or CAP have been inactivated by mutation are unable to grow on a variety of substrates which normally induce enzymes necessary for their catabolism. For example, strains of *E. coli* which bear either type of mutation are unable to grow on lactose, arabinose, maltose, rhamnose, glycerol, or several other substrates as sole sources of carbon. Several other inducible systems are also unable to be expressed in these mutants. It is of interest that the synthesis of flagellin, the protein subunit of flagella, is catabolite repressible. This is the modern explanation underlying the classical admonition of diagnostic bacteriologists that motility tests should never be performed in the presence of a fermentable carbohydrate.

That the promoter is the site of action of the CAP-cAMP protein complex, and also the site at which catabolite repression is exerted, is supported by several lines of evidence. Promoter mutations occur which convert catabolite sensitivity to catabolite insensitivity with a concomitant loss of catabolite repression control. The separation of operator-repressor type of control from catabolite repression and the role of the promoter, can be demonstrated in strains of *E. coli* where a promoterless *lac* operon is fused to the *trp* operon, in which case the expression of the *lac* genes requires readthrough by transcription which is initiated in the *trp* promoter. Although the expression of the *lac* genes remains under control of the *lacI* gene (the *lacI* gene, in this case, must be supplied on an exogenote because it is removed by the genetic engineering which fused the two operons) under these conditions, because of the presence of an intact *lac* operator, it is no longer under control of catabolite repression because the promoter for the *trp* operon is itself catabolite insensitive. The role of CAP and cAMP in transcription control is further demonstrated in an in vitro *lac* mRNA synthesizing system employing DNA from a *lac* operon-containing specialized transducing phage. Synthesis of *lac*-specific mRNA is greatly enhanced by the CAP-cAMP complex.

REGULATION OF BIOSYNTHETIC SYSTEMS

The differential rate of synthesis of enzymes involved in the formation of low-molecular-weight cellular components is generally repressed by a signal which corresponds to an excess of the pertinent end product. As pointed out above, repressor-operator interactions could adequately account for repression phenomena, but very few cases exist where this mechanism of genetic regulation has been definitively demonstrated for biosynthetic systems. The operon which specifies the enzymes specifically involved in tryptophan biosynthesis responds to an operator-repressor type of modulation system, whereas the enzymes involved in the biosynthesis of many other amino acids involve additional complexities.

The Tryptophan Operon

Figure 9-7 depicts the *E. coli trp* operon, which is composed of five structural genes, a promoter-operator region, and an attenuator region. In vivo and in vitro analyses of the regulation of expression of this operon show that the synthesis of *trp*-specific polygenic mRNA is regulated by the interaction of a specific repressor protein with *trpO*. The binding of this repressor protein, which is the product of the *trp R* gene, to *trpO* requires tryptophan, so that when this amino acid is in excess, the differential rate of synthesis of the tryptophan-specific biosynthetic enzymes is curtailed. The effect of interaction of the *trp* repressor protein with the *trp* operator is different from that resulting from the union of *lac* repressor and *lacO*. As was pointed out previously, occupancy of *lacO* by the *lac* repressor impedes the movement of RNA polymerase from the promoter to the structural genes, thereby effecting repression of the *lac* operon. In the case of the *trp* operon, however, the tryptophan-activated repressor prevents RNA polymerase from binding to the *trp* promoter. This competition suggests that in the case of the *trp* operon, promoter and opera-

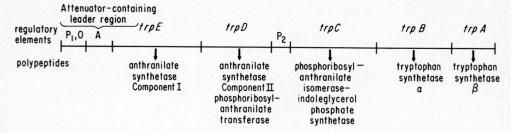

FIG. 9-7. The tryptophan operon of *E. coli* is composed of an operator, an attenuator, and two promoters P_1 and P_2. Promoter P_1 is of relatively high efficiency; the transcript formed from this promoter contains the mRNA for trp E, D, C, B, and A and is under the control of trpO. Promoter P_2 is of low efficiency; the transcript from this promoter contains the mRNA for trp C, B, and A and is not under the control of trpO.

tor functions overlap. It should be pointed out, however, that *cis*-active *trpO^c* mutations exist which cause constitutive operon expression but unperturbed promoter function, thus maintaining the view that operator and promoter function in this system possess some distinction.

The *trp* operon possesses an additional *cis*-active regulatory region, an attenuator, within which the action of RNA polymerase ceases prior to entering the structural genes. This termination responds to a signal which corresponds to excess tryptophan but which is independent of the *trp* repressor. The nature of the element which transduces the excess tryptophan signal to the attenuator region remains obscure. It has been conjectured that the presence of the attenuator region allows a fine control on the rate of synthesis of the tryptophan biosynthetic enzymes.

The *trp* operon possesses an additional feature of interest, namely, an internal promoter (designated P_2, located between *trpD* and *trpC* in Figure 9-7). This promoter, which is not coupled to the normal *trp* regulatory elements, allows production of low levels of RNA containing the message for *trpC*, *trpB*, and *trpA* under conditions of repression. The significance of this low-efficiency promoter is unknown, and it may simply represent an evolutionary vestige.

Other Aspects of Genetic Regulation of Biosynthetic Systems

The regulation of the formation of enzymes involved in amino acid and other biosyntheses has been extensively studied, but to date no unifying principle has been described to suggest a common underlying mechanism. Regulatory regions which are conjoined to clusters of structural genes have been described, and many of these are operatorlike in that they are *cis*-active. However, in most instances, repressor proteins like the product of the *trp R* gene have not been described.

Aminoacyl-tRNA and Repression It has been shown, in several amino acid biosynthetic systems, that aminoacyl-tRNA rather than the free amino acid is involved in repression. The foremost example of this involvement is in the histidine operon of *S. typhimurium*. The histidine operon in this organism consists of a promoter, an operatorlike region, an attenuator, and nine structural genes. Six distinct types of mutations give rise to derepressed rates of expression of this operon. One of these is located in the operatorlike region, while the remaining five types are not linked (by transduction) to the operon. Three of the five unlinked mutations (in *hisR*, *hisU*, and *hisW*) affect the levels of tRNA^{his}, causing formation of approximately 50 percent of that found in the parental strain. Another mutation (in *hisS*) causes formation of a histidinyl-tRNA synthetase which is less efficient in forming *his*-tRNA. The remaining locus (*hisT*) specifies an enzyme which modifies tRNA^{his} by the formation of pseudouridine nucleotides adjacent to the anticodon. It is thought that this modification allows histidinyl-tRNA to participate in repression. It is of interest to note that the *hisT* mutations also cause certain other amino acid-synthesizing enzymes to be depressed, thus indicating that other tRNAs must be similarly modified in order to function in repression.

Autoregulation of Enzyme Synthesis

Several lines of evidence exist to suggest that some enzymes possess ambivalent functions as catalysts and as regulators of gene expression. Examples of this involvement follow. (1) Phosphoribosyl-ATP pyrophosphorylase, the first enzyme specific for histidine biosynthesis, binds histidinyl-tRNA and phage DNA containing the *his* operon. These properties suggest that this enzyme, by some unknown mechanism, participates in regulating the *his* operon. (2) An enzymatically inactive, immature form of biosynthetic threonine deaminase, the first enzyme specific for isoleucine biosynthesis, has been implicated as playing a role in regulating the synthesis of the isoleucine-valine biosynthetic enzymes in a number of organisms. (3) Glutamine synthetase is apparently involved in regulating its own biosynthesis as well as that of a number of other enzymes involved in nitrogen metabolism. Although the mechanism underlying the putative genetic regulatory properties of these and other enzymes remains to be described, their conjectured roles remain attractive because of the failure to implicate other types of repressors, such as described for the *trp* operon.

Gene Organization as Related to Genetic Regulation

Regulons Most of the genetic systems described above are single operons where the genes specifying related functions respond as a unit to a single physiologic regulatory signal. Other systems are known in which the genes specifying related functions are dispersed on the chromosome. An excellent example of this latter situation is the genes which specify the enzymes for arginine biosynthesis in *E. coli*. In this case only three of the eight structural genes are in a single operon. Interestingly, in spite of this dispersal, the various regions respond to a common regulatory element which is coded by the *argR* locus. The *argR* locus apparently specifies a repressor which is capable of recognizing the six operator regions present in the arg system. The type of regulatory system characterized by the *arg* genes has been termed a "regulon," ie, dispersed genes all of which respond to the same regulatory element. (The previously described *ara* system is also, sensu strictu, a regulon because two genes, *araE* and

araF, which are involved in permeation of arabinose, are under the control of the locus, *araC*, which regulates the *ara* operon.)

Multifunctional Pathways The cases cited above involve unifunctional pathways, in which a single end product exerts control. Many other biosynthetic pathways are multifunctional in that they give rise to more than a single end product, all of which serve as regulatory signals. The premier example of such a pathway is that leading to the formation of isoleucine and valine. This pathway, which has been studied extensively in *E. coli* and *S. typhimurium* and which illustrates additional complexities of genetic regulation, is shown in Figure 9-8. Four of the enzymes are involved in both valine and isoleucine formation. An additional function of this pathway is to provide α-ketoisovalerate which is used for leucine biosynthesis; ie, a branch point exists in that α-ketoisovalerate serves as the immediate precursor of valine, as well as a precursor of leucine. The enzymes in the leucine-specific por-

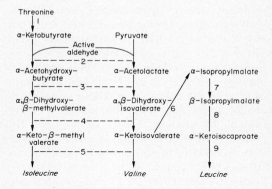

FIG. 9-8. The biosynthetic pathways for isoleucine, valine, and leucine biosynthesis. The enzymes are (1) deaminase, (2) α-acetohydroxyacid synthetase, (3) isomeroreductase, (4) dehydrase, (5) transaminase, (6) synthetase, (7) isomerase, (8) dehydrogenase, (9) transaminase. Enzyme 1 is specifically involved in isoleucine biosynthesis; enzymes 2, 3, 4, and 5 are involved in both isoleucine and valine biosynthesis; enzymes 6, 7, 8, and 9 are specifically involved in leucine biosynthesis. Enzymes 1, 4, and 5 are specified by a single operon, the repression of which requires the simultaneous presence of isoleucine, valine, and leucine. Enzyme 2 is specified by an operon, the expression of which is controlled by valine and leucine. Enzyme 3 is specified by an operon, the expression of which is induced by the α-acetohydroxyacids. Enzymes 6, 7, and 8 are specified by a single operon, the expression of which is repressed by leucine. α-Ketoisovalerate also serves as a precursor of pantothenate (not shown).

tion of the branched pathway are specifically controlled by leucine. However, the enzymes of the isoleucine-valine portion of the pathway are repressed only when isoleucine, valine, and leucine are in excess. This phenomenon is known as multivalent repression. This type of regulation exists also for other multifunctional pathways. The isoleucine-valine pathway exemplifies additional regulatory diversity in that one of the enzymes in this pathway, the isomeroreductase, is induced by its substrate rather than repressed by end product. The manner in which the tripartite regulatory signal represented by excess isoleucine, valine, and leucine is transduced for genetic regulation of this system remains obscure. However, the three cognate tRNAs, as well as threonine deaminase, have been implicated in the regulatory mechanism.

REGULATION OF THE SYNTHESIS OF STABLE RNA

Owing to the fact that the regulation of protein synthesis in bacteria is exerted at the level of mRNA production, the cell must possess a way to rid itself of this template when physiologic conditions dictate cessation of synthesis of its encoded proteins. This removal of needless template is accomplished by RNases present in the cell, so that mRNA is destroyed at such a rate that its half-life represents a fraction of the generation time of the cell. This relatively rapid destruction of mRNA contrasts with the stability of ribosomal-RNA and transfer-RNA, which because of their use in all protein synthesis, are preserved through several generations.

The question arises as to whether or not the synthesis of stable RNA is regulated or whether its concentration in the cell is simply a reflection of gene dosage and the intrinsic capacity of its promoters to support transcription. The rate of synthesis of stable RNA is regulated. The first indication of this regulation comes from the results of measurements of the RNA content of cells growing at different growth rates. As was shown in Chapter 5 (Table 5-2 and Fig. 5-4), the rate of stable RNA synthesis is altered prior to the rate of DNA synthesis in shift-up and shift-down experiments, and the total RNA and DNA contents are not strictly proportional to one another in cells growing at different rates. The results of mutant methodology further demonstrate that the rate of synthesis of stable RNA is controlled by revealing that a single genetic locus is involved in this regulation. This genetic locus, known as *rel*, governs the response of stable RNA synthesis to amino acid starvation. When a culture of an amino acid auxotroph of *E. coli* or other bacteria is starved for an amino acid, stable RNA synthesis is abruptly halted. This behavior is known as the stringent response. If, however, in a *rel⁻* strain a similar experiment is performed, the stable RNA continues to be synthesized, and this is known as the relaxed response (therefore the designation *rel* for the gene which controls this response). These results show that the synthesis of stable RNA is under the control of amino acids. Furthermore, it has been shown that the stringent response is triggered not by lack of free amino acids per se but by the depletion of one or more of the aminoacyl-tRNA pools. The stringent response is accompanied by the intracellular accumulation of guanosine tetraphosphate (ppGpp) and guanosine pentaphosphate (pppGpp). It is now known that these purine nucleotides, which have been termed "magic spots" I and II because of their characteristic chromatographic behavior, are produced by ribosome-associated stringent factor, which is the product of the *rel* gene, when translation is caused to idle by occupancy by an uncharged tRNA molecule of the acceptor (A) site of a ribosome participating in translation. This very complicated feedback regulation provides the cell with an effective mechanism for curtailing the synthesis of stable RNA when its presence is no longer needed for protein synthesis. The role of ppGpp and pppGpp in this response is unknown, but it has been suggested that they may function as inhibitors of initiation of transcription of stable RNA by serving as analogs of purine ribonucleoside triphosphate, with which all stable RNAs are initiated.

METABOLIC REGULATION

The discussion of the biosynthetic capabilities of bacteria in Chapter 5 pointed out that many bacterial species are able to exist by a relatively autotrophic metabolism. Autotrophic metabolism implies the existence of complex enzyme systems which participate in the synthesis of the various types of small molecules required for cell replication. An organism such as *E. coli* or *S. typhimurium,* which can effect its own replication using a compound such as glucose as sole source of carbon, would be expected to possess mechanisms whereby an integration of the various pathways is maintained to allow the efficient use of carbon and energy.

The accrued benefit of efficient regulation of carbon flow through a biosynthetic pathway is apparent when the amphibolic nature of the pathways using primary carbon sources is considered. Figure 9-9 represents the glycolytic pathway and tricarboxylic acid cycle for the aerobic utilization of glucose and illustrates some of the points at which intermediates in this pathway are shunted out of the strictly energy-yielding pathway into biosynthetic

pathways. It is apparent that if a balanced supply of these various end products is to be produced by the cell, some regulatory mechanisms must exist, viz, if an unbridled utilization of the glycolytic intermediates occurred, the TCA cycle would cease to function. One manner in which regulation could possibly be accomplished is by the evolutionary selection of enzymes with appropriate substrate affinities and maximum reaction velocities. Without a doubt this type of regulation does occur to some extent, but it does not represent the quantitatively significant metabolic regulatory mechanism in bacteria. It is apparent that an organism which depended solely upon this type of regulation would be suited for efficient growth in a limited number of environments. The demand for specific end products differs depending upon the environment, and the synthesis of compounds which are already

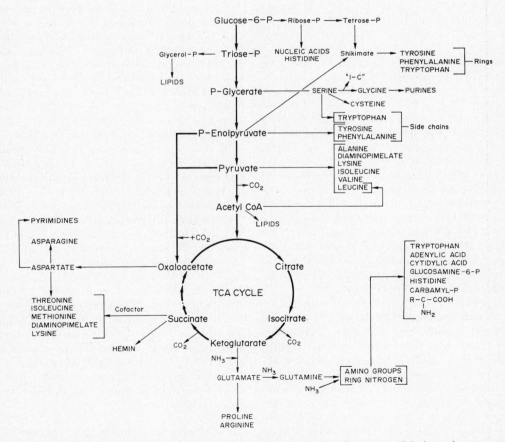

FIG. 9-9. The amphibolic nature of the glycolytic and tricarboxylic acid pathways. Amphibolic pathways are those which serve as energy source and as a source of biosynthetic intermediates.

present represents a waste of carbon and energy.

The genetic regulatory mechanisms described above are also involved to some degree in regulating carbon flow through various pathways, for the differential rate of synthesis of enzymes responds to metabolic regulatory signals. However, genetic regulation is more properly viewed as a regulation of macromolecule synthesis and less as a regulation of intermediary metabolism. For example, when a derepressed biosynthetic pathway receives a signal signifying excess end product, the synthesis of the pertinent enzymes may be curtailed, but carbon will continue to flow through the pathway. In this case, the activity of the pathway will decrease only when the concentration of the enzymes constituting the pathway are diluted by growth of the cells. This obviously would constitute a sluggish and inefficient manner for controlling the flow of carbon. However, inhibition of the activity of the pathway would result in an immediate response to the end product and an efficient utilization of metabolites.

Efficient and highly specific mechanisms have evolved whereby the flow of carbon through the various biosynthetic pathways is regulated. The negative feedback inhibition that end products exert on their own biosynthesis represents the foremost, and conceptually the simplest, example of metabolic regulation. It is known that in virtually all biosynthetic pathways which have been studied in bacteria, one of the enzymes of the pathway is effectively inhibited by the end product. The enzyme upon which this control is exerted is invariably the first enzyme specific for the pathway. This provides efficient control of the entire pathway, since inhibition of an enzyme other than the first would result in accumulation of the pertinent biosynthetic intermediates.

Simple End Product Inhibition Physiologically, the simplest case of end product inhibition is that exerted on a pathway specifically involved in the synthesis of a single end product. There are numerous examples of this pattern of end product inhibition in bacteria, plants, and animals. Historically, one of the most significant examples of this type of control is the inhibition by isoleucine of threonine deaminase, the first enzyme in the isoleucine biosynthetic pathway.

End Product Inhibition in Multifunctional Pathways Other, physiologically more complex patterns of end product inhibition are found in multifunctional pathways, ie, pathways whose intermediates serve as the source of more than one end product. An example of this type of pathway is the synthesis of lysine, methionine, and threonine from aspartic acid (Fig. 9-10). It is clear that if the first enzymatic reaction in this pathway, catalyzed by aspartokinase, was inhibited exclusively by one of the three end products, starvation for the remaining two amino acids would occur. This problem is obviated in E. coli by the presence of three distinct aspartokinases: aspartokinase I is inhibited by threonine, aspartokinase III is inhibited by lysine, and aspartokinase II is not inhibited. The presence of independently regulated enzymes provides for a fractional inhibition of the total activity. Interestingly, this regulatory problem is not solved uniformly by all bacteria. For example, in Bacillus polymyxa and Rhodopseudomonas capsulatus a single aspartokinase is present, and in these organisms lysine, threonine, or methionine alone cannot cause enzyme inhibition, but efficient inhibition is observed in the presence of both lysine and threonine. This type of end product inhibition is known as "concerted" or "multivalent." Figure 9-10 shows the pathway for the synthesis of the aspartate family of amino acids in E. coli. It is noteworthy that regulation of metabolite flow occurs at points other than the first enzyme in the multifunctional portion of the pathway. Each branch point in the pathway is controlled by the ultimate, specific end product. Another interesting feature of this pathway, which illustrates the high degree of integration of the various catalytic steps, is that two homoserine dehydrogenases (aspartate semialdehyde ⇌ homoserine), I and II, are present. (I, like aspartokinase I, is inhibited by threonine, whereas II, like aspartokinase II, is not inhibited.) The ultimate in metabolic integration is demonstrated by these pairs of enzymes. It has been shown that the activity of aspartokinase I and homoserine dehydrogenase I resides in the same protein and that aspartokinase II and homoserine dehydrogenase II are also a single protein.

COOPERATIVE END PRODUCT INHIBITION.
Other patterns for regulating metabolic flow in multifunctional pathways are known. For ex-

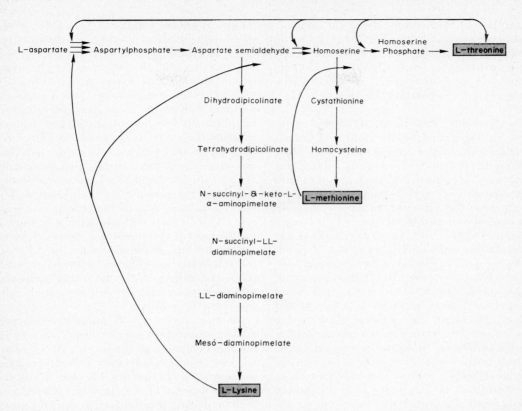

F IG. 9-10. Pathways for synthesis of the aspartate family of amino acids. The enzymes inhibited by the end products are indicated. End product inhibition provides for efficient control of carbon flow through this highly branched pathway.

ample, cooperative end product inhibition is exerted on the first enzyme in purine biosynthesis, glutamine phosphoribosyl pyrophosphate amidotransferase. The products of the purine biosynthetic pathway are 6-hydroxypurine ribonucleotides and 6-aminopurine ribonucleotides. The transferase is inhibited to a greater degree by pairs consisting of hydroxynucleotides and aminonucleotides than by pairs of hydroxynucleotides or pairs of aminonucleotides.

CUMULATIVE END PRODUCT INHIBITION. Another pattern of regulation for multifunctional enzymes has been reported for glutamine synthetase of *E. coli*. Glutamine serves as an amino donor in the biosynthesis of tryptophan, adenylic acid, cytidylic acid, glucosamine-6-phosphate, histidine, and carbamylphosphate. Each of the end products is able to partially inhibit the activity of the synthetase. The degree of inhibition exerted by combinations of the end products is cumulative in that the residual

activity is the product of the fractional activities in the presence of the individual inhibitors. For example, when tested independently, tryptophan, cytidylic acid, carbamylphosphate, and adenylic acid show respective fractional activities of 0.84, 0.86, 0.87, and 0.59. In combination, the total residual activity is 0.84 × 0.86 × 0.87 × 0.59 = 0.37. This type of cumulative effect provides another means whereby the multiple products of a multifunctional enzyme can effectively regulate metabolite flow by modulating the activity of a key enzyme.

The various patterns of end product inhibition described above endow the cell with obvious physiologic advantages. However, this type of modulation of enzyme activity is not reserved strictly to biosynthetic systems. The activity of catabolic enzymes can be regulated in similar fashion. In these cases, however, the physiologic relationship of the inhibiting molecule to the affected enzyme is not always as obvious as it is in cases of end product inhibition. A case where the relationship is apparent is inhibition of the key glycolytic enzyme, phosphofructokinase, by ATP. The relationship between effector molecule and enzyme in this case constitutes, at least partially, the molecular basis of the Pasteur effect, ie, the inhibition of glycolysis by respiration (Chap. 4).

Metabolite Activation Metabolic pathways are integrated by the ability of certain metabolites to stimulate enzymes whose products ensure the efficient use of the stimulating molecule. This type of activation occurs in both biosynthetic and catabolic pathways. Excellent examples of this type of activation occur with the biosynthetic and biodegradative threonine deaminases of *E. coli*. Biosynthetic threonine deaminase, as previously mentioned, is specifically involved in the biosynthesis of, and is inhibited by, isoleucine. Also, the synthesis of isoleucine is coupled to the synthesis of valine by virtue of shared enzymes. It is known that valine stimulates the activity of threonine deaminase in the presence of a low concentration of isoleucine. It would seem that valine exerts a positive control in order to balance isoleucine formation with its own biosynthesis, so that both may be efficiently used for protein biosynthesis. Biodegradative threonine deaminase is a catabolic enzyme produced by *E. coli* when it is grown under relatively anaerobic conditions. Its role is distinct from the biosynthetic enzyme, and it is not inhibited by isoleucine. However, its activity is stimulated by adenylic acid. Since the ultimate function of this enzyme is to provide energy by the degradation of threonine, the role of AMP-stimulation of its activity may be regarded as a regulatory signal to insure metabolite flow through a pathway which will ultimately provide for the utilization of the activator molecule, ie, the formation of ATP from AMP. Although a number of examples of metabolite activation exist, care must be exercised in attributing physiologic significance to them. In many instances the observed activations may be fortuitous.

Mechanism of End Product Inhibition and Metabolite Activation

One of the most striking features of the types of inhibitions and activations described above is that the effector molecules, ie, the inhibitor or activator ligands, bear little if any structural resemblance to the substrates of the enzymes whose activity they modulate. This fact, together with the observation that various treatments, such as exposure to mercurials, high pH, high temperatures, and proteolytic enzymes, can render these enzymes refractory to inhibition by the specific ligand without affecting their catalytic function, indicates that the effector molecule binds to a site other than the active site of the enzyme. Also, mutant enzymes can be obtained which are no longer subject to the action of effector ligands. The term "allosteric" is used to describe this property. The activity of allosteric enzymes is modulated by the binding of low-molecular-weight ligands to stereospecific sites distinct from the active site. Therefore, the basis of this property is different from the strict competitive inhibition by a ligand which is isosteric with respect to the substrate.

Another property of allosteric enzymes which in most cases may be visualized as physiologically significant is that the velocity of the reaction catalyzed increases with a high order concentration of substrate. In other words, the reaction kinetics bear a sigmoidal relationship with increasing substrate or effector concentration. Not all allosteric enzymes exhibit high-order kinetics. Some yield typical Michaelis-Menten kinetics, in which a plot of reaction velocity versus substrate or effector concentration generates a rectangular hyperbola.

Allosteric effects are usually separated into two categories: homotropic effects caused by interactions between identical ligands and heterotropic effects caused by interactions between different ligands. The sigmoid curves obtained for some allosteric enzymes when substrate concentration is plotted against initial reaction velocity are a positive homotropic effect. Inhibition of the enzyme by a stereospecific ligand is a heterotropic effect. Heterotropic effects need not always be antagonistic but can also be positive. An example of this is shown in Figure 9-11, which illustrates the effects of isoleucine and valine on the activity of biosynthetic threonine deaminase. Native threonine deaminase exhibits cooperative homotropic effects with respect to substrate only in the presence of low concentrations of the inhibitor isoleucine. The induction of this homotropic effect by the end product inhibitor is, in itself, a heterotropic effect and is negative.

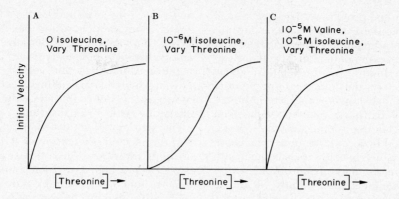

FIG. 9-11. Kinetic analysis of L-threonine deaminase in the presence of allosteric effectors. The initial reaction velocity in the presence of various concentrations of the substrate L-threonine is shown (A). The negative allosteric effector, L-isoleucine, induces (B) a cooperativity which is removed (C) by the positive effector L-valine.

Higher concentrations of isoleucine will completely inhibit the enzyme at the substrate concentrations shown in Figure 9-11. The homotropic cooperativity induced by isoleucine can be reversed by valine, and this action may be considered a positive heterotropic effect with respect to threonine binding and a negative heterotropic effect with respect to isoleucine binding.

Heterotropic effects are usually reciprocal, for example, in the case cited previously, if isoleucine induces cooperativity with respect to substrate binding, the substrate will induce cooperative isoleucine binding. This relationship is illustrated in Figure 9-12.

The high-order kinetics exhibited by many allosteric enzymes probably is of some survival value to the organism. Basically, such a kinetic pattern allows the enzyme to respond in a maximum way to small changes in substrate concentration and permits maintenance of a finite pool of the substrate. It is evident in the case of a substrate such as threonine, which serves as a source of protein as well as a source of isoleucine, that unrestricted threonine deaminase activity would deplete the threonine required for protein synthesis. Similar physiologic significance can be attached to other allosteric enzymes which are endowed with this type of kinetic property.

Several models have been offered to explain how the binding of allosteric ligands modulates the activity of enzymes. All these models are predicated on the observations that (1) effector-ligand binding sites, as mentioned above, are different from catalytic sites and (2) all allo-

steric proteins are oligomeric, ie, composed of identical protomers. A protomer is defined as the smallest subunit possessing, at least potentially, all of the structure necessary for accommodating the stereospecific ligands known to affect the native enzyme. The unifying principle of the various models is that all invoke subunit interaction mediated by conformational

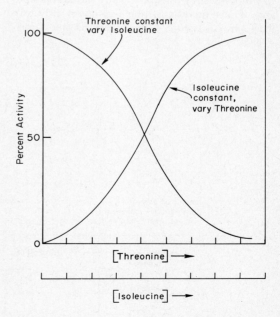

FIG. 9-12. The reciprocal effects of threonine and isoleucine on the activity of threonine deaminase. Threonine is the substrate for the enzyme, and isoleucine is an allosteric inhibitor of enzyme activity. Isoleucine induces cooperativity with respect to enzyme activity, and threonine induces cooperativity with respect to isoleucine inhibition.

changes within the protomers. The question is whether the conformational changes are induced by the binding of the allosteric ligand or whether they occur spontaneously and are stabilized by the binding of the ligands. These two conditions form the basis for the sequential and concerted mechanisms of allosteric transitions, respectively. In a sequential mechanism, ligand binding to one of the enzyme's protomers is attended by a conformational change in the protomer, which because of its contact with adjacent protomers, may change their conformation so as to affect their affinity for the ligand. The concerted transition model, on the other hand, supposes that symmetry among the protomers is constantly preserved and that a spontaneous isomerization between different conformational forms exists. According to this model, in the simplest case (such as that for a simple end product inhibited enzyme), two isomers of the enzyme would exist, one catalytically active and the other inactive. The inhibiting ligand which binds only to the inactive form of the enzyme pulls the equilibrium toward the inactive species, and the substrate or positive effector ligand binds to the active form to pull the equilibrium toward the active species. These models, which are shown in Figure 9-13, are consistent with several of the experimental results obtained with allosteric enzymes. Both models allow effective enzyme activity modulation by either affecting the apparent dissociation constant (km) for substrate or the maximum reaction velocity (V_{max}). Systems in which ligand binding affects the Km are known as K systems, those in which the V_{max} is affected are known as V systems.

The two models outlined previously represent the mechanistic extremes with respect to allosteric transition. Each of these mechanisms, as well as mechanisms which combine features of both, function in certain systems, and, undoubtedly, other mechanisms also exist.

It would be surprising if regulation of all enzymes occurred by identical mechanisms. It seems more probable that a variety of effective regulatory mechanisms exists. The evolutionary selection of regulatory properties would, of course, be secondary to the selection of the enzymatically active protein per se. The added structure which endows an enzyme with the ability to respond to regulatory signals must be compatible with the primitive catalytic structure; any structure which allows efficient regulation ought to be preserved. Aspartate transcarbamylase is composed of two different types of polypeptide chains of which there are six of each in the native enzyme. These are or-

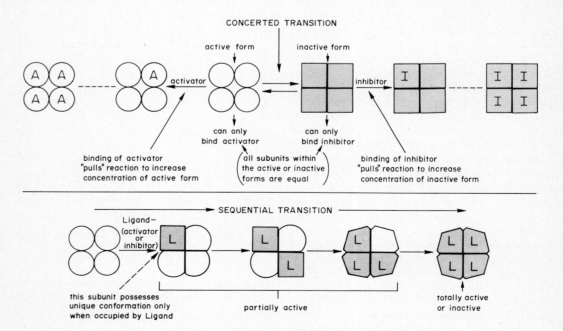

FIG. 9-13. Models for concerted and sequential transitions in allosteric proteins.

ganized into two different types of subunits, one of which contains the catalytically active site, while the other contains the inhibitor (CTP) binding site. There are two trimeric catalytic subunits and three dimeric regulatory subunits in the native enzyme. The role of the two types of subunits can be demonstrated by exposing the native enzyme either to the sulfhydryl reagent, p-hydroxymercuribenzoate, or to high temperatures, in which case the enzyme dissociates into the two types of subunits. The catalytic subunit, when freed of the regulatory subunit, is no longer inhibited by CTP and demonstrates normal (as opposed to sigmoidal) reaction kinetics. Also, the isolated regulatory subunit binds CTP and is able to restore the regulatory property to the catalytic subunit. As opposed to aspartate transcarbamylase, threonine deaminase is composed of four identical polypeptide chains. Nonetheless, this enzyme possesses stereospecific sites for substrate (threonine), isoleucine, and valine. In contradistinction to aspartate transcarbamylase, the primary structure of the single type of polypeptide chains in threonine deaminase provides for the ultimate formation of three different stereospecific binding sites. The comparative anatomy of these two enzymes serves to support the contention that effective regulatory properties are able to reside in grossly different types of structures.

EPIGENETIC MODIFICATION AND REGULATORY MECHANISMS

The foregoing discussion reveals that a common feature, the reversible binding of effector molecules, is involved in genetic and metabolic regulatory mechanisms. An additional feature found in some regulatory systems involves alteration of the participating macromolecules by modifying their covalent structure. These types of alterations fall within the broad category of epigenetic modification.

Phenomena which are explicable in terms of epigenetic modification ultimately are based in the activity of enzymes which are capable of catalyzing the formation or removal of covalent bonds. These modifications yield two general effects with regard to regulation: (1) they influence the ability of macromolecules to participate in genetic regulatory events, and (2) they modulate enzyme activity. An example of the first type, which was discussed above, is modification of tRNA which allows its participation in repression. Other types of epigenetic modifications have an even greater influence on genetic expression. For example, spore formation in *Bacillus subtilis* is preceded by a proteolytic cleavage of the β subunit of RNA polymerase, which reduces its molecular weight from 155,000 to 110,000. This altered polymerase, which is incapable of binding sigma factor, is unable to transcribe the genes required for vegetative functions but acquires the ability to transcribe sporulation-specific genes. A similar consequence, wrought by a different mechanism, occurs when phage T4 infects *E. coli*. In this case the host RNA polymerase is adenylylated and phosphorylated and these modifications apparently cause curtailment of transcription from host genes, while facilitating transcription of phage genes.

The role in metabolic regulation of the modification of enzyme structure by covalently associated adducts is exemplified by the adenylylation of the glutamine synthetase of *E. coli*. The central role of glutamine in the general nitrogen metabolism of the cell is summarized in Figure 9-14 and described in detail in Chapter 4. The previously described cumulative inhibition of the activity of glutamine synthetase exerted by some of the end products for which glutamine serves as an amide donor apparently is, by itself, insufficient for the proper integration of this activity into the general metabolism of the organism. As can be seen in Figure 9-14, one of the functions of glutamine is to serve as a source of nitrogen in the conversion of α-ketoglutarate to glutamic acid. This reaction is catalyzed by glutamate synthase, another key enzyme in nitrogen assimilation. *Escherichia coli* and many other gram-negative cells have evolved an elaborate mechanism which allows glutamine synthetase activity to respond to the levels of α-ketoglutarate and glutamine present in the cells. This mechanism, which involves the adenylylation alluded to above, also causes the catalytic potential of glutamine synthetase to respond to UTP and ATP.

Glutamine synthetase exists in two forms, adenylylated and unadenylylated. The adenylylated form of the enzyme is less active than is the unadenylylated form and also is more sensi-

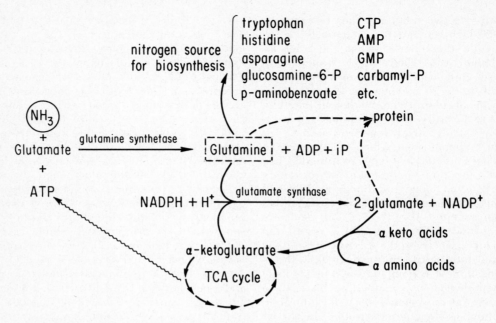

FIG. 9-14. The central role of glutamine in ammonia assimilation by the Enterobacteriaceae.

tive to inhibition by histidine, tryptophan, CTP, and AMP, but less sensitive to inhibition by alanine and glycine. Adenylylation and deadenylylation of glutamine synthetase is catalyzed by a single enzyme (P_I). Adneylylation involves the transfer of AMP from ATP to form a phosphodiester bond with a tyrosyl residue in each of the 12 subunits which constitute the enzyme. Deadenylylation involves phosphorolysis of this bond to form ADP and unmodified enzyme. It is the modulation of these two activities which provides the linkage between glutamine synthetase activity and the metabolic signals mentioned above. The adenylylation activity is stimulated by glutamine and is inhibited by α-ketoglutarate and UTP, so that when a physiologically sufficient quantity of glutamine is present, a less active glutamine synthetase is produced, but when the level of α-ketoglutarate is high, the more active form of synthetase is maintained. (Recall that α-ketoglutarate requires glutamine for its conversion to glutamate via the glutamate synthase reaction.) The effect of UTP may also be significant in that it allows glutamine synthetase to respond to a signal of excess concentration of this nucleotide. (Recall that glutamine is a source of amide nitrogen in this nucleotide.) The deadenylylating activity is

stimulated by α-ketoglutarate, UTP, and ATP and is inhibited by glutamine. The physiologic significance of these effects is as explained above, but an additional feature, stimulation of the conversion of the synthetase to a more active form by ATP, may also have significance. It would provide a signal to ensure that α-ketoglutarate participates in the tricarboxylic acid cycle, rather than being shunted out of this energy-yielding pathway. The adenylylation-deadenylylation activities of P_I are further regulated by an additional protein, P_{II}. This regulatory protein exists in two forms, unuridylylated and uridylylated, which are required, respectively, for the adenylylation and deadenylylation activity of P_I. The uridylylation-deuridylylation of P_{II} is catalyzed by a single protein, uridylyl transferase-uridylyl removing (UT-UR) enzyme. The activity of this enzyme is metabolically regulated. The UT activity requires α-ketoglutarate and ATP and is inhibited by glutamine and inorganic phosphate, while the UR activity requires manganous ions alone, or magnesium ions plus ATP and α-ketoglutarate. These coupled protein modifications (Fig. 9-15), each of which responds to metabolic signals, represent a cascade mechanism whereby the signals are amplified to affect the activity of a key metabolic reaction. The significance

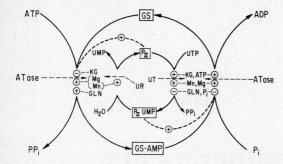

FIG. 9-15. The interrelationship between the adenylylation-deadenylylation of glutamine syntatase and the uridylylation-deuridylylation of the P_{II} regulatory protein and the control of these covalent modifications by various metabolites. Abbreviations are: UT, uridylytransferase; UR, uridylyl-removing enzyme; GS, glutamine synthetase; KG, α-ketoglutarate; $+$ = stimulation; $-$ = inhibition. (From Stadtman and Ginsburg: In Boyer [ed]: The Enzymes, 3rd ed, 1974. Courtesy of Academic Press)

of the proper integration of this key enzyme, glutamine synthetase, is further underscored by the large amount of energy expanded in effecting this regulation.

FURTHER READING

Books and Reviews

Chamberlin JJ: The selectivity of transcription. Annu Rev Biochem 43:721, 1974

Cohen GN: The Regulation of Cell Metabolism. New York, Holt, Rinehart, Winston, 1968

Englesberg E, Wilcox G: Regulation: positive control. Annu Rev Genet 8:219, 1974

Goldberg, RF: Autogenous regulation of gene expression. Science 183:810, 1974

Jacob F, Monod J: Genetic regulatory mechanisms in the synthesis of protein. J Mol Biol 3:318, 1961

Koshland DE Jr: Conformational aspects of enzyme regulation. In Horecker BL, Stadtman ER (eds): Current Topics in Cellular Regulation. New York, Academic Press, 1969, vol 1, p 1

Monod J, Wyman J, Changeux JP: On the nature of allosteric transitions: A plausible model. J Mol Biol 12:88, 1965

Rickenberg HV: Cyclic AMP in prokaryotes Annu Rev Microbiol 28:353, 1974

Stadtman ER, Ginsburg A: The glutamine synthetase of *Escherichia coli*: structure and control. In Boyer PD (ed): The Enzymes, 3rd ed. New York, Academic Press, 1974, vol 10, p 755

Umbarger HE: Regulation of amino acid metabolism. Annu Rev Biochem 38:323, 1969

Zubay G, Chambers DA: Regulating the lac operon. In Vogel HJ (ed): Metabolic Pathways: Metabolic Regulation. New York, Academic Press, 1971, vol 5, p 297

Selected Papers

Bertrand K, Korn L, Lee F, et al: New feature of the regulation of the tryptophan operon. Science 189:22, 1975

Decedue CJ, Hofler JG, Burns RO: Threonine deaminase from *Salmonella typhimurium:* Relationship between regulatory sites. J Biol Chem 250:1563, 1975

DeCrombrugghe B, Chem B, Gottesman M, et al: Regulation of lac mRNA synthesis in a soluble cell-free system. Nature [New Biol] 230:37, 1971

Gilbert W, Maizels N, Maxam A: Sequences of controlling regions of the lactose operon. Cold Spring Harbor Symp Quant Bio 38:845, 1973

Gilbert W, Müller-Hill B: The lac operator is DNA. Proc Natl Acad Sci USA 58:2415, 1967

Haseltine WA, Block R: Synthesis of guanosine tetra- and pentaphosphate requires the presence of a codon-specific, uncharged transfer ribonucleic acid in the acceptor site of ribosomes. Proc Natl Acad Sci USA 70:1564, 1973

Ippen K, Miller JH, Scaife F, Beckwith, J: New controlling element in the lac operon of E. coli. Nature 217:825, 1968

Pardee AB, Jacob F, Monod J: The genetic control and cytoplasmic expression of "inducibility" in the synthesis of β-galactosidase by E. coli. J Mol Biol 1:165, 1959

Rose JK, Squires CL, Yanofsky C, Yang HL, Zubay G: Regulation of in vitro transcription of the tryptophan operon by purified RNA polymerase in the presence of partially purified repressor and tryptophan. Nature [New Biol] 245:133, 1973.

Sekiya T, Khorana G: Nucleotide sequence in the protomer region of the *Escherichia coli* tyrosine tRNA gene. Proc Natl Acad Sci USA 71:2978, 1974

Silverstone AE, Magasanik, B, Reznikoff WS, Miller JH, Beckwith JR: Catabolite sensitive site of the lac operon. Nature 221:1012, 1969

Warren SG, Edwards BFP, Evans DR, Wiley DC, Lipscomb WN: Aspartate transcarbamoylase from *Escherichia coli*: electron density at 5.5A resolution. Proc Natl Acad Sci USA 70:117, 1973

10
The Action of Chemotherapeutic Agents on Bacteria

One of the major triumphs of medical science in the twentieth century has been the virtual eradication of many infectious diseases by the use of chemotherapeutic agents. Two important discoveries revolutionized the therapy of infectious diseases. The first was the discovery in 1935 of the curative effect of the red dye prontosil on streptococcal infections. Prontosil was the forerunner of the sulfonamides. It has no antibacterial activity in vitro, its action in vivo being attributed to the liberation of p-aminobenzenesulfonamide (sulfanilamide). The second discovery, and the discovery that issued in the golden age of antibiotic therapy, was reported in 1940 by Florey and his associates. Although the discovery of pencillin had been made in 1929 by Fleming, it was the Oxford group that demonstrated its unequalled potency and the feasibility of its extraction from culture fluids. A few of the useful antibiotics, like pencillin, were entirely fortuitous discoveries, but from the discovery of streptomycin in 1944 to the present, the search for such agents has been a highly planned, scientifically designed effort.

ANTIBIOTICS

An antibiotic is a chemical substance, derived from or produced by various species of microorganisms, which is capable in small concentrations of inhibiting the growth of other microorganisms. Antibiotics are widely distributed in nature, where they play an important role in regulating the microbial population of soil, water, sewage, and compost. They differ markedly both chemically and in their mechanism of action. There is thus little or no relation between the antibiotics other than their ability to affect adversely the life processes of certain microorganisms. Of the several hundred antibiotics that have been purified, only a few have been sufficiently nontoxic to be of use in medical practice. Those that are currently of greatest use have been derived from a relatively small group of microorganisms belonging to the genera *Bacillus*, *Penicillium*, and *Streptomyces*.

Desirable Properties of an Antibiotic. Selective toxicity is an essential property of a chemotherapeutic agent: It must inhibit or destroy the pathogen without injury to the host. The ideal antibiotic is one that is bactericidal rather than bacteriostatic in its effects. Bactericidal agents kill the organisms against which they are used, whereas bacteriostatic agents exert only an inhibitory effect and rely on the cellular and humoral defense mechanisms of the host for the final eradication of the infection.

The ideal antibiotic is one to which susceptible organisms do not become genetically or phenotypically resistant. It is desirable that it be effective against a broad range of microorganisms. It should not be allergenic, nor should continued administration of large doses cause adverse side effects. It should remain active in the presence of plasma, body fluids, or exudates. It is desirable that the antibiotic be water soluble and stable and that bactericidal levels in the body be rapidly reached and maintained for prolonged periods.

Mechanisms of Action. Chemotherapeutic agents interfere at a number of vulnerable sites in the cell. They interfere with (1) cell wall synthesis, (2) membrane function, (3) protein synthesis, (4) nucleic acid metabolism, and (5) intermediary metabolism. One must keep in mind, however, that there may be a number of stages between the initial or primary effect of the drug and the eventual death of the cell that results. Also, some agents may have more than one primary site of attack or mechanism of action.

Antibiotics Affecting the Cell Wall

The bacterial cell is surrounded by a rigid supportive structure, the cell wall, that protects the fragile protoplasmic membrane beneath from osmotic and mechanical trauma. The assimilation into the cell of soluble substances from the external environment creates an osmotic pressure within the cell that is many times that of the surrounding medium. Any substance that destroys the wall or that prevents the synthesis of wall polymers in growing cells leads to the development of osmotically sensitive cells and death.

The component of the wall that confers rigidity is the murein or peptidoglycan layer. This substance consists of polysaccharide chains composed of alternating units of N-acetylglucosamine and N-acetylmuramic acid. Short peptides linked to the carboxyl group of muramic acid are covalently cross-linked with peptides of neighboring polysaccharide chains (pp. 91 and 92).

The biosynthesis of the bacterial cell wall consists of three stages, each of which occurs at a different site in the cell (Fig. 10-1). The first stage, the synthesis of the uridine nucleotide precursors, UDP-acetylmuramyl-pentapeptide and UDP-acetylglucosamine, takes place in the cytoplasm. In the second stage these precursors are utilized to form a linear peptidoglycan. This is accomplished by transfer of the sugar fragments to a membrane-bound phospholipid carrier with the formation of disaccharide-pentapeptide-P-P-phospholipid. These lipid intermediates are then modified, the nature of the modification depending upon the organism. In *Staphylococcus aureus* the modification consists of the amidation of the α-carboxyl group of glutamic acid and the addition of five glycine residues to form an open pentaglycine chain. This modified disaccharide-pentapeptide moiety is transported through the cell membrane via the phospholipid carrier to the growing peptidoglycan at the outside of the membrane. The third stage in the biosynthesis of the cell wall takes place at this site, outside the cell membrane, and consists of the cross-linking of the linear peptidoglycan strands.

When bacteria are placed in an environment nutritionally complete but containing a substance that inhibits peptidoglycan biosynthesis, nucleoside diphosphate intermediates accumulate within the cells. The nature of these intermediates provides information on the specific reaction site of the drug.

Among the antibiotics that affect the bacterial cell wall are penicillin, cycloserine, ristocetin, vancomycin, bacitracin, and novobiocin. Of these only penicillin and D-cycloserine have a

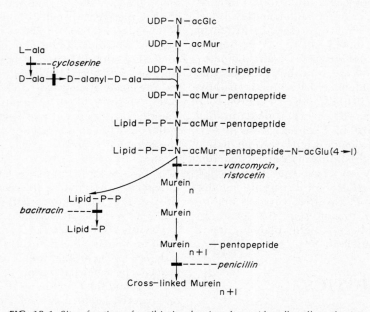

FIG. 10-1. Site of action of antibiotics that interfere with cell wall synthesis.

TABLE 10-1 ANTIBIOTICS AFFECTING THE CELL WALL

Antibiotic	Source	Antibacterial Activity	Major Therapeutic Applications	Toxicity
Penicillin	*Penicillium chrysogenum*	Most gram-positive organisms, gram-negative cocci, spirochetes, actinomycetes	Gram-positive coccal infections, syphilis, gonorrhea, meningococcal meningitis	Nontoxic but sensitization reactions present problem
Cycloserine	*Streptomyces orchidaceus*	Many gram-positive and gram-negative bacteria, *Mycobacterium*	Tuberculosis caused by drug-resistant bacilli	Toxic for central nervous system
Bacitracin	*Bacillus licheniformis*	Many gram-positive species, *Neisseria*	Sterilization of gut before surgery, topical application	Nephrotoxic when given parenterally
Vancomycin	*Streptomyces orientalis*	Gram-positive bacteria, spirochetes	Severe staphylococcal infections resistant to other drugs	Common toxic symptoms: deafness, thrombophlebitis, skin rashes
Ristocetin	*Nocardia lurida*	Gram-positive bacteria, *Mycobacterium*	Severe staphylococcal infections, endocarditis due to enterococci	Highly toxic, causes leukopenia

mode of action directly explicable in terms of their inhibition of cell wall synthesis (Table 10-1).

The Penicillins Penicillin is still the most widely used antibiotic for general therapeutic use. In the years since the first crude product was obtained from *Penicillium notatum* the penicillin molecule has been chemically manipulated, and numerous natural and semisynthetic congeners have been produced, several of which are very useful therapeutically. By greater attention to cultural conditions that provide the chemical precursors of the antibiotic and by substitution of a high-yielding mutant of *Penicillium chrysogenum*, penicillin production has been enhanced manyfold.

The term "penicillin" is generic for the entire group of natural and semisynthetic penicillins. The basic structure (Fig. 10-2) consists of a thiazolidine ring joined to a β-lactam ring, to which is attached a side-chain that determines many of the antibacterial and pharmacologic properties of a particular type of penicillin. Of

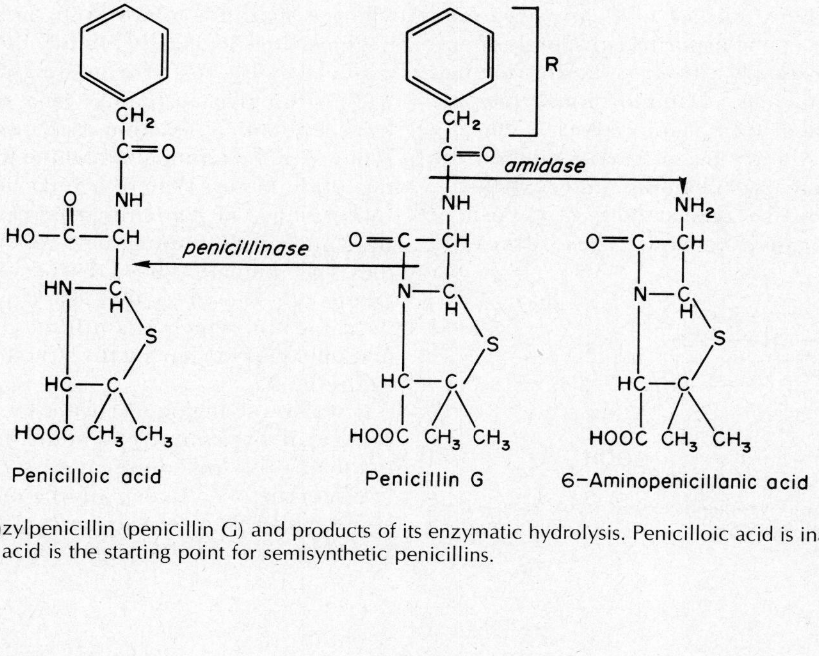

FIG. 10-2. Benzylpenicillin (penicillin G) and products of its enzymatic hydrolysis. Penicilloic acid is inactive. 6-Aminopenicillanic acid is the starting point for semisynthetic penicillins.

the natural penicillins produced, benzylpenicillin or penicillin G is clinically the most useful. Its almost exclusive formation is ensured by the addition of the appropriate precursor, phenylacetic acid, to the medium.

SEMISYNTHETIC PENICILLINS. The penicillin nucleus itself, 6-aminopenicillanic acid, is the primary structural requirement for biologic activity. It can be prepared in quantity from benzylpenicillin or other natural penicillins by the action of an amidase derived from a number of microbial species. Once this penicillin nucleus is available various side-chains can be attached and penicillins of a semisynthetic nature produced. Several of these have been useful in circumventing some of the shortcomings of penicillin G. Among the most useful of the semisynthetic penicillins are the penicillinase-resistant group in which an alteration of the side-chain has provided protection for the β-lactam ring from the action of penicillinase without removing its antibacterial activity. Such penicillins include methicillin, which is acid labile, and the isoxazolyl penicillins (cloxacillin, oxacillin, and nafcillin) which combine resistance to penicillinase with resistance to acid. Of the broad-spectrum penicillins, ampicillin has proved clinically most useful. It is acid stable but is inactivated by penicillinase. Its outstanding property is its greatly increased activity against various gram-negative bacilli.

CEPHALOSPORINS. Antibiotics of this group are formed by a species of *Cephalosporium*. One of these, cephalosporin C, resembles penicillin in possessing a fused β-lactam ring and an active nucleus, 7-amino-cephalosporanic acid, that can also be manipulated chemically (Fig. 10-3). Alterations to it have yielded the useful derivatives cephalothin and cephalexin, compounds active against both gram-positive and gram-negative bacteria. These drugs are resistant to staphylococcal penicillinase but are susceptible to the β-lactamases of certain gram-negative bacteria.

ANTIMICROBIAL EFFECTS OF THE PENICILLINS. Penicillin-sensitive organisms are killed by these antibiotics; the essential requirement for bactericidal action is actively multiplying bacteria. Penicillin G is effective against most gram-positive and gram-negative cocci. Among the least susceptible of the gram-positive cocci are the enterococci and penicillinase-producing strains of S. *aureus*. Although most gram-negative bacilli are resistant to low concentrations of penicillin G, moderate to high concentrations are effective.

MECHANISM OF ACTION. Penicillin interferes with the formation of the organism's protective cell wall. When susceptible bacteria are cultured in the presence of lethal concentrations of penicillin they lyse. If subinhibitory concentrations are used, large, swollen filamentous forms are produced. Such effects, however, are observed only in growing organisms. If growth is prevented by the omission of a nutrient or by the use of a bacteriostatic agent, penicillin is without effect. When rod-shaped organisms are grown in the presence of penicillin in a protective hypertonic medium containing magnesium and a stabilizing concentration of sucrose, large osmotically fragile, spherical forms, spheroplasts, are produced. These forms revert to rod-shaped organisms when penicillin is removed (p. 39).

Penicillin specifically inhibits the last step in cell wall synthesis, the cross-linking of the linear peptidoglycan strands. This reaction is a transpeptidation reaction that results in the removal of the terminal D-alanine from the pentapeptide chain. When bacteria are grown in the presence of penicillin, uncross-linked uridine nucleotide intermediates of cell wall synthesis accumulate. Those that accumulate in S. *aureus* are known as the "Park nucleotides," the largest of which is a uridine-diphosphate-muramyl peptide having the structure shown in Figure 10-4.

A structural analogy between penicillin and the D-alanyl-D-alanine end of the pentapeptide in the uncross-linked precursor of the cell wall has been invoked to explain the molecular basis for the antibacterial action of penicillin. The CO-N bond in the β-lactam ring of penicillin

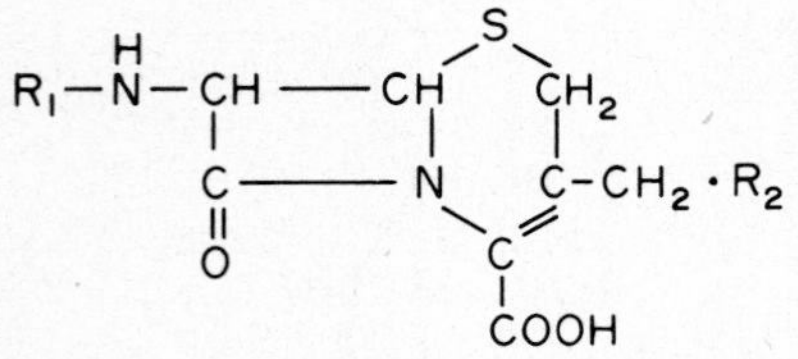

FIG. 10-3. 7-Amino-cephalosporanic acid. Substitutions at the R_1 and R_2 positions have yielded clinically useful derivatives.

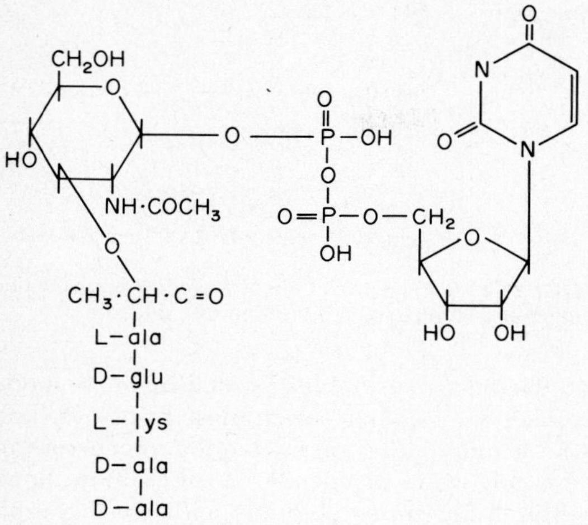

FIG. 10-4. Structure of the Park nucleotide, a uridine nucleotide accumulated by *Staphylococcus aureus* when grown in the presence of penicillin. The muramyl pentapeptide moiety is shown at left.

lies in the same position as the peptide bond involved in the transpeptidation. It has thus been proposed that penicillin, acting as a substrate analog of the normal transpeptidation substrate, combines with the transpeptidase and thereby irreversibly inactivates it.

Another enzyme whose activity is inhibited by penicillin is D-alanine carboxypeptidase. This enzyme hydrolyzes the C-terminal D-alanyl-D-alanine sequence of the uridine nucleotide pentapeptide precursor, and strongly binds ^{14}C-penicillin. Several endopeptidases are also inhibited by penicillin. No correlation, however, appears to exist between inhibition of these enzymes and killing of the organism. At the present time there are conflicting possibilities and hypotheses on the role and existence of these and other penicillin receptor sites in the membrane. Further studies are needed for their clarification.

RESISTANCE TO PENICILLIN. Resistance to penicillin results from a modification of either (1) the antibiotic itself or (2) a specific target structure in the bacterial cell. Modification of the antibiotic structure is effectively achieved by β-lactamases or by penicillin amidases. The major cause of resistance to penicillin is penicillinase, a β-lactamase that opens the β-lactam ring hydrolytically, thus converting the antibiotic to the inactive penicilloic acid. Penicillin

amidase removes the acyl side-chain but leaves the penicillin nucleus intact (Fig. 10-2). The penicillin amidases do not occur widely in bacteria. Their primary importance is in the preparation of the starting material for the synthesis of penicillins refractory to β-lactamase.

β-Lactamases are found in both gram-positive and gram-negative organisms and are responsible for many highly resistant strains. In the development of semisynthetic penicillins one of the primary goals was to find compounds that were insensitive to β-lactamase activity. In this respect methicillin and the isoxazolyl group of penicillins for the gram-positive organisms and carbenicillin for the gram-negative species are extremely useful.

The differential penicillin sensitivity between gram-positive and gram-negative organisms emphasizes major differences in mechanisms of resistance. The β-lactamases of gram-positive bacteria are extracellular and are produced in relatively large amounts. They are inducible and have a very high affinity for their substrates. The enzymes from gram-negative organisms are cell bound and produced in smaller amounts; they are usually constitutive and have a much lower affinity for their substrates. The release by gram-positive species of large amounts of β-lactamase into the immediate environs results in a populational effect. By contrast, however, localization of the enzyme in the periplasmic space of gram-negative species restricts access of the drug to the membrane target sites only after the drug has penetrated the cell wall layer. In these organisms penicillinase resistance cannot be attributed to β-lactamase activity alone but is due to a complex interaction between β-lactamase and a barrier in the outer membrane. Alteration of the carbohydrate composition of the lipopolysaccharide and hydrolysis of the murein skeleton disturb the barrier functions and render the organism sensitive to penicillin.

Further discussion of penicillin resistance, its genetics, epidemiology, and clinical importance is found on pp. 161 and 224 of this Chapter and in Chapters 8 and 24.

D-Cycloserine The structural similarity of D-cycloserine to D-alanine is the basis of its bactericidal activity (Fig. 10-5). It is a competitive inhibitor of two sequential reactions in the synthesis of the peptidoglycan of the cell wall, alanine racemase and D-alanyl-D-alanine syn-

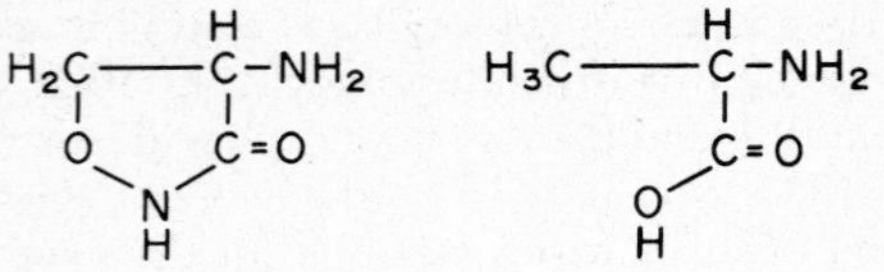

FIG. 10-5. Structural relationship between cycloserine (left) and D-alanine (right).

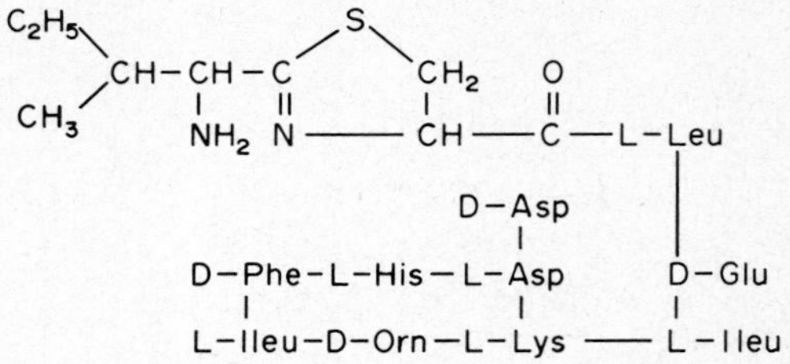

FIG. 10-6. Bacitracin A. One of a group of polypeptide antibiotics containing a thiazoline ring structure.

thetase. The latter enzyme has two binding sites for D-cycloserine, the donor and acceptor sites. The donor site is believed to be the primary site of antibiotic action. The concentration of D-cycloserine required for 50 percent saturation is lowest for this site and is related directly to the minimum inhibitory concentration for growth.

D-Cycloserine has a higher affinity than D-alanine for both of the D-alanine reacting sites of the D-alanyl-D-alanine synthetase. The rigid planar ring structure of D-cycloserine is believed to hold the molecule in the proper conformation for binding to the active sites on the inhibited enzymes.

The inhibition of peptidoglycan synthesis by growth in the presence of minimal inhibitory concentrations of the drug results in the accumulation of an incomplete cell wall precursor lacking the terminal D-alanyl-D-alanine dipeptide. The accumulation of this precursor may be diminished by the addition of D-alanine to the culture broth. Growth inhibition by D-cycloserine also leads to spheroplast formation in a hypertonic medium. This effect is prevented by the addition of D-alanine.

Resistance to D-cycloserine may be attributed to two different mechanisms. In certain organisms such as *E. coli* and *Streptococcus faecalis,* the antibiotic is effective only if a transport system for D-alanine is present. Loss of some component of the alanine transport system can protect the organism against D-cycloserine activity. In other mutants resistance is attributed to elevated levels of both alanine racemase and alanyl-D-alanine synthetase.

Bacitracin Bacitracin is a polypeptide antibiotic that is bactericidal for many gram-positive species. With the exception of *Neisseria,* however, it has little effect on gram-negative organisms (Fig. 10-6). Resistance to the drug does not develop readily, and cross-resistance between it and other antibiotics does not occur either in vitro or in vivo.

Bacitracin resembles penicillin in its mode of action, causing spheroplast formation and the accumulation of nucleotide precursors of the cell wall. Its specific site of action, however, differs from that of penicillin in that it interferes with cell wall synthesis at an earlier stage. It interferes with the second stage of cell wall synthesis in which the linear peptidoglycan is synthesized via a membrane-bound phospholipid intermediate and transferred to an endogenous acceptor. In the last step of this stage of cell wall biosynthesis the pyrophosphate form of the phospholipid is dephosphorylated to yield inorganic phosphate and regenerate the phospholipid.

$$C_{55} \text{ isoprenyl-PP} \rightleftharpoons C_{55} \text{ isoprenyl-P} + P_i$$

It is this reaction that is specifically inhibited by bacitracin. Bacitracin, therefore, inhibits cell wall synthesis by preventing reentry of the lipid carrier into the reaction cycle of cell wall synthesis.

The Vancomycin Group Among the clinically useful members of the vancomycin group are vancomycin and ristocetins A and B. The molecular structure of this amphoteric group of antibiotics has not been fully delineated. The characteristic feature, however, is a complex structure containing sugars and aromatic amino acids in phenolic ether linkage. Antibiotics of this group bind rapidly and irreversibly to sensitive organisms. They interfere with the biosynthesis of peptidoglycan by complexing with the acyl-D-alanyl-D-alanine terminus of the peptidoglycan precursor molecules. In the presence of sufficient vancomycin one would expect that both glycan chain extension and incorporation of new chain by transpeptidation would be curtailed.

Vancomycin and ristocetin are bactericidal. They do not show cross-resistance with other drugs, and the development of resistance is not a problem. Vancomycin is a narrow-spectrum antibiotic active against gram-positive bacteria and spirochetes. Ristocetin has pronounced activity for gram-positive and acid-fast bacteria and has been successfully used in the therapy of severe staphylococcal infections and of bacterial endocarditis due to enterococci.

Antibiotics Affecting the Cell Membrane

The cell membrane plays a vital role in the cell. It poses an osmotic barrier to free diffusion between the internal and external environment. It effects the concentration of metabolites and nutrients within the cell and serves as a site for respiratory and certain biosynthetic activities of the cell. Several antibiotics have been shown to impair one or more of these functions, resulting in major disturbances in the viability of the cell. The action of agents whose primary target of attack is the cell membrane is independent of growth and begins immediately when cells and antibiotic come together. Unlike inhibitors that interfere with cell wall biosynthesis and are relatively innocuous for mammalian tissues, antibiotics that attack the cell membrane distinguish less successfully between microorganisms and mammalian tissues. Few have found a place in clinical medicine because of their toxicity (Table 10-2).

Polymyxins The polymyxins are a family of relatively simple polypeptides characterized by poor diffusibility and significant toxicity. The members of the group are designated by the letters A, B, C, D, E, but of these only polymyxin B and polymyxin E (colistin) are currently used in clinical medicine (Fig. 10-7). The in vivo and in vitro activity of polymyxin is restricted to gram-negative organisms. Clinically it has been especially useful against infec-

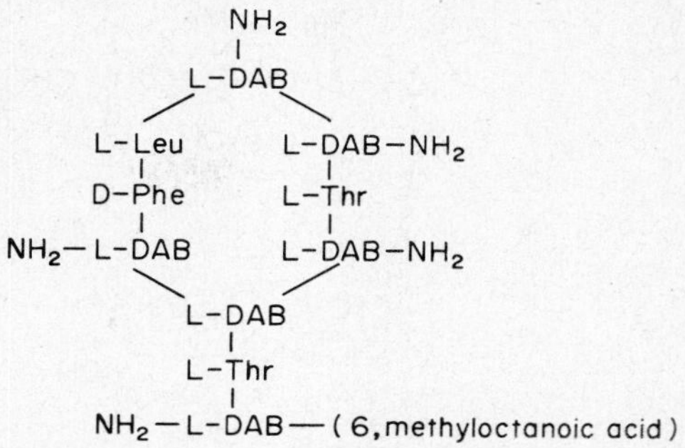

$$
\begin{array}{c}
NH_2 \\
| \\
L-DAB \\
\end{array}
$$

L-Leu   L-DAB-NH$_2$
| |
D-Phe   L-Thr
| |
NH$_2$-L-DAB   L-DAB-NH$_2$

L-DAB
|
L-Thr
|
NH$_2$-L-DAB-(6,methyloctanoic acid)

FIG. 10-7. Polymyxin B. DAB is α, γ-diaminobutyric acid, a component that is present together with L-threonine and D-6-methyloctanoic acid, in all polymyxins.

tions caused by *Pseudomonas aeruginosa*, an organism notoriously resistant to most antibiotics.

Polymyxin binds specifically to the cell membrane, destroying its osmotic properties and causing leakage of metabolites from within the cell. Studies using liposome model membrane systems suggest that phosphatidylethanolamine is the target molecule in a multisite-type mechanism. It has not been demonstrated, conclusively, however, whether other phospholipids, such as phosphatidylglycerol, are also targets for polymyxin action.

Polyenes The polyene antibiotics are selectively active on membranes that contain sterols. The lethal effect on fungi of two of these drugs, amphotericin B and nystatin, is referable to changes in the permeability of the membrane produced by antibiotic-sterol interaction. The nature of this interaction has not been proved unequivocally. In red blood cells the interaction leads to the formation in the membrane of molecular size pores of 5 Å. In the pathogenic fungus, *Epidermophyton floccosum*, however, no pores were observed by electron microscopic examination of membranes treated with amphotericin B. Ultrastructural alterations induced by the drug consisted of

TABLE 10-2 ANTIBIOTICS AFFECTING THE CELL MEMBRANE

Antibiotic	Source	Antimicrobial Activity	Major Therapeutic Applications	Toxicity
Polymyxin	*Bacillus polymyxa*	Gram-negative bacteria	*Pseudomonas aeruginosa* and *Shigella* infections; urinary tract infections	Nephrotoxic
Nystatin	*Streptomyces noursei*	Many fungi	*Candida albicans* infections	Minimal
Amphotericin B	*Streptomyces nodosus*	Many fungi	Histoplasmosis, coccidioidomycosis, North American blastomycosis, cryptococcosis	Nephrotoxic

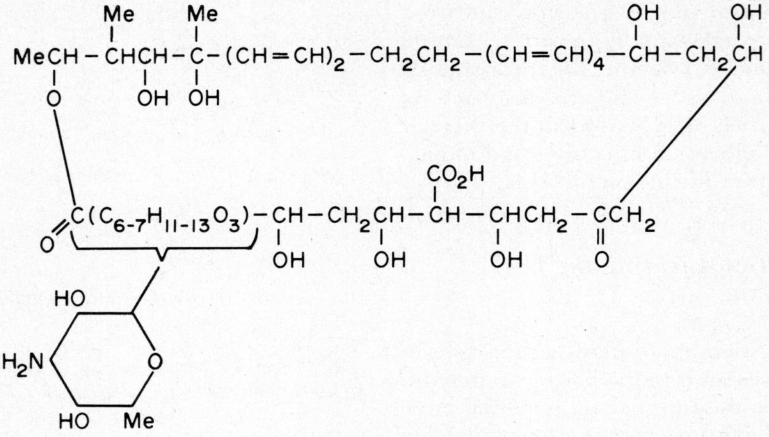

FIG. 10-8. Nystatin, an antifungal agent.

crater formation and vesiculation of the plasma membrane. Bacteria and other prototrophic forms are resistant to the polyenes because their membranes lack sterols.

The basic polyene structure is a large lactone ring containing a flexible hydroxylated portion and a rigid hydrophobic section of unsubstituted conjugated double bonds. In amphotericin B and nystatin there is also an amino sugar, mycosamine (Figs. 10-8 and 10-9).

Antimicrobial Agents that Interfere with DNA Function

A number of antimicrobial drugs specifically interfere with the structure and function of DNA, but few of these agents have shown a selective toxicity acceptable for clinical use. In spite of their limited clinical use these drugs have been very useful as biochemical tools and have contributed significantly to the study of

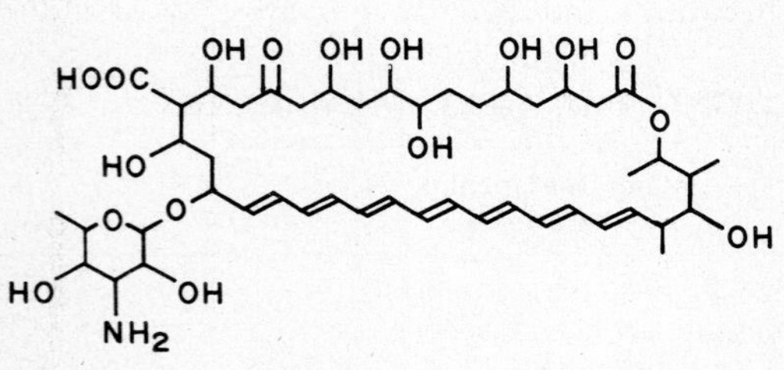

FIG. 10-9. Amphotericin B, a polyene antibiotic with selective activity for fungi.

molecular biology (Table 10-3). The structure of the DNA molecule is intimately related to its two primary roles, duplication and transcription. Any agent that disturbs the structure of the organized double helix of DNA is potentially capable of causing profound effects on all phases of cell growth and metabolism. Among the mechanisms employed by the drugs for altering the structure or function of DNA are cross-linking and intercalation between the stacked bases of the double helix.

Mitomycin   The addition of mitomycin to growing bacterial cells results in inhibition of cell division with the formation of long filamentous forms, bacteriostasis, and death (Fig. 10-10). The bactericidal effect coincides with inhibition of DNA synthesis and usually is accompanied by massive degradation of the preexisting DNA.

Before its inhibitory effects are expressed in vivo, mitomycin is converted enzymatically to a highly reactive hydroquinone derivative that acts as a bifunctional alkylating agent. This active form readily cross-links with DNA by bonding to two sites, one on each of the complementary strands. Guanine residues in DNA are the most probable sites for alkylation. The formation of covalent cross-links in DNA prevents separation of the complementary strands, thereby inhibiting progress of the replicating fork and causing a blockage of DNA synthesis.

Mitomycin exhibits some selectivity in the cross-linking of DNA. Under certain condi-

TABLE 10–3 ANTIMICROBIAL AGENTS THAT INTERFERE WITH DNA FUNCTION

Agent	Source	Clinical Use	Remarks
Mitomycin	*Streptomyces* sp.	None	Useful biochemical tool
Nalidixic acid	Synthetic	Urinary tract infections by *Escherichia, Enterobacter, Proteus*	Useful biochemical tool
Novobiocin	*Streptomyces niveus*	Infections by penicillin-resistant staphylococci	Frequent toxic effects: rashes, fever, intestinal symptoms
Griseofulvin	*Penicillium griseofulvum*	Infections of hair, skin, nails, caused by dermatophytes	Few toxic effects; drug-resistance not a problem

tions it blocks the synthesis of host cell DNA but permits viral DNA synthesis. The reason for the relative resistance of viral DNA is not clear, but the finding has been useful in studies of viral DNA synthesis in the absence of host cell DNA synthesis.

Nalidixic Acid Nalidixic acid is not a natural product but a synthetic derivative of 1,8-naphthyridine. It has been used in the clinical management of urinary tract infections caused by various gram-negative organisms (Fig. 10-11).

In addition to its clinical value it has been a useful tool in studies on the regulation of bacterial cell division. It selectively blocks DNA replication in susceptible bacteria, but the mechanism for this inhibition is unknown.

Novobiocin This antibiotic is bactericidal for gram-positive organisms, and its range of antibacterial activity is very similar to that of penicillin and erythromycin (Fig. 10-12).

At present, the mode of action of novobiocin cannot be explained by any unitary hypothesis. Its primary effect probably is on DNA synthesis, although numerous secondary effects are also induced. DNA polymerase activity is inhibited immediately. Cell wall and protein synthesis are inhibited later. Novobiocin causes an accumulation in *S. aureus* of the same wall precursor nucleotides as does penicillin. This inhibition of cell wall synthesis, however, is not the primary mode of action of the antibiotic, for unlike penicillin, novobiocin does not induce spheroplast formation, and it strongly inhibits the growth of L forms and spheroplasts produced by penicillin. Novobiocin also affects the integrity of the protoplast membrane and causes a leakage of nucleotides into the medium.

Griseofulvin This is a fungistatic agent specific for fungi whose walls contain chitin (Fig. 10-13). It has been successfully used in the treatment of infections caused by the dermatophytes.

The mode of action of griseofulvin is not completely understood, but observations suggest that DNA replication is the primary site of action. Treatment of growing cells with griseofulvin causes such morphologic abnormalities as swelling and branching in the growing tip while old cells distant from the growing point are not affected. It inhibits mitosis in the metaphase, causing multipolar mitosis and abnormal nuclei. Adenylic acid and guanylic acid can partially reverse the growth inhibition caused by griseofulvin, suggesting a metabolite-analog relationship with a purine riboside.

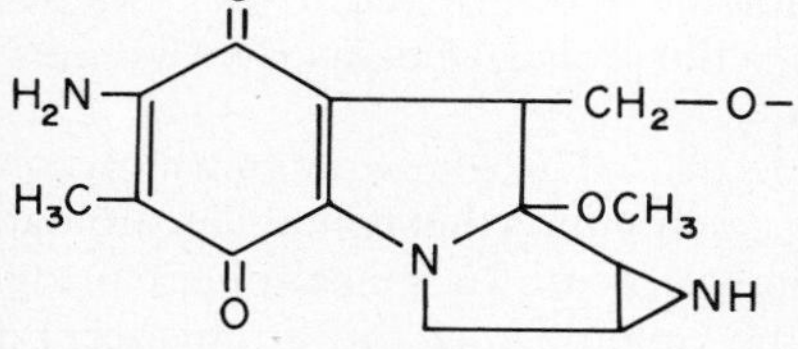

FIG. 10-10. Mitomycin C, an antibiotic that cross-links with DNA.

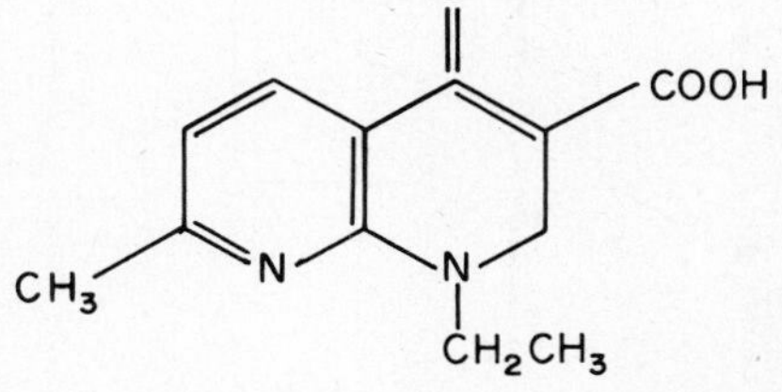

FIG. 10-11. Nalidixic acid, a synthetic compound used in urinary tract infections.

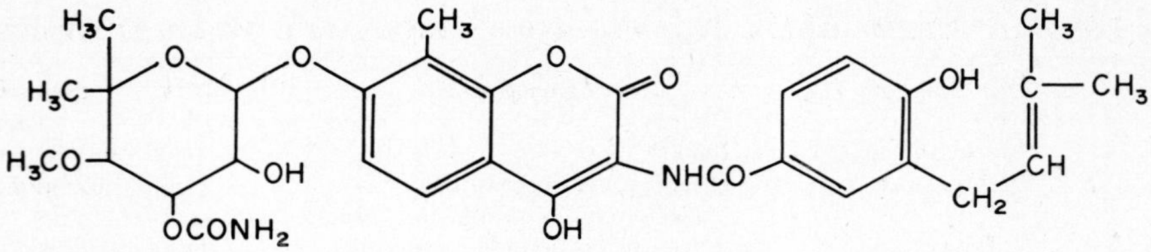

FIG. 10-12. Novobiocin. Its antibacterial spectrum resembles that of penicillin.

Antimicrobial Agents that Inhibit Protein Synthesis

The spectacular advances that have been made in the field of protein biosynthesis have led to a better understanding of the actions of certain antibiotics. In turn, the actions of the antibiotics have shown that with the production of characteristic lesions, one can demonstrate certain detailed features of protein synthesis.

Protein synthesis is the end result of two major processes, (1) DNA-dependent ribonucleic acid synthesis, or transcription, and (2) RNA-dependent protein synthesis, or translation. An antibiotic that inhibits either of these processes will inhibit protein synthesis. Although the antibiotics that primarily inhibit translation are the ones that have been most useful clinically, the agents that inhibit transcription have been useful in studying the steps involved in protein synthesis (Table 10-4).

Agents that interfere at the Level of Transcription During transcription the genetic information in DNA is transferred to a complementary sequence of RNA nucleotides by the enzyme RNA polymerase, a complex protein composed of four subunits, β, β', α, α. Asso-

ciated with this core polymerase which forms the internucleotide linkages is the sigma factor, a dissociable component that acts catalytically in the accurate initiation of RNA chains (Fig. 10-14). Antibiotics that either alter the structure of the template DNA or inhibit the RNA polymerase will interfere with the synthesis of RNA and, consequently, with protein synthesis.

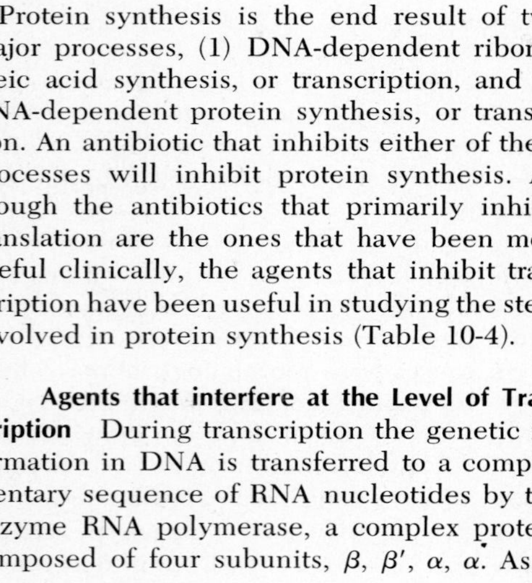

ACTINOMYCIN. The actinomycins are bright red oligopeptides active against many gram-positive and gram-negative organisms as well as mammalian cells. Their prototype is actinomycin D, and others differ only slightly in chemical composition (Fig. 10-15).

Actinomycin forms complexes specifically with DNA, thereby impairing DNA function. This binding is dependent upon guanine residues and helical secondary structure. Two models have been proposed for the structure of the actinomycin-DNA complex. According to one, actinomycin is located in the minor groove of helical DNA, with which it can form as many as seven hydrogen bonds. In the second model the actinomycin chromophore is intercalated into DNA adjacent to guanine-cytosine pairs, thus distorting the helix.

Actinomycin blocks RNA synthesis by preventing the progression of RNA polymerase along the DNA template. Although its toxicity prevents clinical use, actinomycin has been extensively used as a tool for specifically shutting off DNA-directed RNA synthesis. It has been helpful in following the decay of mRNA and for showing the absence of DNA-dependent steps in the growth of many RNA viruses.

RIFAMYCINS. The rifamycins are ansa compounds, ie, compounds that contain an aromatic ring system spanned by a long aliphatic bridge. Some of the members of the group occur in nature, but most are semisynthetic (Fig. 10-16). The most extensively studied member of the

FIG. 10-13. Griseofulvin, a selectively toxic antibiotic for fungi whose walls contain chitin.

TABLE 10—4 ANTIMICROBIAL AGENTS THAT INHIBIT PROTEIN SYNTHESIS

Antibiotic	Source	Antimicrobial Spectrum	Major Therapeutic Application	Remarks
Actinomycin	*Streptomyces* sp.	Many gram-positive and gram-negative bacteria, mammalian cells	None	Useful biochemical tool
Rifampicin	Semisynthetic derivative of rifamycin SV (from *Streptomyces mediterranei*)	Gram-positive bacteria, *M. tuberculosis*	Limited use in tuberculosis therapy	Useful biochemical tool
Streptomycin	*Streptomyces griseus*	Many gram-positive and gram-negative species, *M. tuberculosis*	Tuberculosis, urinary tract infections, *H. influenzae* meningitis, plague, tularemia, *Salmonella* and *Shigella* infections	Common toxic symptoms: damage of eighth cranial nerve and vestibular apparatus
Tetracyclines	*Streptomyces* sp.	Many gram-positive and gram-negative bacteria, rickettsiae, *Mycoplasma*, chlamydiae	Respiratory tract infections, brucellosis, urinary tract infections	Toxic side effects: gastrointestinal irritation, phototoxic skin reaction, liver damage, discoloration of teeth; superinfections of intestinal tract
Chloramphenicol	*Streptomyces venezuelae* (synthetic product now marketed)	Many gram-positive and gram-negative bacteria, rickettsiae, chlamydiae	Typhoid fever	Potentially lethal reactions: bone marrow defects, gray syndrome of infants
Erythromycin	*Streptomyces erythreus*	Spectrum resembles that of penicillin	*S. pyogenes* and *S. pneumoniae* infections	Major toxic effect: liver damage
Lincomycin	*Streptomyces lincolnensis*	Gram-positive cocci (except enterococci), veillonella, bacteroides	Staphylococcal septicemia, osteomyelitis, arthritis	Low toxicity
Puromycin	*Streptomyces alboniger*	Prokaryotic and eukaryotic species	None	Useful biochemical tool
Fucidin	*Fusidium coccineum*	Gram-positive bacteria, gram-negative cocci	Staphylococcal infections by drug-resistant organisms	Few and mild side effects: gastrointestinal disturbances, rashes

group is rifampicin (rifampin). Rifampicin, at very low concentrations, inhibits the growth of gram-positive bacteria and *Mycobacterium tuberculosis*. It selectively inhibits protein synthesis by inactivating the DNA-dependent RNA polymerase. In the first step of transcription the polymerase is bound to a specific site on the DNA template with the formation of a primary enzyme-DNA complex. Rifampicin inactivates this complex by binding specifically and strongly to the β subunit of the RNA polymerase. The binding apparently prevents a

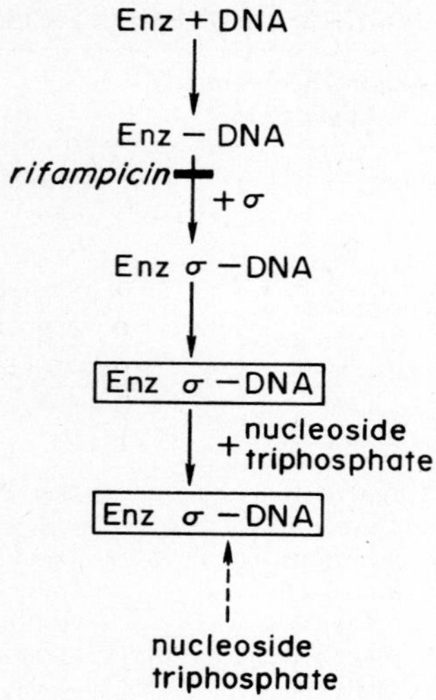

FIG. 10-14. Inhibition of the initiation of transcription by rifampicin. The box indicates a conformational change in the initiation complex, which consists of RNA polymerase, sigma factor, and DNA.

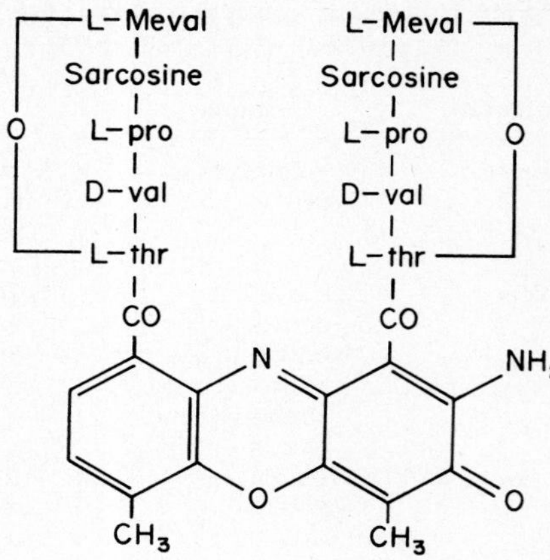

FIG. 10-15. Actinomycin D. This agent forms complexes with DNA by binding to deoxyguanosine residues.

conformational change that is essential for the initiation of RNA synthesis. Only the initiation of RNA synthesis is arrested. There is no effect on chain elongation. The enzyme from resistant mutants does not bind the antibiotic and there

is little inhibition of mammalian RNA polymerase.

Agents that Affect Translation   The translation of mRNA into protein in bacterial cells can be divided into three major phases: the initiation, elongation, and termination of the peptide chain. In the initiation phase mRNA binds to the 30S ribosomal subunit to form a complex

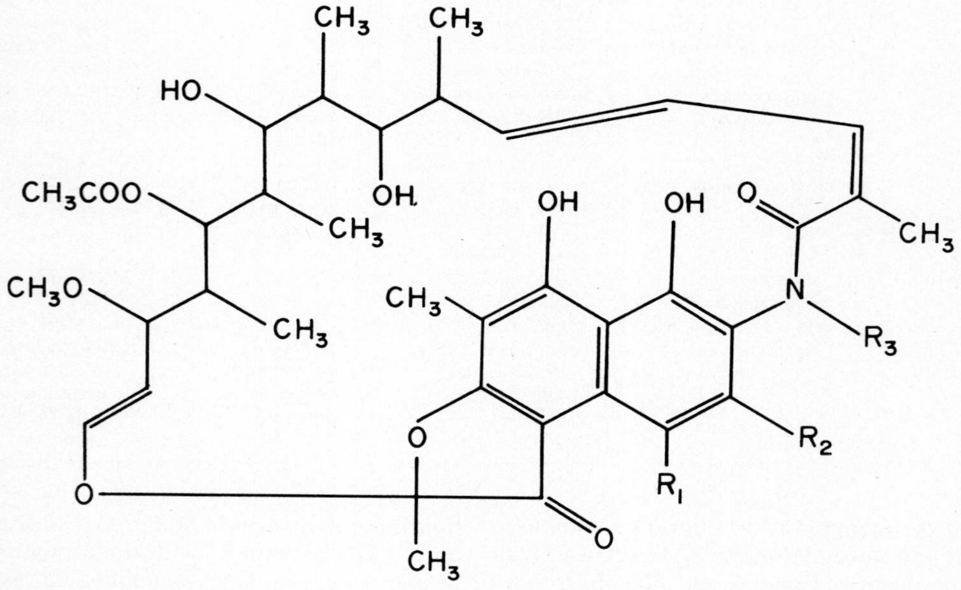

FIG. 10-16. Basic structure of the rifamycins. Various derivatives are substituted in the R_1, R_2, and R_3 positions. In rifampicin, R_1 is —OH; R_2 is —CH=N—N⟨ ⟩N—CH₃; R_3 is H.

to which first the initiator tRNA (fMet-tRNA$_f$) and then the 50S ribosomal subunit bind. Bind-protein initiation factors and GTP. The codon, AUG, is the initiation signal in mRNA and is recognized by the anticodon of fMet-tRNA$_f$. A 50S ribosomal subunit is subsequently added. The fMet-tRNA$_f$ in the complex is bound to the hypothetical peptidyl donor tRNA site on the ribosome.

The first step in the elongation cycle consists of the attachment to the vacant acceptor site of aminoacyl-tRNA specified by the codon that is adjacent to the 3′ site of the initiator codon. In the next step of the elongation phase, the formyl-methionyl residue of the fMet-tRNA$_f$ located at the peptidyl donor site is released from its linkage to tRNA$_f$ and is joined with a peptide bond to the α-amino group of the aminoacyl-tRNA in the acceptor site. The enzyme catalyzing this peptide formation is peptidyl transferase, which is part of the 50S ribosomal subunit. The final step of elongation, translocation, consists of the removal of the discharged tRNA from the ribosome, the movement of fMet-aminoacyl-tRNA from the acceptor site to the peptidyl donor site, and the movement or translocation of the ribosome along the mRNA from the 5′ toward the 3′ terminus by the length of three nucleotides. After translocation, the stage is prepared for the binding of the next aminoacyl residue to the fMet-AA-tRNA, each addition requiring aminoacyl-tRNA binding, peptide bond formation, and translocation. Peptidyl-tRNAs replace the fMet-tRNA in the second and in all subsequent cycles.

The polypeptide chain grows from the amino terminal toward the carboxyl terminal amino acid and remains linked to tRNA and bound to the mRNA-ribosome complex during elongation of the chain. When completed it is released during chain termination. Termination is triggered when a chain termination signal (UAA, UAG, or UGA) is encountered at the aminoacyl-tRNA acceptor site of the 30S subunit. The polypeptide is released, and the messenger-ribosome-tRNA complex dissociates.

It is the elongation phase of protein synthesis that is most susceptible to inhibitors (Fig. 10-17). For a number of these the ribosome is the site of action, and a complex array of inhibitory effects has been observed. A subdivision of antibiotics into major classes has been made on the basis of their binding to the 30S or 50S ribosomal subunits, with the assumption that the

site of fixation provides presumptive evidence for its site of action.

INHIBITORS OF THE 30S RIBOSOMAL SUBUNIT. As noted above, 30S ribosomal subunits provide attachment sites for mRNA and move relative to it during translation. The 30S subunit also provides a binding site for fMet-tRNA$_f$ and aminoacyl-tRNA. Inhibition of protein synthesis on the 30S subunit could result (1) if mRNA is prevented from attaching, (2) if movement of mRNA relative to the 30S subunit is impaired, or (3) if the aminoacyl acceptor site is blocked. Numerous antibiotics, including streptomycin, other aminoglycosides, and tetracyclines, act at the level of the 30S ribosomal subunit.

Streptomycin. Streptomycin is bactericidal for a wide variety of gram-positive and gram-negative species and for the tubercle bacillus. It is an aminoglycoside composed of streptidine, an inositol substituted with two guanido groups, and streptobiosamine, a disaccharide containing a methylamino group (Fig. 10-18). Clinically, the chief merit of streptomycin lies in its ability to attack certain organisms that are not affected by penicillin. Bacterial resistance, however, is a major problem in its clinical use, since some organisms rapidly become resistant to very high concentrations.

MECHANISM OF ACTION. Streptomycin produces a variety of effects when it is added to growing bacterial cells. Its cationic structure results in interaction with anionic components of the cell. The negative charge on the cell surface is reduced, and the cells agglutinate. Streptomycin is readily taken up by microorganisms and causes a rapid efflux of potassium. This is followed, first, by inhibition of protein synthesis and then by impairment of DNA and RNA synthesis, inhibition of respiration, RNA breakdown, excretion of nucleotides, and cell death. Another characteristic effect produced by streptomycin is the phenotypic suppression of certain auxotrophic mutations. In the presence of sublethal concentrations of the antibiotic, cells that carry nonsense or missense mutations can be suppressed (p. 151).

Although streptomycin induces many effects in whole cells, genetic studies and investigations with in vitro polypeptide-synthesizing systems strongly support the hypothesis that the lethal effect of streptomycin results from

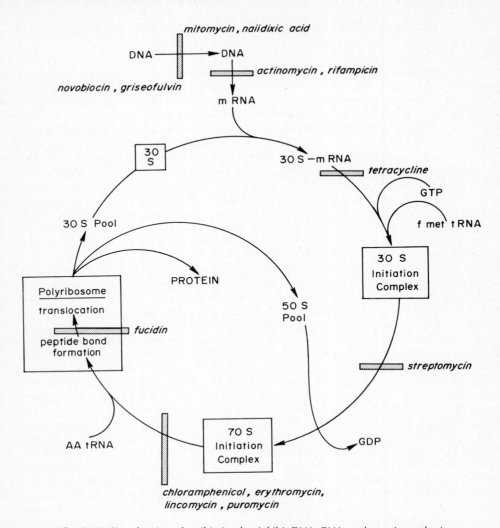

FIG. 10-17. Site of action of antibiotics that inhibit DNA, RNA, and protein synthesis.

irreversible binding of the drug to ribosomes and the subsequent interference with protein synthesis.

When streptomycin is added to in vitro polypeptide-synthesizing systems it has two major effects: (1) it markedly inhibits polypeptide synthesis, and (2) it causes misreading of the synthetic polynucleotide messengers. If ribosomes from streptomycin-resistant strains are used, both of these effects are abolished or greatly reduced.

INHIBITION OF PROTEIN SYNTHESIS. Streptomycin binds irreversibly to the 30S ribosomal subunit, thereby interfering with its proper functioning. In growing cells 30S and 50S

subunits exist either as polyribosomes or in a pool of free particles. During protein synthesis one 30S and one 50S ribosome join together in an initiation complex on a molecule of messenger RNA. This 30S to 50S couple (a 70 S monomer), now part of a polyribosome, moves along the mRNA as a polypeptide chain is formed. After completion of the polypeptide the 70S particles dissociate and return transiently to the pool of free particles. Streptomycin drastically interrupts this ribosome cycle at the initiation of protein synthesis.

The in vitro polypeptide-synthesizing systems that have been most useful in delineating the nature of this inhibition are those employing a natural messenger, such as viral RNA,

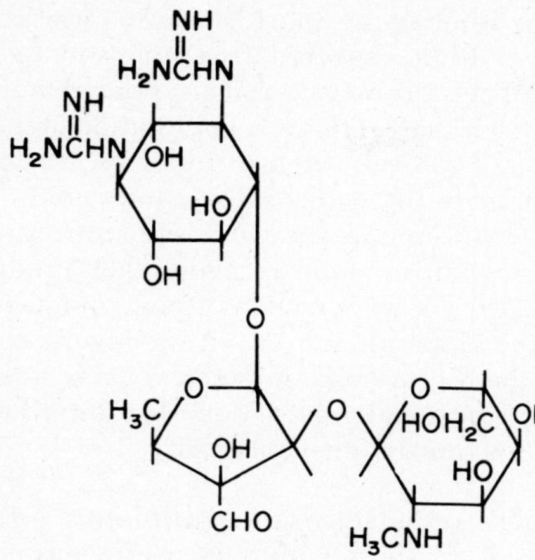

FIG. 10-18. Streptomycin. The streptidine moiety (upper ring structure) is an inositol substituted with two guanido groups linked to the streptobiosamine moiety by a glycosidic bond.

rather than a homonucleotide (poly U). The natural messenger provides a more physiologic in vitro system in which protein synthesis is inhibited almost as effectively as in the cell. The addition of streptomycin to such a system slows down polypeptide synthesis on polysomes but allows ribosomes to leave mRNA either prematurely or at the termination signal. Upon release they dissociate into subunits but subsequently reassociate at the normal initiation sites on mRNA to form streptomycin monosomes, irreversibly inactivated initiation complexes that contain stabilized mRNA. These modified complexes cannot form peptide bonds. Their movement along the mRNA is impeded, thereby blocking the ribosome cycle at an early stage in the initiation of protein synthesis.

STREPTOMYCIN-INDUCED MISREADING. One of the effects produced by streptomycin when added to an in vitro polypeptide-synthesizing system is misreading of messenger. Streptomycin can inhibit the incorporation of certain synthetic polymer-directed incorporations (eg, poly U-phenylalanine) and can stimulate the incorporation of amino acids not coded for by certain synthetic polymers. Although the extensive misreading in in vitro homonucleotide systems is probably an artificial response, it has provided an explanation for the ability of streptomycin to suppress mutations in a class of

mutants that are conditionally streptomycin dependent (CSD). Such mutants can grow in the absence of their specific growth requirement provided streptomycin is present in the medium. This behavior apparently is due to a misreading of the genetic message by streptomycin. The wrong message of the mutant is not corrected physically but is read differently in the presence of streptomycin. The net result of this misreading of an incorrect message is the synthesis of a functional protein. In strains that permit correction by streptomycin, streptomycin mimics the action of a suppressor, a mutation at a second distinct site that reverses the mutant phenotype. Unlike the genetic suppression, however, the correction produced by streptomycin is phenotypic and is not heritable (p. 151).

Although it is difficult to assess the in vivo significance of misreading of the code, an apparent relationship does exist between misreading, killing action, and phenotypic suppression. The streptamine or deoxystreptamine moiety of the aminoglycoside is the chemical structure responsible for misreading. Aminoglycoside drugs, such as spectinomycin, that lack this moiety cause no misreading and are bacteriostatic only.

The chemical basis for all of the in vivo effects of streptomycin is not known, but the major effects observed, inhibition of protein synthesis, misreading, and phenotypic suppression, have been attributed to the irreversible binding of streptomycin to the 30S ribosomal subunit. This binding produces a conformational change at the aminoacyl-tRNA binding site resulting in an interference with both the binding of aminoacyl-tRNA and the fidelity of translation.

STREPTOMYCIN RESISTANCE. In a bacterium, three phenotypically distinct responses to streptomycin are possible: sensitivity, resistance, or dependence. These responses are determined by multiple alleles of a single genetic locus, the *str* locus that codes for protein S12 of the 30S subunit. This protein determines the sensitivity of the entire 30S ribosomal particle to streptomycin. A mutation to resistance would result if this site were eliminated or if it were altered in such a manner that the bound drug could no longer exert its effect. There is evidence for the existence of single-step, high-level mutations to resistance of both of these types. Resistance conferred by mutations in protein S12 can be suppressed by mutations in proteins S4 and S5 of the 30S subunit. The question has been raised whether streptomycin also binds to the nucleic acid moiety of the ribosome.

The amount of misreading observed in a cell-free polypeptide synthesizing system containing ribosomes from a str^r mutant is tenfold less than that observed with ribosomes from str^s strains, even in the absence of streptomycin. This observation may explain the finding that mutations to streptomycin resistance often introduce other phenotypic effects. They may simultaneously confer auxotrophy, change host-prophage relationships, alter control of inducible or repressible enzymes, or alter patterns of genetic suppression (p. 151).

STREPTOMYCIN DEPENDENCE.   When a population of streptomycin-sensitive organisms is plated on a medium containing a high level of streptomycin, a number of the survivors require streptomycin for growth. These mutants are streptomycin dependent and arise from the str^s wild-type strain in a single step. The str^d phenotype is determined by a mutation allelic with or very close to the str^r locus. The genetic basis for streptomycin dependence in these mutants is thus quite different from the conditionally streptomycin dependent (CSD) phenotype discussed previously (p. 211).

As with streptomycin resistance, mutation to dependence also exhibits pleiotropic effects. Unlike streptomycin resistance, however, where phenotypic suppression is restricted, in str^d strains phenotypic suppression is enhanced. In these strains most of the nonsense and missense mutations normally occurring are weakly suppressed, and ambiguity in translation is introduced.

The absolute requirement for streptomycin for growth by str^d mutants can be satisfied by certain other agents that also cause misreading. This would be expected if, as proposed, the str^d mutants represent a special class of str^r mutants in which a change in the configuration of the str protein of 30S subunit prevents correct reading of codons in the cell's mRNA, and certain specific requirements become apparent unless streptomycin or another agent that produces misreading is present. It is thus hypothesized that the dependence on streptomycin represents the requirement for an agent able to overcome ribosomal restriction by introducing selective translational ambiguity.

Other Aminoglycoside Antibiotics.   There are several other aminoglycoside antibiotics that act on protein synthesis at the level of the 30S ribosomal subunit. These include the neomycins, paromomycins, kanamycins, gentamicins, and spectinomycin (Table 10-5). All except spectinomycin are bactericidal. The antibiotics in this group contain both an aminoglycoside and an aminocyclitol moiety joined via a glycosidic linkage. With the exception of gentamicin, which is produced by a species of *Micromonospora*, they are produced by species of *Streptomyces*.

MECHANISM OF ACTION.   All of the aminoglycosides act on protein synthesis at the level of the 30S ribosomal subunit, and most of them also produce ambiguity in translation. Spectinomycin inhibits protein synthesis at the level of the messenger-ribosome interaction but causes no misreading. The level of misreading produced by neomycin, kanamycin, and gentamicin is much greater than that produced by streptomycin. As expected, those aminoglycosides that cause translational errors are all capable of phenotypic suppression of nonsense and missense mutations. Since in spectinomycin the streptamine nucleus, which is the struc-

TABLE 10–5 PROPERTIES OF DEOXYSTREPTAMINE GROUP OF AMINOGLYCOSIDE ANTIBIOTICS

Antibiotics in Group	Antibacterial Spectrum	Major Clinical Application*	Toxicity
Neomycins Paromomycins Kanamycins Gentamicins Spectinomycin	Many gram-positive and gram-negative bacteria, *Mycobacterium*	*E. coli* gastroenteritis, suppression of bowel flora, local application, burn wounds	Renal and eighth nerve toxicity

*Neomycin, kanamycin, gentamicin

ture responsible for misreading, is replaced by a stereoisomer, not only is the misreading property lost but also the agent is bacteriostatic and not bactericidal in its action.

Tetracyclines. The tetracyclines are a family of closely related antibiotics, consisting of tetracycline, the parent compound, chlortetracycline (Aureomycin), demethylchlortetracycline (Declomycin), and oxytetracycline (Terramycin) (Fig. 10-19). The antimicrobial, pharmacologic, and therapeutic properties of all the tetracyclines are similar.

The term "broad-spectrum antibiotic," denoting a wide range of activity, was coined in connection with the tetracycline group. Their antibacterial spectrum is the broadest known and overlaps that of penicillin, streptomycin, and chloramphenicol. It includes a number of gram-positive and gram-negative bacteria, some organisms innately insensitive to other chemotherapeutic agents, and bacteria that have become resistant to other agents.

The tetracyclines are bacteriostatic and inhibit only rapidly multiplying organisms. Resistance appears slowly, and organisms that have become insensitive to one tetracycline always exhibit resistance of approximately the same degree to the others. Resistance usually can be attributed either to alterations in cell membrane permeability or to enzymatic inactivation of the drug.

The tetracyclines produce a variety of side effects, demanding caution in their administration. Among the major problems encountered has been the development of superinfections, the most serious of which involve the intestinal tract. Three types of infectious enteritis, staphylococcal enterocolitis, intestinal candidiasis, and pseudomembranous colitis, may result from treatment with tetracyclines. Such infections are caused by the outgrowth of drug-resistant indigenous bacteria or fungi that normally are kept in check by the growth of the drug-sensitive members of the intestinal flora.

MECHANISM OF ACTION. Tetracycline strongly inhibits protein synthesis. When it is added to growing cultures, nucleic acid synthesis continues for some time in the absence of protein synthesis. Tetracycline interferes with protein synthesis by preventing the binding of amino-acyl-tRNA to the messenger RNA-30S ribosomal subunit. Binding of fMet-tRNA is especially sensitive to tetracycline. As a result initiation and, therefore, polyribosome formation are blocked.

INHIBITORS OF THE 50S RIBOSOMAL SUBUNIT. In the synthesis of protein the 50S ribosomal subunit provides an attachment site for peptidyl-tRNA, the donor site. It also contains the active center for catalyzing the peptide bond-forming reaction of protein synthesis. Inhibition of protein synthesis at the 50S ribosomal subunit could result (1) if attachment of peptidyl-tRNA is prevented, (2) if there is an interference of peptide bond formation, or (3) if the translocation step is inhibited, ie, the movement of peptidyl-tRNA and the ribosome relative to each other. Among the antibiotics that act at the level of the 50S ribosomal subunit are chloramphenicol, lincomycin, and the macrolide group.

Chloramphenicol. Chloramphenicol is a bacteriostatic agent, active against a whole range of gram-positive and gram-negative bacteria, rickettsiae, and chlamydiae (Fig. 10-20). Its clinical use, however, demands cau-

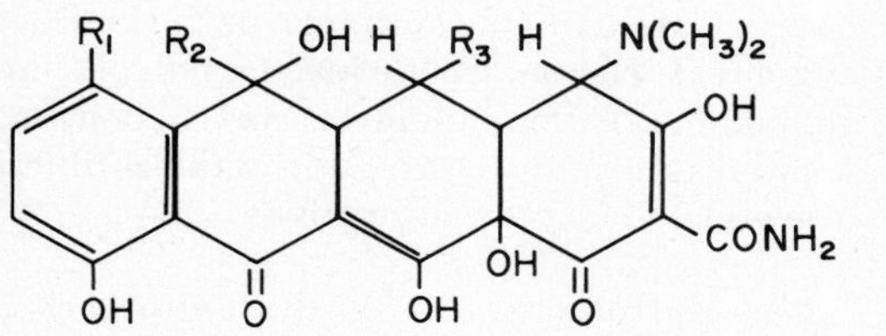

FIG. 10-19. General structure of the tetracyclines. Tetracycline: $R_1 = H$, $R_2 = CH_3$, $R_3 = H$. Chlortetracycline: $R_1 = Cl$, $R_2 = CH_3$, $R_3 = H$. Oxytetracycline: $R_1 = H$, $R_2 = CH_3$, $R_3 = OH$. Demethyl-chlortetracycline: $R_1 = Cl$, $R_2 = H$, $R_3 = H$.

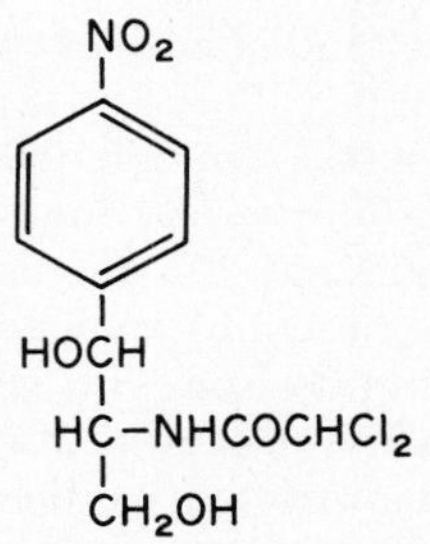

FIG. 10-20. Chloramphenicol, an antibiotic that inhibits peptide bond formation.

tion because of a definite risk of potentially lethal reactions.

MECHANISM OF ACTION. Chloramphenicol inhibits growth of bacteria by interfering with protein synthesis. This action is highly specific, since total RNA continues to be formed at a rate comparable to that of untreated cells. The ribosome cycle is thus dissociated from protein synthesis.

Chloramphenicol binds exclusively to the 50 S ribosomal subunit. The binding is stereospecific, and a 1:1 equivalence exists between the number of ribosomes present and the number of chloramphenicol molecules bound. Other antibiotic inhibitors of the 50S subunit compete with chloramphenicol for this binding.

Since polyribosome formation continues in the absence of protein synthesis, the drug does not interfere with the initiation of protein synthesis. Chloramphenicol inhibits peptide bond formation. Information on the nature of this inhibition, as well as on peptide bond formation in general, has come from the use of model systems. In one of these, the puromycin reaction, peptidyl transfer is uncoupled from other reactions of protein synthesis, making possible the identification of inhibitors that act specifically on the peptidyl transferase. When puromycin is added to a system synthesizing peptides, it is incorporated into the growing peptide chain instead of the next incoming amino acid, and peptidyl puromycin, ie, an incomplete peptide chain terminated by puromycin, is released from the ribosome. A further discussion of this reaction is on p. 217.

Chloramphenicol prevents the formation of peptidyl puromycin at concentrations that inhibit protein synthesis in vivo. This inhibition results from the binding of chloramphenicol in the vicinity of the peptidyl transferase catalytic center, interfering with functional attachment of the aminoacyl end of aminoacyl-tRNA to the ribosome.

Mammalian cells contain 80S ribosomes rather than the 70S variety found in bacteria. Although the 60S and 40S subunits of the 80S ribosomes have functions analogous to the corresponding subunits from 70S ribosomes, differences in the fine structures of the two classes have been demonstrated by their differential susceptibility to antibiotics. Among the most significant of these differences is that between the peptidyl transferase site of the two types of ribosome. Chloramphenicol does not bind to the 60S subunit of the 80S ribosome, indicating that the unique site, the CM site, at which chloramphenicol acts on 70S ribosomes is absent from 80S ribosomes.

RESISTANCE. Chloramphenicol and the macrolide antibiotics, erythromycin and lincomycin, compete for binding at the CM site on the 50S subunit. Since they bind to the same unique site on the ribosome in a 1:1 ratio and are mutually exclusive, a ribosome to which erythromycin is bound is resistant to chloramphenicol. This type of resistance is important in the effective clinical utilization of antibiotics whose activity is related to inhibition of 50S subunit function. Since the simultaneous use of a competitive pair of these agents results in the therapeutic effects of a single agent, there would be no advantage to the simultaneous administration of two or more of the 50S inhibitors.

In some organisms mutation to chloramphenicol resistance may be attributed to an alteration of the 50S ribosomal subunit, resulting in a decreased affinity for the drug. Ribosomes from such mutants have low activity in cell-free protein synthesis and are unable to bind labeled chloramphenicol, erythromycin, and lincomycin.

Resistance to chloramphenicol is not infrequently accompanied by resistance to the tetracyclines. This cross-resistance phenomenon is largely confined to enteric bacteria and is conferred upon the bacterium by episomal transfer. The phenomenon involves the intraspecies or interspecies transfer of hereditary factors, the episomes, that carry, among other genetic properties, genes determining multiple drug resistance, including resistance to chloramphenicol (p. 223). In this type of resistance the biochemical basis is either the acquisition of impermeability to the antibiotic or the ability to degrade it. The enzymatic inactivation of chloramphenicol is dependent on acetyl-coenzyme A and results in the conversion of the antibiotic to acetylated inactive derivatives.

The Macrolides. All of the antibiotics of this group contain a macrocyclic lactone ring of 12 to 22 carbon atoms to which one or more sugars are attached. Included in the macrolide group are erythromycin, oleandomycin, carbomycin, and spiramycin. The antibacterial spectrum is similar for all of these agents and resembles that of penicillin. Erythromycin possesses the highest level of activity and spiramycin the lowest.

ERYTHROMYCIN. Of the macrolide antibiotics erythromycin is clinically the most important (Fig. 10-21, Table 10-4). Although primarily bacteriostatic, it may be either bacteriostatic or bactericidal depending on the organism and the concentration of the drug. Bacteria develop resistance to erythromycin readily both in vitro and in vivo.

MECHANISM OF ACTION. The action of erythromycin is similar in many ways to that of chloramphenicol. As with chloramphenicol, erythromycin causes an uncoupling of the processes of peptide bond formation and ribosome addition and movement along messenger RNA. The formation of peptide bonds is inhibited by erythromycin, but the ribosome cycle appears to continue. This prolonged movement of ribosomes and stabilized mRNA into polyribosomes in the absence of protein synthesis suggests a special drug-induced monosome that bears no peptidyl-tRN but can move along mRNA even in its absence.

The 50S ribosomal subunit is the site of action of erythromycin, but the mechanistic details of its action on protein synthesis are not yet clear. Although both chloramphenicol and erythromycin bind at or near the CM site on the 50S ribosomal subunit, findings obtained by the use of the fragment reaction (p. 217) suggest that their precise effects on peptidyl transfer and protein synthesis differ. Erythromycin does not inhibit this reaction, but chloramphenicol, lincomycin, and certain of the macrolide antibiotics do.

Resistance to erythromycin is a genetically controlled property of ribosomes. The ribosomes from a number of mutants highly resistant to erythromycin have a reduced ability to bind erythromycin and are less active in in vitro polypeptide synthesis than ribosomes from erythromycin-sensitive strains. These differences can be correlated with an altered 50S ribosomal subunit protein component, the conformation of which is less favorable for erythromycin binding.

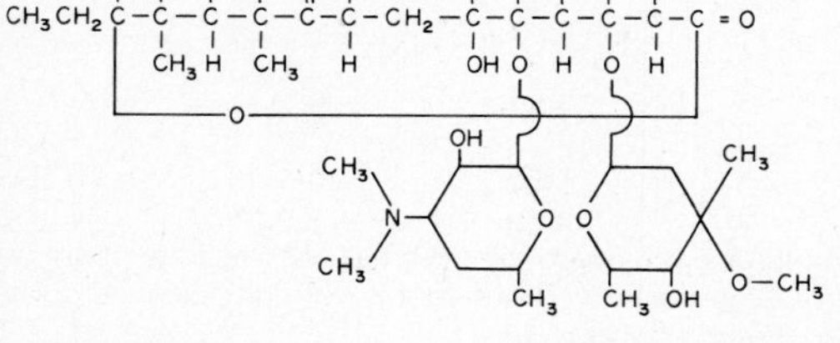

Lincomycin. Lincomycin is structurally unlike any other major antibiotic (Fig. 10-22). Its activity spectrum is similar to that of erythromycin. Gram-positive bacteria are more sensitive than gram-negative species both in vivo and in vitro (Table 10-4). Its antibacterial range, low toxicity, and clinical efficacy make it a suitable substitute for penicillin in the treatment of infections caused by gram-positive cocci, where penicillin is contraindicated.

Lincomycin-resistant strains emerge during the course of therapy. Some of these strains are resistant only to lincomycin and erythromycin, while others show the dissociated type of resistance characteristic of the macrolides, ie, strains sensitive to lincomycin when tested in the absence of erythromycin are resistant to lincomycin when tested in its presence. This type of resistance involving inhibitors of the 50S ribosomal subunit is probably caused by an induced alteration of the ribosome as a result of an adaptation to erythromycin. The addition of erythromycin at a concentration not exceeding the level of the mutant's resistance does not inhibit protein synthesis on these altered ribosomes, but since only one antibiotic molecule can be bound to a given ribosome at a time, lincomycin binding is prevented.

MECHANISM OF ACTION. Lincomycin binds exclusively to the 50S ribosomal subunit. Like

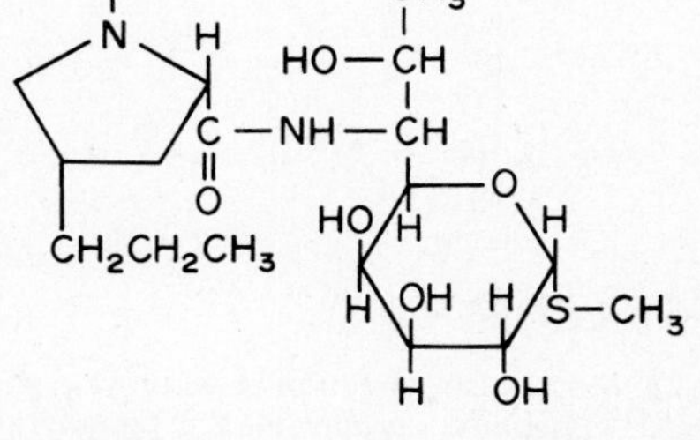

FIG. 10-21. Erythromycin, a macrolide antibiotic.

FIG. 10-22. Lincomycin, an antibiotic that binds to the 50S ribosomal subunit.

erythromycin and a number of other 50S subunit inhibitors, it competes with chloramphenicol for its binding site on the ribosome, and like chloramphenicol and erythromycin, it does not bind to the 60S subunit of mammalian 80S ribosomes. It also resembles chloramphenicol in that it inhibits the fragment reaction (p. 217). Qualitatively, at least, it appears that the mode of action of lincomycin is very similar to that of chloramphenicol and that inhibition of protein synthesis results from interference with the binding of the aminoacyl end of aminoacyl-tRNA to ribosomes. However, certain differences do exist between the mode of action of these two antibiotics. Thus, in vivo in the presence of high concentrations of chloramphenicol, polyribosomes are completely preserved, but in the presence of lincomycin, an extensive and rapid breakdown of polyribosomes occurs at all drug concentrations, and the majority of the ribosomes dissociate to 50S and 30S ribosomal subunits. This breakdown of polyribo-

somes by lincomycin could result from selective inhibition of some aspect of polypeptide initiation.

Puromycin. This antibiotic provides an excellent example of the structural analog concept of antimetabolite action (Fig. 10-23). It is structurally analogous to the terminal aminoacyl adenosine portion of tRNA and therefore inhibits protein synthesis by terminating the growth of polypeptide chains. As a result growth of the cell is prevented.

Since puromycin inhibits protein synthesis at a step that is present in all living cells, it inhibits growth of both prokaryotic and eukaryotic species. As a result it is not clinically useful but is included in this discussion because of its usefulness in elucidating the reactions involved in peptide bond formation.

MECHANISM OF ACTION. As mentioned previously (p. 132) there are two binding sites on

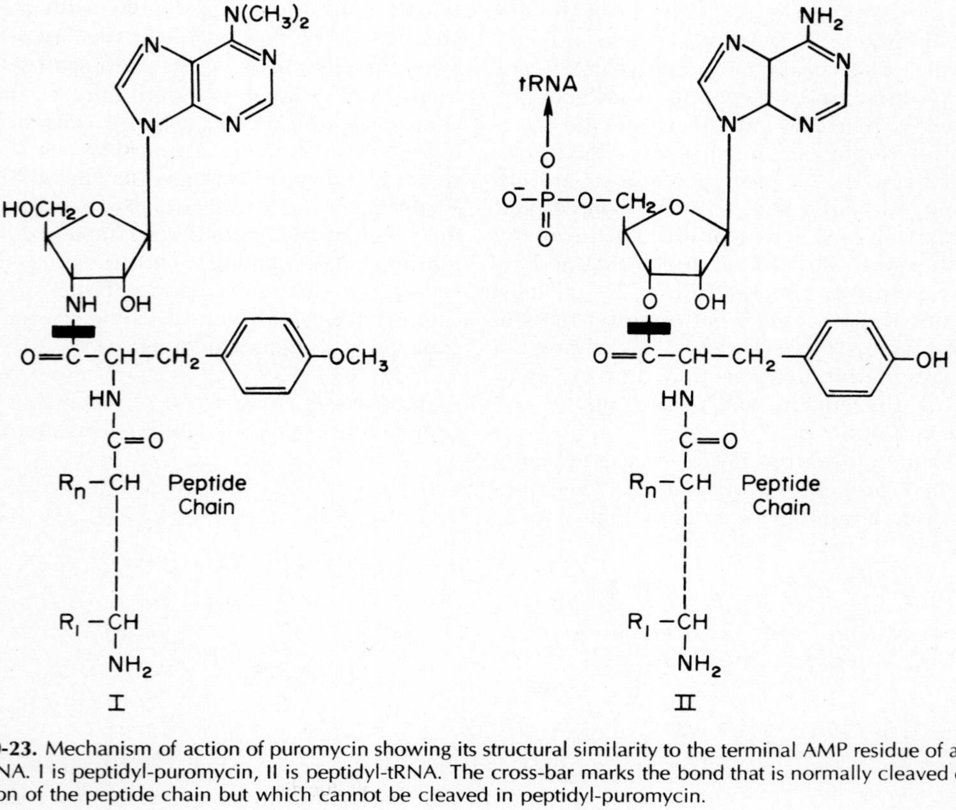

FIG. 10-23. Mechanism of action of puromycin showing its structural similarity to the terminal AMP residue of aminoacyl-tRNA. I is peptidyl-puromycin, II is peptidyl-tRNA. The cross-bar marks the bond that is normally cleaved during extension of the peptide chain but which cannot be cleaved in peptidyl-puromycin.

the ribosome, the peptidyl-tRNA donor site, which is the site where the peptidyl group of peptidyl-tRNA is donated to the incoming tRNA or to puromycin, and the aminoacyl-tRNA acceptor site which accepts aminoacyl-tRNA during chain elongation. When peptidyl-tRNA is on the donor site and the acceptor site is vacant, puromycin can react with peptidyl-tRNA to form peptidyl-puromycin and tRNA. The polypeptide chain is then released, leaving the ribosome with discharged tRNA bound in the donor site. Growth of the peptide chain is reinitiated at frequent intervals as the ribosome moves along the mRNA molecule, resulting in the abortive synthesis of a collection of oligopeptides with random N-terminal amino acids. Puromycin also causes an increase in the rate of subunit exchange, suggesting that the release of 50S subunits bearing tRNA, while only 30S

subunits remain associated with mRNA, which subsequently recombines with 50S subunits to form initiation complexes (Fig. 10-24).

THE PUROMYCIN REACTION. The finding that puromycin becomes linked to the carboxyl group of peptide chains by means of a peptide bond has led to the use of this reaction as a model system for the study of peptide bond formation in protein synthesis (Fig. 10-24B). In a simplified peptide bond-synthesizing system, the N-formyl-methionyl hexanucleotide fragment CAACCA-fMet, obtained by the digestion of N-formyl-methionyl-tRNA with ribonuclease, undergoes a ribosome-catalyzed reaction with puromycin in the presence of methanol to give N-formyl-methionyl-puromycin, a reaction that is analogous to peptidyl transfer in protein synthesis. Supplementation of the system with methanol permits rapid catalysis by isolated 50S subunits and eliminates the requirement for 30S subunits normally required for peptidyl transferase activity. The reduced size of both substrate analogs eliminates other reactions that are normally interlinked with peptidyl transfer and confines the reaction to the immediate vicinity of a catalytic center on the 50S subunit.

Fucidin. Fucidin, the sodium salt of fusidic acid, is the clinically useful form of this antibiotic (Fig. 10-25). It has a rather narrow antibacterial spectrum which includes primari-

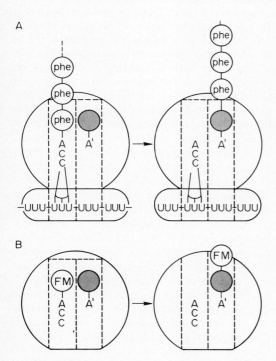

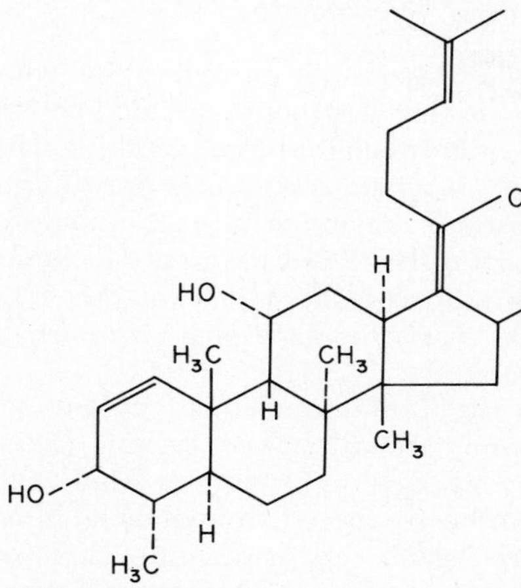

FIG. 10-24. A. Reaction of puromycin (dark sphere) with polyphenylalanyl-tRNA-charged 70S ribosomes. The puromycin occupies the aminoacyl acceptor site. B. Fragment reaction employed in the study of peptide bond formation. The system contains 50S ribosomal subunits, an f-Met-oligonucleotide, puromycin, and alcohol. (Adapted from Monro, Staehelin, Colma, Vasquez: Cold Spring Harbor Symp Quant Biol 34:357, 1969).

FIG. 10-25. Fusidic acid, which is used clinically as its sodium salt, fucidin.

ly gram-positive bacteria and the gram-negative cocci. Fucidin provides a useful addition to the antistaphylococcal armamentarium and has been used successfully in the treatment of a variety of serious staphylococcal infections (Table 10-4).

MECHANISM OF ACTION.   Fusidic acid inhibits protein synthesis in whole cells and in cell-free extracts. Unlike 50S ribosomal subunit inhibitors, however, it neither binds to the ribosome nor inhibits chloramphenicol binding. The fragment reaction is unaffected by its presence. The specific site of attack of fusidic acid is the translocation reaction, the last composite step in peptide bond formation. In this step the discharged tRNA in the peptidyl tRNA donor site is released from the ribosome, the peptidyl-tRNA is shifted from the aminoacyl-tRNA acceptor site to the donor site, and the ribosome moves the length of one codon along the mRNA. In the course of translocation G factor and GTP become attached to the ribosome, the bound GTP is cleaved into GDP and P_i, and the G factor, GDP, and P_i are released from the ribosome. Fusidic acid blocks translocation by inhibiting the GTPase activity of the G factor. As a consequence of inhibition of translocation, ribosome movement on messenger RNA stops, and the polyribosomes freeze as such.

METABOLIC ANTAGONISM

Enzymes are often inhibited by compounds possessing a structure related to the natural substrate. Such inhibitors combine with the enzyme in such a manner as to prevent the normal substrate-enzyme combination and the catalytic reaction. The inhibition of biochemical reactions by specific agents of this type provides the basis for a rational approach to chemotherapy.

Many of the inhibitors of this type are analogs of various growth factors, organic factors required by all bacteria for growth. Many bacteria can synthesize these essential metabolites from simple organic precursors, but others require that they be supplied in a preformed state. Such growth factors include various vitamins, amino acids, purines, and pyrimidines. The enzymes essential in the synthesis and the utilization of certain of these factors can be inhibited by substances structurally related to the metabolites. Such inhibitors are known as "antimetabolites."

Competitive and Noncompetitive Inhibition

The antimetabolites that cause reversible inhibition of enzyme reactions are of two major types, competitive and noncompetitive. Competitive inhibition can be overcome by increasing the substrate concentration; noncompetitive inhibition cannot be reversed by the substrate.

In the competitive type of inhibition both inhibitor (I) and substrate (S) compete for the same enzyme site.

$$E + S \rightleftharpoons ES \rightarrow E + P$$
$$E + I \rightleftharpoons EI$$

The EI complex yields no reaction products, and although the formation of EI is reversible, the continuing competition with substrate reduces the effective free enzyme concentration. In inhibitions of this type the percentage of inhibition of the enzyme is a function of the ratio of the concentrations of inhibitor and substrate rather than a function of the absolute concentration of the inhibitor alone. This relationship may be treated quantitatively by use of the Michaelis-Menten equation, which defines the relationship between the enzyme reaction rate (v) and the substrate (S) concentration. Competitive inhibition is most easily recognized by using Lineweaver-Burk plots, ie, plots of $1/v$ versus $1/S$ at varying concentrations of inhibitor (Fig. 10-26). In competitive inhibition, the plot is characterized by straight lines of differing slope that intersect at a common intercept on the $1/v$ axis. Thus, at any inhibitor concentration, there is a substrate concentration that can evoke full activity of the enzyme.

In noncompetitive inhibition, inhibition depends only on the concentration of the inhibitor, and inhibition is not reversed by increasing the substrate concentration. In contrast to the competitive type of inhibition, the inhibitor binds at a locus on the enzyme other than the substrate binding site. It may bind to the free enzyme, to the ES complex, or to both, resulting in the formation of both EI and ESI complexes.

$$E + I \rightleftharpoons EI$$
$$ES + I \rightleftharpoons ESI$$

The EI and ESI complexes are inactive. The

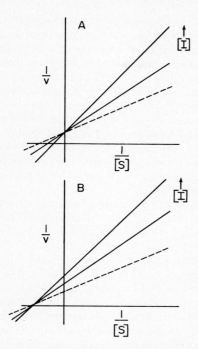

FIG. 10-26. Lineweaver-Burk plots of competitive (A) and noncompetitive (B) inhibition. The reaction in the absence of inhibitor is represented by the dotted line.

rate of conversion of S→P is slowed but not stopped. The effect exerted may be on the affinity of the enzyme for substrate or on the rate of the reaction.

In a Lineweaver-Burk plot of noncompetitive inhibition, the plots differ in slope and do not share a common intercept on the 1/v axis. The intercept on the 1/v axis is greater for the inhibited than for the uninhibited reaction, indicating that the enzyme activity cannot be restored regardless of the substrate concentration.

Usefulness of Competitive Inhibitors in Chemotherapy With the introduction of the therapeutic agent sulfanilamide, attention was focused on the potential value of metabolite analogs in the designing of new chemotherapeutic agents. Although thousands of analogs of the essential metabolites have been designed, and many have been shown to be effective inhibitors in vitro, with the exception of analogs of p-aminobenzoic acid (PABA), most of them have not demonstrated the requisite selectivity necessary for clinical use. The reason for the lack of selectivity lies in the basic similarity between most of the enzymatic reactions present in bacterial and mammalian cells.

In addition to the lack of selectivity, another shortcoming of structural analogs that act as competitive inhibitors of essential metabolites is the following. Although a compound may strongly inhibit an isolated, purified enzyme in vitro, such conditions are nonexistent in vivo. In the living cell, which is analogous to an open system, substrate is continuously supplied to the enzyme by the previous enzyme of the metabolic pathway, and its product is removed by the next enzyme. In this system of balanced growth, a steady state is reached in which the level of substrate is often insufficient to saturate the enzymes. If a competitive inhibitor is added to this system, the competitor is bound by the enzyme, and inhibition of activity results. In the biosynthetic pathway, however, reactions that precede the inhibited reaction continue to supply the natural substrate. In time the concentration of substrate is sufficiently high to reverse the inhibition, and the reaction is resumed at a rate characteristic of the higher level. Therefore, structural analogs, in order to be successful antimicrobial agents, must either have a much higher affinity for the enzyme than has the natural substrate or must function as something more than a simple competitive inhibitor. Most of the competitive inhibitors that have been studied have a lower affinity for the target enzyme. An exception is the antibiotic cycloserine which is an analog of D-alanine. This drug binds to D-alanyl-D-alanine synthetase 100 times more effectively than the natural substrate, which may account for its clinical efficacy.

Whereas structural analogs that inhibit by competing at the substrate binding site of an enzyme are usually only transient inhibitors, these inhibitors may be quite effective when they function as end product inhibitors or repressors. In such cases they mimic the effect of the essential metabolite and inhibit the activity or the synthesis of new enzymes. Their action is thus to reduce the availability of the natural analog.

Analogs of p-Aminobenzoic Acid

Sulfonamides The term "sulfonamide" is a generic name for derivatives of p-aminobenzenesulfonamide or sulfanilamide. First administered in 1935 by Domagk as the red dye Prontosil, sulfanilamide was the first effective chemotherapeutic agent to be used systemically for the prevention and cure of bacterial infections in man. In vitro, Prontosil is inactive against bacteria, but in the body it is broken down to para-aminobenzenesulfonamide, the chemotherapeutic moiety of the molecule.

The introduction of sulfanilamide awakened the medical profession to the new field of bacterial chemotherapy. Numerous derivatives of sulfanilamide were synthesized and tested for their clinical value in various types of infections. Although the advent of the antibiotics detracted from the popularity and usefulness of the sulfonamides, they continue to play an important but smaller role in the control of infectious diseases.

The minimal structural requirement for antibacterial action is that the sulfur be linked directly to the benzene ring and that the NH_2 group in the para position be either retained as such or replaced only by radicals that can be converted in the tissues to a free amino group (Fig. 10-27). Of the thousands of derivatives synthesized, only 12 are clinically useful.

Sulfonamides have a wide range of antibacterial activity against both gram-positive and gram-negative species. Since their action is only bacteriostatic, phagocytosis is required for killing of the organism. Among the organisms most susceptible to the sulfonamides are *Streptococcus pyogenes, Streptococcus pneumoniae, Haemophilus influenzae, Vibrio cholerae, Yersinia pestis, Neisseria meningitidis,* and the *Chlamydiaceae.* Although there is usually a direct correlation between the efficacy in vitro and in vivo, tissues and exudates of sulfonamides contain substances that can neutralize their inhibitory effect. These include such substances as p-aminobenzoic acid, methionine, and the purines. In vivo usefulness also is conditioned by the extent of conjugation of the drug after absorption. The conjugate is therapeutically inactive.

At the present time the principal use of the sulfonamides is for the treatment of uncomplicated urinary tract infections. Although very effective in the control of bacillary dysentery, their use has decreased because of an increasing number of isolates of resistant strains. The emergence of drug-resistant strains has led to the replacement of sulfonamides in the prophylaxis and treatment of meningococcal meningitis. It is still useful, however, in the treatment of *H. influenzae* meningitis and in combination with neomycin for preoperative suppression of the bowel flora.

A number of toxic reactions have been attributed to the various sulfonamides, the most serious of which are renal blockage from crystalluria, some systemic disorders that are probably allergic in origin, and blood dyscrasias.

Some of the clinically useful sulfonamides and their major uses are shown in Table 10-6. In addition, triple sulfonamide mixtures have also been widely used. These preparations always contain sulfadiazine; the second component usually is either sulfamerazine or sulfacetamide, and the third component, sulfamethazine. The triple mixture is less toxic. Since each drug retains its individual solubility in the urine the smaller dose reduces the risk of renal blockage. A higher blood level is also achieved by a combination of drugs absorbed and excreted at different rates.

MECHANISM OF ACTION.   The sulfonamides are structural analogs of p-aminobenzoic acid (PABA), an essential metabolite that functions in the cell as a precursor of folic acid (pteroylglutamic acid). The biologically active form of folic acid is tetrahydrofolic acid (FH_4), a coenzyme important in the transfer and reduction of 1-carbon fragments. Tetrahydrofolate serves as the acceptor of the β-carbon atom of serine when it is cleaved to yield glycine. This reaction is of special significance as a source of active 1-carbon units required in the synthesis of methionine, thymine, and the purines.

Sulfonamides interfere with the synthesis of PABA. The specific reaction inhibited is the condensation of PABA with 2-amino-4-hydroxy-6-dihydropteridinylmethyl pyrophosphate to form dihydropteroic acid. PABA and the sulfonamides are competitive substrates in this reaction (Fig. 10-28).

Organisms that synthesize folic acid are sensitive to sulfonamides, whereas those that have

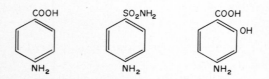

FIG. 10-27. Structural relationship between p-aminobenzoic acid (left), sulfanilamide (center), and p-aminosalicylic acid (right).

TABLE 10-6 SULFONAMIDES OF CLINICAL IMPORTANCE

Drug	Properties	Clinical Use
Sulfadiazine	Rapidly absorbed and excreted	Meningitis
Sulfafurazole (Gantrisin)	Rapidly absorbed and excreted	Urinary tract infections
Sulfamethoxazole (Gantanol)	Rapidly absorbed and excreted	Urinary tract infections
Sulfamethoxypyridazine (Midicel, Kynex)	Rapidly absorbed, slowly excreted	Urinary tract infections, respiratory infections
Sulfadimethoxine (Madribon)	Rapidly absorbed, slowly excreted	Urinary tract infections, respiratory infections
Succinylsulfathiazole (Sulfasuxidine)	Poorly absorbed	Treatment of *Salmonella* and *Shigella* carriers, suppression of intestinal flora before surgery
Phthalylsulfathiazole	Poorly absorbed	Treatment of *Salmonella* and *Shigella* carriers, suppression of intestinal flora before surgery

a requirement for preformed folic acid are insensitive because of the absence of the sulfonamide-inhibited reaction. The addition of either PABA or folic acid to a system in which growth has been inhibited by the sulfonamides neutralizes the inhibitory effect. Certain metabolites involved in folic acid coenzyme-requiring reactions (ie, methionine, serine, thymine, and the purines) also overcome inhibition produced by these drugs.

Man, like certain microorganisms, requires preformed folic acid for growth and cannot synthesize it from PABA. The successful use of the sulfonamide drugs in therapy, in spite of the presence of folic acid in human tissues, is due to the impermeability of the bacterial cell to folic acid as it occurs in the tissues.

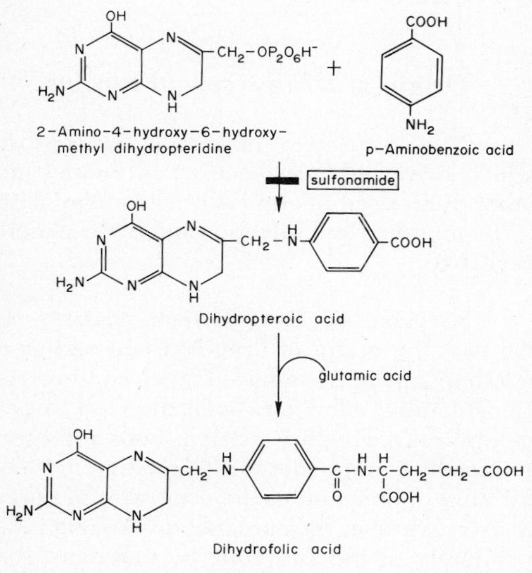

FIG. 10-28. Inhibition of dihydropteroic acid synthesis by the sulfonamides.

Sulfones Derivatives of 4, 4'-diaminodiphenylsulfone (dapsone) form a group of agents that display marked specificity, primarily against the genus *Mycobacterium*. Although they have been employed in the treatment of tuberculosis, their present clinical use is limited to the management of leprosy. They halt progression of the disease, especially when treatment is initiated in the early phases. Toxic side effects of the sulfones include hemolytic anemia, peripheral neuritis, dermatitis, and erythema nodosum. Sulfones interfere with the metabolism of PABA, which antagonizes the drug in vitro.

p-Aminosalicylic Acid (PAS) The antimicrobial activity of PAS is highly specific for *M. tuberculosis*. At present PAS plays a very important role in the chemotherapy of tuberculosis, where it is the most important ancillary agent for the disease when given in combination with either streptomycin or isoniazid. PAS is a bacteriostatic agent structurally similar to PABA and is antagonized by PABA in vitro (Fig. 10-27).

Other Metabolite Analogs

Isoniazid Isoniazid, the hydrazide of isonicotinic acid, is highly specific for *M. tuberculosis* (Fig. 10-29). It is effective in very low concentrations and is bactericidal for only actively growing organisms. Isoniazid does not inhibit growth immediately but only after the organisms undergo one or two divisions. Tubercle bacilli exposed to the drug lose their acid-fast staining property.

Isoniazid penetrates cells with ease and, un-

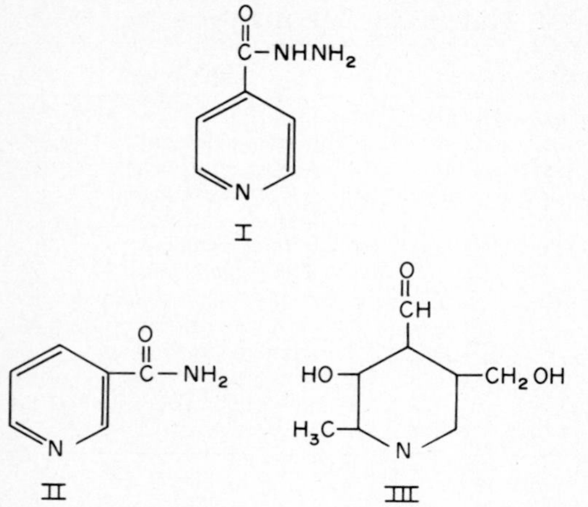

FIG. 10-29. Structural relationship among I, isoniazid (isonicotinic acid hydrazide), II, nicotinamide, and III, pyridoxal.

like streptomycin, is as effective against bacilli within monocytes as against extracellular organisms. At present, isoniazid is the most potent and useful agent in the treatment of tuberculosis. However, resistance to isoniazid develops rapidly, a problem that can be largely circumvented by the simultaneous administration of isoniazid with either streptomycin or PAS. Currently, this combination therapy represents the mainstay in the treatment of tuberculosis. The most important side effects of isoniazid are related to its toxicity for the peripheral and central nervous systems. Peripheral neuritis is the most common of these side effects, resembling that of a vitamin B_6 deficiency. Convulsions may also occur.

MECHANISM OF ACTION.   In spite of extensive studies there is no convincing evidence pinpointing any single mechanism as the primary site of attack by isoniazid. Its structural similarity to both niacin and pyridoxal suggests that the drug might act as an antimetabolite against either of these vitamins. Although pyridoxal reverses competitively the inhibitory action of isoniazid on tubercle bacilli and on various pyridoxal-requiring reactions, the importance of these effects is difficult to evaluate because of the formation of a pyridoxal-isonicotinyl hydrazone.

Alternatively isoniazid may act on nicotinamide adenine dinucleotidase (NADase), the enzyme that breaks down NAD. In the intact cell

the enzyme normally exists in an inactive form. Isoniazid activates NADase by altering the conformation of a protein inhibitor which is normally associated with it. As a result NAD is rapidly broken down, and the cell's supply of NAD, which is required in all phases of metabolism, is depleted.

DRUG RESISTANCE

The introduction of the sulfonamides and penicillin opened a new era in clinical medicine and stimulated a wave of optimism in the fight against infectious diseases. Early in the use of these drugs, however, it was realized that even though devastating epidemics had been curbed, disease caused by infectious organisms remained a major problem. One of the major factors contributing to the persistence of infectious diseases is the tremendous capacity of microorganisms for circumventing the action of inhibitory drugs.

The ability of many microorganisms to develop resistance to the chemotherapeutic drugs offers a serious threat to their future usefulness and demands both resourcefulness and ingenuity in meeting and counteracting this problem. If the use of these agents is to be successful, we must abandon the notions that they affect only those organisms against which they are directed at any particular time, and that regardless of how recklessly they are used, the organisms are powerless to respond.

Origin of Drug-resistant Strains

There are two major mechanisms by which increased resistance to antibiotics and other drugs used in clinical practice may arise: (1) by mutation and selection and (2) by genetic exchange.

Selection of Drug-resistant Mutants In the past the origin of drug-resistant strains of microorganisms has aroused much controversy. Considerable effort has been directed toward determining whether resistant cells represent the products of phenotypic adaptation induced by some interaction of the drug with the organism or whether they are mutants arising independently of the antibiotic by mutation. It is now firmly established that drug resistance arises by the latter mechanism, ie, by a random mutation that results in an altered susceptibility to the drug, the drug serving only as a selective agent favoring the survival of resistant over sensitive organisms once the genetic alteration has taken place and has been expressed phenotypically.

MUTATION RATES. Mutations generally occur at a frequency of about 1 in 10^5 to 10^{10} cell divisions (p. 142). As would be expected, the frequency rate of spontaneous mutation to resistance varies with the bacterial species and the antimicrobial drug. For example, the rate of mutation by *M. tuberculosis* to streptomycin resistance is approximately 10^{-10} and to isoniazid, 10^{-6}. Knowledge of the mutation rate as well as the site of attack of the various drugs is important in a rational approach to chemotherapy. The successful use of combination treatment in tuberculosis provides such an example. Because of the rapid emergence of strains of tubercle bacilli resistant to the drugs commonly used in the chemotherapy of tuberculosis, it is necessary to administer two drugs simultaneously. The success of this combined therapy can be explained by the fact that in a patient on combined streptomycin and isoniazid therapy, the likelihood of an organism mutating to resistance to both streptomycin and isoniazid is very low, about 1 in 10^{16} cell divisions.

Resistance Mediated by Genetic Exchange
Genetic information that controls bacterial drug resistance occurs both in the bacterial chromosome and in the DNA of extrachromosomal plasmids and episomes. The resistance trait may be transmitted from these loci by the transfer of genetic material from a resistant cell to a sensitive one.

INFECTIOUS DRUG RESISTANCE. The transmissibility of drug resistance was first postulated in 1957 to explain the marked increase in the rise of drug resistance in the *Shigella* isolates from bacillary dysentery in Japan. The majority of the strains isolated from patients were resistant not to a single drug but to many drugs used in the treatment of dysentery. These included streptomycin, sulfonamides, tetracycline, and chloramphenicol. When cells of a multiply resistant strain of *Shigella* or *Salmonella* were mixed with cells of a sensitive strain of *E. coli*, multiple resistance was found

to be transferred to the latter organism, usually en bloc. Transfer is now known to occur among all genera of the Enterobacteriaceae.

In multiple drug resistance of this type, the genetic elements that control it have the properties of episomes and are designated resistance factors or R factors. An R factor consists of two components, the R determinant for drug resistance and the resistance transfer factor, or RTF, which is responsible for the transmissibility of the R determinant. The resistance determinants are linked together on an episome and confer resistance only in the cell possessing them unless the RTF is also present. The resistance determinants and the RTFs are independent replicons, each of which is capable of replicating and operating on its own in the bacterial cell. When a resistance determinant and its transfer factor are present in the same cell, association of the two occurs, and an R factor is produced.

For transfer of R factors, cell-to-cell contact or conjugation is required. Resistance transfer factors code for the formation of specific pili through which the transfer of the resistance factors is accomplished. The frequency of transfer of R factors by conjugation varies with the factor to be transferred as well as with the bacterium. Seldom, however, do more than 1 percent of the cells in a donor culture transfer their R factors, because of their inability to form specific pili (Chap. 8).

Infectious drug resistance has far-reaching epidemiologic implications and has been found in many countries throughout the world. The drug-resistant determinants found thus far to be transmitted in this manner include those for streptomycin, sulfonamides, chloramphenicol, tetracycline, neomycin, kanamycin, ampicillin, and furazolidone. Environmental exposure of the normal intestinal flora to antibiotics favors the growth of those organisms that carry the R factor. Following infection with pathogenic species, these drug-resistant saprophytes can transmit resistance to cells of the sensitive pathogen, which may then, if antibiotics are used in treatment, completely replace the initially drug-sensitive organism. There is clear-cut clinical evidence that transfer of drug resistance of this type occurs within the human intestinal tract.

TRANSDUCTION. Resistance to penicillin in *S. aureus* usually is mediated by a penicillinase plasmid. This plasmid is analogous in many ways to a nontransmissible R factor of the enteric bacteria (ie, a resistance determinant in the absence of an RTF), but its transfer is accomplished by transduction rather than by mating.

When a plasmid is transduced into a staphylococcal cell either it can select a specific site that ensures its replication and distribution to daughter cells as autonomous units, or it can become integrated into the bacterial chromosome or into another penicillinase plasmid already located at a maintenance site. The plasmid's first choice is usually to remain an autonomous unit on its own maintenance site. Only rarely does it become inserted into the bacterial chromosome.

The penicillinase plasmids in staphylococci contain the determinants for the enzyme β-lactamase (p. 161). Genetic markers, such as resistance to erythromycin and to a number of inorganic ions, may also be located on this plasmid. Whereas resistance to streptomycin, tetracycline, chloramphenicol, and the macrolides can also be transduced, these determinants are located on different plasmids.

Biochemical Mechanisms of Drug Resistance

Resistance is caused by genetically controlled peculiarities of the metabolism or structure of the cell which enable it to escape the action of the drug. Among the biochemical changes which have been found in bacterial mutants selected for resistance are (1) decreased permeability of the organism to the drug, (2) increased destruction of the inhibitor, (3) increased synthesis of an essential metabolite or drug antagonist, and (4) changes in the properties of enzymes, resulting in a different relative affinity of substrate and antagonist.

In general, the mechanisms of extrachromosomally controlled drug resistance are different from those dependent on chromosomal genes and usually involve either a decrease in the permeability of the cell or enzymatic inactivation of the inhibitor. Transferable sulfonamide resistance and tetracycline resistance result from reduced cell membrane permeability to the drugs. This impermeability mechanism of drug resistance is specific for each drug, since loss of either sulfonamide or tetracycline resistance in lines resistant to both drugs does not impair resistance to the other drug. The determinant concerned must therefore code for a specific protein, probably that of a permease required to transport the inhibitor across the cell membrane.

Specific inactivating enzymes occur in a number of bacteria carrying R factors. In fact, enzymatic inactivation is the predominant mechanism of transferable resistance to penicillin, chloramphenicol, kanamycin, streptomycin, and neomycin. The transferable drug-resistance characters and mechanisms of resistance are shown in Table 10-7.

Resistance controlled by chromosomal genes is usually due to changes in enzymes or active sites involved in essential metabolic reactions in the cell. An example of this mechanism is resistance to streptomycin where differences exist between the ribosomes of streptomycin-resistant and streptomycin-sensitive organisms. As discussed above, streptomycin binds to a specific site on the ribosome, thereby deranging protein synthesis. Any mutation that deletes this site or alters it in such a manner that the drug cannot exert its effect results in a mutation to streptomycin resistance. This site is a protein (S12) on the 30S subunit coded for by the str A gene. Following the exposure of cultures of E. coli to high levels of streptomycin, survivors generally are all mutants in this gene.

In bacterial resistance to the sulfonamides, more than one mechanism is responsible for the resistant state. In some organisms a high degree of resistance is linked to an increased production of p-aminobenzoic acid. In others, such as S. pneumoniae, resistance to the sulfonamides results in an altered dihydropteroate synthetase that displays a reduced binding capacity for the drug.

TABLE 10–7 MECHANISMS OF PLASMID-DETERMINED ANTIBIOTIC RESISTANCE

Antibiotic	Mechanism of Resistance
Penicillin	Hydrolysis of β-lactam ring
Streptomycin	Adenylylation of streptomycin
Neomycin/kanamycin	Phosphorylation of antibiotic
Tetracycline	Reduced permeability
Chloramphenicol	Acetylation of antibiotic
Erythromycin/ lincomycin	Ribosomal modification
Sulfonamides	Probably reduced permeability

FURTHER READING

Books and Reviews

Biochemical Studies of Antimicrobial Drugs. Sixteenth Symp Soc Gen Microbiol. London, Cambridge Univ Press, 1966

Blumberg PM, Strominger JL: Interaction of penicillin with the bacterial cell: penicillin-binding proteins and penicillin-sensitive enzymes. Bacteriol Rev 38:291, 1974

Corcoran, JW, Hahn FE (eds): Antibiotics. Mechanism of Action of Antimicrobial and Antitumor Agents. New York, Springer Verlag, 1975, vol 3

Dowding J, Davies J: Mechanisms and origins of plasmid-determined antibiotic resistance. In Schlessinger D (ed): Microbiology—1974. Washington, DC, Am Soc Microbiol, 1975

Gale EF, Cundliffe E, Reynolds PE, Richmond MH, Waring MJ: The Molecular Basis of Antibiotic Action. New York, Wiley, 1972

Gottlieb, D, Shaw PD (eds): Antibiotics. New York, Springer Verlag, 1967, vol 1

Hamilton-Miller JMT: Chemistry and biology of the polyene macrolide antibiotics. Bacteriol Rev 37:166, 1973

Lacy RW: Antibiotic resistance plasmids of *Staphylococcus aureus* and their clinical importance. Bacteriol Rev 39:1, 1975

Lengyel P, Söll D: Mechanism of protein biosynthesis. Bacteriol Rev 33:264, 1969

Novick RP: Extrachromosomal inheritance in bacteria. Bacteriol Rev 33:210, 1969

Salton MRJ, Tomasz A (eds): Mode of action of antibiotics on microbial walls and membranes. Ann NY Acad Sci 235:1, 1974

Vazquez D: Inhibitors of protein synthesis. FEBS Lett 40: S63, 1974

Wehrli W, Staehelin M: Actions of the rifamycins. Bacteriol Rev 35:290, 1971

Weinstein L: Chemotherapy of microbial diseases. In Goodman LS, Gilman A (eds): The Pharmacological Basis of Therapeutics, 3rd ed. New York, Macmillan, 1965, pp 1144–1342

Weisblum B, Davies J: Antibiotic inhibitors of the bacterial ribosome. Bacteriol Rev 32:493, 1968

Wolstenholme GEW, O'Connor M (eds): Bacterial Episomes and Plasmids, Ciba Foundation Symposium. Boston, Little, Brown, 1969

Selected Papers

Garvin RT, Biswas DK, Gorini L: The effects of streptomycin or dihydrostreptomycin binding to 16 S RNA or to 30 S ribosomal subunits. Proc Natl Acad Sci USA 71: 3814, 1974

Gurgo C, Apirion D, Schlessinger D: Polyribosome metabolism in *Escherichia coli* treated with chloramphenicol, neomycin, spectinomycin or tetracycline. J Mol Biol 45:205, 1969

Helser TL, Davies JE, Dahlberg JE: Changes in methylation of 16 S ribosomal RNA associated with mutation to kasugamycin resistance in *Escherichia coli*. Nature [New Biol] 233:13, 1971

Izaki K, Matsuhashi M, Strominger JL: Biosynthesis of the peptidoglycan of bacterial cell walls. XIII. Peptidoglycan transpeptidase and D-alanine carboxypeptidase: penicillin-sensitive enzymatic reaction in strains of *Escherichia coli*. J Biol Chem 243:3180, 1968

Lawrence PJ, Strominger JL: Synthesis of the peptidoglycan of bacterial cells walls. J Biol Chem 245:3653, 1970

Luzzatto L, Apirion D, Schlessinger D: Polyribosome depletion and blockage of the ribosome cycle by streptomycin in *Escherichia coli*. J Mol Biol 42:315, 1969

Miskin R, Zamir A: Enhancement of peptidyl transferase activity by antibiotics acting on the 50 S ribosomal subunit. J Mol Biol 87:121, 1974

Modolell J, Davis BD: Rapid inhibition of polypeptide chain extension by streptomycin. Proc Natl Acad Sci USA 61:1279, 1968

Monro RE, Staehelin T, Celma ML, Vazquez D: The peptidyl transferase activity of ribosomes. Cold Spring Harbor Symp Quant Biol 34:357, 1969

Nozawa Y, Kitajima Y, Sekiya T, Ito Y: Ultrastructural alterations induced by amphotericin B in the plasma membrane of *Epidermophyton floccosum* as revealed by freeze-etch electron microscopy. Biochim Biophys Acta 367:32, 1974

Ortiz PJ: Dihydrofolate and dihydropteroate synthesis by partially purified enzymes from wild-type and sulfonamide-resistant pneumococcus. Biochemistry 9:355, 1970

Ozaki M, Mizushima S, Nomura M: Identification and functional characterization of the protein controlled by the streptomycin-resistant locus in *E. coli*. Nature 222: 333, 1969

Pestka S: Translocation, aminoacyl-oligonucleotides, and antibiotic action. Cold Spring Harbor Symp Quant Biol 34:395, 1969

Siewert G, Strominger JL: Bacitracin: an inhibitor of the dephosphorylation of lipid pyrophosphate, an intermediate in biosynthesis of the peptidoglycan of bacterial cell walls. Proc Natl Acad Sci USA 57:767, 1967

Tai PC, Wallace BJ, Davis BD: Selective action of erythromycin on initiating ribosomes. Biochemistry 13:4653, 1974

Wallace BJ, Davis BD: Cyclic blockade of initiation sites by streptomycin-damaged ribosomes in *Escherichia coli*: an explanation for dominance of sensitivity. J Mol Biol 75:377, 1973

Waring MJ: Drugs which affect the structure and function of DNA. Nature 219:1320, 1968

Weissmann G, Sessa G: The action of polyene antibiotics on phospholipid-cholesterol structures. J Biol Chem 242:616, 1967

Zillig W, Zechel K, Rabussay D, et al: On the role of different subunits of DNA-dependent RNA polymerase from *E. coli* in the transcription process. Cold Spring Harbor Symp Quant Biol 35:47, 1970

11
Sterilization and Disinfection

Knowledge of the basic principles of sterilization and disinfection is fundamental to the intelligent practice of medicine. Although new techniques of sterilization and disinfection have been introduced as we have gained a better understanding of the dynamics of microbial life and death, some of the procedures and agents now employed were introduced centuries before the concept of infection was formulated. Most of the simple chemical agents once used in therapy have been replaced by the sulfonamides and antibiotics, but many of this group have retained their importance as effective antiseptics or disinfectants in the destruction of microorganisms in the nonliving environment. At the present time no group of chemical agents is more widely used than the antiseptics and disinfectants. The repercussions resulting from the removal of a single antimicrobial agent, hexachlorophene, from the agents currently used in the home and hospital are indicative of our tremendous dependency on such agents (p. 231).

Definitions Various terms have been employed to describe the damaging effects of certain chemical and physical agents on microorganisms. The term "sterilization" is an absolute one, which implies the total inactivation of all forms of microbial life in terms of the organism's ability to reproduce. The suffix -cide is added when a killing action is implied, while -stasis is added when the organism is merely inhibited in growth or prevented from multiplying. A bactericide destroys bacteria. A germicide or disinfectant is an agent that kills microorganisms capable of producing an infection. A bacteriostatic agent is a substance that prevents the growth of bacteria. An antiseptic opposes sepsis or putrefaction either by killing microorganisms or by preventing their growth. The term is commonly used for agents that are applied topically to living tissue. These are only broad definitions, however, since the same agent may act differently under different test conditions.

The selection of an appropriate procedure or agent is determined by the specific situation and whether it is necessary to kill all microorganisms or whether it is necessary to kill only certain species. The complete destruction of all microorganisms present in or on any material is essential in surgical procedures, in the preparation of all media, glassware, and other materials used in the microbiology laboratory, and in the canning of nonacid high-protein foods. About 95 percent of all sterilization is done by steam under pressure in the autoclave. Sterilization by chemicals is less reliable. In the care of patients with communicable diseases, the destruction of the pathogen is necessary in order to prevent the transmission of the infection to susceptible individuals. For this purpose a disinfectant is adequate and is usually employed as a cleaning-up process in order to prevent the spread of a specific infection.

DYNAMICS OF STERILIZATION AND DISINFECTION

THE DEATH RATE OF MICROORGANISMS. Knowledge of the kinetics of death of a bacterial population is helpful in understanding the basis of sterilization by lethal agents. In the case of a microorganism, the only valid criterion of death is the irreversible loss of the ability to reproduce. This is usually determined by plating techniques that quantitate by colony counts the number of survivors.

When a bacterial population is exposed to a lethal agent there is a progressive reduction with time in the number of survivors. The kinetics of death of a microbial population are usually exponential; the number of survivors decreases with time. If the logarithm of the number of survivors is plotted as a function of the time of exposure, a straight line is obtained (Fig. 11-1). Its negative slope defines the death rate. The death rate, however, tells only what fraction of the initial population survives a given period of exposure to the antibacterial agent. In order to determine the actual number of survivors, one must also know the initial population size. The relationship is expressed mathematically by the formula:

$$K = 1/t \log B/b$$

where B is the initial number of organisms, and b is the number after time t. Although the logarithmic curve is mathematically convenient and approximately correct when relatively high concentrations of a disinfectant are used, with lower concentrations the disinfection curve is sigmoidal, the rate being slow in the early stages, then proceeding rapidly for most of the

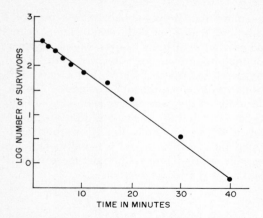

FIG. 11-1. Death rate of *Escherichia coli* when exposed to 0.5 percent phenol at 20C. [From Chick: J Hyg (Camb) 10: 237, 1910]

disinfection process, and finally slowing down at the end. The flattening of the slope toward the end of the process is extremely important from the point of view of sterilization, resulting in the requirement for a more prolonged or intense treatment in order to destroy the resistant survivors that are more likely to be present in an initially large microbial population. Practical experience has shown that under no circumstances can one extrapolate the exponential death rate to zero and assume that the time of exposure so indicated will guarantee sterility.

Because of the exponential form of the survivor-time curve, the larger the initial number of cells to be killed, the more intense or prolonged is the treatment required for sterilization. Also, as might be expected, the rate of disinfection varies with the concentration of disinfectant employed. The effect of concentration on rate, however, is not constant but varies with the different disinfectants, as discussed below.

ANTIMICROBIAL CHEMICAL AGENTS

Factors Affecting Disinfectant Potency In contrast to chemotherapeutic agents that exhibit a high degree of selectivity for certain bacterial species, disinfectants are highly toxic for all types of cells. The relative value of a particular disinfectant depends to a great extent upon the conditions under which it operates.

CONCENTRATION OF BACTERICIDAL AGENT. Many agents are lethal for bacteria when used only in extremely high concentrations. Others may stimulate, retard, or even kill the organism in very low concentrations. Most of the chemical compounds that can kill bacteria exhibit a bacteriostatic effect in concentrations lower than those required to kill. There is also a marked tendency of poisonous agents to stimulate biologic processes when employed in low concentrations. The concentration required to produce a given effect, however, as well as the range of concentrations over which a given effect is demonstrable, varies with the disinfectant, the organism, and the method of testing. A close relationship exists between the concentration of drug employed and the time required to kill a given fraction of the population. This relationship is shown in the expression

$$C^n t = K$$

where C is the drug concentration, t is the time required to kill a given fraction of the cells, and n and K are constants. With phenolic compounds, for example, a change in the concentration of the disinfectant has a pronounced effect on the disinfection rate: Halving the concentration increases approximately 64-fold the time required for sterilization. With most disinfectants, however, there is a much less dramatic effect on sterilizing time.

TIME. When bacteria are exposed to a specific concentration of a bactericidal agent, even in excess, not all of the organisms die at the same time, but rather there is a gradual decrease in the number of living cells. Disinfection is usually considered as a process in which bacteria are killed in a reasonable length of time, but there are varying opinions about what this length of time should be (Fig. 11-1).

pH. The hydrogen ion concentration exerts its influence on bactericidal action by affecting both the bacteria and the chemical agent. When suspended in a culture medium of pH 7, bacteria are negatively charged. An increase of pH will increase the charge and may alter the effective concentration of the chemical agent at the surface of the cell. The pH also determines the degree of ionization of the bactericide. In general, the nonionized form of a dissociable agent passes through the cell membrane more readily than the relatively inactive ionic forms.

TEMPERATURE. The killing of bacteria by chemical agents, like other chemical reactions, increases with an increase in temperature. For each 10C temperature increment there is, at low temperatures, a doubling of the death rate. With some agents, such as phenol, the rate is increased five to eight times, suggesting a more complex reaction and the influence of other factors.

NATURE OF THE ORGANISM. A number of factors relating to the organism itself exert a pronounced effect on the efficacy of the bactericidal agent. These include the species of organism and its chemical composition, the growth phase of the culture, the presence of special structures such as spores and capsules, the previous history of the culture, and the number of bacteria in the test system (Fig. 11-2).

PRESENCE OF EXTRANEOUS MATERIALS. The presence of organic matter and other foreign materials, such as serum, blood, and pus, often influences the activity of many agents used for disinfection and renders inert substances that show high activity in their absence. These foreign materials alter disinfectant activity in a number of ways: surface adsorption of the disinfectant by protein colloids, formation of a chemically inert or less active compound, or a binding of the disinfectant by active groups of the foreign protein.

Among the disinfectants which are inhibited to the greatest extent by organic material with a high protein content are the aniline dyes, the mercurials, and the cationic detergents. The mercurials are markedly inhibited by compounds containing sulfhydryl groups; the quarternary ammonium compounds are inhibited by soaps and lipids.

Highly bacteriostatic disinfectants require the addition of inactivators to the medium used for subculture in order to neutralize any of the disinfectant carried over with the inoculum. The addition of the inactivator is necessary in order to distinguish bacteriostatic from bactericidal activity and to determine whether the organisms have been irreversibly killed.

Evaluation of Disinfectants The standard methods that have been devised for the evaluation of disinfectants employ phenol as the standard reference material. The ratio of the concentration of the disinfectant being tested to the concentration of the reference standard required to kill in a specified time is referred to as the phenol coefficient. The official quantitative test for evaluating disinfectants is that of the Food and Drug Administration of the U.S. Department of Agriculture. This official method specifies standardized conditions for the testing of disinfectants against strains of *Salmonella typhi, Staphylococcus aureus,* and *Pseudomonas aeruginosa* of known susceptibility to phenol. Criticism has been directed against the phenol coefficient test because of the limited information that it provides. It has been recommended that the test be supplemented with a series of additional laboratory methods designed to determine various properties of the disinfectant: the effect of variations in time and temperature on the bactericidal power of the disinfectant against a variety of organisms including spores, its activity both in the absence and in the presence of organic matter, penetrability, the extent of bacteriostasis, tissue toxicity tests, and in vivo testing.

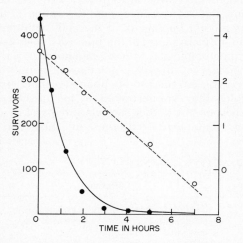

FIG. 11-2. Death rate of anthrax spores treated with 5 percent phenol at 33.3C. Number of surviving spores is plotted on an arithmetic scale and on a logarithmic scale. [From Chick: J Hyg (Camb), 8:92, 1908]

Mechanisms of Antimicrobial Action The mechanisms by which drugs kill or inhibit the growth of microorganisms are varied and complex. Sequential or simultaneous changes often occur which make it difficult to differentiate primary from secondary effects. In general, however, all of the observable effects of chemical agents on bacteria depend on chemical changes in the components of the bacterial cell. Some of these changes result in damage to the cell membrane, some irreversibly inactivate proteins, and others induce extensive breakdown of RNA.

Agents that Interfere with Membrane Function

The cell membrane separates the living protoplasm from the nonliving environment and regulates the flow of solutes into and out of the cell. The structural integrity of the membrane depends upon the orderly arrangement of the proteins and lipids of which it is composed. Exposure of bacteria to organic solvents and detergents results in a structural disorganization of the membrane which prevents its normal function. The net effect is release from the cell of small metabolites and interference with active transport and energy metabolism.

Surface-active Agents   Substances that alter the energy relationships at interfaces, producing a reduction of surface or interfacial tension are referred to as surface-active agents. They are widely used in industry and in the home as wetting agents, detergents, and emulsifiers. Surface-active agents are compounds that possess both water-attracting (hydrophilic), and water-repelling (hydrophobic) groups. The interface between the lipid-containing membrane of a bacterial cell and the surrounding aqueous medium provides a particularly susceptible site for agents of this type. The hydrophobic portion of the molecule is a long-chain hydrocarbon that is fat soluble, while the hydrophilic portion may be either an ionizable group or a nonionic but highly polar structure. Included in the surface-active agents are cationic, anionic, nonionic, and amphoteric substances (Table 11-1).

The most important antibacterial agents are the cationic surface-active agents in which a hydrophobic residue is balanced by a positively charged hydrophilic group, such as a quarternary ammonium nucleus. When bacteria are exposed to agents of this type, the positively charged group associates with the phosphate groups of the membrane phospholipids, while the nonpolar portion of the detergent pentrates into the hydrophobic interior of the membrane. The resulting distortion causes a loss of the semipermeability of the membrane with a leakage from the cell of nitrogen and phosphorus-containing compounds and other important substances, after which the agent itself may enter the cell and denature its proteins. The quarternary ammonium compounds are more active at an alkaline pH. They are bactericidal for a wide range of organisms, although gram-positive species are more actively susceptible.

Among the anionic detergents are the soaps and fatty acids, agents that dissociate to yield a negatively charged ion. These agents, most active at an acid pH, are effective against gram-positive organisms but are relatively ineffective against gram-negative species because of the lipopolysaccharide of their cell wall. The anionic detergents cause gross disruption of the lipoprotein framework of the cell membrane. The primary injury of the bile salts, long used by microbiologists to lyse pneumococci, is dissociation of the cell membrane, permitting autolytic enzymes to act upon substrates from which they are restricted in the intact cell. When used together the two groups of detergents neutralize each other, and the action of

TABLE 11-1   SURFACE-ACTIVE AGENTS

Trade Name	Type of Compound	Structure
Zephiran	Cationic	Alkyldimethylbenzyl ammonium chloride
Triton K-12	Cationic	Cetyldimethylbenzyl ammonium chloride
Cepryn chloride	Cationic	Cetylpyridinium chloride
Duponol LS	Anionic	Sodium oleyl sulfate
Triton W-30	Anionic	Sodium salt of alkylphenoxyethyl sulfonate
Carbowax 1500 dioleate	Nonionic	Oleic acid ester of polymerized polyethylene glycol
Tween 80	Nonionic	Sorbitan monooleate polyoxy-alkylene derivative

both is inhibited by proteins. Nonionic detergents are relatively nontoxic, and a few promote bacterial growth. For example, Tween 80 facilitates a diffuse submerged growth of *Mycobacterium tuberculosis* and provides a source of oleic acid which is stimulatory to the organism. Triton X-100, another nonionic detergent, has a specific solubilizing effect on the cytoplasmic membrane, selectively separating the proteins of the cell wall and membrane.

Phenols The lethal effect of the phenols is due to their ability to orient themselves at interfaces, causing membrane damage, release of cell contents, and lysis. Low concentrations of phenol precipitate proteins. Membrane-bound oxidases and dehydrogenases are irreversibly inactivated by concentrations of phenol that are rapidly bactericidal for the organism.

Following its introduction as a surgical antiseptic by Lister in 1865, phenol was widely used as a disinfectant. At present, however, its use is limited primarily to the testing of bactericidal agents, having been replaced as a practical disinfectant by less caustic and toxic phenol derivatives.

The antibacterial activity of phenol is greatly increased by various substitutions in the phenol nucleus; the compounds of greatest importance are the alkyl- and chloro-derivatives and the diphenyls. Not only do many of these derivatives have a very high antibacterial activity, but also they are considerably less toxic than phenol. Since most phenolic disinfectants have a low solubility in water, they are formulated with emulsifying agents, such as soaps, which also increase their antibacterial action.

The simplest of the alkyl phenols are the cresols. Ortho-, meta-, and paracresol are appreciably more active than are phenol and are usually employed as a mixture, tricresol. Cresols, obtained industrially by the distillation of coal tar, are emulsified with green soap and sold under the trade names of Lysol and Creolin.

The halogenated diphenyl compounds exhibit unique antibacterial properties. Of these compounds the most important is the chlorinated derivative, hexachlorophene, which is highly effective against gram-positive organisms, especially staphylococci and streptococci. The specific mode of action of hexachlorophene is unknown. Like other surfactants, however, it appears to adsorb to and disrupt the cytoplasmic membrane, interfering with membrane-associated functions. Hexachlorophene is bactericidal if used in sufficiently high concentrations and, unlike many disinfectants, retains its antimicrobial potency when mixed with soaps or when added to various cosmetic preparations. It has been used in a wide variety of products, such as germicidal soaps, antiperspirants, toothpastes, and furnace filters. In 1961 routine daily hexachlorophene bathing of newborn infants became an accepted procedure in many nurseries in order to reduce colonization of the umbilical stump with *S. aureus* (Chap. 26). Numerous studies attest to the effectiveness of this procedure in decreasing the incidence of severe staphylococcal disease and hospital-based epidemics. In 1971, however, the Food and Drug Administration placed strict controls on the use of hexachlorophene and curtailed its use in the newborn nursery. This action was prompted by evidence of neurotoxicity following dermal absorption. The concern about hexachlorophene toxicity is timely and is justified. It emphasizes the need for the recognition that no drug should be used indiscriminately and that the benefits of each must be weighed against its potential hazards.

Organic Solvents Chloroform and toluene are often used to keep solutions sterile and to disrupt permeability barriers. Of the organic solvents, alcohols probably provide the best insight into the interaction of solvents with lipid membranes. Alcohols disorganize the lipid structure by penetrating into the hydrocarbon region. Short-chain alcohols produce quantitatively greater changes in membrane organization than do the higher homologs. In addition to their effect on the cell membrane, alcohols and other organic solvents also denature the proteins of the cell.

ALCOHOLS. The aliphatic alcohols, especially ethanol, have been widely employed as skin disinfectants because of their bactericidal action and ability to remove lipids from surfaces. The action of the alcohols as disinfectants, however, is severely restricted by their inability to kill spores at normal temperatures, and for this reason they should not be relied upon for the sterilization of instruments.

Ethanol is used extensively to sterilize the skin prior to cutaneous injections. It is also used for the disinfection of clinical thermometers and is very effective provided a sufficient period of contact is allowed. It is active against gram-positive, gram-negative, and acid-fast organisms. Ethanol is most effective at a concentration of 50 to 70 percent. Isopropyl alcohol is appreciably more active than ethanol and is less volatile. For these reasons it has been recommended that it replace ethanol for the sterilization of thermometers.

Agents that Denature Proteins

Proteins are the most abundant organic molecules in a bacterial cell and are fundamental to all aspects of cell structure and function. In its native state each protein possesses a characteristic conformation that is required for its proper functioning. Agents that alter the conformation of the protein by denaturation cause an unfolding of the polypeptide chain so that the chains become randomly and irregularly looped or coiled. Among the chemical agents that denature cellular proteins are the acids, alkalies, alcohol, acetone, and other organic solvents.

Acids and Alkalies These agents exert their antibacterial activity through their free H^+ and OH^- ions, through the undissociated molecules, or by altering the pH of the organism's environment. The strong mineral acids and strong alkalies have disinfectant properties proportional to the extent of their dissociation in solution. Some hydroxides, however, are more effective than their degree of dissociation would indicate, suggesting that the metallic cation also exerts a direct toxic action on the organism.

The intact molecule of the organic acids is apparently responsible for their activity. Although the extent of their dissociation in solution is less than that of mineral acids, they are sometimes more potent disinfectants. Benzoic acid, widely used as a food preservative, is approximately seven times as effective as hydrochloric acid, showing that both the whole molecule and the organic radical possess disinfectant activity. The formation of lactic acid and other organic acids during bacterial growth slows and finally arrests the growth of many species of bacteria. Salts of propionic acid are frequently added to breads and other foods as a preservative to halt spoilage.

Agents that Destroy or Modify the Functional Groups of Proteins

The catalytic site of an enzyme contains specific functional groups that bind the substrate and initiate the catalytic event. Inhibition of enzyme activity results if one or more of these functional groups are altered or destroyed. Compounds containing mercury or arsenic combine with sulfhydryl groups; formaldehyde, anionic detergents, and acid dyes react with amino and imidazole groups; basic dyes, quarternary ammonium compounds, and cationic detergents react with acidic groups, such as hydroxyl or phosphoric acid residues. The presence of organic matter and other substances containing free reactive groups markedly reduces the effectiveness of agents whose toxicity is due to combination with reactive groups of proteins.

Heavy Metals Soluble salts of mercury, arsenic, silver, and other heavy metals poison enzyme activity by forming mercaptides with the sulfhydryl groups of cysteine residues. The initial reaction is reversible, and if extraneous -SH groups are provided in the form of glutathione or sodium thioglycollate, most of the cells recover.

Various forms of mercury have been employed in medicine for many years. Mercuric chloride, once popular as a disinfectant, is very toxic and has limited use at the present time. Such organic mercurials as Metaphen, Merthiolate, and Mercurochrome are less toxic and, although unreliable as skin disinfectants, are useful antiseptic agents (Table 11-2).

Silver compounds are widely used as antiseptics, either as soluble silver salts or as colloidal preparations. The inorganic silver salts are efficient bactericidal agents, but their practical value is restricted by their irritant and caustic effects. The most commonly employed of the silver salts is silver nitrate, which is highly bactericidal for the gonococcus and is routinely used as required by state law for the prophylaxis of ophthalmia neonatorum in newborn infants. Colloidal silver compounds, in which silver is combined with protein and from which silver ions are slowly released, have been widely used as antiseptics, particularly in ophthalmology. They are primarily bacteriostatic, however, and relatively poor disinfectants.

TABLE 11–2 HIGHEST DILUTION OF MERCURIALS
INHIBITING GROWTH FOR 48 HOURS

Organism	Phenylmercuric Nitrate	Merthiolate	Mercuric Chloride
Staphylococcus aureus	1:120,000,000	1:26,000,000	1:18,000
Streptococcus pyogenes	1:150,000,000	1:28,000,000	1:120,000
Neisseria gonorrhoeae	1:36,000,000	1:12,000,000	1:50,000
Escherichia coli	1:4,000,000	1:860,000	1:34,000

°*From Birkhaug: J Infect Dis 53:250, 1933*

Oxidizing Agents Included in this group of agents are the halogens, hydrogen perixode, and potassium permanganate. The oxidizing agents inactivate enzymes by converting functional -SH groups to the oxidized S-S form. The stronger agents also attack amino groups, indole groups, and the phenolic hydroxyl group of tyrosine.

Chlorine and iodine are among our most useful disinfectants. For certain purposes, iodine as a skin disinfectant and chlorine as a water disinfectant, they are unequaled. They are unique among disinfectants in that their activity is almost exclusively bactericidal and they are effective against sporulating organisms.

Iodine exists principally in the form of I_2 at pH values below 6, where maximal bactericidal action is manifested. The rate of killing decreases as the pH is increased above 7.5. The iodide ion, I^-, formed as a result of iodine hydrolysis in aqueous solutions, has no significant bactericidal effect, and the triiodide ion I_3^-, also present in aqueous solutions, has minimal activity. Iodine tincture, USP, contains 2 percent iodine and 2 percent sodium iodide in dilute alcohol. The principal use of iodine is in the disinfection of the skin, and for this purpose it is probably superior to any other agent. Mixtures of iodine with various surface-active agents that act as carriers for the iodine are known as iodophors. They have been widely used for the sterilization of dairy equipment.

In addition to chlorine itself, there are three types of chlorine compounds, the hypochlorites, the inorganic chloramines, and the organic chloramines. The disinfectant action of all chlorine compounds results from their ability to liberate free chlorine. In aqueous solution the liberated chlorine reacts with water to form hypochlorous acid, which in neutral or acidic solutions is nonionized and is a strong oxidizing agent and an active disinfectant.

$$Cl_2 + H_2O \rightleftharpoons HOCl + H^+ + C^-$$

Although chlorine is one of the most potent bactericidal agents, its activity is markedly influenced by the presence of organic matter. For example, in the disinfection of water it is first necessary to determine its chlorine demand. This is because of the possible presence in water of substances capable of combining with chlorine. It is customary to add sufficient chlorine to the water supply to satisfy the chlorine demand of the water and at the same time to provide enough residual for complete disinfection.

In the food and dairy industries hypochlorite solutions are widely used for sanitizing dairy and food-processing equipment, and in the home and restaurant, hypochlorites, such as clorox and Purex bleach, are employed for household sanitation and the disinfection of food utensils.

Hydrogen peroxide in a 3 percent solution is a harmless but very weak disinfectant whose primary use is in the cleansing of wounds. When hydrogen peroxide is applied to tissues, oxygen is rapidly released by the tissue catalases, and the germicidal action is brief. Another oxidizing agent, potassium permanganate, is used in the treatment of urethritis.

Dyes Some of the coal-tar dyes, especially the aniline dyes and the acridines, not only stain bacteria but are bacteriostatic at high dilutions. Within the usual pH range the basic dyes are more effective. Their affinity for the acidic phosphoric acid groups of nucleoproteins has been demonstrated. The dyes, however, are readily neutralized by serum and other proteins, thereby limiting their use to selective agents in culture media and to the treatment of local lesions on the skin and in the mouth and vagina.

Of the aniline dyes, derivatives of triphenylmethane, brilliant green, malachite green, and crystal violet have been used for many purposes. They are highly selective for grampositive organisms, and staphylococci are particularly susceptible to the violet dyes (Table 11-3). The bacteriostatic activity of some of the triphenylmethane dyes remains ill defined, but the action of gentian violet is attributed to its interference with the synthesis of the peptidoglycan component of the cell wall, where it blocks the conversion of UDP-acetylmuramic acid to UDP-acetylmuramylpeptide. In gram-negative organisms lipopolysaccharide in the outer envelope provides a major penetration barrier for the uptake of gentian violet. This finding explains the selective activity of gentian violet for gram-positive organisms.

The acridine dyes, often referred to as "flavines" because of their yellow color, exert a bactericidal and bacteriostatic effect upon a number of organisms. Among the compounds of clinical use are proflavine and acriflavine which have been employed in wound antisepsis. Unlike the aniline dyes, antimicrobial activity is retained in the presence of serum or pus.

The acridine dyes interfere with the synthesis of nucleic acids and proteins in both bacterial and mammalian cells. They are planar heterocyclic molecules that interact with double-stranded helical DNA by intercalation. Because of its flat hydrophobic structure, acridine is inserted between two successive bases in DNA, separating them physically. When the chain is replicated, an extra base is inserted into the complementary chain opposite the intercalated drug. When the latter chain is then replicated, the new chain will also contain an extra base.

Alkylating Agents   The lethal effects of formaldehyde, ethylene oxide, and glutaraldehyde result from their alkylating action on proteins. Inhibitions produced by such agents are irreversible, resulting in enzyme modification and inhibition of enzyme activity.

FORMALDEHYDE.   Formaldehyde is one of the least selective agents acting on proteins. Carboxyl, hydroxyl, or sulfhydryl groups of protein are alkylated by direct replacement of a hydrogen atom with a hydroxymethyl group. Its reaction with a sulfhydryl group of an enzyme protein is as follows:

$$\text{E---SH} + \text{H---}\overset{\overset{\text{H}}{|}}{\text{C}}\text{=O} \rightarrow \text{E---S---}\overset{\overset{\text{H}}{|}}{\underset{\underset{\text{H}}{|}}{\text{C}}}\text{---OH}$$

Formaldehyde is a gas that is usually employed as its 37 percent solution, formalin. Formalin is used for coagulating and preserving fresh tissues for microscopic study and is the major component of embalming fluids. When used at a sufficiently high concentration, it destroys all organisms including spores.

ETHYLENE OXIDE.   Ethylene oxide is an alkylating agent extensively employed in gaseous sterilization. It is active against all types of bacteria, including spores and tubercle bacilli, but its action is slow. It can be used for sterilizing a wide range of materials, but its greatest applicability lies in the sterilization of materials that would be damaged by heat, such as polyethylene tubing. It has been of special value in the sterilization of heart-lung machines.

TABLE 11-3   MAXIMUM DILUTIONS OF TRIPHENYLMETHANE DYES INHIBITING GROWTH FOR 24 HOURS

Organism	Brilliant Green	Malachite Green	Crystal Violet
Escherichia coli	1:675,000	1:40,000	1:85,000
Salmonella typhi	1:500,000	1:30,000	1:85,000
Shigella dysenteriae	1:1,500,000	1:250,000	1:400,000
Bacillus subtilis	1:15,000,000	1:4,000,000	1:4,000,000
Staphylococcus aureus	1:4,000,000	1:1,000,000	1:1,000,000

From Kliger: J Exp Med 27:463, 1918

The alkylating action of ethylene oxide is responsible for its bactericidal acitvity. It is an epoxy compound with the formula:

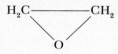

The ethylene oxide ring opens in the presence of a labile hydrogen and forms a hydroxy ethyl radical (CH_2CH_2OH) that then attaches to the position in the protein formerly occupied by the hydrogen. A labile hydrogen is available in carboxyl, amino, sulfhydryl, hydroxyl, and phenolic groups of proteins. Irreversible death of the cell results from blockage of these reactive groups. A number of enzymes are inhibited, among the most sensitive of which are phosphokinases and certain peptidases. In addition to its action on protein, ethylene oxide also reacts with DNA and RNA, possibly by esterification of phosphate groups or reaction with the ring nitrogen of purines and pyrimidines. It is mutagenic for bacteria. Its use as a disinfectant presents some hazard of potential toxicity for man, including mutagenicity and carcinogenicity.

ANTIMICROBIAL PHYSICAL AGENTS

A wide variety of bacterial species have adapted to the great diversity of physical conditions that exist in the various ecologic niches on earth. Bacteria are found in the ocean waters at all latitudes from 20 degrees south to 90 degrees north and at the bottom of the seas at hydrostatic pressures as great as 13,000 pounds per square inch. Some live in natural hot springs at temperatures near boiling; others grow at temperatures near freezing. Perhaps the one large area that most closely approaches sterility is the surface of a sandy desert. Although the dry heat found there is destructive to most bacteria, the greatest sterilizing effect is exerted by the short wave rays from the sun in the near ultraviolet spectrum.

Most of the pathogenic bacteria have limited tolerance to extreme variations in their physical environment and have little survival ability outside the living body. Others, however, produce spores that are highly resistant to deleterious physical conditions in the environment and endow the organism with an increased survival value. In the following discussion attention will be focused primarily on those physical agents that are useful as sterilizing agents.

Heat

Heat is the most reliable and universally applicable method of sterilization and, whenever possible, should be the method of choice. As with other types of disinfection the sterilization of a bacterial population by heat is a gradual process, and the kinetics of death are exponential. The first order inactivation by heat means that a constant fraction of the organisms undergoes an inactivating chemical change in each unit of time and that one such change is sufficient to inactivate an organism.

The time required for sterilization is inversely related to the temperature of exposure. This relationship may be expressed by the term "thermal death time," which refers to the minimum time required to kill a suspension of organisms at a predetermined temperature in a specified environment. Because of the high temperature coefficients involved in heat sterilization, a minimal change in temperature significantly alters the thermal death time. In accordance with the law of mass action, the sterilization time is directly related to the number of organisms in the suspension.

Mechanism of Thermal Injury The mechanism by which organisms are destroyed by dry heat is different from that of moist heat. The lethal effects of dry heat, or desiccation in general, are usually ascribed to protein denaturation, oxidative damage, and toxic effects of elevated levels of electrolytes. In the absence of water, the number of polar groups on the peptide chain decreases, and more energy is required to open the molecules, hence the apparent increased stability of the organism.

The lethal effect of moist heat above a particular temperature of exposure is usually attributed to the denaturation and coagulation of protein. The pattern of thermal damage is quite complex, however, and coagulation undoubtedly masks other, more subtle changes induced in the bacterial cell before coagulation becomes apparent. One of the primary sites of thermal injury in a cell is the cell membrane, which not only controls the passage of solutes into and out of the cell but also is the site of respiratory activity and the initiation of protein synthesis. Damage to the membrane results in the leakage of K^+ ions, amino acids, and 260-nm absorbing material and occurs at temperatures below that which causes coagulation. The 260-nm absorbing material consists of degraded ribosomes that result from the heat treatment. Autodegradation of nucleic acids within bacterial cells occurs frequently and is triggered by a number of physical and chemical agents that exert their effect by activation of ribonucleases. In the normal bacterial cell the activity of ribonuclease is masked by their association with an inhibitor. This inhibitor is inactivated by heat, organic solvents, and ultraviolet irradiation, resulting in an unmasking of ribonuclease activity.

Moist Heat Objects may be sterilized either by dry heat applied in an oven or by moist heat provided as steam. Of the two methods, moist heat is preferred and kills bacteria more rapidly than does dry heat. The exposure of practically all mesophilic nonspore-forming bacteria to moist heat at 60C for 30 minutes is sufficient for sterilization. Among the exceptions are S. aureus and Streptococcus faecalis, which require for sterilization an exposure time of 60 minutes at 60C. A temperature of 80C for 5 to 10 minutes destroys the vegetative form of all bacteria, yeast, and fungi. Among the most heat-resistant cells are the spores of Clostridium botulinum, an anaerobe of medical importance as a cause of food poisoning. Spores of this organism are destroyed in 4 minutes at 120C or 330 minutes at 100C.

The application of moist heat in the destruction of bacteria may take several forms: boiling, live steam, and steam under pressure. Of these, steam under pressure is the most efficient because it makes possible temperatures above the boiling point of water. Such temperatures are necessary because of the extremely high thermal resistance of bacterial spores.

An autoclave is a chamber in which steam sterilization is carried out. The basic essential in this type of sterilization is that the whole of the material to be sterilized be in contact with saturated steam at the required temperature for the necessary period of time. It is important that saturated steam be used, otherwise the process becomes virtually a dry-heat treatment for which different time-temperature relationships hold. As in all heat sterilization processes, there is a well-established temperature-time relationship that must be observed if reliable sterilization is to be achieved. For sterilizing small objects an exposure of 20 minutes at 121C (15 pounds steam pressure per square inch) is used and provides a substantial margin of safety. Attention must be given, however, to the need for sufficient time to allow for the load to reach the required temperature before the actual sterilizing period begins. Also, overloading or incorrect packing of the sterilizer must be avoided in order to permit free access of steam to all of the material to be sterilized.

For the sterilization of certain liquids or semisolid materials that are easily destroyed by heat, a fractional method of sterilization is employed. This process, often called tyndallization, consists of heating the material to 80 or 100C for 30 minutes on three consecutive days. The rationale for this fractional type of sterilization is that vegetative cells and some spores are killed during the first heating and that the more resistant spores subsequently germinate and are killed during either the second or third heating. The method is useful in sterilizing heat-sensitive culture media containing materials such as carbohydrates, egg, or serum.

PASTEURIZATION. As mentioned above, most vegetative bacteria can be killed by relatively short exposures to temperatures of 60 to 65C. The most important application of temperatures in this range is in the pasteurization of milk and in the preparation of bacterial vaccines. Although pasteurization was originally devised by Pasteur as a means of destroying microorganisms that cause spoilage of wine and beer, the process is now used primarily to make beverages and foods safe for consumption by killing any disease-producing microorganisms that they might contain. The most widespread application of this treatment is the pasteurization of milk, which consists of heating to a temperature of 62C for 30 minutes, followed by rapid cooling. This treatment does not sterilize the milk, but it does kill disease-producing bacteria commonly transmitted through milk.

Dry Heat Sterilization by dry heat requires higher temperatures and a longer period of heating than does sterilization with steam.

Its use is limited primarily to the sterilization of glassware and such materials as oils, jellies, and powders that are impervious to steam. The lethal action results from the heat conveyed from the material with which the organisms are in contact and not from the hot air that surrounds them, emphasizing the importance of uniform heating of the whole of the material to be sterilized. The most widely used type of dry heat is the hot air oven, in which sterilizing times of 2 hours at 180C are adequate even for spore-forming organisms.

Other useful forms of dry heat include incineration for objects to be destroyed, and flaming by passage of transfer needles, coverslips, or small instruments through the flame of a Bunsen burner.

Freezing

Although many bacteria are killed by exposure to cold, freezing is not a reliable method of sterilization. Its primary use has been in the preservation of bacterial cultures. Repeated freezing and thawing are much more destructive to bacteria than is prolonged storage at freezing temperatures. Although it was previously believed that the lethal effect of freezing was due to membrane damage by ice crystals, such a mechanism plays only a minor role in the death of frozen organisms. In freezing of bacteria the formation of ice crystals outside the cell causes the withdrawal of water from the cell interior, resulting in an increased intracellular electrolyte concentration and a denaturation of proteins. The cell membrane is damaged, and a leakage of intracellular organic compounds ensues. The leakage material contains inorganic phosphorus, ribose, peptides, and nucleotides that arise as a result of the activation of latent ribonucleases and peptidases.

If bacteria are frozen rapidly to temperatures below −35C, ice crystals that form within the cell produce a lethal effect during defreezing. If cultures are dried in vacuo from the frozen state by a process known as lyophilization or freeze drying the initial mortality is greatly diminished. This method is widely used for the preservation of bacterial cultures.

Radiation

Sunlight possesses appreciable bactericidal activity and plays an important role in the spontaneous sterilization that occurs under natural conditions. Its disinfectant action is due primarily to its content of ultraviolet rays, most of which, however, are screened out by glass and by the presence of ozone in the outer regions of the atmosphere. Other electromagnetic rays of shorter wavelength, such as x-rays and gamma rays and rays produced by radioactive decay and by ion accelerators, also exert a pronounced effect when absorbed by bacteria (Fig. 11-3).

EFFECTS OF RADIATION. Only absorbed light promotes photochemical reactions. As a molecule absorbs light it receives energy in the form of discrete units termed "quanta." The energy of a quantum is inversely related to its wavelength. In the primary reaction only 1 quantum of light is absorbed by each molecule of absorbing substance. The number of quanta absorbed by a biologic system is proportional to the product of the duration and intensity of the radiation as well as to the absorption coefficient of the irradiated material. The absorption of a quantum by an electron in an atom results in activation of the molecule, which then either uses the extra energy for chemical changes such as decomposition and internal rearrange-

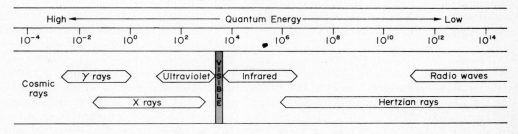

FIG. 11-3. The electromagnetic spectrum. The wavelength in nm is plotted on an exponential scale.

ments or loses it entirely as heat or fluorescence.

Radiation may have sufficient energy to remove an electron completely from an atom and produce an electrical charge (ionization) or only enough energy to raise electrons to states of higher energy (excitation). Energy equivalent to 10 electron volts is required to pull an electron completely out of an atom. This is provided by x-rays and gamma rays that ionize atoms by the ejection of electrons from any atoms through which the radiation passes.

In the visible and ultraviolet range, although the quantum energy absorbed by the molecule cannot remove an electron completely, the excitation produced often leads to photochemical changes. In the infrared range of the spectrum the energy is inadequate to initiate a chemical change in biologic material, and the absorbed energy is dissipated as heat.

Ultraviolet Radiation   EFFECTS OF ULTRAVIO-LET RADIATION.   The effectiveness of ultraviolet light as a lethal and mutagenic agent is closely correlated with its wavelength. The most effective bactericidal wavelength is in the 240 to 280 nm range with the optimum at about 260 nm, which corresponds with the absorption maximum of DNA. The major mechanism of the lethal effect of ultraviolet light on bacteria is attributed to this absorption by, and resultant damage to, the DNA. Ultraviolet radiation leads to the formation of covalent bonds between pyrimidine residues adjacent to each other in the same strand, resulting in the formation of cyclobutane-type pyrimidine dimers. These dimers distort the shape of the DNA and interfere with normal base pairing. This results in an inhibition of DNA synthesis and secondary effects, such as inhibition of growth and respiration. Although other effects have been shown to be produced by ultraviolet radiation, such as photohydration of cytosine and cross-linkage of complementary strands of DNA, the extremely high dose required rules them out as a possible mechanism for ultraviolet damage to cells.

REPAIR MECHANISMS.   If, following treatment with ultraviolet light, cells are immediately irradiated with visible light in the 300 to 400 nm range, both the mutation frequency and the bactericidal effect of ultraviolet light are greatly reduced. This phenomenon, known as photoreactivation, results from the activation

by light of an enzyme that hydrolyzes the pyrimidine dimers. Another mechanism also exists in some cells for the repair of light-damaged DNA. This is a dark-repair mechanism that invokes the activity of an elaborate set of enzymes for the excision of the ultraviolet-induced dimers and repair of the damaged strand. Excision-repair is probably the primary cause of an enhanced resistance to ultraviolet light by some strains of bacteria.

PRACTICAL APPLICATIONS.   Ultraviolet radiation can be produced artificially by mercury vapor lamps. The unit of radiation energy is measured in terms of microwatt/unit area/unit of time. A 15-watt ultraviolet light delivers 38 μw/cm^2/second of radiation at a distance of 1 meter. Ultraviolet radiation is equally effective against gram-positive and gram-negative organisms. The lethal dose for most of the common, non-spore-forming bacteria varies from 1,800 μw/cm^2 to 6,500 μw/cm^2. Bacterial spores require up to 10 times this dose.

Although the bactericidal properties of ultraviolet radiation are indisputable, it cannot be properly classified as a sterilizing agent because of the many uncertainties surrounding its use. Unlike ionizing radiation, the energy of ultraviolet radiation is low, and its power of penetration is very poor. It does not penetrate into solids and penetrates into liquids very slightly. For this reason ultraviolet rays have no effect on organisms shielded or protected from the incident beams.

The primary application of ultraviolet radiation is in the control of airborne infection. It is used for the disinfection of enclosed areas such as entryways, hospital wards, and operating rooms. Whereas the application of ultraviolet radiation has failed to produce uniform results in the control of airborne infections in public places, it has provided a significant reduction in the incidence of secondary infections following surgery.

Ionizing Radiations   PROPERTIES OF IONIZ-ING RADIATIONS.   Ionizing radiations are classified according to their physical properties and fall into two major categories: (1) those that have mass and may be either charged or uncharged and (2) those that are energy only. Some of the ionizing radiations are products of radioactive decay (α-, β-, γ-rays) and others are produced in an x-ray machine, by particle bombardment, or by nuclear reactors. Primary cosmic rays from outer space that bombard the earth and its atmosphere are composed of protons, alpha particles, and heavy atomic nuclei. Few of these rays, however, reach the earth at altitudes of sea level because of the protective blanket provided by the atmosphere. The ionizing radiations that are of greatest practical value for purposes of sterilization are the electromagnetic x-rays and gamma rays and the particulate cathode rays (artificially accelerated electrons). These radiations have a much higher energy content than does ultraviolet radiation and consequently have a much greater capacity to produce lethal effects.

In the passage of ionizing radiations through matter, the energy of the protons is transferred by collisions with an orbital electron in an atom of the absorbing medium. Following such a collision an electron is ejected from the atom with high energy and at great speed. As this electron moves through the medium it will ionize and excite atoms with which it interacts. The energy given to it will be dissipated as it moves through the medium.

The effects of ionizing radiations upon living systems depend upon the amount of energy absorbed. The amount of radiation to which a system is exposed is the exposure dose. For x-rays or gamma rays the exposure dose is measured in roentgens and is equivalent to an energy absorption of about 83 erg/g of air. That portion of the exposure dose which is actually absorbed by the biologic system, the absorbed dose, is the biologically effective dose, the unit of which is the rad. The rad is based on an energy absorption of 100 erg/g of air. For practical purposes the Mrad, equal to 10^6 rad, is used because this is the dosage range required for sterilization. (See p. 240)

Ionizing radiation has both direct and indirect effects on the macromolecules of the cell. The direct effect is exerted by the initial transfer of energy within a limited vital or sensitive area, according to the target theory. However, since biologic systems are composed of large amounts of water, the primary mechanism for the lethal effect of ionizing radiation is an indirect one. As ionizing radiations pass through water, they cause the water molecules to ionize.

$$H_2O \xrightarrow[\text{quantum}]{\text{energy}} H_2O^+ + e^-$$

The resulting positive ion reacts with unionized water to yield another species of charged water molecule and the free hydroxyl radical.

$$H_2O^+ + H_2O \rightarrow H_3O^+ + OH \text{ (free radical)}$$

The ejected electron can also react with unionized water to give an OH^- ion and a free hydrogen radical. The hydroxyl radical is a strong oxidizing agent, and the hydrogen radical is a powerful reducing agent. The hydroxyl radical is highly reactive with macromolecules, especially DNA, and ruptures it by effecting a break in both of the constituent chains.

The presence of oxygen in cells at the time of radiation enhances the magnitude of the radiation effect. The increased effect results from the interaction of oxygen with radiation-produced free radicals, drawing these radicals into destructive autoxidative chain reactions. The presence of oxygen during radiation also promotes the formation of hydrogen peroxide and organic peroxides. Certain chemical compounds, such as those that contain sulfhydryl groups, protect biologic systems from the damaging effects of ionizing radiation by diverting the absorbed energy.

The penetrating power of ionizing radiations contributes to their effectiveness as sterilizing agents. Although cathode rays, because of their particulate nature, have a greater intrinsic energy and consequently the greater power of penetration, x-rays and gamma rays have a relatively greater penetrating ability. Because of the nature of the mechanisms involved, optimum activity never occurs at the surface of the material being treated. With gamma rays, it occurs just below or inside the surface, and with cathode-rays, it occurs a few centimeters deeper.

LETHAL EFFECTS. Most of the pathogenic non-spore-forming bacteria are relatively sensitive to the effects of ionizing radiation. Spores are among the most radiation-resistant microorganisms known. Even among the nonspore-formers, however, considerable variation exists. Gram-positive non-spore-formers are generally more resistant than are the gram-negative organisms, and within the latter group the pseudomonads are among those most readily killed.

The rate or intensity of radiation is of little importance in determining the fraction of organisms killed. It is the total dose administered that is important. The death of microorganisms exposed to ionizing radiation is usually exponential throughout the sterilization period, although in some cases it tends to be sigmoidal. The slope of the time-survivor curve is determined by the intensity of the radiation, but in terms of dose against percentage killed, the relationship is always exponential. Toward the end of the process, however, the tailing effect may become prominent, emphasizing the importance of ensuring that the full dose has been given.

Although the sterilizing dose is dependent upon the initial level of contamination, a dose of 2.5 Mrad of ionizing radiation has been accepted as the sterilizing dose. This dose is sufficient to kill the most resistant microorganisms and also provides an adequate margin of safety under conditions of practical use.

The main areas in which ionizing radiations have been applied for purposes of sterilization are in pharmacy and medicine. They are especially suitable for sterilizing such articles as catgut and silk or nylon sutures and disposable items, such as plastic syringes, needles, surgical blades, catheters, prostheses, surgical gloves, plastic tubing, plastic dishes, and blood transfusion sets.

Ultrasonic and Sonic Vibrations

Sound vibrations at high frequency, in the upper audible and ultrasonic range (20 to 1,000 kc) provide a very useful technique for disrupting cells, especially for the extraction of enzymes. The sound wave generators that are widely employed for disruption of cells operate in the frequency range of 9 to 100 kc per second. No specific frequency has been found to be uniquely effective, but generally ultrasonic waves are more effective as the frequency is increased.

The passage of sound through a liquid produces alternating pressure changes which, if the sound intensity is sufficiently great, cause cavities to form in the liquid. The cavities, which are about 10μ in diameter, grow in size until they collapse violently, with the production of high local velocities and pressures of the order of 1,000 atmospheres. During this violent collapse stage, the cell disintegrates. In addition to disintegrating cells, cavitation produces a number of chemical and physical changes in the suspending medium, which may be deleterious to certain enzymes. Among the most important of these is the formation of hydrogen peroxide when cavitation takes place in a liquid containing dissolved oxygen. Ultrasonic vibrations have also been shown to cause a depolymerization of macromolecules and intramolecular regroupings. Double-strand breaks are produced in transforming DNA by sonic radiation, and integration into the host genome is inhibited.

Microorganisms vary markedly in their sensitivity to sonic and ultrasonic vibrations. The most susceptible are the gram-negative rods, and among the most resistant are the staphylococci which require long periods of exposure. Although sonic vibrations are lethal to many members of the exposed bacterial population, there are many survivors. Consequently, treatment with sonic vibrations is of no practical value in sterilization and disinfection.

Filtration

The principal method used in the laboratory for the sterilization of heat-labile materials is filtration. Although mechanical sieving plays a role in all filtration processes, electrostatic and adsorption phenomena and the physical construction of the filter also exert a pronounced effect.

A number of different types of filters are employed for purposes of sterilization. These include (1) Seitz filters, consisting of discs of an asbestos-cellulose mixture that is discarded after a single filtration, (2) sintered glass filters, prepared by fusing together fine glass fragments, (3) candle filters, which are thick-walled tubes made of diatomaceous earth (Berkefeld filter) or unglazed ceramic (Selas and Chamberland filters), and (4) membrane filters consisting of porous discs of cellulose esters. Candle and membrane filters are available in a wide range of pore sizes. They absorb very little of the fluid being filtered and thus are very useful for the sterilization of certain materials that cannot tolerate, without deterioration, the high temperatures used in heat sterilization.

Membrane Filters Membrane filters, composed of biologic inert cellulose esters, are available in pore sizes ranging from 14 μm down to 0.025 μm. The 0.22-μm filter is the most widely used for sterilization filtration purposes because the pore size is smaller than any known bacteria. It should always be used with solutions containing serum, plasma, or trypsin where species of *Pseudomonas* or other bacteria of a small size are known to occur.

Membrane filters are also useful in microbiology for purposes other than sterilization. Because of their inertness, they provide an optimum method for the collection of microorganisms, since any bacteriostatic agent present in the suspending medium may be easily flushed from the filter. This technique has been invaluable in the sterility testing of disinfectants and antibiotics where it is necessary to overcome the inhibitory effects of the drug. In clinical microbiology it has been useful for the culture of organisms present at a low concentration in in a large volume of fluid.

Membrane filters act essentially as two-dimensional screens, retaining all particles that exceed the pore size. In liquid filtration a large number of particles somewhat smaller than the pore size are retained by van der Waals forces, by random entrapment in the pores, and by buildup on previously retained particles. However, the important characteristic of the membrane filter is that all particles larger than the pore size are positively retained on the filter surface.

FURTHER READING

Books and Reviews

Allwood MC, Russell AD: Mechanisms of thermal injury in nonsporulating bacteria. Adv Appl Microbiol 12:89, 1970

Bellamy WD: Preservation of foods and drugs by ionizing radiations. Adv Appl Microbiol 1:49, 1959

Bennett EO: Factors affecting the antimicrobial activity of phenols. Adv Appl Microbiol 1:123, 1959

Chambers CW, Clarke NA: Control of bacteria in nondomestic water supplies. Adv Appl Microbiol 8:105, 1966

Chatigny MA: Protection against infection in the microbiological laboratory: devices and procedures. Adv Appl Microbiol 3:131, 1961

Él'piner IE: Action of ultrasonic waves on microorganisms, viruses, and bacteriophages. In Ultrasound. Its Physical, Chemical, and Biological Effects. New York, Consultants Bureau, 1964, chap 9

Farrell J, Rose AH: Low-temperature microbiology. Adv Appl Microbiol 7:335, 1965

Harold FM: Antimicrobial agents and membrane function. Adv Microbial Physiol 4:45, 1970

Heckly RJ: Preservation of bacteria by lyophilization. Adv Appl Microbiol 3:1, 1961

Hugo WB (ed): Inhibition and Destruction of the Microbial Cell. New York, Academic Press, 1971

McDade JJ, Phillips GB, Sivinski HD, Whitfield WJ: Principles and applications of laminar-flow devices. In Norris JR, Ribbons DW (eds): Methods in Microbiology. New York, Academic Press, 1969, vol 1, 137-168

Mulvany JG: Membrane filter techniques and microbiology. In Norris JR, Ribbons, DW (eds): Methods in Microbiology. New York, Academic Press, 1969, Vol 1 205-253

Pizzarello DJ, Witcofski RL: Basic Radiation Biology. Philadelphia, Lea & Febiger, 1967

Reddish GF (ed): Antiseptics, Disinfectants, Fungicides, and Chemical and Physical Sterilization, 2nd ed. Philadelphia, Lea & Febiger, 1957

Russell AD, Jenkins J, Harrison IH: The inclusion of antimicrobial agents in pharmaceutical products. Adv Appl Microbiol 9:1, 1967

Sykes G: Methods and equipment for sterilization of laboratory apparatus and media. In Norris JR, Ribbons DW (eds): Methods in Microbiology. New York, Academic Press, 1969, vol 1, pp 77-121

Selected Papers

Beppu T, Arima K: Induction by mercuric ion of extensive degradation of cellular ribonucleic acid in *Escherichia coli.* J Bacteriol 98:888, 1969

Billen D, Bruns L: Relationship between radiation response and the deoxyribonucleic acid replication cycle in bacteria: dependence on the excision-repair system. J Bacteriol 103:400, 1970

Chick, H. An investigation of the laws of disinfection. J Hyg (Camb) 8:92, 1908

Chick H: The process of disinfection by chemical agencies and hot water. J Hyg (Camb) 10:237, 1910

Fried VA, Novick A: Organic solvents as probes for the structure and function of the bacterial membrane: Effects of ethanol on the wild type and an ethanol-resistant mutant of *Escherichia coli* K12. J Bacteriol 114:239, 1973

Gezon HM, Thompson DJ, Rogers KD, et al: Control of staphylococcal infections and disease in the newborn through the use of hexachlorophene bathing. Pediatrics 51:331, 1973

Gustafsson P, Nordström K, Normark S: Outer penetration barrier of *Escherichia coli* K12: Kinetics of the uptake of gentian violet by wild type and envelope mutants. J Bacteriol 116:893, 1973

Hamkalo BA, Swenson PA: Effects of ultraviolet radiation on respiration and growth in radiation-resistant and radiation-sensitive strains of *Escherichia coli* B. J Bacteriol 99:815, 1969

Randolph ML, Setlow JK: Mechanism of inactivation of *Haemophilus influenzae* transforming deoxyribonucleic acid by sonic radiation. J Bacteriol 111:186, 1972

Schnaitman CA: Solubilization of the cytoplasmic membrane of *Escherichia coli* by Triton X-100. J Bacteriol 108:545, 1971

Shew CW, Freese E: Lipopolysaccharide layer protection of gram-negative bacteria against inhibition by long-chain fatty acids. J Bacteriol 115:869, 1973

Silvernale JN, Joswick HL, Corner TR, Gerhardt P: Antimicrobial actions of hexachlorophene: Cytological manifestations. J Bacteriol 108:482, 1971

Sinsky TJ, Silverman GJ: Characterization of injury incurred by *Escherichia coli* upon freeze-drying. J Bacteriol 101:429, 1970

Waldstein EA, Sharon R, Ben-Ishai R: Role of ATP in excision repair of ultraviolet radiation damage in *Escherichia coli.* Proc Natl Acad Sci USA 71:2651, 1974

SECTION 2
IMMUNOLOGY

12
Introduction to Immunology

Some principles which have led to the dramatic success of immunology in preventive medicine were discovered empirically in ancient times. Thucydides, the Greek physician, recorded that during the plague of Athens only those who had recovered from the disease could nurse the sick because they did not suffer a recurrence. In the fifteenth century, Chinese and Arabs applied this knowledge to clinical prophylaxis by infecting persons with material gathered from the pustules of smallpox patients, giving them a mild form of the disease and thereby protecting them against further development of this dread disease. In 1717 a letter from Lady Mary Montague to Sarah Chiswell contained the following description:

The smallpox so fatal and so general amongst us is here entirely harmless. . . . People send to another to know if any of their family has a mind to have the smallpox; they make parties for this purpose and when they are met, the old woman comes with a nutshell full of the matter of the best sort of smallpox and asks what veins you please to have opened. She immediately zips open that you offer to her with a large needle . . . and puts into the vein as much venom as can lie upon the head of a needle and after binds up the wound with a hollow bit of shell . . . .

Nearly 80 years later, in 1796, Edward Jenner conducted his now famous experiment in which he inoculated an 8-year-old boy with cowpox, thus providing protection against the more virulent smallpox.

With the development of the germ theory of disease in the late nineteenth century, the immune state following the injection of bacterial products could be analyzed, and the discipline of immunology soon developed as an adjunct to microbiology. Maturation of the discipline has proceeded since then, and immunology is now recognized as one of the most rapidly developing and pervasive of all the biologic and medical sciences. Modern immunology has made many contributions to the understanding of biologic phenomena and is increasingly involved in the prevention and treatment of disease states. In addition to microbial immunity, such highly specialized subdivisions as immunochemistry, autoimmunity, immunobiology of transplantation, and cancer immunology have arisen. These special topics are discussed in separate chapters of this book.

The underlying basis of any immunologic response is the distinction between self and nonself. An organism with a functional immune system is generally able to recognize foreign substances. Those foreign substances which can trigger a response are designated antigens (Chap. 13). This response is characterized by specificity and memory. Specificity is the ability of the immune system to vary its response to match the stimulus. Memory is the ability to react to a second exposure to the same stimulus more rapidly and more intensely. The secondary response is often sustained longer than that stimulated by the first exposure.

The immune response can be conveniently regarded as having three major types of effector: soluble substances (antibodies) that are released into the bloodstream, certain classes of cells that require or act more effectively in conjunction with the antibodies, and certain classes of cell that are effective in the absence of antibody. Collaboration between the different classes of cells involved is required for the induction of immunity as well as for its regulation and the maintenance of the steady state. Those activities for which antibody is uniquely responsible are called "humoral responses," hence the term "humoral immunity." Those activities for which cellular participation is required are called a cellular responses," and the corresponding state is called "cellular immunity."

Antibodies are globular proteins which bind antigen; an alternative term for antibody is immunoglobulin. The exquisite specificity inherent in all immune responses appears to rest solely in the amino acid sequence of the antibody molecule (Chap. 13). The classes of immunoglobulin include immunoglobulin G (IgG), immunoglobulin M (IgM), and immunoglobulin A (IgA), all of which have well-documented protective functions but differ in the site of activity in the body. The remaining two classes are immunoglobulin E (IgE), which is associated with allergy and parasitic infections, and immunoglobulin D (IgD), about which little is known. These various classes of antibody are secreted by some of the types of lymphoid cells to be described later.

Two major classes of cells dominate cellular immunity, phagocytes and lymphocytes. A role for phagocytosis in protection from disease was suggested in the late nineteenth century by Elie Metchnikoff, but his theory, despite its popularization by Bernard Shaw in "The Doctor's Dilemma," attracted a great amount of criticism, and its acceptance came only gradually. A dispute as to which component of immunity, cellular or humoral, was most important originated with Metchnikoff and still erupts periodically.

We now recognize three major classes of phagocytic cells. Most numerous are the polymorphonuclear leukocytes (PMN), which accumulate in pus and other sites of inflammation. PMN are able to ingest bacteria but do not appear to ingest larger particles. Phagocytosis, which is greatly facilitated by antibody (opsonization), is one of the most potent defenses against many microorganisms. Also found circulating in the blood and wandering in the tissues are the large mononuclear cells. In their resting state, as they travel in the bloodstream, they are designated monocytes. In tissue, although still fully motile, they tend to become larger and are known as macrophages or histiocytes. Macrophages can ingest bacteria, red blood cells, and even tumor cells, and they are scavengers of dead cells and cell debris. Specialized phagocytic cells are found in large numbers in the spleen and other lymphoid organs and in the liver. These cells normally remain in the tissues and are usually referred to as "fixed phagocytic cells."

Lymphocytes are small cells with a relatively large, rounded nucleus and a scanty cytoplasm. When motile in the blood and tissue fluids, they have an elongated cytoplasmic process called a "uropod" or "dag." Some lymphocytes have rough endoplasmic reticulum in their cytoplasm, while others do not. In their resting state, there are few mitochondria, and the golgi apparatus is poorly developed. In their active state, which occurs following immunization, mitochondria and golgi are more pronounced. One form of lymphocyte, generally called a "B cell," is indispensable to the humoral immune response. B cells have antibody on the plasma membrane, and some of them secrete antibody. B cells can divide to form new B cells or can undergo terminal differentiation to form a plasma cell. The plasma cell is morphologically distinctive, since it has an eccentrically placed nucleus and an abundance of rough endoplasmic reticulum. The plasma cell is a highly specialized cell whose function is to secrete antibody. In addition to B cells, another broad class of lymphocytes is crucial to the development of an immune response. These cells have developed under the influence of the thymus gland and are called "T cells." T cells may participate in both humoral and cellular immunity. They are required for a humoral response to many antigens and can also differentiate into those effector cells implicated in transplant rejection, in the defense against fungi and certain viruses, and in a wide variety of disease states, including the autoaggressive or autoimmune diseases and in cancer.

While the science of immunology began as an adjunct to microbiology and the study of infectious diseases, it has expanded to include biologic and medical aspects originally undreamed of. The goals of the modern immunologist are to elucidate the mechanism of molecular and cellular events which occur upon the encounter of an immunocompetent organism with an antigenic substance and then to learn how to manipulate and control them.

13
Immunochemistry

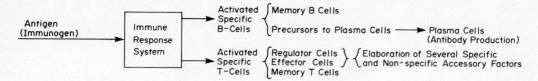

Fig. 13-1. Schematic representation of the immune response system and the products of specific stimulation.

Infectious agents (eg, bacteria, rickettsia, fungi, viruses), certain environmental agents, and neoplastic changes in the host's cells (due to either spontaneous mutation or transformation by chemical carcinogens or tumorigenic viruses) may induce an immune response in the host. The term "antigen" has been used to define both the functional and reactive attributes of such an agent. More recently, a subtle distinction has been made between immunogens, which initiate an immune response, and antigens, which are reactive with and processed by the products of an immune response.

If the immune surveillance network is pictured as a black box, as diagrammed in Figure 13-1 (leaving the mechanism for recognition and activation for later discussion), the products of the immune response can be measured in several ways. Generally, the responses can be divided into two areas, which are not necessarily mutually exclusive. Activation of specific bone marrow-derived lymphocytes (B cells) leads to the production of memory B cells and antibody-forming cells, which are the major elements of the humoral response system. Activation of specific thymus-dependent lymphocytes (T cells) leads to the production of memory T cells, regulator cells (which are helper or suppressor in function), and effector cells, which are the components of the cell-mediated response system.

The production of circulating antibodies is an exclusive function of antibody-forming cells and is, therefore, a B cell function. T cells do not produce substantial amounts of antibody, but for most immunogens their cooperation is usually required for the generation of antibody-forming cells from specific B cells. Effector cells, generated by activation of specific T cells, direct their response through direct cell-immunogen contact, hence, a cell-mediated immunity.

In addition to these direct effects, several accessory systems exist, which will be discussed later (Chap. 16). In this chapter the discussion will center on the types of molecules that initiate an immune response, the nature and function of specific antibodies, the reactions of antigens and antibodies, and the formation of specific antibodies.

IMMUNOGENS

Immunogens, such as bacteria and certain viruses, tend to be very complex, since they consist of proteins, glycoproteins, lipids, glycolipids, polysaccharides (carbohydrates), and nucleic acids. In general, native (or natural) proteins, glycoproteins, and large complex polysaccharides are often immunogenic, while isolated lipids and glycolipids are not. An immune response to nucleic acids is usually difficult to demonstrate, but antibodies to heat-denatured, single-stranded DNA and RNA can be elicited. The sera from patients suffering from the connective tissue disease lupus erythematosus often contain antibodies that react with single-stranded DNA and, in some cases, with double-stranded DNA.

Proteins are, in turn, complex immunogens, since the immune system is usually capable of recognizing several distinct sites (antigenic determinants) on the molecule. Studies of antibodies to these individual sites are difficult, and artificial antigenic determinants, or haptens are often introduced to simplify immunochemical studies. A low-molecular-weight component of known chemical structure (hapten), such as the 2,4-dinitrophenyl moiety, can be covalently coupled to a protein (carrier). The resulting hapten-protein conjugate is often immunogenic, inducing antibodies to the hapten which can be purified and characterized. Using this technique, antibodies specific for penicillin, steroids, hormones, certain lipids, and individual nucleic acid bases may be produced with the appropriate immunogenic hapten-carrier conjugate.

Some components of complex immunogens,

for example, glycolipids, that are nonimmunogenic alone may behave as haptens when they are administered as part of an immunogenic complex. Thus the Forssman hapten is a glycolipid that consists of N-acetyl-galactosamine, galactose, galactose, and glucose joined to a ceramide lipid moiety. In purified form the Forssman hapten is nonimmunogenic. In its natural form it is a potent immunogen, since it is a membrane component of wide and diverse tissue and species distribution. Thus immunization of a Forssman-negative species with Forssman-positive tissue or cells results in the production of hapten-specific antibody.

It must be emphasized that artificial or naturally occurring haptens are nonimmunogenic by themselves and that it is the carrier moiety which determines the immunogenicity.

REQUIREMENTS FOR IMMUNOGENICITY

Foreignness The immune system possesses the ability to distinguish between self and nonself. For example, rabbits do not respond to their own serum albumins, but they do respond to the biologically related but phylogenetically distinct human serum albumins. It is probably during ontogeny that the immune system learns to distinguish self from nonself. In rare instances, components of sites in the body that are poorly drained by the lymphatic system or anatomically sequestered from the immune system are treated as foreign if injury results in access to this site later in life (for example, the lens protein of the eye and certain thyroid proteins). Likewise, many subclinical neoplastic changes may be detected as nonself and dealt with before any serious problem develops.

Size and Shape Molecular shape does not seem to influence immunogenicity. Proteins and polypeptides with globular, rodlike, and random coil configurations are all immunogenic. On the other hand, molecular size does affect immunogenicity: The smaller the molecule, the less immunogenic it is likely to be. For example, bovine and porcine insulin (MW about 6,000) are poor immunogens, but if insulin is polymerized by chemical methods or is heat-aggregated, it may become immunogenic.

Similarly, the H antigen (the flagellar protein) of *Salmonella adelaide* can be prepared in various stages of polymerization: as intact organelles (flagella), as 38,500 dalton monomers (flagellin or MON), or as polymerized flagellin (POL) (prepared from isolated monomers). In terms of immunogenicity, the following relationship holds:

$$Flagella > POL > MON$$

The minimum size for immunogenicity was thought to be about 1,000 daltons. Angiotensin II (1,031 daltons), a native polypeptide hormone, and α-dinitrophenol-hepta-L-lysine (1,200 daltons), a hapten-synthetic polypeptide conjugate, are immunogenic in guinea pigs under certain conditions. Recently, however, a synthetic compound of 450 daltons has been shown to be immunogenic in guinea pigs (Fig. 13-2). Smaller compounds which are apparently immunogenic, such as the catechols from poison ivy (120 to 320 daltons) and picryl chloride (trinitrophenyl chloride), are not truly immunogenic by themselves but become so by virtue of their chemical reactivity with self skin proteins, thereby creating hapten-protein conjugates.

Complexity and Composition Synthetic polypeptides are generally used to study the effect of complexity and composition on immunogenicity. Linear homopolymers, such as poly-L-lys or poly-L-glu, are usually not immu-

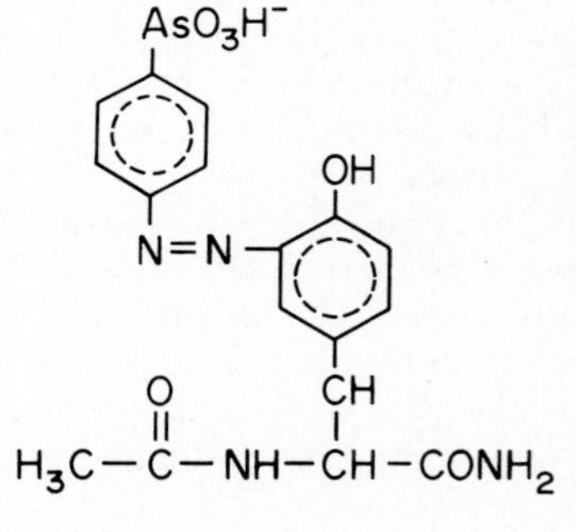

P−azobenzenearsonate −N− acetyltyrosineamide

(RAT)

FIG. 13-2. The structure for a synthetic compound of low molecular weight which has been shown to be immunogenic.

nogenic alone. If they are used as conjugated haptens with a suitable protein carrier, specific antibody responses can be detected. Linear random copolymers are immunogenic. For example, poly-L-(glu$_{60}$lys$_{40}$), where the subscripts denote the mole percent concentrations of initial reactants, is immunogenic in rabbits but not in man, while poly-L-(glu$_{50}$lys$_{30}$ala$_{20}$) is immunogenic in both. Increasing complexity, therefore, contributes to a molecule's immunogenicity. Similarly, branched copolymers, such as poly-L-(tyr,glu)-poly-DL-ala-poly-L-lys, or (T,G) A-L, are extremely potent immunogens (Fig. 13-3). The (T,G) A-L polymer has also been used to demonstrate that the immunodominant groups (T,G) must be readily accessible in order for recognition to take place.

Recognition by Two Lymphocyte Types

Certain immunogens require only stimulation of specific B cells in order for humoral antibodies to be formed (T cell-independent antigens). More often, however, an immunogen will require specific recognition by both B and T cells. While the specific T cells do not produce any detectable antibody, they do function as helper cells in the overall specific activation of B cells (the precursor to the antibody-forming cell, or plasma cell). The mechanism involved in T cell recognition and helper function is presently unknown.

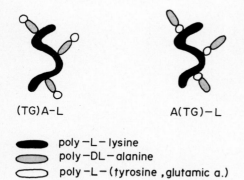

(TG)A–L   A(TG)–L

━━━ poly—L—lysine
▭▭▭ poly—DL—alanine
▱▱▱ poly—L—(tyrosine ,glutamic a.)

FIG. 13-3. Representative structures for two branched copolymers. In both polymers a poly-L-lysine (L) backbone has been used. In one, (T,G)A-L, a poly-DL-alanine (A) branch has been added to available ε-amino groups in the poly-L-lysine backbone, followed by a short copolymer of tyrosine and glutamic acid (T,G). In the other, A(TG)-L, the short copolymer (T,G) was added first, followed by a poly-DL-alanine homopolymer. Several model studies have shown that (T,G)A-L is immunogenic, whereas A(T,G)-L is not.

Other Parameters There are four additional important factors that contribute to a molecule's immunogenicity. First, there is species dependence: for example, dextran (a glucose polymer) is immunogenic in humans and mice but not in rabbits and guinea pigs. Second, within a species there may be differences in the response that are strain dependent and most easily demonstrated in inbred strains of mice or guinea pigs (Chap. 14). The hapten-polypeptide conjugate α-dinitrophenyl-poly-L-lys is immunogenic in strain 2 guinea pigs but not in strain 13. If outbred guinea pigs are tested for their response to this immunogen, one can classify them as responders or nonresponders (which have or do not have a specific immune response gene, *Ir*). Third, the dose administered, the route of injection, and the timing between injections may influence the type of response an animal makes. Indeed, one can induce an immune paralysis or a tolerant state, as opposed to an immune response, by varying these conditions (Chap. 14). Finally, the use of adjuvants can result in increased immunogenicity for a previously demonstrated weak immunogen. Adjuvants are typically water-in-oil emulsions, such as Freund's incomplete adjuvant (mineral oil, water, and lanolin or a synthetic detergent as an emulsifying agent), alum precipitates, or bentonite particles. Their exact mechanism of action is unclear, but adjuvants are thought to protect immunogens from rapid, nonspecific elimination and to give rise to prolonged responses by slow release of the trapped immunogen. Complete Freund's adjuvant contains, in addition, heat-killed mycobacteria; their inclusion results in a local inflammatory reaction and an augmentation of the immune responses.

ANTIGENS AND ANTIGENIC DETERMINANTS

Antigenic determinants are the discrete sites on a molecule to which antibodies or immune cells are specifically directed.

Size of Antigenic Determinants The size of an antigenic determinant can be determined by estimating the minimum size of a fragment of an immunogen which can combine with

TABLE 13–1 ESTIMATED SIZE OF ANTIGENIC DETERMINANTS

Immunogen	Test Component (Hapten) Showing Maximal Inhibition*	Size in Most Extended Form†
Dextran	Isomaltohexaose (6 units of α (1–6) linked D-glucose)	$34 \times 12 \times 7$ A
Polyalanyl bovine serum albumin (polyalanine = hapten; BSA = carrier)	Pentaalanine	$25 \times 11 \times 6.5$ A
Polylysyl rabbit serum albumin (polylysine = hapten; RSA = carrier)	Penta- (or hexa-) lysine	$27 \times 17 \times 6.5$ A

Data from Kabat: J Immunol 97:1, 1966
*Test haptens of increasing size were used. Maximal inhibition of the antibody reactions was observed with the compounds listed in the table. Haptens of greater size showed no further increase in inhibitory capacity.
†Estimated maximal size. The actual size may, in fact, be smaller.

a specific antibody. The assay commonly employed is inhibition by the fragment of precipitation of the intact immunogen by the antibody. For example, a dextran-antidextran precipitin reaction (Chap. 15) can be inhibited by glucose polymers, and polypeptide-antipolypeptide precipitation can be inhibited by oligopeptides. The results of several such studies are summarized in Table 13-1. The extended size of antigenic determinants appears to be about 30 by 15 by 7 A.

Conformation The antibodies elicited with the linear tripeptide copolymer poly-L-(tyr,ala,glu) do not interact with the tripeptide tyrosylalanylglutamic acid. Under physiologic conditions the tripeptide copolymer exists as an α-helix, and it is this conformation that is recognized by the immune system, and not the linear sequence of tyr, ala, glu. Similarly, antibodies to the linear tripeptide unit (presented as a hapten-carrier complex) do not react with the α-helical copolymer. This rather simple example illustrates that the immune system is capable of recognizing and responding to linear sequences and/or specific conformations of amino acids.

Accessibility Antigenic determinants must be accessible to antibodies. For example, antibodies to the branched copolymer (T,G) A-L (Fig. 13-3) do not react with A(T,G)-L because these antibodies are directed largely at the T,G branch, which is sterically blocked by the linear alanine polymer.

Specificity and Cross-reactivity A corollary of the immune system's ability to recognize self from nonself is that both the recognition phase and the response phase are specific for the challenging immunogen. The antibod-

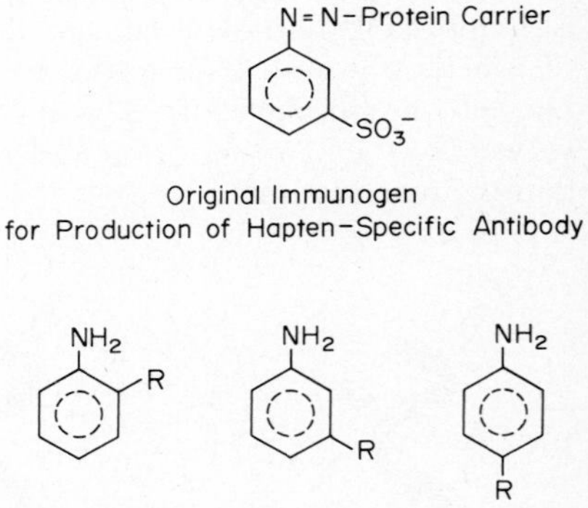

N=N—Protein Carrier

Original Immunogen for Production of Hapten—Specific Antibody

R-group	ortho	meta	para
$-SO_3^-$	$+\pm$	$++\pm$	$\pm$
$-AsO_3H^-$	O	$+$	O
$-COO^-$	O	$\pm$	O

Test Haptens and Reactivity

FIG. 13-4. Specificity of antibodies produced to the m-amino benzene sulfonate hapten. The hapten was coupled through an azo intermediate (via the available amino group) to a protein carrier. The resulting antibodies were tested with the homologous hapten and with several structural analogs coupled to different protein carriers. The extent of precipitation was scored 0, $\pm$, $+\pm$, $++$, in order of increasing reaction. (Data adapted from Landsteiner: The Specificity of Serological Reactions. 1962, p 169. Courtesy of Dover Publications)

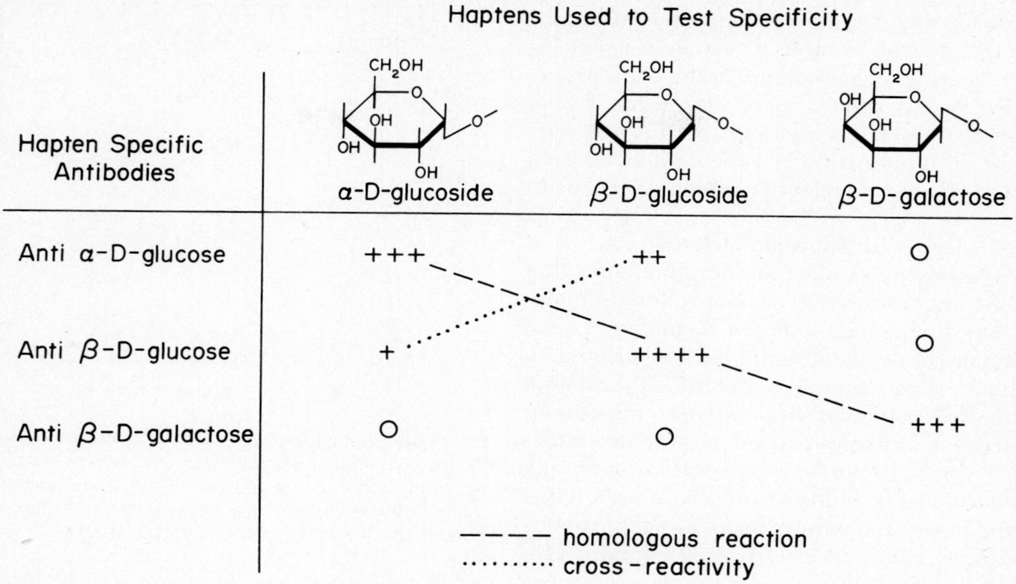

Haptens Used to Test Specificity

FIG. 13-5. The specificity of antibodies produced to individual carbohydrates as haptens. Animals were immunized with α-D-glucosyl-, β-D-glucosyl- or β-D-galactosyl-hapten-protein conjugates. The conjugates were made via an ortho-phenyl azide intermediate. The antibodies were then tested with the homologous hapten and the two analogs. The extent of reaction is scored as described in the legend to Figure 13-4. (Data adapted from Landsteiner: The Specificity of Serological Reactions. 1962, p 176. Courtesy of Dover Publications)

ies elicited to a single antigenic determinant are complementary to that particular determinant. The contributions of Landsteiner and his contemporaries, in which the specificity of antibodies produced to hapten-protein conjugates was demonstrated, are classic. Two often reproduced examples of these exquisite studies are shown in Figures 13-4 and 13-5. In Figure 13-4, where the antibody was produced to the *meta*-sulfonyl derivative, a change in position of the sulfonyl group from *meta* to *para* or *ortho* in the test hapten resulted in complete or partial loss of antibody recognition. Further, slight changes in the nature of the side group from sulfonyl to arsenyl or carboxyl also had a dramatic effect on antibody binding. These latter changes are extremely subtle. In Figure 13-5, carbohydrates were used as test haptens and coupled to a protein carrier through a phenyl azide intermediate. Again, very subtle changes in the conformation of the hydroxyl groups or in the nature of the type of linkage (α vs β) in the test hapten lead to a dramatic decrease in activity.

Cross-reactivity has two primary causes. The first is chemical similarity. This is illustrated by the example just given, in which antibody to α-

D-glucoside hapten cross-reacts with the β configuration. The second cause is the presence of the same antigenic determinant in two different antigens. For example, the membranes of the red blood cells of certain vertebrates and the membranes of certain bacteria cross-react because both contain the Forssman antigen. Cross-reactivity of this type is often quite unexpected.

Carrier Specificity The function of the protein carrier in conferring immunogenicity upon the coupled haptens has been studied intensively. The carrier moiety is not, of course, immunologically inert. The studies of Mitchison and others, in which such haptens as 2,4-dinitrophenol (DNP) were conjugated to a wide variety of proteins, such as bovine serum albumin (BSA), bovine gamma globulin (BGG), ovalbumin (OVA), and keyhole limpet hemocyanin (KLH), demonstrated that animals primed with DNP-BGG conjugates and challenged later with DNP-BGG respond vigorously with antibody directed at DNP as well as at components on the carrier molecule. If, instead, DNP-BGG primed animals are challenged with DNP-KLH, only a small DNP-specific antibody response is elicited. The existence of carrier specificity in an immune response to a hapten is a reflection of cooperation at the cellular level. The carrier specificity resides in the T lymphocyte, and the specificity of the antibody produced is a function of a B lymphocyte. Both are required for an effective immune response.

Isolation of Antigenic Determinants   It is often possible to isolate antigen fragments that retain antigenic activity by controlled proteolytic digestion. A 6,600-dalton fragment derived from human serum albumin has been shown to contain a single antigenic determinant capable of binding a specific subpopulation of antibodies from an antiserum raised to the intact molecule. Similarly, an eicosapeptide comprising residues 93-112 from the tobacco mosaic virus capsid protein contains a major antigenic determinant. Further, the polypeptide hormone glucagon, which is 29 amino acids in length, has been split into several fragments by trypsin digestion. Antibodies raised to intact glucagon with adjuvant in guinea pigs are directed primarily at the amino terminal end of the hormone, while cell-mediated immune recognition sites are confined largely to the carboxyl terminal end.

ANTIBODIES

Electrophoretic Characterization   Early observations demonstrated that sera from animals that had survived an infection were capable of neutralizing the infectious agent when mixed with it in vitro. Similarly, sera from animals previously immunized with the plant toxin from *Ricinus communis* were also capable of neutralizing the toxin in vitro. In addition, immune sera passively administered to nonimmune individuals were capable of neutralizing toxic or infectious agents in vivo. Tiselius and Kabat analyzed the sera from rabbits hyperimmunized with ovalbumin by free-zone electrophoresis (Fig. 13-6) both before and after absorption with the immunizing agent. After absorption there was a pronounced decrease in the molecular species characterized electrophoretically as γ-globulins. As a result of these studies, antibodies were equated with γ-globulins and later designated as immunoglobulins (Ig). The classification of antibodies based upon electrophoretic mobility is, in fact, inade-

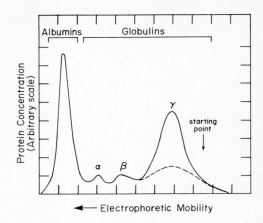

FIG. 13-6. Free-zone electrophoresis of rabbit serum following hyperimmunization with ovalbumin. Data were obtained before (——) and after (----) absorption of the serum with the immunizing antigen. (Data adapted from Tiselius and Kabat: J Exp Med 69:119, 1939.)

quate, since additional classes of immunoglobulins exhibit from α^1 to γ^2 electrophoretic mobilities (Table 13-2).

Immunoglobulin Classes   In man, five major classes of immunoglobulins have been described: IgG, the major serum component, IgM, or macro immunoglobulin, IgA, the immunoglobulin present predominantly in extracellular secretions, IgD, a minor serum component and perhaps an important cell membrane receptor form, and IgE, the immunoglobulin implicated in anaphylactic hypersensitivity. IgG, IgM, IgA, and IgE also occur in most other mammals. Their physicochemical and chemical properties are illustrated in Table 13-2.

One of the striking features of purified immunoglobulins is their inherent electrophoretic heterogeneity. IgG purified from serum shows a broad range of mobilities when electrophoresed (Table 13-2). This electrophoretic heterogeneity is related to a further subclassification of IgG, and to distinct biologic activities. Serum IgG comprises a population of four subclasses (Table 13-3) and, more importantly, individual antibodies specific for unique antigenic determinants. Subclasses have also been described for IgM and IgA (Table 13-2). These subdivisions are based upon slight chemical differences which can often be detected serologically.

The important breakthrough with respect to understanding immunoglobulin structure was

TABLE 13-2 PHYSICAL, PHYSIOLOGIC, AND BIOLOGIC PROPERTIES OF THE HUMAN IMMUNOGLOBULINS

	IgG	IgA	IgM	IgD	IgE
Physical Properties					
Sedimentation coefficient, S_{20w}	6.8–7.0	6.6–14.0	18.0–19.0	7.0	7.9
Molecular weight, daltons	143,000–160,000	159,000–447,000	900,000	177,000–185,000	188,000–200,000
Electrophoretic mobility	$\gamma^2-\alpha^1$	$\gamma^2-\beta^2$	$\gamma^1-\beta^1$	γ^1	γ^1
Carbohydrate content, %	2.3	7.5	7–11	13	11–12
Number of 4-chain units per molecule	1	1–3	5	1	1
Heavy chains	γ	α	μ	δ	ϵ
Light chains	κ or λ	κ or λ	κ or λ	κ or λ	κ or λ
Heavy chain allotypes	Gm	Am	—	—	—
Light chain allotypes	Inv (κ)	Inv (κ)	Inv (κ)	Inv (κ)	Inv (κ)
Heavy chain subclasses	$\gamma_1, \gamma_2, \gamma_3, \gamma_4$	α_1, α_2	$\mu_1, \mu_2(?)$	—	—
Heavy chain molecular weight, daltons	50,000–55,000	62,000	65,000	70,000	75,000
Light chain molecular weight, daltons	23,000	23,000	23,000	23,000	23,000
Physiologic Properties					
Normal adult serum concentration, mg/ml	8–16	1.4–4.0	0.4–2.0	0.03	ng amounts
Percent total immunoglobulin	80	13	6	1	0.002
Synthetic rate, mg/kg/d	26	27	5.7	0.4	0.003
Functional catabolic rate in serum, %/d	6	25	15	37	70–90
(or half-life, d)	(23)	(6)	(5)	(3)	(<3)
Intravascular distribution, %	48	41	76	75	51
Biologic Properties					
Agglutinating capacity	±	++	++++	—	—
Complement-fixing capacity	+	—	++++	—	—
Anaphylactic hypersensitivity (homologous)	—	—	—	—	++++
Guinea pig anaphylaxis (heterologous skin)	+	—	—	—	—
Fixation to homologous mast cells	—	—	—	—	++++
Placental transport to fetus	+++	—	—	—	—
Rheumatoid factor-binding activity	+++	—	—	—	—
Tumor-blocking activity	+	?	?	?	?
Present in external secretions	+	++++	±	—	++

TABLE 13-3 PROPERTIES ASSOCIATED WITH SUBCLASSES OF HUMAN IgG

Combined Properties of IgG Subclasses	IgG_1	IgG_2	IgG_3	IgG_4
Approximate occurrence in total serum IgG	65–75	15–23	7	3
Synthetic rate, mg/kg/d, in serum	25	?	3.4	?
Fractional catabolic rate, %/d, in serum	8	6.9	16.8	6.9
(half-life, d)	(23)	(23)	(7)	(23)
Intravascular distribution, %	51	53	64	54
Allotypic markers (Gm types)	1,2,3,4,17	23	5,6,10,11,13,14,21	?
Complement-fixing capacity	+	+	+	−
Heterologous skin-binding capacity	+	−	+	+
Placental transport to fetus	+	±	+	+
Polypeptide structure and location of interchain disulfide bonds				

KEY:

—— = Light chain

——— = Heavy chain (2X the length of the light chain)

| or / = Interchain disulfide bonds

the discovery of the significance of the paraproteins.

Paraproteins Neoplastic and proliferative diseases of lymphoid and plasma cells often result in the production of large quantities of abnormal immunoglobulins or paraproteins. The paraproteins, unlike normal serum immunoglobulins, behave electrophoretically as homogeneous molecules; they are the products of cell clones. Plasma cells in myeloma patients produce homogeneous serum paraproteins and often Bence-Jones urinary proteins. In Waldenström's macroglobulinemia the lymphoid tumors produce monoclonal IgM serum proteins.

The existence of paraproteins of every immunoglobulin class and subclass has permitted the isolation of large amounts of unique populations of immunoglobulins and their characterization. Antisera can be produced to each class and subclass (in rabbits or goats and so on) and, by appropriate absorption procedures, rendered specific for particular classes and subclasses. The existence of the paraproteins has also allowed a comparison of their biologic functions (Table 13-2) and the determination of their primary amino acid sequence.

Characterization of Antibodies Most of the early physical–chemical studies were done with IgG purified from rabbit, horse, and human sera. Several important structural features

of IgG were predicted from these studies long before amino acid sequences and x-ray diffraction studies were reported. For example, its molecular weight was calculated from sedimentation and diffusion studies, the molecule was predicted to be asymmetrical (or nonglobular) from its viscosity parameters, and its unique susceptibility to proteolytic agents suggested a globular domain structure—enzyme-resistant globular domains linked by enzyme-sensitive regions. Hapten-binding studies by hapten-specific antibodies demonstrated the existence of two antigen-binding sites per IgG molecule, and a third domain was suggested for the binding of complement components once hapten or antigen had bound. Thus these early studies predicted a minimum of three functional and structural domains. This early model has been verified by more recent experiments.

Polypeptide Structure of IgG Edelman and his co-workers showed by zone electrophoresis under denaturing and reducing conditions that rabbit IgG consisted of two types of polypeptide chains, and Porter and coworkers described two sizes of polypeptide chains by gel filtration under similar denaturing and reducing conditions (Fig. 13-7). The heavy (H) chains (50,000 to 53,000 daltons) contain a small amount of covalently coupled carbohydrate; the light (L) chains (22,000 to 25,000 daltons) lack carbohydrate. From the mole/mole and wt/wt ratios and the molecular

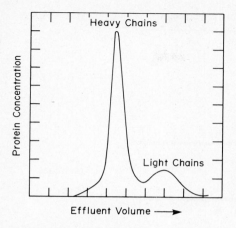

FIG. 13-7. Separation of the heavy (H) and light (L) chains of rabbit IgG by gel filtration column chromatography in the presence of 1N acetic acid (denaturing conditions). (Data adapted from Fleischman, Pain, and Porter: Arch Biochim Biophys [Suppl 1]: 174, 1962.)

weight of the intact IgG, a 4-chain structure (2H plus 2L) was postulated.

Porter and co-workers digested rabbit IgG with the proteolytic enzyme papain and chromatographed the resulting peptides on cation-exchange columns (Fig. 13-8). The peptides I and II (Fab fragments) contained univalent binding sites for hapten or antigen, while fragment III contained no hapten-binding site and was readily crystallizable (Fc fragment). Porter's group later showed that individual IgGs contained either fragment I or fragment II but never both. The difference between I and II was later shown to reside in the type of light chains. The intact IgG was characterized by a sedimentation coefficient of 7S, while both the Fab and Fc sedimented with 3.5S.

Digestion of rabbit IgG with pepsin results in a 5S component that precipitates with antigen and is, therefore, a bivalent fragment F (ab')$_2$. The analogous Fc' fragment is usually completely digested. If disulfide bond reducing agents, such as β-mercaptoethanol, are added to the 5S fragment, two Fab' fragments (3.5S) result. Extensive reduction of Fab' or Fab with β-mercaptoethanol yields an Fd' or Fd fragment, respectively, and free light chain. Taken together, Edelman and Porter's contributions resulted in the postulated structure for rabbit IgG shown in Figure 13-9. Subsequent studies with the different human Ig classes and subclasses have shown that they also possess the same fundamental 4-chain structure. The differences reside in the number of 4-chain units per Ig molecule and the additional appearance of accessory polypeptides. For example, IgM and often IgA (Fig. 13-10) contain a j chain (15,000 daltons) which may stabilize the polymeric structure of these immunoglobulins with disulfide bonds. IgA can also contain an associated T piece (60,000 daltons) that appears to enhance its secretion into extracellular fluids. A summary of the different structures is illustrated in Figure 13-10, and differences in their physiologic and biologic properties are summarized in Table 13-2.

Interchain and Intrachain Disulfide Bonds

From Figures 13-9 and 13-10 and Table 13-3, it is clear that the various species of IgG contain several interchain HL and HH disulfide bonds. These bonds play a role in stabilizing the structure, but they are not essential, since some IgA and IgD molecules do not possess HL disulfide bonds.

The intrachain disulfide bonds are critical for conferring the domain structure upon immunoglobulin molecules. If the polypeptide chains are stretched out and the positions of cysteine residues involved in intrachain disulfide bonds marked, one can see that they generate loops of some 60-80 amino acids (Fig. 13-11). For human IgG, each 110 amino acid segment contains a disulfide-bonded loop of 60-80 amino

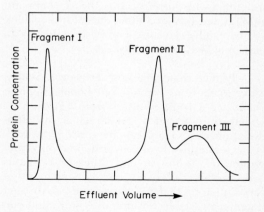

FIG. 13-8. Separation of peptides following digestion of rabbit IgG with the enzyme, papain. Separation was achieved by chromatography over the cation-exchange resin, carboxymethyl cellulose, and elution with an increasing ionic strength gradient. The peaks were labeled I, II, and III in order of their appearance. (Data adapted from Porter: Biochem J 73:119, 1959.)

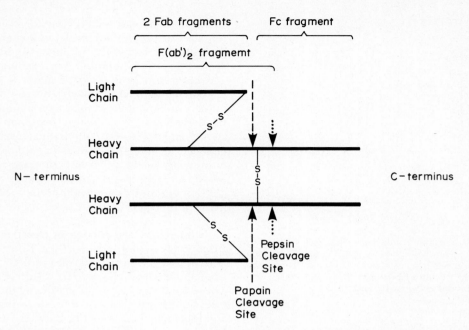

FIG. 13-9. Proposed structure for rabbit IgG showing the 4-chain basic structure, important disulfide bonds and probable sites of enzymatic cleavage by papain or pepsin.

acids, and there are two loop sections per light chain and four loop sections per heavy chain. The disulfide-binding pattern, critical amino acid residues, and overall lengths for various paraproteins are also shown in Figure 13-11.

The differences in the molecular weights of the major immunoglobulin classes are due to differences in the H chains: the H chains for IgM (μ) and IgE (ϵ) contain one additional loop segment. The L chains κ or λ are shared by all classes of heavy chains ($\gamma,\mu,\alpha,\delta,\epsilon$).

Peptide Mapping and Sequence Studies
Since Bence-Jones proteins are homogeneous L chains, chemically identical from a given individual, they are ideal for chemical structure determination. They can be readily purified, characterized by tryptic peptide mapping, and sequenced. When several different L chains had been characterized in this manner, it became apparent that they possessed two distinct regions, a variable (V) amino (N) terminal end (no Bence-Jones proteins from different individuals have identical sequences in this region), and a constant carboxyl (C) terminal end (with only two major variants, κ or λ). The constant regions (C_κ) of all κ Bence-Jones proteins possess 95 to 100 percent sequence homology

in residues 111–214 and little homology with C_λ constant regions. In fact, there are also two types of κ chains: some possess a leucine (Inv 1,2) at position 191, while others contain a valine at this position (Inv 3). This genetic marker, or allotype, follows classic mendelian inheritance patterns and can also be detected by specific antisera. Individuals and families can be typed with respect to this κ Inv marker. In a heterozygote (Inv 1,2/Inv 3) a single Ig molecule contains a single allotype and never both. No allotypic markers have been demonstrated for human λ chains.

The κ chains terminate in cys at residue 214, and λ chains terminate in ser at residue 215, with a penultimate cys residue. These cysteine residues are involved in HL interchain disulfide bonds. By amino acid sequence studies of many Bence-Jones proteins, the N-terminal half of the molecule (V region) has been shown to be variable (in selected areas) and has been implicated as the antigen-binding site, the variability reflecting individual antibody specificities. However, the first 18-20 amino acids of the N-terminal end are actually fairly constant, and based upon these sequences, κ L chains can be subtyped into at least three groups (κ_I, κ_{II}, κ_{III}) (Fig. 13-12), and the λ light chains can be sub-

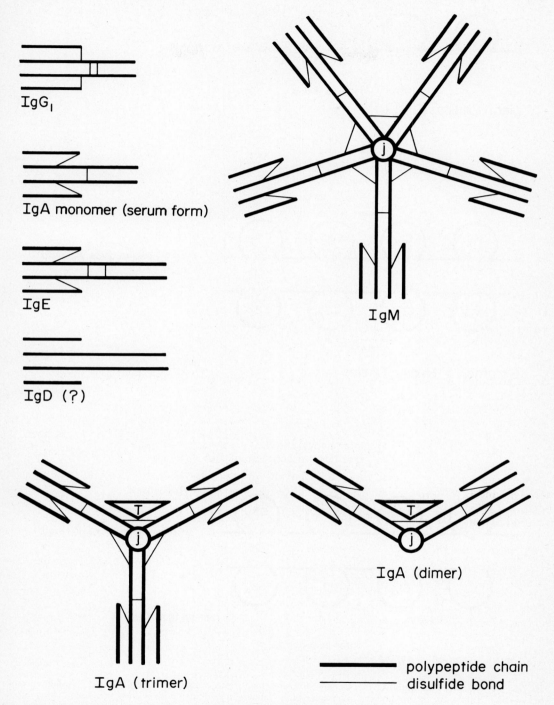

IgG₁

IgA monomer (serum form)

IgE

IgD (?)

IgM

IgA (trimer)

IgA (dimer)

━━━━━━━ polypeptide chain
───────── disulfide bond

FIG. 13-10. Representative structures for the major human immunoglobulin classes. Each contains the basic 4-chain polypeptide unit, and some may exist as polymers (eg, IgM and IgA). The accessory polypeptides j and T may also be present in the polymeric forms.

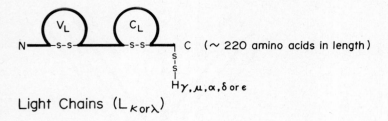

Light Chains (L$_{\kappa \, or \, \lambda}$)

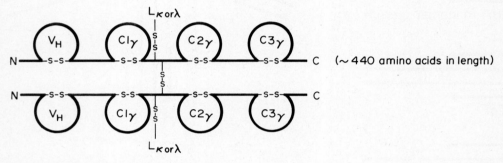

Gamma – 1 Heavy Chains

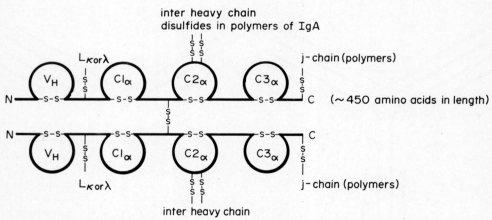

Alpha Heavy Chains

FIG. 13-11. Detailed description of the 4-chain structures for various human immunoglobulins. The differences in heavy chain lengths are shown, and the importance of the intrachain disulfide bonds is illustrated. Some of the important structural and functional attributes are also given in the figure. (Data adapted from Putnam: Progress in Immunology, vol I, p 25, 1974; Bennich and von Bahr-Lindstrom, ibid, p 49.)

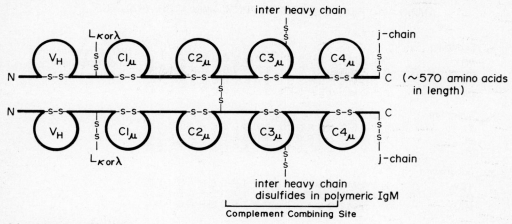

Mu Heavy Chains

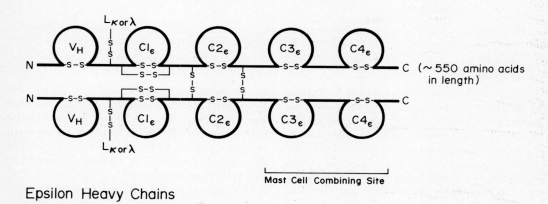

Epsilon Heavy Chains

FIG. 13-11. (cont.)

typed into five groups (λ_I, λ_{II}, λ_{III}, λ_{IV}, λ_V). Therefore, sequencing an unknown Bence-Jones protein through the first $18-20$ amino acids is often sufficient for typing and subtyping, since V_κ is always found with C_κ (and V_λ with C_λ). Other constant or conserved residues that fall within the confines of the variable region include the cysteine residues responsible for the loop structure, which seems to be structurally important.

When the H chains from homogeneous myeloma proteins were similarly characterized, an analogous structural relationship became apparent (Fig. 13-11). In all cases the N-terminal

110 amino acid segment was found to contain variable sequences (V_H), and the remaining segments were found to be constant (C_H). For example, all IgG_1 myeloma H chains (γ_1) share an identical amino acid sequence from residue 111 to the C-terminal end except for a few changes which account for heavy chain allotypic markers (Gm markers). Like the Inv allotypes of κ light chains, these genetic differences can be distinguished serologically. IgG_1 heavy chain constant regions show very little amino acid sequence homology with the H chains of other IgG subclasses (γ_2, γ_3, γ_4). These, in turn, have their own unique constant

AMINO ACID RESIDUE POSITION FROM AMINO TERMINAL END

V_{κ_I} Subgroup

							10													23	

ROY   D I Q M T Q S R S S L S A S V G D R V T I T C   (first cysteine involved
Eu   B I Z M T Z S P S T L S A S V G B R V T I T C   in an intrachain
Ou   D I Q M T Z S P S S L S A S V G B R V T I T C   disulfide bond)
DAV   D I Q M T Q S P S T L S T V V G D R V T I T C

$V_{\kappa_{II}}$ Subgroup

Ti   E I V L T Q S P G T L S L S P G E R A T L S C
B6   Z I V L T Z S P G T L S L S P G Z R A A L S C
DIL   E I V L T Q S P G T L S L S P G D R A T L S C

$V_{\kappa_{III}}$ Subgroup

TEW   D I V M T Q S P L S L P V T P G E P A S I S C
MIL   D I V L T Q S P L S L P V T P G E P A S I S C
MAN   D I V M T Q S P L S L P V T P G E P A S I S C

Code: A alanine   I isoleucine   R arginine
      B asparaginyl (DorN)   K lysine   S serine
      C cysteine   L leucine   T threonine
      D aspartic a   M methionine   V valine
      E glutamic a   N asparagine   W tryptophan
      F phenylalanine   P proline   Y tyrosine
      G glycine   Q glutamine   Z glutamyl (E or Q)
      H histidine

FIG. 13-12. The subtyping of human κ chains based upon amino acid sequence analyses. Three groups of κ chains can be distinguished in this manner. (The data and the one-letter amino acid code are based on Hood and Prahl: Adv Immunol 14:291, 1971.)

regions and allotypic markers (Table 13-3). The Gm allotype markers can, in some cases, be defined by sequence studies, and in the case of Gm1 (or a) of IgG heavy chains this amounts to amino acid changes in two residues (Table 13-4). Allotypic markers on other classes of immunoglobulins have only been described for IgA$_2$. Am$_2^+$ has no HL disulfide bonds, and Am$_2^-$ has one HL disulfide bond.

The N-terminal 18-20 amino acids in the variable regions of the H chains (γ, μ, α, and ϵ) of several human paraproteins have been compared, and an interesting relationship has been found. By analogy with κ or λ light chains, the N-terminal 18-20 amino acids fall into four subtypes (V$_{HI}$, V$_{HII}$, V$_{HIII}$, and V$_{HIV}$), but in contrast to the class association for L chains, the H chain subtypes appear to be shared by all H chain classes and subclasses. In addition, in one case, an individual produced both an IgG and an IgM paraprotein that shared identical amino acid sequences in the variable regions of both γ and μ chains. This case is frequently cited as evidence for separate genes controlling the synthesis of variable and constant regions of immunoglobulins. In this example, the identi-

TABLE 13-4 RELATED SEQUENCE CHANGES
IN THE Gm1 (OR a) ALLOTYPIC MARKER
IN HUMAN IgG$_1$ HEAVY CHAINS

Gm Type	Amino Acid Residues Involved	Residue Positions
1+	-Asn-Glu-Leu-	356 – 357 – 358
1−	-Glu-Glu-Met-	

Data adapted from Waxdal, Konigsberg, and Edelman: Biochemistry, 7:1967, 1968; Frangione, Milstein, and Pink: Nature 221:145, 1969; Burton and Deutsch: Immunochemistry, 7:145, 1970

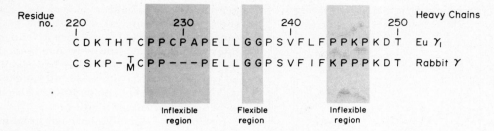

FIG. 13-13. Structural analysis of the immunoglobulin hinge region. Partial sequences in the region of the proposed hinge region are shown for rabbit IgG and the human IgG$_1$ paraprotein Eu. The one letter amino acid code of Figure 13-12 has been used. (Data adapted from Day: Advanced Immunochemistry. 1972. Courtesy of Williams & Wilkins.)

cal variable gene product appears to be associated with two distinct types of constant region gene products (C$_\mu$ and C$_\gamma$).

Hydrodynamic studies suggest that the Fab fragments of rabbit and human immunoglobulins are linked to the Fc domain through a flexible polypeptide region (the hinge region). Chemical studies have confirmed this model: this region contains two relatively inflexible proline-rich sequences connected by a highly flexible glycine-rich region (Fig. 13-13). This primary structure is entirely compatible with the flexible hinge concept.

Several investigators are currently attempting to correlate immunoglobulin amino acid sequence and tertiary structure with biologic function. For example, by comparing the sequences in H chain constant regions known to fix complement components (Table 13-2), the structural features necessary for this effector function may become apparent. Similarly, IgE is known to fix to mast cells through the C-terminal domain of the ϵ heavy chain, and aspects of this recognition site are also currently under investigation.

The Antibody-binding Site Structural studies have centered on the N-terminal 110 amino acids that comprise the variable region in both L and H chains. Since the information for antigenic determinant complementarity must be built into the primary sequence of each chain, and a given antigen initiates the biosynthesis of antibody molecules having complementary receptor sites, these variable regions have all the requirements that one would impose on hypothetical binding sites.

Several lines of evidence indicate that the variable regions are directly involved in the binding sites. It is possible to produce rabbit antisera directed at the binding sites of hapten-specific antibodies produced in other rabbits. The donor and recipient animals must be matched for rabbit immunoglobulin allotypes, so that the specificity detected can only be ascribed to differences in the variable regions (idiotypes). Antiidiotypic antibodies can block the hapten-specific binding of the donor antibody, and the antiidiotypic immunoglobulins only react with intact donor immunoglobulin or the isolated Fab or F(ab')$_2$ fragments. Therefore, the idiotypic specificity must reside in the region of the binding site and, most likely, in the variable regions of the H and L chains.

Further studies have also shown that the proteolytic fragments [Fab and F(ab')$_2$] contain antigen-specific binding sites, thus narrowing the list of possible candidates to the variable regions (V$_L$ and V$_H$) and the first constant domains (C$_L$ and C$_H$). More extensive digestion of the Fab fragments from a mouse myeloma protein (with DNP-lysine specificity) with pepsin yielded an F$_V$ fragment containing only the V$_H$ and V$_L$ regions. The F$_V$ fragment was also capable of binding DNP-lysine.

Indirect evidence that the variable region comprises the antigen-binding site has resulted from the studies of Wu and Kabat and of Capra and Kehoe. In these studies the amino acid sequences of variable regions of both paraprotein L and H chains were analyzed for the extent of variation in each residue. Wu and Kabat studied the variability in human κ chains irrespective of their subtype (V$_{\kappa_I}$, V$_{\kappa_{II}}$, V$_{\kappa_{III}}$) and described three hypervariable regions (residues 24–34, 50–56, and 89–97) (Fig. 13-14). They also found that certain residues were invariant and therefore presumably important structural-

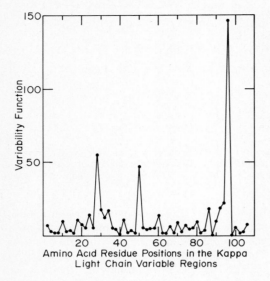

Fig. 13-14. An analysis of human κ chain variable region sequences. Variability in a given residue position is defined as the number of different amino acids found in that position divided by the frequency of the most common amino acid at that position. Variability can theoretically range from a ratio of 1.0 (conserved residue) to 400 (maximal variation). (Data adapted from Wu and Kabat: J Exp Med 132:211, 1970.)

ly (for example, cys 23 and 88, trp 35, and phe 98). By comparing the sequences of only V_{κ_1} light chains, the first hypervariable region was further confined to residues 30–32. They suggested that these hypervariable regions were direct contact residues with antigen, and areas of minimal variability in the V region were necessary for a certain basic tertiary structure and for intersubunit interactions (such as V_H and V_L contact).

The H chain variable regions have been similarly studied by Capra and Kehoe. Regions of hypervariability were assigned to four regions (residues 31–37, 50–52, 86–91, and 101–109). Again the cys residues 22 and 98, responsible for the loop, were invariant, as were trp 38 and ser 30.

Largely due to the work of Singer and co-workers, important residues in the region of the binding site were described by the affinity labeling technique. An antibody with affinity for a hapten is reacted with an analog of the hapten containing a chemically reactive group. As a result of recognition and binding, a covalent bond may be formed between the reactive hap-

ten and an amino acid at or near the binding site (usually tyr or lys). The reactive residue can then be identified by preparing tryptic peptides of the reacted antibody and limited sequence analysis. These studies have implicated tyr residues at positions 30–40 and 80–100 and lys residues at positions 50–52 of H chains as being important for binding.

Recently, the three-dimensional structure for the paraprotein IgG New was reported by Amzel and co-workers. Crystals of the Fab fragments were prepared, and by a combination of amino acid sequencing and x-ray crystallography, the structure was determined at 3.5 A resolution. The New protein binds the γ-hydroxyl derivative of vitamin K_1. X-ray crystallography of the Fab-vitamin K complex is shown in Figure 13-15. The results of these studies are consistent with all the direct and indirect evidence that has accumulated concerning the nature of antibody-binding sites. Their size (15 by 6 by 6 A) had been largely predicted. The positions or roles of the H and L hypervariable regions in the site are now obvious, and the positions of potentially reactive tyr and lys residues identified by affinity labeling technique are also apparent.

Summary of Antibody Structure

Antibody molecules in man are comprised of a basic 4-chain unit of 2L and 2H chains. The class and subclass of immunoglobulin are defined by the H chain (γ_1, γ_2, γ_3, γ_4, μ_1, μ_2, α_1, α_2, ϵ, or δ). All immunoglobulins share either κ or λ light chains. Polymeric forms of IgM contain five basic units linked by inter H chain disulfide bonds and a cysteine-rich j chain. Polymeric forms of IgA (two or more basic units) also contain a j chain and may contain an additional secretory piece (T) if found in extracellular secretions. The domain structure of immunoglobulins is intimately related to its function. There is an N-terminal variable region domain responsible for antigen binding, and there are specialized constant region domains implicated in the binding of complement components and sites on certain types of cells. Antibody function is thought to be mediated through recognition of antigen and subsequent activation of an auxiliary system (eg, complement).

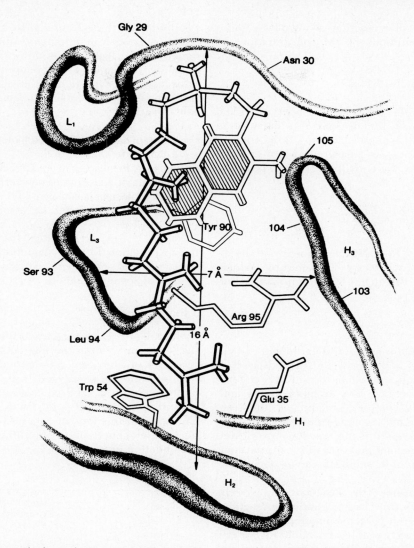

Fig. 13-15. The antibody-combining site of the human IgG$_1$ paraprotein New as determined by x-ray diffraction studies. The position of the hapten, a derivative of vitamin K, has also been determined. (From Amzel, Poljak, Saul, Varga, and Richards: Proc Natl Acad Sci USA 71:1427, 1974.)

ANTIGEN – ANTIBODY REACTIONS

Thermodynamics Theoretically, if an antigen-antibody reaction is truly reversible, it should obey the Law of Mass Action:

$$(1) \qquad Ag + Ab \rightleftharpoons AgAb \text{ complex}$$

It follows that at equilibrium, the following relationship should apply:

$$(2) \qquad K = \frac{[AgAb]}{[Ag][Ab]}$$

where the values in brackets reflect the molar concentrations of reactants and product at equilibrium. Once the equilibrium constant has been determined, the change in the standard free energy, $-\triangle G°$, can be calculated (the free energy of a reaction taking place under standard conditions of 1M concentrations of reactants):

(3) $\qquad -\Delta G° = RT\ln K$

where R is the universal gas constant (1.986 times 10^{-3} kcal/°K/mole), and T is the absolute temperature (in degrees Kelvin). If the equilibrium constant K is measured at two or more temperatures, the enthalpy, $\Delta H°$, can be calculated.

(4) $\qquad \dfrac{d(\ln K)}{dT} = \dfrac{\Delta H°}{RT^2}$

Alternatively, the $\Delta H°$ can be measured directly by microcalorimetry. The entropy change, $\Delta S°$, can be calculated with the measured values of $-\Delta G°$ and $\Delta H°$,

(5) $\qquad -\Delta G° = -\Delta H° + T\Delta S°$

Since antigens are multideterminant and antibodies are at least bivalent, it is difficult to obtain quantitative data for most antigen–antibody reactions. For example, if the antigen-antibody complex precipitates, the reactants and product are not in a true state of equilibrium. However, if the reactions are carried out in extreme antigen excess, where the complexes are soluble, valid data can be obtained.

Hapten–Antibody Reactions It is relatively easy to treat hapten–antibody reactions quantitatively where the hapten is univalent and the antibody is at least bivalent (polymeric forms of immunoglobulin possessing additional binding sites, eg, IgA and IgM). The reaction of antibody site(S) with free hapten (H) can be written as follows:

(6) $\qquad \text{H} + \text{S} \underset{k_r}{\overset{k_f}{\rightleftharpoons}} \text{HS}$

where the equilibrium constant, K, is defined by the ratio of the forward to reverse rate constants ($K = k_f/k_r$). Although the rate constants can, in some cases, be measured, more often K is measured directly by equilibrium dialysis. In principle, the technique involves the dialysis of a mixture of free hapten and specific antibody, where only the free hapten can pass

easily through dialysis tubing. By knowing the initial concentration of hapten and the concentration of free hapten at equilibrium, one can calculate the amount of bound hapten, the association constant, K, and the valence of the antibody (the number of binding sites per molecule of antibody). If

r = moles of hapten-bound/total moles of antibody (calculated)
c = moles of free hapten at equilibrium (measured)
n = valence of antibody (or number of sites/antibody molecule) (calculated)
K = equilibrium constant (or affinity constant) (calculated),

the mass action formula (equation 6) can be rewritten and rearranged according to the method of Scatchard, where

(7) $\qquad r/c = nK - rK$

By plotting r/c against r, K can be obtained from the slope and n from the intercept on the abscissa. In practice, several different concentrations of hapten are dialyzed in individual experiments with a fixed concentration of antibody to generate the points in Figure 13-16. Curvature in this type of data presentation reflects heterogeneity in the binding affinities of a population of antibodies in the serum. Anti-

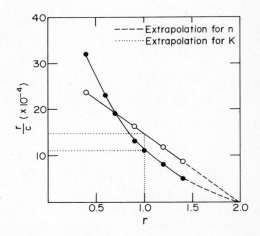

FIG. 13-16. Scatchard plots for two hypothetical hapten-antibody systems. The linear relationship reflects a homogeneous antibody response to the haptenic determinant. The nonlinear relationship reflects a heterogeneous antibody response. Both sets of data can be used to obtain values for n and K (or K_0) by the proper extrapolations.

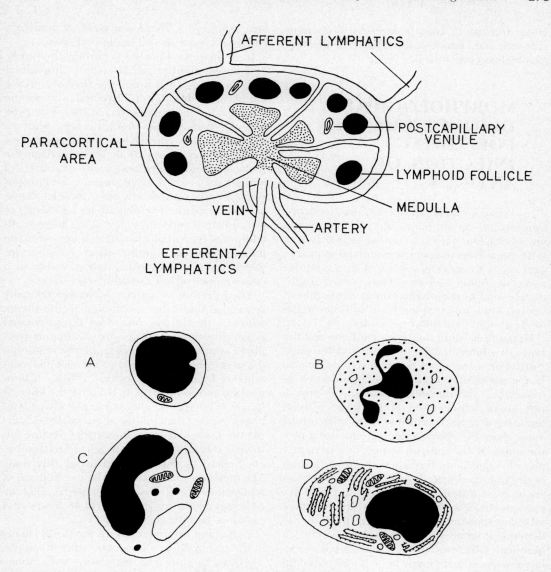

FIG. 14-2. The lymph node contains a number of densely packed lymphocytes in germinal follicles and a looser collection in the paracortical areas, which separate the follicles, and in the central medullary area. The follicles are rich in antibody-forming (B) cells, and the paracortical and medullary areas contain predominantly thymus-derived (T) cells. The lymph flows through sinusoids which are separated by cords of lymphocytes and dendritic macrophages. A lymphocyte, a macrophage, a polymorphonuclear (PMN) neutrophil, and an antibody-forming plasma cell are depicted.

filter and are also phagocytic. The sinuses also provide channels through which lymphoid cells and phagocytic cells can pass from one area of the node of another. The postcapillary venules of lymphoid tissue are distinctive and appear to be involved in lymphocytic migration. In an active lymph node, considerable rearrangement of the cells occurs, and foreign material can pass more freely through the walls of the dilated sinusoids. Postinjection changes are most obvious in the lymph nodes which are normally quiescent, such as the popliteal node. In the absence of stimulation, resting nodes have few primary follicles or nodules in the cortical area. By contrast, nodes from the mesentery or neck are in a constant state of activity, since they are constantly exposed to microorganisms, and changes following immunization may be less pronounced.

MORPHOLOGICALLY DISTINCT CHANGES FOLLOWING INJECTION OF ANTIGEN

When a physician injects a bacterial suspension into an unimmunized patient or when an investigator injects a similar suspension of microorganisms into an experimental animal or exposes it to antigen via the skin, a complex series of changes follows. These changes ultimately lead to the production of antibodies of various kinds and frequently, in addition, to the development of cellular immunity.

Depending upon the type of antigen and the route of administration, the cortex or the paracortical area may show the most active changes. If the antigen is a contact allergen, such as oxazalone, dinitrochlorobenzene, or poison ivy, all of which elicit almost pure cellular hypersensitivity responses, the paracortical areas show the greatest degree of cellular proliferation. If the antigen is one that primarily provokes antibody formation, such as dextran or polymerized flagellin, the germinal centers show great mitotic activity, and new follicles may appear. The great majority of antigens give mixed responses and thus affect both the T-dependent paracortical area and the B cell-rich germinal follicles. Within 72 hours the stimulated nodes contain many large lymphoblastoid cells which stain intensively with the dye, pyronin. Hence, they are often referred to as large pyroninophilic cells. With time, these cells divide to form small lymphocytes and plasma cells.

Intradermal, subcutaneous, intramuscular, intraperitoneal, and intravenous routes are frequently used experimentally. The intradermal route appears to be highly effective in inducing cellular immunity. The intramuscular and subcutaneous routes characteristically give good antibody responses. In clinical use, the inhalation of antigenic aerosols or the injection of antigenic solutions is used to modify preexisting and unwanted immunity or to induce a state of local immunity. These are novel approaches, and their success is still being evaluated.

If the material injected is particulate, it may first be distributed rather widely throughout the phagocytic cells lining the sinusoids of the lymph node draining the injection site. In the follicles, the most numerous of the phagocytic reticular cells is the dendritic cell, with its elongated and convoluted cytoplasmic processes. Antigen appears to be located on the surface of such cells, and small quantities of antigen may persist in this manner for long periods. In the paracortical area, the phagocytic cells more nearly resemble tissue histiocytes or macrophages and tend to ingest the antigen. An additional type of phagocytic cell appears to be most active in trapping dead lymphocytes which accumulate during, and probably as a consequence of, intense proliferation.

The injection of antigen is characteristically somewhat traumatic. As studied in the sheep, which is docile and can stand the prolonged immobilization necessary for continuous lymphatic cannulation, the afferent lymph draining the injection site, typically in the foot pad, contains red cells, lymphocytes, PMN, macrophages, and cell debris. In contrast, the efferent lymph is composed almost exclusively of lymphocytes, and the number of lymphocytes leaving the node may show a transient decline following the injection of antigen. PMN tend to congregate in the lymph node at this time. Macrophages enlarge and show evidence of phagocytosis (activated macrophages), and lymphocytes begin to divide 24 to 48 hours after exposure to antigen.

Following the induction of immunity, many of the responding cells remain within the node. This can be shown by expressing cells from a teased node and testing for antibody production in a plaque assay, or by showing that they can confer immunity when transferred to a non-immunized and incompetent host (Fig. 14-3). The earliest detectable antibody response is by cells producing high-molecular-weight (IgG) antibody followed a few days later by a more mature, lower-molecular-weight (IgG) antibody. These cells are B type lymphocytes, some of which do enter the circulation, while others differentiate into plasma cells, which tend to remain within the node and are rarely seen in the bloodstream. In addition to B cells, specifically reactive T cells are also generated following the original stimulus, and again there

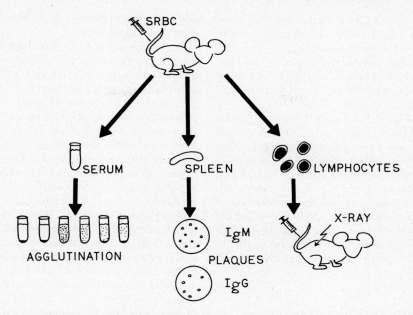

FIG. 14-3. Antibody production can be conveniently followed by procedures such as the hemolytic plaque assay, hemagglutination with serum dilution, and transfer of antibody-forming capacity to another animal. In the illustration, a mouse receives sheep red blood cells. Serum can be removed at intervals and titrated. A suspension of spleen cells can be used in a plaque assay to determine the actual number of IgM (direct) or IgG (indirect) plaques, or cells can be treated in various ways and transferred to an irradiated recipient to determine the long-term changes induced by the treatment.

is a tendency for some of the activated T cells to remain within the node. This tendency is most marked after primary exposure to antigen, and many studies have used very sensitive assays against tumor cells to detect the appearance of effector T cells. With time, some of the specific T cells migrate to other lymphoid organs. Since both T and B cells tend to persist within the node, it is not surprising that the response to a second exposure to the same, or to a closely related, antigen is more rapid and more intense than in the primary response. It is possible that the regulation of migration of lymphoid cells is determined by the expression of the differentiation antigens to be described below. Thus, the possession of the markers, such as T1[a] or PC, could prevent a cell from escaping from the thymus or lymph node, respectively.

The sequence of events occurring in the draining node, then, begins with a generalized proliferation and a diminution of cellular traffic through the node, the emergence of 19 S IgM antibody-producing cells and of cells capable of suppressing the growth of a transplant, followed by the formation of cells making 7S IgG antibodies. After the third day, many of those cells from the lymph node escape into the

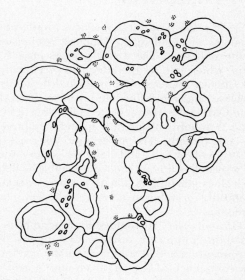

FIG. 14-4. While most of the particulate antigen injected is taken up by macrophages and is degraded and lost, some persists on the surface of dendritic macrophages within the lymph node. Quantities of antigen remaining are minute, and sensitive procedures, such as electron microscopy of autoradiographs, as in the illustration, are required for their detection. (Adapted from Nossal and Ada: Antigens, Lymphoid Cells, and the Immune Response, 1971. Courtesy of Academic Press)

draining or efferent lymphatic and find their way into the bloodstream and thence into the tissues and other lymphoid organs. This explains why the contralateral nodes develop immunity which appears later and because of the dispersion of immune cells, is weaker than that shown in the draining node.

Most of the antigen originally injected leaves the node within 24 hours and, unless degraded or excreted, may be sequestered in the Kupffer cells of the liver. While much of the antigen is thus lost to the lymphoid system, Nossal and his colleagues have, through special autoradiographic techniques, shown the persistence of antigen molecules on the surface of dendritic cells within the lymph node (Fig. 14-4). Presumably this antigenic material is presented to the surface of lymphocytes passing through the sinusoids.

CELLULAR INTERACTION IN INDUCTION OF IMMUNITY

Exactly how antigen causes proliferative changes involved in the immune response is quite unknown. The actual process of activation, which follows the adequate presentation of antigen, appears to be mediated by adenylcyclase, and rapid fluctuations of cyclic AMP and GMP have been reported following activation. A minority of antigens appear to influence B cells directly. The majority do not react directly with B cells and need the intervention of a second cell type, the helper cell. The helper cell is generally a T cell, but macrophages, dendritic or otherwise, may also share this function.

One necessary attribute of the macrophage is its ability to process antigen. An antigenic determinant (or active site) is generally confined to a sequence of five or seven amino acid or carbohydrate molecules (Chap. 13). The material originally injected may have a molecular weight of over 2 times 10^6 daltons and must be partially degraded before it can be appropriately presented to the specific responding lymphocyte. Processing can best be conceived as a function of the macrophage. Presentation is also of importance; presumably either the T cell or the macrophage can present antigen to a B cell in optimal form.

Communication between different cells of the lymphoid system is a subject of topical interest to the immunologist, and it appears probable that a variety of cell-surface markers aid in recognition between cell types. An ever-increasing number of candidates for this function are being described. They fall into two broad categories: differentiation antigens and histocompatibility antigens. By a differentiation antigen, we imply that a cell-surface marker is exposed only at certain stages of development or differentiation. Examples are antigens of differentiating embryos which appear only transiently and are otherwise only expressed abnormally, as in malignant tumors (eg, teratomas), organ-specific antigens of which those of the thyroid are perhaps best documented, and antigens of lymphoid cells which have become specialized, for example B cells, T cells, and plasma cells. While the most intensive investigation has been conducted on the cellular antigens of mice, there is increasing evidence that the finding in man and other species will be essentially similar.

The first differentiation antigen to be described in mice was originally designated θ and is now referred to as Thy-1 (Table 14-1). Two allelic forms are known. Thy-1 antigens are expressed on thymocytes and also on T cells outside the thymus. Two distinct subpopulations of murine T cells are distinguished: The thymocyte, designated T1, is rich in Thy-1 and poor in histocompatibility-2 antigen; T2 has reciprocal levels. A second murine thymic marker, $T1^a$, is expressed only on thymocytes and on some, but not all, tumors of thymic origin. $T1^a$ is not expressed on normal T cells that have left the thymus. An expanding number of antigens designated Ly (presently Ly1-8), found on lymphocytes, are also predominantly on the T cell series. The B cell series of lymphocytes carry at least two sets of markers: one is immunoglobulin, which may be present on the surface of nonantibody-secreting cells, and the other is often referred to as "MBLA." MBLA thus appears to be related to the differentiation of B cells, while another marker, called "PC," reflects the differentiation of plasma cells. Additional subclasses of lymphocytes are being described; one is called an "Fc cell," since it has receptors for the Fc region of the antibody molecule. This cell is being studied in relation

**TABLE 14–1 DISTRIBUTION OF SOME
ANTIGENS OF THE MOUSE, INCLUDING
ANTIGENS FOUND ONLY IN
DIFFERENTIATED CELLS**

Antigen	Distribution
H-2	All lymphocytes, tissues, red cells, tumors
H-5	Lymphocytes, red cells, tumor cells, and many tissues
H-6	Lymphocytes, red cells, tumor cells, and many tissues
Ia	B lymphocytes (weakly on T cells ?)
Thy-1	T lymphocytes, thymus, and tissues
TL	T lymphocytes in thymus, some leukemias
Ly-1	Some T lymphocytes but not T cytotoxic cells
Ly-2, 3	Another subset of T cells including T cytotoxic cells
Ka	Cytotoxic effector cells, not in thymus
Ly-4	B lymphocytes
MBLA	B lymphocytes
PC	Plasma cells, not found on B or T cells
T	Sperm, teratoma
HY	Sperm, epithelial cells, some lymphocytes

to its possible role in tumor immunity (Chap. 23). Another is called the "null cell," as it has neither Ig surface molecules nor T cell markers and has no Fc receptors. Delineation of the biologic function of the many subclasses of lymphocytes is a subject of very intensive investigation, especially in cancer immunology and studies on immunologic deficiency, immune responsiveness, and histocompatibility.

The means whereby T cells recognize and bind to their appropriate antigen has been a matter of very intensive controversy. Serious claims have been made that T cells carry a special class of immunoglobulin, IgT, and that this subserves a similar binding function to the immunoglobulin on B cell surfaces. Other investigators have denied this and reported that the antisera defining IgT, usually raised in rabbits, were contaminated with small quantities of highly avid xenoantibody to H antigens. This is a reasonable objection, since serum does contain small quantities of free histocompatibility antigen. It was then reported that T cells, which had only a small quantity of IgT on their surface, could release IgT in the form of a complex with antigen. Undoubtedly the supernatant after reaction of T cells and antigen has some highly potent immunobiologic properties which are now being investigated. Investigations by Binns and Wigzell may offer a new perspective. These investigators studied the reactions of sera made in F_1 hybrids between two inbred strains of rat, Lewis and DA. The (Lewis × DA)F_1 hybrids were immunized

against T cells from Lewis rats (Fig. 14-5). The resultant antiserum could suppress graft-versus-host and MLC reactions and could also be shown to bind to Lewis T cells, using fluorescent-labeled antirat globulin as an indicator. The specificity is believed to be against idiotypic determinants expressed on the homozygous lymphocytes of inbred animals but absent from the F_1 hybrid. Antigens of this type had been postulated earlier from experiments in mice by Ramseier and Lindermann. In mice, the relevant antibodies were very difficult to detect. Interestingly, the antibody produced by Binns and Wigzell cross-reacts with the heavy chain of immunoglobulin, and the investigators believe that the IgT molecule has the same structure in the variable region as the immunoglobulin heavy chain. One reason for the success reported by Binns and Wigzell, as compared to the difficulties encountered by other investigators, was the change to the rat as a test animal. Earlier in this section, it was explained that various fragments of information could be best obtained from highly selected experimental situations. The rat is, under certain conditions, able to produce unusually high titered antibodies. Following skin graft rejection, rat serum may often give detectable reactions when diluted 5,000-fold, whereas the titer reached in mice is rarely more than 50, and antibodies are rarely, if ever, detected following rejection of a single small skin graft in man.

The histocompatibility (H) antigens were detected by their role in inducing an immune

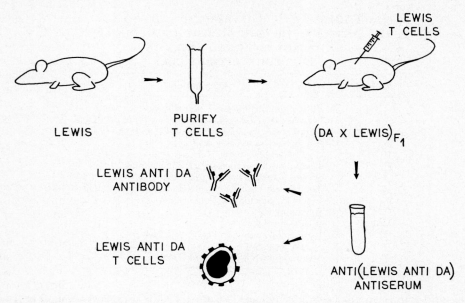

FIG. 14-5. F_1 hybrid animals can be attacked by cells from either parent. This may lead to death, or the animal may recover. Since the F_1 possesses all the H antigens of each inbred parent, it is proposed that the parental cells carry special idiotypes not present on the F_1. Lewis rat lymphocytes are injected into (Lewis × DA)F_1 hybrid recipients. The F_1 rat makes an antibody which was found to react with Lewis immunoglobulin and with Lewis T cells.

response to transplanted tissues (Chap. 22). The most potent of these antigenic systems in the mouse is called H-2. At first, only one genetic locus was detected. However, with time, at least eight genetic loci with a wide variety of functions have been demonstrated to lie close to each other in what is now called the "H-2 region." These functions all appear to be related to immunologic reactivity. Amazingly, exactly the same functions are carried out by a comparable set of closely linked genes in what is called the "HLA region" in man. These genes are implicated not only in the rejection of transplanted tissues and cells but also in controlling the levels of immunologic response and the levels of some, but not all, of the complement components, the best documented being the C2 and C3 proactivator (Chap. 16).

Histocompatibility antigens are expressed on all lymphoid cells, on platelets, and, to a lesser or more variable extent, on macrophages and PMN. Although an increasing number of H antigens and differentiation antigens expressed only on some subclasses of lymphocyte are being recognized, their functions are unclear. However, they are known to be relevant to cellular cooperation in the immune response.

Currently, the most intensively studied of

the antigenic markers associated with H-2 are called the "Ia antigens." The genetic loci coding for them are located within the H-2 system in the same general location (I region) as a series of genes regulating the immune responses, Irl genes.

That different individuals respond differently to the same antigen has been known for a very long time. Immunochemists would frequently inject the same antigen into four rabbits in the expectation that at least one of the four would produce a good antibody. That the capacity to respond was a genetic function was shown in randomly bred mice selected for high or low antibody and then mated to produce high and low responding lines. Maurer, McDevitt, and their colleagues, among others, conducted many experiments in inbred lines using linear or branched synthetic copolymers of several amino acids. The study was later extended to include a variety of natural antigens. From studies with mice derived from ancestors in which crossing over (recombination) had occurred within the H-2 region (recombinant lines), it was possible to identify the location of the regulatory genes. These genes do not necessarily regulate recognition, since an IgM response can usually be detected, but rather regulate the switch from IgM to IgG production that occurs after a few days. Antisera produced against cells from the recombinant lines were found to react with subpopulations of lymphoid cells. Because of the large numbers of different recombinant lines available, rather precise mapping has been possible. The antisera react with the products of I region genes. From various immune response studies, the I region can be subdivided into IA, IB, and IC subregions. The antisera are usually against the products of genes within the IA region, hence the designation Ia antigens. The Ia genes do not themselves appear to be directly responsible for regulation of the immune response and may frequently be expressed predominantly on B cells. From cell transfer experiments to x-irradiated and T cell-depleted recipients, it has been shown that restoration of the capacity to respond to antigen is a T cell function. These experiments have clearly demonstrated the need for collaboration between T helper cells and B cells for the production of antibody. Because cells from animals differing at certain genes within the H-2 region are unable to collaborate, T-T collaboration and the involvement of H-2 region genes in the immune response have been delineated.

IMMUNOLOGIC FUNCTION

Having established (1) that the lymphoid organs are the seat of the response to antigen, (2) that antibody of several classes and various activated cells are produced, and (3) that specific antibodies and activated cells may leave the node through the efferent lymphatics or the venous circulation, we can consider the immunobiology of the host and the functioning of the various components of the immune system.

The individual living in a normal environment is constantly mounting a defense against foreign agents. These range from the many varieties of microorganisms to unicellular and multicellular parasites. The individual is also constantly subjected to other environmental agents, including foods, pollens, danders, and other dusts. Thus, even in the absence of controlled immunization, the individual is constantly responding to environmental factors. There is a background level of immunity to an enormous repertoire of antigens. Even the germ-free animal is not in an antigen-free environment and has a certain amount of so-called natural antibody. Natural antibodies to such diverse substances as blood group antigens, bacterial flagella, many viruses, and somewhat surprisingly, to a host of antigens present on the tissue and red cells of other species have been demonstrated. Some of these antibodies have an apparently high specificity for antigens the individual has never experienced. This can be accounted for by the phenomenon of cross-reactivity. An antibody, besides binding to its homologous ligand can, not infrequently, bind to other ligands. The binding is frequently weaker than to the homologous ligand, but on occasion a proportion of the antibody produced or some of the responding cells bind more strongly to a different ligand. This is called "heteroclitic reactivity." Almost all immune responses involve the formation of certain amounts of cross-reactive antibody by stimulating related clones, and this feature, which is also discussed as it relates to infectious diseases (Chap. 18), undoubtedly increases the versatility of the immune system.

It is relatively easy to grasp how antibodies function in defense, since they are so important in promoting phagocytosis (opsonization) and have a variety of direct effects. Conceptualization of cellular immunity is less simple. Certain types of infection tend to give rise to chronic inflammatory states. This is best typified by the tuberculin reaction, which is described in detail in Chapter 18. The normal host, animal or man, treated with an extract of tubercle bacilli (tuberculin) develops little or no reaction at the injection site. The presensitized individual develops an accumulation of large mononuclear cells at the injection site which can be palpated as an area of induration. This accumulation, which characteristically takes 36 to 72 hours to develop, is a delayed hypersensitivity reaction.

While it is easy to extract antibody from blood or body fluids and to test for activity, it was not easy for the early immunologist to extract the reactive cells from the site of a delayed hypersensitivity reaction or to measure their activity. Within the last few years, many in vitro techniques for determining cellular reactivity have been developed, and various procedures for the recovery of active cells are now available. Already mentioned were extraction and transfer of effector cells from regional or draining lymph node. If antigen is injected into the peritoneal cavity, or if suitable sponge matrices are impregnated with antigen, the reactive cells can be recovered in the ascitic fluid or from the sponge. Although the full extent of cellular reactivity remains to be realized, it is known that tuberculinlike or delayed-type responses are involved in the rejection of transplants and in many autoimmune diseases. The involvement of cellular immunity in the response to viruses and fungi is inferred from the prevalence of these infections in T cell-deficient humans or animals. However, the way in which effector lymphocytes exert their powerful effects has not been fully elucidated, unless it is through the mediation of IgT as discussed earlier.

Most of our recent knowledge of the effector properties of T cells comes from studies with plant extracts called "lectins" or "mitogens" or from reactions observed when lymphocytes from two individuals are allowed to interact in mixed culture (MLC). The most commonly used mitogens are phytohemagglutinin from the red kidney bean, which reacts predominantly but not exclusively with T cells, or with concanavallin A from jack beans. Poke weed berries and roots contain a mitogen which stimulates B cells; the events in B cell stimulation appear to be essentially similar to the changes to be described for T cells.

The T cell stimulated by mitogen shows no morphologic changes for about the first 24 hours. This is, however, a very active period metabolically. Among the fluctuations reported are changes in levels of cyclic AMP and GMP, the phosphorylation of histones, changes in cation flux across the cell membrane, increase in the number of lysosomes, and incorporation of purines into RNA. By the thirty-sixth hour the cell has begun to enlarge. Thymidine incorporation into DNA provides a convenient quantitative measure of the response. The nucleus enlarges, nucleoli become predominant, and the cell divides. Provided stimulation is maintained, repeated divisions occur.

Similar changes, but affecting a smaller proportion of responding cells, are observed in MLC, and the reaction often takes considerably longer to reach its maximum level. Stimulation is by B cells, and the responding cells develop the property of killing nucleated cells from the stimulating donor. These are the cytotoxic

effector cells described in the chapter on tumor immunity (Chap. 23). The proliferation gradually dies down, and the responding cells revert to a resting population of small lymphocytes by about the twelfth day. If new medium and a fresh population of stimulating cells are added, the response is more rapid and the cytotoxic potential much greater. Of considerable interest is the finding that cells, stimulated by autologous lymphoid cells from a donor of the same inbred (syngeneic) strain, that have been modified by exposure to virus (ectromelia or lymphocytic choriomeningitis, for example) or by various haptens respond vigorously but can attach only to cells of similar H-2 type and modified in the same way. The possible importance of the H antigens in the response to virus is under investigation.

Effector lymphocytes can also be generated in vivo by the injection of allogeneic tumor cells or by the transfer of impregnated sponges. If the peritoneal route is employed, the transplanted tumor proliferates briefly and then dies. The residual cellular population is very rich in cytotoxic effector cells that can react with fresh tumor cells in vivo or in vitro and kill them. From such studies it has been learned that divalent (Mg^{++} and Ca^{++}) ions are necessary for the binding of the effector cell to its target. Killing is initiated within 6 minutes after contact is established but may take 30 minutes to complete.

During lymphocyte activation, many substances which affect immunologic reactivity are produced and released into the supernatant. These include factors which can themselves induce lymphocyte transformation (blastogenic factors), factors which can be cytotoxic for target cells in the absence of effector cells or antibody (lymphotoxins), and factors which can induce macrophages to migrate more actively (macrophage migration factor) or inhibit their motility (macrophage migration inhibition factor). These factors probably play a very important role in vivo, but because they are produced in trace quantities and may be highly labile, direct in vivo studies are very difficult.

REGULATION OF IMMUNITY

The immunologist must explain many unusual features of regulation of the level of the immune response and even of the capacity to respond at all. For example, the level of immunity reached is not a simple function of the amount of antigen injected. Giving 100 times as much antigen does not mean that 100 times the amount of antibody will be found. Indeed, there may be a lower level of response, or the larger dose may not only fail to induce a detectable response but may impair reactivity to a subsequent exposure to the same antigen. This refractory state is usually referred to as "immunologic paralysis."

Critical to the outcome of exposure to antigen is, besides the dose, the structure of the antigen (Chap. 13). In general, antigens appear to have two functional components: part of the molecule or the antigenic complex relates to the helper cell and is called the "carrier," and part of the molecule stimulates specific responding lymphocytes and is called the "hapten," or sometimes the active site or "ligand." Frequently, the carrier elicits a T cell response, while the hapten elicits a B cell response.

Regulation of the level and duration of response is both a B cell and a T cell function. Antibody of high affinity for antigen can inhibit immune responsiveness, presumably by competing for available antigen with antibody of lower binding affinity. Characteristically, antibody formed soon after immunization is of low affinity, while the antibody which appears late in the response has higher affinity. The administration of hyperimmune serum can completely inhibit antibody formation or can reduce the amount of antibody formed and can also impair the generation of effector T cells. This offers an approach to the suppression of the immune response to a transplant. The administration of antibody has frequently been used experimentally in the study of tumor immunity (Chap. 23) and, less frequently, to prevent the rejection of skin or kidney grafts. This form of treatment is variously called passive enhancement (because it can enhance the growth of a tumor), antibody-mediated suppression, facilitation, or even antibody-mediated tolerance. There is a very extensive literature on this subject, and in part, this reflects the differing test situations and amount and type of antibody used. Antibody appears to be capable of interfering with the induction of immunity (afferent inhibition), with the immune response proper (central inhibition, as discussed in Chap. 23), or with the functioning, probably the binding, of cytotoxic

effector cells to their target (efferent inhibition). Besides its clinical application in regulating responsiveness, immunosuppression by antibody is valuable in the experimental dissection of various immune processes.

Also of great theoretical and potential practical importance is immunologic tolerance. As with antibody-mediated suppression, there is a bewildering variety of forms of tolerance. One form results from overdosage of antigen, especially polysaccharide antigen, the pneumococcal polysaccharides being a classic example. Another form appears to operate in the developing fetus. The existence of this form of tolerance was postulated by Burnet and Fenner, who reasoned that lymphocytes should respond against antigens present on tissues and organs of the body (self-antigens) unless there was a mechanism to prevent this from happening. They suggested, in the clonal selection hypothesis, that lymphocytes were descended from highly mutable precursors. Each mutation was random and gave rise to daughter cells of differing specificity. In this phase, development of cells that met their appropriate antigen was suppressed. Since the only antigens likely to be encountered in intrauterine life were self-antigens, the deletion of self-reacting clones prevented autoaggression. After maturation, at the time of birth, the high mutation rate was lost, and the response of the mature cells to antigen was proliferation. The hypothesis was tested by Medawar and his colleagues by injecting foreign tissue cells (nonself) into prenatal mice. Mice injected in utero with cells from another strain of mice were unable to respond to skin grafts from the second strain when grafted in adult life. This confirmation of Burnet's hypothesis led to the award of the Nobel prize. However, while most immunologists accept some variant of the clonal selection hypothesis, in its original form it is untenable, since the fetus was later found to be quite capable of responding to a wide variety of antigens, while in some species, tolerance could be induced after birth.

The form of unresponsiveness induced by Medawar is now known as chimerism, and its permanence depends upon the persistence of viable lymphoid cells from the tolerizing donor in the bloodstream and tissues of the recipient. Other forms of tolerance are frequently less long-lasting. Since the early studies of Medawar, many immunologists, most notably Weigle and his colleagues, have studied the induction of tolerance to nonliving antigens. They have been able to distinguish between T cell tolerance and B cell tolerance, to show that minute as well as massive doses of antigen can tolerize, and that aggregated antigen is usually immunogenic, whereas disaggregated antigen is more characteristically tolerogenic. Tolerance may frequently be broken by the injection of lymphoid cells from a normal and especially from a hyperimmunized donor, and it is easier to break B cell tolerance than T cell tolerance.

Tolerance induction is now most frequently studied through the injection of hapten-carrier conjugates. Interesting results are obtained when the same hapten is attached to a different carrier or vice versa and a tolerant host is challenged with the new antigen. From such studies, it has been learned that the nature of the carrier is critical in establishing tolerance and that tolerance can be broken by changing the carrier. Further, animals genetically unresponsive to an antigen for lack of the appropriate *Ir* allele respond well to the same hapten placed on a different carrier. From such experiments it has become abundantly clear that the T cell tolerance to the carrier and B cell tolerance to the hapten are separate states that can be induced independently and that persist for different time periods. Such experiments also led to the conclusion that helper cells have specificity in their ability to handle antigen. Helper function can be an attribute of T cells, although some helper functions are exhibited by macrophages, and regulation of the ability to respond is believed to reside in the T cell. T lymphocytes from immunized donors can also suppress responsiveness, hence their designation, T suppressor cells. Thus, antigen drives the immune response forward; antibody and T suppressor cells damp it down. The net result is the steady state of immunity usually observed as a consequence of immunization.

Interestingly, although perhaps predictably, autologous proteins make excellent carriers for the induction of tolerance to a hapten. Predictability would be based on the failure of the immune system to react against the rest of the body. This is a fundamental prerequisite for the immune system. It must be able to distinguish self from nonself. How this is achieved has baffled immunologists for many years. Ehrlich recognized the problem but glossed over it by coining the self-explanatory descriptive term "horror autotoxicus." Other immunologists generally followed his example and teleologically assumed that the system recoiled from reacting against self. With the recognition that a wide variety of diseases were indeed due to immunologic self- or autoaggression, theoreticians have produced several schemes other than the clonal selection hypothesis to explain the discrimination between self and nonself. Experimentalists, however, have inevitably produced evidence that cannot be readily explained by any one theory.

IMMUNOLOGIC RESPONSIVENESS AND THE GENERATION OF DIVERSITY

Basically, most immunologists do support, at least in part, Burnet's clonal selection hypothesis, but a rather different theory has been proposed by Jerne. Jerne was fascinated by the immense complexity of the major histocompatibility locus, which, incidentally, is known to have many additional components that Jerne was originally unaware of. He suggested that an essential function of the histocompatibility antigens was to serve as a reference standard during the differentiation stage. The theory is a fascinating one and attempts to reconcile many apparently unrelated facts, including the success of the soma of interspecies mules but their gametic failure, the complexity of the MHC, the observation that over 2 percent of lymphocytes respond in MLC but less than 0.1 percent respond to antigen, and the inordinately high turnover of cells (10^8/day) in the thymus. Jerne proposed two subsets of V gene stem cells all directed against alloantigens; one (S) recognizing self-(H)- antigens, the other (A) directed at H antigens of other members of the species. The more polymorphic the H antigens, the larger the A subset would be. The S subset was deleted as per Burnet, and the A subset was encouraged to mutate by discarding thymic cells that were nonmutant while allowing mutant cells to escape from the thymus. Like Burnet's hypothesis, some features were less attractive than others, and several important differences were later suggested.

Burnet's and Jerne's hypotheses are two well-known examples of the general class of somatic mutation theory. The other major class of hypotheses is called the germ line theory. This suggests that all lymphoid cells possess a library of V gene information. The responding cells carry not only genes for the H and L chain constant regions, but also the thousands of genes coding for each V region. The irrelevant V region genes are excluded by formation of a DNA loop that places the selected V gene in apposition to the Fc gene(s).

Two other concepts need to be mentioned. One is the instructional theory proposed by Pauling. At one time, this was almost universally accepted. The nascent immunoglobulin was believed to gain its specificity by the manner of folding around the antigenic template. This theory was made untenable when the amino acid sequence variability and the dependence of specificity on sequence were proven by Tanford, Porter, and Edelman and their colleagues.

Many ingenious experiments have been designed to provide a definitive answer to the enigma of the genetic and molecular bases for the extreme diversity of humoral and cellular immune responsiveness. The question has not yet been resolved. All immunologists accept clonal expansion, which is, that in the great majority of responses, proliferation of specifically responsive cells follows exposure to antigen. However, there is no unanimity about the original state of the cell before it encounters antigen. It is possible that the final answers will only be provided by studies on lymphoid cells from the primitive vertebrate with its simpler immune system or from the fetal animal, especially the fetal sheep or the fetal pig. The fetus in these animals is more completely protected from the environment than in most species because of the unusual form of the placenta. The question is not entirely academic. Had we adequate knowledge of the processes leading to the initiation of immunity, we would be in a better position to plan a rational attack on tumors or to prevent the inception of autoimmune or atopic states.

FURTHER READING

Books and Reviews

Amos DB (ed): Progress in Immunology. New York, Academic Press, 1971

Bach FH, Good RA (eds): Clinical Immunobiology. New York, Academic Press, 1972, vol 1

Bach FH, Good RA (eds): Clinical Immunobiology. New York, Academic Press, 1974, vol 2

Bellanti JA, Dayton DH (eds): The Phagocytic Cell in Host Resistance. New York, Raven Press, 1975

Brent L, Holborow J (eds): Progress in Immunology II. New York, American Elsevier, 1974, vols 2-5

Burnet FM: The Clonal Selection Theory of Acquired Immunity. Nashville, Vanderbilt, 1959

Cooper MD, Lawton AR: The development of the immune system. Sci Am 231:59, 1974

Good RA, Fisher DW: Immunobiology. Stamford, Ct, Sinauer, 1971

Greaves MF, Owen JJT, Raff MC: T and B Lymphocytes: Origins, Properties, and Roles in Immune Responses. New York, Academic Press, 1973

Katz DR, Benacerraf B: The regulatory influence of activated T cell or B cell responses to antigen. Adv Immunol 15:2, 1972

McClusky RT, Cohen S (eds): Mechanism of Cell-Mediated Immunity. New York, Wiley, 1974

Möller G (ed): Transplantation Proceedings, 1972, vol 13

Möller G (ed): T and B Lymphocytes in Humans. Transplantation Reviews, 1973, vol 16

Möller G (ed): Components of Immune Recognition: Detection and Analysis. Transplantation Reviews, 1974, vol 18

Möller G (ed): Concepts of B Lymphocyte Activation. Transplantation Reviews, 1975, vol 23

Nossal GJV, Ada GL: Antigens, Lymphoid Cells and the Immune Response. New York, Academic Press, 1971

Porter R, Knight J: Ontogeny of Acquired Immunity. Amsterdam, Holland, Associated Scientific Publishers, 1972

Samter M (ed): Immunological Diseases, 2nd ed. Boston, Little, Brown, 1971, vols 1 and 2

Sercarz EE, Williamson AR, Fox C (eds): The Immune System: Genes Receptors, Signals. New York, Academic Press, 1974

Shreffler DC, David CS: The H-2 major histocompatibility complex and the I immune response region: Genetic variation, function and organization. Adv Immunol 20:125, 1975

Unanue ER: The regulatory role of macrophages in antigenic stimulation. Adv Immunol 15:95, 1972

Weigle WO: Immunobiological unresponsiveness. Adv Immunol 16:61, 1973

Yoffrey JM, Courtice FC: Lymphatics, Lymph and the Lymphomyeloid Complex. New York, Academic Press, 1970

Selected Papers

Binz H, Wigzell H: Shared idiotype determinants on B and T lymphocytes reactive against the same antigenic determinant 1. J Exp Med 142:197, 1975

Jerne N: The somatic generation of immune recognition. Eur J Immunol 1:1, 1971

Lindahl-Kiessling K, Osoka D: Lymphocyte recognition and effector mechanisms. Proc 8th Leukocyte Culture Conference. New York, Academic Press, 1974

Marshall WH, Valentine FT, Lawrence HS: Cellular immunity in vitro. J Exp Med 130:327, 1969

Ramseier H, Lindermann J: Cellular receptors. Effect of alloantibodies on the recognition of transplantation antigens. J Exp Med 134:1083, 1972

Triplett EL: On the mechanism of immunologic self recognition. J Immunol 89:505, 1962

15
Methods of Detecting and Quantitating Antigen and Antibody Reactions

This chapter is concerned with the various in vitro methods of detecting and quantitating antigen–antibody interactions. The techniques used for detecting antigens differ depending on whether the antigen in question is soluble or cell bound.

SOLUBLE ANTIGENS

Quantitative Precipitation Most techniques examining the reactions of soluble antigens with their antibodies depend upon precipitation. This occurs when a multivalent antigen reacts with divalent IgG antibody. Precipitation depends upon the formation of large insoluble lattices of multiply connected antigen and antibody molecules. A typical quantitative precipitin curve is shown in Figure 15-1. This curve is the result of a quantitative assay which involves adding increasing amounts of an antigen to constant volumes of antiserum. The precipitates formed are washed, and the total protein in the precipitates is determined for each point, commonly by using the Kjeldahl nitrogen estimation method. The curve is linear initially, from zero antigen added to a peak known as the equivalence point. When antigen is added in excess, the amount of protein precipitated usually decreases, since adequate cross-

linking no longer occurs. An antiserum characterized in this way can subsequently be used to determine the amount of antigen in unknown samples, always working in the linear portion of the quantitative precipitin curve, ie, in antibody excess.

Ouchterlony Analysis This is a powerful yet simple technique which allows qualitative detection of antigens in solution and also allows one to determine antigenic relationships between different antigens. A 2 percent w/v solution of hot agar in isotonic saline is poured into a petri dish or onto a microscope slide to a depth of 1 to 2 mm. Using a commercially available punch, various patterns of circular holes can be cut into the agar layer after it is cooled. A commonly used pattern consists of six holes in a hexagonal arrangement around a central hole. When an antiserum and its antigen in solution are placed in adjacent wells, both diffuse through the agar layer and eventually into each other. A band of precipitated antigen forms between the wells. Typical precipitation patterns seen using related and unrelated antigens with a polyspecific serum are shown in Figure 15-2. If the two antigens, A and B, are identical (Fig. 15-2a), a continuous precipitin line is formed between the two antigen wells and the antiserum well. Two unrelated antigens produce the result shown in Figure 15-2b, where the line produced with one antigen completely crosses that produced with the other. This also implies, of course, that the antiserum contains two unrelated populations of antibodies, specific for antigen A and for antigen B, respectively. An interesting pattern is seen when A and B have some antigenic determinants in common. In Figure 15-2c, for example, the antiserum primarily reacts with antigen B, but some of the antigenic determinants are shared by A. The result is a spur of precipitation with antigen B, resulting from diffusion of antibodies which fail to react with A through the zone of precipitation given by A and their subsequent reaction with B.

Radial Immunodiffusion This is a quantitative gel immunoprecipitation technique derived from the older simple linear immunodiffusion technique of Oudin. In the Oudin technique, agar containing the antiserum is allowed to solidify in a test tube, and the antigen,

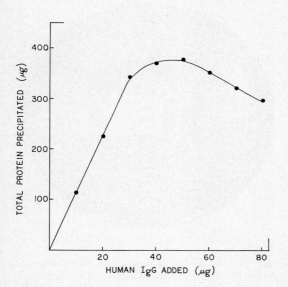

FIG. 15-1. A quantitative precipitin assay of a goat antiserum to human IgG with human IgG as antigen.

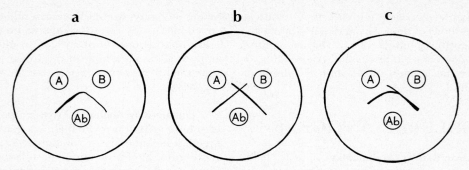

FIG. 15-2. Ouchterlony analysis of a precipitating antiserum (Ab) to two antigens A and B. a. A and B are antigenically identical, and the antiserum reacts equally well with both, showing a line of identity. b. A and B are antigenically unrelated, and separate crossed lines of precipitation are produced with the antiserum. c. A and B are antigenically related, with antigen A possessing only a portion of the antigenic determinants of B, resulting in a spur of precipitation with B.

in solution, is placed on top. A precipitate is formed at the boundary and migrates into the agar. In radial immunodiffusion, the agar containing the antiserum is poured onto a plate, as in the Ouchterlony method, and wells are cut into it. A solution of antigen is introduced, and a circular zone of precipitation forms around the well as the antigen diffuses into the agar and reacts with the antibody. The greater the amount of antigen, the larger the zone of precipitation. In fact, the square of the diameter of the zone of precipitation, or the surface area, is proportional to the antigen concentration when a fixed volume of antigen solution is used. Radial immunodiffusion plates are commercially available for the quantitation of levels of various human serum proteins. In general, standards containing known amounts of the protein in question are placed in the same plate as the unknown sample, and a standard curve is constructed from them. Figure 15-3 shows a radial immunodiffusion plate for the determination of human IgG.

Electroimmunodiffusion In this quantitative technique of immunoprecipitation devised by Laurell, the principle, used in radial immunodiffusion, of incorporating antiserum into the agar layer is again employed. However, instead of relying upon diffusion to establish zones of precipitation, antigen migration is induced electrophoretically. Agarose (ion-free agar prepared by removing the charged agaropectin component) is used in order to reduce the cathodal migration of incorporated IgG seen with agar. The buffer commonly used is one first described by Michaelis; it contains sodium di-

ethylbarbiturate and sodium acetate and has a pH of 8.2 and an ionic strength of 0.1. The samples (1 to 3 μl) are introduced into wells cut into the plate, and electrophoresis is performed with a potential gradient of 3 to 4 volts per cm. Cooling the plate during electrophoresis is usually necessary. Rocket-shaped precipitin lines are formed, their height being proportional to the antigen concentration under standard conditions. Figure 15-4 shows examples of the kinds of patterns produced.

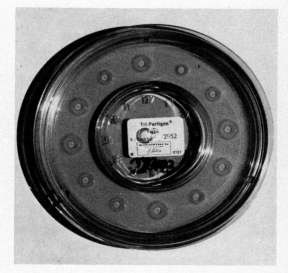

FIG. 15-3. Radial immunodiffusion used to determine human IgG levels. The outer annulus of the plate contains agarose with incorporated goat antiserum to human IgG. In the wells are samples containing various amounts of IgG. Circular areas of precipitation can be seen around each well. (Courtesy of Hoechst A.G.)

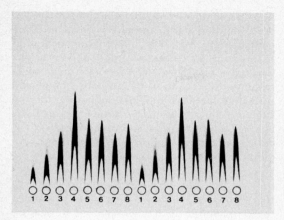

FIG. 15-4. Electroimmunodiffusion used for albumin determination. Duplicate samples (1 to 8) containing varying amounts of human albumin were subjected to electrophoresis through agarose containing goat antiserum to human albumin. (Courtesy of Hoechst A. G.)

Immunoelectrophoresis The immunoprecipitation method of Ouchterlony gives an incredible confusion of precipitated lines when a complex antiserum and a complex antigen mixture (eg, human serum and goat antiwhole human serum) are placed in adjacent wells. The immunoelectrophoresis technique of Grabar and Williams overcomes this problem by electrophoretically separating the complex

antigen mixture before antiserum is added. Figure 15-5 shows the result of a typical immunoelectrophoretic analysis.

The method involves allowing a 2 percent agar solution containing a sodium barbital buffer, pH 8.2, with an ionic strength of 0.1, to solidify on a microscope slide. A die is then used which cuts the pattern shown in Figure 15-5, with wells for the sample adjacent to a trough for antiserum. A sample (2 to 5 μl) is then introduced into the sample well, and electrophoresis is performed for about 45 minutes at 6 volts per cm (for serum). Subsequently, the antiserum (40 to 50 μl) is introduced into the trough, and diffusion of separated antigens and the antiserum gives rise to the arcs of precipitation visible in Figure 15-5. About 30 different human serum proteins can be differentiated using rabbit or goat antiwhole human serum, using this method. By using antisera to pure human serum proteins any arc of questionable identity can usually be unambiguously identified. Immunoelectrophoresis is a frequently used diagnostic tool in medicine, useful in the detection of monoclonal gammopathies, in the detection of Bence-Jones proteins (light chain-dimers) in serum or urine, or for the characterization of many serum protein deficiencies or disorders.

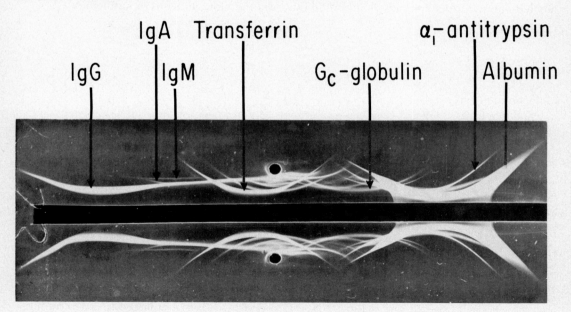

FIG. 15-5. Immunoelectrophoresis of normal human serum. The electrophoretic separation and precipitation with a goat anti-serum to whole human serum were performed as described in the text. The precipitin arcs corresponding to some serum proteins are indicated. (Courtesy of Hoechst A. G.)

Two-dimensional Immunoelectrophoresis This technique can be regarded as a combination of the electrophoretic separation method used in conventional immunoelectrophoresis and electroimmunodiffusion. The antigen mixture is first separated electrophoretically in agarose as described for immunoelectrophoresis. The strip of agarose containing the separated antigens is then placed on a second slide, and an antibody-containing agarose solution is allowed to solidify adjacent to it. Electrophoresis as described for electroimmunodiffusion is then performed at right angles to the original electrophoretic separation, giving rise to peaks such as those shown in Figure 15-6. Quantitation is possible with this technique by comparing the surface area of the precipitated arcs with those given by known amounts of standard antigens.

Radioimmunoassays The most sensitive techniques in use in immunology are the various kinds of radioimmunoassays for the detection and quantitation of antigens. Radioimmunoassays have been developed for the determination of many diverse substances, from hormones to immunoglobulin allotypes. The principle of quantitation used is that of the inhibition assay. Binding of a radioactively labeled antigen to its antibody is inhibited by known amounts of unlabeled antigen to generate a standard curve, and unknown samples are compared to this. The quantitation of bound labeled antigen can be accomplished in various ways. Systems have been devised using electrophoretic separation of antibody-bound and unbound labeled antigen, separation of the immune complex from free antigen on the basis of size by gel filtration, and precipitation of the antigen-antibody complex by an antiimmunoglobulin serum or by the addition of saturated ammonium sulfate. However, the most convenient is the solid-phase radioimmunoassay. In this technique, antibody is covalently attached to an insoluble matrix, commonly to agarose beads which have been activated to bind amino groups using cyanogen bromide. Antibody-bound, radioactively labeled antigen can then be separated from free antigen by centrifugation or filtration. An example of the kind of data obtained in a solid-phase radioimmunoassay is shown in Figure 15-7.

Complement-fixation Tests Complexes of antibodies and antigens, both soluble and cell bound, have the ability to fix the various components of serum complement. Thus, measurements of complement fixation can be used to determine the presence of immune complexes and therefore antigens or antibodies.

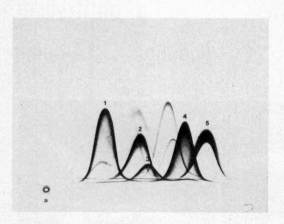

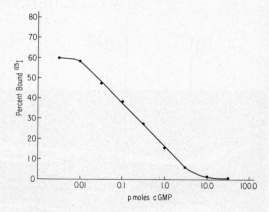

FIG. 15-6. Two-dimensional immunoelectrophoresis. The application well (a) of the first dimension (electrophoresis from left to right) contained normal human serum. The agarose gel of the second dimension (from bottom to top) contained an oligospecific antiserum. The numbered precipitates belong to the following proteins: (1) transferrin, (2) α_2-macroglobulin, (3) ceruloplasmin, (4) α_1-antitrypsin, (5) α_1-acid glycoprotein. (Courtesy of Hoechst A. G.)

FIG. 15-7. A solid-phase radioimmunoassay for guanosine 3'-5'-cyclic monophosphate (cyclic-GMP). Shown is a standard curve obtained by measuring the binding of a radioactive derivative of cyclic-GMP (^{125}I-succinyl-cyclic-GMP-tyrosine methyl ester) to agarose beads with covalently attached rabbit antibody to cyclic-GMP, in the presence of known amounts of unlabeled cyclic-GMP. Unknown samples are quantitated by comparison with this standard curve.

Complement levels are usually measured by adding to aliquots of the complement (normally from guinea pigs) sheep erythrocytes presensitized with rabbit antisheep erythrocyte antibodies. Upon incubation at 37C, hemolysis occurs and can be quantitated by centrifuging the samples and estimating the hemoglobin released into the supernatant by reading its optical density at a wavelength of 541 nm.

The complement-fixation protocol for a soluble antigen involves incubating dilutions of antigen with its antiserum in the presence of an amount of guinea pig complement which will give 90 percent hemolysis of subsequently added sensitized sheep erythrocytes if no fixation occurs. After incubation, usually at 4C for periods up to 18 hours, the sensitized sheep erythrocytes are added and hemolysis is measured after 1 hour at 37C. If complement fixation by antigen–antibody complexes has occurred, it is manifested in reduced hemolysis. The protocol for cellular antigens is the same, except that the antigen–antibody–complement complexes (ie, cells) can be removed by centrifugation before the sensitized sheep erythrocytes are introduced. By comparing them with known standard amounts of antigens, unknown samples of antigen can be quantitated.

CELLULAR ANTIGENS

Agglutination Reactions Hemagglutination as a method of determining human blood groups has been in use since the days of Landsteiner. The principle requires little description. Divalent antibodies cause agglutination by simultaneously binding to two adjacent cells. An extension of the process leads to clumping of many cells, a process easily detectable for red cells by mixing the cells with antisera to A, B, or H specificities on a white tile. Some antisera induce agglutination in isotonic saline (saline agglutinins), while others (albumin agglutinins) require the addition of albumin to the solution. This reduces the repulsive force (the zeta potential) which exists between cells caused by the presence of negatively charged groups on their surfaces.

A refinement of the simple agglutination test described above is the antiglobulin or Coombs test. This method is used in situations where an antibody on the surface of a red cell fails to induce agglutination, by virtue of insufficiency of antigen or antibody. Agglutination is induced by the addition of an antiimmunoglobulin reagent, eg, an antiserum to human immunoglobulin prepared in goats, which reacts with the bound antibody.

A further refinement of hemagglutination assays is the use of passive agglutination of erythrocytes with soluble antigens bound to their surface. The method of attachment depends upon the nature of the antigen. Bacterial lipopolysaccharides bind to red cells upon simple incubation, as do some proteins. Red cells treated with tannic acid will bind protein antigens and are more easily agglutinable than are untreated red cells. Reactive haptens, such as trinitrobenzene sulfonic acid, will covalently attach to red cell membranes. Bifunctional cross-linking agents, such as bisdiazobenzidine, or 1,3-difluoro-4,6-dinitrobenzene can also be used to bind protein antigens to erythrocytes. Cells with bound antigen form a convenient method of detecting and assaying antibodies to almost any hapten or soluble antigen. Inhibition of passive agglutination can also be used to quantitate haptens or antigens in solution.

Hemagglutination is a commonly used technique for detecting red cell antigens, and its usefulness led to attempts to use leukocyte agglutination for the detection of white blood cell antigens, eg, HLA. Such attempts have been largely unsuccessful, and cytotoxicity assays are commonly used for tissue typing.

Cytotoxicity Assays Natural blood group antibodies which lyse erythrocytes in the presence of complement are uncommon, and hemolytic systems are not used for red cell typing. HLA typing of lymphocytes relies almost exclusively upon cytotoxicity. Lymphocytes can be easily prepared from human blood by the technique of Ficoll-Hypaque gradient centrifugation. Ficoll is a commercial high-molecular-weight polysaccharide which induces spontaneous red cell agglutination. Hypaque is a radiopaque dye which is used to vary the density of the Ficoll-Hypaque solution in water. The density of the solution is adjusted to 1.078, at which density agglutinated erythrocytes sink, while lymphocytes float. By simply layering diluted defibrinated blood on the Ficoll-Hypaque solution and centrifuging, lymphocytes can be isolated from the interface.

For HLA typing, the lymphocytes are incubated in small typing trays with human alloantisera specific for the different HLA antigens. Following a wash step to remove unbound antibody, rabbit complement is added to effect lysis. To differentiate between live and dead cells, a vital dye, commonly trypan blue, is added. Such dyes penetrate the membrane of cells lysed by complement but fail to stain living cells. By testing lymphocytes with a battery of sera, unambiguous HLA typing can usually be achieved.

A more quantitative assay of cell death induced by antibody and complement is the chromium[51] release assay. Lymphocytes are prelabeled by incubating with $Na_2{}^{51}CrO_4$, which is rapidly taken up by lymphocytes but released from a viable cell at a rate of only about 5 percent per hour. A cell which has suffered membrane damage due to antibody and complement will release the ^{51}Cr-label very rapidly. Figure 15-8 shows a titration of an anti-HLA antiserum upon human peripheral blood lymphocytes labeled with ^{51}Cr. Dilutions of the serum were added to the cells, followed by the addition of rabbit complement.

Yet another assay of cell death by antibody and complement involves adding fluorescein diacetate (FDA) to the cells. FDA is itself membrane-permeable and nonfluorescent. On entering a cell, natural esterases convert FDA into fluorescein, thus causing the cells to become visibly fluorescent under ultraviolet light. Fluorescein itself is nonmembrane-penetrable and is retained by the cell until lysis occurs. Thus, after a cytotoxicity assay,

dead cells are nonfluorescent and live cells fluorescent.

Immunofluorescence This is a very sensitive technique for the detection of cellular antigens, whether they are cytoplasmic, nuclear, or on the plasma membrane. Direct immunofluorescence requires an antibody which is conjugated to a fluorescent dye, such as fluorescein or rhodamine. The isothiocyanate derivatives of the dyes are used to bind them covalently to IgG preparations of the antisera. Free or fixed cells are then incubated with the fluorescent antibodies, washed, and examined under a microscope with an ultraviolet light source. Cells which have bound the antibody are brightly fluorescent and easily visible.

Indirect immunofluorescence operates in a similar way, except that the fluorescent dye is conjugated to IgG from an antiimmunoglobulin serum. The cells under study are first incubated with the specific antiserum, washed, and then incubated with the fluorescent-conjugated antiimmunoglobulin serum. Stained cells are again detected by observation under an ultraviolet microscope (Fig. 15-9).

The availability of fluorescent dyes of different colors greatly increases the flexibility of the technique, particularly for examining membrane antigens using the technique of capping. Capping is an energy-requiring process whereby certain membrane molecules accumulate over one pole of a cell (particularly a lymphoid cell) when specific antibody mole-

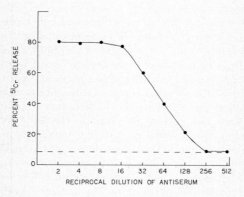

FIG. 15-8. A titration of a cytotoxic anti-HLA-A2 alloantiserum against human peripheral blood lymphocytes from an HLA-A2-positive individual, using the ^{51}Cr-release assay. The dashed line indicates the background release of ^{51}Cr by cells in the absence of antiserum but with added complement.

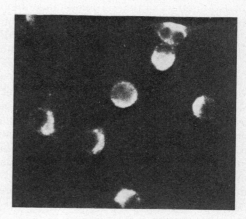

FIG. 15-9. Cytoplasmic staining of a tumor-associated-embryonic antigen in acetone-fixed mouse L-cells, using indirect immunofluorescence. The specific antibody is a rabbit antiserum to a mouse teratoma, and the developing serum is a goat antiserum to rabbit IgG conjugated with fluorescein. (Courtesy of Dr. Linda R. Gooding)

cules bind to them. When a fluorescent antibody is used to induce capping, a brightly fluorescent cap can be observed on the cell under ultraviolet light. If an antiserum conjugated with fluorescein is used to induce capping, the cap is green. A second antibody, conjugated with rhodamine (which emits a red fluorescence) can be added to the capped cells at OC, where capping no longer occurs, and a second stain introduced. If the two antisera react with the same membrane antigenic complex, the rhodamine-labeled antibody will also be visible in the cap. If the two antibodies react with different membrane markers, the rhodamine fluorescence will be visible on the rest of the cell and not isolated in the cap. This technique has been used to prove that membrane immunoglobulin on mouse B cells is not associated with H-2 antigens and that H-2 antigens coded by different genes are not associated with each other on the membrane.

Immunoferritin Techniques The use of specific antibodies to detect cellular antigens by electron microscopy is a technique of increasing value. The principle is similar to that of immunofluorescence, except that the antibody is conjugated to an electron-dense molecule, such as the iron-containing molecule, ferritin. Cells are incubated with ferritin-conjugated antibody, and sections are examined by electron microscopy. Ferritin molecules can be observed on the cell surface where antibodies are bound. Other markers, such as viruses, have been used in place of ferritin and can be distinguished from ferritin morphologically, allowing the detection of two antigens on the same cell using antisera conjugated to ferritin and, for example, to tobacco mosaic virus.

Hemolytic Plaque Assays and Rosette Tests These techniques differ from the others described in that, rather than seeking to detect antibodies or antigens, they serve to detect and enumerate antibody-producing cells.

In the plaque assays, cells producing hemolytic antibodies are the most readily detected. Antibody-secreting lymphoid cells, for example, spleen cells from an immune mouse, are mixed with target erythrocytes in a warm (46C) isotonic 0.6 percent w/v agarose solution. This cell-containing agarose is then overlayered on a preformed 1.2 percent w/v agarose layer in a petri dish. The plates are then incubated at 37C in a humid atmosphere for two hours, during which time IgM and IgG secreted by the antibody-producing cells diffuse and bind to the target erythrocytes. On addition of complement and further incubation, the erythrocytes which have bound IgM antibody will lyse, causing visible clear plaques in the otherwise red agarose, with a plasma cell at the center of each plaque. IgG antibodies do not cause lysis because of their lower lytic and complement-fixing activity, but including an antiimmunoglobulin serum in the top agarose layer enhances complement binding and hemolysis. IgM-secreting cells give direct plaques. IgG-secreting cells requiring development with antiimmunoglobulin serum give indirect plaques.

As an alternative to plaque assays, cells producing antierythrocyte antibodies can be detected by the rosette test. Mixtures of immune lymphoid cells and target erythrocytes are incubated together, and a slide is made of the mixture. Microscopic examination reveals many free erythrocytes and lymphoid cells, but a proportion of the lymphoid cells will have clusters of red cells around them apparently bound to the membrane. These lymphoid cells are the antibody-secreting plasma cells with erythrocytes bound to them by surface antibody.

The flexibility of both the hemolytic plaque assay and the rosette test can be increased to include antigens other than erythrocytes by modification of erythrocytes with haptens or protein antigens, as described for passive hemagglutination.

FURTHER READING

Books and Reviews

Faulk W, Hijmans W: Recent developments in immunofluorescence. Prog Allergy 16:9, 1972

Jerne NK, Nordin AA, Henry C: The agar plaque technique for recognising antibody-producing cells. In Amos DB, Kaprowski H (eds): Cell Bound Antibodies. The Wistar Institute Press, 1963, p 109

Kabat EA, Mayer MM: Experimental Immunochemistry. Springfield, Ill, Thomas, 1961

Laurell CB: Electrophoretic and electroimmunochemical analysis of proteins. Scand J Clin Lab Invest 29[Suppl]: 124, 1972

Weir DM (ed): Handbook of Experimental Immunology. Philadelphia, Pa, Davis, 1967

Selected Papers

Kennedy JC, Axelrod MA: An improved assay for haemolytic plaque-forming cells. Immunology 20:253, 1971

Laurell CB: Quantitative estimation of proteins by electrophoresis in agarose gels containing antibodies. Anal Biochem 15:545, 1966

Mancini G, Carbonara AO, Heremans JF: Immunochemical quantitation of antigens by single radial immunodiffusion. Immunochemistry 2:235, 1965

Mittal KK, Mickey MR, Singal DP, Terasaki PI: Serotyping for homotransplantation, XVIII. Refinement of micro-droplet lymphocyte cytotoxicity test. Transplantation 6: 913, 1968

Ressler N: Two-dimensional electrophoresis of serum protein antigens in an antibody containing buffer. Clin Chim Acta 5:795, 1960

Sanderson AR: Cytotoxic reactions of mouse isoantisera. Br J Exp Pathol 45:398, 1964

16
Inflammation and the Complement System

INTRODUCTION

A primary biologic function of the immune system is protection of the host against microbial invasion and perhaps against the development and spread of neoplasms. To subserve this function, components of the immune system must discriminate self from nonself, then efficiently localize and destroy material recognized as nonself. The discrimination of self from nonself requires the recognition of foreign substances and is mediated by immunoglobulins and by lymphoid cells containing surface (perhaps immunoglobulin) receptors. The interaction of host recognition factors with foreign materials results in a modification of the recognition factor, which in turn leads to the production or release of biologically active molecules. These products enhance vascular permeability locally, produce vascular stasis, and chemotactically attract phagocytic wandering cells, such as polymorphonuclear leukocytes and macrophages, to the local sites of the immune reaction. The generation of biologically active phlogistic products amplifies the initial immune reaction and permits the rapid influx of inflammatory cells capable of localizing, ingesting, and degrading antigenic materials. The production of biologically active molecules and the attraction and activation by these molecules of phagocytic wandering cells is termed an "immune effector function." The inflammatory process is a biologic mechanism by which the immune system mediates the actual localization and destruction of antigens.

The sequence of events leading to an immunologically mediated inflammatory reaction is (1) binding of an antigen to a recognition component, (2) modification of the recognition component, which results in the activation or release of immune effector molecules, which (3) produce a local inflammatory reaction by altering vascular permeability, producing vascular stasis, and chemotactically attracting and activating immune effector cells.

The type of inflammatory process produced by an antigen depends on the amount of antigen present, its chemical nature and biodegradability within phagocytes, its route of entry, and the type of immune recognition factor which detects its presence. For example, antigens which bind to IgE on the surface of mast cells or basophils lead to alterations in cellular cyclic adenosine monophosphate (AMP) levels and selective release by the mast cells of immune effector molecules, such as histamine, slow-reactive substance, and a factor termed "eosinophil chemotactic factor of anaphylaxis" (ECF-A). These molecules can produce vasodilatation, edema, bronchoconstriction, rhinorrhea, and influx of eosinophils. The inflammatory reaction occurs immediately (immediate hypersensitivity) and is maximal within 15 minutes after the interaction of antigen with IgE bound to mast cells (see Chap. 17). Detection of antigens by IgG or IgM molecules results in activation of the complement (C) system and cleavage of biologically active peptides from C components. These products increase vascular permeability, induce vascular stasis, and chemotactically attract polymorphonuclear leukocytes and macrophages. This type of inflammatory reaction, the Arthus type of hypersensitivity, is maximal at 12 to 24 hours after interaction of antigen and antibody (Chap. 19). Antigens recognized as foreign by sensitized T lymphocytes lead to lymphocyte activation and production by the lymphocytes of mediators of inflammation termed "lymphokines" (see Chap. 23). These products enhance vascular permeability, attract and activate macrophages, and produce blastogenesis of other lymphocytes. This type of inflammation, delayed hypersensitivity, is maximal at 24 to 48 hours after the introduction of antigen and is characterized histologically by the accumulation of predominantly macrophages and lymphocytes.

The factors that control the magnitude of an inflammatory response are complex and poorly understood, but they depend in part on the efficiency with which inflammatory cells are mobilized, the amount of antigenic material present, and its digestibility by polymorphonuclear leukocytes or macrophages. It should be emphasized that immunologically mediated inflammatory reactions are normally subclinical and probably continuously ongoing in areas of the body where foreign materials penetrate the internal milieu. Clinically apparent inflammation is usually indicative of a suboptimally effective immune response.

THE COMPLEMENT SYSTEM

During the later part of the nineteenth century it became apparent that microbial invasion produced a number of human diseases and that specific immunization could provide an effective means to prevent certain infections. Studies of immunologic mechanisms of host defense against bacteria demonstrated that microorganisms injected into the peritoneal cavities of immune animals underwent rapid dissolution. Bacteria were similarly lysed in vitro when added to the cell-free serum of immunized animals. Serum that had been aged for a few weeks or had been heated at 56C, however, no longer supported a bactericidal reaction despite the fact that it still contained antibacterial antibody. The bactericidal reaction therefore required antibody and a heat-labile serum factor initially termed "alexin" (Greek, to ward off) and now called "complement."

Complement is a series of proteins which interact as an enzyme cascade and function as an immune effector of the acute inflammatory response (Table 16-1). Activation of the complement system on the surface of cells results in the production of structural and functional membrane alterations which lead to cell death. During sequential activation of complement (C), a number of biologic events are initiated which facilitate the localization and destruction of foreign material by immune effector cells.

The C system can be activated by two synergistic pathways. The classical pathway, which consists of three components, C1, C4, and C2, is activated by immune complexes of antigen and IgG or IgM antibodies. The first component, C1, functions as a naturally occurring antiglobulin and, under appropriate conditions, binds to the Fc portion of IgG or IgM molecules. Following binding, C1 acquires esterase activity and can cleave its natural substrates, C4 and C2, which bind to the immune complex and have proteolytic activity capable of cleaving C3. The second pathway, the properdin or alternative pathway, bypasses C1, C4, and C2 and enters the reaction sequence at the level of C3.

The Classical Complement Pathway

The first component of C, C1, is composed of three separate proteins, C1q, C1r, and C1s, which dissociate in the absence of calcium. C1q is the recognition subunit of the classical C system. This protein is chemically similar to collagen and combines with the Fc portion of either IgM or IgG antibody which has been altered by attachment to an antigen or by heat aggregation. The secretory (IgA) and

TABLE 16-1 THE HUMAN COMPLEMENT SYSTEM

Component	Concentration in Serum (μg/ml)	Molecular Weight	Sedimentation Coefficient	Relative Electrophoretic Mobility
Classical Pathway				
C1q	180	400,000	11.1	γ_2
C1r	—	180,000	7.5	β
C1s	110	86,000	4.5	α
C4	640	206,000	10.0	β_1
C2	25	117,000	4.5	β_1
Properdin Pathway				
Properdin	25	184,000	5.4	γ_2
Factor D(C3PAse)	—	24,000	3.0	α
Factor B(C3PA, GBG)	200	93,000	5.6	β
C3b	—	171,000	9.0	α_2
Terminal Components				
C3	1,500	180,000	9.5	β_2
C5	80	180,000	8.7	β_1
C6	75	95,000	5.5	β_2
C7	55	110,000	6.0	β_2
C8	80	163,000	8.0	γ_1
C9	230	79,000	4.5	α
Inhibitory Components				
C1 INH	180	90,000	—	α_2
C3b INA (KAF)	25	100,000	—	β_2
C6 INA	—	—	—	β_1
Anaphylatoxin INA	—	310,000	—	α

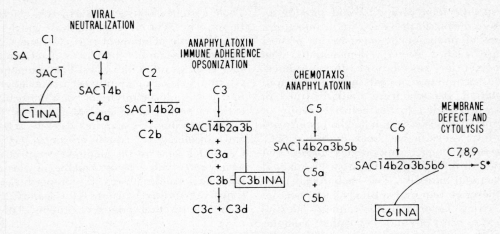

FIG. 16-1. The complement cascade and biologic activities mediated by the complement system. S indicates an antigenic site, and A indicates antibody of the IgG or IgM class; *indicates a lytic site.

reagenic (IgE) immunoglobulins are not normally capable of binding C1q. In the case of IgM, a single molecule of antibody complexed with antigen is capable of binding C1q, whereas two adjacent IgG molecules on the surface of an antigen are necessary for C1q fixation. The active site of the C1 enzyme (C$\overline{1}$)° has esterase activity and is on the C$\overline{1}$s subunit of the molecule. It has been suggested that C1r plays the role of an intermediate agent between C1q and C1s in the C1 activation process. The subunits of C1 are bound by one molecule of calcium, and classical pathway activation will not proceed in the presence of chelating agents such as EDTA.

The next step in the C sequence is the enzymatic cleavage of C4 by C1s into a large fragment, C4b, and a smaller fragment, C4a (Fig. 16-1). The C4b fragment has an active site which can bind to cell membranes or other antigen surfaces. As many as 20 C4b sites can cluster around a single C1 site, thus producing amplification at this step. The next reaction involves magnesium-dependent absorption of C2 to the cell-bound C4b. Following absorption, the C2 molecule is cleaved by the C1s enzyme into two fragments, one of which, C2a, becomes bound to the C4b. The C$\overline{4b2a}$ enzyme (C3 convertase) then can cleave C3 into two fragments, C3a, which is released into the fluid

°*A bar over a C component indicates that it is in its enzymatically active form.*

phase and possesses anaphylatoxinlike activity (see below), and C3b, which binds to the surface of the antigen. The C$\overline{4b2a}$ enzyme can cleave many thousand C3 molecules, but only the C3b fragments which become bound adjacent to C$\overline{4b2a}$ participate in the cleavage of C5. It should be noted that C3b molecules can interact with elements of the properdin pathway, leading to cleavage of additional C3 and C5 (see below). As a consequence of the enzymatic cleavage of C5, the C5a fragment is released into the fluid phase and functions as a mediator of inflammation. The C5b fragment may remain bound to the C$\overline{4b2a3b}$ complex and combine with C6 and C7, on the antigen surface, or it may form a C5b6 complex, dissociate from the earlier components and combine with C7 in the fluid phase. This C5b67 complex can in turn bind to membrane surfaces. C8 then binds to the C5b subunit of the C5b67 complex and then C9 combines with C8. It is believed that C8 initiates and C9 accelerates complement-mediated membrane damage.

Mayer has provided evidence that only one complement lesion is necessary for cell lysis. This hypothesis has become known as the one-hit theory. In order to prove it, it was necessary to determine whether the number of cells destroyed by complement activation was directly proportional to the amount of C present. By varying the number of available effective molecules of C1, C4, and C2, a direct correlation between the number of cells destroyed and the amount of C utilized was demonstrated, thereby supporting a one-hit theory of complement lysis.

The Properdin Pathway

Early in the 1950s Pillemer described a factor in serum which combined with zymosan, a yeast cell wall polysaccharide, and selectively consumed C3 while apparently not requiring C1, C4, and C2. Pillemer termed the factor which bound to zymosan "properdin" (Lat. *perdere:* to destroy). Other workers subsequently demonstrated a similar bypass of the early acting C components when serum was incubated with a factor derived from cobra venom or with bacterial lipopolysaccharides (endotoxins). The action of the properdin pathway required magnesium, a hydrazine-sensitive factor called factor A, and a heat-labile factor termed factor B. Since these factors bore striking chemical similarities to C4 and C2, the properdin system was at first disputed to be a function of efficient utilization of natural antibody and C1, C4, and C2. Subsequent investigation has clearly established the existence of an alternative (properdin) C pathway. In recent years, components of the properdin system have been isolated and purified and are distinct from the early acting proteins of the classical complement sequence.

The exact reaction sequence of the properdin pathway, as well as its mode of activation, including the role of antibody and properdin, is not yet clear. What is presently established is that factor B (also called C3 proactivator [C3PA] or glycine-rich beta-globulin [GBG]) provides the catalytic subunit for C3 cleavage (Fig. 16-2). Factor B exists in serum as an inactive precursor and may be cleaved by factor $\overline{D}$ (also called C3Pase or GBGase) into two subunits, $\overline{B}$ and a small inactive subunit. Factor B may also be cleaved by plasmin or trypsin. C3b is essential for the production of the biologically active cleavage-product of factor B ($\overline{B}$). It appears that C3b is required for the assembly of properdin system enzymes and provides a binding site for factor B which allows its proper cleavage by factor $\overline{D}$ or by other proteolytic enzymes. In any case, C3b, factor $\overline{D}$, and factor $\overline{B}$ form a C3 cleaving unit with similarities to $C\overline{4b2a}$. The role of properdin may be to stabilize the factor D,B,C3b complex. The C3b requirement of the properdin pathway may be produced by cleavage of C3 by the $C\overline{4b2a}$ enzyme from the classical pathway or by cleavage of C3 by proteolytic enzymes, such as plasmin or trypsin. Destruction of C3b is mediated by a C3b inactivator (KAF) which cleaves C3b

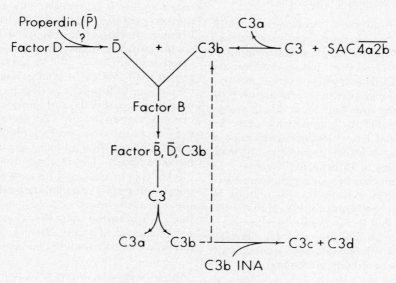

FIG. 16-2. The properdin pathway.

into the biologically inactive fragments, C3c and C3d. In the absence of the C3b inactivator, an autocatalytic, positive feedback loop would drive the properdin pathway until all available C3 was consumed.

The relative biologic importance of the properdin system, as compared to the classical C pathway, is unclear at this time. It is apparent however, that the two pathways act synergistically in whole serum, since selective blockage of the classical pathway depresses the rate of C3 cleavage by such properdin pathway activators as endotoxin, zymosan, and inulin. This synergism may reflect the role of $\overline{C4b2a}$ in producing the C3b required for the properdin pathway function. In addition, C1s itself may function independently of C4 and C2 in the activation of the properdin pathway.

Biologic Activities Mediated by the Complement System

VIRUS NEUTRALIZATION. The binding of antibodies to certain viruses results in the formation of infectious virus-antibody complexes (VA). The addition of C1 and C4 to VA produces virus neutralization. Sequential addition of the later acting C components produces additional virus neutralization. The mechanism of virus neutralization by C may be due to steric hindrance produced by virus-bound C, which prevents the attachment of the virus to cells.

IMMUNE ADHERENCE. Nelson, in 1953, demonstrated that immune complexes that had reacted with C1, C4, C2, and C3 adhered to cells which possessed an immune adherence (IA) receptor. Cells that possess the IA receptor include nonprimate platelets, primate erythrocytes, polymorphonuclear leukocytes, macrophages, and some B lymphocytes. The IA phenomenon may have biologic significance in enhancing phagocytosis (opsonization) by leading to the binding of antigens to phagocytes. IA may also be a mechanism for rapid clearance of immune complexes from the circulation by fixed phagocytic cells (macrophages) in the liver and spleen, and it may permit localization of nonphagocytized complexes at B lymphocyte-rich areas of the spleen and lymph nodes, facilitating additional antibody production.

OPSONIZATION. Antigens that have bound antibody and C1, C4, C2, and C3 are far more easily phagocytized than antigen alone. The addition of C5 further enhances the phagocytosis of immune complexes. Complement-dependent opsonization may be important in limiting bacterial infections, particularly by bacteria such as pneumococci which are poorly opsonized in the absence of C.

ANAPHYLATOXIN ACTIVITY. In 1910 Friedberger found that guinea pigs injected intravenously with serum that had been incubated with immune precipitates developed systemic anaphylaxis. Removal of the immune precipitates, before injection did not prevent anaphylaxis, and Friedberger, therefore, proposed that a toxic factor, anaphylatoxin, was produced by the interaction of serum with immune complexes. It is now realized that anaphylaxis can be produced by IgE-mediated reactions (Chap. 17) as well as by C activation, but the term anaphylatoxin has persisted. It is used to describe a pharmacologically active substance derived from serum which (1) causes hypotension when injected intravenously, (2) causes abrupt contraction of guinea pig ileum with subsequent tachyphylaxis, (3) is blocked from producing ileum contraction by antihistamines, (4) fails to contract estrous rat uterus, (5) increases vascular permeability in guinea pig skin, and (6) degranulates mast cells from guinea pigs but not rat mesenteric preparations. It is now clear that the production of anaphylatoxin activity in serum requires C activation. Two complement-derived peptides, C3a and C5a, have activities in common with classical anaphylatoxin, that is, anaphylatoxin purified from complement-activated serum. C5a is 100 to 1,000 times more potent than is C3a in contracting guinea pig ileum, and C3a produces degranulation of rat mesenteric mast cells, a property not shared by classical anaphylatoxin. C5a therefore appears to be identical to classical anaphylatoxin, while C3a, although less potent, produces similar biologic effects. The biologic function of anaphylatoxins in vivo may be to induce vascular permeability and vascular stasis, thus allowing the efflux of serum proteins, including antibodies, into surrounding tissues and permitting establishment of stable chemotactic gradients necessary for recruitment of phagocytic cells.

CHEMOTACTIC ACTIVITY. Chemotaxis is the unidirectional migration of cells toward an increasing concentration of a chemical attractant.

Leukocytes, such as polymorphonuclear leukocytes and macrophages, are capable of chemotactic migration, while less evidence suggests that small lymphocytes can also migrate chemotactically. Leukocyte chemotaxis can be quantified in vitro using a chamber with two compartments separated by a porous filter. The cells are placed on one side of the filter, and the substances to be tested for chemotactic activity are placed on the other side. The number of cells migrating through the filter can then be counted. Activation of C in serum by inflammatory agents, such as immune complexes or endotoxins, produces chemotactic activity for polymorphonuclear leukocytes and macrophages (Fig. 16-3). The greatest amount of chemotactic activity isolated from activated serum is due to the production of C5a. C3a and an activated macromolecular complex of C5, C6, and C7 also are reported to have chemotac-

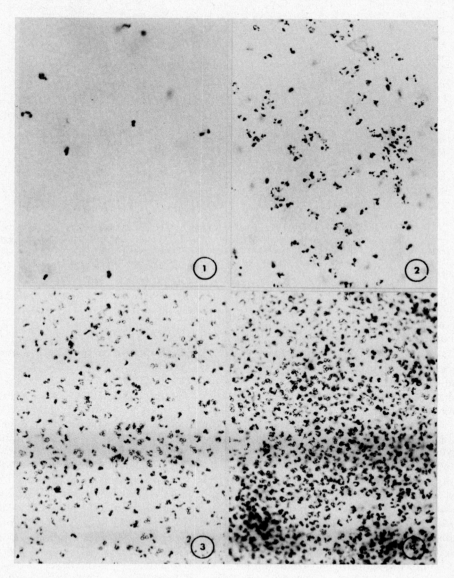

FIG. 16-3. Neutrophil response to chemotactic factor generated by graded doses of *Veillonella alcalescens* endotoxins incubated in guinea pig serum. 1. Serum alone. 2. Serum plus 0.05 μg endotoxin. 3. Serum plug 0.5 μg endotoxin. 4. Serum plus 5.0 μg endotoxin. ($\times$325) (from Snyderman et al: J Exp Med 128:259, 1968)

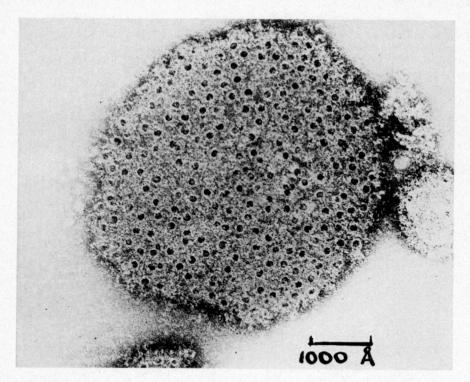

1000 Å

FIG. 16-4. Complement-mediated membrane damage demonstrated by electron microscopy. Human erythrocytes were lysed with anti-I antibody and human complement. Multiple dark round membrane defects measuring approximately 100 Å are present. (× 117,600 Courtesy of Drs. W. R. Rosse and R. Dourmashkin)

tic activity for polymorphonuclear leukocytes. Injection of C5a into the skin produces vasodilatation, vascular stasis, and local accumulation of polymorphonuclear leukocytes and macrophages. The histologic picture looks quite similar to an Arthus reaction (Chap. 19), and indeed C5a is an important mediator of the acute inflammatory response initiated by immune complexes.

MEMBRANE DAMAGE. The interaction of erythrocytes, nucleated cells, or gram-negative bacteria with antibody and C produces cell lysis. Electron microscopic examination of cells that have undergone complement-mediated lysis reveals membrane defects of approximately 90 to 110 Å (Fig. 16-4). There is evidence to suspect that these defects represent the insertion of the activated terminal C components C5 through C9 into the lipid bilayer of the membrane. This hydrophilic core through the membrane produces cell lysis by permitting free movement of water but not of proteins across the cell membrane.

Modulation of the Complement System

Complement activation is modulated by the enzymatic instability of certain C intermediates and by specific inhibitors of certain components. Examples of enzyme instability are the rapid decay of C2a from the $\overline{C4b2a}$ enzyme (half-life about 7 minutes) and of C3b from the SAC $\overline{14b2a3b}$ complex. C1 esterase inhibitor, a normal serum constituent, combines stoichiometrically with $C\overline{1}$, resulting in inactivation of its esterase activity. An inherited deficiency of this inhibitor is associated with hereditary angioneurotic edema. (See below.) A C3b inactivator present in serum destroys the hemolytic, immune adherence, and opsonic activity of C3b by cleaving it into two fragments, C3c and C3d. An inactivator of bound C6 has also been described but is not yet well characterized. In addition to the inhibitors regulating the complement sequence, an anaphylatoxin inactivator has been described which cleaves the C-terminal arginine from the C3a and C5a fragments, rendering them biologically inactive.

Deficiencies of the Complement System and Their Relationship to Human Diseases

Complete or partial deficiencies of all the classical C components, with the exception of C9, and several of the C inhibitors have been described in man or animals (Table 16-2). Some of these deficiencies are associated with severe diseases, while in others clinical manifestations are sporadic. Defects in the C system could result in the inability of the host to efficiently eliminate microbial antigens or circulating immune complexes. Indeed, C deficiencies have been associated with recurrent bacterial and fungal infections as well as with collagen-vascular inflammatory diseases.

A deficiency or dysfunction of the C1 esterase inhibitor results in hereditary angioneurotic edema, an autosomal dominant heritable disease. It is characterized by acute and transitory local accumulations of edema fluid, which, when localized in the larynx, can become life threatening by causing obstruction of the tracheal airways. During attacks, hemolytic C activity in these individuals is markedly depressed due to consumption of C4 and C2 by unregulated C1 esterase. The edema may be

TABLE 16-2 DEFECTS OF THE COMPLEMENT SYSTEM IN MAN

Defective Component	Associated Disease(s)
C1q	Combined immunodeficiency disease
C1r	Glomerulonephritis, polyarthritis
C2	Collagen-vascular diseases
C3	Recurrent infections
C5	Recurrent infections
C6	Septic arthritis
C7	Raynaud's phenomenon, acrosclerosis
C1 inhibitor	Hereditary angioneurotic edema
C3b inactivator	Recurrent infections

produced by a kinin cleaved from C2 by the action of $C\overline{1}s$. Attacks appear to proceed after activation of Hageman factor (factor XII, the plasma protein that initiates clotting), which leads to the formation of plasmin and kallikrein. These proteases cleave and activate C1, resulting in activation of the C system. An approach to the control of this disease has been the use of plasmin inhibitors, such as ε-aminocaproic acid, which reduce the frequency and severity of attacks.

Partial C1q deficiencies have been found in several patients with combined immunodeficiency disease. Normal levels of C1q were restored upon bone marrow transplantation. Selective deficiency of C1r has been found in a few patients with glomerulonephritis and polyarthritis. Deficiencies of the second component of complement have been found in a number of patients with collagen-vascular diseases, particularly systemic and discoid lupus erythematosus.

Individuals with defects or dysfunction of C3 or C5 suffer from severe recurrent bacterial infections. Sera from these patients generate less chemotactic activity and support less phagocytic activity than do normal sera. It should be noted that an almost complete deficiency of these components is required to produce clinically apparent disease. A defect of the C3b inactivator has also been described. A patient with this deficiency had very low levels of C3, because of hypercatabolism of this component, presumably because of constant activation of the alternative C pathway by C3b. This patient suffered from bacterial infections, and serum from this individual was not able to generate chemotactic activity, possibly because C3 is required for the activation of C5. The depression of C3 could be reversed in vivo by the administration of C3b inactivator.

Deficiencies of the late-acting C components have been described recently. Abnormalities of C6, C7, and C8 have been found in several patients. However, the relationship of these terminal C component defects to the pathogenesis of disease is as yet uncertain. C6 deficiency is associated with minimally delayed blood clotting and an increased incidence of septic arthritis. A patient with a C7 deficiency developed a disease similar to progressive systemic sclerosis.

The association of C defects with infectious

diseases could certainly be anticipated, but the high frequency of collagen-vascular inflammatory diseases with deficiencies of C, in particular C1r and C2, was less predictable. This latter association suggests that patients with isolated deficiencies of the early acting classical C components are more susceptible to subtle infections that cause systemic inflammatory diseases, or that elimination of antigens and immune complexes in general by these individuals is suboptimal, thus producing chronic stimulation of the immune response. In any case, understanding the intriguing relationship of C defects with inflammatory diseases will lead to a better understanding of the pathophysiology of these diseases, as well as of the biologic role of the C system.

FURTHER READING

Books and Reviews

Mayer MM: The complement system. Sci Am 229:54, 1973

Nelson RA Jr: The complement system. In Zweifach BW, Grant L, McClusky RT (eds): The Inflammatory Process, 2nd ed. New York, Academic Press, 1974, vol 3, p 37

Rapp HJ, Brosos T: Molecular Basis of Complement Action. New York, Appleton-Century-Crofts, 1970

Samter M (ed): Immunological Diseases, 2nd ed. Boston, Little, Brown, 1971, vols 1 and 2

Selected Papers

Gewurz H, Shin HS, Mergenhagen SE: Interactions of the complement system with endotoxic lipopolysaccharides. Consumption of each of the six terminal complement components. J Exp Med 128:1049, 1968

Jensen J: Anaphylatoxin in its relation to the complement system. Science 155:1222, 1967

Klebanofof SJ: Antimicrobial systems of the polymorphonuclear leukocyte. In Bellanti JA, Dayton DH (eds): The Phagocytic Cell in Host Resistance. New York, Raven Press, 1975, p 45

Muller-Eberhard HJ: Complement and phagocytosis. In Bellanti JA, Dayton DH (eds): The Phagocytic Cell in Host Resistance. New York, Raven Press, 1975, p 87

Muller-Eberhard HJ: Complement. Annu Rev Biochem 44:697, 1975

Pillemer L, Blum L, Lepow IH, et al: The properdin system and immunity: Demonstration and isolation of a new serum protein, properdin, and its role in immune phenomena. Science 120:279, 1954

Ruddy S, Gigli I, Austen KF: The complement system of man. Activation, control and products of the reaction sequence. New Engl J Med 287:489, 1972; Phylogeny, ontogeny, and biology. New Engl J Med 287:545, 1972; Inherited abnormalities. New Engl J Med 287:592, 1972; Acquired abnormalities. New Engl J Med 287:642, 1972

Shin HS, Snyderman R, Friedman E, Mellors A, Mayer MM: Chemotactic and anaphylatoxic fragment cleaved from the fifth component of guinea pig complement. Science 162:361, 1968

Snyderman R, Phillips JK, Mergenhagen SE: Biological activity of complement in vivo: Role of C5 in the accumulation of polymorphonuclear leukocytes in inflammatory exudates. J Exp Med 134:1.131, 1971

Snyderman R, Pike MC: Interaction of complex polysaccharides with the complement system: Effect of calcium depletion on terminal component consumption. Infect Immun 11:273, 1975

Vogt W, Schmidt G, Dieminger L, Lynen R: Formation and composition of the C3 activating enzyme complex of the properdin system. Sequential assembly of its components on agarose. Z Immunitaetsforsch 149:440, 1975

17
Allergy

Allergy is an important part of the host response to infection. Allergic reactions occur as a part of many immune disorders. The most prevalent immune disorder of man is a consequence of allergy to harmless environmental antigens. The classic definition of allergy, altered reactivity to antigen, applies to all immune responses. This definition was devised in 1906 by von Pirquet, who suggested that the definition of immunity be restricted to protective reactions to antigens. Instead, medical use has restricted the definition of allergy to those harmful antigen reactions associated with disease.

An allergic reaction is also a hypersensitivity reaction. Immunologists recognize two general types of allergic reactions. Each is named with respect to the time interval between antigen challenge and the appearance of the reaction. Immediate hypersensitivity reactions occur shortly after antigen exposure and are initiated by the combination of antigen and antibodies. Delayed hypersensitivity reactions occur several days after antigen challenge and are initiated by the combination of antigen and immune cells.

There are two kinds of immediate hypersensitivity reactions. Anaphylactic hypersensitivity occurs within seconds to minutes and is initiated by IgE antibodies. The anaphylactic form of immediate hypersensitivity receives its name from anaphylaxis, the most sudden and violent of all allergic reactions. A second kind of immediate hypersensitivity occurs within hours after antigen challenge. This form of immediate hypersensitivity is named for the immunologist who described it and is called Arthus hypersensitivity. Arthus hypersensitivity is initiated by complement-fixing IgG antibodies.

Anaphylactic hypersensitivity is the principal concern of this chapter. The antibodies responsible for human anaphylaxis are also called reagins and skin-sensitizing and homocytotropic antibodies. Reagin has also been used to describe complement-fixing antibodies; IgE antibodies do not fix complement through the classic (C1) pathway. Homocytotropism, the capacity to sensitize the skin of animals belonging to the homologous species, is shared by IgE and antibodies belonging to other immunoglobulin classes. Anaphylaxis and related allergic diseases are the only known important biologic consequences of IgE antibodies. Therefore, anaphylactic antibodies will be used as the exclusive synonym for IgE antibodies in this chapter.

Allergic reactions are harmful. They occur in susceptible individuals who have been previously exposed to an antigen. Subsequent exposure of the individual to the same antigen can cause inflammation, disease, and death. The immune system of allergic individuals responds to antigen by activating accessory systems which cause inflammation. A hypersensitivity reaction is an immunologically initiated inflammatory reaction. Mobile cells and protein components of the body fluids and other tissues make up the accessory systems recruited by hypersensitivity reactions. The accessory system responsible for anaphylactic hypersensitivity is composed of tissue mast cells and circulating basophils. Mast cells and basophils secrete enriched quantities of chemicals called "mediators," which produce the tissue changes characteristic of anaphylactic allergic reactions.

Important differences exist between the two immediate types of hypersensitivity and delayed hypersensitivity. Different immune mechanisms initiate each type of allergic reaction, and the accessory systems activated by each mechanism are different. Each type of hypersensitivity produces a characteristic type of inflammation. Anaphylactic hypersensitivity produces extensive anatomic change but very little tissue destruction. Arthus-type hypersensitivity produces cell death and destruction of normal anatomic structures. Delayed hypersensitivity causes cell death and less anatomic destruction. Differences in the immune and accessory systems involved in hypersensitivity reactions provide a basis for clinical intervention in allergic diseases.

HYPERSENSITIVITY REACTIONS

Allergens Certain antigenic products of the natural environment are clinically important because of their ability to produce allergic disease. Antigens that provoke spontaneous hypersensitivity reactions are called "allergens" in order to suggest the expectation of a harmful immune reaction. These include (1) microbiologic organisms and their products, (2) airborne products of plant, animal, and insect origin, (3) drugs and other chemicals, and (4) certain foods. This classification of allergens includes polysaccharides, proteins, and small hapten molecules of natural and synthetic origin. Classifications of allergens can be based on (1) their frequent association with a specific allergic disease, (2) the ecologic probability of harmful exposure, and (3) the immunogenic properties of the particular allergen.

ALLERGIC REACTIONS.   Immediate and delayed allergic reactions can occur in healthy persons and in patients. Severe reactions cause symptoms and occur in allergic diseases. Skin tests provide a clinically useful way of evaluating allergen hypersensitivity. The tuberculin or Mantoux skin test is a classic example of a clinically useful skin test. A small quantity of tuberculin allergen is injected into the dermis of the skin. Clinical and histopathologic examination of the sequence of changes at the site of allergen challenge in tuberculin-sensitive patients usually reveals immediate and delayed hypersensitivity reactions. Alternately, one or the other type of hypersensitivity reaction may dominate the test site. The anaphylactic portion of the allergic reaction to tuberculin appears within seconds to minutes. Itching and burning at the skin test site are followed by the development of erythema and a central area of edema. Microscopic examination reveals local vascular congestion and edema and an absence of inflammatory cells and cell death. Local swelling and redness increase over the next 6 to 12 hours. With certain protein allergens, this intermediate portion of the reaction can reveal a mononuclear cell infiltrate and eosinophils followed by infiltration of basophilic mononuclear cells and lymphocyte cuffing about postcapillary venules. This unusual intermediate portion of the skin test reaction is called "Jones-Mote hypersensitivity" after the investigators who described it (Fig. 17-1). Some of the histopathologic events of this intermediate basophilic allergic reaction appear to be initiated by antibodies. Other portions involve the participation of immune cells. During this interval, swelling and redness increase. The reaction site becomes tender and ecchymotic and exhibits surrounding petechiae. Severe reactions exhibit central softness and become necrotic. These destructive changes are mediated by complement-fixing IgG and IgM antibodies. The destructive portion of the immediate

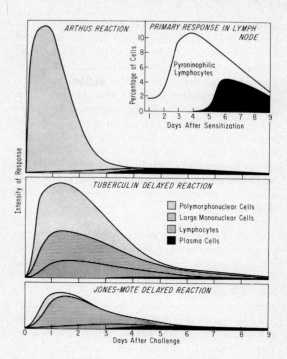

Fig. 17-1. A comparison of the time course of changes in the cell composition of several cutaneous hypersensitivity reactions and the primary response to antigen in the lymph node. Note the prominence of lymphocytes and mononuclear cells in the typical Jones-Mote reaction and the similarity of this response to the primary response in lymph nodes. In contrast, polymorphonuclear leukocytes predominate in the Arthus reaction. The typical cutaneous response to tuberculin reveals a cell composition that lies between these two extremes. Differences in the cutaneous response to antigen reflect differences in the kind of hypersensitivity responsible for the skin test reaction.

hypersensitivity reaction reaches a maximum 24 to 36 hours after antigen challenge. This portion of the immediate reaction is called an "Arthus reaction" after the investigator who described this form of hypersensitivity. Microscopically, edema, cell death, thromboses of small blood vessels, and tissue necrosis with destruction of anatomic boundries are evident. An intense infiltrate of polymorphonuclear leukocytes is present (Fig. 17-1). A severe Arthus reaction can obscure other portions of the immediate and delayed response.

The typical delayed cutaneous hypersensitivity reaction appears as the immediate reaction subsides. Residual portions of severe immediate hypersensitivity reactions are often superimposed on the delayed response. Delayed reactions exhibit less warmth and tenderness and are much less red and swollen. The typical delayed reactions feel firm or indurated to the touch. Microscopically, the delayed hypersensitivity response reveals a mononuclear cell infiltrate composed of lymphocytes, large mononuclear cells, a few plasma cells, and a small number of polymorphonuclear cells (Fig. 17-1). Although many of the histopathologic changes of the delayed hypersensitivity reaction begin during the intermediate cutaneous basophilic reaction, the delayed reaction reaches maximum intensity 48 to 72 hours after allergen challenge and can persist for more than a week.

ALLERGEN RESPONSIVENESS.   The ability of an individual to respond to an allergen is dependent upon prior exposure and an innate capacity to recognize and respond to the specific allergen. Normal subjects become sensitized to many common allergens. In healthy persons, modest immediate and delayed hypersensitivity reactions occur to allergens prepared from the streptococcus, mumps virus, *Candida albicans*, and many other microorganisms. Skin test reactions can be used clinically as a quantitative measure of immune function. Allergic patients exhibit increased reactions to many common allergens. Differences between normal and allergic patients can be detected either (1) as increased reactivity to allergens which provoke small reactions in normal persons or (2) as reactivity to allergens which fail to elicit responses in exposed normal persons. At the other extreme of responsiveness, patients can fail to react to allergens which cause responses in most normal people, despite known exposure and the ability to respond to other allergens. Individuals who exhibit innate specific unresponsiveness are called "nonresponders." Care must be taken to distinguish between patients who are unresponsive because of disease activity or drug therapy and patients who are nonresponders to a specific allergen. Positive responses to other allergens help distinguish between nonresponders to specific allergens and general unresponsiveness.

Approximately one person in five exhibits an innate capacity to develop exquisite anaphylactic hypersensitivity. These individuals often develop severe allergic diseases. This unusual constitutional tendency toward allergic disease is called "atopy," and the allergic diseases caused by anaphylactic hypersensitivity are atopic diseases. Anaphylaxis is an atopic disease. Collectively, atopy and the atopic diseases probably represent the most common immune disorder of man. Atopy is a familial disorder, and a family history of atopy and other immune disorders is important in the evaluation of allergic patients. Transient increases in anaphylactic hypersensitivity occur in nonatopic patients following antigen stimulation. For example, cutaneous anaphylactic hypersensitivity to the type-specific pneumococcal polysaccharide occurs during the recovery phase of pneumococcal pneumonia. This transient hypersensitivity differs from the persistence of anaphylactic hypersensitivity characteristic of atopic patients.

Hypersensitivity and Infection   Relationships among immunity, allergy, and unresponsiveness are shown in Figure 17-2. At one end of the spectrum of host responsiveness, the immune individual eliminates microorganisms without the penalty of extensive tissue disruption. The immune host remains healthy despite exposure to potentially infectious agents. An unresponsive host is illustrated at the opposite end of the same spectrum. Unresponsiveness results in an immunologically compromised host, who is susceptible to infection with nonpathogenic microorganisms. In these patients, tissue injury and disease result from the toxic effects of the replicating microorganism.

Allergic hosts lie between these two extremes. The allergic patient is responsive but cannot eliminate the microorganism or its toxic products without the penalty of extensive tissue disruption. Hypersensitivity is responsible for many of the symptoms and tissue changes produced by infectious diseases. The clinical severity of the infection is often proportionate to the intensity of the hypersensitivity reaction. Hypersensitivity to infectious agents represents an intermediate level of immune function, between unresponsiveness and a completely protective response. Quantitative studies indicate that normal immune function is decreased in allergic patients.

Figure 17-2 presents a simplification of the response of allergic patients to microorganisms. Immunity, hypersensitivity, and unresponsiveness to different antigens of the same infectious agent can occur simultaneously. For example, a patient who is immune to toxins and

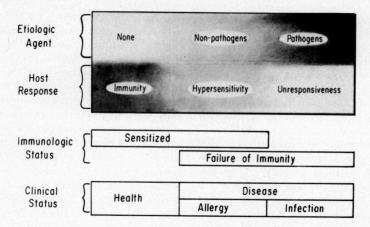

Fig. 17-2. A schematic representation of the relationships among etiologic agents, host responsiveness, and the immunologic and clinical status of the individual.

other antigenic components of an infectious agent can be allergic to harmless antigenic components of the same organism. Under these circumstances, the infection behaves as an allergic disease.

An allergic component of an infectious disease is suspected when the patient's symptoms are unusually severe or protracted. This expectation becomes reinforced when the infection occurs in a known allergic patient. Modification of the hypersensitivity reactions becomes an important part of treatment. Improvement after treatment for hypersensitivity provides additional evidence of an allergic basis for the patient's symptoms. Direct evidence that the patient's symptoms or disease can be caused by a hypersensitivity reaction is needed to confirm an allergic component of the infectious disease.

Allergic Diseases Hypersensitivity reactions can also be caused by allergens which are neither infectious nor otherwise harmful. An allergic disease is suspected when a harmless substance provokes inflammation in patients but not in similarly exposed healthy individuals. Production of a hypersensitivity response in some but not all allergen-exposed individuals is one requirement of an allergic disease. This attribute can be demonstrated by in vivo allergen testing in patients and normal subjects. The direct skin test is the classic method for detection of allergic reactions. In vitro tests which measure various components of hypersensitivity reactions can also be used to detect allergic reactions. Occasionally, it is necessary

to know that an allergen-induced hypersensitivity reaction can cause the actual symptoms of an allergic disease. Allergen provocation tests are used to provoke characteristic symptoms and physiologic changes consistent with the allergic diseases. In a provocation test, naturally occurring allergen exposure is simulated. Allergen exposure is carefully controlled and stopped when symptoms or disease-related changes are detected. The provocation of respiratory symptoms by inhalation of airborne allergens represent an example of this test procedure. Provocation tests involve considerable risk and are not used unless the potential gain to the patient outweighs the risk.

Participation of an immune mechanism is the second requirement of a hypersensitivity disease. Evidence is needed that the hypersensitivity reaction can be initiated by specific antibodies or immune cells. The passive transfer of the reaction with antibodies or immune cells provides a critical means for confirming an immunologic basis for an allergic reaction. Allergic reactions can be passively transferred from a sensitized donor to a normal recipient with antibodies or immune cells. In vitro tests with adoptively sensitized normal cells can be used to detect the immunologic initiation of an allergic reaction.

ANAPHYLAXIS

Anaphylactic death was first clearly described in 1839 by Magendie, who reported the sudden death of rabbits following several injections of egg albumin. An awareness of the lack of protection provided by certain kinds of exposure developed after the studies of Richet and Portier in 1902, who observed the unexpected death of dogs previously insensitive to the toxin principle of a sea anemone. Richet identified the condition as the opposite of protection (phylaxis) and coined the term "anaphylaxis." Prausnitz and Küstner reported the passive transfer of anaphylactic hypersensitivity to fish proteins in 1921. Küstner was allergic to fish proteins. Intradermal injection of small quantities of Küstner's serum passively transferred fish allergen hypersensitivity to the skin of nonallergic human recipients but not to guinea pigs. The serum antibody responsible for anaphylaxis remained elusive until 1967 when biochemical studies by the Ishizakas identified IgE as the carrier of anaphylactic hypersensitivity.

Systemic anaphylaxis occurs within seconds after antigen challenge. Death occurs when the allergic reaction impairs the function of a physiologic system necessary for life. Anaphylactic death can be experimentally induced in guinea pigs, rabbits, dogs, rats, mice, horses, calves, pigeons, and monkeys. Anaphylactic reactions occur in man. The physiologic consequences of anaphylaxis differ among animal species, probably because of variation in the distribution of chemical permeases responsible for anaphylaxis. If life can be sustained and the allergic reaction stopped, the tissue changes induced by anaphylaxis can be reversed, and complete recovery is possible.

Anaphylaxis in Man In man, anaphylaxis usually begins with intense itching about the ears and scalp. Clinical recognition of pruritis as a first symptom of anaphylaxis is important, since prompt parenteral treatment with 0.1 to 0.3 ml of 1:1,000 adrenalin can prevent death and modify the severity of the reaction. If untreated, the pruritis is followed rapidly by angioedema, urticaria, asthma, malaise, and weakness. Although fatal anaphylaxis is rare, syncope, cyanosis, shock and death can occur. Anaphylactic death usually results from respiratory failure and occurs most often in atopic patients who have a constitutional predisposition to severe allergic reactions.

Instances of human anaphylaxis have decreased in the past four decades. This trend is a result of the use of antibiotic therapy instead of passive immunization with sera for infectious diseases. The passive immunization of human beings with immune sera raised in rabbits, horses, and other animal species formerly provided an effective means of therapy for severe infections. Exposure of patients to heterologous serum also causes sensitization to the foreign serum proteins. The heterologous serum protein antigens persist in the passively immunized patient and cause anaphylaxis and the serum sickness syndrome. This hypersensitivity disease usually begins 6 to 10 days following the sensitizing dose of the heterologous serum. Symptoms begin when the patient produces antibodies to the passively administered foreign serum proteins. IgE antibodies are produced and cause anaphylaxis. Complement-fixing antibodies are produced and cause the serum sickness portion of the illness. The time required to generate antibodies is different for each of the antigenic proteins of a heterologous serum. Protracted symptoms can occur when the patient generates anaphylactic and complement-fixing antibodies to several serum proteins, resulting in recurring episodes of anaphylactic hypersensitivity. Heterologous serum therapy should not be used without precautions to avoid fatal anaphylaxis.

Recently, hyperimmune human sera against toxins and infectious agents have become available. Human serum is homologous, and the risk of anaphylaxis from passive immunotherapy is small. Hyperimmune human serum can be used in the treatment of tetanus, mumps, measles, and other infectious agents which cannot be treated with antibiotics.

Despite this trend, certain forms of therapy result in antigen exposure and anaphylaxis in man. Heterologous antihuman lymphocyte and thymocyte sera are used in the experimental suppression of immunity in transplant patients. Hypersensitivity to antibiotics and other drugs is a frequent cause of anaphylactic hypersensitivity in patients. Penicillin allergy has replaced heterologous serum therapy as a frequent cause of anaphylactic hypersensitivity in patients. Wasp and bee stings also cause unexpected anaphylaxis. An awareness of the reversibility of this violent form of hypersensitivity is clinically important.

Experimental Anaphylaxis Guinea pigs can be sensitized for anaphylaxis with as little as 0.1 mg of protein. Injection of the same dose of antigen three weeks later produces anaphylaxis. Within 30 to 60 seconds after challenge, the sensitized animal exhibits agitation, pilorection, coryza, and sneezing, and often defecates and/or urinates and makes a few spasmodic jumps. Respiration becomes slowed and forceful as the animal becomes cyanotic and appears preoccupied with breathing. Convulsions occur, and respiratory death follows within minutes. Necropsy reveals distention of the lungs with air. Bronchospasm is the primary cause of anaphylactic death in the guinea pig.

Rabbits are more difficult to sensitize for anaphylaxis than are guinea pigs. Allergen challenge provokes arrhythmic respiration, panting, and hyperemia of the ears, which characteristically blanch when the animal falls, convulses, exhibits exophthalmos and head retraction, and dies. Necropsy reveals dilatation of the right auricle and ventricle and engorgement of the inferior vena cava, portal vein, and liver. Heart failure and death result from smooth muscle constriction in the pulmonary arterioles.

Anaphylaxis in dogs begins with agitation, salivation, and emesis, which may be followed by bloody diarrhea. Blood pressure and body temperature fall, respirations become slow and labored, muscle tone is lost, and the animal dies of vascular collapse. Blood coagulability, neutrophil counts, and complement activity are decreased. Necropsy reveals accumulated leukocytes in the lungs, enlargement of the liver, and pooling of blood in the liver and gastrointestinal tract.

Anaphylactic hypersensitivity is difficult to induce in rats and mice. Repeated doses of antigen with adjuvants, potentiating factors (cold, endotoxins, x-ray, and other forms of shock), and adrenalectomy have been used. Anaphylaxis in mice results in circulatory shock with hemoconcentration and death. Death may be prevented by the use of plasma expanders.

THE ATOPIC DISEASES

The atopic diseases were defined in 1923 by Coca and Cooke. Atopy is defined as a predisposition toward an abnormal hypersensitiveness. Cooke included patients with anaphylaxis, asthma, angioedema, urticaria, certain forms of acute gastroenteritis, and allergy to infectious agents among those considered atopic. Studies of the clinical epidemiology of atopy reveal a tendency of certain atopic diseases to cluster in families. This finding prompted Cooke to suggest that genetic influences control anaphylactic hypersensitivity and the susceptibility to the atopic diseases.

Constitutional Susceptibility Atopy occurs with varying severity in 10 to 30 percent of the population of the United States. Atopic individuals are susceptible to anaphylaxis and other allergic disorders which cause conjunctivitis, rhinitis, sinusitis, bronchitis, asthma, angioedema, urticaria, and certain types of gastrointestinal disturbances. Pollen hay fever and allergen-induced asthma are the most prevalent atopic diseases. Atopic patients with allergic diseases make up a large portion of the practice of ambulatory medicine. The incidence of atopy in families increases with the number of kin surveyed. For example, approximately 25 percent of atopic patients have at least one atopic parent. This incidence increases to more than 40 percent when grandparents are included and to more than 50 percent when the patient's siblings are also included. The prevalence of similar atopic diseases in families is greater than chance expectation. Shared environmental influences or a genetic predisposition toward atopic disease could account for this remarkable clustering of similar illnesses within certain families.

Evidence of a genetic component of atopy stems from recent studies of the associated segregation of the immune response to specific allergens and genetic markers in human families. The size of the skin test response to pollen allergens appears associated with the haplotype chromosome responsible for the histocompatibility (HLA) antigens inherited by family members. Analogous studies of the immune response in experimental animals suggest that this family association of tissue antigens and specific immune responses represents linkage between genes controlling the response to the specific allergen and the transplantation antigens of man. Evidence of similar HLA-associated immune response (Ir) genes controlling the specific response to bacteria and viruses can also be detected in man. These recent observations suggest that genetic mechanism controlling allergen recognition are located on the chromosome that is responsible for the major histocompatibility complex of man.

Allergen exposure results in sensitization and production of IgE by cells proximate to the skin and mucosal surfaces of the body. In contrast to evidence of the genetic control of atopic predisposition, studies of monozygotic twins reveal more than 70 percent discordance in the development of clinically significant atopic disease. Environmental factors, such as allergen exposure, contribute to the selection of atopic individuals who develop allergic diseases. The route of allergen exposure and quantity of allergen reaching a particular mucosa may be important. Local exposure can predispose to restricted forms of atopic disease. For example, pollen hay fever is restricted to the upper respiratory tract.

Skin Tests   The direct skin test provides the most practical method for detecting anaphylactic hypersensitivity in man. Allergen skin tests can be accomplished in atopic patients. When used properly, skin tests provide a reasonably safe, simple, reliable assessment of hypersensitivity to specific allergens. The results of skin tests are immediately available. Although similar information can be obtained by in vitro assays of hypersensitivity and by measurement of IgE antibodies, in vitro tests are less economical and the results are not immediately available. A high degree of correlation exists between the results of direct skin tests, provocation tests such as allergen-inhalation challenge, and experimental in vitro assay of IgE antibodies.

The risk of inducing anaphylaxis during skin testing increases with the dose of allergen used and the number of positive responses elicited during the test procedure. Patients should not be tested without continued observation and the availability of drugs to counteract anaphylaxis. The least dose of allergen to which hypersensitive patients will respond is used. The epicutaneous scratch or prick test provides the most reliable and safest method for clinical assessment of cutaneous anaphylactic hypersensitivity. An example of this method is illustrated in Figure 17-3. Less sensitive patients can be tested with an intradermal injection of 0.03 ml of a sterile dilution of allergen. The concentration of allergen used for intradermal testing is usually 1:1,000 or less than the concentration used for epicutaneous tests. Positive reactions begin within seconds. Local itching is followed by the development of an erythematous flare. Intense reactions are accompanied by pale, edematous, elevated wheals at the test site. Positive reactions reach maximum size in 15 to

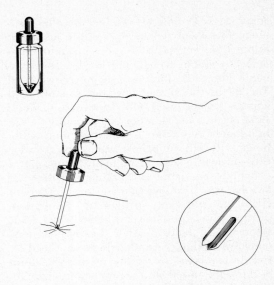

Fig. 17-3. The epicutaneous skin test. This form of the direct skin test makes use of a two-tined solid needle to make a minute circular scratch on the outer surface of the skin. The small hollow space between the barbs carries a microdrop of allergen to the scratched skin surface. Measurements of the flare response induced by this technique yield reproducible estimates of allergen responsiveness. Measurable differences detected by this technique in atopic patients are 10 to 20-fold better than the conventional 1 to 4-plus method of scoring skin tests. The direct skin test is clinically useful and can be used as a quantitative measure of anaphylactic hypersensitivity.

30 minutes and subside in 2 to 6 hours. Anaphylactic hypersensitivity reactions can also be elicited by local applications of allergen to the mucous membranes of the respiratory tract and the conjunctival sac.

It is difficult to quantify anaphylactic antibodies by direct skin tests or by conventional serologic tests. The classic method for quantification of anaphylactic antibodies is based on a modification of the passive transfer experiment described by Prausnitz and Küstner. Dilutions of serum from a sensitive donor are injected into test sites in the skin of a nonatopic recipient. After a period of 24 hours or longer, each adoptively sensitized site is challenged with allergen. Sites previously sensitized with sufficient anaphylactic antibodies exhibit a positive reaction. Allergen challenge of normal skin or challenge with a different allergen fails to yield a wheal and flare response. The lowest dilution of donor serum yielding a positive response provides a measure of the concentration of anaphylactic antibodies in the donor serum.

This method of detecting and/or quantifying anaphylactic antibodies is called the Prausnitz-Küstner reaction or P-K reaction. The P-K reaction can be used to detect atopic hypersensitivity in patients who cannot be subjected to direct skin tests. The possibility of infecting the recipient with serum hepatitis limits the clinical usefulness of P-K tests. In vitro assays of IgE antibodies have replaced this clinical use of the P-K test. Until the identification of IgE, this adoptive hypersensitivity reaction provided the only experimental evidence that anaphylaxis and the atopic diseases were caused by the same antibody.

When blood is transfused from an atopic donor to a normal recipient, the P-K titer of anaphylactic antibodies in the serum of the recipient decreases within a few hours. In the first few hours following transfusion, allergen challenge of the recipient does not cause a reaction. During this latent period, anaphylactic antibodies become fixed to the tissues of the recipient. Direct allergen skin tests become positive after a 4-hour latent period and reach a maximum in 24 to 48 hours. The passively transferred anaphylactic antibodies can be detected in the normal recipient for six to eight weeks. Allergen inhalation during this period

can cause hay fever and asthma. The transfused normal recipient responds to allergens like an atopic patient. Adoptive sensitization with human anaphylactic antibodies can cause adoptive disease in transfused nonatopic patients.

PASSIVE CUTANEOUS ANAPHYLAXIS. Direct and adoptive skin tests can also be accomplished in experimental animals. Positive test reactions are less easily detected. This difficulty can be overcome by the prior intravenous injection of Evans blue dye (Fig. 17-4). The dye binds to serum albumin and is retained within blood vessels. A positive skin test increases vascular permeability at the reaction site. Extravasation of serum and the dye at the test site facilitates detection of a positive reaction. Passive cutaneous anaphylaxis (PCA) can be detected in experimental animals in a manner similar to the P-K reaction in man. Serum from a sensitive animal is used to adoptively sensitize the skin of a normal animal. Direct or intravenous allergen challenge produces reactions at the sensitized skin sites.

HOMOCYTOTROPISM. Prausnitz and Küstner observed the passive transfer of anaphylactic antibodies to nonallergic humans but not to

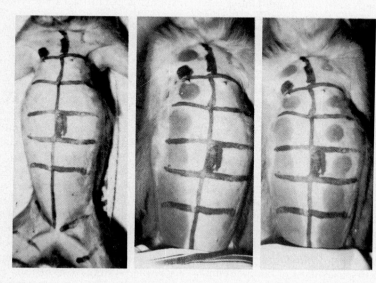

Fig. 17-4. Monkey passive cutaneous anaphylaxis with human anaphylactic antibody. The figure on the left shows unreacted skin sites sensitized with human serum from patients sensitive to two different pollen antigens. Intravenous challenge with ragweed antigen in the middle figure results in bluing of sites passively sensitized with human serum containing anaphylactic antibodies to ragweed pollen but not at sites sensitized with orchard grass on the left side of the animal's abdomen. Challenge with orchard grass antigen shown in the figure on the right results in bluing of sites sensitized with human anaphylactic antibody to orchard grass, demonstrating the specificity of the reaction. (Adapted from Buckley and Metzgar: J Allergy 36:382, 1965)

guinea pigs. Passive transfer of anaphylactic hypersensitivity was possible only in the homologous species. Adoptively sensitized skin test sites become responsive after an appreciable latent period and remain responsive for prolonged periods of time, suggesting that anaphylactic antibodies become fixed at the skin test site. Because of this property, anaphylactic antibodies have been called "skin-sensitizing antibodies." Recent evidence suggests that binding to basophils and mast cells is responsible for this cytotropism. These two observations identify important properties of anaphylactic antibodies; collectively, these properties are called "homocytotropism."

BLOCKING ANTIBODIES. Parenteral immunization with allergens produces serum IgG antibodies which block passive anaphylactic sensitization. IgG antibodies are produced in greater quantity than IgE antibodies. Serum and extracellular fluid antibodies can compete with cell-bound antibodies for allergen and decrease mediator release. Serum antibodies of the IgG class which decrease the release of the chemical mediators of anaphylaxis are called blocking antibodies. Parenteral injections of allergens are used in the treatment of patients with atopic diseases. Blocking antibodies generated by injection therapy may contribute to the clinical modification of allergic diseases.

In contrast to the possible protective effect of human blocking antibodies, certain subclasses of IgG antibodies in experimental animals exhibit homocytotropism and induce adoptive sensitization. Guinea pig IgGla, mouse IgGl, and rat IgGa are less homocytotropic than anaphylactic antibodies from the same animal species. The latent period during which tissue binding occurs is shorter, and passively sensitized skin sites remain reactive for no more than a few days. Evidence suggests that homocytotropic IgG subclasses and anaphylactic antibodies utilize the same mast cell surface receptor and initiate mediator release in the same way. A role of homocytotropic human IgG subclasses in naturally occurring anaphylaxis and other atopic diseases has not been demonstrated.

Experimentally, heterologous adoptive local systemic anaphylaxis can be caused by IgG antibodies. Human IgG antibodies do not cause homologous anaphylaxis but can cause adoptive local and systemic anaphylaxis in a heterol-ogous species, such as the guinea pig. This type of passive sensitization also persists for a relatively short period of time. Heterologous passive cutaneous anaphylaxis provides an experimentally useful method for detecting low concentrations of human IgG antibodies. In contrast, human IgE antibodies cause P-K reactions and anaphylaxis in man and in closely related higher primates (Fig. 17-4) but do not cause anaphylaxis in unrelated species, such as the guinea pig. Similarly, mouse IgE antibodies cause anaphylaxis and homologous PCA reactions in mice and closely related rodents, such as the rat, but not in unrelated animal species. The homocytotropic properties of anaphylactic antibodies were ignored for many years. IgE and IgG antibodies are produced by patients with anaphylaxis and the serum sickness syndrome, and conventional immunoserologic tests detected precipitating IgG antibodies in sera from these patients. The demonstration of heterologous PCA reactions with serum from patients with anaphylaxis and serum sickness led to the erroneous assumption that precipitating antibodies cause human anaphylaxis. The anaphylactic phenomenon detected by passive sensitization of guinea pigs with human IgG antibodies is not initiated by the antibodies responsible for human anaphylaxis.

MECHANISMS RESPONSIBLE FOR ATOPIC HYPERSENSITIVITY

The prevalence of patients with atopic diseases has stimulated many studies of anaphylactic hypersensitivity. In the past two decades, investigations have yielded useful information about the biologic mechanisms responsible for atopic diseases. Clinically useful information includes the structure, function, and distribution of IgE, the immune mechanisms by which anaphylactic antibodies initiate allergic reactions, and the components of the accessory system responsible for atopic disease. Many informative studies have been accomplished in man, but because of the risks of certain types of experimental studies in man, additional important information has been obtained in experimental animals. Although this assessment of mechanisms is presented in relation to human atopic diseases, an awareness of the comparative biology of anaphylactic hypersensitivity is important.

IgE Immunoglobulin E (γE) is responsible for the atopic diseases. IgE occurs in nanogram quantities in serum and other body fluids, and it binds to tissue mast cells and circulating basophils and initiates the tissue changes characteristic of anaphylactic hypersensitivity. It is not presently possible to isolate sufficient IgE from the serum of healthy human beings to study the structural properties of the molecule. IgE myeloma proteins provide the main source of immunoglobulin for physicochemical studies. IgE has a sedimentation coefficient (S_{20w}) of 7.9, weighs approximately 188,000 Daltons, migrates electrophoretically as a γ_1-globulin, and contains 10.7 percent carbohydrate. IgE contains 40 half-cysteine residues per molecule and is sensitive to sulfhydryl reducing agents. Heating at 56C for 30 minutes results in irreversible thermal denaturation of the Fc portion of the molecule, and this change results in the loss of the skin-sensitizing property of the molecule within four hours. Similar heat treatment of the Fab portion of the molecule causes no appreciable conformation change, and the antigen-binding activity of the Fab fragment is retained. IgE is multivalent with respect to antigen-binding sites. Complement is not fixed by IgE through the classic (C1) pathway. IgE does not pass the placental barrier to the fetus. Half of the IgE in serum is replaced every 2 to 3 days, and half of the IgE bound to skin is replaced every 11 to 12 days.

SITES OF IgE PRODUCTION. Gastrointestinal and respiratory tract secretions contain measurable quantities of IgE. Seasonal exposure produces an enrichment of IgE in the nasal secretions of pollen-sensitive patients. The levels of IgE detected in secretions and fluids expressed from allergic nasal polyps can exceed serum IgE levels, suggesting that IgE is synthesized locally in the mucosal tissues. Adenoidal and tonsillar tissues, peribronchial and peritoneal lymph nodes, and the lamina propria of the gastrointestinal and respiratory tract mucosa contain IgE-laden plasma cells. In contrast, relatively few IgE-containing cells are found in the peripheral lymph nodes and spleen. Although IgE molecules do not contain a secretory piece, the distribution of IgE-producing cells near to mucosal surfaces and the portals of entry to the body identify IgE as a secretory antibody.

MEASUREMENT OF IgE LEVELS. The low concentration of IgE in serum and body secretions can be measured by a radioisotope modification of the antiglobulin reaction. The most widely used method depends upon the ability of IgE in an unknown serum to inhibit the binding of isotope-labeled IgE to anti-IgE antibodies (Chaps. 15 and 21). In order to facilitate separation of the reactants after specific binding, antibody to IgE is covalently linked to an insoluble polymer particle. The unlabeled IgE in the unknown serum competes with the isotope-labeled IgE, resulting in a decrease in the binding of the isotope-labeled IgE to the insoluble particle. The decrease in binding of the isotope-labeled IgE is proportional to the quantity of IgE in the unknown serum.

IgE LEVELS. Cord serum contains detectable quantities of IgE, which, however, do not correlate with levels detected in maternal serum. Serum IgE averages a sevenfold increase between birth and early adult life and does not change appreciably with advancing age. The distribution of IgE levels in healthy persons appears multimodal and ranges between 5 and 1,200 nanograms per ml of serum. Rarely, exceptionally high levels (10,000 ng/ml) may be detected in apparently healthy individuals. Studies in monozygotic twins reveal up to 84 percent concordance between serum IgE levels. This suggests that serum IgE levels are under genetic control. This degree of concordance contrasts sharply with the discordance of asthma and other atopic diseases in similar twin studies.

Serum IgE levels in atopic patients overlap the range observed in normal nonatopic controls. Although measurements of IgE levels are not usually helpful in the individual patient, patients with atopic disease average higher levels than controls. Experimentally, production of IgE antibodies is facilitated by low doses of allergen, a finding which is consistent with the dose ranges of naturally occurring pollen exposure. In pollen-sensitive patients, serum IgE levels tend to increase as a result of seasonal exposure. Levels in patients with infected atopic eczema are generally higher than in patients with uncomplicated atopic eczema, asthma, or allergic rhinitis. Diagnostically useful levels of IgE are found in atopic patients with pulmonary allergic aspergillosis. This syndrome is characterized by asthma, peripheral blood eosinophilia, transient x-ray lung infiltrates, *Aspergillus fumigatus* in the sputum, positive immediate and late skin test reactions, precipitating serum antibodies to the asperigillus antigen, and extreme (>6,000 ng/ml) elevations of serum IgE. Elevated IgE levels have been reported in patients with eosinophilic gastritis and in certain forms of polyarteritis. Parasitic infections cause marked elevation of serum IgE; this trend is most marked during the tissue phase of infection. Among patients with immunodeficiency diseases, those with the Wiskott-Aldrich syndrome, advanced Hodgkin's disease, and other disorders of T cell-dependent immune function frequently have elevated serum IgE levels. Reduced serum IgE levels occur in patients with generalized defects in immunoglobulin synthesis, in certain patients with IgA deficiency, and in patients with ataxia telangectasia.

IgE Binding to Mast Cells.   The chemical mediators or tissue permeases secreted by tissue mast cells or circulating basophils are responsible for the tissue changes initiated by the reaction of allergens and IgE antibodies. Mast cells contain enriched quantities of the chemical mediators of anaphylaxis. Quantitative studies of the release of a mediator, histamine, by peripheral blood leukocytes indicate that the contribution by other white blood cells is insignificant. IgE molecules bind to receptor sites on the surface of the basophil. Attachment is through the Fc portion of the molecule. The number of receptor sites on basophils from different persons varies between 30,000 and 100,000 per mast cell. The number of IgE molecules bound per cell varies between 10,000 and 40,000. The avidity of the basophil receptor site for IgE is comparable to the specific binding of antigen and antibody. Permease release is activated by the bridging effect of a polyvalent allergen between two adjacent receptor site-bound IgE molecules.

Anaphylactic Antibody Activity   In addition to the P-K reaction and the homologous PCA reaction in experimental animals, components of the allergic reaction initiated by IgE antibodies can be measured by several in vitro methods. The Shultz-Dale bioassay of mediator release (Fig. 17-5) and chemical measurements of histamine released by passively sensitized

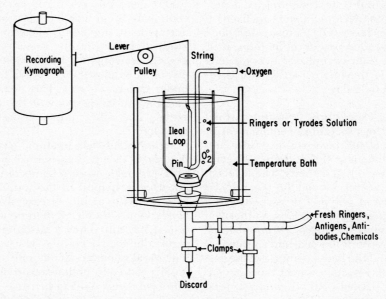

Fig. 17-5. Apparatus for Schultz-Dale type of in vitro reaction. Introduction of antigen into the water bath results in the release of histamine, which causes contraction of the smooth muscle of the ileal loop and displacement of the lever and scribe on the revolving recording kymograph drum.

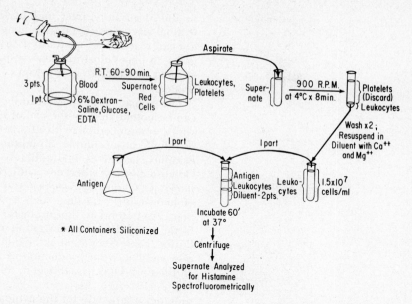

Fig. 17-6. Leukocyte in vitro histamine release method for assay of anaphylactic antibody. Careful assays with this complex procedure have provided direct evidence of seasonal changes and of the effect of treatment on anaphylactic antibody in human disease.

peripheral blood leukocytes (Fig. 17-6) represent two important in vitro experimental methods for quantifying anaphylactic antibodies. When the Schultz-Dale technique is used with guinea pig uterus as the passively sensitized tissue, anaphylactic antibodies can be detected in guinea pig serum. Passive sensitization of the guinea pig uterus with serum from a heterologous species detects IgG antibodies. A modified form of the Schultz-Dale technique, using passively sensitized human or monkey smooth muscle-containing tissues, detects human anaphylactic antibodies. Assay of the histamine released from passively sensitized human leukocytes has been used to study the anaphylactic antibody response to seasonal pollen exposure and the outcome of specific immunotherapy in ragweed hay fever patients. Serum anaphylactic antibody titers to ragweed allergen increase following seasonal exposure and after specific immunotherapy. Injection therapy results in decreased hay fever symptoms, but this clinical trend shares no consistent relationship with anaphylactic antibody titers or the production of IgG blocking antibodies.

Identification of IgE as the immunoglobulin responsible for anaphylactic antibody activity has made possible measurement of the serum concentration of IgE antibodies. Methods for measurement of IgE levels make use of an antiglobulin reaction similar to the Coombs' test (Fig 17-7). This method has been used to confirm the seasonal increase in serum IgE antibodies to ragweed previously detected by histamine release from passively sensitized human leukocytes. The seasonal increase in IgE antibodies to ragweed allergen in ragweed allergen-immunized patients appears less than the seasonal increase in untreated control patients. This tendency is proportional to the total allergen dose used for treatment. Patients immunized with high allergen doses exhibited a maximum increase in IgG blocking antibodies.

ATOPIC SENSITIZATION. The presence of IgE in cord sera suggests that naturally occurring sensitization and production of anaphylactic antibodies begins prior to birth. Surveys suggest that IgE antibodies to common allergens in children are directed predominantly toward foods during the first year of life. IgE antibodies to egg albumin and cows' milk are most prevalent. Nothing is known of IgE antibodies to the intestinal microbial flora during

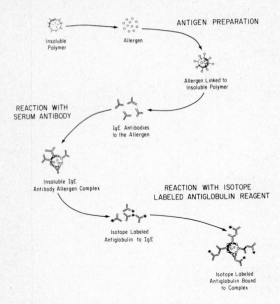

ANTIGEN PREPARATION

Insoluble Polymer

Allergen

Allergen Linked to Insoluble Polymer

REACTION WITH SERUM ANTIBODY

IgE Antibodies to the Allergen

Insoluble IgE Antibody Allergen Complex

REACTION WITH ISOTOPE LABELED ANTIGLOBULIN REAGENT

Isotope Labeled Antiglobulin to IgE

Isotope Labeled Antiglobulin Bound to Complex

Fig. 17-7. Measurement of IgE antibody to an allergen. An allergen is linked chemically to an insoluble polymer. The washed insolubilized allergen is mixed with serum containing IgE antibodies to the allergen. The insoluble allergen-polymer is washed free of serum proteins not specifically bound to the allergen, and the complex is mixed with a solution containing an isotope-labeled antiglobulin (antibodies to IgE). The polymer-allergen-IgE complex binds isotope-labeled antiglobulin. The insoluble reactants are washed and counted. The isotope counts bound to the insoluble polymer provide a measure of serum IgE antibodies to the allergen. (Adapted from Aas and Johansson: J Allergy Clin Immunol 48:143, 1971)

this period of development. Antibody levels to foods decrease as the infant matures, and anaphylactic antibodies to pollens and animal danders became detectable during the second year of life.

Although the immediate burden of low-dose exposure to airborne allergens falls on the mucosal surfaces of the respiratory tract, evidence suggests that mucociliary clearance mechanisms carry most of this antigen burden into the pharynx. The contents of the pharynx are swallowed and the gastrointestinal tract probably bears the primary burden of exposure to sensitizing doses of allergens. This route of dominant allergen exposure does not alter the subsequent sensitization of all mucosal surfaces and later involvement in allergic reactions. Sensitized cells generated in gastrointestinal mucosal lymphoid aggregates reach the lymphatic circulation and home preferentially to other submucosal lymphoid structures

in the respiratory tract and in the gastrointestinal tract. Sensitized cells generated in the gut can reach other secretory lymphoid aggregates in the colostrum and respiratory tract without measurable production of serum antibodies.

The primary anaphylactic antibody response can be potentiated by the use of specific adjuvants. Immunization with allergens adsorbed on alum, an insoluble aluminum hydroxide complex, facilitates IgE antibody production. Combinations of allergens with *Haemophilus pertussis, Corynebacterium parvum* or extracts of helminthic parasites, such as *Ascaris* antigen, also potentiate the production of anaphylactic antibodies. Immunization early in life, during the development of the immune system, also facilitates the production of anaphylactic antibodies. Once established, this tendency can persist into adult life. This observation provides a rationale for the avoidance of allergenic foods by infants of atopic parents. IgE antibodies have been detected in adults during the course of human trichinosis and appear before the generation of antibodies in other immunoglobulin classes. Radiation exposure and radiomimetic immunosuppression at the time of allergen sensitization facilitates the production of anaphylactic antibodies.

Recently, Tada and his colleagues reported an incisive series of experiments in which thymectomy, radiation, and radiomimetic immunosuppression were used in hapten carrier-sensitized rats to evaluate mechanisms regulating anaphylactic antibody production. In these experiments, cooperative interactions between carrier-specific T cells and hapten-specific B cells appeared necessary for IgE antibody production. Carrier-specific T cells elaborate soluble factors which either initiate or inhibit IgE antibody production. Passively administered IgG antibodies to the carrier and the hapten are also capable of inhibiting IgE antibody synthesis. Radiation and radiomimetic immunosuppression appear to impair the function of those T cells which promote IgG production and suppress IgE production. T cells which facilitate IgE production are relatively unaffected.

FUNCTION OF ANAPHYLACTIC ANTIBODIES. Little is known of the normal function of IgE anaphylactic antibodies. The preservation of the capacity to produce anaphylactic antibodies during the evolution of man and other animals suggests anaphylactic hypersensitivity has intrinsic survival value. Clear evidence of the nature of this survival value is not available. The location of IgE-producing cells proximate to mucosal surfaces and the presence of IgE in external secretions suggest that IgE is a secretory antibody. An awareness of the possible importance of IgE antibodies can be deduced from their distribution and pathologic function. The reaction of IgE antibodies and allergens initiates local changes in vascular permeability and blood flow and produces local edema and smooth muscle contraction. These changes could retard the local extension of allergen into exposed tissue and facilitate the migration of immunocompetent cells and eventually other antibodies into challenged tissues. In this sense, the local changes induced by anaphylactic antibodies have been viewed as a gatekeeping activity which modulates reactions between allergens and more destructive components of the immune system.

The nondestructive nature of the tissue changes induced by anaphylactic antibodies and the localization of IgE-producing cells near secretory membranes suggest a primary role in the defense of important mucosal surfaces, such as the adsorptive surface of the gut. Protection of the adsorptive lining of the gastrointestinal tract by mechanisms which cause destructive inflammation could impair nutrient assimilation. Failure of immune mechanisms to retard the excessive local microorganism growth and prevent toxic injury to the adsorptive surface of the gastrointestinal tract can also cause maladsorption. As an alternative, the nondestructive changes induced by a local anaphylactic reaction provide specific advantages. An allergen-induced increase in local mucus production would facilitate sequestration of allergens in the gut lumen and minimize the chance of injury to the adsorptive surface. Allergen-induced smooth muscle contraction and activation of gut motor function would hasten the elimination of the allergen from the adsorptive surfaces of the gastrointestinal tract. Preservation of the capacity to initiate local anaphylactic hypersensitivity reactions may provide an intrinsic survival value in the protection and maintainence of the adsorptive function of the nonrigid bowel. A capacity for accelerated clearance of specific microflora and their products form important gut adsorptive

surfaces would facilitate the effectiveness of the neutralizing capacity of IgA coproantibodies.

A similar anaphylactic hypersensitivity reaction in a semirigid structure, such as the respiratory tract, would place the responding host at a disadvantage. The route of allergen exposure, the site of the hypersensitivity reaction, and alternative types of responses may be important considerations in assessing the function of anaphylactic antibodies.

PARASITISM. A protective role of anaphylactic antibodies has been identified in experimental studies of certain parasitic diseases. These experiments identify mechanisms of possible importance in the maintainance of hemostasis between the host and gut microflora. Following subcutaneous injection, the larvae of the rat hookworm (*Nippostrongylus brasiliensis*) migrate through the tissues of the infected animal to the lungs, molt, and then continue to the small intestine via the trachea and the esophagus. The nemotode matures in the small intestine and mates, and egg production begins approximately one week after infection. A self-cure of the infestation begins two weeks later and results in a sharp reduction in egg production and in the expulsion of the adult worms from the intestine. This self cure occurs coincident with the development of anaphylactic hypersensitivity to worm allergens. The self-cure can be blocked by antihistamines, antiserotonin compounds, and corticosteroids. Sensitized cells and antibody are needed to transfer passively this capacity for self-cure. Active immunization with the nemotode allergen in Freund's complete adjuvant and generation of precipitating antibodies fail to produce anaphylactic antibodies or protection against worm infestation.

The complexity of this experimental model becomes apparent in similar studies of nematode infection in mice. Using *Nematospiroides dubius*, immunity is induced by the larval stage of the infection. Following oral ingestion of the larvae, the parasite burrows into the wall of the small intestine, matures, and returns to the gut lumen in 7 to 8 days. The adult worms persist for months, but expulsion can be induced within 2 to 4 hours by superimposing a second infection. In germ-free mice, fewer *N. dubius* larvae develop into adult worms, and worm survival in the intestine and egg production are reduced. Germ-free mice develop a marked eosinophilia during worm infection, and mononuclear cell infiltrated nodules persist at the site of larval implantation in the small intestine. Conventionally reared mice develop leukocytosis without eosinophilia, and the intestinal nodules at the site of larval implantation become infiltrated with neutrophils and disappear. Bacterial monocontamination of the germ-free mouse reduces the number of persisting intestinal nodules and facilitates worm development and survival. This trend is most pronounced with species of bacteria that infest the small intestine. Experimentally, the anaphylactic antibody response to bacteria and other allergens is potentiated during infection with nematode worms. Although a protective role of anaphylactic antibodies in certain parasitic diseases cannot be excluded, reactions to other gut allergens and activation of other host defense mechanisms appear important.

Chemical Mediators of Anaphylaxis The tissue changes initiated by anaphylactic antibodies are produced by chemical compounds released by passively sensitized mast cells or basophils. These compounds are the chemical mediators of anaphylaxis. The mediators of anaphylaxis produce local changes in the permeability of blood vessels and are, therefore, also called "permeases." The compounds responsible for anaphylactic reactions include (1) histamine, (2) serotonin, (3) bradykinin, (4) slow-reacting substance-A (SRS-A), (5) heparin, and possibly (6) acetylcholine. Mediator release is accompanied by the release of an eosinophil chemotactic factor (ECF), which directs the local infiltration of eosinophils into the area of allergic injury. Histamine, serotonin SRS-A, and heparin occur in enriched concentrations in human mast cells and blood basophils.

Figure 17-8 illustrates the events which can initiate mediator release and the pharmacologic mechanisms which can modify anaphylaxis. Formation of an allergen bridge between two mast cell-bound IgE antibodies activates a series of enzymatic mechanisms, which result in the release of SRS-A, histamine, and other mediators. The release of mediators from the

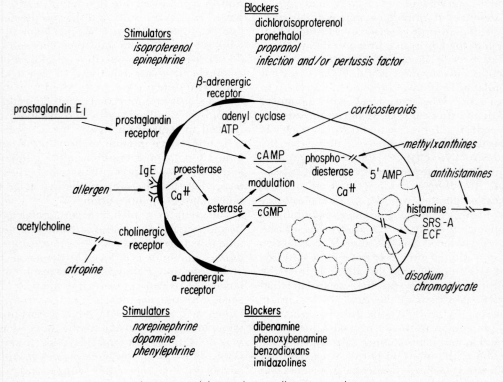

Fig. 17-8. Modulation of mast cell permease release.

granules of the mast cell is modulated by the intracellular concentration of cyclic adenosine monophosphate (cAMP) and cyclic guanosine monphosphate (cGMP). Increased concentrations of cAMP retard mediator release. Increased concentration of cGMP counteract the effects of cAMP. Locally active hormones, such as prostaglandin E_1, corticosteroids, and stimulators of β-adrenergic receptors on the cell increase intracellular cAMP. Infection and medications, such as propanol, block the β-adrenergic receptor and interfere with drugs used to treat anaphylaxis. Stimulation of cell α-adrenergic receptors increases modulation by cGMP and facilitates mediator release. Methyl xanthines, such as aminophyllin, inhibit the activity of an enzyme, phosphodiesterase, which inactivates cAMP. Disodium chromoglycolate has a direct stabilizing effect on cell membranes and prevents release of the permeases from the mast cell granules. Antihistamines block the activity of histamine at a site distant from the mast cell.

The quantity of histamine that can be released varies among different tissues and cells. Mast cells, basophils, platelets, and eosinophils contain large quantities of histamine. Histamine causes arteriolar and capillary dilatation, increases tissue permeability, provokes smooth muscle contraction, and increases gastric acid secretion. Methylation, acetylation, and oxidation by monoamine oxidase inactivate and degrade histamine.

Serotonin (5-hydroxytryptamine) is structurally related to the amino acid tryptophan and is important in rat and mouse anaphylaxis. The mouse uterus is 1,000 times more sensitive to serotonin than to histamine. Serotonin, histamine, and heparin are released from mast cells and the chromaffin cells of the intestine. Serotonin is present in platelets, spleen, gastrointestinal tract, brainstem, mast cells, and lung tissue. The pharmacologic effects of serotonin are increased intestinal peristalsis, respiratory rate, and smooth muscle contraction and decreased central nervous system activity. Serotonin produces local pain and erythema and provokes histamine release when injected into the skin. Serotonin is degraded by monoamine oxidase.

Slow-reacting substances are divided into two classes on the basis of their physical properties and the tissue of origin. Slow-reacting substance-A (SRS-A) is representative of the first class of compounds. SRS-A is an acidic compound which is soluble in organic solvents. Its release occurs coincident with and is primarily responsible for the bronchial constriction of asthma. SRS-A has been isolated following the in vitro addition of allergen to sensitized human lung tissue. This mediator is unstable at room temperature and is rapidly inactivated by exposure to heat, oxygen, or hydrogen. Although the chemical structure of SRS-A is not known, it is inactivated by an enzyme, aryl sulfatase, which is found in enriched quantities in the eosinophil. This suggests that the eosinophil may have a role in modifying the extent of tissue injury induced by anaphylactic reactions.

Bradykinin is representative of the second class of slow-reacting substances. Bradykinin is a small peptide which is produced by the action of peptidases on serum globulin and other proteins. Tissue changes induced by bradykinin occur more slowly than changes caused by histamine. Bradykinin causes smooth muscle contraction, enhances capillary permeability, and may also enhance the migration of leukocytes through blood vessel walls. Local cutaneous injection of bradykinin causes pain but does not produce a pruritic wheal or erythema.

Heparin is an acid mucopolysaccharide found in high concentrations in mast cells. It decreases the coagulability of blood by altering the surface charge of formed elements of blood and blood vessel walls. Prolonged clotting times are observed in anaphylaxis and may be a consequence of the release of heparin from mast cells.

Acetylcholine causes peripheral vasodilatation and is primarily localized at neural synaptic connections. A possible role of acetylcholine in cholinergic urticaria is the basis for its inclusion among the chemical mediators. Acetylcholine is inactivated by cholinesterase.

FURTHER READING

Books

Amos DB (ed): Progress in Immunology. New York, Academic Press, 1971

Brent L, Holborow J (eds): Progress in Immunology II. New York, American Elsevier, 1974

Goodfriend L, Sehon AH, Orange RP (eds): Mechanisms in Allergy. New York, Marcel Dekker, 1973

Ishizaka K, Dayton DH Jr (eds): The Biological Role of the Immunoglobulin E System. Washington, DC, US Government Printing Office, 1973

Reviews

Bienenstock J: The physiology of the local immune response and the gastrointestinal tract. In Brent L, Holborow J (eds): Progress in Immunology II. New York, American Elsevier, 1974, vol 4

Bloch KJ: The anaphylactic antibodies of mammals including man. Prog Allergy 10:84, 1967

Cochrane CG: Mediators of the Arthus and related reactions. Prog Allergy 11:1, 1967

Movat HZ (ed): Cellular and Humoral Mechanisms in Anaphylaxis and Allergy. New York, Karger, 1969

Ogilvie BM: Immunity to parasites. In Brent L, Holborow J (eds): Progress in Immunology II. New York, American Elsevier, 1974, vol 4

Selected Papers

Austen KF: Reaction mechanisms in the release of mediators of immediate hypersensitivity from human lung tissue. Fed Proc 33:2256, 1974

Buckley CE III, Dorgey FC, Corley RB, et al: HL-A linked human immune-response genes. Proc Natl Acad Sci USA, 70:2157, 1973

Ishizaka K, Ishizaka T: Identification of E antibodies as a carrier of reaginic activity. J Immunol 99:1187, 1967

Kniker WT, Cochrane CG: The localization of circulating immune complexes in experimental serum sickness. The role of vasoactive amines and hydrodynamic forces. J Exp Med 127:119, 1968

Levine BB, Vaz NM: Effect of combinations of inbred strain, antigen, and antigen dose on immune responsiveness and reagin production in the mouse. Int Arch Allergy 31:156, 1970

Levy DA, Lichtenstein LM, Goldstein EO, Ishizaka K: Immunologic and cellular changes accompanying the therapy of pollen allergy. J Clin Invest 50:360, 1971

Taniguchi M, Tada T: Regulation of homocytotrophic antibody formulation in the rat. X IgT-like molecule for the induction of homocytotrophic antibody response. J Immunol 113:1757, 1974

Wescott RB: Metazoa-protozoa-bacteria interrelationships. Am J Clin Nutr 23:1502, 1970

Immunologic Responses to Infectious Disease

A discussion of the immune response to infectious disease provides a logical bridge between a description of basic immunologic mechanisms and a discussion of the role of these mechanisms in various clinical states. Indeed, almost every type of immunochemical and immunobiologic response plays a role in the immune reaction to some infectious agent and may even have evolved primarily to perform this role. This concept is reflected in immunologic deficiency states (Chap. 20), where the immune deficit is expressed primarily as an increased susceptibility to infection. On the other hand, it may be an aberrant use of the host's defense against infectious disease that leads to many autoimmune phenomena (Chap. 19).

A CENTRAL CONCEPT: MICROORGANISMS ARE MULTIANTIGENIC UNITS

The antigenic components of the individual microorganisms have been discussed in their respective chapters. Even the simplest of viruses are composed of multiple antigenic subunits, and some of the bacteria, with their numerous structural components and secretory products, can present to the infected host dozens of different immunogens. Recognition of the multiple antigenic nature of microorganisms is the most important step toward understanding the immune response to infectious disease. This recognition may help explain why antibodies of many different specificities appear in a host challenged with a single infectious agent and why the presence of an immune response to an organism does not assure immune protection.

A few generalizations, to which numerous exceptions do exist, are helpful in categorizing multiple antigens. First, most antigens associated with infectious agents are either proteins or polysaccharides. The latter induce almost exclusively a humoral response, which is frequently thymus independent and of restricted heterogeneity. Protein antigens, on the other hand, are thymus dependent and can induce the full spectrum of immunologic reactions.

Second, the virulence of a microorganism is generally dependent upon only one, or a few, of its many components or products, and it is an immune response against these critical components which provides the host with its best protection against the organism. For example, the streptococcal M protein (Chap. 27) is singly responsible for the organism's virulence, acting, presumably, to help abort the phagocytic activity of the host. Antibody against the M protein provides more effective host protection than antibody against any other streptococcal antigen. Viral neutralization, on the other hand, does not usually depend on the presence of antibody to any critical site but simply to any viral surface determinant. There are exceptions, however. With T-even bacteriophage, antibody to the end plate assembly, with its constituent tail fibers, induces neutralization, whereas antibody to the head piece of the virus does not. Third, not only may an infectious agent expose the host to its own structural components and secretory products, but it may alter the antigenicity of the infected cell and thereby initiate an immune reaction against the host's own tissues.

Original Antigenic Sin   Usually there are many different strains of a microorganism. Frequently the different strains bear antigenic determinants which are similar, and hence cross-reactive, but not identical. Thus, antibody raised against one strain may bind to a different strain, but with lower affinity. For example, infection of an individual with one of the four serotypes (say, type 1) of the group B arbovirus dengue virus (Chap. 62) leads to the expansion of that clone of lymphocytes that produces antibody specific for it. Upon infection with a dengue virus strain of one of the other three closely related serotypes (say, type 3), both the expanded type 1-specific clone and the unexpanded type 3-specific cells are stimulated. Because of the previous expansion of the type 1-specific clones, the dominant antibody produced will be type 1-specific. This antibody will bind to type 3 virus, but with lower affinity than to type 1 virus. The phenomenon where the primary infecting virus determines the dominant antibody specificity elicited by secondary infection is referred to as "original antigenic sin."

MECHANISMS OF HOST DEFENSE

Immunologic Defenses at the Mucous Membranes

Most infectious agents enter the host through portals lined with mucous membranes. While nonimmunologic anatomic factors play a major role in defending the mucous surfaces against microorganisms, both cellular and humoral antimicrobial mechanisms are operative at the mucosal surface. Specific antibody of the IgG, IgM, and IgA classes can be isolated from the secretions of infected mucosal surfaces, but the dominant antibody species is secretory IgA. In vitro a complex of secretory IgA and its antigen can activate the alternate (but not the classical) complement sequence (Chap. 16) and thus initiate opsonization, and if both complement and lysozyme are present, it can also induce bacteriolysis. In vivo, however, the predominant function of mucosal IgA appears simply to be prevention of microbial adherence to the mucosal surface. Thus, in experimental cholera, antibody does not decrease the number of viable organisms in the gut but does greatly increase the proportion of them that are free in the lumen. Again, enteropathic strains of *Escherichia coli* adhere to intestinal mucosa better than do nonenteropathic strains; in one model this adherence is dependent upon a bacterial surface protein, K-88. Antibody specific for K-88 is protective, while antibody against other bacterial surface antigens is not.

Lymphocytes, predominantly T cells, are found in the lamina propria of several mucosal surfaces. These cells are able to initiate and mediate a local cell-mediated immune reaction to many mucosal pathogens, including tubercle bacilli, listeria, and pneumococci, and this reaction may proceed without evidence of systemic immunity.

Immunologic Defenses against Extracellular Organisms

Many bacteria, most notably streptococci, staphylococci, and pneumococci, exist primarily in an extracellular environment, whether in the circulation or within infected tissues. The immunologic system attacks such organisms in three ways: inactivation of toxins, bacteriolysis, and phagocytosis. Of these, the first and last mechanisms are most important.

Inactivation of Toxins Some organisms exert their major pathogenic effects by the elaboration of soluble exotoxins, such as the lecithinase C of *Clostridium perfringens* and the ADP-ribosylation enzyme of *Corynebacterium diphtheriae*. These toxins are generally quite immunogenic and can stimulate IgG, IgM, and IgA production. However, only IgG can inactivate the biologic activity of most exotoxins. Inactivation occurs principally by steric inhibition, by the antibody, of the toxin-binding site. This effect, of course, depends upon the antibody's having a greater affinity for the toxin than the toxin has for its substrate and explains the need for hyperimmune serum to achieve effective antitoxin activity.

The role of antibody in the inactivation of endotoxins is unclear. Some endotoxins, like those of the plague bacillus, *Yersinia pestis*, do induce inactivating antibody, but the classic endotoxins, like the salmonella lipopolysaccharides (LPS), generally do not induce inactivating antibodies in the infected host. LPS, however, is a potent activator of the alternate complement pathway, and there is some evidence that this is facilitated by natural antibody to LPS. Complement-mediated opsonization may thus occur and may provide an explanation for the allegedly nonimmune clearance of LPS by the reticuloendothelial system. Also, normal serum contains alpha-2-globulins, which can bind and inactivate LPS in vitro. However, their in vivo significance is unknown.

Bacteriolysis Many infected hosts develop antibody that, with complement, can lyse the infecting organism, especially gram-negative bacilli, in vitro. IgG or IgM can generate such lytic complement activity, although bacteriolysis proceeds best when both the classic and alternate complement pathways are utilized. Secretory and aggregated serum IgA can activate the terminal complement components through the alternate pathway but require the additional presence of lysozyme to effect bacteriolysis. It is unlikely, however, that secretory IgA-mediated bacteriolysis could represent a significant host defense in vivo, since most sites of secretory IgA elaboration have little, if any, complement activity. Indeed, the bactericidal effects of complement activation seem in general to be far less important in vivo than do the opsonins, chemotactic factors, and so on generated from various complement components (Chap. 16).

Immune lymphocytes and some lymphokines can directly destroy cells (Chap. 23) and thus might be expected to have direct bactericidal effects as well, but little is known about this potential mechanism.

Phagocytosis Effector Cells. Phagocytosis is the principal host mechanism for the elimination of most microorganisms and is a function of both monocytes, which in the tissues differentiate into macrophages, and polymorphonuclear leukocytes (PMNs). Both PMNs and monocytes are derived from a common stem cell in the bone marrow, where they normally mature. Upon release from the marrow, PMNs circulate for six to seven hours and then pass into the tissues, where they survive for four or five days. Monocytes remain in the circulation for one to three days prior to entering the tissues. Here, as macrophages, they survive for several months and may either migrate within the tissues or become fixed macrophages, such as the hepatic Kupffer cells. Both PMNs and monocytes, once released from the marrow, normally do not undergo mitosis. Thus an increased need of the host for more phagocytes to meet an infectious challenge is met initially by increased release from marrow stores and then by increased phagocyte production within the marrow. Proliferation of stem cells and release of both PMNs and monocytes are regulated by neurologic mechanisms and by serum factors, some of which increase during bacterial and viral infections.

Chemotaxis. The first role of the immunologic system in phagocytosis is to attract PMNs and monocytes to the site of interaction between antibody or immune lymphocytes and either the microorganism itself or infected cells. This function is mediated by chemotactic factors (Chap. 16), either released from immune T lymphocytes or formed from complexes or cleavage products of complement components. Complement–dependent chemotactic factors may be generated by both the classic and alternate pathways, as well as by plasmin, trypsin, and bacterial and tissue proteases.

Attachment. The first step in phagocytosis itself is the attachment of the microorganisms to the phagocyte. Many pathogens owe their virulence to their ability to resist such attachment. Consequently, a major function of several facets of the immune response to an infectious agent is opsonization (Gr. *opsonein*, to prepare food for). Attachment is facilitated by the following.

(1) Both monocytes and PMNs have receptors for the Fc fragment of certain subclasses (in man, IgG_1 and IgG_3) of antigen-bound IgG but not for the other IgG subclasses, IgM, or IgA. Appropriate types of IgG specific for a microorganism may thus facilitate attachment of this organism to a phagocyte.

(2) Both monocytes and PMNs also have receptors for activated C3. Thus, in the presence of complement, a complex of any complement-fixing antibody with its antigen can initiate opsonization (Chap. 16). C3-mediated opsonization may be particularly important in the early stages of infection, when IgM antibody predominates. Likewise, since endotoxin itself, or perhaps in complex with natural antibody, can initiate alternate pathway activation, C3-mediated opsonization of endotoxin-containing organisms may proceed in nonimmune individuals. Aggregated IgA and some denatured proteins can also activate the alternate pathway, but their role in opsonization is unknown.

(3) Organisms bearing activated C3 also can adhere to erythrocytes by immune adherence (Chap. 16). Since C3 can directly mediate opsonization, this mechanism seems redundant. In vivo, however, potent serum C3 inactivators may destroy bacterium-bound C3 before opsonization can occur. Since erythrocytes are so abundant, however, immune adherence may occur before C3 inactivation. The erythrocyte-bacterium complex is then readily phagocytosed. This mechanism seems most important against circulating gram-negative bacteria.

(4) In contrast to the binding of an antigen-antibody complex to a phagocyte, uncomplexed cytophilic antibody (Chap. 23) may bind, by its

Fc receptor, to macrophages. If the antibody is directed against a microbial antigen, subsequent encounter of the macrophage-antibody complex with the microbe may facilitate attachment.

(5) Certain bacterial components, such as the streptococcal M protein and staphylococcal protein A (Chaps. 26 and 27) can inhibit attachment even in the presence of opsonins. The activity of protein A, at least in part, is due to its capacity to bind, with great affinity, to the Fc fragment of IgG. Such binding to the Fc fragment of bacterium-bound antibody would inhibit IgG-mediated opsonization and, by blocking complement fixation, C3-mediated opsonization as well. Antibody specific for staphylococcal protein A itself, however, can render the bacteria susceptible to opsonization by either IgG or C3.

INGESTION AND DESTRUCTION OF THE MICROORGANISM. Following attachment, pseudopodia extend from the phagocyte and fuse around the organism, thus forming a phagocytic vesicle or phagosome within the cell. The phagosome fuses with cytoplasmic lysosomal vesicles to form a phagolysosome. Within the phagolysosome the microorganism is killed and digested by both oxygen-dependent and oxygen-independent mechanisms. The oxygen-independent mechanisms include the effects of low intravacuolar pH (as low as 4.0 in PMNs), lactoferrin, lysozyme, granular cationic proteins, proteases, lipases, and glycosidases. Lactoferrin chelates iron necessary for the growth of certain organisms. Lysozyme itself is lytic to few organisms, but it does facilitate and amplify the microbicidal effects of other mechanisms. Granular cationic proteins have been found only in PMNs. In vitro they have potent bactericidal effects, but their relative importance in vivo is unclear.

The oxygen-dependent mechanisms of the PMN can be divided into the myeloperoxidase (MPO)-mediated and the MPO-independent systems. In the macrophage, however, MPO is either absent or present in very low amounts. Both groups of oxygen-dependent mechanisms rely heavily on the presence of intracellular peroxide, generated principally from nicotinamide adenine dinucleotide (NADH) and oxygen by NADH oxidase. The precise microbicidal mechanism of MPO is a subject of current controversy, but it involves, at least in part, the production of highly reactive singlet oxygen (0^-) radicals by the oxidation of chloride ions in the presence of excess peroxide. The MPO-independent mechanisms involve the direct microbicidal effects of peroxide, as well as the production of reactive hydroxyl (OH^-) and singlet oxygen radicals and superoxide anions $(O_2{}^-)$. Patients with chronic granulomatous disease (Chap. 20) generally are deficient in their ability to generate intracellular peroxide, and, thus, their phagocytes have diminished microbicidal activity. These patients are particularly sensitive to those organisms which possess either catalase or superoxide dismutase but normally handle infections with organisms, such as pneumococci, enteric streptococci, and *Haemophilus influenzae*, which both lack catalase and themselves produce peroxide.

Immunologic Defenses against Intracellular Organisms

Certain bacteria, most notably the mycobacteria, and most pathogenic fungi and protozoa replicate and remain within the host's cells and are thus inaccessible to many of the defense mechanisms useful against extracellular organisms. The infected cells must thus be lysed and the infectious agents contained therein released into an area with abundant microbicidal and phagocytic activity. The major effector of both host cell lysis and microbial destruction is the activated macrophage.

Initiation of the Response: Lymphocyte Stimulation and Macrophage Recruitment Although intracellular pathogens induce an antibody response and its associated direct and complement-mediated antitoxic, phagocytic, and microbicidal effects, it is principally the immune T lymphocyte that initiates the host defense against intracellular organisms. Upon primary exposure to the microbe, specific antigen-reactive, recirculating T cells in the spleen, lymph nodes, Peyer's patches, and so on undergo mitosis and either differentiate into, or stimulate the production of, antigen-specific effector T cells. Within two or three days, these cells enter the blood and subsequently the infected tissues. Early, and with acute infections, such as listeria infections, these effector cells are short-lived and rapidly dividing, but, with more indolent infections, such as leishmaniasis and tuberculosis, long-lived, radioresistant cells eventually predominate.

Within the tissues the immune T effector cells encounter microbial antigens and are stimulated to elaborate various lymphokines, most notably monocyte chemotactic factor and macrophage migration inhibition factor (MIF), which attract macrophages and retain them within the infected area.

The Activated Macrophage PMNs and normal macrophages have little cytolytic capacity. Likewise, intracellular pathogens, such as the tubercle bacillus, may be readily ingested by PMNs or normal macrophages but are resistant to the cells' internal microbicidal effects. While the PMN is usually an end stage cell, with limited capacity for de novo protein synthesis, the monocyte or macrophage does retain considerable RNA and protein-synthetic poten-

tial. Through a number of mechanisms (Chap. 23), the macrophage can be activated to secrete collagenase, plasminogen activator, and lysosomal hydrolases into the extracellular environment, where they may destroy adjacent cells. Activation, likewise, greatly augments macrophage spreading and phagocytic and microbicidal activity by increasing aerobic metabolism and peroxide production and inducing synthesis of additional lysosomal and nonlysosomal enzymes (Fig. 18-1). It is not known whether macrophages activated by T cell products, such as SMAF (Chap. 23), differ from those activated by other means, but activated macrophages do manifest both specific and nonspecific cytolytic and microbicidal effects. Thus, the site of the host response to an intracellular organism is characterized by local tissue necrosis, numerous lymphocytes at various stages of blastogenesis, and abundant activated macrophages, containing digested cellular and microbial debris. In some cases, there are also large multinucleate cells formed from fusion of several macrophages.

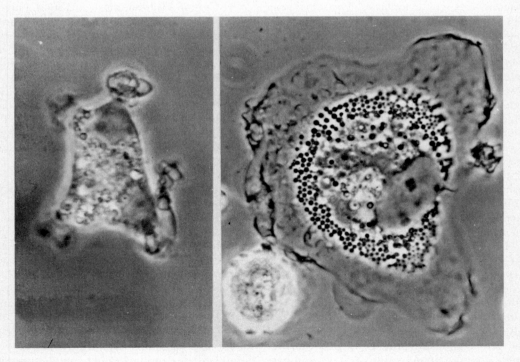

FIG. 18-1. Phase photomicrograph of macrophage activation. Left: Unactivated macrophage with well-developed pseudopodia but few lysosomes. Right: Macrophage activated by incubation for one day with immune lymphocytes and antigen. The cell is much enlarged and shows increased spreading, prominent nucleoli, and a large ring of phase-dense lysosomes. Both ×1560. (Courtesy of Dr. D. O. Adams)

RESISTANCE OF VIRULENT ORGANISMS. The virulence of an extracellular pathogen is largely a function of its resistance to attachment. Intracellular pathogens, on the other hand, are readily ingested by phagocytes, but their virulence is dependent upon resistance to the microbicidal effects of the activated macrophage. Some organisms can disrupt the phagosomal membrane, inhibit lysosome–phagosome fusion, resist phagolysosomal enzymes, or inhibit the metabolism of the macrophage. This resistance is frequently species specific; for example, *Leishmania enreittii,* which is lethal to guinea pigs but not mice, is readily phagocytosed by activated macrophages from both species but is destroyed only by murine cells.

Immunologic Defenses against Extracellular Viruses

Although viruses replicate only within the cell, generally exist only briefly in the extracellular state, and do not elaborate soluble exotoxins, the immunologic defense against viral infection shares many similarities with that against bacteria or fungi. Figure 18-2 illustrates the three modes by which viruses may

spread from cell to cell. Several mechanisms are available to prevent Type I dissemination. These are particularly important against infections with picornaviruses and flaviviruses, whose spread from the primary infection site to vital organs, like the heart and central nervous system, is frequently dependent upon the development of a high titer of extracellular virus in the circulation.

Secretory IgA Secretory IgA plays little role in the defense against a primary viral infection, but for many years thereafter, lymphocytes and plasma cells of the tonsils, adenoids, and mucosal lamina propria may persistently elaborate high levels of specific secretory IgA. Such antibody production is best initiated by local immunization through the oral or aerosol route but may also be stimulated by parenteral administration of live or killed virus. Secondary viral challenge at the mucosal surface, however, is met by a rapid, vigorous increase in local secretory IgA production. The increase is detectable within seven hours of infection, and in two to three days, the gut alone may produce over 3 g of antibody per day. Individuals with selective IgA deficiency (Chap. 20), although they are well able to clear virus from the circu-

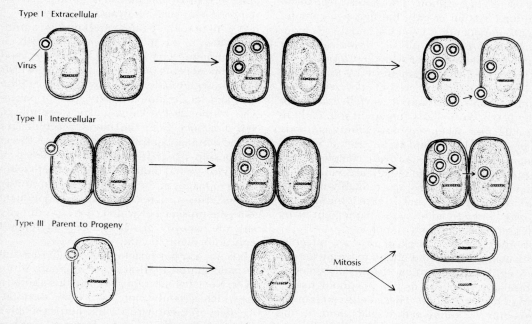

Type I Extracellular

Virus

Type II Intercellular

Type III Parent to Progeny

Mitosis

FIG. 18-2. Three modes of virus dissemination. It should be emphasized, however, that most viruses capable of Type II or Type III spread also lyse infected cells and thus utilize Type I spread as well. (From Notkins: Hosp Practice 9:65, 1974)

lation, frequently are unable to rid the mucosal surfaces of viruses. Likewise, although infants do not produce secretory IgA for one to three months after birth, breast-fed babies enjoy a decreased incidence of infantile diarrhea because of colostral IgA. Words of warning concerning secretory IgA are in order, however. Because the lung is a primary shock organ in man (Chap. 17), aerosol vaccines, despite their superior ability to induce local IgA secretion, should be avoided in atopic individuals. Likewise, oral vaccination of breast-fed infants should be delayed until after weaning, due to the potential interference of colostral IgA.

Viral Neutralization   Neutralization refers to the loss of infectivity and may be induced by interaction of specific antibody of either the IgG, IgM, or IgA class with the virion (Chap. 64). Such neutralization may occur in two ways: (1) The antibody, in some cases only a single immunoglobulin molecule, may bind to certain critical sites on the virion surface and thereby so distort the structural conformation of the viral coat as to prevent adsorption, penetration, or uncoating, or (2) binding of antibody to noncritical viral determinants may fix large amounts of complement on the virion surface and sterically impair some phase of infectivity, usually adsorption. The latter mechanism requires fixation of only the first two complement components, C1 and C4, and thus is independent of either virolysis, opsonization, or mediator release, all of which require fixation of more terminal components. C1,4 fixation not only coats the viral surface but may increase the avidity of antibody binding as well, and thus it may play a particularly important role early in the infection, when only low affinity antibody is present. Rheumatoid factor (RF) is an IgM that binds to antigen–antibody complexes and is present in the serum of patients with certain chronic viral infections, most notably hepatitis B. The role of RF in viral disease is unclear, but it may generate additional complement-fixing sites on virus–antibody complexes.

Within the first week of primary infection with many viruses, and often preceding detectable antibody production, specifically immune lymphocytes appear in the lymphoid tissues and in the circulation. These cells can transfer immunity to uninfected animals, and, in the presence of viral antigen, are stimulated in vitro to undergo blastogenesis and elaborate lymphokines, including interferon (Chap. 68). The ability of these lymphocytes to lyse infected cells and to recruit and activate macrophages is discussed below, but their role as direct mediators of viral neutralization is unclear. Some studies have shown a reduction in viral infectivity after incubation in vitro with immune lymphocytes, but this effect has not been proven independent of antibody secreted by the lymphocytes. On the other hand, immune lymphocytes, when stimulated to blastogenesis by viral antigen, may actually augment the titer of infectious virus, since several viruses are unable to replicate in normal lymphocytes but can do so in dividing lymphocytes.

Destruction and Clearance of Viruses   Viral neutralization does not necessarily destroy or eliminate the infectious agent. Antibody and complement may dissociate from the virus or be digested by serum or intracellular proteases, thus restoring viral infectivity. Clearly, additional mechanisms must be available for the destruction and clearance of neutralized virus. In vitro studies have shown that fixation of the complete complement sequence can induce structural lesions in certain enveloped viruses. These lesions do not themselves destroy the virus but, rather, expose internal viral components to lysis by nucleases and proteases. The in vivo role of such virolysis is unknown.

As with nonviral pathogens, however, a principal effect of the interaction of virus with either immune lymphocytes or antibody and complement is the potentiation of phagocytosis through agglutination and opsonization of the virus and localization and activation of phagocytes. Although PMNs may play some role in viral clearance from the blood, macrophages are the dominant antiviral phagocytes. A direct relationship exists between the virulence of many viruses and their ability to replicate within macrophages of the host. Host susceptibility to some viruses segregates as a single dominant gene, the presence of which correlates directly with the capacity of macrophages to support replication of the specific virus.

It is unclear how macrophages from resistant hosts do inhibit replication of internalized viruses. Neonatal macrophages lack this ability, a fact which certainly contributes to the devastating effect of certain viruses, like herpes simplex and rubella, on the neonate. Maturation of macrophage virucidal capacity seems dependent upon an intact thymus-derived immune system. Evidence suggests that, within the first few weeks of life, T cells are stimulated by various ubiquitous nonviral antigens to elaborate soluble factors that induce macrophage maturation. Whether one of these maturation factors is interferon (Chap. 68) is a subject of current controversy.

Immunologic Defenses against Intracellular Viruses

Some viruses, especially the herpesviruses, myxoviruses, paramyxoviruses and poxviruses, although they do lyse infected cells, are also able to employ Type II dissemination (Fig. 18-2), against which extracellular mechanisms are ineffective. As with intracellular bacteria and fungi, the immune response to these viruses focuses on both destruction of infected cells and elimination of the infectious agent. The antigenic stimulus may be either the virus or the altered antigenicity of the infected cell itself. Host cell antigenicity may be altered by (1) appearance of viral structural antigens on the cell surface, (2) expression of virus-coded, nonstructural antigens at the cell surface, (3) modification or unmasking of host-directed cell surface antigens by the infectious process. Where the response is directed at an altered cellular surface, the full spectrum of immune effectors active against allografts and tumor cells (Chap. 23 for descriptions of the individual mechanisms) may thus be deployed, including (1) cytotoxic antibody, (2) lymphocyte-dependent antibody (LDA), (3) activated macrophages, (4) lymphokines, and (5) direct lymphocyte-mediated cytotoxicity (DLMC). Likewise, these effector mechanisms are subject

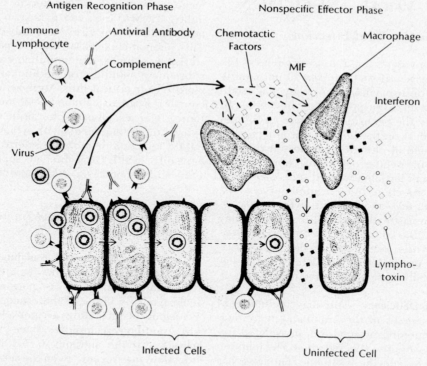

FIG. 18-3. The host immune response to viral infection consists of two phases. In the antigen recognition phase, immune lymphocytes, antibody, and complement react with virus and virus-infected cells. This response can lyse infected cells and neutralize extracellular virus. It also generates immunologic mediators which recruit and activate macrophages. These cells phagocytose viruses and also destroy infected and uninfected cells. In concert with interferon, elaborated by lymphocytes, infected cells, and macrophages themselves, as well as with various lymphokines, such as lymphotoxin, the macrophages halt intercellular viral spread by inhibiting viral replication and breaking contact between adjacent cells. (From Notkins: Hosp Practice 9:65, 1974)

to various inhibitory effects, such as abrogation of DLMC by free antigen, blocking antibody, and immune complexes.

Although these various mechanisms are well able to lyse the infected cells and destroy virus so released, in vitro studies with herpes simplex virus have shown that lysis of the infected cells may occur too slowly to prevent Type II dissemination to adjacent cells. These studies suggested that two additional mechanisms are operative (Fig. 18-3): (1) inhibition of viral replication in adjacent cells by interferon secreted by immune lymphocytes and, perhaps, activated macrophages and (2) disruption of contact between adjacent cells by nonspecific, soluble factors generated from the complement system, immune T cells, and activated macrophages.

IMMUNOPATHOLOGY OF VIRAL INFECTION

Persistent Viral Infection

Some viruses are able to circumvent the host's defenses. If such viruses do not rapidly infect and destroy vital tissues, they may establish long-term, even permanent, infections. In some cases, the persistent infection has no detectable effect on the host, but in others it induces a state of chronic or recurrent disease. Examples of such persistent infections include recurrent herpes labialis (cold sores), so-called slow viral infections of the central nervous system (Chap. 82), and, indeed, even virally induced neoplastic disease. Three factors may account for the failure of host defenses to eliminate the virus: deficiency of the host, virus-mediated abrogation of the defenses, and immunologic abrogation of the defenses.

Host Deficiency This may include general deficiencies of the immunologic system, either congenital or acquired, or isolated unresponsiveness to a specific virus. The immune response to specific synthetic antigens has been shown to be controlled by Ir genes linked to the major histocompatibility complex (Chaps. 16 and 22), and recent studies have suggested that similar genes may control the immune response to certain viral pathogens.

Virus-mediated Abrogation of Host Defenses Normal lymphocytes do not support the replication of many viruses but can do so while undergoing blastogenesis. A virus may thus produce specific unresponsiveness to its own antigens by exploiting its ability to induce blastogenesis of the specific antigen-reactive T cells and, thereby, facilitate lytic infection and depletion of these cells. Some viruses, such as the Friend leukemia virus, can produce generalized immunosuppression by infection of stem cells or peripheral lymphoid tissues.

A viral genome that has been integrated into host germ cell DNA may be vertically transmitted to the offspring. Subsequent production of virus-coded proteins by fetal or neonatal cells may induce tolerance. Similarly, transplacental or neonatal infection with the virus itself, as in the case of the murine mammary tumor viruses, may also induce tolerance to viral antigens.

Immunologic Abrogation of Host Defenses Some viruses, such as lymphocytic choriomeningitis (LCM) virus, can persist in the circulation as infectious virus–antibody complexes. This phenomenon is, at least in part, due to steric inhibition by nonneutralizing antibody of subsequent binding of additional antibody molecules to critical sites. Antibody or immune complexes can also abrogate cell-mediated antiviral defenses, for example, serum or cerebrospinal fluid from patients with cytomegalovirus (CMV) infection or subacute sclerosing panencephalitis (SSPE) can abrogate specific virus-induced blastogenesis or MIF production.

Autodestructive Host Immune Reactions

Systemic Effects of Circulating Virus-Antibody Complexes FACILITATION OF VIRAL INFECTIVITY. Some cells, such as peripheral blood leukocytes, by virtue of their receptors for the Fc region of IgG, allow greater adsorption by virus–antibody complexes than by free viral particles. If the antibody is nonneutralizing, infection may occur, even in normally nonpermissive cells.

TISSUE DAMAGE. Immune complexes in the circulation and their deposition in tissues, especially the end-arterioles of the glomerulus and vascular intima, can initiate severe inflammatory diseases (Chap. 19). Infectious virus-antibody complexes have been found in the circulation of animals infected with a number of different viruses, including LCM virus, Aleutian mink disease virus, lactic dehydrogenase virus (LDV), and the murine leukemia viruses. Some of these infected animals developed immune complex diseases, all cases of which were associated with deposition in the affected tissues of viral antigen, specific antiviral antibody, and complement. It is noteworthy, however, that the mere presence of circulating virus–antibody complexes did not assure the production of immune complex disease. Host genetic factors and the ability of the virus to replicate within the tissue sites of complex deposition also influenced the frequency, severity, and tissue location of the disease.

In man, virus–antibody complexes also seem able to induce inflammatory disease. Glomerulonephritis, arthritis, and arteritis, with deposition of viral antigen, antibody, and complement in the glomeruli, arteries, and synovia, have been reported in several cases of hepatitis B infection. Moreover, hepatitis B antigen has been found in 60 percent of patients with periarteritis nodosa. The severity of respiratory syncytial viral infection is increased by the administration of killed vaccine, which stimulates the production of circulating IgG and, presumably, leads to the formation of circulating virus–antibody complexes.

Perhaps the most striking example of virus-induced immune complex disease in man is the dengue hemorrhagic shock syndrome (DHSS). Dengue fever is endemic in Southeast Asia and is caused by several antigenically similar flaviviruses. DHSS is a frequent complication of a secondary bout of dengue fever caused by infection with a virus of a different serotype from that causing the initial infection. Because of the phenomenon, original antigenic sin, large amounts of antibody against the initial virus are produced. This antibody combines with, but does not neutralize, the cross-reactive second virus. The presence of bound antibody allows the virus to adsorb to the Fc receptors of peripheral blood leukocytes and, thereby, replicate to high titer in the circulation. Virus–antibody complexes activate the complement system, which, in turn, generates massive amounts of inflammatory mediators (Chap. 16)

and initiates widespread intravascular coagulation. In severe cases, over 80 percent of the serum C3 and C5 may be activated.

Excessive Local Tissue Destruction The formation of circulating infectious virus–antibody complexes, with its resultant pathologic effects, represents a qualitative abnormality of the host response to viral infection. In some cases, however, the normal inflammatory response to infection may induce significant tissue destruction — in essence, a quantitative abnormality of the host response. The clearest example of this phenomenon is seen with lymphocytic choriomeningitis (LCM) viral infection.

LCM virus itself usually induces very little cytopathology. In some in vitro cell cultures it may replicate and be released into the medium indefinitely without destruction of the cells. Inoculation of LCM virus into newborn mice leads to generalized infection of all tissues, where the virus persistently replicates and establishes a lifelong, largely asymptomatic, carrier state. Neurons of the brain and peripheral nervous system are extensively involved, but no neurologic abnormalities are observed. Newborn mice, however, are immunologically immature, and the neonatal infection establishes a state of immunologic unresponsiveness to the viral antigens.

In marked contrast, infection of adult mice with LCM virus, particularly by intracerebral inoculation, induces massive infiltration of lymphocytes and macrophages throughout the meninges, ependyma, and choroid plexus. This inflammation is accompanied by extensive cerebral edema, which kills the animal within two weeks of infection. Mice may be completely protected from the disease by the elimination of circulating T cells, but inhibition of antibody production has no effect. Affected animals have circulating and tissue-associated T cells that are cytotoxic in vitro to LCM virus-infected cells, but it is likely that the in vivo cytopathology is produced both by direct lymphocyte-mediated cytotoxicity and by macrophages recruited and activated by the immune lymphocytes.

With LCM, because the virus itself is so benign, the immunopathologic effects can be easily appreciated. It is likely, however, that the tissue destruction associated with many viral infections is due to a combination of virus and host effects. It may thus be expedient, in those clinical settings where inflammatory effects predominate, such as some viral encephalopathies, to suppress all or part of the patient's immune response. This consideration makes it incumbent upon the physician to assess, early in the course of serious infectious disease, the extent and significance of inflammatory lesions, even if it entails biopsy of involved tissues. Similarly, he must know the mechanism of the immunologic damage in order to choose an appropriate immunosuppressive modality—for example, the T cells responsible for fatal LCM viral infection are resistant to corticosteriods.

FURTHER READING

Books and Reviews

Almeida JD, Waterson AP: The morphology of virus-antibody interaction. Adv Virus Res 15:307, 1969

Atkins E: Pathogenesis of fever. Physiol Rev 40:580, 1960

Brent L, Holborow J (eds): Progress in Immunology II. New York, American Elsevier, 1974, vol 4

Cowan KM: Antibody response to viral antigens. Adv Immunol 17:195, 1973

Klebanoff SJ: Antimicrobial systems of the polymorphonuclear leukocyte. In Bellanti JA, Dayton DH (eds): The Phagocytic Cell in Host Resistance. New York, Raven Press, 1975, pp 45–49

Larsh JE, Weatherly NF: Cell-mediated immunity in certain parasitic infections. Curr Top Microbiol Immunol 67:113, 1974

Lyampert IM, Danilova TA: Immunological phenomena associated with cross-reactive antigens of microorganisms and mammalian tissues. Prog Allergy 18: 423, 1975

Mackaness GB, Blanden RV: Cellular immunity. Prog Allergy 11:89, 1967

Möller G (ed.): The immune response to infectious diseases. Transplant Rev 19: 1, 1974

Notkins AL: Viral infections: Mechanisms of immunologic defense and injury. Hosp Practice 9:65, 1974

Notkins AL (ed.): Viral Immunity and Immunopathology. New York, Academic Press, 1975

Reed WD, Eddleston ALWF, Williams R: Immunopathology of viral hepatitis in man. Prog Med Virol 17:38, 1974

Wheelock EF, Toy ST: Participation of lymphocytes in viral infections. Adv Immunol 16:124, 1973

Selected Papers

Ashe WK, Daniels CA, Scott GS, Notkins AL: Interaction of rheumatoid factor with infectious herpes simplex virus-antibody complexes. Science 172:176, 1971

Gibbs DL, Roberts RB: The interaction in vitro between human polymorphonuclear leukocytes and Neisseria gonorrhoeae cultivated in the chick embryo. J Exp Med 141:155, 1975

Greenberg LJ, Gray ED, Yunis EJ: Association of HL-A 5 and immune responsiveness in vitro to streptococcal antigens. J Exp Med 141:935, 1975

Jones TC, Len L, Hirsch JG: Assessment in vitro of immunity against Toxoplasma gondii. J Exp Med 141:466, 1975

Lafferty KJ: The interaction between virus and antibody. Virology 21:61,76, 91, 1963

Rosen FS: The endotoxins of gram-negative bacteria and host resistance. N Engl J Med 264:919, 1961

Rossen RD, Kasel JA, Couch RB: The secretory immune system: Its relation to respiratory viral infection. Prog Med Virol 13:194, 1971

Shin HS, Smith MR, Wood WB Jr: Heat labile opsonins to pneumococcus II. Involvement of C3 and C5. J Exp Med 130:1229, 1969

Zinkernagel RM, Doherty PC: H-2 compatibility requirement for T-cell-mediated lysis of target cells infected with lymphocytic choriomeningitis virus. Different cytotoxic T-cell specificities are associated with structures coded for in H-2K or H-2D. J Exp Med 141:1427, 1975

19
Autodestructive Immune Reactions Initiated by Antibody

TABLE 19-1 AUTODESTRUCTIVE DISEASES INITIATED BY ANTIBODY

Initiating Factor	Example
Immune complexes	
Local	Arthus reaction
Systemic	Serum sickness, NZB/W disease, systemic lupus erythematosus
Antibody to self	Idiopathic thrombocytopenic purpura (ITP), Goodpasture's syndrome, Hashimoto's thyroiditis
Antibody to antigen bound to self	Quinine- or Sedormid-induced thrombocytopenia
Antibody to neoantigens	Antiviral antibody mediated destruction of virus-infected cells
Antibody to cross-reactive antigens	Rheumatic fever, hemolytic anemia following anti-pneumococcus type XIV anti-serum

The inflammatory process, by destroying antigens, provides an important mechanism by which the immune system mediates host defense (Chap. 16). However, inflammation can also produce severe host morbidity or mortality under certain conditions. Persistent inflammatory reactions that occur in specialized tissues, such as the heart, kidney, lungs, synovium, and central nervous system, may lead to marked functional impairment of vital organs. Immunologically mediated tissue destruction directed by antibody can be initiated by (1) immune complexes of antigens and antibodies, (2) antibodies directed to the host's own tissues, (3) antibodies directed to antigens bound to host tissues, (4) antibodies directed to neoantigens on the host tissues, or (5) antibodies directed toward antigens that cross-react with the host's tissues (Table 19-1).

INFLAMMATORY DISEASES PRODUCED BY IMMUNE COMPLEXES

Arthus Reaction The introduction of a nontoxic foreign protein into the skin of an animal results in no inflammatory reaction unless the animal is sensitive to the antigen. Cutaneous administration of antigen to animals with circulating antibody to the antigen produces a local inflammatory reaction characterized by increased vascular permeability, vascular stasis, and the local accumulation of polymorphonuclear leukocytes and macrophages. Hemorrhage, necrosis, and sloughing of the skin occur in severe reactions (Fig. 19-1). The local inflammatory response to immune complexes is termed the "Arthus reaction." Edema and hyperemia begin 3 to 6 hours after antigen challenge, and the inflammatory response is maximal by 12 to 24 hours. Immunofluorescence studies of lesions from Arthus reactions demonstrate vascular localization of antigen, antibody (predominantly IgG or IgM), and complement. Activation of the complement cascade by the immune complexes results in the local accumulation of leukocytes and platelets (Chap. 16). The immune complexes are phagocytosed and digested, but during phagocytosis lysozomal enzymes released locally destroy host tissue.

Experimental Serum Sickness The intravenous injection of a nontoxic foreign protein into a nonimmune animal causes no deleterious effects until antibody is produced. Five to ten days after the administration of the antigen, its rate of clearance from the circulation is markedly increased and circulating immune complexes can then be detected (Fig. 19-2). At first, the complexes are in great antigen excess, but as

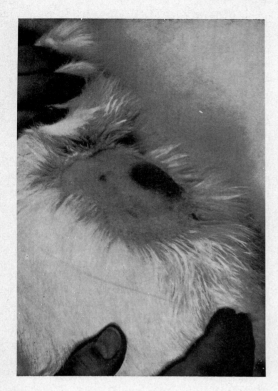

FIG. 19-1. A moderately severe Arthus reaction in the skin of a rabbit sensitized to serum albumin. (Courtesy of Dr. Gil Eiring)

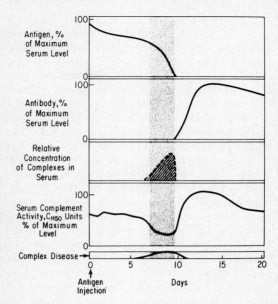

FIG. 19-2. Relationships between the serologic events and experimental immune complex disease. Injected antigen is equilibrated with body fluid and undergoes gradual catabolic attrition until day 6, when antibody production begins. Rapid attrition of antigen characteristic of immune elimination occurs between day 7 and day 10. During this interval, antibody production results in the presence of identifiable antigen-antibody complexes in the serum, depression of complement activity, and tissue changes in kidney glomeruli and blood vessel walls characteristic of immune complex disease. Free antibody appears after antigen elimination and is followed by a rebound in serum complement activity.

antibody production increases, the immune complexes increase in size, and the ratio of antigen to antibody decreases. The most pathogenic immune complexes are those formed in slight antigen excess with a size of approximately 22S and a circulation time of approximately 90 minutes. The formation of immune complexes in slight antigen excess is associated with a number of pathophysiologic events. The animal becomes febrile, thrombocytopenic, and leukopenic and develops carditis, arthritis, and glomerulonephritis. This phenomenon is called "experimental one-shot serum sickness." At the onset of these signs, the complement titer falls precipitously, and immune complexes and complement can be detected in the affected organs. As antibody production increases further, the immune complexes become still larger and are more easily phagocytosed (and cleared) by the reticuloendothelial cells of the liver and spleen. Once all antigen is removed from the circulation, free antibody can

be detected in the serum, and the signs and symptoms of the immune complex disease resolve. Complement activation and the local accumulation of polymorphonuclear leukocytes and platelets appear to be necessary for the tissue damage produced by one-shot serum sickness reactions.

The repeated daily administration of antigens at a level estimated to produce circulating immune complexes in slight antigen excess is termed "experimental chronic serum sickness" and produces chronic glomerulonephritis. The pathogenesis of chronic serum sickness glomerulonephritis, in contrast to one-shot serum sickness, involves glomerular damage which cannot be completely blocked by inhibition of the complement system or by depletion of circulating polymorphonuclear leukocytes.

NZB/W Disease The F_1 hybrid of a cross between New Zealand Black (NZB) and New Zealand White (NZW) mice spontaneously develops an immunologic disease which closely resembles serum sickness as well as human systemic lupus erythematosus. At about four months of age, the F_1 hybrids begin to develop a Coombs-positive hemolytic anemia, glomerulonephritis, vasculitis, antinuclear factors, and antibody to DNA and RNA. Autoimmune hemolytic anemia is most severe in NZB mice, whereas glomerulonephritis is most severe in female NZB/W-F_1 mice. This disease illustrates the contribution of genetic, infectious, and immunologic factors to the production of a spontaneous inflammatory disease. Genetically, multiple autosomal genes seem to be involved. Immunologically, these animals have heightened B cell responsiveness and depressed T cell function. They produce excessive levels of antibody to many experimental antigens and have delayed skin graft rejections as well as depressed lymphoproliferative responses in vitro to T cell stimulants. Many strains of normal mice harbor Gross leukemia virus and develop no overt disease. NZB/W mice, however, produce unusually large amounts of antibody to this virus, and viral antigen-antibody complexes can be detected in glomerular deposits at the time when they develop glomerulonephritis. As in experimental serum sickness, serum complement levels fall during the development of glomerulonephritis. NZB/W disease thus appears to be a naturally occurring systemic immune complex disorder involving a genetic predisposition for abnormal immunologic responsiveness and an infectious agent to which the animals respond immunologically. Its similarity to human immune complex diseases makes it a very important experimental model, since the histopathology and serology of NZB/W disease is quite similar to human systemic lupus erythematosus. Moreover, some human beings with hepatitis B virus infection develop a systemic inflammatory disease with widespread vasculitis. This illustrates the potential importance of virus-antibody complexes in the pathogenesis of human disease (Chaps. 18 and 23).

Human Counterparts of Immune Complex Diseases Rheumatoid arthritis is an inflammatory disease that involves the synovial lining of joints. It produces symmetrical cartilage destruction and often leads to crippling. Inflammation associated with rheumatoid arthritis may also involve blood vessels in many areas of the body, but tissue destruction is usually most severe in the synovium. Complexes of rheumatoid factors (immunoglobulins that bind to the Fc portion of other immunoglobulins), IgG antibody, and complement are present in the synovial fluid, as are large numbers of polymorphonuclear leukocytes. Rapid local consumption of complement takes place within the joint, and complement breakdown products are present in the synovial fluid. The synovial tissue contains abundant numbers of plasma cells that secrete immunoglobulins. Rheumatoid arthritis appears to be, at least in part, an immune reaction of the Arthus type occurring in multiple joints. Complement activation is important in mediating the inflammatory process. The antigen or antigens that initiate the immune reaction remain unknown.

A human counterpart of experimental serum sickness can be seen following injection of patients with heterologous serum. This syndrome was quite prevalent when patients were treated with antiserum raised in animals to various toxins, such as tetanus toxin. Six to ten days after injection with heterologous antitoxin, treated individuals developed fever, malaise, arthritis, hematuria, and leukopenia. The pathophysiology of human serum sickness appears to be identical to the experimental animal counterparts, in that antibody directed against the foreign serum proteins initiates the disease.

Systemic lupus erythematosus is a multisystem inflammatory disease and is most common in young women. It is characterized by the development of fever, rash, arthralgias, arthritis, glomerulonephritis, serositis, leukopenia, circulating antibody to DNA, and depressed serum complement levels. Immune complexes of DNA-anti-DNA, and complement can be eluted from glomerular deposits. The similarities of the serologic findings and the histopathologic lesions in lupus with those of NZB/W disease of mice is striking. No common infectious agent has yet been recovered from patients with systemic lupus erythematosus. They have, however, been noted to have depressed T cell function and heightened antibody responsiveness. A higher incidence of inflammatory diseases is present in the families of patients with lupus erythematosus, but no direct inheritance pattern has yet been found.

DISEASES MEDIATED BY ANTIBODY DIRECTED TO A HOST'S OWN TISSUES

Several human diseases are thought to be initiated by the development of antibodies to components of the host's own tissues. Idiopathic thrombocytopenic purpura (ITP) serves as a good example. This disease is more common in women than in men and usually develops during the third decade of life. ITP is characterized by the development of hemorrhage and purpura. The circulating platelet counts are profoundly depressed, but examination of the bone marrow demonstrates heightened platelet production. Serum from these individuals contains antibody to human platelets and produces thrombocytopenia when injected into another individual. The antibody responsible for platelet destruction is of the IgG class, but the factors that lead to its formation are unknown. Autoimmune hemolytic anemias are also produced by the development of antibody to the host's own erythrocytes (Chap. 21). These may be initiated by either IgG or IgM type antibodies.

Inflammatory diseases of the thyroid (Hashimoto's thyroiditis) and hypofunction of the adrenal cortex (idiopathic Addison's disease) are associated with a high frequency of circulating antibodies to the target organ. In the case of Hashimoto's thyroiditis, antibody and complement can be found deposited within the inflamed thyroid gland.

Goodpasture's syndrome is another example of devastating host tissue destruction that may be produced by the development of antibody to certain self-components. This condition, more common in men, is associated with pulmonary hemorrhage, acute, rapidly progressive glomerulonephritis, and profound anemia. Antibody to pulmonary and glomerular basement membrane appears to be responsible for this disorder. Antibody and complement can be detected in the affected organs, and eluted antibody binds specifically to the basement membrane

of the lung and renal glomeruli. A similar disease can be produced in experimental animals by immunization with lung tissue or by the administration of antibody eluted from the kidneys of patients with Goodpasture's syndrome.

DISEASES PRODUCED BY ANTIBODY DIRECTED TO ANTIGEN BOUND TO HOST'S TISSUES

Hemolytic anemia and/or thrombocytopenia may be produced in susceptible individuals by the ingestion of certain drugs. Drugs can produce hemolytic anemia or thrombocytopenia by several mechanisms. One such mechanism involves the binding of the drug and antibody to the erythrocyte or platelet. Antibody which develops to the drug then forms an immune complex that becomes bound to the circulating cell and leads to its destruction by the reticuloendothelial system. Thrombocytopenia induced by quinine or Sedormid appears to be caused by the development of antibody to the drug. Serum from affected individuals does not destroy normal platelets unless the responsible drug is added, at which time antibody and the drug bind to the platelets.

TISSUE DESTRUCTION BY ANTIBODY DIRECTED TO NEOANTIGENS ON THE HOST'S CELLS

The infection of cells with certain viruses is followed by the development of viral antigens on the infected cell's membranes. For example, following infection of rabbit kidney cells with herpes simplex virus, herpes-associated antigens appear on the kidney cell membranes (Chap. 65). Antibody directed to herpes simplex virus then binds to the neoantigens on the rabbit kidney cells, and, in the presence of complement, cell lysis occurs. This laboratory phenomenon may be a prototype for many idiopathic autoimmune diseases that appear to follow viral infections. The infected host produces antibody to viral antigens, and antibodies then bind to and destroy cells containing virus-associated neoantigens on their surface (Chap. 64).

TISSUE DESTRUCTION BY ANTIBODY THAT CROSS-REACTS WITH THE HOST'S ANTIGENS

Many microbial products have antigens that cross-react with antigenic components of human tissues. For example, several components of streptococci share antigens with components of human heart and kidney. Antibodies directed to the streptococcal antigens can then cross-react with the host's myocardial or renal tissues. The contribution of this type of cross-reactivity to the development of poststreptococcal diseases, such as rheumatic fever or glomerulonephritis, is presently uncertain but may play some part in the pathogenesis of these diseases. Another example of cross-reactivity between bacterial antigens and human tissues can be found in pneumococcal disease. Polysaccharide capsular antigens of *Streptococcus pneumoniae* type XIV cross-react with human blood group antigens. When antipneumococcal antiserum was used for therapy in pneumococcal pneumonia, treatment of patients with antiserum to type XIV pneumococcus frequently produced hemolytic anemia due to cross-reactivity of the antiserum with the patient's erythrocytes. Cross-reactivity between microbial agents and erythrocytes may also be responsible for the formation of cold agglutinating antibody to blood group substances following mycoplasma infections and infectious mononucleosis. The same phenomenon may be related to the development of hemolytic reactions in syphilis.

SUMMARY

In summary, autodestructive diseases mediated by the immune system are an important cause of human morbidity and mortality. Immunologic reactions play a central role in protecting the host against microbial invasion and perhaps the development and spread of neoplasms. Under some circumstances, however, the inflammatory process initiated by immune reactions can be detrimental to the host. In some diseases the offending antigen is well characterized, but in most human inflammatory diseases the initiating agent remains to be identified. There is increasing awareness that genetic predisposition, perhaps related to histocompatibility-linked immune response genes, and exposure to infectious agents or other environmental antigens can produce inflammatory diseases. This awareness can be expected to lead to new insights concerning the etiology and treatment of these diseases.

FURTHER READING

Books and Reviews

Cochrane C, Koffler D: Immune complex disease in experimental animals and man. Adv Immunol 16:186, 1973

Samter M (ed): Immunological Diseases, 2nd ed. Boston, Little, Brown, 1971, vol 1 and 2

Selected Papers

Dixon FJ, Vazquez JJ, Weigle WD, Cochrane CG: Pathogenesis of serum sickness. Arch Pathol 65:18, 1958

Dixon FJ, Feldman JP, Vazquez JJ: Experimental glomerulonephritis: the pathogenesis of a laboratory model resembling the spectrum of human glomerulonephritis. J Exp Med 113:899, 1961

Koffler D, Schur PH, Kunkel HG: Immunological studies concerning the nephritis of systemic lupus erythematosus. J Exp Med 126:607, 1967

Lambert PH, Dixon FJ: Pathogenesis of the glomerulonephritis of NZB/W mice. J Exp Med 127:507, 1968

Mellors RC: Autoimmune disease in NZB/BL mice. J Exp Med 122:25, 1965

Porter DD, Larsen AG: The immunopathology of Aleutian disease of milk. In Miescher PA (ed): Immunopathology VI International Symposium. New York, Grune & Stratton, 1970, p. 404

Snyderman R, Pike MC, Altman LC: Abnormalities of leukocyte chemotaxis in human disease states. Ann NY Acad Sci 256:386, 1975

Talal N, Steinberg AD, Jacobs ME, Chused TM, Gazdar AD: Immune cell cooperation, viruses, and antibiotics to nucleic acids in New Zealand mice. J Exp Med 134:52S, 1971

Ziff, M: Pathophysiology of rheumatoid arthritis. Fed Proc 32:131, 1973

20

Normal and Abnormal Development of the Immune System

THE DEVELOPMENT OF NORMAL IMMUNE FUNCTION

Certain well-known attributes of the human fetus and newborn infant suggest abnormal immune function. These include diminished lymphoid tissue, an increased incidence of and often poor response to infection, and low to absent immune responses to certain types of antigens. These features led to the misconception that the human fetus and newborn are immunologically inactive. Although very little is yet known about the ontogeny of human specific immune responsiveness, information is rapidly accumulating that the fetus is immunologically competent from a very early age. It has been possible to gain information about the development of capacities for various types of specific immune responses in certain lower species through extensive studies of the fetus while in utero. The most ambitious and successful work of this type has been accomplished through hysterotomy and immunization of sheep and monkeys in utero. In this way it was learned that sheep can respond to antigens such as bacteriophage when they are immunized as early as the thirty-fifth day of their 149-day gestation period. This corresponds to a period of very minimal lymphoid development, when only an epithelial thymus is evident in the embryo. Later in development sheep embryos can respond to other antigens, such as ferritin and ovalbumin, but they never achieve the adult sheep's ability to respond to some other antigens, such as *Salmonella typhi*. Similar types of observations were made in the monkey. These findings support the concept that the capacity for specific immunologic responsiveness does not develop as an all-or-none phenomenon but rather that it appears in stepwise fashion for different types of antigens.

Although the time course of immunologic responsiveness appears to be genetically programmed for any given species, the question has arisen whether various morphologic and phenomenologic changes that occur in the lymphoid system of developing embryos might be related to antigen exposure. Studies in newborn piglets tend to support such a concept. In this species there is a six-layered placenta and no placental transfer of immunoglobulin takes place. In germ-free colostrum-deprived piglets no surface Ig-bearing B lymphocytes, plasma cells, natural antibodies. or germinal centers can be found, and the total lymphoid mass is extremely small. Nevertheless, such newborn piglets appear to be fully immunologically competent, since antibody production can be detected within 48 hours after immunization.

In studies with the chick embryo, however, a somewhat different picture has emerged. In this species, Lawton and Cooper found that cells containing IgM could be detected 24 hours after yolk sac stem cells enter the bursa of Fabricius at the thirteenth day of embryonation (when the embryo presumably has not encountered antigen). IgG-containing cells could first be found at 21 days of embryonic life, and they appeared in follicles which had prior to that time been engaged only in IgM synthesis. Therefore, since both IgM- and IgG-producing cells were normally found in the chick prior to hatching, these workers postulated that the first stage of B cell maturation, that is, development of the capacity to become antigen reactive and to bear surface Ig, is a clonal developmental stage and is thus antigen independent. The second stage, the clonal proliferation stage, begins when B cells encounter antigen. Lawton and Cooper hypothesized that IgG-producing cells are derived from IgM-producing cells through a genetic switch mechanism controlling immunoglobulin heavy-chain synthesis. This thesis was supported by the fact that injection of anti-μ chain antiserum into the chick embryo at the thirteenth day consistently led to agammaglobulinemia involving all classes of immunoglobulins.

Ontogeny in the Human Fetus

The human immune system, like that of other species, arises in the embryo from gut-associated tissue. The thymus first appears as a proliferation of epithelial cells lining the third and fourth branchial pouches at about the sixth or seventh week of embryonic life. Lymphoid tissue first appears in the thymus at about the eighth week of gestation, presumably as a result of a thymic microenvironmental influence on pluripotential stem cells which have migrated there from the yolk sac, fetal liver, or spleen. There, in the cortical area, these cells acquire surface alloantigenic markers analogous to θ (found on both thymocytes and T cells in the peripheral blood of mice) and TL (found only on thymocytes and leukemic cells) and immunocompetence. Fetal cortical thymocytes are among the most rapidly dividing cells in the body, with a mean generation time of six to eight hours. Many of these very immature cells die in situ, and the remainder migrate to the medulla. The more mature medullary thymocytes have a greater capacity to mediate cellular immune reactions and are resistant to the lytic effects of corticosteroids. They leave the thymus via the bloodstream and are distributed throughout the body, with heaviest concentrations in the paracortical areas of the lymph nodes, the periarteriolar areas of the spleen, and thoracic duct lymph. Thymic cells forming spontaneous sheep erythrocyte rosettes (E) have been noted as early as 8 weeks. Lymphocytes with membrane markers characteristic of T cells comprise 65 to 100 percent of thymus cells at this age. By 20 to 22 weeks T cells represent 10 to 30 percent of the fetal splenic lymphocyte population. Reactivity to phytohemagglutinin first appears in the thymus at 10 weeks, in the spleen at 13 weeks, and in the peripheral blood at 14.5 weeks. Mixed leukocyte reactivity is first detected in the thymus at 12.5 weeks and antigen-binding cells at 20 weeks. Evidence of specific cellular immune responsiveness appears even earlier in the fetal liver, as cells from this organ have been found to be capable of responding in mixed leukocyte culture as early as 7.5 weeks, and mild but definite graft-versus-host disease is observed following infusion of liver cells from 8- to 9-week fetuses into patients with severe combined immunodeficiency disease. Precursors of phagocytes and macrophages are also present in the liver at 8 weeks.

The first evidence of development of the humoral limb of the immune system is found in the appearance of surface Ig-bearing cells in the fetal liver as early as 9.5 weeks and in the peripheral blood, bone marrow, and spleen by 11.5 weeks. By 14 weeks the percentages of blood cells bearing surface Ig of the three major classes are similar to those found in normal adult blood. B cells appear in fetal spleen by 12 to 13 weeks, and by 15 to 25 weeks 30 to 45 percent of spleen cells bear surface Ig. The synthesis and secretion of IgM and IgE may occur as early as 10.5 weeks of gestation and IgG as early as 12 weeks, as shown by the incorporation by cultured fetal lymphoid cells of radio-labeled amino acids into immunoglobulins. Cultured spleen cells synthesize the most immunoglobulin, but small amounts can also be detected in cultures of thymus, liver, and gastrointestinal tract between 12 and 18 weeks gestation. No evidence of IgA or IgD synthesis is found in normal noninfected fetuses. Free secretory piece has been found in the urine of premature infants, however, indicating the normal fetal synthesis of this protein. Despite the capacity of fetal B lymphocytes to differentiate into immunoglobulin-synthesizing and secreting B plasma cells, plasma cells are not normally found in lymphoid tissues of the fetus until about 20 weeks' gestation, then only rarely. Peyer's patches have been found in significant numbers by the fifth intrauterine month, and plasma cells have been seen in the lamina propria by 25 weeks' gestation. At birth there may be primary lymphoid nodules, but usually secondary follicles are not present, and typical plasma cells are extremely few in number. These follicles appear shortly after birth as a result of antigenic stimulation afforded by extrauterine life. Intrauterine infection with *Treponema pallidum*, cytomegalovirus, rubella virus, toxoplasma, or other agents does, however, result in abundant fetal plasma cell formation and in development of mature reaction centers in the lymphoid tissues.

Normally the human fetus begins to receive significant quantities of maternal IgG transplacentally at around 12 weeks' gestation, although small amounts have been detected in the fetus as early as 7.5 weeks. The quantity increases steadily until, at birth, cord serum contains a concentration of IgG comparable to or greater than that of maternal serum (Fig. 20-1). IgG is the only class of immunoglobulin to cross the placenta to any significant degree, and all four subclasses appear to cross with ease. Complement components do not cross the placenta. The young of other species receive maternal antibodies by other routes, such as across the fetal yolk sac or via colostrum or ova. A small amount of IgM (10 percent of adult levels) and a few nanograms of IgE are usually found normally in cord serum, and since neither IgM nor IgE cross the placenta in any significant quantity, these proteins are presumed to be of fetal origin. The detection of maternal isoantibodies to fetal IgG, the finding of small amounts of IgG of fetal allotype in some cord sera, and the in vitro synthesis already mentioned are evidence

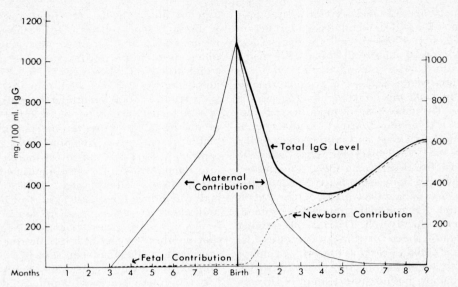

FIG. 20-1. Schematic representation of IgG concentrations in the fetus and newborn. [From Allansmith: In Falkner (ed): Human Development, 1966. Courtesy of W. B. Saunders]

for the normal fetal production of small quantities of this immunoglobulin as well. These observations raise the possiblity that certain antigenic stimuli normally cross the placenta to provoke responses even in noninfected fetuses. Indeed, some atopic infants frequently have reaginic antibodies to antigens (such as egg) to which they have had no known exposure during postnatal life, suggesting that synthesis of these IgE antibodies could have been induced in the fetus by placentally transmitted antigens ingested by the mother.

Ontogeny in the Infant and Child

T cells are present in cord blood in roughly the same quantity as in adults, although the percentage of E rosette-forming cells is somewhat less. These cells have the capacity to respond normally to the two T cell mitogens, phytohemagglutinin (PHA) and concanavalin A (Con A), and they are capable of mounting a normal mixed leukocyte response (a response considered to be mediated only by T cells). Thus, the absence of these responses in tests of cord blood lymphocytes is evidence a priori of profound primary dysfunction of the T cell system. The capacity of the newborn human infant to develop delayed hypersensitivity in vivo is

also present at birth, as demonstrated by experimentally induced rhus sensitivity and by BCG-induced tuberculin reactivity. Both premature and full-term infants were not, however, sensitized as regularly by the topical application of dinitrofluorobenzene as were older infants. Studies of homograft rejection in newborns have found first set homograft rejection time somewhat prolonged — 12 to 96 days as opposed to a normal adult rejection time of 10 to 11 days. The number of infants studied was small, however, and all of the skin grafts were either from parents to their infants or from the donors of fresh blood used in exchange transfusions of the infants, factors which could have accounted for the prolonged rejection times.

The newborn infant is quite susceptible to infections with gram-negative organisms, since he has not received IgM antibodies (eg, heat-stable opsonins) to these organisms from his mother. Quantities of certain heat-labile opsonins, C3b and C4b, are also lower in newborn serum than in adult serum. These factors probably account for the finding of impaired phagocytosis of some organisms by newborn polymorphonuclear cells, whereas in the presence of normal adult serum these cells phagocytize and kill such bacteria normally.

Maternally transmitted IgG antibodies serve quite adequately as heat-stable opsonins for gram-positive bacteria, and IgG antibodies to viruses afford adequate protection against those agents. Since premature infants have received less maternal IgG at the time of birth than full-term infants, their serum opsonic activity is low for all types of organisms. B lymphocytes are present in normal percentages and numbers in cord blood. A majority of these bear both surface IgM and IgD, in contrast to adult B cells which have more nearly equal proportions of IgM-IgD-bearing and IgG-bearing cells. The ability of cord blood cells to act as effectors in antibody-dependent lymphocyte cytotoxicity tests employing HLA antibody-coated lymphocytes as targets appears to be fully developed, however, and this function is thought to be mediated by Fc receptor bearing lymphocytes. The neonatal human being ordinarily begins to synthesize antibodies of the IgM class at an increased rate very soon after birth, in response to the immense antigenic stimulation of his new environment. Premature infants appear to mature immunologically at about the same rate as term infants. At about six days after birth, the serum concentration of IgM rises sharply. This rise continues for about a month, diminishes somewhat, then continues to rise until adult levels are achieved by approximately 1 year of age (Fig. 20-2). Cord serum usually does not contain detectable IgA. Serum IgA normally first becomes detectable at around the thirteenth day of postnatal life. The serum concentration of IgA gradually increases during early childhood until adult levels are achieved and preserved between the sixth and seventh years of life (Fig. 20-2). Cord serum contains an IgG concentration comparable to or greater than that of maternal serum. As indicated in Figure 20-1, maternal IgG gradually disappears during the first six to eight months of life. At the same time, an increased rate of synthesis of IgG by the newborn takes place. The total immunoglobulin level in the infant usually reaches a low point at approximately the fourth to fifth month of postnatal life. IgG synthesis continues at an increased rate until adult concentrations are reached and maintained by 6 to 7 years of age (Fig. 20-2). IgD is detectable at least as early as the sixth postnatal week, and adult concentrations are achieved by age 4 to 5 years. The rate of development of mature levels of IgE during childhood has been found to follow generally that of IgA. After adult concentrations of each of the three ma-

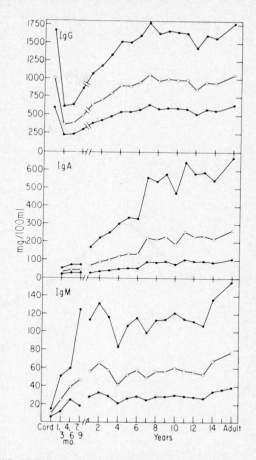

FIG. 20-2. Immunoglobulin concentrations in 201 normal subjects from infancy to adulthood. The lines connecting the open circles represent the geometric means, while the boundaries are obtained by taking the antilogs of the mean logs ± two pooled standard deviations of the logs. (From Buckley, Dees, and O'Fallon: Pediatrics 41:600, 1968)

jor immunoglobulins are reached, these levels remain remarkably constant for a given individual. Studies of serum immunoglobulin levels in identical twins suggest that hereditary factors play a major role in maintaining the constancy of serum immunoglobulin concentrations in normal individuals.

Lymphoid tissue is proportionally small but rather well developed at birth and matures rapidly in the postnatal period. The thymus is largest relative to body size during fetal life and at birth is ordinarily two-thirds its mature weight, which it attains during the first year of life. It reaches its peak mass, however, just before puberty, then gradually involutes there-

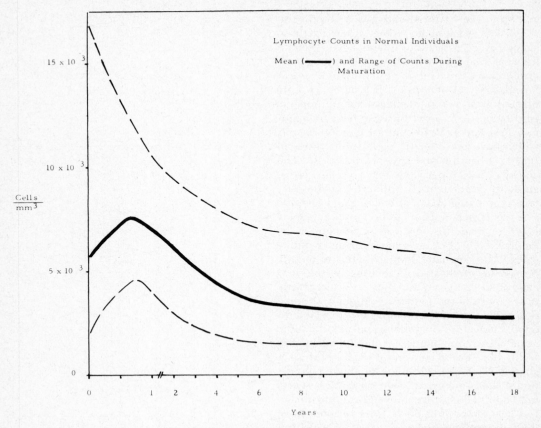

FIG. 20-3. Absolute lymphocyte counts in normal individuals during maturation. (From Altman: Blood and other body fluids. Biological Handbook, Fed Amer Soc Exp Biol, Washington, D.C., 1961, p 125)

after. By 1 year of age all lymphoid structures are mature histologically. Absolute lymphocyte counts in the peripheral blood also reach a peak during the first year of life, and the maturation curve of circulating lymphocytes (Fig. 20-3) parallels strikingly the serum IgM maturation curve (Fig. 20-2). Peripheral lymphoid tissue (including lymph nodes, tonsils, adenoids, appendix, and the lamina propria plasma cell system) increases rapidly in mass during infancy and early childhood. It reaches adult size by approximately 6 years of age, exceeds those dimensions during the prepubertal years, and then undergoes involution coincident with puberty. It may be pertinent that the adult-sized peripheral lymphoid mass is achieved at essentially the same age that adult concentrations of serum IgG and IgA are reached. The spleen, however, gradually accrues its mass during maturation and does not reach full weight until adulthood. The mean number of

Peyer's patches is one-half the adult number at birth and gradually increases until the adult mean number is exceeded during adolescent years.

THE IMMUNODEFICIENCY DISEASES

Examples of defective development of the human immune system were first recognized over two decades ago, and since that time reports of clinical immunodeficiency syndromes have appeared in the literature at an almost exponential rate. The classification presented in Table 20-1 is a revision of one formulated by the World Health Organization in 1970 to facilitate recognition and understanding of these disorders. It lists 11 forms of primary im-

TABLE 20-1 REVISED WHO CLASSIFICATION OF PRIMARY IMMUNODEFICIENCIES

Deficiency	Suggested Cellular Defect			Inheritance		
	B lymphocytes*		T lymphocytes	X-linked	Autosomal Recessive	Other†
	(a)	(b)				
X-linked agammaglobulinemia	X	(X)‡		X		
Thymic hypoplasia			X			X
Severe combined immunodeficiency	X	X	X	X	X	X
With dysostosis	X	?	X		X	
With ADA§ deficiency	X		X		X	
Immunodeficiency with generalized hematopoietic hypoplasia	X		X		X	
Selective Ig deficiency:						
IgA	?	X	(X)			X
Others (IgM, IgE)		?				X
X-linked immunodeficiency with increased IgM		X		X		
Immunodeficiency with ataxia telangiectasia		X	X		X	
Immunodeficiency with thrombocytopenia and eczema (Wiskott-Aldrich syndrome)			X	X		
Immunodeficiency with thymoma		X	X			X
Immunodeficiency with normal or hypergammaglobulinemia	X	X	(X)			X
Transient hypogammaglobulinemia of infancy		X				X
Variable immunodeficiencies (largely unclassified and very frequent)	X	X	(X)		(X)	X

From New Engl J Med 288:966, 1973
°(a) indicates absent or very low, (b) easily detectable or increased, (X) less frequent occurrence than X.
†Other implies multifactorial or unknown genetic basis or no known genetic basis.
‡Some cases with circulating B lymphocytes without detectable surface immunoglobulins have been found.
§Adenosine deaminase.

munodeficiency that appear to be separate clinical syndromes and a twelfth category which includes all other forms of deficiency involving specific immune responses. These latter conditions were judged not classifiable because of lack of consistent patterns. For each category, a suggestion is given concerning the possible cellular deficit (T or B cells, see Chap. 14) and type of inheritance, based on information derived from studies of clinical and immunologic function in patients with these disorders. It should be noted, however, that the original and revised versions of this classification were drawn up before much information had been accumulated regarding the numbers of T and B cells usually present in the peripheral blood of these patients, since methods for detecting and enumerating these cells in man were not developed until the early 1970s. Studies with these techniques have since shown that cells having surface markers characteristic of T or B cells are rarely completely lacking in any of these conditions. Nevertheless, the classification still provides a useful framework if the diseases are thought of in terms of their functional deficiencies rather than according to the presence or absence of particular cell types. It is also important to keep in mind that, with one or two possible exceptions (eg, failure of development of the thymus gland in DiGeorge syndrome and profound deficiencies of key enzymes in purine catabolism in some forms of severe combined immunodeficiency), the primary biologic error is not known for any of these defects.

B Cell Functional Deficiencies

The deficiency states characterized primarily by deficits in B cell function include x-linked and non-x-linked (common variable or B lymphocyte type, see p. 352) agammaglobulinemia, selective IgA deficiency, x-linked immunodeficiency with hyper-IgM, and transient hypogammaglobulinemia of infancy. The general clinical characteristics of this group of deficiency states are presented in Table 20-2 and are consistent in each except that (1) in selective IgA deficiency, antibodies are usually made in normal quantity in immunoglobulin classes other than IgA, and (2) specific antibody production appears to be normal in infants with transient hypogammaglobulinemia of infancy despite low serum immunoglobulin concentrations, and these infants have fewer infections than patients in the other three groups.

X-linked Agammaglobulinemia Commonly referred to as "Bruton's agammaglobulinemia" (a misnomer because a small amount of immunoglobulin can usually be detected), this was the first described of the deficiency states. It was discovered in 1952 when a serum electrophoretic analysis revealed an apparent absence of gamma globulin in a young boy who had had repeated infections for several years.

TABLE 20-2 CLINICAL CHARACTERISTICS OF PRIMARILY B CELL FUNCTIONAL DEFICIENCIES

1. Recurrent infections with high-grade extracellular encapsulated pathogens.
2. Chronic sinopulmonary disease.
3. Antibody deficiency in serum and secretions.
4. Few problems with viral or fungal infections.
5. Absence of cortical follicles in lymph node and spleen (except in B lymphocyte type, selective IgA deficiency, or x-linked immunodeficiency with hyper IgM).
6. May or may not lack B lymphocytes with surface immunoglobulins or complement receptors.
7. Usually a paucity of palpable lymphoid and nasopharyngeal tissue (except in conditions listed under 5).
8. Growth retardation not striking.
9. Compatible with survival to adulthood or for several years after onset.

After gamma globulin therapy was instituted, the frequency and severity of his infections decreased. The study of a number of kindreds with multiple apparently similar cases has favored an x-linked mode of inheritance. A majority of boys afflicted with this malady remain well during the first six to nine months of life, presumably by virtue of maternally transmitted immunoglobulin. Thereafter, they repeatedly acquire infections with extracellular pyogenic organisms, such as pneumococci, streptococci, and haemophilus, unless given prophylactic antibiotic or gamma globulin therapy. Infections with other organisms, such as meningococci, staphylococci, and pseudomonas, occur less frequently. The most frequent types of infections include sinusitis, pneumonia, otitis, furunculosis, meningitis, and septicemia. Viral infections (including live virus vaccinations), on the other hand, are usually handled normally, with the notable exceptions of hepatitis, polio, and other enteroviruses. Several examples of prolonged polio vaccine virus shedding have occurred in hypogammaglobulinemic patients, and paralytic polio has occurred, presumably due to mutation of the vaccine virus to a more neurotropic form.

Marked deficiencies of all classes of immunoglobulins are found (Fig. 20-4). Moreover, antibody formation is severely impaired, as evidenced by low to absent isohemagglutinin titers, positive Schick tests, and either no or a very small amount of antibody to viruses and phage particles. Polymorphonuclear functions are usually normal if heat-stable opsonins (eg, IgG antibodies) are provided, but some patients with this condition have had transient, persistent, or cyclic neutropenia.

Lymphopenia is ordinarily not present, and the percentage of T cells has been found to be normal or elevated in most of these patients. In contrast, surface Ig-bearing cells are absent or present in very low number, but cells with two other B cell markers, the receptor for C3 and one for the Fc portion of IgG, are usually present in normal number. In vitro lymphocyte responses to the mitogens, PHA, Con A, and pokeweed, are usually normal, but cyclic impairment in PHA responsiveness has been noted. Mixed lymphocyte responsiveness and the DNA synthetic response to antigens are normal. Cell-mediated immune responses can be detected in vivo, and the capacity to reject allografts is intact, although in a number of in-

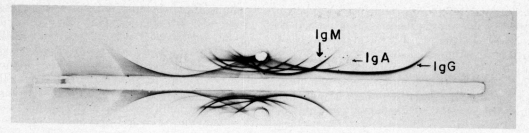

FIG. 20-4. Immunoelectrophoretic analysis of normal human serum (upper well) and serum from a patient with congenital agammaglobulinemia (lower well) using goat antiwhole human serum in the trough. Note absence of arcs in the gamma globulin region in the lower pattern.

stances skin graft rejection time has been greatly prolonged. The thymus has appeared morphologically normal in all autopsied cases, and lymphoid cells are abundant in thymus-dependent areas of peripheral lymphoid tissues. Conversely, germinal centers are not found in these tissues, and plasma cells are lacking or rarely found. Hypoplasia of adenoids, tonsils, and peripheral lymph nodes is the rule, and follicles are not present in Peyer's patches.

Associated conditions frequently seen in this entity are rheumatoid arthritis (30 to 50 percent of cases), dermatomyositis, vasculitis, and lymphoreticular malignancy. Systemic infection can be prevented by gamma globulin (primarily IgG) injections (loading dose 1.2 ml/kg, maintenance 0.6 ml/kg every three to four weeks), but many patients go on to develop crippling sinopulmonary disease. Lack of secretory IgA could well account for this, since presently no effective means exists for replacing this immunoglobulin at the mucosal surface.

Selective Immunoglobulin Deficiency (Isolated IgA Deficiency) The term "dysgammaglobulinemia" refers to conditions in which there are deficiencies of one or more, but not all, of the immunoglobulin classes. An isolated absence or near-absence of IgA is thought to be not only the most common type of dysgammaglobulinemia but also the most frequent type of immunodeficiency. It has an observed incidence of 0.2 percent in normal populations and of over 1 percent among patients referred for recurrent infections or allergic respiratory problems. There is a strong familial occurrence of this defect, and though an autosomal mode of inheritance appears certain, it is unclear whether the trait is recessive or dominant with

variable expressivity. Synthesis of other immunoglobulins is usually normal, accounting for the fact that this diagnosis is missed when gamma globulin levels are determined by serum electrophoresis. IgD is undetectable in serum more often than in normals, but IgM is often elevated, as is IgE, which, like IgA, is produced predominantly by paramucosal lymphoid tissue. Until recently it was thought that this defect rarely changes with time. The author has, however, observed the spontaneous development of normal serum IgA concentrations in eight children who were documented for several years to have absent or extremely low IgA. The fact that all patients with absent serum IgA studied thus far have been found to have circulating IgA-bearing B lymphocytes supports the concept that this is a defect in terminal differentiation of the B cell, but a defect that is apparently not always permanent. While IgA deficiency has been reported in apparently healthy individuals, there is abundant evidence to indicate that it is more commonly associated with ill health. Among the various clinical entities with which it has been associated are atopic hypersensitivity, recurrent sinopulmonary and ear infections, recurrent urinary tract infections, sprue, rheumatoid arthritis, lupus erythematosus and other collagen diseases, idiopathic pulmonary hemosiderosis, and ataxia telangiectasia. In addition, a high frequency of autoantibody formation has been reported, as well as a peculiar propensity of these patients to produce antiruminant antibodies. The latter often interfere with accurate performance of immunologic studies employing ruminant heteroantisera. Of much greater clinical importance is the fact that a majority of these patients produce anti-IgA antibodies which have caused severe or fatal anaphylactic reactions when these patients have been given blood or plasma transfusions from normal donors. For this reason, only blood products lacking IgA (eg, from other such patients) should be administered to these patients, and gamma globulin (which contains a small amount of IgA) is contraindicated. The high frequency of atopy (55 percent) noted among a group of patients with this disorder is intriguing and may carry implications pertinent to the development of the atopic state. It is possible that IgA antibodies are important in limiting the absorption of foreign antigens through mucosal surfaces, thereby preventing stimulation of other types of immune responses, such as formation of IgG or IgE antibodies.

X-linked Immunodeficiency with Hyperimmunoglobulinemia M A second distinct variety of dysgammaglobulinemia or selective immunoglobulin deficiency was first described in 1961, and since then many examples have been recorded. In this condition, serum concentrations of IgG and IgA are either totally absent or markedly diminished, and the concentration of IgM is usually extremely elevated but may be normal. Despite these findings, membrane immunofluorescence studies of peripheral blood lymphocytes from these patients have revealed normal percentages of B lymphocytes bearing all five classes of immunoglobulins on their surfaces. Children afflicted with this defect are unduly susceptible to the same types of extracellular pyogenic organisms that plague patients with Bruton's agammaglobulinemia. A clinically misleading feature is the frequent occurrence of generalized lymphadenopathy, tonsillar and adenoidal hypertrophy, and splenomegaly. Normal lymphoid follicles may be observed, but fluorescent antibody studies demonstrate positive staining of plasma cells only by anti-IgM reagents. Because of the hyperimmunoglobulinemia M, gamma globulin concentrations determined by electrophoresis have been frequently reported to be normal. Quantitative immunochemical measurement of the individual immunoglobulins is the only accurate means of detecting this and the other types of dysgammaglobulinemias. No M band is seen on electrophoresis, indicating that the IgM hyperglobulinemia is polyclonal rather than monoclonal (as in Waldenström's macroglobulinemia). It has been suggested that the increased IgM may be due to the deficit of 7S immunoglobulins which normally inhibit overproduction of antibodies of the IgM class either by antigen binding or by a feedback mechanism. High titers of IgM antibodies to blood group substances and to salmonella O antigen have been found in some patients, but often little or no antibody can be detected in their sera. Administration of exogenous gamma globulin, the treatment of choice for patients with this condition, has in many instances resulted in a decrease in IgM concentration, while in others the IgM level was unaffected. Thymic-dependent lymphoid tissues are most often normal, as are T cell functions, but several examples of this type of dysgammaglobulinemia have also been recorded in infants with thymic abnormalities. Neutropenia occurs more commonly in this condition than in any of the primarily B cell functional deficiency states, and, when it does, it is frequently persistent. This plus the occasional coexistence of impaired cell-mediated immunity in these patients may account for the fact that this is the only disorder affecting primarily humoral immune functions in which *Pneumocystis carinii* pneumonia is seen with any frequency. This dysgammaglobulinemia has occurred in children and in adults and in both congenital and acquired forms. A sex-linked mode of inheritance has been proposed for this familial defect, since it has been observed most commonly in males, but several apparent examples in females now seem to make this less certain.

Transient Hypogammaglobulinemia of Infancy This is a frequently mentioned entity that has seldom been documented in the literature. Affected infants have an apparent delay in onset of normal immunoglobulin synthesis until well after maternally transmitted immunoglobulin has been catabolized. The deficiency may last until 15 to 18 months of age, during which time the infant may or may not be unduly susceptible to infection. It has been postulated that maternally produced antibodies to gamma globulin, stimulated by passage of allotypically different fetal immunoglobulins into the maternal circulation, may cross into the fetal circulation and suppress immunoglobulin synthesis. Although no direct evidence for this has been found in cases of human transient hypogammaglobulinemia, experimental models of this phenomenon have been described. This defect has been observed in relatives of infants with severe combined immunodeficiency disease (SCID), and it has been suggested that the condition may represent a heterozygous state or variable expression of SCID. Since infants of both sexes are affected, an autosomal mode of inheritance is suggested.

T Cell Functional Deficiencies

The only immunodeficiency disease thought to be primarily a T cell functional disorder is the thymic hypoplasia or DiGeorge Syndrome. Even in this condition, however, B cell function is compromised due to the absence of T helper cells. The clinical characteristics of patients with T cell functional deficiencies are presented in Table 20-3.

Thymic Hypoplasia (Pharyngeal Pouch or DiGeorge Syndrome) Embryologically the thymus and parathyroids arise from the third and fourth pharyngeal pouches and are fused for a time during development. This disorder is thought to represent a failure of development of these pouches. The thymic hypoplasia syndrome is usually manifested in the newborn period by hypocalcemic tetany and by the early appearance of mucocutaneous moniliasis, which persists despite conventional therapy. Additionally, afflicted infants have characteristic facies as well as associated anomalies of the trachea, esophagus, heart, or great vessels. DiGeorge patients are usually unable to survive beyond infancy because of their extreme susceptibility to opportunistic agents which afflict those with an absence of T cell-mediated immunity (ie, fungi, viruses, *P. carinii,* and gram-negative bacteria). Affected infants fail to

TABLE 20-3 CLINICAL CHARACTERISTICS OF T CELL FUNCTIONAL DEFICIENCIES

1. Recurrent infections with low-grade or opportunistic infectious agents such as fungi, viruses, or *Pneumocystis carinii.*
2. Delayed cutaneous anergy.
3. Accompanied by growth retardation, short life span, wasting, and diarrhea.
4. Susceptible to graft-versus-host (GVH) disease if given fresh blood, plasma, or unmatched allogeneic bone marrow.
5. Fatal reactions from live virus or BCG vaccination.
6. High incidence of malignancy.

manifest cell-mediated immune reactions in vivo, and allograft rejection is markedly impaired. Circulating lymphocyte counts may be normal early in infancy, but the lymphocytes of most such patients respond poorly if at all to the T cell mitogens, phytohemagglutinin (PHA), and concanavalin A (Con A). This is undoubtedly related to the fact that the majority of the circulating lymphocytes in these patients have been found to carry B cell differentiation markers. Lymphoid follicles appear normal, but lymph node paracortical areas and thymus-dependent regions of the spleen are depleted. Antibody formation may occasionally appear to be normal early in infancy but usually diminishes with time, despite persistence of normal immunoglobulin concentrations, probably due to the deficiency of T helper cells.

Combined Immunodeficiency

Patients with combined immunodeficiency have, with varying degrees of severity, clinical problems seen both in patients with primarily B cell functional deficiencies and in those with primarily T cell dysfunction. The combined system defects include immunodeficiency with normal or hyperimmunoglobulinemia (Nezelof syndrome), the ataxia telangiectasia syndrome, immunodeficiency with thrombocytopenia and eczema (Wiskott-Aldrich syndrome), immunodeficiency with thymoma, the various forms of severe combined immunodeficiency disease (SCID), and immunodeficiency with generalized hematopoietic hypoplasia.

Immunodeficiency with Normal or Hyperimmunoglobulinemia This thymic dysplasia syndrome, first described by Nezelof, has immunologic features similar to but quantitatively less severe than those of the DiGeorge syndrome. Affected individuals do not, however, have parathyroid abnormalities, and the thymus gland is present, though abnormal. The clinical courses of these patients have been quite variable, with some dying in infancy from viral or fungal infections and others remaining relatively well as late as 8 years of age. These individuals experience unduly severe infections with vaccinia and varicella viruses, remain lymphopenic, and have markedly depressed cell-mediated immune responses. Half of the reported cases have also had neutropenia. There is often continuous diarrhea, which responds to treatment with disaccharide-free diets. At postmortem examinations the thymus glands are extremely small and lack corticomedullary distinction or Hassall's corpuscles. Thymus-dependent peripheral lymphoid tissues are also depleted. Although immunoglobulin concentrations remain normal or elevated, antibody formation is depressed or even lacking for certain antigens. The condition has a familial occurrence, affects members of both sexes, and is thought to be an autosomal recessive trait.

Immunodeficiency with Ataxia Telangiectasia   This clinical syndrome is characterized by progressive cerebellar ataxia, recurrent sinopulmonary infections, and oculocutaneous telangiectasia. While its neurologic and cutaneous features have been recognized for 40 years, the associated immunodeficiency was not appreciated until just over a decade ago. Affected patients appear normal during the first 12 to 18 months of life but thereafter develop progressive cerebellar ataxia and repeated respiratory infections. The telangiectatic lesions may not appear until 6 to 8 years of age and appear to be related to exposure to sunlight. The immune deficit involves both cellular and humoral aspects of immunity. An isolated deficiency of serum IgA has been reported in from 50 to 80 percent of these patients, but other types of dysgammaglobulinemia, normogammaglobulinemia, and hyperimmunoglobulinemia have also been found. Antibody formation is poor to some antigens but apparently normal to most. A constant feature of this defect is impaired cell-mediated immunity, as manifested by delayed cutaneous anergy and prolonged allograft survival. Peripheral blood lymphocyte responsiveness to mitogenic and antigenic stimulation has been reported to be impaired by some workers and to be normal by others. Absolute lymphocyte counts are usually normal, although lymphopenia has been present in some, and granulocytopenia has also been observed. All thymus glands examined at postmortem were small, lacked Hassall's corpuscles, and exhibited poor organization. Peripheral lymphoid tissues are depleted in thymus-dependent areas and often replaced by reticulum cells. Despite depressed cell-mediated immune responses, many patients have

received live virus vaccinations or had viral infections without experiencing graft-versus-host disease. This suggests that the T cell defect is not as severe as in some other syndromes with thymic abnormalities. A high frequency of malignancy has been reported in this condition. The tumors are usually of the lymphoreticular type, but adenocarcinomas of the stomach and brain tumors have also been seen. Gonadal agenesis, abnormal liver function, and an unusual form of diabetes with associated hyperinsulinism are additional characteristics of many patients with this syndrome. As yet no satisfactory explanation has been found for the simultaneous occurrence of these seemingly unrelated features. The condition affects both sexes approximately equally and is thought to have an autosomal recessive mode of inheritance.

Immunodeficiency with Thrombocytopenia and Eczema (Wiskott-Aldrich Syndrome)   This syndrome is characterized by megakaryocytic thrombocytopenic purpura, atopic eczema, undue susceptibility to infection, low to absent isohemagglutinins, and a progressive acquisition of cellular immunodeficiency. This sex-linked recessive trait usually leads to death in childhood, primarily from infection. Like patients with ataxia telangiectasia, children with the Wiskott-Aldrich syndrome have a high incidence of lymphoreticular malignancy, and this is also often a cause of death. Abnormal immunoglobulin concentrations have been reported in this syndrome, the predominant dysgammaglobulinemia characterized by a low IgM, an elevated IgA, and a normal or slightly low IgG concentration. The dysgammaglobulinemia is not constant even with the same patient, however, and thus is not a reliable diagnostic criterion. The immunoglobulin deficiencies, when they occur, may be due in part to the hypercatabolism of IgG and IgM that has been documented in these patients along with hypercatabolism of albumin and IgA. A failure of immune recognition of polysaccharide antigens has been demonstrated in this condition, and undue susceptibility to bacterial infections has been attributed to inability to respond to bacterial polysaccharide antigens. The thymus and lymphoid tissues are morphologically normal early in life, but a progressive depletion of cells occurs in thymus-dependent areas of peripheral lymphoid tissues and susceptibility to viral and fungal agents develops. The in vitro responses of cultured peripheral blood lymphocytes to phytohemagglutinin and antigens have been variable.

Immunodeficiency with Thymoma This syndrome occurs in adults and is looked upon as an acquired type of primary immunodeficiency, though a genetic influence is likely. Its characteristics include the almost simultaneous development of hypogammaglobulinemia, deficits in cell-mediated immunity, and benign thymoma. Concentrations of all five classes of immunoglobulins are low, antibody formation is poor, and progressive lymphopenia develops. Other inconstantly associated features include eosinophilia, anemia, thrombocytopenia, or pancytopenia. Commonly these patients develop arthritis or other types of collagen diseases, and an autoimmune basis has been suggested for both the hematologic and mesenchymal abnormalities. Studies of peripheral blood lymphocytes from these patients have generally revealed normal percentages of immunoglobulin-bearing B lymphocytes. Recently some patients with this disorder, similar to those with common variable hypogammaglobulinemia, have been shown to have an excess of peripheral blood suppressor T cells capable of inhibiting immunoglobulin synthesis not only by their own B cells but by normal B cells as well. Interestingly, benign thymoma has also been described in association with pure red cell aplasia, thrombocytopenia, or pancytopenia without demonstrable immunodeficiency.

Severe Combined Immunodeficiency Disease (SCID) This defect, the most severe deficiency involving specific immune mechanisms, occurs in at least two genetic forms: autosomal recessive (Swiss type) and x-linked recessive (Gitlin type, the predominant form in this country). In addition, sporadic cases have been described. Evidence of marked heterogeneity with respect to immunologic features is also rapidly accumulating, and it now seems apparent that several different primary biologic errors may give rise to the same clinical syndrome. Recent identification of deficiencies of adenosine deaminase (ADA) or nucleoside phosphorylase, key enzymes in purine catabolism, in some but not all of these patients is strong evidence in favor of this. Regardless of

the primary cause, affected individuals have a marked susceptibility to both high-grade and low-grade pathogens, and death usually occurs in infancy. Like infants with the DiGeorge syndrome, they often have extensive candidiasis, are extremely susceptible to other mycotic and viral agents, and frequently die of *P. carinii* pneumonia. Intractable diarrhea is a typical and early finding and can be either infectious in etiology or the result of a secondary disaccharidase deficiency. Growth may appear normal for the first few months of life, but extreme wasting (runting) occurs after infections and diarrhea begin. SCID, described by the Swiss in the 1950s, was not recognized in this country until the 1960s, possibly because such infants succumbed to generalized vaccinia when immunized against smallpox (commonly performed in the United States at five to six months of age in the past). Similarly if these patients are exposed to measles or measles vaccine, they usually do not manifest a rash but may die from Hoecht's giant-cell pneumonia. Death has also occurred following BCG immunization in infants afflicted with this condition.

Typically, these patients have very small thymuses (less than 2 g), which usually fail to descend from the neck, contain few thymic lymphocytes, lack corticomedullary distinction, and usually lack Hassall's corpuscles. Both the follicular and paracortical areas of the peripheral lymph nodes are depleted of lymphocytes. Tonsils, adenoids, and Peyer's patches are absent or extremely underdeveloped. These infants usually lack or have only small amounts of immunoglobulin in their sera, fail to make antibodies, and are usually markedly lymphopenic, although a few have been described with normal lymphocyte counts. Whereas most normal infants and children manifest delayed hypersensitivity when challenged with candida antigens, these infants do not react. In addition, contact sensitization cannot be accomplished, and homograft rejection does not take place. Peripheral blood lymphocytes do not respond or respond only feebly in cultures stimulated with PHA, Con A, pokeweed mitogen, allogeneic cells, or antigens. A deficiency in a portion of the first component of complement, C'lq, has been noted in several infants with this syndrome.

A variant of this syndrome has been described, consisting of SCID plus a distinctive form of short-limbed dwarfism (not achondroplasia) and/or ectodermal dysplasia. Such infants have redundant skin, absence of hair and eyebrows, ichthyosiform skin lesions, and erythroderma. The occurrence of this variant of SCID in a brother and a sister suggests an autosomal recessive mode of inheritance.

Gamma globulin injections have failed to halt the progressively downhill course of SCID. Fatal graft-versus-host disease is an invariable accompaniment of transplants of bone marrow or transfusions of nonirradiated blood or plasma from any but HL-A-compatible sibling donors.

Immunodeficiency with Generalized Hematopoietic Hypoplasia This very rare condition, originally referred to as reticular dysgenesis by de Vaal, is characterized by failure of development of the granulocytic series as well as other hematopoietic elements in infants with SCID. Death from infection usually occurs within the first few weeks of life, in contrast to the somewhat longer survival of patients with SCID who have normal granulocyte formation. Although the primary biologic error remains unknown in this condition, it has been postulated that it lies in a defective stem cell, the putative precursor of hematopoietic elements as well as of immunocompetent cells.

Variable Immunodeficiency This category in the WHO classification embraces what will eventually probably be several separate entities, including common variable (acquired, non-x-linked, or B lymphocyte) hypogammaglobulinemia, chronic mucocutaneous candidiasis with immunodeficiency, the hyper IgE syndrome, and all other varieties of dysgammaglobulinemia (except selective IgA deficiency and x-linked immunodeficiency with hyper-IgM). Although many of the defects have been thought to be acquired, studies demonstrating familial immunologic abnormalities and consanguinity in various of these patients have strongly implicated genetic influences on the development of most of these conditions. There is also the alternate possibility that in some cases environmental agents might cause the defects. This possibility is supported by the observation that several infants with the congenital rubella syndrome have had dysgammaglobulinemias. Both males and females and children and adults have manifested abnormalities included under this broad category. The types of infections experienced by most patients in this group are similar to those seen in patients with primarily B cell functional deficiencies, although patients with the hyper IgE syndrome and those with chronic mucocutaneous candidiasis also have problems seen in T cell dysfunction.

Patients with common variable (or B lymphocyte) hypogammaglobulinemia resemble those with x-linked agammaglobulinemia from both a clinical and an immunologic standpoint. They experience very similar types of infections, and the serum and secretory immunoglobulin deficiency is usually just as severe. They differ, however, in several other respects. Most such patients have peripheral blood Ig-bearing B lymphocytes, and their lymphoid tissues appear to have normal cortical follicle formation (Table 20-2). Because of this, the peripheral lymphoid tissues (including tonsils) may appear to be normal or even increased in size. There is, however, a deficiency or absence of plasma cells surrounding the follicles. Thus, the disorder appears to be another example of an abnormality in terminal differentiation of the B cell line. Further evidence that patients with x-linked hyper-IgM, selective IgA deficiency, and this disorder represent a spectrum of this type of defect is seen in the fact that this variety of hypogammaglobulinemia has occurred in the same sibship with selective IgA deficiency, and some patients with hyper-IgM have later been noted to become panhypogammaglobulinemic or vice versa.

Insight into one possible reason for failure of differentiation has recently come from the work of Waldmann and co-workers, who found an excessive number of suppressor T cells in these patients. These T cells were capable of inhibiting immunoglobulin synthesis not only of their own pokeweed mitogen-stimulated B cells but also of those of normals. Moreover, treatment of some such patients' peripheral blood lymphocytes with antilymphocyte globulin, corticosteroids, or physical removal of the T cells resulted in synthesis of immunoglobulin by the patients' B cells. This information may thus have important therapeutic implications. Older patients and adults with this disorder have a spruelike syndrome, with or without nodular lymphoid hyperplasia of small intestinal lymphoid tissues and of the germinal centers of the spleen and lymph nodes. Many of these patients also have an increased tendency to develop autoimmune disorders, such as hemolytic anemias, gastric atrophy, and pernicious anemia. Noncaseating granulomas of the lungs, spleen, skin, and liver have also been seen, as well as amyloidosis.

Not all patients with chronic mucocutaneous candidiasis have been found to have immunodeficiency. When defects have been found, they have usually been disorders of T cell function. Even in those cases, however, it has not been clear whether the deficient cell-mediated immune function was primary or secondary to the extensive fungal disease (eg, an antigen overload mechanism). Reversal of delayed cutaneous anergy has occurred following high-dose intravenous amphotericin B and clearing of the fungal lesions and also following transfer factor therapy (which has also usually been given in conjunction with amphotericin B). Lymphocyte DNA synthetic responses in vitro have generally been normal in these patients, but lymphokine production has frequently been abnormal, suggesting that the latter may be a major cause of in vivo anergy when it does occur.

The hyper IgE syndrome is a recently recognized entity characterized by recurrent severe staphylococcal abscesses involving the skin, lungs, and joints from early life and by extremely high serum concentrations of IgE (some over 40,000 IU/ml). Concentrations of other immunoglobulins have usually been normal or only slightly elevated, except for IgD which has also frequently been high. Despite this, antibody responses to recall antigens have often been found to be impaired. Most of these patients have also had deficient cell-mediated immune function, as manifested by delayed cutaneous anergy, impaired lymphocyte DNA synthetic responses to antigens, and abnormal responses in mixed leukocyte culture. Abnormalities have also been noted in both mononuclear and polymorphonuclear chemotaxis, and serum from several such patients has been found to inhibit monocyte responses to lymphocyte-derived mononuclear chemotactic factor. Extensive studies of the complement system and of phagocytosis and killing by polymorphonuclear (PMN) cells from these patients have all been normal, as have studies of PMN metabolism. Recurrent infections with other organisms, mainly *Haemophilus influenzae*, pneumococci, *Candida albicans*, trichophyton, and aspergillus, have also been noted in these individuals.

The mainstay of therapy in these patients is chronic antistaphylococcal penicillin therapy, although chronic ampicillin and nystatin therapy has also been required in some.

The immunoglobulin abnormalities in the milder forms of dysgammaglobulinemia have been highly variable. Studies of the IgG class in a number of these individuals have revealed restricted electrophoretic mobility in some, unusual ratios of the two different types of light chains in others, and deficiencies of certain of the IgG subtypes in others.

IMMUNOLOGIC RECONSTITUTION

Immunologic competence has been successfully restored in experimentally produced deficiency states of animals by infusions of syngeneic thymus, fetal liver, spleen, and lymph node cells. Injection of allogeneic histoincompatible immunocompetent cells, however, has usually been followed by graft-versus-host reactions. Until the past decade, all efforts to correct human immunodeficiency were either unsuccessful or resulted in fatal graft-versus-host disease. The latter reaction invariably occurs if patients with severe T cell defects (who are unable to reject allografts) are given transplants of HLA-incompatible bone marrow or blood cells capable of responding to foreign HLA antigens of the host. Within the past eight years, more than 30 infants with severe combined immunodeficiency have been successfully reconstituted immunologically by transplants of HLA-compatible sibling marrow cells and are now alive and chimeric. In addition, 3 infants with SCID were partially or fully reconstituted by transplants of fetal liver cells, and 3 were partially corrected by fetal thymus transplants. These cases of successful reconstitution do not help to clarify the natures of the underlying genetic errors in SCID, since both the ADA-negative and ADA-positive forms of SCID have been corrected by transplants of bone marrow or fetal liver. One infant with SCID became partially reconstituted by histoincompatible bone marrow cells from her mother. Graft-versus-host disease was circumvented in that instance by the phenomenon of immunologic enhancement. The immunologic deficits of four infants with DiGeorge syndrome were improved after transplants of fetal thymic tissue. There are, however, DiGeorge patients who appear to have had spontaneous improvement in their immunologic function, so the latter cannot be excluded as the mechanism of improvement in those transplanted with thymus, particularly since chimerism was not demonstrated. Transplantation of bone marrow cells from an HLA-identical sibling also resulted in improved immunologic capacity and partial chimerism in a case of Wiskott-Aldrich syndrome. The thrombocytopenia was not improved by this measure, however. Immunologic and clinical improvement occurred in other patients with Wiskott-Aldrich syndrome who were treated with transfer factor.

The infrequent availability of HLA-compatible donors for infants with lymphopenic immunologic deficiency makes bone marrow transplantation an effective form of therapy for only a select few at the present time. While fetal liver and thymus transplants have met with some measure of success, they do not appear to be nearly so effective as bone marrow, so the latter remains the treatment of choice for those infants with SCID who have sibling donors compatible at the major histocompatibility complex (MHC). For those who are not so fortunate, further advances in the understanding of transplantation immunology and in modification of the immune response will be necessary before the barrier of graft-versus-host disease can be surmounted in MHC-incompatible allogeneic marrow grafts. Fetal liver and/or thymus transplants thus appear to offer the only hope for those without compatible donors at present.

PHAGOCYTIC CELL DISORDERS

The essential role of phagocytic cells in host defense is seen in those patients who, although fully endowed with all of the necessary components and functions needed for specific immune responsiveness, have either an insufficient number or inadequate function of polymorphonuclear cells and/or macrophages. The types of infections experienced by such individuals are similar in many respects to those that plague the patient with antibody deficiency, eg, primarily infections with high-grade encapsulated pathogens. Their severity can, and often does, equal or surpass those in the agammaglobulinemic host. Similar types of infections are seen in patients with hereditary deficiencies of components or inhibitors of the complement system (Chap. 16).

Disorders of Production

Hereditary Neutropenia   This is an autosomal trait that occurs in both recessive and dominant forms and is characterized by the absence of granulocytes from the peripheral blood from birth. Arrested myeloid differentiation is the apparent cause of this condition, for the bone marrows of these patients contain an increased number of granulocyte precursors. The recessive form is invariably fatal in the first year of life, but the dominant form is a benign condition in which the life span is normal and the abnormality is detected only as an incidental finding. No explanation for the latter paradox is apparent.

Cyclic Neutropenia or Periodic Myelodysplasia   This entity is characterized by a periodic diminution in the number of peripheral blood polymorphonuclear leukocytes. The rhythmicity of the disorder is remarkably uniform, the neutropenia occurring every 21 days in the majority of instances. Fever, malaise, and ulcers on the oral mucous membranes and occasionally arthritis, abdominal pain, sore throat, lymphadenitis, and cutaneous ulceration accompany the neutropenia. Patients with this disorder typically are sick for one week, then well for two before the cycle repeats. Serial bone marrow studies have shown that intermittent failure of bone marrow neutrophil maturation was basic to the peripheral blood neutrophil fluctuations. During this time, promyelocytes are increased in the marrow. All other aspects of immunity are usually normal in these patients. Interestingly, splenectomy has relieved the clinical symptoms of some of these patients even though it did not alter the neutropenic episodes in the slightest. The condition occurs in both sexes with approximately equal frequency, and in females the rhythmicity ordinarily has no relation to menstruation. Cyclic neutropenia has been familial in a few instances, but there is no clear evidence for inheritance of the disorder.

Neutropenia with Immunodeficiency   As noted earlier, neutropenia may occur in association with several of the primary immunodeficiency disorders, but it is seen most often in the two x-linked defects, infantile x-linked agammaglobulinemia and x-linked immunodeficiency with hyper-IgM. When neutropenia occurs, it may be transient, persistent, or cyclic in nature, with the transient variety being most common. Whether the neutropenias are related to the intrinsic unresponsiveness of polymorphonuclear neutrophils to normal chemotactic stimuli observed in one such patient with x-linked agammaglobulinemia is unknown. Gitlin noted that, in the transient type, neutropenia often occurred at the onset of a severe infection but ordinarily gave way to leukocytosis later in the course of the illness. The cyclic variety is different from the periodic myelodysplasia described above, in that the periodicity is usually not uniform. Persistent neutropenia from birth is also seen in immunodeficiency with generalized hematopoietic hypoplasia (reticular dysgenesis).

Acquired Neutropenia   This may occur secondary to toxic effects of drugs, pollutants, or irradiation or as a consequence of autoimmune reactions involving leukocytes. The latter may be seen as a transient phenomenon in the newborn as a consequence of maternal isoimmunization by fetal leukocytes during pregnancy. Neutropenia has also been noted in patients with neoplasms, overwhelming infections, or endotoxemia. It is well known in those conditions characterized by hypersplenism, in aplastic anemia, and in certain forms and/or stages of leukemia.

Disorders of Function

In these disorders, the number of peripheral blood leukocytes is usually normal (a few exceptions are noted below), but their function may be impaired at one or more of the following phases of the phagocytic process: (1) chemotaxis, (2) opsonization, (3) ingestion of particles, or (4) intracellular killing.

Chemotactic Defects   These occur in two forms: (1) those in which the blood chemotactic activity is diminished and (2) those in which the cellular response is impaired in the face of normal chemotactic stimuli. In the first instance, the diminished chemotactic activity has been attributed by some to the presence of plasma or serum inhibitors of chemotaxis in children with recurrent staphylococcal infections, in alcoholics with advanced liver disease, in Hodgkin's disease, and in agammaglobulinemia. Controversy exists as to whether the inhibitors are abnormal constituents or a normal factor that is unopposed by an absence of a normal antagonist to the inhibitor, since the inhibitor could be neutralized by normal plasma in some instances. Certain drugs, such as colchicine and steroids, can also act as inhibitors of chemotaxis. Chemotactic factors per se can be diminished in conditions in which C3 and/or C5 are diminished or dysfunctional (Chap. 16). Other examples of such deficiencies are seen in the normal newborn, where both components are low, and in acute glomerulonephritis, where C3 is markedly reduced.

The newborn's polymorphonuclear cells have also been noted to have an intrinsic impairment in their ability to respond to normal chemotactic stimuli. As mentioned above, this type of abnormality has also been seen in one boy with x-linked agammaglobulinemia. It has also been found transiently in patients with diabetes mellitus, in patients in terminal shock, in rheumatoid arthritis, and in alcoholics.

Depressed responsiveness of polymorphonuclear cells to normal chemotactic stimuli has also been noted in the Chediak-Higashi-Steinbrink syndrome. This is a rare disorder of man, Aleutian mink, and cattle, which is characterized by gigantism of cytoplasmic lysosomes in white cells, melanocytes, Schwann cells, and possibly a number of other tissue cells. Clinically, affected individuals have partial (oculocutaneous) albinism with resultant photophobia, a marked undue susceptibility to viral and enteric bacterial infections, hepatosplenomegaly, lymphadenopathy, anemia, leukopenia, cutaneous ulcers, and neurologic changes. Peripheral blood smears show abnormally large peroxidase-positive granules in the neutrophils and eosinophils. In addition to the above-mentioned impaired responsiveness to chemotactic stimuli, an intracellular microbicidal defect has also been demonstrated in the granulocytes of such patients. All aspects of adaptive immunity are normal. Death from infection generally occurs before the fifth year of life, but a few patients have survived until the late teens, and some deaths have been attributed to lymphoma. A simple autosomal recessive mode of inheritance has been postulated. Heterozygous carriers have been identified by the presence of the granulation anomaly in leukocytes.

Another type of intrinsic polymorphonuclear abnormality is that seen in the lazy leukocyte syndrome, where the neutrophils not only fail to respond normally to chemotactic stimuli but also have slower than normal random motility. Patients afflicted with this disorder have mild but recurrent infections characterized by gingivitis, stomatitis, otitis, and low-grade fever associated with severe neutropenia and poor mobilization of granulocytes from the marrow, even though the serum does not contain inhibitors of chemotaxis of normal leukocytes and the phagocytic and killing capacities of the polymorphonuclear cell are normal. A somewhat similar disorder has been described in two kindreds in which afflicted members had congenital ichthyosis and recurrent fungal infections. Neutropenia was not present in these individuals, however, and random mobility of the leukocytes was normal.

Recently a defect in monocyte chemotactic responsiveness was discovered in a patient with chronic mucocutaneous candidiasis and delayed cutaneous anergy. This was reversed following therapy with transfer factor. Similarly, patients with the Wiskott-Aldrich syndrome were found to have depressed monocyte chemotactic responsiveness. In this situation the defect was thought to be due to chronic in vivo release of lymphocyte-derived mononuclear chemotactic factor, since excess amounts of this lymphokine were produced by unstimulated cells in vitro.

Opsonic Defects These may be due to deficiencies of the heat-labile (complement-derived C3b) or heat-stable (specific IgM and IgG antibodies) serum factors (called opsonins) that alter the surfaces of bacteria so that they are more readily phagocytosed. As pointed out earlier, newborn serum is deficient in C3 and C5. Thus, not only is it incapable of generating normal quantities of C3a and C5a chemotactic factors, but it also cannot provide adequate quantities of the opsonin, C3b. In addition to this deficiency of heat-labile opsonin, it is virtually devoid of one of the important types of heat-stable opsonins, eg, specific IgM anti-

bodies to gram-negative bacteria. Patients with congenital deficiencies of C3 or C3b inactivator or with dysfunction of C5 (Leiner's syndrome, Chap. 16) produce inadequate quantities of heat-labile opsonins and may have recurrent, often severe infections. The patients with B cell functional deficiencies are, of course, the classic examples of patients deficient in heat-stable opsonins, accounting to a large extent for their special tendency to develop pyogenic infections. Sickle cell disease is accompanied by a special type of opsonin defect, where inadequate C3b is generated due to an abnormality of alternate pathway activation.

Ingestion Defects The capacity of the phagocytic cell to ingest bacteria is determined by the maturity of the cell, the presence of specific cell membrane receptors, and the energy potential of the cell. In acute myelocytic leukemia the ingestion capacity of the cells is severely limited due to their immaturity. Phagocytic cell membrane receptors for C3b and the Fc portion of the IgG are often saturated in conditions such as systemic lupus erythematosus, rheumatoid arthritis, multiple myeloma, and macroglobulinemia, where circulating immune complexes or immunoglobulin aggregates interact continuously with the cells. A familial deficiency of a phagocytosis-promoting tetrapeptide, tuftsin, has also been reported to result in diminished ingestion of staphylococcal organisms by polymorphonuclear cells. The negative surface charge of the phagocyte membrane can be altered by such drugs as levorphanol, a morphine analog, or by viruses, such as the influenza virus, that bind to the membrane. Any condition in which there is an associated inhibition of glycolysis, such as that due to hypophosphatemia of malnutrition, can produce a phagocytic defect on the basis of diminished cellular energy potential.

Killing Defects A variety of disorders can alter the phagocytic cell's ability to kill bacteria even though the cells may have responded normally to chemotactic stimuli and the bacteria have been well opsonized and ingested normally. Among the best known of these conditions is chronic granulomatous disease of childhood (CGD). This is a fatal disorder characterized by chronic suppurative infections, draining adenopathy, pneumonia, hepatomegaly with liver abscess, osteomyelitis, splenomegaly, hypergammaglobulinemia, and dermatitis, with onset of symptoms usually before 1 year of age. Adaptive immunity is usually entirely normal in this condition, although rarely IgA deficiency or hypogammaglobulinemia has been seen. The neutrophils from patients with this disease have been shown to be defective in their ability to kill catalase-positive bacteria (such as *Staphylococcus aureus*, klebsiella-enterobacter organisms, proteus, and *Serratia marcescens*) and some fungi (candida and aspergillus) despite a normal ability to phagocytize these organisms. Moreover, the ingested bacteria enjoy protection from antibiotics that do not penetrate the phagocytic cell membrane and seed out into the body fluids again as soon as the cells die. These intracellular organisms evoke granulomatous reactions in the liver and spleen and other organs which they invade, and pigmented histiocytes are found in such reactions. In contrast, catalase-negative organisms, which generate their own peroxide, such as streptococci and pneumococci, are killed normally by these cells. Metabolic studies of leukocytes from these patients show normal increments of glucose consumption, lactate production, Kreb's cycle activity, and lipid turnover during phagocytosis of latex particles. In contrast, their leukocytes fail to show normal oxygen consumption, direct oxidation of glucose, and hydrogen peroxide formation. The inability of leukocytes from patients with chronic granulomatous disease to lyse bacteria appears to be related to their inability to stimulate the direct pathway of glucose metabolism to form hydrogen peroxide during phagocytosis. The myeloperoxidase—iodide (or other halide)—hydrogen peroxide system has been shown to be an important bactericidal system of human polymorphonuclear cells. Hence, it is speculated that the failure of CGD cells to generate peroxide during phagocytosis is the explanation for their impaired microbicidal activity. Recent evidence has suggested, however, that the superoxide anion radical and/or singlet oxygen may be even more important for microbicidal activity, and generation of both of these is impaired in CGD cells. The precise enzymatic defect or defects in these patients have not yet been defined, although a glutathione peroxidase deficiency was reported in some affected females and an NADH oxidase deficiency in some patients with the x-linked form. The disease has occurred both as a sex-

linked recessive and as an autosomal disorder. In the x-linked form, neutrophils from female heterozygotes are intermediate between normals' and homozygotes' in intracellular bactericidal capacity. A useful screening test for this disorder is based upon the failure of polymorphonuclear cells from affected individuals to reduce the redox dye nitroblue tetrazolium (NBT) to purple formazan during phagocytosis.

In vitro fungicidal and bactericidal activity is also markedly diminished in the neutrophils and monocytes of patients with congenital absence of the lysosomal enzyme, myeloperoxidase. Only one of the five individuals (from three pedigrees) known to have this defect had increased susceptibility to infection, however. In contrast to the situation in CGD, leukocyte metabolism during phagocytosis was normal, as was NBT dye reduction, but granulocyte iodination of bacteria was markedly diminished. As noted above, intracellular killing is also defective in Chediak-Higashi leukocytes, presumably on the basis of delayed degranulation and decreased deposition of lysosomal enzymes into the phagocytic vesicles. Bactericidal capacity may be depressed in patients with severe (< 1 percent of normal) deficiencies of G-6-PD, but most individuals with this hereditary defect (that involves both erythrocytes and leukocytes) have between 20 and 50 percent of the normal amount of G-6-PD and hence no clinical problems with infection. Acquired but transient defects in phagocytic killing have been noted in patients with severe thermal injuries and in children undergoing craniospinal irradiation for treatment of acute lymphoblastic leukemia. Large doses of corticosteroids can depress NADH oxidase activity, and leukocytes from such patients show diminished NBT dye reduction. Finally, newborn leukocytes, despite their unresponsiveness to chemotactic factors and inadequate amounts of heat-labile and heat-stable opsonins, have no intrinsic microbicidal defects. They do, however, have increased resting rates of oxygen consumption, HMP activity, and NBT dye reduction.

FURTHER READING

Books and Reviews

Baehner R L: Molecular basis for functional disorders of phagocytes. J Pediatr 84:317, 1974

Bergsma D, Good RA, Finstad J, Paul N W (eds): Immunodeficiency in Man and Animals. Birth Defects:

Original Article Series. Sunderland, Mass, Sinauer Associates, 1975, vol 11

Cooper MD, Keightley RG, Wu LYF, Lawton AR: Developmental defects of T and B cell lines in humans. Transplant Rev 16:51, 1973

Fudenberg H, Good RA, Goodman HC, et al: Primary immunodeficiencies. Report of a World Health Organization committee. Pediatrics 47:927, 1971

Gelfand EW, Biggar WD, Orange RP: Immune deficiency: evaluation, diagnosis, and therapy. Pediatr Clin North Am 21:745, 1974

Good RA, Quie PG, Windhorst DB, et al: Fatal (chronic) granulomatous disease of childhood: A hereditary defect of leukocyte function. Semin Hematol 5:215, 1968

Kauder E, Mauer AM: Neutropenias of childhood. J Pediatr 69:147, 1966

Park BH, Good RA: Principles of Modern Immunobiology: Basic and Clinical. Philadelphia, Lea and Febiger, 1974

Reimann HA: Recurrent mucosal and dermal ulceration. In Periodic Diseases. Philadelphia, Davis, 1963, chap 6, p 94

Sterzl J, Silverstein AM: Developmental aspects of immunity. Adv Immunol 6:337, 1967

Stiehm ER: Fetal defense mechanisms. Am J Dis Child 129:438, 1975

Stiehm ER, Fulginiti VA (eds): Immunologic Disorders in Infants and Children. Philadelphia, Saunders, 1973

Selected Papers

Buckley RH, Wray BB, Belmaker EZ: Extreme hyperimmunoglobulinemia E and undue susceptibility to infection. Pediatrics 49:59, 1972

Buckley RH, Amos DB, Kremer WB, Stickel DL: Incompatible bone marrow transplantation in lymphopenic immunologic deficiency: circumvention of fatal graft-versus-host disease by immunologic enhancement. N Engl J Med 285:1035, 1971

Giblett ER, Ammann AJ, Wara DW, Sandman R, Diamond LK: Nucleoside-phosphorylase deficiency in a child with severely defective T-cell immunity and normal B-cell immunity. Lancet 1:1010, 1975

Gitlin D, Biasucci A: Development of γG, γA, γM, $B_1C/B_1A,C_1$ esterase inhibitor, ceruloplasmin, transferrin, hemopexin, haptoglobin, fibrinogen, plasminogen, α_1-antitrypsin, orosomucoid, β-lipoprotein, α_2-macroglobulin, and prealbumin in the human conceptus. J Clin Invest 48:1433, 1969

Hayward AR, Ezer G: Development of lymphocyte populations in the human fetal thymus and spleen. Clin Exp Immunol 17:169, 1974

Maugh TH: Singlet oxygen: a unique microbicidal agent in cells. Science 182:44, 1973

Meuwissen HJ, Pollara B, Pickering RJ: Combined immunodeficiency disease with adenosine deaminase deficiency. J Pediatr 86:169, 1975

Miller ME, Oski FA, Harris MD: Lazy leukocyte syndrome. Lancet 1:665, 1971

Schiff RI, Buckley RH, Gilbertsen RB, Metzgar RS: Membrane receptors and in vitro lymphocyte responsiveness in immunodeficiency. J Immunol 112:376, 1974

Stites DP, Carr MC, Fudenberg HH: Ontogeny of cellular immunity in the human fetus: development of responses to phytohemagglutinin and to allogeneic cells. Cell Immunol 11:257, 1974

van Furth R, Schuit H, Hijmans W: The immunological development of the human fetus. J Exp Med 122:1173, 1965

Waldmann TA, Durm M, Broder S, et al: Role of suppressor T cells in pathogenesis of common variable hypogammaglobulinemia. Lancet 2:609, 1974

Wolff SM, Dale DC, Clark RA, Root RK, Kimball HR: The Chediak-Higashi Syndrome: Studies of host defense. Ann Intern Med 76:293, 1972

Yount WJ, Hong R, Seligmann M, Good RA, Kunkel HG: Imbalances of gamma globulin subgroups and gene defects in patients with primary hypogammaglobulinemia. J Clin Invest 49:1957, 1970

21
Immunohematology

BLOOD GROUPS AND IMMUNOHEMATOLOGY

Experiments in blood transfusion were first undertaken seriously in the middle of the seventeenth century but were not successful. Several of the recipients died, and the practice was outlawed in both France and England. It was revived early in the nineteenth century by Blundell, a Scottish obstetrician, for saving patients with postpartum bleeding. It was sometimes successful, but often the patient became hypotensive, passed dark urine, and became oliguric, and frequently died.

The reason for these adverse reactions remained mysterious until 1904, when Landsteiner discovered that the serum of some normal human donors agglutinated the red cells of other donors. He defined the major blood groups (A, B, and O) by a series of cross-reactions. Blood could usually be transfused safely when the groups of the donor and recipient were the same. Serious reactions occurred when the serum of the recipient agglutinated the donated cells. Since that time many other blood groups have been described after finding an antibody in the serum of a patient that reacts with antigens present on the red cells of others. These antigens, isoantigens or alloantigens, number more than a hundred. The antibodies to these antigens (isoantibodies or alloantibodies) are often encountered in two clinical situations: in pregnancy, when the fetus has different antigenic components than the mother, and following blood transfusion, when the transfused blood has different antigens than the recipient.

The blood group antigens may be used as individual identifying markers, since they are present at birth and remain intact throughout the life of the individual. Antigens that are characteristic of certain ethnic groups have been used to trace migrations of peoples and intermixture of races. Since the blood group antigens are passed on by genetic mechanisms, they may be used to test the laws of heredity in human beings in a way almost unavailable by any other means. Finally, the chemical characteristics of some of these antigens are now being elucidated and may give important information concerning the nature of the antigen-antibody interaction.

GENERAL PRINCIPLES OF IMMUNOHEMATOLOGY

Antigens

Antigens on the surfaces of cells are usually not defined by their chemical characteristics (at least when first recognized) but rather by their interaction with antibodies. Thus, all cells reacting with a given antibody are said to possess the antigen against which that antibody was made. For example, cells reacting with an antibody called anti-X are said to be X-positive, those not reacting to be X-negative. If another antibody is found that reacts with human red

TABLE 21-1   THE ASSIGNMENT OF SPECIFICITY TO NEW ANTIBODIES BY AGGLUTINATION REACTIONS WITH CELLS OF SEVERAL DONORS

	Donor 1	Donor 2	Donor 3	Donor 4	Donor 5
Anti-X	+	+	−	−	+
Anti-Y	−	−	+	−	+
Anti-Z	+	−	+	−	−
Unknown antisera					
1	+	+	−	−	+
2	−	−	−	+	−

The cells of five donors were reacted with serum previously denoted anti-X, anti-Y, and anti-Z (hypothetical designations). New antibody 1 has the same reactions as anti-X; if no differences were found when other cells were tested, this antibody would be also called anti-X. New antibody 2 does not give the same reactions as anti-X, anti-Y, or anti-Z, and, therefore, it does not react with the X, Y, or Z antigen. If its reactions are not the same as any known antibody, it is said to define a new specificity, and a name, for example, anti-Q, is assigned. The antigen is then called the Q antigen, and cells are said to be Q-positive or Q-negative.

cells it may be tested on several samples of X-positive and X-negative cells, and if it gives the same reactions as the first antibody with these cells, it also is called anti-X. If it gives different reactions, it is clearly not anti-X and has specificity for another antigen. The reactions of this new antibody with a panel of red cells containing many different antigens are then compared with those of other defined antibodies, for example anti-Y and anti-Z, until it is seen that its reactions are identical to those of some previously defined antibody. If an identical pattern of reaction is not found, the antibody is said to define a new blood group antigen (Table 21-1).

CHEMISTRY. Chemical determinants of the blood group antigens are either polysaccharide or protein. The polysaccharide antigens occur on either glycoproteins or glycolipids, and the determining structure usually consists of more than one sugar moiety. The sugars commonly involved are glucose, galactose, fucose, N-acetyl glucosamine, N-acetyl galactosamine, and N-acetylneuraminic acid (sialic acid). The latter moiety is of great importance, since it imparts most of the charge to the cell surface.

The protein antigens are less well characterized, since they do not survive removal from the membrane. This implies that they are so-called integral proteins and are fixed to the hydrophilic lipid layers of the membrane. To date the specific chemical determinants have not been identified in any case.

It is also possible for antigens to be peripheral to the main structure of the membrane, as if passively adsorbed. Such antigens may be removed by relatively simple chemical techniques (eg, washing, change in pH, change in ionic strength). Although they are less firmly attached to the membrane than the more integral antigens, they can nevertheless take part in immunologic reactions that can result in the destruction of the cell.

GENETICS. Almost all blood group antigens are determined genetically, and in most instances they are dominant or codominant in inheritance. Hence, once an antigen has been identified, its occurrence in the family members can be determined. The genetic locus that codes for the antigen usually has more than one allele. The gene products of these alleles can usually be identified by family or population studies, if appropriate antisera are available.

Some antigens appear to be closely associated (linked) with other antigens. Thus the N antigen and the S antigen (p. 366) occur more frequently together than one would expect if both were randomly distributed throughout the population. Further, they are inherited together. Hence, they and other alleles at the same loci are said to comprise a blood group system bound together by genetic linkage. Most antigens are a part of such systems, which may be very complex indeed.

Antibodies

The antibodies directed against the antigens on the red cell surface are usually IgG or IgM. When they are IgG, they are usually of the IgG_1 and IgG_3 subclasses. IgA antibodies can also occur, but to date no IgD or IgE antibodies have been found.

In general, the antibodies directed against the polysaccharide antigens have the following characteristics: (1) they are usually, but not always, IgM, (2) they usually react better at colder temperatures than 37C, (3) they may occur without sensitization by injection of human blood during transfusion or during pregnancy. The antibodies directed against protein antigens on the red cell surface have the following characteristics: (1) They are usually IgG, (2) they react equally well or better at 37C than at lower temperatures, and (3) they do not occur without prior sensitization with human blood (except in the case of autoimmune disease).

The tests used to detect the presence of the antibody depend in large part upon the immunoglobulin type of the antibody. The easiest way to detect the presence of the antibody is by its ability to agglutinate red cells. In its simplest form, this occurs when one antigen-binding site of the antibody is attached to an antigen site on one cell and the other to an antigen site on another cell (Fig. 21-1). When this occurs, a lattice of cells is bound together as an agglutinate. In forming this lattice the antibody must overcome or bridge the repulsive forces which keep red cells apart. More than one antibody molecule must make the bridge, and the red cell must be able to deform. Red cells in saline suspension are mutually repelled by two forces: (1) the negative charge at the red cell

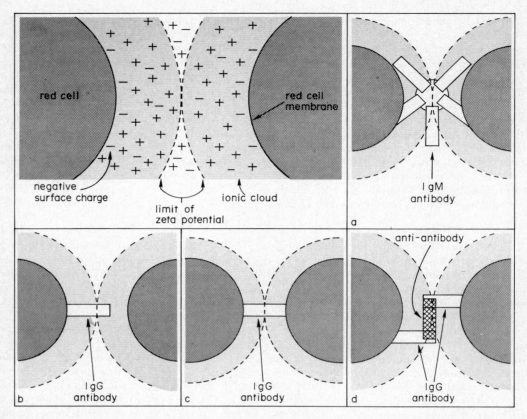

FIG. 21-1. The repulsive forces between red cells. The combination of a negative surface charge and a surrounding ionic cloud tend to keep red cells in saline suspension apart. a. Agglutination by an IgM molecule. b. An IgG molecule cannot interact with two cells because of their mutual repulsion. c. Reduction in the mutual repulsion by dissipation of the zeta potential allows an IgG molecule to react with two cells and agglutinate them. d. An antiantibody reacts with two IgG antibodies, one on each cell, resulting in agglutination.

surface and (2) the cloud of positive ions that accompanies the red cell when it is suspended in saline solution, the so-called zeta potential. Of these, the latter is the more important force. When an antibody reacts with a red cell the negative surface charge is reduced. IgM antibodies are sufficiently large to bridge the gap imposed by the zeta potential, and agglutination usually occurs. If the antigen is located at the outer surface of the membrane, IgG antibodies may also be able to bring about agglutination. More frequently, however, IgG molecules are too small to bridge the gap between the mutually repelled cells, and no agglutination occurs.

In these circumstances IgG antibodies may be demonstrated in one of three ways: (1) The force of the zeta potential may be overcome by

centrifugal force, (2) the zeta potential may be dissipated by suspending the cells in some anisotropic medium, such as 22 percent albumin or polyvinylpyrrolidone (PVP), after which the cell-to-cell gap is small enough to be spanned by IgG molecules, or (3) antibody molecules on each cell may be joined together by antiglobulin molecules (antibody against the antibody made by injecting human immunoglobulins into rabbits or goats). This antiglobulin reaction is sometimes known as the direct Coombs reaction.

The presence of an antibody reacting with the antigen but incapable of bringing about agglutination may be detected by the blocking reaction. In this case, the cell is coated with the IgG blocking antibody, and the coated cells are then reacted with the agglutinating (IgM) antibody of the same specificity. No agglutination occurs because the nonagglutinating antibody has covered or blocked the antigen sites, preventing reaction with the agglutinating IgM antibody.

The presence of antibody can sometimes be detected by its ability to bring about lysis of the cell through the activation of hemolytic serum complement. For this to occur, the first component of complement must by fixed and activated, a process that requires the presence of only one IgM molecule on the red cell surface but two IgG antibody molecules in some geometric juxtaposition (a doublet). Hence IgM molecules are generally more efficient in the fixation of complement than are IgG molecules. In some instances, however, complement may not be fixed under any circumstances, as with the antibodies to antigens of the Rh system. This is thought to be because of the spacing of antigen sites on the red cell surface in such a way that the doublet cannot be formed.

Since human red cells are resistant to the hemolytic action of complement, uncompleted sequences may accumulate on the surface and can be detected by the use of antibody against the components of complement. Since the third component of complement (C3) tends to accumulate in the largest amount, anti-C3 may be used to detect the fact that an immunologic reaction has taken place on the red cell surface.

As noted above, the reaction of the antibody and the antigen on the red cell may be strongly dependent on the temperature. Thus some reactions may not occur at all at 37C but may be very strong at 0C (the so-called cold-reacting antibodies). Others may occur equally well at the two temperatures. This phenomenon may be crucial to the detection of the antibody.

Mechanisms of Lysis In Vivo

Destruction of the red cell in vivo appears to occur as the result of one or more of three processes. Destruction may occur because of the presence of the IgG antibody on the red cell surface. This has been shown to be caused by adherence of such coated cells to macrophages, especially in the spleen. These macrophages may then ingest either the whole cell or only a part of it. When only part of the cell is taken, a spherocyte (globular red cell) results, which may then be destroyed by mechanical entrapment in the spleen. This mechanism can obtain only when there is a warm-reacting antibody and IgG_1 or IgG_3.

Destruction may occur by the direct lytic action of complement. When the complement sequence is completed as the cell circulates, the membrane is ruptured and intravascular hemolysis occurs. For unknown reasons, the human red cell is remarkably resistant to the lytic action of complement; hence destruction by this process occurs only when many sequences are initiated. Since two IgG antibodies in juxtaposition are required for the fixation of the first component of complement ($C\bar{1}$) and thus for the initiation of the complement sequence, these antibodies are relatively inefficient in initiating complement lysis.

The addition of complement to the sensitized red cell membrane may result in the sequestration of the cells by erythrophagocytosis. The activated third component (C3) is required but is readily placed on the membrane if sequences are initiated.

IgM antibodies are relatively more efficient in bringing about lysis by complement-dependent mechanisms. When IgM antibodies are warm reacting, as in incompatible transfusions in the ABO groups, marked intravascular lysis occurs. When these antibodies are cold reacting, particularly in autoimmune disease, they are able to initiate these reactions only when the temperature in the peripheral parts of the body are lowered by exposure to cold ambient temperatures.

BLOOD GROUPS

The ABO, Lewis, and Secretor Systems

In 1902 Landsteiner discovered the ABO blood group system by mixing the red cells of each of the laboratory assistants with the serum of all the others. From these reactions he defined the groups as follows:

Current nane	Patient serum agglutinates cells of donor in the group
O	A, B, and AB
A	B and AB
B	A and AB
AB*	none

*Discovered two years later.

The cause of the agglutination was found to be naturally occurring antibodies to the antigens of the system. These antibodies accounted for many of the reactions which occurred when blood was transfused (Table 21-2). Since that time subgroups of A and B have been described. The most important of these is A_2, which was first recognized because cells of this type reacted with many examples of anti-A less strongly than did cells of most (90 percent) group A donors. By cross-absorption experiments, it was found that the usual A cells had two closely related antigens, designated A and A_1. A_2 cells had only one of these antigens, the A antigen. Most anti-A antisera contained antibodies to both antigens, but absorption of such antiserum with A_2 cells left only anti-A_1.

The antibodies to the antigens of the ABO(H) system regularly occur in the serum of people lacking the antigen, even though they have been neither transfused nor pregnant. These antibodies are not present at birth and gradually develop during early childhood. Their presence has been attributed to antigenic stimulation from oligosaccharides of the same chemical conformation as the A or B antigens. Such oligosaccharides abound in nature. The quantity of the isoantibody may be markedly increased, however, by the antigenic stimulation of incompatible blood.

The antigens of the ABO blood groups are inherited characteristics. According to the theory of their transmission proposed in 1924, the allelic A and B genes give rise to their respective gene products, the A and B antigens, whereas the allelic O gene gives rise to no gene product, ie, it is an amorph. Thus, the phenotype (detectable antigens on the red cell) of a person whose genetic makeup is AO will be group A, but he may pass the O gene to his offspring.

It became apparent that O red cells did contain an antigen which was related to their O-ness. These cells were more strongly agglutinated than were A, B, or AB cells by certain animal sera and plant products (lectins), as well as by certain isoantibody-containing sera. The antigen responsible for these reactions was called the H antigen, and it was expressed on the cell surface in inverse proportion to the amount of A and/or B antigen expressed on the cell.

Rarely, the A, B, and H antigens may all be lacking. This rare blood type is called "Bombay" and is due to the absence of the gene responsible for the formation of the H antigen, which is a precursor of the A and B antigens (p. 366). Patients with this blood type have anti-A, anti-B, and anti-H in their serum.

The antigens of the ABO(H) system are present on many other tissues in addition to red blood cells. They may appear in water-soluble form in the secretions of the body (with the exception of the cerebrospinal fluid). Their presence in water-soluble form appears to be under separate genetic control by the so-called secretor gene (Se) which is inherited as a mendelian dominant. People who lack the gene may have the cellular ABO(H) antigens on their red cells but not the water-soluble forms in their saliva or in other secretions.

The antigens of another blood group system which is closely related, the Lewis system, may also be found in the secretions. There are two recognized antigens in the Lewis system, Lewis a (Le^a) and Lewis b (Le^b). Individuals

TABLE 21-2 THE ABO BLOOD GROUPS

Group	Specific Antigens on cell	Quantity of H Antigen	Antibodies in Serum	May Receive Blood from*	May give Blood to*
O	None	High	Anti-A Anti-B	O	O, A, B, AB
A	A, A_1	Low	Anti-B	A, O	A, A_2, AB
A_2	A	More than A	Anti-B occ. anti-A_1	A (usually), A_2, O	A, A_2, AB
B	B	Like A	Anti-A	B, O	B, AB
AB	A, A_1, B	Less than A or B	None	AB, A, B, O	AB
A_2B	A, B	More than AB	None	AB, A, B, O	AB

*In most instances, type-specific blood is given (eg, type A to type A patient, and so on). Occasionally this rule may be broken in special circumstances, but the groups must be selected from these columns. When, for instance, type-O blood containing anti-A is infused into a person whose cells are type A, the antibodies are normally diluted so that no reaction takes place.

CELLULAR ANTIGENS   *GENES*   SOLUBLE ANTIGENS

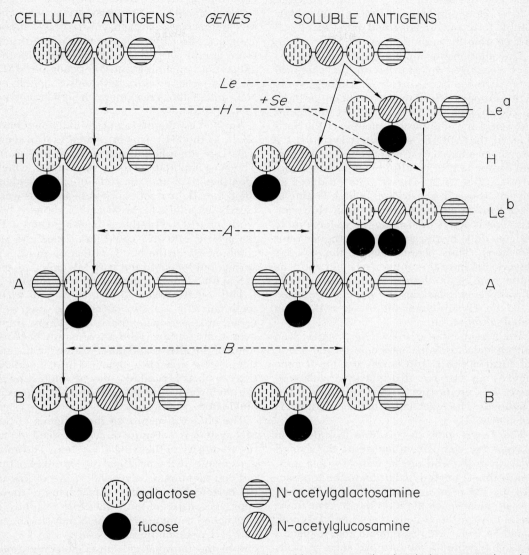

galactose   N-acetylgalactosamine

fucose   N-acetylglucosamine

FIG. 21-2. The antigens of the ABH and Lewis systems are formed from a tetrasaccharide, which is connected to other saccharides, to lipid moieties, or to protein moieties. This basic tetrasaccharide, shown on the top line, is acted upon by enzymes which are determined by the presence of specific genes.

The Lewis gene codes for a fucosyl transferase, which adds a fucose molecule to the second sugar (an N-acetylglucosamine). This gene is active only in cells forming soluble antigen and not in the red cell precursors. When this is the only sugar added to the tetrasaccharide, the antigen formed is Le^a. This antigen is passively absorbed to red cells.

The *H* gene codes for a fucosyl transferase which adds a fucose to the terminal sugar (a galactose), forming the H antigen. In cells forming soluble antigen, this occurs only in the presence of another gene, the secretor *(Se)* gene, but can occur in the absence of this gene in cells forming cellular antigen (eg, the red cells). If a fucose is present on both terminal sugars (both the *Le* gene and the *H* gene are active), the result is the Lewis^b (Le^b) antigen.

The *A* gene codes for an N-acetylgalactosamine addition to the terminal sugar of H substance, forming the A antigen. This occurs in cells forming either soluble or cellular antigens. Similarly, the *B* gene codes for a galactosyl transferase, which places a galactose molecule in the same spot, forming the B substance.

may have either antigen or neither, in a complex genetic pattern that will be explained below. These antigens occur only in water-soluble form and are adsorbed onto the red cell surface from the serum.

The relationship among these systems has been suggested by studies on the chemical nature of the antigens involved. Although some of the suppositions have not yet been verified, no known serologic facts contradict the theory that states that the basic structure of the antigens of the ABO(H) and Lewis systems is a four-sugar oligosaccharide attached to the protain component or to a lipid component (a globoside) (Fig. 21-2). The *H* gene produces an enzyme (fucosyl transferase), which is able to place a fucose on the terminal sugar. However, this gene is active in forming the water-soluble antigen only in the presence of the secretor *(Se)* gene. Thus people lacking the secretor gene do not have this antigen or other antigens made from it in their secretions (especially saliva). Persons lacking the *H* gene (Bombay) make no H substance either on cells or in water-soluble form.

The *A* gene induces an enzyme that places an N-acetylgalactosamine molecule on the terminal sugar of the H substance; and the *B* gene induces an enzyme that places a galactose there, thus producing, respectively, the A and B antigens. The exact nature of the A_1 antigen is not known.

The Lewis gene *(Le)* is able to induce an enzyme that can place a fucose on the second sugar from the end of the water-soluble antigen. If this is the only addition to the tetrasaccharide, the resulting antigen is Le[a]. This occurs in the absence of either the *Se* gene (most commonly) or the *H* gene (very rarely). If both *H* and *Se* genes are present and able to place a fucose molecule on the terminal sugar as well, the resulting antigen is Le[b]. This theory adequately explains the complex relationship among the ABO(H) system, the Lewis system, and the secretor system.

The MNSs System

For about 20 years the A and B antigens were the only two known on human red cells. In 1927 Landsteiner and Levine injected rabbits with human red cells and tried to determine the nature of the antigens to which the

antibodies had been produced. From these experiments there emerged two new antigen systems, the MN system and the P system. The MN system was thought to consist of two allelic antigens, M and N. People were divided into three groups: (1) those reacting only with the antiserum containing anti-M (genotype MM), (2) those reacting only with anti-N (genotype NN), and (3) those reacting with both (genotype MN).

Antibodies identifying other antigens either allelic to the MN locus or related to it in some way were identified during the next few years. The most important of these were anti-S, which identified the S antigen, and anti-s, which identified the allelic s antigen. These antigens were clearly not allelic to the M and N antigens but were inherited with them. Thus a person with the genotype Ms/NS could pass either the Ms combination or the NS combination to his offspring, but he could not pass MS or Ns; ie, the MN and Ss genetic loci were closely linked.

This sytem, although not usually of great importance in transfusion therapy, was very useful in assessing genetic relationships. However, some problems did arise, mainly because some of the alleles and modifications of the antigens were difficult to detect. These modifications, such as M_g and M_k, may be interesting as the chemical nature of the M and N antigens is elucidated.

The chemical nature of the antigens of the MN system is not quite so well worked out as the chemistry of the ABO(H) system. The antigens reside on the principal glycoprotein of the red cell membrane, glycophorin. According to the current hypothesis, the backbone of these antigens consists of three galactose residues in a branched configuration. The N antigen has an N-acetyl neuraminic acid residue (NANA) on one of the terminal galactose molecules, and the M antigen has a NANA molecule on both galactose molecules. The genetic theory previously held may need to be revised to accommodate these facts.

The P System

The other major system defined by the animal experiments of Landsteiner and Levine is called the P system. When the antisera obtained from rabbits injected with human red cells were absorbed with a series of cells, two types of cells were defined: P+ (80 percent of donors), which reacted with an antibody remaining after absorption with the second type of cell, and P- (20 percent of donors). The system was found to be more complex when it was discovered that an antibody, anti-Tj^a, reacted with P+ cells and most P- cells: the few cells with which this antibody did not react were all P-. Since this would not occur if the anti-Tj^a were not related to the P system, it could be shown that the P system is complex and resembles the A antigen system. Cells originally called P+ are now called P$_1$ cells and contain only the P antigen. Rare cells containing neither antigen, which did not react with anti-Tj^a, are called pp; and no antibody reacting with this antigen has been found. A fourth, very rare antigen, P^k, was later found.

			Reaction with anti-Tj^a	
Old name	New name	Antigens	Unabsorbed	Absorbed with P$_2$ cells
P+	P^1	P + P$_1$	+	+
P-	P$_2$	P	+	-
	pp	none	-	-

The antigens of the P system are polysaccharides and occur elsewhere in nature, as in the fluid of the hydatid cyst formed by *Echinococcus*. Curiously, the antibodies to these antigens are often IgG. They are not often involved in transfusion reactions but are thought to cause early fetal death in women lacking the P and P$_1$ antigens. The Donath-Landsteiner antibody seen in paroxysmal cold hemoglobinuria, a disease complicating syphilis and certain viral syndromes, is anti-P.

The Rh System

The most important of the blood group systems, other than the ABO system, is the Rh system, since it is within this system that the major difficulties of transfusion and of fetomaternal incompatibility occur. This system was first discovered by Levine and Stetson when transfusion of the mother of a baby with hemolytic disease of the newborn (erythroblastosis fetalis) with the blood of the father resulted in an acute hemolytic reaction. An antibody was found in her serum that was not related to the ABO, MN, or P systems but that agglutinated the father's cells, the baby's cells, and the cells of 85 percent of all random donors. This antibody did not agglutinate the cells of the mother and was thus clearly isoimmune. The authors suggested that the baby had on his cells an antigen lacking in the mother, which had passed from the baby to the mother and had caused antibody to be formed. Since the baby had inherited the antigen from the father, the father's cells injected into the mother also were rapidly destroyed in an acute hemolytic reaction.

When other instances of hemolytic disease of the newborn were investigated, it was found that no agglutinating antibody could be demonstrated. However, blocking antibody (p. 362) could be demonstrated on the cells of the babies and in the serum of the mothers. Further, antibodies reacting with these new antigens appeared to be involved in many previously incomprehensible transfusion reactions. The antibodies were demonstrated with much greater ease by the use of the antiglobulin (Coombs) test. With this adjunct, a new era in investigating the nature of the blood groups was opened. It soon became apparent that the original antigen (called somewhat erroneously the Rh antigen, since the same antigen was thought to occur on the cells of Rhesus monkeys) was part of a complex system of antigens that were identified with antibodies occurring as the result of sensitization by transfusion. Five different antigens appeared to be related in this system, and considerable confusion occurred because of the variant nomenclature evolved by different investigative groups. According to Wiener, eight different gene complexes were possible at a single locus, and the five antigens occurred in these complexes in different combinations. According to the interpretation of Race and Fisher, three tightly linked loci, each with two alleles, were responsible for the expression of the genetic information. The alleles were named *C, c, E, e,* and *D, d.* Since the antibody for the d antigen was never identified, the existence of this allele cannot be affirmed. In a modest attempt to resolve these problems in nomenclature, Rosenfield and his associates suggested a new system of nomenclature which assigned numbers to the antibodies and did not try to explain the relationship between the antigens. The different names used in each classification system are shown in Table 21-3.

Each person has two of these gene complexes, one inherited from each parent; and, in turn, one or the other is passed to each of his children. However, careful family studies or the

TABLE 21-3   ALTERNATIVE NOMENCLATURE OF ANTIBODIES AND GENE COMPLEXES OF THE RH SYSTEM

		Antibodies					
Rosenfield ⟶		Anti-Rh1	Anti-Rh2	Anti-Rh3	Anti-Rh4	Anti-Rh5	Frequency in whites
Wiener ⟶		Anti-Rh$_0$	Anti-rh′	Anti-rh″	Anti-hr′	Anti-hr″	
	Fisher	Anti-D	Anti-C	Anti-E	Anti-c̄	Anti-e	
R^1	CDe	+	+	−	−	+	0.408
r	cde	−	−	−	+	+	0.39
R^2	cDE	+	−	+	+	−	0.14
R^0	cDe	+	−	−	+	+	0.025
r''	cdE	−	−	+	+	−	0.011
r'	Cde	−	+	−	−	+	0.009
R^Z	CDE	+	+	+	−	−	0.001
R^Y	CdE	−	+	+	−	−	Very rare

Genes or Gene Complexes

use of special antibodies is needed to determine the gene complex from the antigens present on the cell surface; eg, a person DCe/DcE (R^1R^2) could not be distinguished readily from one DCE/Dce (R^ZR^o), since the same antigens would be present on the cells of both.

The antigens of the Rh system vary considerably in their antigenicity as measured by the chances of eliciting antibody when injected into a person lacking the antibody. The D (Rh_o) antigen is clearly the most potent and in common parlance is the antigen referred to when speaking of Rh-positive or Rh-negative cells. This antigenicity is manifested by the fact that it is the antigen most commonly involved in sensitization by transfusion or pregnancy. Nevertheless sensitization occurs in only 70 percent of Rh-negative recipients even when fairly large amounts of blood are repeatedly injected.

The antibodies to antigens of the Rh system are commonly IgG, although IgM antibodies are not rare and usually occur early in the immune response. Since the antigens are complex proteins, the antibodies from different patients are not uniform, a fact that has caused considerable confusion in defining the system. The antibodies do not appear naturally, although autoimmune antibodies may have specificity for this complex.

The other antigens of the Rh system are very much less potent and consequently cause less difficulty in transfusion or fetomaternal incompatibility. Antibodies to these antigens are sometimes found as a cause of autoimmune hemolytic anemia.

Variations in the Rh Antigens D^u. In some patients the expression of the D antigen appears to be particularly weak, since anti-D antibodies react with these cells rather poorly. In most instances this is due to the presence of a variant form of the antigen called D^u. The D^u antigen is fairly common in blacks and not rare in whites. It is important because its presence may be missed unless special care is taken in typing the cells with the use of antiglobulin reactions or proteolytic enzyme treatment of cells.

The current interpretation of D^u states that the D antigen actually consists of several (probably four) parts and that D^u is determined by the presence of some, but not all, of these parts of the D antigen. Thus the D^u antigen may stimulate antibodies in D-negative recipients, and the usual D antigen may stimulate antibodies to the missing parts in D^u recipients.

THE F ANTIGEN. Antibodies have been described that react with cells from patients with the c and e antigens present on the same genetic complex. This antibody, designated anti-ce or anti-f, will not react with cells whose genotype is DCe/DcE or (d)cE/(d)Ce, but will react with cells of the genotype (d)ce/(d)ce or (d)ce/DCE. This antibody is important because it suggests that the order of the antigens on the red cell surface is D(d) Cc Ee.

SUPPRESSIONS. Certain cells have been found in which neither of the alleles at one or more of the three loci is expressed on the membrane surface. Cells expressing only the D antigen (D−/D−) have been shown to react so strongly with anti-D that antibodies which do not ordinarily agglutinate cells in saline suspension are able to do so. Rarely, there may be no expression of any of the Rh antigens on the cells surface, and these cells are called Rh$_{null}$. This condition may occur in the products of consanguineous matings, suggesting a recessive inheritance. These cells are defective in other ways. Their life span is shortened, and the expression of antigens that are not part of the Rh system may be altered. It is possible that some membrane defect brings about changes that do not permit the expression of the Rh antigens or that these cells lack some complex genetic precursor of the Rh antigens. Many antibodies formed in autoimmune hemolytic anemia react with all cells except Rh$_{null}$ cells.

Other Blood Group Systems

The Kell Group In 1946 an antibody was found in a case of hemolytic disease of the newborn that was not related to the Rh system. The antibody was called anti-Kell or anti-K. The allelic antigen was described by another antibody called anti-Cellano or anti-k. The Kk genetic locus is closely linked to two other loci, Kp and Js. The alleles of Kp are Kp^a (rare) and Kp^b (very common). The alleles of Js are Js^a (Sutter^a), which exists only in blacks, and Js^b, which occurs in all whites and most blacks. These three closely linked genetic loci are similar in some respects to the three loci present in the Rh complex. Anti-K is frequently involved in cross-matching difficulties and hemolytic disease of the newborn. Anti-k is much rarer, since homozygotes for the K antigen (the only people who could make anti-k) constitute only 0.2 percent of all people.

The Duffy Group An antibody describing a new antigen system was found in a patient named Duffy and was called anti-Duffy or, more commonly, anti-Fy^a. Soon the allelically determined antigen was found and named Fy^b. The cells of all whites are either Fy(a$^+$, b$^-$), Fy(a$^-$, b$^+$), or Fy(a$^+$, b$^+$). About 60 percent of all blacks are Fy(a$^-$, b$^-$), and they run a greater risk of sensitization by transfusion. Fortunately the antigens of this system are not particularly good antigenic stimuli, so that difficulties in transfusion or pregnancy are rare.

The Kidd (JK) System Two antigens have been described belonging to this system: Jk^a and Jk^b. The antibodies to these antigens are particularly unstable on storage and do not remain in the serum of sensitized patients. Hence, at the time of subsequent transfusion, the antibody cannot be detected at cross-match. However, antibodies capable of destroying the red cells that were transfused are formed in an anamnestic response within five to seven days. Hemoglobinemia and hemoglobinuria result as the transfused cells are destroyed. This type of delayed transfusion reaction has been described in other blood group systems.

Other Systems Many other antigens have been defined on the red cell surface by the fact that antibodies have been produced to them. In some instances the antigens are rare, and in others, the antigens are found in over 99.9 percent of the population. Because of their frequency distribution, these so-called private and public blood groups do not often cause trouble in the clinical setting. They do, however, add to the antigenic complexity of the red cell surface.

Paternity Exclusion One of the uses of blood groups is to exclude paternity where this is contested. Paternity is excluded (1) if the child has an antigen which both the supposed father and the mother lack or (2) if the child does not have an antigen which the father must pass to his progeny. In no instance can paternity be established by blood groups, but in the instance of some of the rare blood groups, the statistical chances of paternity being real can be very high. The interpretation of blood groups in paternity testing requires considerable expertise. The precision with which paternity can be excluded will be greatly increased when the HLA leukocyte antigens are added to the battery of antigens examined.

TRANSFUSION THERAPY AND TRANSFUSION REACTIONS

Blood can normally be transfused with relative safety if it can be demonstrated that antibodies do not exist in the serum of the patient which will react with antigens on the transfused red cells. Donors are selected so that the ABO and Rh$_0$(D) groups are the same as those of the patient. In emergencies, group O blood may be used for all patients even though anti-A and anti-B may be present in the plasma. Further tests of compatibility (the cross-match) are performed by mixing the donor's cells and the patient's serum and observing for three reactions: (1) agglutination of the cells in saline suspension, (2) agglutination of the cells when suspended in 22 percent albumin, and (3) testing for the presence of antibody on the red cells using antiglobulin screen. If no evidence of antibody is found, the blood may be transfused.

These tests are not foolproof, and blood may be transfused which contains an antigen reacting with an antibody present in the plasma of the patient. When this occurs, the red cells are destroyed by the mechanisms outlined above. The clinical consequences of this may range from little or no reaction to death, depending upon the concentration of the antibody and its ability to stimulate the hemolytic mechanisms. Transfusion reactions are divided into three main types.

Major Hemolytic Reactions

When the destruction of the transfused blood is sudden and massive, several reactions take place which may result in serious morbidity or death of the patient. (1) Hemoglobin is released into the blood and filtered by the kidneys, resulting in hemoglobinuria. (2) The blood pressure may fall, and this combined with the massive hemoglobinuria may result in renal failure, which may clear only very slowly. (3) The coagulation system may be activated so that it no longer functions, resulting in hemorrhage. Reactions of this type are usually due to incompatibility within the ABO system and are frequently due to clerical errors, such as mislabeling the blood, using the blood from the wrong patient in compatibility testing, and so on.

Minor Hemolytic Reactions

When the rate of destruction is less rapid, the results may be only a falling hematocrit as the transfused blood is destroyed and the appearance of jaundice as the hemoglobin is me-

tabolized. Little needs to be done except to find compatible blood for transfusion.

Delayed Transfusion Reaction

Certain blood group antibodies do not persist in the serum (particularly the Kidd and Duffy antibodies). Thus, at the time of compatibility testing before transfusion, no incompatibility is found even though the patient has been previously sensitized. When the blood is transfused, it elicits an anamnestic response, and the concentration of antibody rises rapidly. This results in the destruction of the transfused blood 5 to 10 days later. Frequently the destruction is manifest by hemoglobinuria. The reaction is usually not serious.

HEMOLYTIC DISEASE OF THE NEWBORN

In the preceding discussion many allusions have been made to hemolytic disease of the newborn (erythroblastosis fetalis or HDN), a disease first recognized in the early 1930s. As detailed above, its explanation came with the discovery of the Rh groups, and although they are by no means the only cause of the problem, they account for a vast majority of all cases.

The problem occurs when antigens are present on the red cells of the child that are lacking on those of the mother. If cells from the baby cross the placenta, antibodies are produced in the mother. These antibodies recross the placenta and cause the destruction of the cells of the infant. The effects may be mild or may be severe enough to cause death, even before birth.

THE TIMING OF SENSITIZATION. Sensitization does not generally occur during the first pregnancy, but a rise in antibody titer is seen shortly after the birth of the child. With the next pregnancy, the titer of antibody may increase slowly during the pregnancy but again may rise sharply after delivery. It is thought that a transfusion of sufficient cells from the infant to the mother to initiate antibody production occurs at delivery. Once the mother is immunized, small transplacental leaks of cells during subsequent pregnancies may increase the antibody titer. Thus the disease is usually manifest only during the second and subsequent incompatible pregnancies.

CLEARANCE OF THE IMMUNIZING DOSE. Even when the infant is Rh positive and the mother is Rh negative, sensitization to Rh is much less common when the mother's serum contains antibodies to A or B antigens on the infant's cells. It is thought that the immunizing dose of fetal cells is cleared by the anti-A or anti-B before the Rh incompatibility can be recognized.

TYPE OF ANTIBODY PRODUCED. Only IgG antibody molecules are able to cross the placenta. Therefore, if antibodies of other immunoglobulin types are made, they cannot reach the infant. Further, it has been postulated that those IgG antibodies with the greater affinity for the antigen are more likely to be responsible for the onset of the hemolytic reactions.

ANTIGENICITY OF THE ANTIGEN. Some of the antigens on the red cell are able to elicit an antibody response more readily (or, rather, more frequently in a random population) than others. The $D(Rh_o)$ antigen is a particularly strong antigen, but injection studies have shown that many D-negative people are not sensitized when D-positive cells are injected. Other potentially immunizing antigens, such as those of the Duffy, Kidd, and MNSs groups, are injected regularly in transfusions, but antibody response is seen only rarely.

EXPRESSION OF THE ANTIGEN ON FETAL CELLS. The antigens of the ABO(H) system are poorly expressed on fetal cells. This may account in part for the rarity of hemolytic problems in cases where the mother's serum contains IgG antibodies to either the A or B antigens. Whatever the reason, less than 1 in 3,000 of such incompatible mother-infant combinations results in serious hemolytic anemia.

Hemolytic disease of the newborn due to the $D(Rh_o)$ antigen now appears to be preventable. If the mother has not been previously sensitized, she is given a large dose of anti-D shortly after delivery. This in some way prevents the initiation of an immune response, sensitization does not occur, and the next pregnancy cannot result in an erythroblastotic infant.

AUTOIMMUNE DISEASE OF THE HEMATOPOIETIC SYSTEM

The foregoing discussion is mainly concerned with isoantibodies. However, in certain instances, immunologic tolerance is apparently broken, and the patient begins to make antibodies to antigens present on his own (autologous) cellular blood elements. Classically, this process has involved the red cells in the form of autoimmune hemolytic anemia, but more recently the occurrence of thrombocytopenia (lack of platelets) and leukopenia (lack of white cells) has been ascribed to the same process.

Autoimmune Hemolytic Anemia

ANTIBODIES. The antibodies causing autoimmune hemolytic anemia are usually of either the IgM or IgG immunoglobulin class. They are further divided into those that react only at temperatures below body temperature (cold-reacting antibodies) and those that react at body temperature (warm-reacting antibodies). In general, the warm-reacting antibodies are IgG, while the cold-reacting ones are IgM. The most notable exception to this rule is the Donath-Landsteiner antibody of paroxysmal cold hemoglobinuria, which is cold-reacting but IgG. The reasons why some antibodies react only in the cold are not clear, but a probable cause is the state of the cellular membrane and the availability of the antigen at these temperatures as opposed to its availability at higher temperatures. The mechanism of hemolysis and the resultant clinical syndrome both are related to the immunoglobulin class and the temperature of reactivity of the antibody molecule.

ANTIGENS. The antigens present on the red cells that react with self-made antibody may or may not belong to groups defined by isoantibodies (alloantibodies). Thus some warm-reacting IgG autoantibodies may react with cells of only specific Rh antigens, while others may react with all cells that contain any

Rh antigens but not with Rh$_{null}$ cells which contain no Rh antigens. Rarely, antibodies to specificities outside the Rh system (Kell, P, and so on) have been reported. However, nearly half of all warm-reacting IgG antibodies that occur in autoimmune hemolytic anemia react with all available red cells. Thus, although they have specificity for some antigen on the red cell surface, this antigen cannot be defined serologically, since negative cells cannot be found. In no instance has the antigen been chemically defined.

The cold-reacting IgM antibodies (cold agglutinins) appear to react with polysaccharide antigens that reside on the glycophorin molecule in red cells. All cold agglutinins react with all cells under appropriate conditions. Specificity of these antibodies is denominated by the reactivity with adult cells or newborn cells (or the rare examples of adult cells that behave like newborn cells). Thus those antibodies that react with adult cells most strongly are called anti-I; and those that react with newborn or newborn-like cells most strongly are called anti-i. Those that react equally well with adult and cord cells are called anti-Pr, since the antigen is destroyed by proteolytic enzymes. These antigens are clearly heterogeneous.

SEROLOGIC DIAGNOSIS OF THE SYNDROMES. The diagnosis of autoimmune hemolytic anemia depends upon the demonstration of the fixation of antibody or complement to the red cell membrane. This is best done by the antiglobulin (Coombs) technique (p. 362) by using specific antisera, such as anti-IgG, anti-IgM, anti-C3, and so on. The pattern of reaction will depend upon the material remaining on the patient's red cells after thorough washing. In patients with disease due to warm-reacting antibody, IgG alone, IgG and C3, or C3 alone may be demonstrated by antiglobulin (Coombs) reaction. In these patients, antibody may or may not be demonstrable in the serum, and the antibody can be eluted from the red cells even when not detectable in the serum, and its characteristics can be investigated.

In patients with cold agglutinin disease, IgG antibodies are not usually involved, and the IgM which may have coated the red cells is readily washed off. Often a heavy coating of C3 is present on the cells. More significantly, however, the antibody in the serum is readily demonstrated by the agglutination of normal red cells at 0C in saline dilutions of the serum. In some cases dilutions of serum of 1 part in 50,000 still cause agglutination of the cells.

The Donath-Landsteiner antibody is demonstrated by the bithermic hemolytic reaction. Cells, antiserum, and fresh serum as a source of complement are reacted together at 0C and then at 37C. If the antibody is present, hemolysis occurs. Two temperatures are needed, since the antibody will not fix to the cell at 37C and the terminal steps of complement will not be completed at 0C.

ETIOLOGY. The mechanisms that bring about the production of self-destructive antibodies against red cells are not at all clear. Warm-reacting IgG antibodies are often associated with other abnormalities of the immune system in patients with systemic lupus erythematosus, chronic lymphocytic leukemia, and Wiskott-Aldrich syndrome, but just as frequently, no such underlying disease is discernible. Since cold-reacting antibodies are usually monoclonal, they have been thought to be related to benign monoclonal gammopathy. Why this particular clone should be selected for autonomous proliferation is not clear. Both warm-reacting IgG and cold-reacting IgM antibodies may follow certain infections, including mycoplasma infection, infectious mononucleosis, and other less well defined viral infections. In these instances the antibody production may be related to the presence of the invading organism.

TREATMENT. The principal objective of treatment is to bring about the cessation of synthesis of antibody or at least interruption of the mechanisms of hemolysis. When the antibody is IgG, hemolysis occurs largely in the spleen, and splenectomy is often useful. Adrenocorticosteroids and cytotoxic agents may reduce the rate of antibody production. These steroids may also inhibit the ability of the reticuloendothelial cells to phagocytose the altered red cells.

Immune Thrombocytopenia

An apparently entirely analogous syndrome to autoimmune destruction of red cells by warm-reacting IgG antibody also occurs with regard to platelets. However, the antibody-mediated nature of the destruction has been hard to define, since it has been difficult to use antiglobulin reagents to detect the presence of IgG on the platelet surface. New techniques have shown that these antibodies are IgG, and are quantitatively related to the rate of destruction of the platelets.

This problem appears to be analogous to that of warm-reacting IgG-mediated hemolytic anemia, since (1) in both instances the major destruction appears to occur in the spleen; hence, both syndromes may be benefited by splenectomy, (2) in both instances remission may often be induced by corticosteroids, which may be due in part to suppression of antibody or suppression of sequestration, and (3) both are commonly seen in patients with systemic lupus erythematosus.

Leukopenia

Although neutropenia due to autoimmune destruction has often been suspected, especially in patients with systemic lupus erythematosus, the demonstration of the antibodies or of cellular destruction has been singularly difficult to obtain. Recently techniques similar to those used for platelets have demonstrated such antibodies.

ANIMAL BLOOD GROUPS

The erythrocytes of all animals are characterized by an array of antigens as complex as those found in man. Through the use of red cell agglutination and lysis, animal blood groups have been shown to include examples of complex antigens (phenogroups), soluble blood group substances, mosaicism, and gene interaction, as well as numerous antigens controlled by simple mendelian genetics.

The appearance of complex antigens (many antigenic factors apparently determined by one locus) is relatively common in animals. The mouse H-2 system, an erythrocyte blood group as well as the major histocompatibility locus, is probably the best known because of its importance in transplantation research. This group is discussed in Chapter 22. Two other examples of complex antigens in animal systems are the B group of cattle and the Hg system in rabbits. In the bovine B system, blood group factors B and G may be inherited separately as alleles *B* and *G* or together as BG. Another alternate allele in this system, *BGK*, produces a factor K as well as B and G. Eighteen other factors have also been reported for this blood group. The Hg system in rabbits consists of four alleles that control the production of nine factors. Animals homozygous for the Hg^A allele show blood group factors A, P, and R. Animals homozygous for the Hg^D allele have factors D, J, K, N, and R. The other blood groups known in rabbits consist of two codominant alleles, each represented by one blood group factor, or of one dominant gene that controls the presence of a factor and a recessive gene that apparently controls the absence of the factor.

There are several soluble blood group substances known in animal systems: J in cattle, R in sheep, and A in pigs. Of these the J group is probably the most thoroughly studied. The level of J substance in the red cells is influenced by the level of the substance in the serum and also by an allele determining the type of erythrocyte: J^{cs} (J present in the serum and on the cells), J^s (J present only in the serum), and J^a (J not present). The erythrocytes of newborn J^{cs} cattle are apparently J-negative until the age of one month, although the serum contains high levels of J at birth. J-negative animals (J^aJ^a) can make a natural antibody to J. The strength of this antibody varies during the year, with the highest titers occurring in the late summer and early fall. The reasons for this are not clearly understood.

Cattle also provide examples of chimerism in utero, leading to erythrocyte mosaicism in the adult. Approximately 90 percent of bovine twins have anastomosed blood vessels in utero. This results in migration of primordial blood cells and hormones between twins. If the pair are male and female, the female twin will become a sterile freemartin because of the transfer of male hormones to the female before birth. When the blood cells of such pairs are typed by hemolysis, only part of the cells will lyse if the blood group is not shared by both twins. The proportion of cells in each twin showing the foreign blood group can vary widely. The original observations by Owen on chimerism in freemartins led directly to the development of the original concept of tolerance.

Animal blood group factors usually appear on

erythrocytes if either or both parents possess the factor. Exceptions to this rule arise from cases of genetic interaction. Examples of this interaction in animal blood groups include the R system in sheep, hybrid antigens in doves, and interaction or hybrid antigens in rabbits. The R system of sheep is defined by two antibodies, anti-R and anti-r, whose reactions are mutually exclusive and which react with the red cells of almost all sheep. The R gene is dominant over r. The few sheep that do not react with either anti-R or anti-r are thought to have no r substance because they lack a gene at a second locus that is necessary for the production of r substance from some precursor. The recessive genotype ii is epistatic for R and r, so that the genotype of a sheep in group R is I-/R-, and the genotoype of an r sheep is I-/rr. A sec-

ond type of gene interaction was observed on erythrocytes from hybrids between two species of doves, *Streptopelia chinensis* and *Streptopelia risoria*. Antiserum prepared in rabbits against the red cells of the hybrid birds reacted with cells from both parents and from the hybrids. After absorption with erythrocytes from both parents, the rabbit antiserum still reacted with red cells from the hybrid. A third type of gene interaction occurs in the Hg system in rabbits, when heterozygotes for certain alleles at the Hg locus show interaction products. A rabbit of the type Hg^4Hg^F will show all the factors associated with each allele in the homozygous state plus the factor J. In this case the J factor is a normal constituent of the Hg^D-animal and also appears as an interaction product in the Hg^4Hg^F heterozygote.

FURTHER READING

Books and Reviews

Allen FH, Diamond LK: Erythroblastosis Fetalis. Boston, Little, Brown, 1958

Cohen C (ed): Blood groups in infrahuman species. Ann NY Acad Sci 97:1-328, 1962

Dacie JV: The Haemolytic Anaemias—Congenital and Acquired. Part II. The Autoimmune Haemolytic Anaemias. New York, Grune & Stratton, 1962

Mollison PL: Blood Transfusion in Clinical Medicine, 4th ed. Philadelphia, Davis, 1967

Pirofsky B: Autoimmune Hemolytic Anemias. Baltimore, Williams & Wilkins, 1969

Race RR, Sanger R: Blood Groups in Man, 5th ed. Philadelphia, Davis, 1968

Stone WH, Irwin MR: Blood groups in animals other than man. Adv Immunogenetics 3:315, 1963

Wiener AS: Advances in Blood Groupings. New York, Grune & Stratton, 1961, Vol 1

Zmijewski CM: Immunohematology. New York, Appleton-Century-Crofts, 1968

Selected Papers

Cohen C, Tissot R: Blood groups in the rabbit: two additional isoantibodies and the red cell antigens they identify. J Immunol 95:148, 1965

Landsteiner K: Über Agglutinationserscheinungen normalen menschlichen Blutes. Wien Klin Wochenschr 14: 1132, 1901

Landsteiner K, Levine, P: On the inheritance of agglutinogens of human blood demonstrable by immune agglutinins. J Exp Med 48:731, 1928

Levine P, Stetson RE: An unusual case of intragroup agglutination. JAMA 113:126, 1939

LoBuglio AF, Cotran RS, Jandl JH: Red cells coated with immunoglobulin G: binding and sphering by mononuclear cells in man. Science 158:1582, 1967

Mollison PL, Crome P, Hughes-Jones NC, Rochna E: Rate of removal from the ciculation of red cells sensitized with different amounts of antibody. Br J Haematol 11: 461, 1965

Pollack W, Hager HJ, Reckel R, Toren DA, Singher HO: A study of the forces involved in the second stage of hemagglutination. Transfusion 5:158, 1965

Watkins W: Blood group substances. Science 152:172, 1966

22
The Immunobiology of Transplantation

A great many persons who would otherwise be healthy suffer from prolonged illness or die from malfunction or failure of a single organ. Included in this group are persons with end-stage renal disease, many heart conditions, congenital malformations of the liver, diabetes, especially juvenile diabetes, bone marrow aplasias, and thymic deficiencies. Many or all of these conditions are correctable by the substitution of normal tissue for that which is diseased or malfunctioning.

The surgical techniques for this substitution have been developed over a period of many years. Indeed, sporadic attempts at transplantation have been reported since 700 BC, the serious study having been advanced by the experiments of Bert in which skin grafts placed on another part of the same individual (autografts) were successful, while similar grafts transferred to another individual (allografts) were rejected. The technique of vascular suturing was developed by Carrell and Guthrie early in this century. Numerous advances have enabled the technically successful transplantation of viscera and tissues. Unfortunately, the applicability of transplantation is greatly limited by the difficulty in overcoming the immune response to foreign tissue. This reaction, if untreated, leads to rejection of the transplant.

A consideration of transplantation immunity is thus relevant to a text on microbiology and immunology for two reasons. First, it is one of the most intensively studied models of immune responsiveness. Second, it offers great challenges and opportunities for students of infectious disease, since the drugs used to control transplant rejection interfere with the immunologic defenses against microorganisms and hence predispose to a wide variety of infections, some common, some rare outside the immunodeficient patient. Transplantation of tissues and organs is one of the triumphs and frustrations of the surgeon and the immunologist—triumph when the function can be restored to a dying patient, frustration when the transplant ceases to function because of the processes of immunologic rejection.

ANTIGENIC INDIVIDUALITY

The immunologic reaction against a transplant is directed against a multiplicity of protein and glycoprotein molecules of varying structure and function, the hydrophobic portions of which are inserted into the membranes of mammalian cells. While these molecules are accepted as self by the lymphoid system of the original host, many of them function as highly potent antigens when transferred or transplanted to another individual. Cell surface molecules which are recognized in this way are known as transplantation or histocompatibility (H) antigens. They present the greatest barrier to the successful transplantation of tissues and organs.

Many cell surface molecules are constant for all individuals of the same species but may be different from similar molecules present on the cells of another species. They are then called species specific or xenoantigens. One classic example is the Forssman antigen, present on the red cells of sheep but absent from the rabbit. Rabbit antibodies against sheep red blood cells are highly hemolytic for sheep red cells when complement is added, providing a highly sensitive assay for determination of complement fixation (Chap. 15).

Other cell surface markers, alloantigens, differ from individual to individual within the species. The antibodies they provoke are alloantibodies. Familiar to everyone are the red cell antigens and antibodies discussed in Chapter 21. Less familiar and considerably more complex are the antigens of the major histocompatibility complex (MHC) of each species, typified by the H-2 system of the mouse and the HLA system of man, mentioned briefly in Chapter 14.

Similarities between the mouse H-2 system and the human HLA system are very striking. Each system occupies a considerable segment of chromosome (a haplotype), and each includes a number of genetic loci of varying functions, all of which appear to have some relevance to the functioning of the immune system. The major components include genes determining serologically detectable cell surface marker antigens (H antigen), genes controlling the immune response (IR) capacity of the individual, and genes controlling the ability to stimulate proliferative or cytotoxic responses in foreign lymphocytes. These are often called lymphocyte activating determinants (LAD). The MHC also includes genes that appear to be activated only at certain stages of lymphocyte differentiation, which, in the mouse, determine

THE 17TH CHROMOSOME AND H-2 REGION OF THE MOUSE

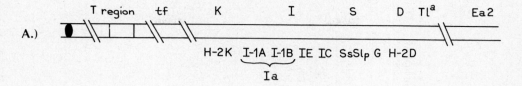

THE C6 CHROMOSOME AND HLA REGION OF MAN

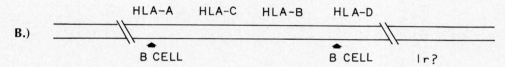

FIG. 22-1. The mouse seventeenth chromosome carries genes for embryonic differentiation in the complex T region. Products of some genes in this region are antigens on sperm and teratoma cells. The H-2 region includes genes controlling immune responses (Ir), antigens of lymphocyte subpopulations (Ia), complement C4 levels (SS), MLC stimulation (I region), and antigens of red cells and tissues (H-2K, H-2G, and H-2D). The human C6 chromosome may carry genes analogous to T and Ir (not shown). The HLA region includes the HLA-D locus corresponding to the MLC of the mouse and genes regulating antigens of tissues HLA-A, B, and C. HLA-D probably includes two loci. Antigens expressed on lymphocyte subpopulations are mapped in the HLA-A and HLA-B regions.

antigens designated Ia antigens. Genes regulating the serum levels of some complement components can also be found. The order of genes on the chromosome has been deduced from studies of recombinant individuals in whom crossing over is believed to have occurred between two homologous chromosomes during meiosis. A diagrammatic representation of the H-2 and HLA regions is depicted in Figure 22-1, together with an example of recombination.

THE HLA SYSTEM OF MAN

The MHC of man is located on the C6 chromosome. The most easily detected markers are the HLA antigens included in what are generally referred to as the first and second segregant series. These are glycoproteins of MW 56,000 and comprised of two chains, often called light and heavy. The light chain is antigenically indistinguishable from a globular protein, β-2 microglobulin (MW 11,750), isolated from serum or urine. On the cell surface this

light chain is noncovalently bound to a heavy chain of MW 45,000 which is inserted into the membrane by a hydrophobic portion. The remainder of the molecule can be freed from the cell surface by digestion with papain. The fragment thus released is thought to have two domains (Chap. 13), each of which includes an internal disulfide bond. The antigenic specificity is believed to be determined by the amino acid sequence rather than by any variability in the carbohydrate side-chain.

The serology of HLA is exceedingly complex. Some 20 distinct specificities in each of the first and second series have been identified by an international group of serologists and geneticists (Table 22-1). Thus, since each chromosome determines one first series and one second series specificity (now called HLA-A and HLA-B, respectively) and since each individual has two homologous chromosomes, the number of possible combinations is extremely high. To compound the complexity, each haplotype is also believed to carry a third locus determinant, now called HLA-C. The HLA-C products are also believed to be cell surface protein, their chemistry is less well under-

TABLE 22-1 ANTIGENIC SPECIFICATIONS OF HLA

New Terminology	Old Terminology	New Terminology	Old Terminology	New Terminology	Old Terminology	New Terminology	Old Terminology
HLA-A	1st segregant series, 1st locus, or 4A series antigen	HLA-B	2nd segregant series, 2nd or FOUR locus antigens	HLA-C	3rd segregant series, 3rd locus, or AJ series antigen	HLA-D	MLR-S1, LAD, or LD determinant
HLA-A 1	HL-A 1	HLA-B 5	HL-A 5	HLA-CW 1	T1	HLA-DW 1	LD 101
HLA-A 2	HL-A 2	HLA-B 7	HL-A 7	HLA-CW 2	T2	HLA-DW 2	LD 102
HLA-A 3	HL-A 3	HLA-B 8	HL-A 8	HLA-CW 3	T3	HLA-DW 3	LD 103
HLA-A 9	HL-A 9	HLA-B 12	HL-A 12	HLA-CW 4	T4	HLA-DW 4	LD 104
HLA-A 10	HL-A 10	HLA-B 13	HL-A 13	HLA-CW 5	T5	HLA-DW 5	LD 105
HLA-A 11	HL-A 11	HLA-B 14	W 14			HLA-DW 6	LD 106
HLA-A 28	W28	HLA-B 18	W 18				
HLA-A 29	W29	HLA-B 27	W 27				
HLA-AW 23	W23	HLA-BW 15	W 15				
HLA-AW 24	W24	HLA-BW 16	W 16				
HLA-AW 25	W25	HLA-BW 17	W 17				
HLA-AW 26	W26	HLA-BW 21	W 21				
HLA-AW 30	W30	HLA-BW 22	W 22				
HLA-AW 31	W31	HLA-BW 35	W 5				
HLA-AW 32	W32	HLA-BW 37	—				
HLA-AW 33	W19.6	HLA-BW 38	W 16.1				
HLA-AW 34	—	HLA-BW 39	W 16.2				
HLA-AW 36	—	HLA-BW 40	W 10				
HLA-AW 43	—	HLA-BW 41	—				
		HLA-BW 42	—				

stood, and they mey be less stable than the other HLA antigens. Only five HLA-C specificities have so far been described.

At a little distance from the HLA-B locus, but still closely linked and on the same chromosome, is the polymorphic HLA-D' locus. This locus differs from the others in that no antigenic product has to date been identified, and the activities of the HLA-D locus are known only through the ability of lymphocytes of one individual to stimulate those of another to blast transformation and DNA synthesis in mixed lymphocyte culture (MLC). The process of identification of alleles of HLA-D is somewhat unusual. Most individuals have two different alleles of HLA-D and thus tend to stimulate all other individuals except those siblings who inherit the same two HLA haplotypes. Only some children of first cousin marriages and certain other exceptional individuals carry the same allele on both chromosomes. Lymphocytes from these individuals cannot stimulate lymphocytes from other persons carrying the same allele (Fig. 22-2). Having obtained such a typing cell, it is possible to identify other persons sharing that particular allele and thus to define its distribution and frequency in a population. Using this laborious approach, six alleles have currently been recognized at HLA-

D, although it has been deduced that another nine or more alleles have yet to be identified.

Mentioned earlier (Chap. 14) were a number of antigens, such as Thy-1, TL, and Ia antigens, present only on subpopulations of lymphocytes. First described in the mouse, similar antigens have now been identified in man. At least two genetic loci for B cell antigens have been located in the HLA region, one close to the gene for HLA-A, the other close to HLA-B. While information on these new antigens is still incomplete, there is a correlation between some antigens of this type and the HLA-D alleles. Certain antisera react with lymphocytes carrying a specific HLA-D allele and can block stimulation by such cells in MLC.

In both mouse and man, genes regulating immune responses are located in or near the MHC. The mouse data are much more detailed than are those on the human being. While the evidence is far from complete, loci have been suggested in man regulating the levels of antibody to several viruses, including parainfluenza and cytomegalovirus, in addition to genes controlling the atopic responses to a variety of allergens, including ragweed and house dust. Studies on human beings are difficult because of the heterogeneity of HLA in populations, the small size of human families, and the

GENERATION

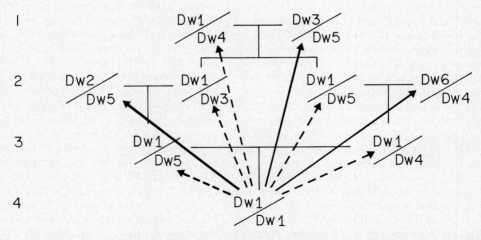

FIG. 22-2. Illustration of the way in which an individual can inherit two HLA haplotypes each carrying the same HLA-D determinant. In this case, the great grandfather transmitted the haplotype carrying the gene for Dwl. In turn each transmitted the gene to his children in the third generation. These descendants of 101 are first cousins. Their child has a probability of 0.25 of inheriting Dwl from each parent and thus becoming homozygous at the HLA-D locus. This child's lymphocytes would not stimulate those family members who share Dwl ‒‒, but would stimulate individuals who do not carry this determinant ——.

variations introduced by the marked age differences in family members. Many atopic responses are not developed until adolescence and fade in late middle age. Many disease states also show an association with HLA. This association may be very close, and linkage may be clearly recognized, as with ankylosing spondylitis and Reiter's syndrome, or less constant, as in gluten enteropathy or juvenile diabetes. Many investigators suspect a casual relationship.

HLA AND TRANSPLANTATION

The involvement of HLA in transplant rejection has been proven in two ways: by intrafamilial kidney or skin transplants and by skin grafts placed on an unrelated recipient previously sensitized against a given HLA specificity.

While HLA is a multiantigenic complex, and two unrelated individuals are rarely exactly alike, the situation is relatively simple within the family, since the entire complex is inherited as a gametic unit. The importance of HLA has been demonstrated by skin grafts exchanged between family members. It is convenient to designate the paternal haplotypes by symbols as A and B and the maternal haplotypes as C and D. The children must inherit either A or B from the father and C or D from the mother, and the only possible HLA genotypes of the children are AC, AD, BC, or BD. If there are five children, two of them must inherit the same pair of haplotypes, for example, AC (Fig. 22-3). This type of sibling pair is designated HLA identical. In the absence of incompatibility for A and B blood group antigens, skin grafts between HLA identical siblings persist for an average of 23 days (range 14 to 40) before rejection occurs. The majority of sib-sib pairs and parent-sib pairs share one haplotype, for example, AC and AD, AB and AC. These pairs are said to be haploidentical. Skin grafts between haploidentical pairs persist for an average of 13 to 14 days. The range of rejection times is wide, from 6 to 40 days. Some sib pairs differ at both haplotypes, AC and BD, and these are HLA nonidentical, with skin grafts persisting on the average for about 12 days, with a range of 6 to 14 days. Evidently the MHC has a very strong influence on skin graft rejection.

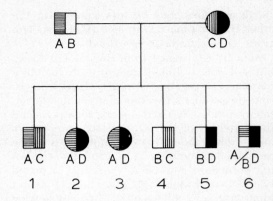

FIG. 22-3. Inheritance of HLA in a family. The code letters A B C D represent the haplotypes which could be formally written, for example, HLA-A1B8CwlDw3, A2B12Cwl-Dw5, A9B13Cw3Dwl, and A10Bw15Cw3Dw4. Sibs 2 and 3 are HLA identical; 1 and 2, 3 and 5, and so on are haploidentical; 3 and 4, 1 and 5 are nonidentical. Sib 6 is a recombinant, having inherited part of the A haplotype (for example, A1) and part of the B (for example, B12Cw1Dw5).

But because HLA-identical grafts are ultimately rejected, non-HLA antigens must also be segregating in the family. Because of the wide range of rejection times observed in haploidentical grafts, the immunogenicity of different haplotypes must vary greatly.

The influence of HLA is also observed in the behavior exhibited by kidney grafts and in reactions observed in bone marrow transplants. Kidney grafting is a common therapeutic procedure for end-stage renal disease. The techniques for kidney transplantation, including the optimal preparation of the patient and implantation, of the ureter, have become well established. While a few recipients do have problems associated with surgery, this would not be a major source of morbidity or mortality without the additional stresses imposed by immunosuppressive drugs.

All renal transplant recipients recieve immunosuppressive agents to prevent rejection. Since HLA-identical kidneys differ only with respect to minor antigens, the amount of immunosuppression required by recipients of an HLA-identical kidney is minimal and complications are unusual. When there are major HLA differences between donor and recipient, greater amounts of immunosuppressive agents are required, and rejection crises may occur, the reversal of which may require life-threatening amounts of drugs. This difficulty is most frequent with organs from cadavers and HLA-nonidentical sibs but may also occur with haploidentical kidneys. The three major difficulties encountered as a consequence of attempted rejection are (1) infection due to the level of (suppressive) therapy required to prevent rejection, (2) degenerative changes resulting from the rejection reaction, and (3) other side effects from the drugs, liver damage, Cushing's syndrome, and so on.

Transplantation, therefore, urgently requires advances in two different areas before it can become a safe and predictable treatment: (1) ways of assessing the immunogenicity of a given kidney and (2) more selective methods of immunosuppression.

IMMUNOGENICITY OF TRANSPLANTS

In some instances, notably with A and B or Rh blood group antigens, incompatibility for some specificities is demonstrably more likely to elicit a strong immune response than others. Unfortunately, there is no evidence that any single HLA specificity is a stronger transplantation antigen than any other.

In mice, repeated studies showed that the transplanted tissues from a donor of a given H-2 genotype would readily be accepted by a recipient of the same H-2 type, whereas transplants from donors of other H-2 types would not. The early approach to human donor selection followed this precedent. It was thought that a recipient having, for example, HLA antigens A1, A3, B5, B8 would accept a kidney from a donor of phenotype A1, A3, B5, B8 more readily than a kidney carrying antigens A2, A3, B7, B8. While there is some evidence for the validity of this concept, in practice, because of the large number of alleles, it has been extremely difficult to find donors compatible for four antigens. While there does appear to be a statistical improvement in results when donor and recipient are matched for both A and both B series antigens, the results are by no means as uniformly favorable as those obtained with genetically identical sibling transplants. There are two likely explanations for this: One is that very few transplant pairs have been characterized for HLA-C specificities and thus may differ in these antigens, and the other is that products of

the HLA region that cannot presently be typed for may also be immunogenic. In face of these uncertainties, research must proceed in several different directions. Some laboratories are concentrating on identifying new alleles of known loci, others are concentrating on the immune response potential of the recipient, and still others are attempting to induce a selective unresponsiveness in the recipient.

Transplantation of Bone Marrow

Patients with immunodeficiency disease, bone marrow aplasias, metabolic deficiencies, and leukemias and other malignancies are candidates for bone marrow transplantation. The three special problems faced in bone marrow transplantation are (1) reactions of lymphoid cells in the transplanted marrow against the host (2) rejection or failure of engraftment, and (3) lack of adequate stimulus for differentiation. Of these, we need only be concerned with reactions of the graft against the host (GvH) (Chap. 20).

Mention has been made of the HLA-D locus and its effects in MLC stimulation. In the immunodepressed recipient, whether the immunodepression is drug induced or idiopathic, marrow from a donor who stimulates the recipient in vitro in MLC is likely to cause a fatal GvH reaction in vivo. It appears probable that a separate genetic locus is responsible for GvH effects, since, in mice, combinations stimulating strongly in MLC may fail to give GvH reactions. Tentative identification of a GvH locus has been reported. In the mouse, at least one additional locus, not related to H-2, can induce wasting, especially when the transplanted marrow is from a presensitized donor. A similar locus or loci are probably represented in man, where fatal GvH disease has frequently been reported when the marrow donor was an apparently HLA-identical sibling.

Transplantation of Cornea

Successful corneal transplants have been performed without recourse to tissue typing or immunosuppression. This is not because the cornea lacks antigens but because the anterior chamber of the eye is one of a limited number of what are known as immunologically privileged sites. Other such sites include poorly vascularized areas of the brain and the testes. These sites lack lymphatic drainage, and the small amount of antigen released into the bloodstream from experimental grafts in these sites is not sufficient to trigger a cellular response. Interestingly, it has recently been found that HLA may be very important in corneal transplantation in those cases where the eye of the recipient is inflamed. In a large series of corneal transplants, failure was rare where the recipient site was not inflamed but quite common when there was even a moderate state of inflammation. In this situation, a direct correlation was observed between the degree of incompatibility and the incidence of failure of the transplant.

IMMUNOSUPPRESSION AND IMMUNOLOGIC TOLERANCE

Renal transplantation would be impossible without immunosuppression. The drug most extensively used is a purine analog derived from 6-mercaptopurine, azathioprine, which inhibits the conversion of inosine monophosphate to adenosine and guanosine monophosphate. It has an additional feedback inhibition in the early biosynthesis of purines. Less often used clinically are the folic acid antagonist, methotrexate, and the alkylating agents, such as cyclophosphamide. Cyclophosphamide

is used in the preparation of bone marrow recipients. Adrenocorticosteroids are also given to most recipients. In addition to their general anti-inflammatory actions, the steroid hormones, especially prednisolone, have powerful immunosuppressive actions when given in large quantities. Amount up to 200 mg daily are not unusual in attempts to reverse severe rejection crises. The mode of action of steroids is unknown; their action is partly to prevent cellular proliferation.

Of special relevance to transplantation immunology is antiserum raised in horses or rabbits to human thymocytes or lymphocytes (Fig. 22-4). In one special experimental situation, the effect of antithymocyte serum or globulin prepared from it (ATG) is most dramatic. Mice thymectomized soon after birth and treated with ATG not only lose their ability to reject allografts but can freely accept xenografts from other mammalian species and even from birds. The nude (athymic) mouse has the same inability to reject xenografts. Thus, in the absence of T cells, graft rejection does not occur. Thymectomy is less effective in older animals, and even with larger doses of ATG, the same dramatic effects may not be achieved, presumably because ATG is unable to prevent the activity of precommitted T cells. However, ATG does deplete the paracortical areas of lymph nodes and provides a useful adjunct to other methods of immunosuppression.

All the preceding forms of immunosuppression are nonselective, that is, besides suppressing the response to the transplant, they also

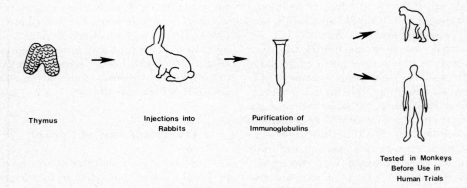

Thymus   Injections into Rabbits   Purification of Immunoglobulins   Tested in Monkeys Before Use in Human Trials

FIG. 22-4. The production and use of antithymocyte globulin. Cadaveric or surgically excised thymus is homogenized and injected into rabbits or horses. Two or three injections are usually given. The serum is tested for potency, often in monkeys, before being used as an adjunct immunosuppressive together with suppressive drugs in recipients of transplanted kidneys.

suppress the response to bacterial and other antigens. While the immunologic system is normally so powerful that many microorganisms rarely cause infection, a host of organisms rarely encountered in clinical practice may be recovered from the transplant recipient. These include cryptococcus, aspergillus, and cytomegalovirus.

It is obviously desirable to find a means of selectively avoiding, inhibiting, or deleting those cells capable of responding to the transplant. There are three possible approaches to this end: one is based on the immune response capacity of the recipient, one is based on immunologic tolerance, and the other is based on immunologic enhancement. At the present time none is readily available clinically.

Response avoidance is theoretically possible, either by avoiding antigenic differences through donor selection or by avoidance of antigens recognizable by the Ir allele of the recipient. Pretreatment of the recipient with donor antigen presented in such a manner as to induce tolerance is also a possibility. Donor antigen could be presented on an autologous (cellular or serum protein) carrier. This procedure is successful for synthetic antigens and is being attempted with transplantation antigens. Since many of the components of the HLA region are still being defined, progress is likely to be slow. Immunologic enhancement should be entirely practicable. It has proven brilliantly successful in modifying some tumor and skin graft rejection. In mice, antibody pretreatment directed against donor skin to enhance recipient skin graft survival has been most successful in congenic strains (identical except for differences at H-2). A few clinical transplant recipients have received alloantibody against the donor in conjunction with conventional therapy, and results from two centers are encouraging. Certainly this form of immunosuppression has been effective in rats, especially when used in conjunction with donor spleen cells. To some extent, clinical transplantation is being stifled by its own success. While results fall far short of those desired by the immunologist and surgeon, present procedures are successful enough to discourage any novel approach. The exception may be the patient who has rejected two or more kidneys and who is unsuitable for dialysis, but here the obstacles created by strong preexisting immunity are formidable.

FETOMATERNAL RELATIONSHIPS

In view of the potency of the MHC in inducing graft versus host disease in newborn rodents or immunodeficient humans, it is surprising that human embryos are not destroyed in utero. The fetus can be regarded as a natural model of transplantation! The human placenta is not a barrier impermeable to HLA antigens nor, indeed, to cells. About one-third of multiparous women have circulating anti-HLA antibodies against their offspring, and a similar number have antibodies detectable by reactions against B lymphocytes. Anti-HLA antibodies are not infrequently found during the first pregnancy, even by the twenty-fourth week of gestation. Lymphocytes and PMN from the fetus frequently pass into the maternal circulation, as do fetal red cells. The lymphocytes may persist for at least several days.

There is no evidence that antibodies to HLA can pass the placenta. Whether this is because of placental impermeability or absorption of antibodies by the ubiquitous HLA antigens of the fetal tissues and placenta is unknown. Lack of penetration is more likely, since a sudden increased antibody level in the maternal circulation is not observed after termination of pregnancy. Such an increase has been reported following the rejection of a transplanted kidney. However, antineutrophil antibodies appear to pass through as readily as do anti-Rh antibodies, and they can produce a transient neonatal granulopenia.

Protection against GvH disease may be partly by the placenta and partly by protective substances that reduce lymphocyte-mediated cytotoxicity (LMC). The placenta of hybrid animals is markedly larger than is the placenta of inbred strains. The placenta acts in part as a mechanical barrier. It is also thought to act in part as a target for local GvH reactions. The cytotoxic cells would thus bind to placental sites and therefore not be free to pass to the fetus. In many experimental situations, certain types of targets are highly resistant to LMC, and the placenta may provide such a target. The protective effect of serum may be twofold. Many maternal antibodies are capable of blocking MLC reactions and may block GvH by competing for sites on the target cell. Anti-HLA alloantibodies, although themselves cytotoxic in the presence of rabbit complement, are often only feebly lytic using human serum as a complement source. The other immunosuppressive agent in maternal serum is not specific and does not appear to be an immunoglobulin. There is some evidence it may be an alpha-2 macroglobulin. Alpha-2 macroglobulins have been found capable of suppressing a variety of immune responses.

The level of blocking activity in maternal serum has been reported to rise steadily until term and then decline. This may also be a reflection of the aberrations reported in many immunologic parameters during pregnancy.

FURTHER READING

Books and Reviews

Amos DB, Ward FE: Immunogenetics of the HL-A system. Physiol Rev 55:206, 1975

Dausset J, Colombani J (eds): Histocompatibility Testing 1972. Copenhagen, Munksgaard, 1973

Diczfalusy E (ed): Immunological Approaches to Fertility Control. Stockholm, Karolinska Institute, 1974

Kissmeyer-Nielsen F (ed): Tissue Antigens. Copenhagen, Munksgaard, 1975

Klein J: An attempt at an interpretation of the mouse H-2 complex. Contemp Topics Immunobiol In press, 1975

Klein J: Biology of the Moust Histocompatibility-2 Complex. New York, Springer Verlag, 1975

Lengerová A, Vojtišková M (eds): Immunogenetics of the H-2 System. Basel, Karger, 1971

Najarian J, Symonds R: Transplantation. Philadelphia, Lea and Febiger, 1972

Yunis EJ, Gatti RA, Amos DB (eds): Tissue Typing and Organ Transplantation. New York, Academic Press, 1973

Selected Papers

Doughty RW, Gelsthorp K: An initial investigation of lymphocyte antibody activity through pregnancy and in eluates prepared from placental material. Tissue Antigens 4:291, 1974

Jørgensen F, Lamm LU, Kissmeyer-Nielsen F: Mixed lymphocyte cultures with inbred individuals: an approach to MLC typing. Tissue Antigens 3:323, 1973

Lalezari P, Bernard GE: A new neutrophil-specific antigen. Its role in the pathogenesis of neonatal neutropenia. J Clin Invest 45:1741, 1966

Mann DL, Abelson L, Harris S, Amos DB: Detection of antigens specific for B lymphoid cultured cell lines with human alloantisera. J Exp Med 142:84, 1975

Pedersen NC, Morris B: The role of the lymphatic system in the rejection of homografts. A study of lymph from renal transplants. J Exp Med 131:936, 1970

Porter KA, Andres GA, Calder MW, et al: Human renal transplantation. II. Immunofluorescent and immunoferritin studies. Lab Invest 18:159, 1968

Shearer GM, Rehm TG, Garbarino CA: Cell mediated lympholysis of triphenyl-modified autologous lymphocytes. J Exp Med 141:1348, 1975

Seigler HF, Gunnells JC Jr, Robinson RR, et al: Renal transplantation between HL-A identical donor-recipient pairs: functional and morphological evaluation. J Clin Invest 51:3200, 1972

Zinkernagel RM, Doherty PC: H-2 compatibility requirement for T-cell-mediated lysis of target cells infected with lymphocytic choriomeningitis virus. J Exp Med 141:1427, 1975

23
Tumor Immunology and Immunotherapy

Two central concepts, one related to the tumor, the other to the host, form the basis of tumor immunology. The first states that cells from many, if not all, tumors have, on their surface, antigenic moieties not found on autogenous normal cells. The second postulates that the host possesses an immunologic defense system directed toward the elimination of aberrant cells, most notably those cells recognized as aberrant by the presence of nonself surface antigens.

GENERAL CHARACTERISTICS OF CANCER

As a prelude to a discussion of the immune system's interaction with neoplastic tissue it is well to introduce briefly four general characteristics of most cancers. Hyperplasia refers to an uncontrolled proliferation of cells, in which the tissue's normal architectural patterns are defied. It is important to realize, however, that this does not necessarily imply an increased rate of proliferation. Indeed, many normal cell types replicate much more rapidly than even the most deadly cancers. Anaplasia refers to structural and functional abnormalities of cells in which they resemble their primitive or embryonic counterparts. While both hyperplastic and anaplastic changes can be seen in so-called benign neoplasms, whose growth can expand and distort the normal size and configuration of the tissue or organ in which they arose, the hallmark of cancer is its ability to burst the confines of its site of origin and invade neighboring or distant tissues. This may be by invasion of local sites, such as erosion by a uterine cancer into the bladder wall or a pulmonary cancer into the bronchial artery, or invasion of distant sites, called "metastasis." Metastases generally arise by spread via hematogenous or lymphatic routes but may traverse virtually any of the extracellular compartments. Most primary tumors are able to seed the circulation with tumor cells, but why only a portion of these tumors are able to form metastatic deposits remains an enigma.

Cancers are divided into two broad categories, carcinomas and sarcomas. Carcinomas are derived from epithelial tissue and hence are of either ectodermal or entodermal origin. They comprise the vast majority (about 85 percent) of all cancers. Sarcomas are derived from mesoderm and thus, by strict definition, include the lymphomas and leukemias. It is perhaps unfortunate to realize that, while these tumors comprise only about 10 percent of all human cancers, almost all the research on animal tumor systems has employed sarcomas. There is a third category of mixed tumors that contains both mesodermal and epithelial elements, and the prototype of such neoplasms is the teratoma.

TUMOR ANTIGENS

The concept of tumor-specific transplantation antigens (TSTA) was developed at the end of the nineteenth century, but it was not until inbred mice became available that one could truly distinguish between tumor-specific and normal histocompatibility antigens. Ludwik Gross in 1943 induced a methylcholanthrene sarcoma in C_3H mice. In about 15 percent of the mice the tumor underwent spontaneous regression, and when these mice were challenged with the tumor, they were highly resistant. In addition, two mice in the resistant group developed spontaneous mammary tumors, which grew despite continued immunity to the sarcoma and emphasized the specificity of the sarcoma resistance.

It was not until 1960, however, that George and Eva Klein, together with two students, Hans Olaf Sjögren and Karl Erik Hellström, demonstrated clearly that an animal could be made resistant to its own original tumor, thereby providing final proof to the concept of tumor-specific immunity. They induced a primary methylcholanthrene sarcoma in inbred mice. They then removed a portion of the tumor and preserved its viability by transplantation to another mouse of the same strain while tying a ligature around the remaining primary tumor. When the ligated primary tumor had become necrotic, the transplanted portion was reinjected into the original host and was rejected. The animal was not resistant to other tumors, however, emphasizing the specificity of the immune resistance. This work was followed closely by the demonstration of TSTA on virus-induced and spontaneous tumors. Soon there arose the intriguing generalization that tumors induced by the same virus were antigenically cross-reactive, while the TSTA of chemically (or physically) induced tumors were individually distinct. Thus two tumors induced by a virus, such as polyoma or SV40, though in different species and of different histologic types, would share TSTA, while two fibrosarcomas induced simultaneously on different sides of the same animal with a single preparation of a chemical agent such as methylcholanthrene would have distinct TSTA. Recently it has become apparent, however, that some chemically induced tumors do show weakly cross-reacting antigens. Likewise, at least some virus-induced tumors that bear common TSTA have been shown to possess, in addition, individually distinct transplantation antigens. The most notable example of the latter lies in the murine mammary tumor virus system, where the induction of tolerance to the group-specific antigen allows the expression, in transplantation experiments, of individual antigens otherwise masked by the stronger reaction to the common antigen.

The genesis of TSTAs has been controversial, since it is unclear whether the oncogenic process alters the antigenic nature of the cell or merely unmasks antigens that are already present. Support for the latter concept comes from the exposure of so-called cryptic antigens on normal cells by treatment with such enzymes as trypsin and neuraminidase. On the other hand, both viral and chemical carcinogens do have the capacity to induce neoantigens not found on nonneoplastic cells and, likewise, to induce structural changes in certain normal cell surface components (Chap. 69). Finally, as a hallmark of its anaplastic nature, the tumor cell frequently secretes or expresses on its surface antigens that are characteristic of fetal cells but are normally absent or barely detectable on normal adult cells. Some of these fetal antigens provide the basis for immunodiagnostic procedures discussed below.

THE HOST RESPONSE TO NEOPLASIA

Immunologic Surveillance

In 1959 Thomas suggested that adaptive immunity had evolved specifically as a defense mechanism against cancer. It was Burnet, however, who coined the term "immunologic surveillance" and who has developed the concept that a large segment of the immune system, most notably the circulating T lymphocyte, has the primary function to detect and destroy any cells bearing nonself markers, such as TSTA.

Arguments for Immunologic Surveillance Support for the concept and importance of immunologic surveillance comes from several sources. Abrogation of immune competence by neonatal thymectomy, irradiation, or antithymocyte serum greatly augments the susceptibility of animals to virus-induced tumors and, to a lesser extent, to chemically induced and spontaneous tumors. Similarly, in man, the use of chronic immunosuppressive regimens, particularly in transplant recipients, has led to a hundredfold increase in the incidence of cancer, and there are reports that some of the malignancies disappear following cessation of immunosuppression. In patients with immunologic deficiency diseases, the incidence of cancer is greatly increased. Patients with the most severe deficiencies have not survived long enough to study the incidence of cancer, but with sex-linked infantile agammaglobulinemia, ataxia telangiectasia, and Wiskott-Aldrich syndrome, the incidence of cancer is greater than 10 percent. It is noteworthy that all three of these diseases have somewhat different aberrations of the immune system. Furthermore, strong evidence for some, perhaps immunologic, anticancer surveillance system comes from spontaneous regression of human cancers. There are numerous documented cases of disappearance of histologically proven cancer, and postmortem examination of infantile accident victims under the age of three months revealed small in situ neuroblastomas 40 times as frequently as would have been expected from the incidence of clinically overt neuroblastoma. That the immunologic system is a primary component responsible for the normal regression of tumors is suggested by the direct correlation between clinical survival and the magnitude of lymphocytic infiltration of the tumor.

Arguments against Immunologic Surveillance Several workers, most notably Prehn and Fidler, have argued, not against the existence of immunologic surveillance, but against its playing the central role in the host's defense against cancer. Indeed, were the immunologic system of paramount importance, we might expect the incidence of neoplasia, in the face of immunosuppression or immunologic deficiency disease, to be even higher than the observed 5 to 10 percent. For surveillance to be effective, all tumors must be antigenic; yet many tumors, especially those that arise spontaneously, appear to lack TSTA. It might be argued that these tumors had simply lost their antigens under the pressure of in vivo immunoselection, but similar tumors arising in the absence of immunoselection, either in vitro or in immunosuppressed animals, are likewise nonantigenic. On the other hand, the immune system is often incapable of eliminating incipient neoplasms even when they are composed of highly antigenic cells.

Prehn and his co-workers suggest that the host's principal defenses against cancer are nonimmunologic factors inherent in the normal tissue milieu itself. They noted that chemically induced murine skin papillomas routinely underwent spontaneous regression. When skin containing a papilloma was grafted onto a highly immunosuppressed allogeneic mouse, although the normal component of the incompatible skin survived, the papilloma regressed. Other experiments showed that premalignant, hyperplastic mammary nodules grew to a certain size and then were restrained both from further growth and from turning into carcinomas. This was in spite of the fact that these nodules had elicited no detectable immune response.

IMMUNOSTIMULATION. The most significant blow to the theoretical role of immunologic surveillance, however, comes from the evidence that immune lymphocytes can, under certain circumstances, stimulate the tumor's growth rather than mediate its destruction. The effect can be demonstrated both in vivo and in vitro and is specific in that the stimulating lymphocytes must be obtained from animals immunized against the specific tumor. Immunostimulation, unlike the cytotoxic reactions discussed below, is seen at low lymphocyte:tumor cell ratios, the very condition expected during the incipient phase of a cell-mediated immune response to a tumor. These observations relate principally to the emergence of the primary tumor, while Fidler has shown that the coating of circulating tumor cells with immune lymphocytes may be a significant factor that enables these cells to form metastatic deposits. Thus, the immune lymphocyte, in a number of ways, may function more as an ally than as a foe of the emerging and invading tumor mass.

Components of the Host's Immune Response to Neoplasia   Regardless of its role in preventing the emergence of tumors, the immune system is able to mount a response against neoplastic tissue, and this response seems to pervade the entire immunologic orchestra (Fig. 23-1).

CELL-MEDIATED IMMUNE RESPONSES.   Transfer of lymphoid cells from an animal immunized against a tumor to a second unimmunized animal protects the latter against challenge with the tumor. Similar transfer of serum, however, except in some cases of experimental leukemia, affords no such protection. Such passive transfer experiments are responsible for the tumor immunologist's focus on cell-mediated mechanisms. Within the cell-mediated system the immune lymphocyte has drawn the most attention, and it manifests its antitumor effects in a number of ways.

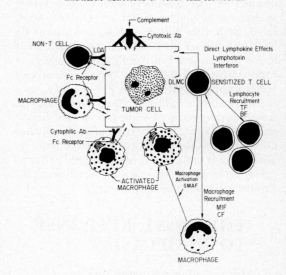

FIG. 23-1. Immunologic mechanisms of tumor cell destruction. DLMC = direct lymphocyte-mediated cytotoxicity. TF = transfer factor. BF = blastogenic factor. MIF = migration inhibition factor. CF = chemotactic factor. LDA = lymphocyte-dependent antibody.

Direct Lymphocyte-mediated Cytotoxicity. DLMC implies a mechanism whereby the immune lymphocyte destroys or inhibits the multiplication of tumor cells by direct contact and without the participation of humoral substances or secondary effector cells. DLMC has been studied in two different in vitro assay systems, each of which seems to detect a different type of DLMC reaction. In one, tumor cells are radiolabeled with chromium[51] and then incubated with immune lymphocytes, and cytotoxicity is measured by the release of isotope. The reaction proceeds rapidly: Cytotoxicity is detectable in less than six hours. In most studies the effector cell has been a radioresistant T lymphocyte that becomes undetectable in the tumor-bearing host shortly after tumor removal. This type of rapid DLMC has been demonstrated only in experimental tumor systems, especially with tumor allografts, however, and there is some question whether it is of importance in man.

In the second assay system, developed primarily by the Hellströms, tumor cells are allowed to adhere to plastic culture vessels and are then incubated for 40 to 72 hours with immune lymphocytes. Immune reactivity is manifested by a detachment of the tumor cells from the plastic and by a decreased proliferation of those tumor cells that do remain adherent. This long-term assay system has been used to demonstrate DLMC against both experimental and human tumors. This type of effector cell persists in the host long after tumor excision, and there is at present no agreement on whether it resides in the T or non-T cell population. This slow-acting DLMC has been detected in patients with almost every type of human neoplasm. Of additional interest was the observation that histologically similar tumors from different individuals cross-reacted. For example, lymphocytes from a patient with a breast carcinoma were cytotoxic to the patient's own tumor cells and to cells from other patients' breast carcinomas but not to colon, brain, or lung tumor cells. It was initially felt that this cross-reactivity was due to a common viral etiology, but it seems unlikely that each histologic tumor type would be induced by a different virus. Recently, Levy has observed cross-reactivity among melanoma, glioblastoma, and normal fetal glial cells. Melanoma and glioblastoma are quite distinct histologically but do share a common embryonic origin in the neural crest.

It thus seems possible that at least some of the cross-reactions detected by DLMC are based on reactivity to recapitulated embryonic antigens.

Lymphokines. Immune lymphocytes not only manifest direct cytotoxicity for tumor cells but also have the capacity, especially T cells, to secrete substances called "lymphokines." Some, such as lymphotoxin, proliferation inhibition factor, and interferon, themselves exert inhibitory effects on the tumor cell. It should be emphasized, however, that the antitumor activity of such lymphokines has been demonstrated only in vitro and that their significance in the host's defense against neoplasia is uncertain. Other lymphokines, such as transfer factor and blastogenic factor, may stimulate noncommitted lymphoid cells to enter the immune attack on the neoplasm. The final class of lymphokines, most notably macrophage migration inhibition factor and monocyte chemotactic factor, amplify the antitumor response by recruiting and activating potent nonlymphoid effector cells. This group of lymphokines is the only one for which a significant in vivo antitumor role has been demonstrated, and there is considerable evidence that the primary function of the immune lymphocyte is not its direct cytotoxic effect but rather its capacity to focus the attack by secondary effector cells, principally macrophages. Indeed, recent studies have shown that some tumors elaborate low-molecular-weight substances that block monocyte chemotaxis and may provide an important mechanism whereby tumors escape immune destruction.

Macrophages. Macrophages themselves may exhibit either specific or nonspecific antitumor effects. As with DLMC, direct contact between the effector and target cells is required, but the activated macrophage cannot divide and, unlike the cytotoxic lymphocyte, seems able to kill only once. Thus, to be effective against an established tumor, a massive macrophage infiltration may be required. Macrophages may acquire cytotoxic or cytostatic activity specific for a particular tumor in several ways. Tumor-specific cytophilic antibody may bind to the macrophage through the cell's receptor for the Fc portion of the antibody molecule. A subsequent combination of the antibody with the tumor cell will activate the cytolytic potential of the bound macrophage. Cytophilic antibody has been found in both the IgG and IgM classes, and some evidence exists that macrophages may themselves secrete material with cytophilic antibody activity. A second, and perhaps more important, mode of specific macrophage activation is mediated by a substance released from immune T lymphocytes that is called "specific macrophage activating factor" (SMAF). This substance possesses a moiety cytophilic for macrophages as well as a recognition site for the specific tumor cell. SMAF appears to consist of at least two components, one with a molecular weight greater than 300,000, the other with a molecular weight between 50,000 and 60,000. There is some speculation that SMAF is the specific T cell receptor shed during the interaction of immune T cells and the tumor.

Macrophages from animals immune to certain microorganisms, most notably mycobacteria and certain fungi and protozoa, acquire nonspecific cytolytic activity when incubated in vitro with the organisms alone. Similar nonspecific activity may be elicited by certain lymphokines and various substances, such as endotoxin and poly I · poly C. Of particular interest is the observation that such macrophages, though activated against no specific tumor type, are cytotoxic only to neoplastic cells and not to their normal analogs.

HUMORAL IMMUNE RESPONSES. Like the cell-mediated component, the antibody-mediated portion of the tumor-directed immune response has several facets.

Cytotoxic Antibody. Cytotoxic antibody binds to cell surface determinants, and the resultant antigen-antibody complex activates the complement sequence, the terminal components of which are lytic to the cell. Most studies argue, however, that although cytotoxic antibody may be demonstrable in vitro, it is of little importance to the host's defense against neoplasia, particularly against solid tumors. This may be explained, in part, by observations made in vitro that cytotoxic antibody is relatively ineffective when assayed with homologous complement.

Lymphocyte-dependent Antibody (LDA). LDA is another manifestation of the humoral antitumor response. Tumor cells treated with LDA are susceptible to lysis by normal, nonimmune lymphocytes. These lymphocytes, which are non-T cells, acquire their cytotoxic activity by binding to the tumor cell-antibody complex by receptors that interact with the Fc region of the antibody molecule. This is quite distinct from direct lymphocyte-mediated cytotoxicity, which requires immune lymphocytes, and cytotoxic antibody, which requires complement. Of particular interest is that only a minute amount of LDA is necessary to render a cell susceptible to lysis. While the in vivo significance of LDA is unknown, it does represent a potentially important component of the antitumor immune response.

Enhancement. Certain humoral components appear to be antagonists of the tumor-directed immune response. In 1907, Flexner and Jobling noted that the growth of a transplantable rat sarcoma was augmented if the recipient had been injected several days before with heat-killed sarcoma cells. Kaliss, Snell, and their co-workers gave some definition to this phenomenon, called "enhancement," when they showed that the potential for augmented growth could be transferred with specific isoantiserum. In the mid 1960s the Hellströms presented what they felt was an in vitro analog of enhancement. They had noted that tumor patients had circulating lymphocytes with in vitro cytotoxic activity against their tumor cells. Such lymphocytes were present whether the patients had been cured of their tumor or had active, progressive disease. Patients with progressive tumors, however, had in their serum blocking factors that could specifically inhibit the cytotoxic activity of their immune lymphocytes. Since clinical studies associated the presence of blocking factors with rapid tumor growth and a poor prognosis, it was postulated that in vivo enhancement was caused by the abrogation of host defenses by blocking factors.

The precise nature of in vitro blocking factors and their relation to in vivo enhancement, however, remains uncertain. Various studies have suggested that blocking can be mediated by soluble tumor antigen, antitumor antibody, or complexes of the two. Since enhancement is an in vivo phenomenon, it has been more difficult to pinpoint the active moieties, but two observations made it unlikely that enhancement and blocking are uniformly mediated by identical factors. First, in some systems enhancement can be produced by minute doses of antiserum, while in vitro blocking always requires large amounts of relatively undiluted serum. Second, sera with in vivo enhancing activity frequently lack in vitro blocking activity, and vice versa.

Moreover, the mechanisms of blocking factor and enhancement seem dissimilar. The former acts on lymphocytes already immune to the tumor, presumably by binding to the tumor cell itself and either competing with the lymphocyte for surface determinants or causing an alteration or disappearance of these determinants. Alternatively, it may interact with the tumor cell and generate another substance inhibitory to the immune lymphocyte. Enhancement may also use such mechanisms, but its primary mode of action seems to be one of preventing the development of immune lymphoid cells rather than of blocking those cells that are already immune.

Just as patients with progressively growing tumors frequently have serum blocking factors, so the Hellströms reported that some patients who had been cured of their tumors had in their serum unblocking factor that could counteract the in vitro effects of blocking factor. Fascinating was their additional observation that normal blacks frequently had serum unblocking factor specific for melanoma, a tumor of the body's pigment-producing cells. Although the concept of unblocking factor is interesting and its potential as a clinical tool great, it has yet to be confirmed.

FETAL ANTIGENS AND IMMUNODIAGNOSIS

Carcinoembryonic Antigen

Gold and Freedman raised a rabbit xenoantiserum against pooled perchloric acid extracts from several human carcinomas. After the antiserum had been absorbed with normal colon tissue, it formed a single precipitin line with extracts from other colon carcinomas. Subsequent studies showed this antiserum to be reactive with a common determinant on all adenocarcinomas of the entodermally derived digestive system epithelium, as well as fetal gut and gut-derived tissues. This determinant, called "carcinoembryonic antigen" (CEA) is a glycoprotein with a molecular weight of 200,000 to 300,000 daltons that consists of 50 to 70 percent carbohydrate. Unlike TSTA, CEA is not an integral component of the cell membrane but rather is loosely carried in the mucinous coating of the cell. Similarly, unlike TSTA, it elicits no immune response in man.

CEA was detected in the serum of several patients with colon cancer, and sensitive radioimmunoassays for serum CEA were therefore developed in the hope that such tests would provide a simple diagnostic screening procedure for early gut cancers. Unfortunately, these hopes were not realized for two major reasons (Table 23-1). A large percentage of normal individuals and patients with nonneo-

TABLE 23-1 OCCURRENCE OF ELEVATED SERUM CEA LEVELS IN VARIOUS CLINICAL STATES

Diagnosis	Percent with Elevated CEA*
Colonic carcinoma	
Localized to bowel wall	19†
Extended to pericolic tissues	53†
Distant metastases	100†
Pancreatic carcinoma	92†
Breast carcinoma	52†
Leukemia	22†
Ulcerative colitis	30‡
Pulmonary emphysema	57‡
Alcoholic cirrhosis	70‡
Normal nonsmoker	3‡
Normal smoker	19‡

Upper limit of normal: 2.5 ng/ml
†*From Zamcheck: Adv Intern Med 19:413, 1974*
‡*From Terry et al: Transplant Rev 20:100, 1974*

plastic diseases have circulating CEA, often at higher levels than tumor patients. More importantly, patients with colonic neoplasms localized to the bowel wall, and thus the ideal target for an early detection system, usually had undetectable CEA levels. Despite these problems, CEA does seem to be the best preoperative diagnostic procedure for pancreatic carcinoma, a lesion for which radiographic techniques are notoriously ineffective. Pancreatitis has produced false-positive results but only in alcoholics. The most significant use for CEA assays, however, is in the postoperative follow-up of cancer patients. Serial determinations showing a rising CEA level have proven to be a very ominous prognostic sign and have frequently preceded the clinical or radiographic indicators of tumor recurrence.

Alpha-1-fetoprotein

Alpha-1-fetoprotein (AFP) is an alpha-globulin secreted by normal embryonic hepatocytes. In the first trimester of fetal life it comprises 90 percent of the total serum globulin. By birth, its level has fallen to 1 to 5 mg/100 ml, and thereafter its concentration decreases by about 50 percent every three days. AFP is a glycoprotein with a molecular weight of 70,000. Unlike CEA, it contains only 4 percent carbohydrate and is not a cell surface antigen but rather is secreted by the cell. Like CEA, however, it is not immunogenic in the homologous species.

The arbitrary normal limit of serum AFP in an individual over 1 year of age is 40 ng/ml. Over 70 percent of patients with hepatic carcinoma have elevated AFP levels, and over half of these have levels above 3,000 ng/ml. About 40 percent of patients with embryonal carcinoma, 20 percent with pancreatic carcinoma, and 5 to 10 percent with hepatic metastases of nonhepatic bowel cancers also have elevated AFP, but their levels are almost always less than 3,000 ng/ml. About 25 percent of patients with active cirrhosis or acute viral hepatitis have AFP levels of 40 to 500 ng/ml, but, unlike CEA, AFP is almost never elevated in patients with other nonneoplastic diseases or normal controls.

There are two useful exceptions to this rule, however. Complications of pregnancy that allow fetomaternal protein transfer, such as placental infarction, or high-risk pregnancies, especially those associated with Rh incompatibility or maternal diabetes, are frequently associated with elevated maternal AFP levels. Secondly, all patients with ataxia telangiectasia have elevated AFP, suggesting that they have abnormal liver as well as thymus development, and leading to the hypothesis that their primary defect is in the differentiation of tissues that require the interaction of entodermal and mesodermal germ lines.

Other fetal antigens with properties similar to CEA or AFP have been associated with gastric and uterine neoplasms.

IMMUNOTHERAPY AND IMMUNOPROPHYLAXIS

Adoptive Transfer

Lymphocytes Transfer of immune lymphocytes has been shown to protect animals against tumor challenge, and, therefore, attempts have been made to immunize two tumor patients each against the other's tumor and then transfer immune lymphocytes between the two patients. Similar transfers have been made from cured patients to patients with progressively growing tumors. No significant antitumor effects have been seen. The transferred lymphocytes, since they were allogeneic, elicited an immune response against their own histocompatibility antigens and were rejected by the recipient or, in some cases where the recipient was anergic, induced a GvH reaction. Transfers between identical twins, where these complications could be obviated, have also failed, however. Adoptive transfer between inbred animals had generally been effective only against tumor challenges of 10^5 to, at very best, 10^7 cells. Since a gram of tumor contains approximately 10^9 cells, the failure in man of adoptive transfer of immune lymphocytes is hardly surprising.

Two other approaches have used syngeneic or autogenous lymphocytes. In one, lymphocytes were activated in vitro by exposure to mitogens, such as phytohemagglutinin (PHA), and reinjected. This procedure has induced regressions of some small tumor deposits and slight decreases in the size of pulmonary metastases but no long-term cures. In the other, the patient's own lymphocytes have been exposed in vitro to autogenous or allogeneic tumor cells in hopes of overcoming a hypothetical in vivo block to sensitization. Reinjection of such cells has had little or no therapeutic effect.

Antibody Injection of hyperimmune antiserum has afforded protection against some tumors, most notably murine leukemia, but attempts at serum therapy in man have been uniformly unsuccessful. Antibody may be useful, however, as a vehicle to transport tumoricidal agents to the neoplasm. Toxins, such as glucose oxidase, diphtheria toxin, and ricin, and high-energy isotopes, such as ^{131}I, have been conjugated to tumor-specific antibody and injected into animals. Some localization of the agents has been achieved, but no significant therapeutic effects have yet been seen.

Active Nonspecific Immunotherapy

Bacille Calmette-Guérin (BCG) It had long been known that injection of animals with certain bacteria or bacterial products could augment the immune response and occasionally induce tumor regression. Thus, the therapeutic effects of injecting live bovine tubercle bacilli (BCG) were tested on a guinea pig hepatoma by Zbar and Rapp and on human melanoma by Morton. In both cases significant tumoricidal effects were seen. Several requirements for a positive effect were noted. The recipient had to develop skin test reactivity to the tubercle bacillus, direct contact between the injected BCG and the tumor was essential, and direct intratumor injection of the agent was the best mode of administration. It was noted, however, that after intratumor injection, uninjected lesions also frequently regressed. The tumor must itself be immunogenic, and the tumor burden small. Over 80 percent of guinea pigs with tumors weighing less than 100 mg, but only 20 percent of those with 500 mg tumors, could be cured with intratumor BCG. In animals, the therapeutic effect seems to be directly proportional to the number of live BCG organisms injected, but this has not yet been convincingly shown in man. Nonviable organisms are clearly ineffective, although Ribi has found that isolated BCG cell walls conjugated to oil droplets retained therapeutic activity. The best method of culturing the bacillus and the most effective strain are currently being debated.

BCG is the only immunotherapeutic agent that has shown convincing therapeutic effects in man. In 25 percent of patients who have had a postoperative recurrence of melanoma and, thus, a very dismal long-term prognosis, intratumor BCG has induced total regression of all clinical disease. When those patients whose recurrences were localized to the skin, subcutaneous tissue, and local lymph nodes were considered separately, the success rate climbed to between 40 and 75 percent. Since these studies have continued on a large scale for no more than four years and since melanoma is itself a very unpredictable tumor, optimism for BCG therapy must still be tempered with caution. It is also clear that BCG is totally ineffective against metastatic melanoma of the bone, brain, or viscera. Indeed, such disease may actually be worsened by BCG, perhaps through the induction of enhancement.

BCG has also been part of an immunotherapeutic regimen that, when given with chemotherapy, has induced more frequent and longer remissions of acute myelogenous leukemia (AML) than has chemotherapy alone. The BCG was administered by multiple subcutaneous injections. Since the immunotherapy also included the injection of irradiated allogeneic tumor cells, however, the effects of BCG alone cannot be assessed. BCG has also been combined with intensive chemotherapy and radiotherapy in acute lymphocytic leukemia and does seem to have increased the remission rate and duration, although the studies have not been as well controlled as those with AML.

Recent studies have attempted to expand the use of BCG. It has been given to animals, both by aerosol and intravenously, in an effort to treat metastatic lesions but so far with only minor therapeutic effect. In man, several trials are now underway to determine whether BCG given immediately before or after surgical excision of various tumors, especially melanoma, will decrease the incidence of recurrence. No significant data are yet available on these studies.

The mechanism of BCG action is unclear. It has been thought to activate lymphocytes immune to the bacillus and thus stimulate these lymphocytes to recruit nonspecifically and activate macrophages, which then presumably exert the primary antitumor effect. BCG may also activate the macrophages directly. Recent studies have shown, however, that the

BCG organism is antigenically cross-reactive with both the guinea pig hepatoma and human melanoma. It is thus possible that some of the effects of BCG are due to activation of immune components specific for the tumor itself.

Corynebacterium parvum   This is another bacterium that is capable of stimulating a vigorous cellular immune response. It has been used intralesionally in studies similar to those with BCG and appears to induce lymphocytes and activated macrophages and to exert effects against experimental tumors comparable to those of BCG. When given parenterally, however, it exerts paradoxical effects, producing activated macrophages but depressed general T cell function. The latter effect appears to be due to a stimulation of the spleen, which then sequesters T cells. The major advantage of *C. parvum* over BCG is that nonviable organisms are employed, thus obviating the generalized infection occasionally induced by BCG. Its proponents have remarked that the ideal role for *C. parvum* may be as an adjunct to chemotherapy, since, in animal studies, it both augments the drugs' antitumor effects and, perhaps more importantly, diminishes their toxic side effects. Its use in man has been too brief to evaluate, but it does seem to be without major harmful side effects.

Dinitrochlorobenzene   (DNCB)   Patients with superficial tumors, mostly skin cancers, have been sensitized to DNCB, and, a few weeks later, their tumors were painted with the agent. A vigorous cellular immune response was generated in and around the tumor, often leading to complete regression of the neoplasm.

Tumor Necrosis Factor   This agent has only recently been described, but it seems potentially important. Normal tumor-free mice were injected with BCG and two weeks later were injected with endotoxin. One or two days later they were bled, and the serum was injected intraperitoneally into animals with various types of established tumors. Within a few days the tumors became necrotic and soon regressed. Furthermore, in vitro their serum was toxic to neoplastic but not normal cells. The factor was not immunoglobulin; it was sensitive to proteases but heat stable. Little more is known about its chemical nature or its mode of action.

Active Specific Immunotherapy

Immunization with Tumor Cells   Several attempts have been made to induce tumor regression by immunization with autogenous or allogeneic tumor cells. Recently, such procedures have been combined with other immunotherapeutic modalities, such as BCG, with some early encouraging results, especially in leukemia, but it is impossible to assess whether the immunization component was itself useful. In those earlier studies where immunization was employed alone, no clinical benefits were realized.

Immunization with Modified Tumor Cells or Antigens   It has been noted above that the tumor-directed immune response is an aggregate of many types of biologic activities, some protective of the host and some deleterious. The nonspecific immunotherapeutic modalities or immunizations with unmodified tumor cells may thus induce both helpful and harmful responses without any apparent control over which will predominate. The inconsistent clinical results may well reflect variations in the net effect of the different components of the immune response. Effective immunotherapy must, therefore, operate with two levels of specificity. It must stimulate a tumor-directed immune response, but, equally important, it must control the type of immune response evoked.

Several workers have attempted to modify the tumor cell so as to render it a more active inducer of a host-protective immune response. Immunization with neuraminidase-treated tumor cells has induced regression of established tumors in several experimental systems where similar immunization with untreated cells had no effect. In man the use of neuraminidase-treated tumor cells has usually been part of a combined immunotherapy protocol, and it has, therefore, not been possible to assess directly its isolated effects. The effect of neuraminidase has generally been ascribed to its unmasking of cryptic antigens, thus rendering the cell more immunologic, but recent studies have shown that neuraminidase-treated cells bind, and thus presumably induce, different classes and subclasses of tumor-directed antibody from those induced by untreated cells. The effect of neuraminidase may thus not be simply to increase immunogenicity but to direct it toward the induction of protective immune responses.

Several nonenzymatic agents have also been used to modify tumor cells. Small haptens, such as dinitrophenol and iodoacetamide, have been bound covalently to tumor cell surfaces and have increased the protective immunogenicity of various experimental tumors. Tumor cells have also been infected with various viruses in order to induce new viral antigens or modify preexisting antigens on the cell surface. In other studies, immunization with hypotonically lysed tumor cells has induced in vivo enhancement and the appearance in the serum of in vitro blocking factors. When the lysed cells were conjugated to lipid prior to injection, however, they induced protective immunity and no serum blocking factors.

A most exciting prospect for immunotherapy

MULTIPLE ANTIGENS OF HUMAN GLIOMAS AND MELANOMAS

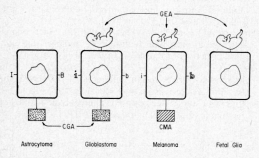

FIG. 23-2. Multiple tumor-associated antigens on the surface of human neoplasms. Both anaplastic (glioblastoma) and well-differentiated (astrocytoma) tumors of glial cell origin, but no other normal or neoplastic cells, bear a common glioma antigen (CGA). Similarly, melanomas share a common melanoma antigen (CMA). A glioembryonic antigen (GEA) is found on fetal glial cells and is recapitulated on melanomas and anaplastic gliomas because of the common origin of the glial cell and melanocyte from the embryonic neural crest. Such embryonic antigens are not recapitulated on well-differentiated tumors. CGA, CMA, and GEA induce cell-mediated but not blocking antibody responses. Each tumor type, however, does bear blocking determinants, designated by the letter B, which induce blocking antibody but not cell-mediated responses. Finally, each patient's tumor bears individual specific determinants designated by the letter I, which are found on no other tumors, even those of the same histologic type.

has emerged from the recent observation that there are several different tumor-associated antigenic determinants on a single tumor cell (Fig. 23-2). Some of these determinants do seem to induce protective immunity, others evoke responses measurable in vitro but not in vivo, and still others seem to be associated with in vitro blocking and, perhaps, in vivo enhancement. Current efforts are directed at isolating, from preparations of soluble tumor-associated antigens, those specific antigens that induce only protective immune responses. Such an antigen would provide an ideal immunotherapeutic or immunoprophylactic agent.

Transfer Factor and Xenogeneic Immune RNA A dialyzable substance extracted from the lymphocytes of donors sensitive to tuberculin has been used to transfer tuberculin sensitivity to unsensitized individuals. Similar transfer of immunity to other antigens has also been demonstrated. The mechanism of action of transfer factor (TF) remains obscure, but it has been proposed that TF is a derepressor of lymphocytes precommitted to the specific antigen. Of particular interest to the tumor immunotherapist, however, is the fact that TF induces only a cell-mediated immune response. Tumor-directed TF might thus be an ideal immunotherapeutic agent, since it would induce no humoral blocking factors and would confine its effects to that component of the immune response that is most often associated with host protection against tumor challenge.

Several clinical trials of TF antitumor therapy have been launched, particularly in patients with melanoma, sarcoma, and acute leukemia. It seems that TF may be administered in large doses without untoward side effects. Of particular note, there have been no reports of accelerated tumor growth in patients receiving TF. This is in contrast to some of the other immunotherapeutic modalities. Likewise, many of the recipients did develop cell-mediated tumor-directed immunity as measured by various in vitro assays. Clinical effects of TF have been less impressive, however. Although there have been anecdotal reports of tumor regression associated with TF therapy, most TF recipients have shown no significant clinical improvement. This may be partly because most TF recipients had extensive disease that may have been unassailable even by a maximally stimulated immune system. A major problem, and perhaps the major reason for TF treatment failure, has been that of obtaining a source of appropriate TF itself. Since the transfer factor phenomenon has been convincingly demonstrated only in man, all TF must be obtained from human donors. The problem has been selecting the proper donor, that is, someone with known immunity to the tumor.

A significant recent advance in TF research is the observation that TF adheres to cross-linked dextrans and thus may be considerably purified by adsorption chromatography on Sephadex G-25. This finding will facilitate studies on the chemical nature of TF and allow standardization of TF doses for clinical trials.

Various studies had shown that RNA extracted from immune macrophages or lymphocytes could transfer sensitivity to nonimmune lymphoid cells. Recent studies have attempted to apply this phenomenon to tumor immunotherapy. Animals, generally sheep, were immunized with human tumor cells. RNA was then extracted from the lymph nodes and spleen of the immunized animals. In vitro incubation with this RNA endowed normal, nonimmune human lymphocytes with in vitro cytotoxic activity against the immunizing tumor cells. The tumor specificity of this immunization transfer remains to be proven, however. Superficially, immune RNA and TF seem to be quite similar. The RNA, however, is nondialyzable, sensitive to ribonuclease, and, of course, not species specific. Most importantly, animal studies have shown that immune RNA, unlike TF, induces both humoral and cellular immunity. Immune RNA has been injected into a limited number of tumor patients. It has induced no serious untoward effects, but its clinical usefulness has not yet been assessed.

FURTHER READING

Books and Reviews

Cerottini JC, Brunner KT: Cell-mediated cytotoxicity, allograft rejection, and tumor immunity. Adv Immunol 18: 67, 1974.

Hellström KE, Hellström I: Lymphocyte-mediated cytotoxicity and blocking serum activity to tumor antigens. Adv Immunol 18:209, 1974.

Herberman RB, Gaylord CE (eds): Conference and workshop on cellular immune reactions to human tumor-associated antigens. Natl Cancer Inst Monograph 1973, vol 37

Möller G (ed): Tumor associated embryonic antigens. Transplant Rev 20:1, 1974

Prehn RT: Immunological surveillance: Pro and con. In Bach FH, Good RA (eds): Clinical Immunobiology. New York, Academic Press, 1974, vol 2, 191-203

Proceedings of the American Cancer Society and National Cancer Institute National Conference on Virology and Immunology in Human Cancer. Cancer 34:1343, 1974

Smith RT, Landy M (eds): Immune Surveillance. New York, Academic Press, 1970

Selected Papers

Cole WH: Spontaneous regression of cancer: The metabolic triumph of the host? Ann NY Acad Sci 230:111, 1974

Fauve RM, Hevin B, Jacob H, Gaillard JA, Jacob F: Antiinflammatory effects of murine malignant cells. Proc Natl Acad Sci USA 71:4052, 1974

Fidler IJ: In vitro studies of cellular-mediated immunostimulation of tumor growth. J Natl Cancer Inst 50:1307, 1973

Folkman J: Tumor angiogenesis: A possible control point in tumor growth. Ann Intern Med 82:96, 1975

Kim U, Baumler A, Carruthers C, Bielat K: Immunological escape mechanism in spontaneously metastasizing mammary tumors. Proc Natl Acad Sci USA 72:1012, 1975

Klein G, Klein E: Are methylcholanthrene-induced sarcoma-associated, rejection-inducing (TSTA) antigens, modified forms of H-2 or linked determinants? Int J Cancer 15:879, 1975

Piessens WF, Churchill WH Jr, David JR: Macrophages activated in vitro with lymphocyte mediators kill neoplastic but not normal cells. J Immunol 114:293, 1975

Plescia OJ, Smith AH, Grinwich K: Subversion of the immune system by tumor cells and role of prostaglandins. Proc Natl Acad Sci USA 72:1848, 1975

Stutman O: Tumor development after polyoma infection in athymic nude mice. J Immunol 114:1213, 1975

SECTION 3
MEDICAL BACTERIOLOGY

24
Host-Parasite Relationships

Infectious disease is the result of an unsuccessful relationship between parasite and host. It is the summation of the vectors of both agents and ranges in severity from human rabies, which is almost invariably fatal, to the common cold, which is almost invariably nonfatal. The most successful human host–parasite relationships, our own microbial flora, are only now being fully appreciated. Indeed with the development of public health services, vaccines, antibiotics, and improved nutrition, it is man's inability to control his own microbial flora that has become one of the most significant components of infectious diseases. Although there are many general principles regarding host defense mechanisms and determinants of microbial pathogenicity, each specific patient and each specific pathogen must be carefully studied for clues as to why that specific combination produced a particular illness. In many instances, however, the specific reasons why a particular individual is infected at a specific time resulting in a given clinical picture are not clearly discernible. New problems have been introduced as a result of therapeutic discoveries in fields of medicine outside of infectious diseases, which have resulted in a partially compromised host susceptible to the resulting infectious diseases of medical progress. This chapter discusses the various host factors that may modify infection, the compromised host, clinical manifestations of infectious diseases, and those attributes of a parasite that permit it to produce disease.

THE HOST

To a considerable extent chance plays a role in any infectious disease. An individual must be at the wrong place at the wrong time—in the center of a typhoid epidemic, living with someone who has active tuberculosis, being bitten by a tick infected with rickettsiae, or using a blanket previously used by a patient with smallpox. What then ensues depends upon a number of host factors. All infectious diseases begin at the surface of the host, with the exception of certain intrauterine transmitted infections. The first barrier, therefore, is the gross surface area, and the intact skin presents a remarkably effective barrier to infection. The spraying of a suspension of bacteria on the skin usually produces no untoward effect. The simple drying effect of skin is sufficient to elimi-

nate most bacteria, and the fatty acids on the surface layers and the skin pH exert an antibacterial effect. The infection of volunteers with intradermal injections of virulent bacteria may require up to 5 to 10 million organisms. There are exceptions, however, such as *Francisella tularensis*, which in human volunteers requires very small numbers of bacteria to produce infection. Any break in the integrity of the skin will, of course, remove the physical barrier. A burn or drug-related exfoliative dermatitis is a notorious setting in which infection can take place. Introducing a foreign body, such as a suture or an indwelling intravenous needle or an intravenous plastic catheter, into the skin can provide a nidus for initiation of infection.

The gastrointestinal surface is protected to a great extent by the acid in the stomach which is inimical to most microbial forms of life. This acid condition, however, can be modified by the ingestion of food or other substances that neutralize the acid. Indeed, the normally unfavorable environment can be overcome by sheer numbers of microorganisms. Production of disease by feeding volunteers salmonella by mouth requires at least a million organisms. However, patients who have had surgical removal of parts of their stomach may have partial or complete achlorhydria resulting in increased susceptibility to infection. Another important feature of the gastrointestinal surface is the fairly rapid motility of the gastrointestinal tract, resulting in bacteria's remaining in certain segments for a very short period of time before being expelled. In addition, the lower parts of the gastrointestinal tract have an enormous bacterial flora of their own that plays a competitive role in the establishment of an extraneous pathogenic organism.

The respiratory surface has as its physical protection a mucous coating that can entrap most microbial forms of life. This mucous coating is swept up from the respiratory tree by cilia where it is coughed and swallowed reflexly, thereby depositing the potentially infectious material into the sterilizing setting of the stomach. Finally, the surface of the urinary tract—the ureter, bladder, urethra—has as its protective barrier the simple flow of urine. Installation of organisms capable of causing urinary tract infections into the healthy bladder is followed by their prompt excretion in the urine with no untoward effects. Obstruction in any of these areas—the gastrointestinal tract, the respiratory tract, and the genitourinary tract—can alter these gross physical barriers in such a way that either resident microbial flora or invasive organisms can replicate and produce disease.

Once microbial forms of life breach these gross physical barriers, they meet an extremely hostile environment. At this point they encounter a very complex cellular response defined as inflammation. This response is as old as recorded history—*rubror et tumor cum calore et dolore*. It should be pointed out, however, that this response may be triggered by many events other than microbial invasion, with a clinical picture that is very difficult to differentiate from that of infection. In bacterial infections the first 20 minutes of the host response usually determines whether or not a given invading organism will produce disease. At the cellular level, one of the earliest cellular responses is that of the polymorphonuclear leukocyte. Chemotaxis, the attraction of phagocytic cells to the site of infection or tissue injury, is one of the earliest events in response to infection. Activation of proesterases is apparently the initial event triggered by a chemotactic factor. Both calcium and magnesium are required for a maximal chemotactic response. In the phagocytosis of the offending pathogen, a change occurs in the plasma membrane of the phagocytic cell resulting in invagination around the bacterial cell with subsequent fusion to produce a phagocytic vacuole. Biochemical changes within the leukocyte at the time of phagocytosis may kill the ingested organism. In addition, fusion of lysosomes with the phagocytic vacuole to produce a phagolysosome may result in digestion of the organism by the enzymatic contents of the lysosome.

In general, the antimicrobial systems of the polymorphonuclear leukocyte are of two types, the oxygen-dependent and the oxygen-independent systems. The oxygen-dependent systems can be further subdivided into (1) myeloperoxidase (MPO)-mediated systems, which, when combined with hydrogen peroxide and appropriate oxidizable cofactor (iodide, bromide, or chloride), have marked antimicrobial activity, and (2) myeloperoxidase-independent systems, which include the production of hydrogen peroxide, superoxide anion, hydroxyl radicals, and singlet oxygen. Oxygen-independent microbial systems include the acid pH within the phagocytic vacuole and the release of lysozyme, lactoferrin, and granular cationic proteins. Antimicrobial systems similar to this have been described in macrophage cell cultures. Complement possesses a dual role in the phagocytic process. Fission of fragments C3 and C5a generates chemotactic factors, and bound C3b has primarily the function of opsonization. This opsonic function is based on the ability of these fragments to bind bacteria or other microbial forms to sites that can specifically interact with receptors on the surface of phagocytic cells. The presence of preformed antibody to the invading agent tremendously improves the efficacy of phagocytosis. This preformed antibody may be from previous infection or from stimulation by a related but not necessarily microbiologic source of antigen.

In addition to the classical stimulation of specific antibody globulin, infection with most microbial forms generates a delayed type of hypersensitivity. We are just beginning to understand this type of host reaction and its role in the way infectious diseases present clinically. The study of patients with specific defects in this type of host response has demonstrated that delayed hypersensitivity may indeed be one of the major mechanisms of host defense against certain types of invading microorganisms. Specifically how this response interferes with the replication of microbes is not clear. Any event that interferes with the inflammatory sequence will obviously allow microbes to become established. These defects range from simple gross vascular insufficiency preventing adequate polymorphonuclear response to blatant leukopenia due either to natural disease or to the effects of drug therapy. With better understanding of the subcellular and biochemical changes in polymorphonuclear leukocytes it has been possible to define certain diseases, such as chronic granulomatous disease, a disease characterized by recurrent bacterial infections in childhood in which specific defects in the production of hydrogen peroxide by the polymorphonuclear leukocytes have been demonstrated. In addition defects in chemotaxis associated with repeated infections in childhood have been described.

Should the invading organism survive the immediate localizing effect of inflammation, the next barrier is the lymphatic system with its filtering lymph nodes with phagocytic capacity. Surviving this allows the organism to gain access to the bloodstream. Bacteremia (fungemia or viremia) signals a failure of local barriers and usually portends more significant illness. Another remarkably effective clearance mechanism, the reticuloendothelial system, is scattered throughout the body but concentrated in the liver and spleen. This system can phagocytose microorganisms with great efficiency. If, however, the number of invading organisms is too great or the organisms are too virulent, or if the system is not functioning, the pathway to metastic disease is open for involvement of the brain, heart, joints, and other organ sites.

The Compromised Host

Every patient with an infectious disease is to some extent a compromised host. In some instances we know enough about the defense mechanisms to pinpoint the area compromised, but in many instances we are unable to define the weakness. With continued observations of infectious diseases, however, it has been possible to define certain settings in which increased infection may be expected. Among the most common compromised hosts are the very young and the very old. Certain prevalent basic diseases, such as alcoholism and diabetes, are often associated with infection. Less commonly the uremic patient is a source of host–parasite problems. Natural diseases involving the hematopoietic system, Hodgkin's disease and other lymphomas, leukemias, and multiple myeloma, are notoriously associated with high attack rates of infections. Various solid tumors, such as carcinoma and sarcomas, also present problems with increased attack rates of infection. Inherited and acquired primary immunodeficiency diseases present problems. In addition to these basic diseases are superimposed conditions which in some respects are the diseases of medical progress. Physical barriers may be altered by the use of indwelling intravenous and urethral catheters. One can change the normal indigenous flora by the use of broad-spectrum antibiotics, thereby leaving a void to be filled by drug-resistant microorganisms, which in themselves have a low degree of pathogenicity but in the compromised host are capable of producing significant illness. Decrease in the total circulating pool of phagocytic cells can be caused by immunosuppression, cytotoxic chemotherapy of cancers, and irradiation. Recently, altered leukocyte responses, such as decreased migration, diminished phagocytosis, and de-

creased bactericidal capacity, have presented problems. Finally, interference with the classic immune globulin production or impairment of delayed hypersensitivity by therapy with steroids or cytotoxic drugs, irradiation, or anti-lymphocyte globulin can lead to infection. In the compromised host, one does not necessarily have problems with the usual pyogenic cocci. Instead, one may see organisms usually selected for by prior chemotherapy, such as *Pseudomonas* species, enterobacteria, and *Serratia*. Problems with viruses, such as cytomegalovirus, hepatitis virus, *Herpesvirus hominis*, and varicella-zoster virus, may be encountered. Fungi, an increasing problem in compromised hosts, range from such common contaminants as *Rhizopus* species to *Cryptococcus*. An increasing number of serious parasitic manifestations also have cropped up in this same setting.

CLINICAL MANIFESTATIONS OF INFECTIOUS DISEASES

Most infectious diseases are evaluated by obtaining a history from the patient, doing a complete physical examination, and then employing selected laboratory procedures. Fever is almost always an accompaniment of clinical infectious disease. It may be subtle or abrupt in its onset, and it may move with great speed or at a very slow tempo. It is usually the inflammatory response that brings the patient to the physician because of the attendant pain and failure to function. It is generally possible, by history and/or physical examination, to localize the site of infection. By virtue of the tempo and clinical appearance of the infection, a differentiation among the usual subdivisions of microbiology is made, ie, whether it is a bacterial, viral, fungal, or parasitic infection. The specific etiology of any given infectious disease, however, can be unequivocally proven only by demonstrating the infectious agent in smears and cultures and by demonstrating an appropriate antibody response. Because the number of antimicrobial drugs is so great and their spectrum so varied, the proper practice of infectious disease demands that some attempt be made to identify specifically the etiologic agent. X-rays may be use to define infectious diseases more precisely. Most infectious diseases of a bacterial nature stimulate the excessive production of polymorphonuclear leukocytes, and study of the peripheral blood for total circulating white cells and types of circulating white cells can provide additional information. Such nonspecific tests as the sedimentation rate and C-reactive protein are sometimes used to substantiate findings in an inflammatory process. The absence of an inflammatory response in terms of white cell count and sedimentation rate is sometimes used as supporting evidence for viral infections. The presence of increased numbers of circulating eosinophils may suggest parasitic infestation. Finally, most bacterial infectious diseases will respond in a resonably predictable way to an effective antimicrobial agent, thereby assisting in the final diagnosis.

THE PARASITE

Of the many thousands of known microorganisms, less than 300 have acquired the ability to produce disease in man and animals. A microorganism is classified as a pathogen if it has the ability to incite disease in susceptible animals. Virulence is a term used to designate the degree of pathogenicity of a given type of microorganism and of a specific strain. Virulence is measured by the number of organisms required to kill members of a particular animal species under standardized conditions. The term "communicability" may be defined as the ability of the organism to spread under natural conditions from animal to animal, man to man, or animal to man.

Most infectious diseases require that the parasitic agent replicate within the host or on the surface in order to initiate a disease process. This may vary from the limited replication of attenuated organisms, such as the live poliomyelitis vaccine or the BCG antituberculosis vaccine, to a fulminant, rapidly progressive, necrotizing cellulitis, such as the clostridial infection, gas gangrene. Some attributes of the offending microbe must permit that organism to replicate in an otherwise hostile environment of the human host. In some instances this mechanism is the only mechanism known for the explanation of clinical illness. In the realm of bacterial infectious diseases the surface antigens of the bacterial cell play a very important role in this initial survival. Examples of this are the surface antigens of *Streptococcus pneumoniae, Streptococcus pyogenes,* and *Bacillus anthracis.* These antigens interfere with phagocytosis, thus allowing the organisms to replicate within the human host. Indeed the development of specific antibodies to these surface antigens results in tremendously increased phagocytosis with the result that individuals with such circulating antibodies are completely resistant to clinical disease caused by the specific bacterium.

Toxins

Products released by invading microorganisms may either interfere with host defense mechanisms or damage host cells. Among the extracellular products are the exotoxins. These are heat-labile protein antigens usually found in culture filtrates of the organism. They are extremely toxic, can be toxoided and are neutralized by homologous antibody. The tetanus and diphtheria toxins are examples of bacterial exotoxins.

Some toxic products of certain bacteria are intimately associated with the bacterial cell and are separated from it only with difficulty. These are the endotoxins produced by gram-negative organisms. Endotoxins are antigenic complexes of protein, polysaccharide, and lipid derived from the cell wall. They are more stable to heat than are the exotoxins and are less toxic and less specific in their action. They do not form toxoids and are therefore not useful immunizing agents. Endotoxins elicit a variety of pharmacologic effects, the most important of which are related to their pyrogenicity, their ability to induce irreversible shock, and their effect on nonspecific immunity.

In addition to the classic exotoxins, a number of cytolytic toxins are produced by certain bacterial species. Most of these toxins are proteins, are found extracellularly, and induce formation of neutralizing antibodies. They are separated from the classic exotoxins, however, on the basis of their ability to cause in vitro physical dissolution of cell membranes. The streptolysin O produced by *S. pyogenes* and the α-toxin of *Staphylococcus aureus* are examples of cytolytic toxins that contribute to the virulence of the organism.

With both the cellular and extracellular products of bacteria, a wide spectrum of disease may result from the host-parasite interaction. Diseases may range from such localized infections as tetanus and diphtheria, which are accompanied by profound systemic intoxication resulting in death, to rapidly invasive infection with systemic spread of the organism and profound intoxication, as seen with *S. pyogenes* and *Clostridium perfringens.* Finally, we still encounter infectious diseases for which a specific pathogen is isolated but for which we have no clear-cut explanation of why that pathogen makes a patient sick. With some of these infections, increased attention is focused on the role of delayed sensitivity as a mechanism for producing cell injury. Such diseases as tuberculosis, mycotic infections, and many helminthic infections belong in this category.

FURTHER READING

Books and Reviews

Bellanti JA, Dayton DH (eds): The Phagocytic Cell in Host Resistance. New York, Raven Press, 1975

Cluff LE, Johnson JE: Clinical Concepts of Infectious Disease. Baltimore, Williams & Wilkins, 1972

Hoeprich PD (ed): Infectious Diseases. Hagerstown, Md, Harper & Row, 1972

Smith H, Pearce JH (eds): Microbial Pathogenicity in Man and Animals. Cambridge, Cambridge Univ Press, 1972

Selected Papers

Armstrong D, Young LS, Meyer RD, Blevins AH: Infectious complications of neoplastic disease. Med Clin North Am 55:729, 1971

Boggs DR: The kinetics of neutrophilic leukocytes in health and disease. Semin Hematol 4:359, 1967

Boggs DR, Frei E: Clinical studies of fever and infection in cancer. Cancer 13:1240, 1960

Douglas SD: Analytic review: disorders in phagocyte function. Blood 35:851, 1970

Frenkel JK: Role of corticosteroids as predisposing factors in fungal diseases. Lab Invest 11:1192, 1962

Gatti RA, Good RA: The immunological deficiency diseases. Med Clin North Am 54:281, 1970

Hart PD, Russell E Jr, Remington JS: The compromised host and infection. II. Deep fungal infection. J Infect Dis 120:169, 1969

Hill RB Jr, Rowlands DJ Jr, Rifkind D: Infectious pulmonary disease in patients receiving immunosuppressive therapy for organ transplantation. N Engl J Med 271: 1021, 1964

Jonston RB Jr, Lawton AR III, Cooper MD: Disorders of host defense against infection: Pathophysiologic and diagnostic considerations. Med Clin North Am 57:421, 1973

Lawrence HS: Transfer factor and cellular immune deficiency disease. New Engl J Med 283:411, 1970

Mankowski ZT, Littleton BJ: Action of cortisone and ACTH on experimental fungus infections. Antibio Chemother 4:253, 1954

Miles AA, Miles EM, Burke J: The value and duration of defense reactions of the skin to the primary lodgement of bacteria. Br J Exp Pathol 38:79 1957

Montgomerie JZ, Kalmanson GM, Guze LB: Renal failure and infection. Medicine 47:1, 1968

Rifkind D, Marchioro RL, Waddell WR, Starzl TE: Infectious diseases associated with renal homotransplantation. II. Differential diagnosis and management. JAMA 189:402, 1964

Silver RT: Infections, fever, and host resistance in neoplastic diseases. J Chronic Dis 16:677, 1963

Smith H: Biochemical challenge of microbial pathogenicity. Bacteriol Rev 32:164, 1968

Spain DM, Molomut N, Haber A: Studies of the cortisone effects on the inflammatory response. I. Alterations of the histopathology of chemically induced inflammation. J Lab Clin Med 39:383, 1952

25
Microbial Ecology and Normal Flora of the Human Body

Ecology is the study of the interactions between living organisms and their environment. Disease in man and animals caused by microorganisms is only a small segment of this constantly changing balance of forces. Microorganisms are ubiquitous. They are present under all conditions that permit the existence of any form of life and are constantly engaged in synthesizing new organic compounds and in breaking down to simpler elements the complex substances that compose plant and animal tissues. Here, as among the higher forms, there is a constant struggle for survival between individuals and species.

The complex relationship between the different microbial species may be classified as neutral, antagonistic, or synergistic. Few species are strictly neutral in their reactions because they interfere in a passive manner by utilizing the available food supply or excreting toxic materials with their waste products. The majority of microbial species exhibit positive antagonism arising from alterations in the physical environment or the elaboration of antibiotics and bacteriocins that are specifically inhibitory for certain organisms. These factors are important in both soil and water ecology and in animal ecology. Antagonism between the gram-positive cocci and gram-negative bacilli of the respiratory tract and their independent and mutual antagonism to fungi was not suspected until the clinical introduction of antibiotics. Following treatment with penicillin, for example, the normal flora (predominantly streptococci, *Neisseria*, and *Haemophilus* species) are replaced by gram-negative enteric bacilli or *Pseudomonas*. On the other hand, broader spectrum antibiosis (as achieved by chloramphenicol and tetracyclines or combinations of penicillins, cephalosporins, and aminoglycosides) may result in the emergence of resistant bacteria or overgrowth by *Candida* species.

Synergism may be described as a cooperative effort by two or more microbial species that produces a result that could not be achieved individually. This phenomenon may be relatively frequent in nature but is uncommon in disease states. Examples of the latter are the synergistic gangrene described by Meleney and some forms of anaerobic lung abscess caused by organisms that are ordinarily normal mouth flora (Chap. 48).

Various ecologic relationships exist between microorganisms and the human host with whom they are associated: commensalism, symbiosis, parasitism, or opportunism. Commensalism refers to the mutual but almost inconsequential association between bacteria and higher organisms. Symbiosis refers to a mutually beneficial relationship between two species. Parasitism refers to that complex spectrum of relationships whereby one organism derives benefits at the expense of another. These relationships were analyzed in a monograph by Theobald Smith in 1934. He stressed that the phenomenon of disease caused by infectious agents is largely a by-product of evolving parasitism, that is, violent reactions between host and parasite tend to lessen as parasitism approaches a biologic equilibrium. The rapid and destructive actions of some microorganisms are expressions of bungling parasitism. The skillful or well-adapted parasite enters its host with ease and may produce lesions only as a means of securing exit in order to infect a new host. In a sense, commensalism represents an ideal form of parasitism.

The terms "pathogen" and "opportunist" require definition. In general, a pathogen is a microorganism that is capable of infecting or parasitizing normal individuals. As medical science becomes more sophisticated we may find that no one is normal and that this terminology is artificial, but at present the terms are useful. Organisms, such as *Staphylococcus aureus*, *Streptococcus pyogenes*, and *Steptococcus pneumoniae*, among the bacteria, *Histoplasma capsulatum* and *Coccidioides immitis* among the fungi, and the plethora of common cold viruses and viruses that cause childhood diseases (measles, mumps, varicella, rubella), appear to represent bona fide pathogens in that their hosts are sufficiently large numbers of the general population who lack demonstrable underlying disease. On the other hand, such organisms as *Pseudomonas aeruginosa*, *Serratia marcescens*, *Candida albicans*, *Pneumocystis carinii*, and *Nocardia asteroides* uncommonly cause de novo disease but are almost always encountered under unusual circumstances, either in abnormal hosts or in situations where the normal flora has been supplanted. These factors relating to the pathogenic potential of various microorganisms will be discussed in the chapters that follow.

NATURAL HABITATS

The diversity of physical and chemical conditions present in different environmental situations results in a segregation of microorganisms in different geographic regions and in animate or inanimate bodies depending on the available nutrients, temperature, moisture, and other environmental conditions. The organism becomes adapted to a certain environment or finds the environment suitable to its existence. In this broad sense, the term "habitat" may be appropriately applied to the places of abode of microbial species. It often is convenient to group bacteria according to their habitats because such information is helpful in orientation.

Soil   The soil is a great reservoir of microorganisms, the majority of which are nonpathogenic. Some microorganisms reach the soil in the excreta or cadavers of animals. Others, such as the autotrophic bacteria, actinomycetes, and fungi, are indigenous. Among the pathogens that may be present in soil are *Clostridium tetani* and *Clostridium perfringens,* the etiologic agents of tetanus and gas gangrene. These organisms have been cultured from virgin soil and thus are able to grow in this environment as well as being introduced via animal and human feces. Another species of *Clostridium, C. botulinum,* whose toxin is responsible for the symptoms of botulism, is also present in the soil and from this source may find its way into improperly processed foods or contaminated wounds. *Bacillus anthracis,* the causative agent of anthrax, is deposited in the soil when animals die of the disease. It infects herbivorous animals and occasionally man by entering the body through the skin or mucous membranes. Species of *Clostridrium* and *Bacillus* produce endospores that are resistant to adverse environmental conditions and are therefore of survival advantage to the cell. Certain of the pathogenic fungi, *C. immitis, H. capsulatum, Cryptococcus neoformans,* and *Blastomyces dermatitidis,* have been grown from the soil which thus provides a reservoir of infection by these agents.

Water   Most bodies of salt and fresh water contain microorganisms, many of which are adapted to extremely adverse conditions (eg, psychrophilic and thermophilic bacteria). Pathogenic bacteria, however, are usually not present except in water that is directly contaminated by the urinary and fecal excretions of man and animals. Among the pathogenic organisms that often reach water that is used for drinking or recreational purposes are *Salmonella* and *Shigella* species, the cholera vibrio, the hepatitis virus, and the poliovirus and other enteroviruses. These organisms, however, are infrequently isolated directly from water. In the feces, they are always accompanied by large numbers of *Escherichia coli*, which is more hardy and persists in the water for a longer period. Culture of *E. coli* from the water serves as an index of fecal contamination.

Milk   Milk from normal cows, even when drawn under aseptic conditions, usually contains from 100 to 1,000 nonpathogenic organisms per milliliter. Other organisms may be added during collection or when cows are diseased. Diseases that may be transmitted by diseased cows or milk handlers include tuberculosis, salmonellosis, streptococcosis, diphtheria, shigellosis, brucellosis, and staphylococcal food poisoning. Pasteurization processes and destruction of diseased cattle have decreased the incidence of milk-borne infections.

Animals   Animals are hosts for many of the microorganisms that produce disease in man (eg, tularemia, brucellosis, psittacosis, salmonellosis, plague, anthrax, insect-born viral and rickettsial diseases). These diseases may be transmitted directly, by vectors, or by contamination of soil, water, or other materials.

Air   While microorganisms are frequently found in air, they do not multiply in this medium. The outdoor air rarely contains pathogens, probably because of the bactericidal effects of desiccation, ozone, and ultraviolet irradiation. Indoor air, on the other hand, may contain pathogenic viruses and bacteria that are shed by man from the skin, hands, clothing, and, especially, the upper respiratory tract.

Talking, coughing, and sneezing produce progressively larger numbers of respiratory droplets, many of which contain bacteria and viruses. A sneeze (Fig. 25-1) may produce as many as 106 particles from 10 μm to 2 mm in

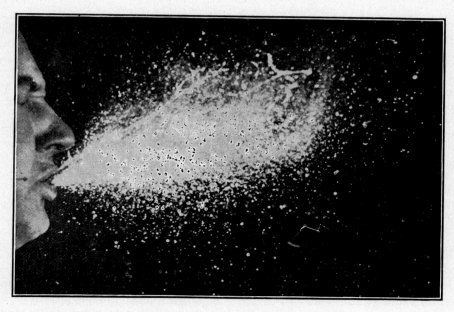

FIG. 25-1. Droplet disperal following a sneeze. The patient had a cold; note strings of mucus. (From Jennison: Aerobiology. Washington, DC, Publ AAAS 17:102, 1947)

diameter. The larger droplets may travel a distance of 1 to 2 meters before reaching the ground. These larger droplets rapidly settle to the floor and dry, leaving organisms attached to dust particles. The smaller droplets remain suspended in air and evaporate rapidly, leaving behind droplet nuclei a few micrometers in diameter, which may or may not contain organisms. These droplet nuclei settle very slowly, and in an ordinary room filled with people they are wafted about in air currents and remain suspended almost indefinitely. Under such conditions great accumulations of potentially infective particles may occur.

MICROBIAL FLORA OF THE NORMAL HUMAN BODY

Man is constantly bombarded by the myriads of microorganisms that occupy his environment. Fortunately, however, man does not provide a favorable habitat for most of these saphrophytes that must compete with the commensal flora that are already adapted to the human environment.

Normal Flora of the Skin

Human skin normally contains a varied microbial population. One animal, the mite *Demodex folliculorum*, is commonly found in sebaceous glands and hair follicles, especially on the face. Two lipophilic yeasts, *Pityrosporum ovale* and *Pityrosporum orbiculare*, are present on the scalp or chest and back, respectively. Nonlipophilic yeasts, *Torulopsis glabrata* and *C. albicans*, are variably present. The bacterial flora are predominantly *Staphylococcus epidermidis*, micrococci, aerobic and anaerobic diphtheroids, and sarcinae. *S. aureus* regularly inhabits only the nose and perhaps the perineum, but transient colonization by this and other bacteria may occur at any site. Saprophytic mycobacteria occasionally are found on the skin of the external auditory canal and the genital and axillary regions.

Most organisms inhabit the stratum corneum and the upper parts of hair follicles. A small number, however, are present deeper within follicles and serve as a reservoir for replenishing flora after washing. Washing may decrease skin counts by 90 percent, but normal numbers are found again within eight hours. Abstinence from washing does not lead to an increase in numbers of bacteria on the skin. Many of the fatty acids found on the skin may be bacterial products which inhibit colonization by other species. Normally 10^3 to 10^4 organisms are found per square centimeter. However, counts may increase to $10^6/cm^2$ in more humid areas, such as the groin and axilla. Small numbers of bacteria are dispersed from the skin to the environment, and certain individuals may shed up to 10^6 organisms in 30 minutes of exercise. The flora of the hair are similar to those of the skin. The relative freedom of the normal conjuctiva from infections may be explained by the mechanical action of the eyelids, the washing effect of the normal secretions that contain the bacteriolytic enzyme, lysozyme, and the production of inhibitors by the normal flora of the eye.

Normal Flora of the Nose, Nasopharynx, and Accessory Sinuses

Innumerable bacteria are filtered from the air as it passes through the nasopharynx, trachea, and bronchi. The majority of these organisms are trapped in mucous secretions and are swallowed. The trachea, bronchi, lungs, and sinuses are usually sterile. The nasopharynx is the natural habitat of the common pathogenic bacteria and viruses that cause infections in the nose, throat, bronchi, and lungs. Man is the primary host for these bacteria, and convalescent patients and healthy carriers maintain the reservoir from which others become infected. Certain individuals become nasal carriers for streptococci and staphylococci and discharge these organisms in enormous numbers from the nose into the air. Efforts to eradicate S. aureus from the nares of such individuals by the use of antibiotics have met with only limited success.

The pharynx usually contains a mixture of viridans (alpha-hemolytic) streptococci, Neisseria species, and S. epidermidis. These streptococci and staphylococci are inhibitory to S. aureus and Neisseria meningitidis. Many strains of viridans streptococci are inhibitory to S. pyogenes. Children infected with S. pyogenes may have fewer inhibitory strains than those who are not infected. The normal flora of the pharynx may be eradicated by high doses of penicillin, resulting in colonization of over-growth with gram-negative organisms, such as E. coli, Pseudomonas, and Proteus. If the viridans streptococci, however, are made resistant to penicillin by stepwise increases in dosage, no abnormal colonization occurs.

The nasopharynx of the infant is sterile at birth, but within two to three days it has acquired the common commensal flora and the pathogenic flora carried by the mother and nursing staff. The carrier rate of pathogens may be almost 100 percent in infants and is higher in children than in adults.

Normal Flora of the Mouth

Streptococcal species comprise 30 to 60 percent of the bacterial flora of the surfaces within the mouth. These are primarily viridans streptococci: S. salivarius, S. mitis (mitior), and S. sanguis. Bacterial plaques developing on teeth may contain as many as 10^{11} streptococci per gram in addition to actinomycetes, Veillonella, and Bacteroides. Anaerobic organisms, such as Bacteroides melaninogenicus, Treponema, Fusobacterium, Clostridium, and Peptostreptococcus, are present in gingival crevices where the oxygen concentration is less than 0.5 percent. Many of these organisms are obligate anaerobes and are killed by higher oxygen concentrations. These organisms, when aspirated into the tracheobronchial tree, may play a role in the pathogenesis of anaerobic pneumonia and lung abscess. The natural habitat of the pathogenic species Actinomyces israeli is the gums. Among the fungi, species of Candida and Geotrichum are found in 10 to 15 percent of individuals.

The mouth of the infant is not sterile at birth but, in general, contains the same types of organisms as those present in the mother's vagina. This usually is a mixture of lactobacilli, corynebacteria, staphylococci, micrococci, coliforms, yeasts, and streptococci. Among the streptococci are enterococci, microaerophilic and anaerobic species, and, of specific importance in neonatal sepsis and meningitis, group B streptococci. These organisms diminish in number during the first two to five days after birth and are replaced by the types of bacteria present in the mouth of the mother and nurse. Mouth flora fully resemble those of adults only after the eruption of teeth.

Normal Flora of the Intestinal Tract

In normal fasting individuals the stomach is usually sterile or contains less than 10^3 organisms per milliliter. Organisms swallowed from the mouth are either killed by the hydrochloric acid and enzymes in gastric secretions or passed quickly into the small intestine, where forward peristalsis is of primary importance in maintaining sterility or keeping the number of organisms less than 10^3 per milliliter. When organisms are present in the duodenum or jejunum, they usually consist of small numbers of streptococci, lactobacilli, and yeasts, especially *C. albicans*. Under abnormal conditions, such as gastric achlorhydria, scleroderma, diabetes, or blind loops following gastric surgery, bacterial overgrowth may occur, resulting in megaloblastic anemia due to consumption of vitamin B_{12} or fat malabsorption and diarrhea secondary to deconjugation of bile salts.

In contrast to the small intestine, the colon is the major reservoir of microorganisms in the body. Approximately 20 percent of the fecal mass consists of bacteria, or 10^{11} organisms per gram wet weight. Distribution of bacteria in the colon is as follows: bacteroides $10^{10\text{-}11}$, bifidobacteria $10^{10\text{-}11}$, eubacteria 10^{10}, lactobacilli $10^{7\text{-}8}$, coliforms $10^{6\text{-}8}$, enterococci $10^{7\text{-}8}$, clostridia 10^6, and variable numbers of yeasts. Thus, greater than 90 percent of the fecal flora consists of bacteroides and bifidobacteria, both of which are obligate anaerobes. Factors which determine the balance of these bacterial species are poorly understood. Enterobacteria produce colicins, substances that are inhibitory to a small number of similar strains of bacteria, perhaps accounting for the predominance of a few serotypes of these species. Flora may be altered by the administration of antibiotics — eg, cephalosporins decrease aerobic and anaerobic streptococci and lactobacilli, while clindamycin may totally eradicate most of the anaerobic species (bacteroides, bifidobacteria, lactobacilli).

Colonic flora may play a role in disease when the integrity of the gut is compromised as in appendicitis, diverticulitis, intestinal perforation, and postoperative infections. It may supply the coliforms, which are the major cause of urinary tract infection and gram-negative bacteremia.

The intestinal tract of the newborn child is usually sterile, but a few organisms may be acquired during delivery. Under normal circumstances intestinal flora are established within the first 24 hours after delivery, primarily with the previously listed organisms. The stool of the breast-fed infant is soft, light yellowish brown in color, and has a faintly acid odor. *Lactobacillus bifidus* is the predominant organism in these stools, others being enterococci, coliforms, and staphylococci. In contrast, artificially fed infants have hard, dark brown, foul-smelling stools and contain *Lactobacillus acidophilus*, coliforms, enterococci, and anaerobic bacilli, including clostridial species. *L. bifidus* may return following addition of 12 percent lactose to cow's milk or other formulas.

The significance of the intestinal flora has been a controversial issue since the time of Pasteur. Are the microorganisms essential for life, a natural but inevitable handicap, or an asset although not essential? Pasteur's studies on microbial fermentations suggested that the intestinal organisms might play an essential role in the metabolism of foodstuff analogous to that of the protozoa in the gut of termites. However, subsequent studies of germ-free animals have shown that these organisms are not essential.

The bacteria of the intestinal tract possess a variety of constitutive and inducible enzyme systems. Examples include glycosidases that are active against dietary sugars or glucuronide metabolites excreted by the liver. When the small intestine is deficient in lactase (as exists in over 80 percent of some populations), lactose is metabolized by colonic bacteria, resulting in abdominal discomfort, flatulence, and diarrhea because of increased water retention and lowered pH. Also, many bacteria produce urease, resulting in the hydrolysis of urea to CO_2 and NH_3. Other reactions occurring with nitrogen compounds include deamidation of amino acids, N-esterification, dealkylation, and hydrolysis and reduction of diazo compounds. Bile acids (cholanic acids conjugated with taurine or glycine) are dehydroxylated or hydrolyzed to free bile acids by intestinal bacteria. Bilirubin is metabolized to urobilinogen, which is reabsorbed by the intestine and excreted in the urine or bile.

The role of bacteria in the metabolism of drugs is poorly studied. However, an interesting phenomenon is known to occur with salicylazosulfapyridine, a drug used in the treatment of inflammatory bowel diseases. This compound is metabolized to sulfapyridine and 5-aminosalicylate by the intestinal microflora but not in germ-free animals. It is possible that the anti-inflammatory effects of this drug are related to this intraluminal cleavage and high local levels of 5-aminosalicylate. Many antibiotics are inactivated by the intestinal flora, which serves as the major reservoir for the generation of antibiotic resistance transfer factors.

Intestinal bacteria manufacture a number of vitamins, including niacin, thiamine, riboflavin, pyridoxine, folic acid, pantothenic acid, biotin, and vitamin K. Broad-spectrum or poorly absorbable oral antibiotics may greatly reduce or alter normal flora and induce vitamin deficiencies in patients with poor nutrition.

Normal Flora of the Genitourinary Tract

The secretions around the urethra of the female and the uncircumcised male frequently contain *Mycobacterium smegmatis*, a harmless commensal that, when found in voided specimens of urine, may be confused with *M. tuberculosis*. The outermost portions of both the male and female urethra may contain many bacteria, generally diphtheroids, nonhemolytic streptococci, and *S. epidermidis*. In addition the female flora contains a large number of anaerobic lactobacilli (Döderlein's bacillus). The sterility of the internal urethra is generally maintained primarily by the normal flow of urine and evacuation of the bladder. Urine aspirated from the bladder with a needle is normally sterile.

The vulva of the newborn child is sterile, but after the first 24 hours of life it gradually acquires a rich and varied flora of nonpathogenic organisms, such as diphtheroids, micrococci, and nonhemolytic streptococci. After two to three days, the estrogen from the maternal circulation induces the deposition of glycogen in the vaginal epithelium, which facilitates the growth of lactobacilli. These organisms produce acid from glycogen, and the flora resembles that of the adult female. When the passively transferred estrogen is excreted through the urine, the glycogen disappears, the lactobacilli are lost, and the pH again becomes alkaline. At puberty the glycogen reappears, and the adult flora again returns. This flora, when aerobic and anaerobic cultures are performed, usually consists of diphtheroids, lactobacilli, micrococci, S. epidermidis, Streptococcus faecalis, microaerophilic and anaerobic streptococci, and yeasts. Despite the close proximity of the anus, the vaginal flora of normal women only rarely shows even small numbers of coliforms. It has been shown, however, that women who are prone to recurrent urinary tract infection generally demonstrate vaginal and urethral colonization with coliforms prior to the invasion of the bladder by these organisms. During pregnancy, a few women demonstrate the presence of group B streptococci (Streptococcus agalactiae), an agent assuming increased importance in the etiology of neonatal sepsis and meningitis. After the menopause the flora resembles that found before puberty.

Bacteria in the Blood and Tissues

Occasionally commensals from the normal flora of the mouth, nasopharynx, and intestinal tract are carried into the blood and to tissues. Under normal circumstances they are eliminated by normal defense mechanisms, particularly phagocytosis. A few organisms may remain viable for a time in lymph nodes and may be cultured from biopsies of such tissues. Any unusual organisms of questionable pathogenicity that appear in only one of a series of blood cultures should be regarded as a contaminant from the skin or a stray transient. Simple manipulations, such as chewing, toothbrushing, dental work, genitourinary catheterization or instrumentation, and proctosigmoidoscopy, may also be associated with transient bacteremia. This phenomenon is generally of little consequence in the normal host, but in the presence of abnormal heart valves, prosthetic heart valves, or other prosthetic devices made of foreign materials, it may lead to colonization and infection by pathogenic organisms or saprophytes of low pathogenicity. The incidence of bloodstream invasion also increases following irradiation and cancer or leukemia chemotherapy. Several studies have shown that the administration of oral, nonabsorbable antibiotics to such patients may sufficiently reduce and control the intestinal flora and, therefore, decrease the mortality from infectious complications.

ACQUISITION OF INFECTIOUS AGENTS

Infectious agents may be acquired by a variety of routes, including foods and water, respiratory secretions, venereal contact, inoculation via foreign materials, disruption of normal skin and mucosal barriers, animal vectors, or invasion of normal flora. These pathogenetic mechanisms will be discussed in more detail in the following chapters dealing with bacterial, fungal, and viral diseases.

Of particular interest to the medical and nursing professions, however, are hospital-acquired (nosocomial) infections. These infections are transmitted to patients either by hospital personnel or by other patients. Modes of acquisition include surgical procedures, indwelling intravenous or bladder catheters, endotracheal tubes, intravenous fluids, and equipment used for respiratory support. Of particular importance is the seemingly innocuous acquisition of pathogenic or opportunistic organisms into the pool of normal flora, predisposing compromised individuals to subsequent invasion by their own flora. This is particularly true of postoperative patients and individuals treated with immunosuppressive or antineoplastic agents. These organisms include the usual pathogens, such as *S. aureus* and *E. coli*, as well as *Pseudomonas*, other enterobacteria, and opportunistic fungi.

Infection committees with surveillance programs to insure that unusual levels of infection do not occur must be an integral part of the modern hospital. Nosocomial infections occur in approximately 5 percent of all patients admitted. These rates vary depending upon the type of hospital (eg, acute vs extended care facilities). Over 80 percent of these infections involve the urinary and respiratory tracts and surgical wounds. The use of antibiotics in hospitals predisposes to the selection of resistant organisms that may be inadvertently passed from patient to patient by the mechanisms described previously.

FURTHER READING

Books and Reviews

Drasar BS, Hill MJ: Human Intestinal Flora. New York, Academic Press, 1974

McDermott W: Conference on air borne infections. Bacteriol Rev 25:173, 1961

Meleney L: Treatise on Surgical Infection. New York, Oxford Univ Press, 1948

Rosebury T: Microorganisms Indigenous to Man. New York, McGraw-Hill, 1962

Skinner FA, Carr JG: The Normal Microbial Flora of Man. New York, Academic Press, 1974

Smith DT: Oral Spirochetes and Related Organisms in Fusospirochetal Diseases. Baltimore, Williams & Wilkins, 1932

Smith T: Parasitism and Disease. Princeton, NJ, Princeton Univ Press, 1934

Selected Papers

Carter B, Jones CPA: A study of the vaginal flora in the normal female. South Med J 30:298, 1937

Cohen R, Roth FJ, Delgado E, Adhearn DG, Lolser MHN: Fungal flora of the normal human small and large intestine. N Engl J Med 280:638, 1969

Crowe CC, Sanders WE, Longley S: Bacterial interference. II. Role of the normal throat flora in prevention of colonization by group A streptococcus. J Infect Dis 128: 527, 1973

Donaldson RM: Normal bacterial populations of the intestine and their relation to intestinal function. N Engl J Med 270:938, 994, 1050, 1964

Drasar BS, Shiner M, McLeod GM: Studies on the intestinal flora. I. The bacterial flora of the gastrointestinal tract in healthy and achlorhydric persons. Gastroenterology 56:71, 1969

Gossling J, Slack JM: Predominant gram-positive bacteria in human feces: Numbers, variety, and persistence. Infect Immun 9:719, 1974

Jennison MW: Atomizing of mouth and nose secretions into the air as revealed by high-speed photography. Aerobiology. Washington DC, Publ AAAS 17:106, 1947

Schimpff SC, Green WH, Young VM, et al: Infection prevention in acute nonlymphocytic leukemia. Laminar air flow room reverse isolation with oral, nonabsorbable antibiotic prophylaxis. Ann Intern Med 82:351, 1975

Sprunt K, Leidy GA, Redman W: Prevention of bacterial overgrowth. J Infect Dis 123:1, 1971

26
Staphylococcus

Staphylococci are responsible for over 80 percent of the suppurative diseases encountered in medical practice. They cause most suppurative infections of the skin, but they also may invade and produce severe infections in any other tissue or organ of the body. In their adaptation to parasitism they have been among the most versatile and successful of the pathogenic bacteria. Although numerous antistaphylococcal antibiotics have been introduced during the past 35 years, the control of staphylococcal infections remains a major medical problem.

Most of the serious staphylococcal infections currently encountered are seen in patients whose normal host defenses are severely impaired. Hospitalized, debilitated patients who have been subjected to extensive surgery or who have serious underlying diseases are especially susceptible to infection with staphylococci. Such problems stem from the compromised status of the host rather than the virulence of the organism and will continue to arise as long as approaches used in the management of many previously fatal diseases prolong the lives of individuals who are unable to cope with their indigenous flora, including the staphylococcus.

Staphylococcus is the only genus of medical importance in the family Micrococcaceae (Table 26-1). It contains gram-positive cocci that are facultatively anaerobic and grow in irregular clusters. Properties distinguishing staphylococci from members of the genus *Micrococcus* that are often present in soil, water, and on the skin of man are shown in Table 26-2. The name "staphylococcus," derived from the Greek nouns *staphyle* (a bunch of grapes) and *coccus* (a grain or berry), was introduced to describe the organisms seen by a number of early investigators in pus from surgical infections. Since most strains freshly isolated from staphylococcal disease produced a golden yellow pigment, the organism was named *Staphylococcus aureus* to distinguish these strains from nonpathogenic staphylococci that produce white (albus) or lemon yellow (citreus) colonies. Pigment production, however, is a variable trait of staphylococci, and its correlation with pathogenicity is unreliable. For this reason other properties are now used for their differention. Three species are currently recognized: *S. aureus, S. epidermidis,* and *S. saprophyticus.* Of these, *S. aureus* is the most significant pathogen for man and is the best defined species in the genus. Useful properties for distinguishing the three species are shown in Table 26-3. Coagulase production is the most useful single criterion for the recognition of *S. aureus;* a staphylococcus that produces coagulase is *S. aureus* irrespective of colonial pigmentation.

Morphology

Staphylococcus aureus is a nonmotile coccus, 0.8 to 1.0 μm in diameter, which divides in two planes to form irregular grapelike clus-

TABLE 26-1   DIFFERENTIAL PROPERTIES OF THE GENERA OF THE FAMILY MICROCOCCACEAE[*]

	Micrococcus	Staphylococcus	Planococcus
Cells: spherical, gram positive	+	+	+
Arrangement: Irregular clusters	+	+	−
Tetrads	v	−	+
Glucose fermentation[†]	−	+	−
Cytochromes	+	+	+
Catalases: Heme	+	+	+
Non-Heme	−	−	−
Hydrogen peroxide formation	−	−	−
Motility	−	−	+
Yellow brown pigment	−	−	+
G + C content of DNA (moles %)	66−75	30−40	39−52

Adapted from Baird-Parker: In Buchanan and Gibbons (eds): Bergey's Manual of Determinative Bacteriology, 8th ed., 1974. Courtesy of Williams & Wilkins Co
[*] *+ = most (90% or more) strains positive; − = most (90% or more) strains negative; v = inconstant—in one strain may sometimes be positive, sometimes negative*
[†]*Growth and acid production anaerobically from glucose with exception of strains of S. saprophyticus which only weakly ferment glucose*

TABLE 26-2 Characters Distinguishing Members of the Genera Staphylococcus and Micrococcus*

	Staphylococcus	Micrococcus
Anaerobic growth; fermentation of glucose	+	−
Cell wall:		
Glycine-containing penta- or hexapeptide cross-bridges	+	−
Ribitol or glycerol teichoic acids	+	−
DNA: G + C content (moles %)	30–40	66–75

From Baird-Parker: Ann NY Acad Sci 236:8, 1974
° + = 90% or more strains positive; − = 90% or more strains negative

ters of cells. In smears from pus the cocci appear singly, in pairs, in clusters, or in short chains. The irregular clusters are found characteristically in smears from cultures grown on solid medium. In broth cultures short chains and diplococcal forms are common, and a resemblance to pneumococci often is observed. A few strains produce a capsule or slime layer that enhances virulence of the organism. The capsule can be visualized by negative staining, phase contrast microscopy, or electron microscopy. *S. aureus* is gram positive, but old cells and phagocytosed organisms stain gram negative.

Ultrastructure and Cell Composition The architecture of a staphylococcus varies with conditions of culture but appears to be very similar to that of other gram-positive organisms. Log phase cells of a standard strain as seen in thin section reveal nucleoids, mesosomes, and a trilaminar cytoplasmic membrane that is separated from the cell wall by a periplasmic region. The thickness of the wall of young cells normally varies between 18 and 25 nm. In encapsulated strains a loose fimbriate or capsular layer also may be seen. As in other bacteria the cell wall gives shape and integrity to the organism and protects the fragile protoplasmic membrane and protoplast from rupture. The osmotic pressure within a staphylococcus is approximately 20 atmospheres. Anything that impairs the structure of the wall will render the cell osmotically sensitive and result in lysis of the cell. Studies with staphylococci have provided much of the extensive information now available on cell wall chemistry and the role of selective inhibitors such as penicillin on wall synthesis.

The cell wall of *S. aureus* consists of three major components: peptidoglycan, teichoic acids, and protein A. The composition of these materials has been used for taxonomic purposes in distinguishing *Staphylococcus* from *Mi-*

TABLE 26-3 Characters Distinguishing Species of the Genus Staphylococcus*

	S. aureus	S. epidermidis	S. saprophyticus
Coagulase	+	−	−
Anaerobic growth and fermentation of glucose	+	+	−
Mannitol: Acid aerobically	+	v	v
Acid anaerobically	+	−	−
α-Toxin	+	−	−
Heat-resistant endonucleases	+	−	−
Biotin for growth	−	+	NT
Cell wall: Ribitol	+	−	+
Glycerol	−	+	v
Protein A	+	−	−
Novobiocin sensitivity†	S	S	R

From Baird-Parker: Ann NY Acad Sci 236:9, 1974
° + = 90% or more strains positive; − = 90% or more strains negative; v = some strains positive; some negative; NT = not tested
†R = MIC > 2.0 μg/ml; S = MIC < 0.6 μg/ml

crococcus and *S. aureus* from *S. epidermidis* (Tables 26-2 and 3). The peptidoglycan comprises 40 to 60 percent of the weight of the cell wall, and the amount of the other major components varies.

The primary structure of the staphylococcal peptidoglycan, as shown in Chapter 6, possesses a distinctive composition unique for the species. The glycan portion of the molecule is similar to that of other bacteria and consists of regularly alternating N-acetylglucosamine and N-acetylmuramic acid residues joined together through β-1,4 glycosidic linkages. In staphylococci, however, all of the N-acetylmuramic acid residues carry tetrapeptide chains that are cross-linked by pentaglycine bridges. The extensive cross-linking of the peptide moiety gives the staphylococcal wall a tight structure that aids the cell in its quest for survival in the hostile environment of the host tissues.

Another major component of the staphylococcal wall is teichoic acid, which in *S. aureus* consists of a water-soluble linear polymer of ribitol phosphate to which either α- or β-linked N-acetylglucosamine residues and ester-linked D-alanine are attached. The walls of *S. epidermidis* contain a glycerol teichoic acid, whereas in micrococci there is another type of teichoic acid or usually no teichoic acid at all. Teichoic acid is an essential component of the phage receptor of *S. aureus* and is characteristic of the species. It plays an important role in the maintenance of normal physiologic functions. Teichoic acids regulate the cationic environment of the bacterial cell and, in so doing, control the activity of autolytic enzymes that function in the growth of the wall and separation of the daughter cells. Although mutants completely lacking teichoic acid do exist, showing that the polymer is not essential, such mutants are phage resistant, grow more slowly than wild-type organisms, and produce large, bizarre, nonseparating cells with abnormal crosswall structure.

The major protein component of the cell wall of *S. aureus* is protein A. This is a group antigen specific for most strains of *S. aureus* and not found in other staphylococci or the micrococci. Purified protein A contains a preponderance of basic amino acids, and its removal from the bacterial cell increases the negative charge on the wall. It is loosely bound to the cell wall, probably to the peptidoglycan. The antigenic importance of protein A is discussed on page 419.

Physiology

Cultural Characteristics The staphylococcus is a facultative anaerobe, but more abundant growth is obtained under aerobic conditions, and some strains require an increased CO_2 tension. Growth occurs over a wide temperature range, 6.5 to 46C, with an optimum for *S. aureus* at 30 to 37C. The pH optimum is 7.0 to 7.5 with growth over a range of pH 4.2 to 9.3. For growth on chemically defined media, staphylococci require a number of amino acids, thiamine, and adenine. Under anaerobic conditions uracil and pyruvate (or acetate) are also required. In spite of their complex nutritional requirements staphylococci grow well on most routine laboratory media, such as nutrient agar or trypticase soy agar. Sheep blood agar is recommended for primary isolation from clinical materials. In the preparation of blood agar human blood should not be used because of the presence of nonspecific inhibitors or antibodies in blood that interfere with the development of staphylococcal colonies.

On agar plates individual colonies are smooth, circular, low-convex, and vary in size from 1 to 4 mm, depending on the strain and medium employed. The colonies are more opaque than those of the streptococcus and pneumococcus. Colonies of most strains of *S. aureus* are golden yellow upon primary isolation. Colonial pigmentation, caused by carotenoid pigments and ranging in color from deep orange to pale yellow, is extremely variable. It depends on growth conditions and is not a valid criterion for the separation of *S. aureus* from *S. epidermidis* organisms. White colonies of *S. aureus* frequently are cultured from clinical materials, and pigmented colonies of *S. epidermidis* are not uncommon. Pigment production may be best observed by growth on agar plates at 37C for 24 hours, followed by incubation at room temperature for an additional 24 to 48 hours. No pigment is produced under anaerobic conditions.

On blood agar a zone of β-hemolysis surrounds colonies of organisms that produce soluble hemolysins. Although primarily associated with *S. aureus*, β-hemolysis also may be produced by strains of *S. epidermidis* and, as with pigmentation, is a variable property of the staphylococcus.

Metabolism Energy is obtained via both respiratory and fermentative pathways. Intact pathways for glycolysis, the pentose phosphate and citric acid cycles, are operative under appropriate growth conditions. The ability of the organism to exist under conditions of both high and low oxidation-reduction potential is an obvious advantage to the organism in its battle for survival in its natural habitat on mucosal surfaces and in competition with other bacterial species in the mixed microflora at the site of an infection.

Catalase is produced by aerobically grown cells. In testing for this enzyme, precaution must be taken to avoid carryover of blood cells with the colony if the colony is taken from a blood agar plate. Catalase is present in red blood cells, and if they are present in the bacterial mixture, they may lead to a false positive reaction.

A wide range of sugars and other carbohydrates are utilized by staphylococci, especially under aerobic conditions. Under anaerobic conditions the principal product of glucose fermentation is lactic acid. In the presence of air the major product is acetic acid with small amounts of CO_2. Acetoin also is usually formed as an end product of glucose fermentation. The fermentation of mannitol by most strains of S. aureus is helpful in its differentiation from S. epidermidis.

Identification   Major characteristics for distinguishing S. aureus from S. epidermidis are shown in Table 26-3. Of these the most convenient and reliable property for diagnostic purposes is the production of coagulases, enzymes that cause the coagulation of plasma. Approximately 97 percent of staphylococci isolated from pathologic processes elaborate these enzymes. In testing for coagulase, carefully controlled conditions and the test tube methods should be employed. The slide coagulase test, although useful for screening purposes and usually correlating well with test tube results, detects a clumping factor that is distinct from the free coagulase. It is less reliable than the test tube method and should not be used in the routine diagnostic laboratory. In performing the coagulase test it is important to remember that certain bacteria other than S. aureus may produce coagulase and that false positive reactions may be elicited by such citrate-utilizing bacteria as the enterococci and Pseudomonas.

Another property of S. aureus useful in its identification is the production of heat-resistant nucleases (phosphodiesterases). These enzymes are unique to S. aureus and differ from the nucleases of S. epidermidis and other microorganisms in that they are resistant to boiling.

For epidemiologic and ecologic studies the staphylococcal species are separated into varieties. In the scheme shown in Table 26-4 six biotypes or ecotypes of S. aureus are recognized. Further differentiation of the biotypes may be accomplished by serotyping and bacteriophage typing.

Although procedures are available for the classification of staphylococcal isolates into specific serologic types, at present the systems are complex and empirical and unsuitable for routine diagnostic use. Serotyping, however, has certain advantages over other marker systems and promises to be a useful tool in the future. It is more stable than either phage typing or antibiotic sensitivity and can identify markers for most human strains of S. aureus, including those nontypable by phages.

Bacteriophage Typing   Most strains of S. aureus are lysogenic; they carry phages to which they themselves are immune but which will lyse some of the other members of the species. Susceptibility of S. aureus strains to the various temperate bacteriophages provides the basis for a phage typing system that has been useful in epidemiologic studies. The system is based on patterns of sensitivity shown by each strain to various phages. The phage patterns of different strains fall essentially into four broad groups, phage groups I to IV. The term "group" refers to strains of S. aureus with related phage patterns, as well as to corresponding groups of phages with host range for these strains. The phages within a group are unrelated and possess different morphologic and serologic properties. The grouping of strains appears to be less fortuitous. For example, group II strains of staphylococci are often associated with skin infections, such as impetigo and pemphigus of the newborn, and the production of enterotoxin is confined primarily to phage groups III and IV. Resistance to penicillin and methicillin first appeared in group III before it developed in other strains. Hospital epidemics started with strains of a few phage patterns (phages 75, 77) in group III and group I (phage 80) but soon shifted to resistant strains of the 52/52A/80/81 complex (group I), to be followed by strains

TABLE 26-4 SUBDIVISION OF STAPHYLOCOCCUS AUREUS INTO BIOTYPES*

	Biotypes					
	A	B	C	D	E	F
Origin of biotype	Human	Pigs, poultry	Cattle, sheep	Hares	Dogs	Pigeons
Fibrinolysin	+	−	−	−	−	−
Pigment	+	+	+	v	−	−
Coagulation of:						
Human plasma	+	+	+	+	v	+
Bovine plasma	−	−	+	−	+	+
α-Hemolysin	+	v	v	−	−	v
β-Hemolysin	v	v	+	+	+	+
Reduction of tellurite	+	+	+	+	+	−
Clumping factor	+	+	+	+	W	−
Growth on crystal violet agar	−	v	v	−	+	+
Typed by adapted phages	H	H	H,B	H	C	−

Data from Hájek and Maršálek: From Baird-Parker: Ann NY Acad Sci 236:10, 1974
° + = more than 80% of strains positive; − = more than 80% of strains negative; v = some strains positive, some negative; W = weak reaction; H = basic international human phage set; B = bovine phage set; C = canine phages

lysed by phage 83A (group III) and strains of the 83A/84/85 complex. Strains untypable by the typing scheme currently in use are now being isolated with increasing frequency. Although incompletely understood at present, the basis of phage patterns would appear to lie in the strain-dependent restriction-modification systems on which lysogenic immunity and phage-dependent restriction are superimposed (Chap. 8).

Techniques currently in use for staphylococcal phage typing are rigidly controlled by the Subcommittee on Phage Typing of the International Committee on Nomenclature of Bacteria. This group is responsible also for the maintenance of stocks of typing phages and their propagating strains, for establishing the composition of basic phage sets, and varying the composition of the set as new phage types emerge. The 22 phages that now constitute the basic set are shown in Table 26-5. In some countries additional phages are useful for typing strains limited to that country.

Only coagulase-positive staphylococci may be typed with the basic set of phages. For typing, each specific phage of the basic set is grown on its homologous propagating strain of staphylococcus and separated from the bacterial cells by centrifugation and filtration, and after proper dilution, a single drop is placed on each separate square of an agar plate previously seeded with a young broth culture of the organism to be typed. The plate is air-dried and incubated at 30C overnight. Phage typing results are recorded by listing only the phages that exhibit strong lysis (ie, a ++ reaction indicating more than 50 plaques).

Genetics In no other genus are the problems associated with the definition of a typical organism within a species more acutely recognized than in the characterization of a typical *S. aureus*. The extreme flexibility of the organism has long been recognized, but its medical implications were not fully realized until the rapid emergence of antibiotic-resistant strains, first

TABLE 26–5 LYTIC GROUPS OF STAPHYLOCOCCUS TYPING PHAGES IN THE BASIC SET OF TYPING PHAGES

Lytic Group	Phages in Group									
I	29	52	52A	79	80					
II	3A	3C	55	71						
III	6	42E	47	53	54	75	77	83A	84	85
IV	42D									
Unassigned		81	187							

to penicillin and then to each antibiotic successively as it was included in the therapeutic regimen. The serious epidemiologic and therapeutic problems created by these drug-resistant strains prompted genetic studies on the staphylococcus similar to those in the enteric organisms. It now appears that most antibiotic resistance in S. aureus, as in the Enterobacteriaceae, is plasmid mediated, and that the genetics of the staphylococcus are analogous to the genetics of Escherichia coli. In S. aureus, however, transfer of plasmids between cells is mediated exclusively by bacteriophages, and conjugation has not been demonstrated.

Most clinical isolates of S. aureus harbor one or more prophages that presumably are integrated into the bacterial chromosome. Of the large number of staphylococcal phages, only those of serologic group B are transducing. In S. aureus, lysogenic conversion, specialized transduction, and generalized transduction have been observed. All of the naturally occurring phages of S. aureus that can transduce are general transducing phages. Almost any character can be transduced at a frequency of about 10^{-4} to 10^{-10} per plaque-forming unit of phage.

About 10 percent of the total cell DNA in naturally occurring organisms is plasmid DNA. These elements contain genetic information that is dispensable for the organisms under ordinary cultural conditions. Since such genes have the capacity to evolve rapidly, they impart to the population of cells carrying them a better ability to survive under changing environmental conditions than cells with a uniform DNA content.

The plasmids in S. aureus that have been studied in greatest detail are those carrying determinants for penicillinase production. Although four different types of penicillinase plasmid have been recognized, no naturally occurring strain carries more than one type. Some penicillinase plasmids carry markers conferring resistance to erythromycin, mercury, and other metal ions, and a group of plasmids carrying resistance determinants for tetracycline, chloramphenicol, and neomycin/kanamycin also have been detected. These, however, appear to be independent entities, and with the exception of plasmids displaying resistance to both penicillin and erythromycin, no tendency to build up multiple antibiotic-resistant plasmids of S. aureus has been detected.

Some strains of S. aureus carry genetic determinants for bacteriocin production. These genes are extrachromosomal and in many ways are analogous to the colicinogenic factors of the enteric bacteria. Staphylococcin production is limited to phage group II strains of S. aureus and varies quantitatively with the strain and growth conditions. Staphylococcin is a heat-stable protein different from other extracellular products of S. aureus and is a distinct phage product. Its spectrum is wide and includes β-hemolytic streptococci, pneumococci, other staphylococci, corynebacteria, and several Bacillus species. Gram-negative bacteria and producer strains are resistant to the action of staphylococcin. For a further discussion of bacteriocins see Chapter 8.

In vitro pigment production is a remarkably unstable property of staphylococci. Nonpigmented clones arise with high frequency in pigmented clones. Although there is strong suggestion of a plasmid location for the genes coding for pigment production, attempts to locate these genes have been inconclusive.

Certain virulence factors, such as beta toxin, delta toxin, and the exfoliative toxin produced by phage group II strains of S. aureus, also are probably specified by plasmid genes. It is hoped that genetic studies in this area will provide a better understanding of the mechanisms governing the synthesis of staphylococcal toxins and other virulence factors.

Resistance Staphylococci are more resistant than most nonsporulating bacteria to adverse environmental conditions and therefore require no special precautions for preservation of clinical materials for culture. They survive for weeks in dried pus and sputum, and on sealed agar slants either at 4C or at room temperature, cultures remain viable for several months. Most strains are relatively heat resistant. Exposure to a temperature of 60C for one hour is usually required for killing. Staphylococci also are more resistant than most bacteria to chemical disinfectants, such as the phenols and mercuric chloride, but they are quite sensitive to low concentrations of basic dyes. Advantage is taken of this susceptibility to dyes in the designing of selective media for the culture of enterobacteria from fecal specimens that also contain many gram-positive organisms, including staphylococci.

Antigenic Structure

The phagocytic response of the host is a crucial factor in determining the initiation and the outcome of staphylococcal infections. In this process of host recognition and immunity the cellular antigens of the staphylococcal cell, especially the more superficial surface ones, are major determinants. The antigenic structure of *S. aureus* is very complex, and of the more than 30 antigens observed, the biologic and chemical properties of only a few have been well characterized.

Polysaccharide A A major antigenic determinant of all strains of *S. aureus* is the group-specific polysaccharide A of the cell wall. The serologic determinant of this polysaccharide is the N-acetylglucosaminyl ribitol unit of teichoic acid; specificity resides in the alpha or beta configuration of the glucosaminyl substituents. Polysaccharide A occurs with the mucopeptide in the cell wall in an insoluble state and requires lytic enzymes for release. Most adults have a cutaneous hypersensitivity reaction of the immediate type to polysaccharide A, and low levels of precipitating antibodies are found in their sera. This group-specific polysaccharide A is not found in the nonpathogenic *S. epidermidis*, which contains instead glycerol teichoic acid with glucosyl residues rather than ribitol teichoic acid. In *S. epidermidis* the group-specific antigen is referred to as polysaccharide B.

Protein A This antigen is the major protein component of the wall of *S. aureus*. It is found in over 90 percent of *S. aureus* strains, but different strains vary greatly in the amount of protein A produced. It is located on the surface of the cell and appears in the culture medium. Protein A is a group-specific antigen present only in *S. aureus* strains, and it is of special interest because it is precipitated by all normal human sera. This property first was thought to be due to the presence of normal antibodies that were formed as a result of constant contact with *S. aureus*. Subsequent findings indicate, however, that the reaction with normal sera is nonspecific. Protein A precipitates with sera from germ-free mice. It precipitates 45 percent of a pooled normal human IgG and reacts with H chains from both normal and myeloma IgG

and with the Fc fragment of normal IgG. In both rabbit and guinea pig normal and immune IgG, the combining site for protein A is the Fc fragment rather than the Fab fragment of classical antibody reactions. Since the Fc part of the IgG molecule does not contain antigen-binding sites, the reaction appears to be nonspecific. Protein A provokes a variety of biologic effects in experimental animals. It is anticomplementary, antiphagocytic, and causes hypersensitivity reactions and platelet injury.

Capsular Antigens Although staphylococci are rarely encapsulated, a few strains have been isolated that carry immunologically significant surface antigens. It appears that encapsulation in vivo is not a rare phenomenon and that the capsular material produced under these conditions imparts to the organism an antiphagocytic advantage. The capsular antigen is found only in mucoid untypable strains of *S. aureus* that lack bound coagulase (clumping factor). A further discussion of this antigen is found on page 420.

Determinants of Pathogenicity

One of the essential attributes of a successful parasite is the ability to survive in the animal host. In this respect the staphylococcus has exhibited exceptional adaptive potential, as evidenced by its unequaled versatility. Much of this versatility may no doubt be attributed to its possession of enzymes that can hydrolyze a wide range of substrates including native animal proteins. Proteases, lipases, esterases, and lyases are among the more important enzymes in facilitating establishment of the organism on the skin and mucous membranes of the host. In order to survive in a hostile environment, however, the successful parasite must counteract host defenses. For more than half a century investigators have systematically examined a wide array of extracellular enzymes, toxins, and cellular components of the staphylococcus in an attempt to define a specific virulence factor responsible for its pathogenicity. Unfortunately, although much has been learned about a wide variety of factors that are often present in the more pathogenic strains, at the present time no single factor can be equated with virulence. It is probable that this most sought-after factor may be produced only in vivo and cannot be demonstrated by our current in vitro approaches. It has been emphasized and ably expressed by Abramson that although it is not always possible to correlate the various enzymes and toxins with pathogenicity, their significance is not decreased. Each of these "may constitute a link in a complex chain of innumerable, presently undetermined, pathogenic factors that combine only in vivo to precipitate the staphylococcal phenomenon as it is currently understood."*

Surface Antigens   In its initial establishment in host tissue, surface properties with antiphagocytic activity are of obvious advantage to the staphylococcus. Although the ability to produce a capsule is limited in S. *aureus* to a few strains, studies with these strains have demonstrated the greater virulence for mice of the encapsulated organisms. Vaccines prepared with these strains stimulate the production of protective antibodies. Purified surface polysaccharide elicits the production of opsonic and skin-sensitizing antibodies. During the infectious process it is likely that most strains of staphylococci elaborate in the in vivo environment surface antigens similar to or identical with the polysaccharide surface antigens of the prototype encapsulated Smith strain.

Extracellular Enzymes   COAGULASES.   In the diagnostic laboratory pathogenic staphylococci are distinguished from nonpathogenic strains by their production of extracellular coagulases that clot plasma. Whereas correlation between coagulase production and pathogenicity is a convenient virulence marker, its use as the sole indicator of pathogenicity leaves much to be desired. The pathogenicity of coagulase-negative strains is well documented both clinically and experimentally. One is therefore not justified in assuming that every coagulase-negative isolate is a secondary contaminant. There is likewise no definite evidence that coagulase is directly involved in pathogenicity, and the earlier theory that coagulase production protects staphylococci from phagocytosis by the deposition of a fibrin layer on their surface remains unproved. Also, although coagulase is antigenic and multiple molecular forms have

*Abramson C: Staphylococcal Enzymes: In Cohen J O (ed): The Staphylococci. New York, Wiley-Interscience, p 235, 1972

been detected, there is no evidence for the importance of these antibodies in acquired resistance to staphylococcal infections.

The action of coagulase in the clotting of plasma is similar to the thrombin-catalyzed conversion of fibrinogen to fibrin. To achieve full enzymatic activity coagulase requires the participation of a plasma component, either prothrombin or a modified prothrombin structure, referred to as coagulase reacting factor (CRF). The coagulase-thrombin product (CT) not only causes fibrinogen clotting but also possesses proteolytic and esterolytic activity similar to that of thrombin. The fibrinopeptides released are indistinguishable from thrombin-induced fibrinopeptides, some of which possess pharmacologic activity comparable to that of bradykinin on smooth muscle. This activity together with defibrination could, perhaps in the absence of anticoagulase, contribute to the overall manifestations of staphylococcal disease.

LIPASES.   Staphylococci produce several lipid hydrolyzing enzymes collectively referred to as lipases. The lipases are active on a variety of substrates, including plasma, and the fats and oils that accumulate on the surface areas of the skin. The utilization of these materials is of survival value to the organism and explains the intense colonization of staphylococci in the sebaceous areas of greatest activity. The production of lipase apparently is essential to the invasion of healthy cutaneous and subcutaneous tissues. In primary human isolates there is a close correlation between in vitro production of lipase and the ability to produce boils. The decreased virulence of hospital staphylococci observed during the last 20 to 30 years parallels a decrease in staphylococcal isolates that produce large amounts of the enzyme. The decrease apparently is due to the presence of a prophage that blocks lipase production.

HYALURONIDASE.   Over 90 percent of S. *aureus* strains produce hyaluronidase. This enzyme hydrolyzes the hyaluronic acid present in the intracellular ground substance of connective tissue, thereby facilitating spread of the infection. Since inflammation antagonizes the spreading action by hyaluronidase, its importance in staphylococcal infections is limited to the very early stages of infection. The staphylococcal enzyme is similar to the hyaluronidase extracted from pneumococci, streptococci, and *Clostridium perfringens* and consists of several enzymatically active components.

STAPHYLOKINASE. One of the proteolytic enzymes of staphylococci has fibrinolytic activity but is antigenically and enzymatically different from the streptokinase of the streptococcus. The dissolution of clots by the staphylococcal enzyme is mediated by its activation of plasma plasminogen to the fibrinolytic enzyme, plasmin. Although it is produced by most strains of *S. aureus*, there is little evidence that it is an important factor in pathogenicity.

NUCLEASE. The elaboration of a heat-resistant nuclease appears to be uniquely associated with *S. aureus* strains. It is found in 90 to 96 percent of the many hundreds of coagulase-positive strains of staphylococci tested and is absent from most coagulase-negative strains. The staphylococcal nuclease has been purified and well characterized. It is a compact globular protein consisting of a single polypeptide chain. Structural disruptions are caused by heat (65C), but they are rapidly and completely reversible. The nuclease is a phosphodiesterase with both endo- and exonucleolytic properties and can cleave either DNA or RNA to produce 3′-phosphomononucleotides. Antisera produced in rabbits against the staphylococcal nuclease inhibit completely its enzymatic activity. It does not precipitate streptococcal nuclease.

Toxins A variety of toxic manifestations are associated with certain of the extracellular proteins produced by staphylococci. Three major groups of staphylococcal toxins have been defined on the basis of their biologic activity: cytolytic toxins (hemolysins and leukocidin), enterotoxins, and epidermolytic toxin. With the improved techniques now available an investigation of the numerous other bands observed by gel electrophoresis may reveal additional components with toxic manifestations.

CYTOLYTIC TOXINS. A number of bacteria produce toxins that cause physical dissolution of mammalian or other cells in vitro. Most of these are proteins, are extracellular, and induce the formation of neutralizing antibodies. There is considerable diversity, however, in the manner in which the various cytolytic toxins interact with the cell surface. It is these differences that make the staphylococcal toxins useful probes in studies on the molecular organization of biomembranes. The hemolysins and leukocidin elaborated by *S. aureus* are among the best defined members of this group of cytolytic toxins, a group that also includes streptolysin O and S and various toxins of *Clostridium*. The staphylococcal cytolytic toxins are antigenically distinct from other staphylococcal toxins.

ALPHA TOXIN (α-HEMOLYSIN). This extensively studied toxin exhibits a wide range of biologic activities, including the hemolytic, lethal, and dermonecrotic effects observed following the injection of broth culture filtrates of certain strains of the organism. Alpha toxin disrupts lysosomes and is cytotoxic for a variety of tissue culture cells. Human macrophages and platelets are damaged, but monocytes are resistant. There is injury to the circulatory system, muscle tissue, and tissue of the renal cortex. No other bacterial toxin is so versatile in its effects. Although it was once thought to be responsible for the pathogenicity of the staphylococcus, current evidence makes this unlikely. Together with the other virulence factors described above, however, the alpha toxin probably does play an important role at certain stages in the development of staphylococcal disease.

Pure alpha toxin has a sedimentation coefficient (S_{20w}) of 3.0 and a molecular weight of about 28,000. It consists of four different conformational forms, separable by electrophoresis. Rapid interconversion of these forms occurs upon storage and is reversible in both directions. The alpha toxin molecule readily polymerizes and aggregates reversibly to form both soluble and insoluble 12S products. These forms are biologically inactive and have been referred to as toxoids. Toxoiding of a 3S toxin with formaldehyde, however, does not change the molecular size, possibly because the reagent reacts with active groups essential for both toxicity and polymerization. The reaction with erythrocytes involves two sequential steps: (1) an initial interaction between toxin and cells that results in the prelytic release of K^+, followed by (2) the actual lysis of the cell and release of hemoglobin. The precise mechanism by which α-toxin damages the cell membrane has not been established. The formation of ring structures upon addition of α-toxin to liposomes and to membranes of a variety of mammalian cells suggests that the lytic activity may be due to its capacity to penetrate and disrupt hydrophobic regions of membranes. The possibility has also been suggested, however, that an enzymatic action is involved and that α-toxin is converted from an inactive protease precursor to an active protease by an enzyme in the membrane.

BETA TOXIN (STAPHYLOCOCCAL SPHINGOMYE-LINASE).   The most striking activity of this toxin is its ability to produce a hot–cold lysis, ie, an enhanced hemolytic activity if incubation at 37C is followed by a period at 4C or at room temperature. The toxin is an enzyme with substrate specificity for sphingomyelin (and lysophosphatides). Sphingomyelin degradation is the membrane lesion that leads to hemolysis when the cells are chilled.

$$\text{Sphingomyelin} + H_2O \xrightarrow{\beta\text{-toxin}}$$
$$\text{N-acylsphingosine} + \text{phosphorylcholine}$$

Erythrocytes from different animal species exhibit impressive differences in their sensitivity to β-toxin activity. A correlation exists between toxin sensitivity and content of sphingomyelin.

DELTA TOXIN.   This toxin is a nonantigenic protein with strong detergentlike activity. It is heterogeneous with respect to charge and size, composed of subunits of approximately 10,000 daltons and with a molecular weight of 103,000. It has a high content of hydrophobic amino acids, which if localized in one area could make the molecule amphipathic and strongly surface active. Delta toxin is inhibited by phospholipids and by dilute normal sera. It exhibits a broad spectrum of biologic activity and does not display large preferences for cells of particular species. Erythrocytes, macrophages, lymphocytes, neutrophils, and platelets are damaged by delta toxin, as are spheroplasts and protoplasts of other bacteria.

LEUKOCIDIN.   The Panton-Valentine leukocidin produced by most pathogenic staphylococci attacks polymorphonuclear leukocytes and macrophages but no other cell type. The toxin is composed of two proteins which are electrophoretically separable, the F component and the S component. At physiologic ionic strength, both components of leukocidin ex-ist in different conformational states. They act synergistically, not additively, and each component is inactive alone. An understanding of the molecular basis of leukocidin activity has been provided by studies on its interaction with phospholipids and with isolated cell membranes. Membrane–leukocidin interaction results in the conversion of leukocidin to a soluble inactive form and in the stimulation of potassium and ouabain-sensitive acylphosphatase. The inactivation of leukocidin is stimulated by triphosphoinositide, which is probably present at the active site on the membrane. Leukocidin can interact reversibly with the hydrophobic regions of other phospholipids. It is probable that the toxin interacts with esterified fatty acid on the membrane surface and thereby stimulates acylphosphatase activity. In the leukocyte-treated cell there is an increased permeability to cations and an accumulation in the cytoplasm of orthophosphate at the expense of ATP. In the presence of calcium large amounts of protein derived from the cytoplasmic granules are secreted. This degranulation may be observed microscopically. Both components of leukocidin are highly antigenic and have been toxoided. Although leukocidin alone is not responsible for the pathogenicity of the staphylococcus, it protects the organism from the leukocytes of the host.

ENTEROTOXINS.   Approximately one-third of all clinical isolates of coagulase-positive staphylococci produce toxins that cause food poisoning in man. These toxins are a major cause of bacterial food poisoning and also have been implicated in pseudomembranous enterocolitis. Five different enterotoxins (A, B, C, D, E) have been identified and differentiated on the basis of their reactions with specific antibodies. Enterotoxin B is the toxin most likely to be associated with hospital infection; enterotoxins A and D are most frequently associated with staphylococcal food poisoning. Although a close association of enterotoxin B production with methicillin resistance has been observed, proof of an actual genetic linkage is lacking. The mechanism of action of staphylococcal enterotoxin is unknown. The major hindrance to research on its pathogenesis and mode of action has been the lack of a practical and sensitive assay system. Except for man, the only reliable experimental animal for testing enterotoxin activity is the monkey. The emetic receptor site for staphylococcal enterotoxin is the abdominal viscera, and the sensory stimulus for this action reaches the vomiting center via the vagus and sympathetic nerves. Enterotoxin-induced diarrhea has been attributed to inhibition of water absorption from the lumen of the intestine and to increased transmucosal fluid flux into the lumen. The enterotoxin is a potent mitogen for lymphocytes; it is pyrogenic and enhances gram-negative lethality. The similarity of enteritis in severe food poisoning to pseudomembranous enterocolitis in patients after antibiotic therapy suggests that the cause in both cases is staphylococcal enterotoxin.

EXFOLIATIVE TOXIN (EPIDERMOLYTIC TOXIN). Strains of staphylococci belonging to phage group II are etiologic agents of a spectrum of dermatologic disease that includes generalized exfoliation (Ritter's syndrome), toxic epidermal necrolysis in older individuals, localized bullous impetigo, and generalized scarlatiniform eruption. Since the clinical similarities of these diseases overlap and they share a common etiology, the term staphylococcal scalded-skin syndrome (SSS) is used for this syndrome. An exotoxin, exfoliative toxin, is responsible for the diverse clinical manifestations. Not all phage group II staphylococci produce exfoliative toxin, but all phage group II staphylococci isolated from patients with the scalded-skin syndrome do possess the capacity for toxin production. There is suggestive evidence that the genetic determinant controlling exfoliative toxin production in *S. aureus* is located on the same plasmid as the bacteriocin gene but that this plasmid is different from the penicillinase plasmid.

The development of an animal model made possible the identification and subsequent purification of exfoliative toxin. The toxin is distinct from the alpha and delta toxins. It has a molecular weight of approximately 24,000 and is antigenic. In the experimental animal model using newborn mice the most severe exfoliative form of the syndrome is reproduced. The clinical picture, histologic findings, and electron microscopy of the experimental disease are indistinguishable from those of the human disease. The characteristic histologic change is the development of an intraepidermal cleavage plane at the stratum granulosum. This property of inducing intraepidermal separation appears to be unique to phage group II staphylococci.

The scalded-skin syndrome is observed primarily in children under four years of age. Its relatively rare occurrence in adults, except in the immunologically compromised patient, suggests the importance of neutralizing antibodies in a majority of the population. Of all the staphylococcal toxins and extracellular products studied, only enterotoxin and the exfoliative toxin have a specific clinically recognizable effect. The effects of exfoliative toxin are separable from the effects of the staphylococcal infection itself.

Clinical Infection

Epidemiology The epidemiologic patterns of infection with *S. aureus* are complex. The organism is a normal component of man's indigenous microflora and is carried asymptomatically in a number of body sites. Its transmission from these sites causes both endemic and epidemic disease.

An understanding of the origin and epidemiology of antibiotic-resistant organisms was provided by extensive studies in the 1950s. These studies were prompted by the appearance during this period of epidemics caused by strains of the 80/81 complex. The appearance of epidemics at that time apparently was a result of a set of new circumstances that had evolved with medical progress. One of the most dramatic triumphs of penicillin when it was first introduced for clinical use was in the treatment of staphylococcal infections. By 1946, however, an increasing number of penicillin-resistant strains were isolated from hospital infections. As penicillin became less useful other antibiotics were introduced, but resistance to these also rapidly appeared. Resistance to the new antibiotics was associated almost exclusively with penicillinase production and the development of multiple resistance in a few strains, which then became established endemically in the hospitals. The increasing number of highly susceptible individuals now congregated in hospitals contributed to the epidemic appearance of staphylococcal disease. Also, a greater dependency on antibiotics and a concomitant neglect of aseptic techniques caused multiresistant staphylococci to become more prevalent. Group III phage types and strains within the 80/81 complex are most often incriminated in outbreaks of infection among newborn infants, older surgical and medical patients, and hospital personnel.

The source of staphylococcal infection is a person with a staphylococcal lesion, who may be either a patient or a member of the hospital personnel. Patients with lesions draining pus externally are dangerous to others because they can disseminate the organisms by contamination of the environment. Direct contact via the hands is the single most important route of transmission. A number of cases have been reported of hospital personnel who have developed lesions following contact with patients. There are documented cases of hospital personnel with mild staphylococcal lesions, such as furuncles, paronychia, or styes, who have served as the source of epidemics. An infected surgeon is a common source of infection in surgical patients and newborn infants.

The acquisition and carriage of *S. aureus* is a complex problem that is incompletely understood. The infant is colonized with staphylococci within a few days after birth, but because of antibodies passively received through the placenta, the carrier rate drops during the first two years of life. By the age of six the child has acquired an adult carrier rate of approximately 30 percent. Some individuals who harbor staphylococci are chronic or persistent carriers, but most are intermittent carriers harboring the organism for only a few weeks. *S. aureus* is found in the asymptomatic carrier in a number of body sites, but the anterior nares is considered the major reservoir of infection and source of disease. The perineum is also an important carriage site. The frequency of isolation from the skin reflects the density of colonization of the nose and rectum.

The carrier problem is a serious one in certain groups of hospitalized patients, especially in newborn nurseries. The umbilicus and the groin are usually the sites of primary colonization. Nasal carrier rate can be markedly reduced by maintaining sterility of the umbilical stump. The carriage rate is determined by the presence or absence in the nursery of an epidemic strain. If such a strain is present, most of the infants will be colonized; if a number of different strains are present, less than 20 percent will be colonized. Many of the staphylococcal lesions developed during early infancy are thus due to nursery-acquired strains. Staphylococci are disseminated from these newborns with lesions to other infants and nursery personnel and to their families. Also, since lesions may not develop until after hospital discharge, newborns and patients with postoperative wound infections may transmit hospital strains of staphylococci into the community.

Bacterial Interference Clinical and epidemiologic observations suggest that colonization of one strain of coagulase-positive staphylococci prevents colonization with a second strain. These observations have been examined experimentally by inoculating infants, medical students, and nurses with a selected strain S. *aureus* 502A, a coagulase-positive organism of low virulence, sensitive to penicillin, and unable to produce β-lactamase. An impressive correlation was observed between the prior presence of S. *aureus* in the nose and failure to implant the 502A strain; coagulase-negative staphylococci were less effective in this respect than were coagulase-positive strains. Observations on adults directly colonized with marker strains demonstrated that heavy colonizers of nasal mucosa with S. *aureus* interfered with subsequent colonization with other S. *aureus* strains, that interference between strains is site specific, and that this interference is not restricted to a single type of S. *aureus*. Removal or suppression of the original strain by the use of antibiotics renders the nasal mucosa increasingly susceptible to artificial colonization. The principle of bacterial interference has been used clinically in a number of select nursery situations where the staphylococcal colonization rate and disease rate were high. The data obtained from these studies support the conclusions that this approach is an effective and safe method of curtailing epidemics, provided reasonable precautions are taken.

Pathogenesis In the typical staphylococcal skin infection the organisms penetrate a sebaceous gland or hair shaft where they find an environment nutritionally suitable for growth. The defense mechanisms of the host and the number and virulence of the invading organisms determine the likelihood of development of a staphylococcal infection. Although benign skin infections are common, serious staphylococcal disease is infrequent, emphasizing the excellent protective barrier to invasion provided by the skin and mucous membranes. Any condition that destroys the integrity of these surface areas predisposes the individual to infection. Third-degree burns, traumatic wounds, surgical incisions, decubitus or trophic ulcers, and certain viral infections are only a few of the many precipitating causes of staphylococcal disease. Abdominal surgical procedures account for the largest proportion of postoperative wound infections. Prolonged surgery predisposes to these infections that in most cases are caused by indigenous skin and fecal staphylococci. Foreign bodies, such as intravascular prostheses and intravenous plastic catheters, provide a medium for vascular infection and bacteremia. Influenza virus infections and cystic fibrosis render the patient more susceptible to staphylococcal pneumonia, and bacteremia develops most commonly in individuals with diabetes mellitus, cardiovascular disease, granulocyte disorders, and immunologic deficiency. In fact, it is uncommon to observe staphylococcal bacteremia in individuals who do not have an associated disease that predisposes to infection. By altering the normal flora of the patient, antibiotics may provide the proper setting for the increased proliferation of staphylococci. For example, the appearance of staphylococcal enterocolitis following the oral administration of tetracycline is precipitated by the replacement of indigenous organisms by antibiotic-resistant enterotoxigenic staphylococci.

Phagocytosis of Staphylococci The granulocyte is largely responsible for resistance to staphylococcal infections. Once the organisms have penetrated the skin or mucous membranes, mobile phagocytes migrate into the area in response to the stimulus of chemotactic factors. Chemotactic activity is generated by a number of different mechanisms, each of which is probably of significance at a different stage of the infection. Early in the infection staphylococcal proteases generate their own chemotactically active fragments of complement components. Later in the course of infection or with repeated antigenic challenge, specific antibody may generate chemotactic activity through the classic pathway (Chap. 16).

The inflammatory reaction induced following the accumulation of phagocytes at the site of the bacterial invasion facilitates contact between organisms and phagocytic cells. This interaction of staphylococci with phagocytic cells plays a central role in the critical early stages of infection. Phagocytosis of nonencapsulated strains of staphylococci is promoted by either complement or antibody. For efficient phagocytosis of the more resistant encapsulated strains, however, both antibody and complement are required. In most normal individuals, as well as many with staphylococcal infections, complement is the primary source of opsonic factors. Specific antibodies are present in the IgG fraction of the serum of most individuals as the result of subclinical infection with staphylococci, but the titer of these antibodies is relatively low.

Once the staphylococci have been engulfed and are within the phagocytic vacuole they are killed very rapidly. Many different mechanisms and bactericidal factors are involved. A key role is played by the myeloperoxidase-peroxide-mediated halogenation system. The burst of metabolic activity that occurs following phagocytosis leads to the accumulation of hydrogen peroxide within the phagocytic vacuole. The bactericidal potential of H_2O_2 is greatly increased by myeloperoxidase and oxidizable cofactors, such as iodide or chloride. The peroxidase is present in high concentrations in cytoplasmic granules and is released into the phagocytic vacuole during degranulation. Deficient bactericidal capacity against staphylococci has been demonstrated in the phagocytic cells of patients with chronic granulomatous disease of childhood. Leukocytes of these patients do not exhibit the normal metabolic response to phagocytosis, ie, increased oxygen uptake, increased activity of the hexosemonophosphate shunt, and accumulation of hydrogen peroxide. As a result of this failure of metabolic response engulfed staphylococci remain viable within phagocytic vacuoles. Catalase-negative organisms, however, such as streptococci and pneumococci, accumulate hydrogen peroxide and are therefore readily killed by chronic granulomatous disease leukocytes because they provide the reagent for the myeloperoxidase-halide-hydrogen peroxide bacterial system.

A small number of organisms survive for long periods within the phagocytic cell. Their role in establishing and perpetuating persistence is uncertain. The close association of the organism with man throughout his lifetime, however, is well established, as is the production of chronic, latent or smoldering infections. An important aspect of this host-parasite relationship is the development of a delayed hypersensitivity to staphylococcal antigens. Exaggerated hypersensitivity, however, may interfere with immunity. The success that has been encountered by many clinicians in the use of autogenous vaccines for the treatment of patients with recurrent boils has been attributed to a hyposensitization of the patient who has an excessive amount of delayed hypersensitivity to staphylococcal products.

Clinical Manifestations The characteristic feature of staphylococcal infection is abscess formation. This can occur in any part of the body, but in each area the basic lesion consists of inflammation, leukocyte infiltration, and tissue necrosis. In a fully developed lesion there is a central necrotic core filled with dead leukocytes and bacteria, separated from the surrounding tissue by a relatively avascular fibroblastic wall. In general, staphylococcal disease may be divided into three major groups: (1) infections occurring locally or involving contiguous sites, (2) infections that are spread primarily via the bloodstream, and (3) food poisoning.

SKIN INFECTIONS. Staphylococcal infection of the skin is the most common of all bacterial infections in man. The most superficial of these is folliculitis, in which there is infection of the hair follicle. An extension into the subcutaneous tissue results in the formation of a focal suppurative lesion, the boil or furuncle. A carbuncle is similar to a furuncle but has multiple foci and extends into the deeper layers of fibrous tissue. Carbuncles are limited to the neck and upper back where the skin is thick and elastic.

No pain is associated with folliculitis, but as the infection penetrates into the subcutaneous tissues, swelling, redness, and some pain occur within a few hours. During the next three to five days an increase of necrotic material and liquefaction in the lesion causes a rise in tension, exquisite pain, and tenderness. At the apex of the swelling the skin glistens, becomes thinned, and will shortly drain spontaneously. The pus is creamy yellow. Following rupture of the abscess, pain is relieved almost immediately. About 20 percent of the patients with furuncles have one or more recurrences during the ensuing year, and a small number have chronic recurrent furunculosis for months or years. Dissemination from cutaneous lesions occurs by contiguous extension or hematogenous spread.

Cutaneous lesions in children are less well localized than in adults. In the newborn infant, pustules or impetiginous lesions are the most frequent staphylococcal skin manifestation, and staphylococcal impetigo is common also in young children. It is characterized by the formation of encrusted pustules on the superficial layers of the skin. Removal of crusts exposes a red weeping surface. The disease is highly contagious and, when introduced into a nursery or school, spreads in an epidemic manner.

The staphylococcus also is the cause of a recently described severe skin infection of young infants, the scalded-skin syndrome. The disease, which begins as a localized lesion, progresses to widespread erythema and exfoliation of the skin. The characteristic symptomatology is attributable to a specific exfoliative toxin (p. 423).

RESPIRATORY INFECTIONS. Primary staphylococcal pneumonia is rare except during epidemic periods of influenza. It is a serious infection, however, because of the organism's tendency to produce abscesses and destruction of pulmonary lung parenchyma. The pneumonia usually is patchy and focal in nature, characteristic of a bronchopneumonia rather than lobar pneumonia. Staphylococcal pneumonia is also likely to occur in young children with mucoviscidosis, patients with underlying illnesses, and hospitalized patients receiving antibiotics. Staphylococci may produce infections in any of the paranasopharyngeal areas, and acute sinusitis is especially common.

OSTEOMYELITIS AND PYOARTHRITIS. Osteomyelitis, an infection of the growing bone, is most frequently caused by S. aureus. It occurs primarily in children under the age of 12 years and, in most cases, follows hematogenous spread from a primary focus, usually a wound or furuncle. The organisms localize at the diaphysis of long bones, probably because the arterial circulation in this area consists primarily of terminal capillary loops. As the infection progresses pus accumulates and emerges to the surface of the bone, raising the periosteum and producing a subperiosteal abscess. Clinical symptoms of acute osteomyelitis include fever, chills, pain over the bone, and muscle spasm around the area of involvement. When the infection occurs near a joint, staphylococcal pyoarthritis is a common complication. Pyoarthritis also may result directly from hematogenous spread or by direct inoculation of staphylococci into the joint during intraarticular injections, especially in patients with rheumatoid arthritis receiving corticosteroids. Staphylococcal joint infection destroys the articular cartilage and may result in permanent joint deformity.

METASTATIC STAPHYLOCOCCAL INFECTIONS. One of the characteristic features of S. *aureus* bacteremia is the production of metastic abscesses. Infections of the skin, respiratory tract, or genitourinary tract provide the primary focus for most of these lesions. Trauma and debilitating diseases predispose to the seeding of the bloodstream with staphylococci. The most frequent sites of the metastatic abscesses are the skin, subcutaneous tissues, and lungs. Internal abscesses of the kidneys, brain, and spinal cord are not uncommon. Infection of the pleural, peritoneal, and pericardial cavities accounts for less than 10 percent of the cases.

STAPHYLOCOCCAL ENTEROCOLITIS. This infection is an iatrogenic acute colitis clinically distinguishable from the food poisoning described below. It is observed primarily in hospitalized patients whose normal bowel flora has been suppressed by the oral administration of wide-spectrum antibiotics that selectively permit overgrowth by drug-resistant enterotoxin-producing strains of staphylococci. S. *aureus* often can be isolated in pure culture from the feces of these patients. Clinical manifestations of staphylococcal enterocolitis include abdominal cramps, copious diarrhea, fever, dehydration, and electrolyte imbalance.

FOOD POISONING. In the United States staphylococcal food poisoning is the most common form of bacterial food poisoning. It is caused by the ingestion of food that contains the preformed toxin elaborated by enterotoxin-producing strains. The food is usually contaminated by food handlers who have the organisms on their hands. The foods most commonly involved are improperly refrigerated custard or cream-filled bakery products. Ham, processed meats, ice cream, cottage cheese, hollandaise sauce, and chicken salad are foods that are often implicated. Foods containing the enterotoxin are normal in odor, appearance, and taste. Sufficient toxin is produced in four to six hours at 86F, but not at refrigerator temperatures, to produce symptoms of food poisoning.

Symptoms which appear abruptly two to six hours after ingestion of the food consist of severe cramping, abdominal pain, nausea, vomiting, and diarrhea. Sweating and headache are seen, but fever is not a common feature. Recovery is usually rapid, within six to eight hours.

Laboratory Diagnosis Because of the widespread distribution of staphylococci, meticulous care must be taken in the collection of specimens for laboratory diagnosis. If the material for culture requires aspiration, it is essential that the skin in the area be properly sterilized. The finding of typical irregular clusters of gram-positive cocci upon direct microscopic examination of purulent material is presumptive evidence of the presence of staphylococci. Definitive identification, however, requires laboratory isolation.

Pus, purulent fluids, sputum, and urine specimens should be streaked directly on a blood agar plate and inoculated into a tube of thioglycolate broth. Specimens from patients receiving penicillin should be treated with penicillinase to inactivate the drug. For blood cultures, 10 ml of venous blood should be inoculated into 50 ml of tryptose-phosphate broth. Identification of staphylococci and differentiation of S. *aureus* from S. *epidermidis* is based on colonial and microscopic morphology, catalase and coagulase production, and mannitol and glucose fermentation. Staphylococci and micrococci are catalase positive; pneumococci and streptococci are catalase negative. By definition, all strains of S. *aureus* are coagulase positive.

Antibiotic sensitivity testing of the isolate is useful for clinical and epidemiologic purposes. Bacteriophage typing and serologic testing are not practical procedures for the routine diagnostic laboratory.

Treatment In the management of localized staphylococcal infections the basic principle of therapy is adequate drainage. Foreign bodies at the site of infection should be removed. Although antibacterial agents may control spread of the organisms from the abscess, they are less effective upon bacteria within the abscess and do not facilitate its resolution.

Antibiotic sensitivity testing is important in the selection of the appropriate antibiotic and in evaluating its effectiveness during the course of the infection. Erythromycin and novobiocin are effective outside the hospital against most staphylococcal skin infections. Since the organism usually develops resistance to these antibiotics after 7 to 10 days of treatment, another antibiotic must be used if treatment is extended beyond this time. Serious staphylococcal disease, such as bacteremia, pneumonia, endocarditis, and osteomyelitis, requires the prompt administration of large doses of antibiotic over a long period and should begin with a penicillinase-resistant antibiotic, such as methicillin, oxacillin, or cephalothin. Lincomycin has been used successfully in the treatment of osteomyelitis. Since approximately 80 percent of the staphylococcal infections acquired in the hospital and about 30 percent acquired in the community are caused by penicillin-resistant organisms, penicillin should not be selected initially for therapy of serious infections. If, however, upon sensitivity testing the staphylococcal isolate proves to be sensitive to penicillin, this drug is the drug of choice for continued treatment. Resistance to penicillin usually is not acquired by a penicillin-sensitive organism during the course of treatment. Treatment of most serious staphylococcal infections should be continued for at least four to six weeks to prevent the later emergence of a staphylococcal metastatic abscess.

Prevention   Staphylococcal infection will never be controlled completely because of the carrier state in man. Control of spread of infection both in the home and in the hospital requires proper hygienic care and proper disposal of pus-contaminated materials.

Because of the large number of hospital-acquired staphylococcal infections, prevention and control have been directed primarily toward control of the disease in the hospital, where one is more likely to encounter a more virulent organism as well as a group of very susceptible individuals. Persons with staphylococcal lesions should be segregated from newborns and from highly susceptible adults, such as those with agranulocytosis. Indiscriminate use of antibiotics should be avoided in order to prevent establishment and spread of resistant strains throughout the hospital. All surgical procedures and instrumentation should be performed with maximal attention to aseptic techniques. In the newborn, proper care should be given the umbilical stump, and personnel in the nursery should be screened for staphylococcal carriers. Infection committees that have been set up in hospitals to

control nosocomial infections should provide effective surveillance and follow-through of problems that are uncovered. These committees should be given the authority to carry out their recommendations.

FURTHER READING

Books and Reviews

Bernheimer AW: Cytolytic toxins of bacteria. In Ajl SJ, Kadis S, Montie TC (eds): Microbial Toxins. New York, Academic Press, 1970, vol 1, pp. 183–212

Bernheimer AW: Interactions between membranes and cytolytic bacterial toxins. Biochim Biophys Acta 344: 37, 1974

Buchanan RE, Gibbons NE (eds): Bergey's Manual of Determinative Bacteriology, 8th ed. Baltimore, William & Wilkins, 1974

Cohen JO (ed): The Staphylococci. New York, Wiley-Interscience, 1972

Hughes WT, Feldman S, Cox F: Infectious Diseases in Children with Cancer. Pediatr Clin North Am 21:583, 1974

Lacey RW: Antibiotic resistance plasmids of Staphylococcus aureus and their clinical importance. Bacteriol Rev 39:1, 1975

Lennette EH, Spaulding EH, Truant JP (eds): Manual of Clinical Microbiology, 2nd ed. Washington, DC, American Society for Microbiology, 1974

Mudd S: A successful parasite: Parasite-host interaction in infection by Staphylococcus aureus. In Mudd S (ed): Infectious Agents and Host Reactions. Philadelphia, Saunders, 1970, pp 197–227

Novick R, Wyman L, Bouanchaud D, Murphy E: Plasmid life cycles in Staphylococcus aureus. In Schlessinger D (ed): Microbiology—1974. Washington, DC, American Society for Microbiology, 1975, pp 115-129

Rammelkamp CH Jr: Staphylococcal disease. In Beeson PB, McDermott W (eds): Textbook of Medicine, 12th ed. Philadelphia, Saunders, 1967, pp 180-186

Sheehy RJ, Novick RP: Penicillinase plasmid replication in Staphylococcus aureus. In Schlessinger D (ed): Microbiology—1974. Washington, DC, American Society for Microbiology, 1975, pp 130-140

Yotis WW (ed): Recent advances in staphylococcal research. Ann NY Acad Sci 236:1-520, 1974

Selected Papers

Bailey RR: Significance of coagulase-negative Staphylococcus in urine. J Infect Dis 127:179, 1973

Cluff LE, Reynolds RC: Management of staphylococcal infections. Am J Med 39:812, 1965

Coulter JR, Mukherjee TM: Electron microscopic localization of alpha toxin within the staphylococcal cell by ferritin-labeled antibody. Infect Immun 4:650, 1971

Dean BA, Williams REO, Hall F, Corse J: Phage typing of coagulase-negative staphylococci and micrococci. J Hyg (Camb) 71:261, 1973

Gezon HM, Thompson DJ, Rogers KD, et al: Control of staphylococcal infections and disease in the newborn through the use of hexachlorophene bathing. Pediatrics 51:331, 1973

Grinsted J, Lacey RW: Ecological and genetic implications of pigmentation in *Staphylococcus aureus.* J Gen Microbiol 75:259, 1973

Karakawa WW, Kave JA: Immunochemistry of an acidic antigen isolated from a *Staphylococcus aureus.* J Immunol 114:310, 1975

Lillibridge CB, Melish ME, Glasgow LA: Site of action of exfoliative toxin in the staphylococcal scalded-skin syndrome. Pediatrics 50:728, 1972

Mandell GL: Staphylococcal infection and leukocyte bactericidal defects in a 22-year-old woman. Arch Intern Med 130:754, 1972

Melish ME, Glasgow LA: The staphylococcal scalded-skin syndrome: Development of an experimental model. N Engl J Med 282:1114, 1970

Melish ME, Glasgow LA, Turner MD: The staphylococcal scalded-skin syndrome: Isolation and partial characterization of the exfoliative toxin. J Infect Dis 125:129, 1972

Melly MA, Duke LJ, Liau DF, Hash JH: Biological properties of the encapsulated *Staphylococcus aureus* M. Infect Immun 10:389, 1974

Nordström K, and Forsgren A: Effect of protein A on adsorption of bacteriophages to *Staphylococcus aureus.* J Virol 14:198, 1974

Okabayashi K, Mizuno D: Surface-bound nuclease of *Staphylococcus aureus:* Localization of the enzyme. J Bacteriol 117:215, 1974

Warren R, Rogolsky M, Glasgow LA: Isolation of extra-chromosomal deoxyribonucleic acid for exfoliative toxin production from phage group II *Staphylococcus aureus.* J Bacteriol 122:99, 1975

Yoshida K, Nakamura A, Ohtomo T, Iwami S: Detection of capsular antigen production in unencapsulated strains of *Staphylococcus aureus.* Infect Immun 9:620, 1974

27
Streptococcus

Man is one of the most susceptible of all animals to streptococcal infections, and no organ or tissue of the body is completely immune. Among the diseases of major importance caused by these organisms are streptococcal pharyngitis, scarlet fever, impetigo, and endocarditis. In addition, infections caused by group A streptococci may lead to the postinfection syndromes of acute rheumatic fever, rheumatic heart disease, and acute glomerulonephritis.

Pasteur described chains of streptococci in patients with puerperal sepsis, and Koch identified them in pus from wound infections. Pure culture of the organism was first obtained in 1883, but a long delay followed before there was full recognition and understanding of the multifaceted role of streptococci in disease production. The introduction in the 1930s by Rebecca Lancefield of a serologic method for the classification of streptococci into groups (A, B, C . . . N), based upon the antigenic characterization of the carbohydrates of the cell wall, provided the stimulus needed for the unraveling of the whole spectrum of streptococcal respiratory infection and its nonsuppurative complications.

The genus *Streptococcus* is the only one of the five in the family Streptococcaceae that contains organisms pathogenic for man. The most important of these pathogens are *Streptococcus pyogenes* (group A), *S. agalactiae* (group B), *S. faecalis* (group D), *S. pneumoniae* (pneumococcus, Chap. 28), and the viridans group.

Streptococci are gram-positive organisms, spherical to ovoid in shape, and less than 2μm in diameter. Cell division occurs in one plane, resulting in pairs or chains. They are homofermentative organisms and are catalase negative.

One of the most useful schemes for the classification of streptococci is based on their action on blood agar plates. Beta-hemolytic streptococci are those that produce a completely clear zone around the colony as a result of the formation of extracellular hemolysins. Alpha-hemolytic organisms produce a zone of incomplete hemolysis and greenish discoloration of the medium. Many streptococci are not hemolytic and produce no reaction, a gamma-reaction, on blood agar.

GROUP A STREPTOCOCCI (STREPTOCOCCUS PYOGENES)

Morphology

Group A streptococci are spherical to ovoid microorganisms 0.6 to 1.0 μm in diameter (Fig. 27–1). Many strains form long chains especially in liquid media, a phenomenon which may be enhanced by the addition of type-specific antibody to the growth medium. Although usually staining gram positive, organisms may become gram variable or gram negative as the culture ages.

The ultrastructure of the group A streptococcus is typical of other gram-positive bacteria in that there is a rigid cell wall, an inner plasma membrane with mesosomal vesicles, an electron-dense teichoic acid layer, cytoplasmic ribosomes, and nucleoid. In addition, external to the cell wall, are fimbriae that constitute the type-specific M protein (Fig. 27-2). Some strains produce a capsule of hyaluronic acid which may be demonstrable during the first two to four hours of growth. Since most of these strains also produce hyaluronidase, capsules cannot be demonstrated in older cultures. With the exception of M protein, the ultrastructure is identical to that of other groups of streptococci.

L Forms Protoplasts may be induced by penicillin or phage-associated lysin and may be

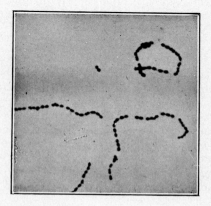

FIG. 27–1. *Streptococcus pyogenes.* Gram stain. ×1,200.

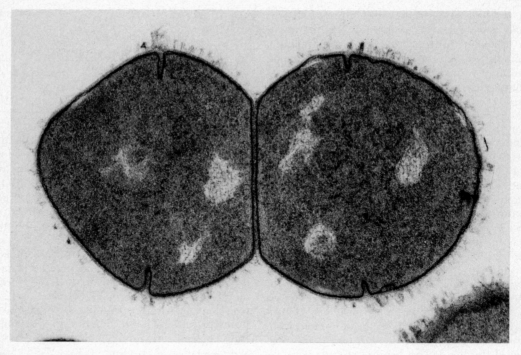

FIG. 27–2. Electron micrograph of group A streptococcus, M type 23, showing external fimbriae with M protein, and cell wall with electron-dense inner layer and closely adherent plasma membrane. The cytosol shows numerous homogeneous ribosomes and lighter nucleoid areas. This pair of organisms demonstrate one complete crosswall and the beginning of secondary septations. Glutaraldehyde-osmium fixation. ×84,000. (Courtesy of Dr. Roger M. Cole.)

propagated on hypertonic media to produce L forms or L colonies. Removal of penicillin usually allows reversion to the parent strains. However, there are many stable L form strains that are no longer capable of reversion. The role of L forms in disease states or in persistence of streptococci in tissues is unknown.

Physiology

All members of the genus *Streptococcus* are facultative anaerobes. Their metabolism is fermentative, and the principal product of their metabolism is lactic acid. They are catalase negative and oxidase negative and do not contain any of the heme compounds. The minimal nutritional requirements of the streptococcus are very complex because of the organism's inability to synthesize many of its amino acids, purines, pyrimidines, and vitamins.

Group A streptococci are killed in 30 minutes at 60C in contrast to certain streptococci, especially members of group D, that are not killed under such conditions.

Cultural Characteristics Growth of *S. pyogenes* is optimal at pH 7.4 to 7.6 at 37C. Primary isolation media usually contain blood or blood products, and growth may be enhanced at reduced oxygen tension. Most of the group A streptococci are beta hemolytic on sheep blood agar (Fig. 27-3), but amounts of fermentable carbohydrate as small as 0.05 percent glucose may decrease this reaction. Sheep blood is preferred for primary isolation, since it is inhibitory to the growth of *Haemophilus haemolyticus*, an organism whose colonial morphology and beta reaction may be confused with hemolytic streptococci. Human blood is generally not used unless known to be free of inhibitory substances.

Laboratory Identification For primary culture, clinical specimens should be processed by both pour and streak plate tech-

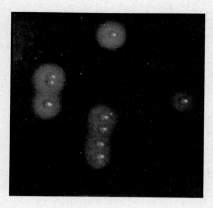

FIG. 27–3. Hemolytic streptococcus. Yeast blood agar. ×3. Note β type hemolysis. (From Li, Koibong: J Bacteriol 69:326, 1955)

niques. Characteristically after 18 to 24 hours of growth on blood agar S. *pyogenes* colonies are domed, grayish to opalescent, and approximately 0.5 mm in diameter. They are surrounded by a defined zone of beta hemolysis several times greater than the colony. Beta hemolysis serves as the marker for primary isolation and may be enhanced by subsurface inoculation or incubation at reduced oxygen tension. Group A streptococci must be distinguished from other beta-hemolytic streptococci (primarily groups B, C, and G) that are often present in the pharynx and other sites. A fluorescent antibody technique is available for group identification. Also useful for distinguishing between β-hemolytic group A streptococci and other β-hemolytic streptococci is the bacitracin test. This test, based on the sensitivity of group A streptococci to bacitracin, predicts with 95 percent accuracy the presumptive identification of this group. Streptococci may be differentiated from staphylococci on the basis of cellular and colonial morphology and on the catalase test. Streptococci are catalase negative, whereas staphylococci are catalase positive.

Lysogeny Among the group A streptococci, lysogeny is very common, as in other streptococcal groups. At least 25 to 30 percent of all organisms in this group are lysogenic, with the percentage increasing to 70 to 100 percent during epidemics. There is suggestive evidence that bacteriophages play a role in alterations of cellular components, but only in the case of phage-directed production of scarla-

tinal toxin is the influence of bacteriophages in streptococci well established. The role of lysogeny in the induction of poststreptococcal syndromes (p. 438) is unclear, but many patients with these diseases possess phage-neutralizing antibodies. A phage-associated muralysin is produced by group C virulent phage during infection of group C streptococcal cells. This lysin is released during cell lysis and has been detected both in mature virus particles and in fragmented phage tails. The enzyme is an N-acetyl-muramyl-L-alanine amidase and is capable of lysing streptococci of group A. The presence of this enzyme has important implications with respect to the in vivo production of L form variants and the release of streptococcal antigens bound within the wall or membrane of these strains.

Antigenic Structure

Carbohydrates The work of Rebecca Lancefield in 1933 laid the groundwork for the serologic classification of streptococci. Antigens (wall polysaccharides or teichoic acids) may be extracted from whole cells by dilute hydrochloric acid, formamide, dilute nitrous acid, autoclaving, or lytic enzymes. The extracts thus obtained are then tested against group-specific antisera by capillary tube precipitation reactions. This is the method employed for defining the various serologic groups. However, presumptive identifications may be made (group A vs nongroup A) on the basis of fluorescent antibody staining or bacitracin sensitivity, as mentioned above.

The group-specific antigen or C polysaccharide is composed of a branched polymer of L-rhamnose and N-acetyl-D-glucosamine in a 2:1 ratio, the latter being the antigenic determinant. This carbohydrate is linked to the peptidoglycan, which consists of N-acetyl glucosamine, N-acetyl muramic acid, glutamic acid, lysine, and D- and L-alanine. The cell also contains a teichoic acid, composed of polyglycerol phosphate and D-alanine, and another polymer, G polysaccharide, which probably contains glucose.

Proteins Group A streptococci produce three surface protein antigens (M, T, and R) that are useful in serologic typing. M protein is the major virulence factor of group A streptococci, and over 60 types have been described. Organisms producing M protein are resistant to phagocytosis in whole blood lacking specific antibody. M protein is acid and heat stable and trypsin digestable, and removal from the cell does not alter viability. M typing is performed by capillary tube precipitin tests using type-specific antisera and hydrochloric acid extracts. Electron microscopy using ferritin-labeled antibody has shown M proteins to be associated with the fimbriae on the outer surface of the cell wall (Fig. 27-2). M protein is destroyed during growth by a proteinase if the pH of the medium falls below 6.5. Some strains lack detectable M protein on initial isolation or lose it with repeated subculture. Such organisms may be identified by their T proteins.

T antigens are resistant to pepsin and trypsin but are acid and heat labile. T typing is done by a slide agglutination test, using trypsin-treated whole streptococci. Some T antigens are restricted to a single M type, while others may be shared by several M types (Table 27-1). Over 90 percent of streptococcal strains may be classified by the use of M and T antisera.

R antigens are destroyed by pepsin but not trypsin, but typing systems using these antigens are not commonly employed.

M-associated protein is found in all M-protein-containing group A streptococci and some strains of groups C and G but not in M-negative strains. Antibody responses to M-associated proteins are usually highest in patients with acute rheumatic fever, however, and levels do not correlate well with anti-SLO or anti-DNase B titers.

Capsule   Many group A streptococci produce a hyaluronic acid capsule that is of little antigenic significance but which may enhance the virulence of the organism.

TABLE 27-1   RELATION OF T PATTERNS TO M TYPES

T Complex	M Types Bearing T Complex
1	1
2	2
3/13/B3264	3,13,33,39,41,43,52,53,56
8/25/Imp 19	2,8,25,55,57,58
5/11/12/27/44	5,11,12,27,44,59,61
14/49	14,49
15/17/19/23/47	15,17,19,23,30,47,54

Determinants of Pathogenicity

M Proteins   In the nonimmune host, group A streptococci produce disease following inoculation onto the surface of the pharynx or into the skin. Virulent strains containing M protein resist phagocytosis and proliferate. They may remain localized in the pharynx or skin or invade the blood and other tissues, causing serious suppurative complications. Antibodies are induced and organisms are eradicated or locally contained. Natural infection may induce long-lasting type-specific (M protein) immunity. Other factors that enhance virulence are discussed below. Several of these (streptolysin O, NADase, DNase B, streptokinase, and hyaluronidase) are of practical importance in the serologic confirmation of streptococcal infection. Others have been postulated to play a role in the induction of organ lesions at distant sites (streptolysin O, erythrogenic toxin, cardiohepatic toxin).

Hemolysins   Streptolysin O (SLO) is produced by most strains of group A streptococci and many strains of groups C and G. SLO and streptolysin S (SLS) are responsible for the beta-hemolytic reaction on blood agar. SLO is inactivated by oxygen, but this can be reversed by reducing agents, such as cysteine or beta-mercaptoethanol. It is also irreversibly inactivated by cholesterol. It has immunologic cross-reactivity with and properties similar to the oxygen-labile hemolysins of pneumococci, clostridia, and bacilli. It is a large molecule, with a molecular weight of approximately 50,000 to 60,000. SLO is toxic for red and white blood cells and for myocardial cells in tissue culture and may cause cardiac death in animals following intravenous injection. Following pharyngeal or systemic infection this toxin is a potent antigen, although not in skin infections, probably because of its inactivation locally by lipids. Antibody responses generally occur within 10 to 14 days but, following repeated infection, may be observed earlier. Titers of 300 to 500 may be normally seen in pediatric populations at high risk of streptococcal infection but are considerably lower in adults or protected populations of children.

Streptolysin S is an oxygen-stable, nonantigenic toxin that is extractable from streptococcal cells by albumin, RNA, or detergents. It has not been isolated free of a carrier molecule.

SLS produces hemolysis by direct cell-to-cell contact and thus is nondiffusable except when transported by carrier. The molecular weight is probably considerably less than 20,000, which may account for its lack of antigenicity. It is lytic for red and white blood cells and for bacterial protoplasts and L forms. SLS is responsible for the surface hemolysis seen on blood agar, and those occasional strains lacking SLS may appear nonhemolytic on surface growth. SLS is inhibited by phosphatidylcholine and phosphatidylethanolamine.

Erythrogenic Toxin (Pyrogenic Exotoxin) A majority of strains of group A streptococci produce this toxin, which, as in the case of diphtheria toxin, appears to be synthesized as a consequence of infection with a temperate bacteriophage. Erythrogenic toxin is responsible for the rash of scarlet fever, produces a pyrogenic response and liver, heart, and diaphragmatic lesions in the rabbit, has immunosuppressant properties, causes reticuloendothelial blockade and lymphocyte transformation, and increases the susceptibility of rabbits to lethal endotoxin shock. It has a molecular weight of approximately 29,000. There appear to be at least three different serologic types (A, B, and C). Classically it has been thought that this toxin caused a red reaction in the skin of nonimmune individuals (positive Dick test) and no reaction in individuals with immunity (negative Dick test). Antitoxin injected into the skin of a patient with scarlet fever causes localized blanching due to neutralization of erythrogenic toxin (Schultz-Charlton reaction). Recently it has been proposed, however, that the rash in some individuals may be more related to hypersensitivity than lack of immunity, and the occurrence of rash may depend on an interplay between cellular and humoral factors.

DNases A, B, C, and D These extracellular enzymes, which presumably assist in the generation of substrates for growth, are produced by most group A streptococci. Nucleases A and C have only DNase activity, while B and D possess RNase activity also. All have a molecular weight of 25,000 to 30,000 and require calcium and magnesium for optimal activity. Antibody titers to DNase B are of great value in the serodiagnosis of pharyngeal or skin infection, especially the latter, where the SLO response may be blunted.

Other Enzymes Streptokinase is an enzyme catalyzing the conversion of plasminogen to plasmin, thus leading to lysis of fibrin and protein hydrolysis. Streptococcal hyaluronidase hydrolyzes hyaluronic acid, both in animal tissues and in the capsule surrounding streptococci. Both of these proteins are antigenic and are of value in serodiagnosis. Many strains of streptococci also produce a proteinase (especially as the environmental pH falls), NADase, phosphatase, esterases, amylase, N-acetylglucosaminidase, neuraminidase, and a cardiohepatic toxin, possibly distinct from erythrogenic toxin. Many strains of streptococci produce a lipoproteinase that causes opacification in horse serum. This test is especially useful in the identification of certain M types of streptococci associated with impetigo.

Clinical Infection

Streptococci produce a variety of important diseases. In the preantibiotic era streptococci were among the most frequent pathogens and produced significant mortality. Since the introduction of sulfonamides and penicillin in the 1930s and 1940s, streptococcal diseases have been well controlled, and deaths are uncommon. The major pathogen for man is the group A streptococcus (*S. pyogenes*) which is the agent responsible for the nonsuppurative sequelae of rheumatic fever and glomerulonephritis.

Acute Streptococcal Infection EPIDEMIOLOGY. Diseases caused by group A streptococci are possibly the most frequent bacterial infections encountered by man. Streptococcal pharyngitis and impetigo are the most common clinical manifestations. The true incidence of these infections is unknown, but it is unlikely that a child reaches the age of 10 years without having encountered the group A streptococcus. Surveys of school children for antibody to streptolysin O or other exoproducts have shown that the majority have significant titers, indicating infection within the preceding three to six months. Upper respiratory infections occur most frequently during the winter months when nasal and pharyngeal carriage also is increased. Group A streptococci are primarily transmitted via droplets from respiratory secretions. Transmission in milk and milk products has been largely controlled by pasteurization, although explosive common source epidemics may occur following contamination of foodstuffs by infected individuals. Hospital-acquired infections occasionally are caused by anal carriers or medical personnel with minimal cutaneous lesions. Streptococcal pyoderma (impetigo) is predominantly a disease of temperate climates and occurs with highest frequency in late summer and early fall. The exact mode of transmission is unknown. Organisms first colonize the skin prior to clinically apparent infection and then secondarily colonize the pharynx. Insect vectors, such as mosquitoes and flies, have been suspected but are unproved vectors in transmission.

Pathogenesis. Group A streptococci possess numerous factors that enhance virulence and allow the organisms to establish themselves in the host. Many strains have a predilection for the upper respiratory tract as opposed to the skin, but the mechanisms responsible for this tissue specificity are unknown. Group A streptococci with their surface M protein antigen are resistant to phagocytosis. The presence of type-specific antibody, however, promotes uptake by neutrophils and monocytes. Streptococci are rapidly killed following ingestion, and disintegration of most organisms occurs within one to four hours. The cell wall, however, is resistant to lysozyme and lysosomal enzymes and may persist in cells or tissues indefinitely. Cell walls and peptidoglycan of group A streptococci produce chronic inflammatory lesions in animal tissues and may induce in rabbits nodules in the skin and myocarditis. In addition, cell walls and peptidoglycan induce complement activation in vitro, with generation of chemotactic factors capable of producing inflammation. The role of these phenomena in the induction of poststreptococcal diseases has been postulated but is unproved.

Clinical Manifestations. *Pharyngitis and Scarlet Fever.* Streptococcal pharyngitis usually is associated with group A organisms, although sporadic cases and epidemics have been reported with groups C and G. When infection is caused by a strain infected with a temperate bacteriophage, scarlet fever may ensue. In the preantibiotic era, streptococcal pharyngitis frequently was associated with suppurative (tonsillar abscess, septicemia, mas-

toiditis, osteomyelitis) as well as nonsuppurative (acute rheumatic fever and glomerulonephritis) complications. Whether associated with the earlier administration of antibiotics or with changes in virulence, the incidence of serious sequelae has progressively declined.

Pharyngeal infection may be asymptomatic or may be associated with all gradations of the syndrome of sore throat, fever, chills, headache, malaise, nausea, and vomiting. Occasionally abdominal pain is seen in children and may be confused with appendicitis. The pharynx may be mildly erythematous or beefy red with grayish yellow exudates which frequently bleed when swabbed for culture. Anterior cervical adenopathy and leukocytosis usually are present. Clinical syndromes indistinguishable from streptococcal pharyngitis may be seen in diphtheria, infectious mononucleosis, and infection with many respiratory viruses (adenovirus, Coxsackie virus, rhinovirus, and *Herpesvirus hominis.*)

The association of a scarlatinal rash (erythema which blanches on pressure, initially involving the trunk and neck, spreading to the extremities) is almost diagnostic of streptococcal infection. Desquamation may occur during convalescence. Individuals may have several episodes of scarlet fever, as there are at least three different erythrogenic toxins (A, B, and C).

Immunity. Pharyngeal infection probably confers lifelong type-specific immunity. Early treatment, however, may abort natural infection and prevent or modify the immune response.

Skin Infection. Group A streptococci and, to a lesser extent, groups B, C, D, and G frequently are isolated from skin lesions. Group A streptococci produce impetigo, cellulitis, erysipelas, wound infection, and gangrene.

Impetigo is a very superficial infection of the skin characterized by crusting and amber lesions that may begin as small vesicles. The early lesions usually contain only streptococci. However, staphylococci may also be found or may subsequently superinfect streptococcal lesions. Many serotypes have been implicated, and several of these so-called pyoderma strains have been associated with nephritis outbreaks (eg, M types 2, 49, 55, and 57) (Table 27-2). In addition, many isolates either lack detectable M protein or, more likely, represent as yet un-

TABLE 27-2 ASSOCIATION OF CERTAIN SEROTYPES WITH ACUTE NEPHRITIS

M Type	Pharyngitis-associated	Pyoderma-associated
1	+++	
2	0	+++
3	++	±
4	+++	±
12	++++	±
25	++	±
49	++	++++
55	0	+++
57	0	++

From Wannamaker: N Engl J Med 282:81, 1970
++++ = Strong evidence of association
± or 0 = questionable or no evidence

described M types. Types 59 through 63 have recently been designated. T agglutination patterns have been of great use in categorizing strains that could not be M typed (Table 27-1).

Cellulitis with lymphangitis and local adenopathy may occur following deeper invasion by streptococci. Systemic symptoms, such as fever, chills, and malaise, are seen, and bloodstream invasion may occur. Erysipelas is an infection of the skin and subcutaneous tissues usually occurring on the face. The lesion is characterized by erythema, edema, and induration, which usually has a distinct advancing border. Streptococci may be isolated from the skin and occasionally from the blood. Some patients are prone to recurrences, usually in the same site. Superficial cellulitis may spread to cause gangrene, especially in patients with peripheral vascular disease or diabetes. In addition to group A, groups B, C, and D and anaerobic streptococci may be involved. Sporadic outbreaks of omphalitis occasionally are seen in newborn infants. Acute glomerulonephritis may follow any of these infections when caused by group A streptococci; however, rheumatic fever occurs only following respiratory infection.

IMMUNITY. The development of type-specific immunity is not well documented in streptococcal impetigo. Antibody to M protein of many of the pyoderma strains has been demonstrated only infrequently.

Puerperal Sepsis. Puerperal sepsis or childbed fever was a common cause of maternal mortality in the preantibiotic era. Streptococci may be normal vaginal flora or are introduced during delivery, occasionally by the attending physician or nurse. Outbreaks still occur occasionally, even in hospitals, and some may be traced to respiratory or anal carriers of streptotocci. In recent years, with better obstetric techniques, puerperal infections are uncommon. The classical syndrome is characterized by chills, fever, facial flushing, and abdominal distention, with pelvic tenderness and serosanguineous vaginal discharge. Group A streptococci are frequently isolated from the lochia or blood. Mortality has been significantly reduced with antibiotics, but even with therapy, recovery may be complicated and prolonged.

LABORATORY DIAGNOSIS. The definitive diagnosis of streptococcal pharyngitis can be made only by direct culture of the posterior pharynx and tonsils. Swabs may be inoculated into broth and examined by fluorescent antibody or onto blood agar with subsequent grouping by bacitracin disk sensitivity or serologic techniques. Differentiation between the carrier state and true infection is difficult but is not of practical importance in the symptomatic patient.

Streptococci are best recovered from impetigo lesions early in the course. Vesicular or pustular fluid inoculated onto blood agar may reveal a pure growth of streptococci. As lesions become older, streptococci and staphylococci may be isolated concomitantly. Cellulitis and erysipelas are best cultured by needle aspiration of tissue fluids, especially from the advancing border in erysipelas, or by subcutaneous injection of a small amount of sterile saline followed by reaspiration. Streptococci also may be isolated from the blood in patients with deeper infections.

TREATMENT. Streptococcal pharyngitis is usually a self-limited disease which may resolve without complication or antibiotics. However, therapy is directed primarily at prevention of rheumatic fever and at decreasing the incidence of glomerulonephritis. The treatments of choice are intramuscular benzathine penicillin given in a single dose or oral penicillin V for 10 days. Alternatives for therapy in the penicillin-allergic patient include erythromycin, and cephalexin (Table 27-3). Tetracyclines and sulfonamides are contraindicated because of increased resistance of streptococci to the former and lack of prevention of rheumatic

TABLE 27-3 TREATMENT OF STREPTOCOCCAL PHARYNGITIS OR IMPETIGO

Parenteral benzathine penicillin	Children: 600,000 to 900,000 units Adults: 1,200,000 units
Oral penicillin V, erythromycin, or cephalexin	15 mg/kg/day in 4 divided doses

fever by the latter. Recurrences of streptococcal infection in patients with previous rheumatic fever may be prevented by monthly injections of benzathine penicillin, by oral penicillin V, or sulfonamides given twice daily (Table 27-4). Sulfonamides are effective in prevention but not in therapy.

Impetigo is best treated with parenteral benzathine penicillin or by oral penicillin V, erythromycin, or cephalexin (Table 27-3). However, parenteral high-dose therapy may be required for deeper, more invasive lesions. Surgical debridement and even amputation may be required in severe infections, especially when complicated by peripheral vascular disease.

PREVENTION. Infection may be prevented by prompt therapeutic intervention during epidemics or prophylactic therapy given to individuals at high risk, such as military recruits or patients with rheumatic heart disease. Immunization with M protein vaccines has been shown to be effective, but the use of such vaccines in general or selected populations remains to be explored.

Impetigo is commonly observed in hot humid climates, especially where crowded living conditions exist. A majority of these infections could be prevented by improved skin hygiene. Epidemics are best halted by improving hygiene and treatment of all cases with effective antibiotic regimens.

Puerperal sepsis may be prevented, for the most part, by strict attention to aseptic techniques.

Sequelae of Acute Streptococcal Infection

ACUTE RHEUMATIC FEVER [ARF]. Rheumatic fever has been described by Feinstein as "an arbitrarily designated portion of the spectrum of inflammatory complications that may follow group A streptococcal infections . . . manifested by the appearance, either alone or in various combinations, of arthritis, carditis, chorea, erythema marginatum or subcutaneous nodules."* This constellation of symptoms usually occurs within two to three weeks after the onset of streptococcal infection, although chorea and erythema marginatum may be seen as late as six months. The diversity of the manifestations of rheumatic fever, the delay in onset after infection, and the inability prior to the 1930s to classify streptococci, led to considerable difficulty in understanding this illness. The clinical experience of T. Duckett Jones led to the establishment of the Jones criteria for the diagnosis of acute rheumatic fever (Table 27-5). In addition to the clinical criteria, the documentation of recent streptococcal infection by culture or serology is of utmost importance. Since the causative streptococcal infection may have resolved or may have been asymptomatic, it is necessary to detect an increase in antibody titer to at least one of several streptococcal antigens (streptolysin O, DNase B, hyaluronidase, or streptokinase). The ability to document a change in titer depends upon the length of the latent period, since many patients will have a maximal response at the time of acute illness.

Rheumatic fever may occur in up to as many as 3 percent of individuals during epidemic

*Feinstein AR: In Wintrobe MM (ed): Principles of Internal Medicine. New York, McGraw-Hill, 1974, p 1171

TABLE 27-4 PROPHYLACTIC REGIMENS AND RECURRENCE RATES OF RHEUMATIC FEVER

	Parenteral Benzathine Penicillin	Oral Penicillin	Oral Sulfadiazine
Number of patient years	560	545	576
Rate of recurrence*	0.4	5.5	2.8

From Wood et al: Ann Intern Med 60:31, 1964
Rate per 100 patient-years (patient-year = number of patients × number of years followed)

TABLE 27-5 MODIFIED JONES CRITERIA FOR THE DIAGNOSIS OF RHEUMATIC FEVER*

Major Manifestations	Minor Manifestations
Carditis	Fever
Arthritis	Arthralgia
Chorea	Elevated sedimentation rate or C-reactive protein
Erythema marginatum	Electrocardiographic changes
Subcutaneous nodules	History of previous rheumatic fever or rheumatic heart disease

Plus *evidence of preceding streptococcal infection (scarlet fever, culture-proven group A streptococcal pharyngitis, or elevated streptococcal antibody test)*
Two major or one major and two minor manifestations with evidence of previous streptococcal infection indicate a high probability of rheumatic fever.

pharyngitis. Milder poststreptococcal inflammatory states (fever, arthralgia without arthritis, erythema nodosum) may also be seen but are not classified as rheumatic fever unless associated with major manifestations (carditis, arthritis, chorea). The major morbidity and mortality associated with rheumatic fever are the subsequent development of rheumatic valvular heart disease, which accounts for about 15,000 deaths per year in the United States. The incidence of this complication depends primarily on the incidence and severity of carditis during ARF and subsequent bouts of ARF.

Pathogenesis. The pathogenesis of rheumatic fever is poorly understood. A variety of theories have been proposed, including antigenic cross-reactivity between streptococcal antigens and heart tissue, direct toxicity due to streptococcal exotoxins, actual invasion of the heart by streptococci, or localization of antigens within damaged muscle or valvular tissues. Needless to say, the streptococcus produces many potentially damaging exotoxins, and the components of its cell wall have been shown to produce inflammation in mammalian tissues. The true pathogenesis of ARF may never be elucidated because of the lack of a suitable experimental model.

Treatment. The duration and vigor of treatment depend upon the severity of the illness. Prolonged bed rest is no longer recommended unless necessary to control heart failure. Salicylates and corticosteroids are of equal benefit in reduction of acute symptoms and control of long-term sequelae. Corticosteroids are usually administered to patients with moderate to severe heart failure. Penicillin does not alter the course of ARF but usually is administered once the diagnosis is definite or if group A streptococci are cultured from the pharynx.

Prevention. The prevention of streptococcal infections prevents rheumatic fever. In addition, prompt treatment of patients with streptococcal pharyngitis within 10 days of onset reduces the incidence of rheumatic fever. Patients who have had previous episodes of rheumatic fever should be placed on continuous antibiotic prophylaxis. The therapy for streptococcal pharyngitis and prophylaxis of streptococcal infection are outlined in Tables 27-3 and 27-4.

ACUTE POSTSTREPTOCOCCAL GLOMERULONEPHRITIS (AGN). AGN is a complication of group A streptococcal pharyngitis or skin infection. In contrast to rheumatic fever, which may follow pharyngeal infection with any serotype, AGN is caused by a limited number of nephritogenic strains. Type 12 has been most frequently associated with AGN following pharyngitis, and a variety of strains, many of them newly defined M types, have been associated with pyoderma nephritis (Table 27-2). The incidence of AGN in epidemics or sporadic streptococcal infection may vary from less than 1 percent to as high as 10 to 15 percent.

AGN is most often seen in children and is characterized by the acute onset of edema, oliguria, hypertension, congestive heart failure, and, frequently, seizures. Laboratory findings include dark or smoky urine with red blood cells, red blood cell casts, white blood cells, proteinuria, depressed serum complement, decreased glomerular filtration rate, and serologic evidence of recent streptococcal infection. In addition less severe cases frequently occur and may be associated with minimal urinary sediment changes or depressed serum complement without symptoms. These changes are frequently seen in the siblings of patients with AGN. Renal biopsy in the typical case shows edema and hypercellularity of the glomerular tuft with red blood cells in Bowman's space or in the tubular lumens. Immunofluorescent examination may show complement components with or without immunoglobulins in a granular pattern.

In order to establish a streptococcal etiology it is necessary to document previous or concurrent streptococcal infection or immune response to streptococcal products. A great majority of patients will show a serologic response either to SLO or to DNase B. It is important that the latter be sought in patients with impetigo, as the SLO response is poor following skin infection. The latent period between streptococcal infection is one to two weeks following pharyngitis and two to three weeks following skin infection. Hematuria may occur during the latent period both in patients who do and who do not develop clinical AGN.

Pathogenesis. Immunofluorescent staining classically shows granular accumulations of immunoglobulin and complement which correspond to the subepithelial deposits seen by electron microscopy. The inflammatory response is possibly due to the deposition of immune complexes within the kidney, although the localization of streptococcal cellular components or exotoxins may also play a role.

Treatment. Therapy is directed at the secondary phenomena of volume excess, hypertension, and seizures. This consists mainly of sodium restriction, diuretics, and anticonvulsants. Recovery is usually complete in children, but fatalities may occur during the acute phase. AGN in adults may be associated with a poorer prognosis and a higher incidence of chronic renal disease.

Prevention. Treatment of streptococcal pharyngitis perhaps lowers the subsequent incidence of AGN. Therapy of impetigo, however, has no effect on the prevention of AGN. Therapy, therefore, is directed toward the prevention of transmission of infection, especially when known nephritogenic strains are involved. Effective regimens are presented in Table 27-3.

OTHER STREPTOCOCCI PATHOGENIC FOR MAN

Group B Streptococci (Streptococcus agalactiae)

Morphology and Physiology These organisms cannot be distinguished on a morpholog-

ic basis from other beta-hemolytic streptococci. In liquid media however, they tend to grow as diplococci or in short chains. Beta hemolysis is produced by an unidentified hemolysin (not SLO) that may cause a double zone of hemolysis on rabbit blood agar when refrigerated after initial incubation. Colonies are usually large and mucoid (greater than 2 mm) with a relatively small zone of beta hemolysis and are occasionally pigmented yellow, orange, or red. This species may be presumptively identified by its ability to hydrolyze sodium hippurate. A majority of strains can grow in 6.5 percent sodium chloride, and a few may grow in the presence of 40 percent bile. Esculin is not hydrolyzed. A small percentage are bacitracin sensitive and may be falsely identified as group A by this screening procedure.

Antigenic Structure The group-specific carbohydrate of *S. agalactiae* is composed of D-glucosamine, D-galactose, and L-rhamnose, with the latter being the major antigenic determinant. There are five serotypes, four based on capsular polysaccharieds (Ia, Ib, II, and III), and a fifth (Ic) that is presumably a protein.

Group C Streptococci (Streptococcus equisimilis, Streptococcus zooepidemicus, Streptococcus equi, Streptococcus dysgalactiae)

Morphology and Physiology The morphology of group C streptococci is similar to that of group A organisms. The species of group C are beta hemolytic, with the exception of *S. dysgalactiae*, which produces the alpha reaction. *S. equisimilis* produces SLO, streptokinase, and other extracellular products and, thus, may induce a rise in antibody titers following infection. The nature of the beta hemolysin of the other two species in unknown.

Antigenic Structure The group-specific carbohydrate is a polymer of L-rhamnose and N-acetyl-D-galactosamine, the latter being the major antigenic determinant. Serotypes within species may be conferred by surface protein antigens that are similar to M protein. Group C streptococci differ from group A streptococci primarily in the substitution of N-acetyl-D-galactosamine for N-acetyl-D-glucosamine, yet the former are not associated with rheumatic fever or glomerulonephritis, perhaps because of the general absence of virulence factors, such as M protein.

Group D Streptococci (Streptococcus faecalis, Streptococcus faecium, Streptococcus durans, Streptococcus bovis, Streptococcus equinus)

Morphology and Physiology Group D streptococci commonly grow as diplococci or short chains, and rare motile strains are encountered. The species of this serologic group are divided into enterococci (*S. faecalis, S. faecium,* and *S. durans*) and nonenterococci (*S. equinus* and *S. bovis*) based upon the ability of the former to grow in the presence of 6.5 percent sodium chloride. Group D streptococci differ from most other streptococci in their capacity to grow at 45C and to withstand temperatures above 60C. In addition, they grow in the presence of 40 percent bile and hydrolyze esculin. All give the alpha or gamma reaction on blood agar, with the exception of *S. faecalis* var. *zymogenes,* which is beta hemolytic. The species within this group may be separated on the basis of their biochemical reactions, which are given in Table 27-6. An occasional nongroup D viridans streptococcus (*S. mutans*) may grow on bile and hydrolyze esculin but will not grow in the presence of 6.5 percent sodium chloride. Such strains may be separated from *S. bovis* and *S. equinus* by their inability to hydrolyze starch.

Antigenic Structure In contrast to most of the other groups of streptococci, the group D antigen is not a wall carbohydrate but is a glycerol teichoic acid containing glucose and D-alanine. This antigen appears to be associated with the cytoplasm or plasma membrane. The cell wall polysaccharides in these species serve as type-specific antigens. Variations in peptidoglycan structure exist among the species of group D, specifically as additions to the peptide portion: *S. faecalis* contains only glutamic acid, lysine, and alanine, while *S. faecium* and *S. durans* also contain aspartic acid, and *S. bovis* and *S. equinus* contain threonine.

Group G Streptococci (Streptococcus anginosus, Streptococcus sp.)

Morphology and Physiology The strains containing the group G antigen, for the most part, do not have species designations. Group G contains the minute or small colony and small cell variants of the species *S. anginosus* and other strains that tend to produce larger beta-hemolytic colonies. Group G streptococci produce SLO, streptokinase, NADase, DNase, and hyaluronidase and may elicit antibody rises, especially to SLO, following infection.

Antigenic Structure The group G carbohydrate is composed of galactose, galactosamine, and rhamnose, with the latter being the major antigenic determinant. There are several serotypes within the group, but the antigens are poorly studied. Strains have been isolated that contain an antigen similar to, or identical with, group A type 12 M protein.

Other Groupable Streptococci Other species of streptococci bearing group antigens have been described but are of lesser clinical importance. These consist of group E, group F (*S. anginosus*—alpha, beta, or gamma reaction), group H (*S. sanguis*—alpha reaction), group K (*S. salivarius, Streptococcus* sp.—alpha reaction), and group N (*S. lactis* and *S. cremoris*), whose group antigen is a glycerol-alanine-galactose teichoic acid.

TABLE 27-6 BIOCHEMICAL AND GROWTH CHARACTERISTICS OF GROUP D STREPTOCOCCI

	S. faecalis	S. faecium	S. durans	S. bovis	S. equinus
Bile esculin	+	+	+	+	+
6.5% NaCl	+	+	+	−	−
Sorbitol	+	−	−	±	−
Mannitol	+	+	−	±	−
Lactose	+	+	+	+	−
Starch	−	−	−	+	+

± = *variable within species*
S. faecalis *var.* zymogenes *is beta hemolytic, and* S. faecalis *var* liquefaciens *liquefies gelatin.*

Viridans Streptococci The designation "streptococcus viridans" or viridans group has been assigned to a large number of alpha-reacting streptococci that resist classification by group-specific carbohydrates. This heterogeneous collection of streptococci, generally found in the mouth or upper respiratory tract, includes the following species: *S. pneumoniae* (Chap. 28), *S. mitior*, *S. milleri*, *S. sanguis*, and *S. mutans*. They are usually classified by fermentation patterns, cell wall sugar composition, and production of dextrans (glucose 1-6 polymers) or levans (fructose 2-6 polymers) from sucrose. Strict criteria for speciation have yet to be evolved. *S. mutans*, an organism perhaps important in the formation of dental plaque, has been subdivided into four serologic groups (a, b, c, and d). This organism possesses a cellular and extracellular dextransucrase that produces an insoluble dextran polymer from sucrose. This dextran is an important component of dental plaque, which, in addition, may contain up to 10^{11} streptococci per gram wet weight.

INFECTIONS BY NONGROUP A STREPTOCOCCI

Although most of the serious streptococcal infections in man are caused by members of group A, there is increasing awareness of the medical importance of streptococci of other groups as causes of human infection. The clinical and epidemiologic features of some of these infections are presented below.

Group B Infections EPIDEMIOLOGY. Group B streptococci are commonly found among the flora of the pharynx, gastrointestinal tract, and vagina. Approximately 5 to 10 percent of pregnant women are vaginal carriers. The exact rates of transmission of group B streptococci to the newborn infant are unknown, as is the incidence of clinical infection following colonization. Other means of transmission have been poorly studied.

CLINICAL MANIFESTATIONS. Group B streptococci cause wound infection, endocarditis, puerperal infection, neonatal septicemia, and meningitis. Wound infections are most commonly seen in patients with diabetes mellitus and peripheral vascular disease. In the last 15 years, group B streptococci have been noted with increased frequency as causes of neonatal septicemia and meningitis. A majority of these infections are encountered following obstetric complications, such as prolonged labor, premature rupture of membranes, and obstetric manipulation. The mortality is approximately 50 percent and is higher when the onset is within 10 days of delivery.

TREATMENT. Penicillin G is the treatment of choice for group B streptococcal infections. A majority of strains are also sensitive to erythromycin, chloramphenicol, cephalosporins, lincomycin, and clindamycin.

Group C Infections Streptococci of group C are important causes of disease in animals. They infect a wide variety of animal species and are responsible for suppurative as well as nonsuppurative infections. The species of major interest in human infections is *S. equisimilis*, which has been isolated from the upper respiratory tract of normal and diseased swine, cows, horses, and man. It has been recovered from streptococcal pharyngitis, but, except for one reported epidemic in which group C pharyngitis was followed by acute glomerulonephritis, poststreptococcal sequelae do not occur even in severe infections. Group C organisms are occasionally associated with erysipelas and puerperal fever.

Group D Infections EPIDEMIOLOGY. Group D streptococci commonly inhabit the skin and the upper respiratory, gastrointestinal, and genitourinary tracts. A majority of infections are apparently caused by invasion by these normal flora. Person-to-person transmission is not of documented importance.

CLINICAL MANIFESTATIONS. Group D streptococci, most commonly *S. faecalis*, are frequently associated with urinary and biliary tract infections, septicemia, endocarditis, wound infection, and intra-abdominal abscess complicating diverticulitis, appendicitis, and other diseases which alter the integrity of the gastrointestinal tract. Group D streptococci are a frequent cause of bacterial endocarditis, especially in the elderly or in patients with underlying valvular heart disease who undergo manipulation of the genitourinary or gastrointestinal tracts.

TREATMENT. The proper identification of group D streptococci is of practical importance in that the enterococcal strains are generally resistant to penicillin G and the penicillinase-resistant penicillins. However, many infections may show a synergistic response when treated with penicillin and an aminoglycoside, such as gentamicin or streptomycin. Among the penicillins, ampicillin is the single most effective agent. Other antibiotics useful in the penicillin-allergic patient are vancomycin and erythromycin. The nonenterococcal strains *(S. bovis* and *S. equinus)* are generally sensitive to penicillin G.

Other Streptococcal Infections INFECTIVE ENDOCARDITIS. Infective endocarditis may be defined as implantation of bacteria or fungi on the endocardial surface of the heart. Endocarditis is most frequently encountered on damaged heart valves or in congenital heart disease. The majority of cases are caused by streptococci (viridans, pneumococci, group D) and staphylococci. Endocarditis may follow a fulminant course (acute) or be a prolonged insidious illness (subacute). Streptococci are more commonly associated with the latter presentation. Endocarditis may complicate infection at other sites, such as pneumonia, abscesses, or urinary tract infection, or may be a result of transient bacteremia, such as that associated with dental manipulation.

The symptoms and signs of endocarditis are fever, weight loss, anemia, heart murmur, splenomegaly, and peripheral embolization. The diagnosis is confirmed by repeated blood culture (aerobic, anaerobic, and fungal). In most cases over 90 percent of the blood cultures taken are positive. The duration of therapy and choice of antibiotic are determined by the sensitivity of the isolated organism to various antimicrobial agents. Parenteral therapy is given for three to six weeks. Many cases of endocarditis may be prevented by prophylactic administration of antibiotics to patients with underlying heart disease who undergo procedures associated with transient bacteremia (dental work or genitourinary manipulation).

DENTAL CARIES. The production of dental plaque and dental caries is a complex phenomenon and will not be discussed in detail here (Chap. 56). The role of streptococci, particularly *S. mutans*, is currently under investigation. This organism possesses a cellular and extracellular dextransucrase and produces an insoluble dextran polymer using sucrose as its substrate. Dental caries may be produced in animals by infection with *S. mutans* combined with the introduction of sucrose into the diet, and may be prevented by the addition of dextranases. *S. mutans*, in addition to *S. sanguis, S. mitis*, and various actinomycetes and other bacteria, appears to play a complex role in cariogenesis in man. Oral streptococci also play a significant role in the pathogenesis of bacterial endocarditis, as discussed above.

MISCELLANEOUS. Streptococci of all groups, and those that are not identified by species or group, may cause pneumonia, septic arthritis, biliary or intra-abdominal infection, urinary tract infection, cellulitis or wound infection, meningitis, osteomyelitis, or sinusitis. Recently, with improved techniques of anaerobic bacteriology, microaerophilic and anaerobic streptococci (Peptococcaceae) are frequently isolated from patients with lung abcess, septic abortion or puerperal infection, endocarditis, empyema, and intra-abdominal infection (Chap. 48).

FURTHER READING

Books and Reviews

Hoeprich PD (ed): Infectious Diseases. Hagerstown, Md, Harper & Row, 1972, pp. 255-268, 745-752, 1045-1060

Markowitz M, Gordis L: Rheumatic Fever. Philadelphia, Saunders, 1972

Uhr JW: The Streptococcus, Rheumatic Fever, and Glomerulonephritis. Baltimore, Williams & Wilkins, 1964

Wannamaker LW, Matsen JM: Streptococci and Streptococcal Diseases. New York, Academic Press, 1972

Wintrobe MM (ed): Harrison's Principles of Internal Medicine. New York, McGraw-Hill, 1974, pp. 761-765, 778-784, 1171-1176, 1388-1396

Selected Papers

Duma RJ, Weinberg AN, Medrek JF, Kunz LJ: Streptococcal infections: bacteriologic and clinical study of streptococcal bacteremia. Medicine 48:87, 1969

Fox EN, Waldman RH, Wittner MK, Mauceri AA, Dorfman A: Protective study with a group A streptococcal M protein vaccine. J Clin Invest 52:1885, 1973

Freedman P, Meister HR, Lee HJ, Smith EC, Co BS, Nidus BD: The renal response to streptococcal infection. Medicine 49:433, 1970

Ginsburg I: Mechanisms of cell and tissue injury induced by group A streptococci: relation to post-streptococcal sequelae. J Infect Dis 126:294, 419, 1972

Lancefield RC: Current knowledge of type-specific M anti-gens of group A streptococci. J Immunol 89:307, 1962

Stollerman GH: Rheumatogenic and nephritogenic strep-tococci. Circulation 43:915, 1971

Wannamaker LW: Differences between streptococcal infections of the throat and of the skin. N Engl J Med 282:23, 78, 1970

Weinstein L, Schlesinger JJ: Pathoanatomic, pathophys-iologic and clinical correlations in endocarditis. N Engl J Med 291:832, 1122, 1974.

Zabriskie J: The role of streptococci in human glomerulo-nephritis. J Exp Med 130:180s, 1971

28
Streptococcus Pneumoniae

Streptococcus pneumoniae is an encapsulated gram-positive coccus that typically occurs in pairs and short chains. It is an inhabitant of the upper respiratory tract of man and certain animals and causes infection primarily of the respiratory tract and contiguous areas. It is the etiologic agent of pneumococcal pneumonia, an acute bacterial infection of the lungs characterized by abrupt onset, chills, fever, chest pain, and productive cough. Pneumococcal pneumonia is the classic prototype from which our present concepts of the pathogenesis of pneumonia have evolved.

The pneumococcus was isolated independently in France in 1881 by Pasteur, and by Sternberg in the United States, but its causative role in acute lobar pneumonia was not recognized until several years later. Referred to in American literature as *Diplococcus pneumoniae* since 1920, the pneumococcus has been recently reclassified as *Streptococcus pneumoniae* because of its genetic relatedness to the streptococci.

Some of the most important achievements in medical science have resulted from studies on this organism. The recognition of different types of pneumococci based on serologic differences in capsular material provided the basis for specific serum therapy and for the classic studies of Heidelberger, Avery, and Goebel on the immunologic and chemical properties of the capsular polysaccharides. In the area of molecular biology, the study of transformation in pneumococci led to the discovery that DNA is the transforming material, a discovery that has been revolutionary in its implications.

Pneumococcal pneumonia is no longer the "captain of the men of death" described by Sir William Osler in his famous textbook before the advent of the sulfonamides and the introduction of penicillin. Although many factors, such as antimicrobial therapy, increasing age of our hospitalized population, and modern immunosuppressive or tumor chemotherapy, have altered its clinical and epidemiologic manifestations, pneumococcal pneumonia remains an important cause of morbidity and mortality. Pneumonia is the only infectious disease among the 10 most common causes of death in the United States today.

Morphology

The pneumococcus is an encapsulated gram-positive coccus, oval, or spherical in

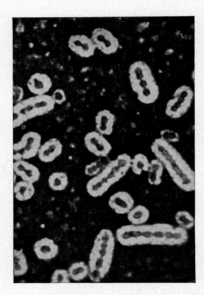

FIG. 28-1. Pneumococcus from spinal fluid. Preparation stained by P. Bruce White method to show capsules. ×1,8000. (Courtesy of Dr. Josephine Bittner and Dr. C.F. Robinow)

shape and 0.5 to 1.25 μm in diameter. Characteristically the organism is lancet shaped, and as observed in direct smears of sputum and body fluids it occurs singly, in pairs, and in short chains (Fig. 28-1). Continued laboratory cultivation, especially on unfavorable media, leads to the formation of longer chains. Pneumococci are very sensitive to the products of their fermentative metabolism, resulting in a gram-negative staining reaction as the culture ages. Capsules may be readily demonstrated by examination of wet mounts of the organisms in India ink or by the use of homologous typespecific antibody in the quellung reaction (p. 447).

Physiology

S. pneumoniae is a facultative anaerobe that can use a fairly wide range of fermentable carbohydrates. Its energy-yielding metabolism is primarily of the lactic acid type, but the amount of acid accumulating is small unless the culture is periodically neutralized. Under aerobic conditions a significant amount of hydrogen peroxide is formed, along with acetic and formic acids. Since *S. pneumoniae* does not produce catalase or peroxidase, the accumulation of hydrogen peroxide kills the organism unless catalase is provided in the culture medium. Erythrocytes are an excellent source of the enzyme.

Cultural Characteristics The pneumococcus has complex nutritional requirements, and although chemically defined synthetic media are available, primary isolation and routine work employ such media as brain-heart infusion agar or trypticase soy agar and broth enriched with 5 percent defibrinated blood. The optimum pH for growth is 7.4 to 7.8. Since 5 to 10 percent of pneumococcal strains require an increased CO_2 concentration for primary growth on solid media, a candle jar or CO_2 incubator should be used for these strains. On blood agar plates pneumococci have a characteristic appearance. Young cultures of encapsulated organisms produce circular, glistening, dome-shaped colonies about 1 mm in diameter. Colonies incubated aerobically are surrounded by a zone of alpha hemolysis similar to the greenish hemolysis observed with the viridans streptococci. Under anaerobic conditions colonies are surrounded by a zone of beta hemolysis due to oxygen-labile pneumolysin O. Colonies produced by type 3 organisms are usually larger and more mucoid than those produced by the other types, a reflection of the greater size of its capsule. As pneumococcus colonies on blood agar become older, autolytic changes result in the collapse of the center of the colony.

Unlike other streptococci, *S. pneumoniae* has a nutritional requirement for the nitrogenous alcohol, choline. Although ethanolamine may be substituted for choline in the culture medium, a number of physiologic defects are observed in the organisms produced. Most of these defects can be directly attributed to changes in the teichoic acid of the surface layers of the organism. About 85 percent of the cell's choline is found in the teichoic acid of the cell wall, and the remaining 15 percent is localized in the membrane lipoteichoic acid.

Laboratory Identification Because of their alpha hemolysis on blood agar, the viridans streptococci may be confused with *S. pneumoniae*. The procedures used for the laboratory identification of the pneumococcus are designed primarily to distinguish it from the alpha-hemolytic streptococci. One of the most useful of these is the bile solubility test, which is based on the presence in pneumococci of an autolytic amidase that cleaves the bond between alanine and muramic acid in the peptidoglycan. The amidase is activated by surface-active agents, such as bile or bile salts, resulting in dissolution of the organisms. The test should be carried out at neutral pH using deoxycholate and live young cells in a saline suspension. In contrast to the pneumococci, viridans streptococci are not bile soluble.

The test most widely used at present for the presumptive identification of the pneumococcus is the optochin disk sensitivity test. Optochin (ethyl hydrocuprein hydrochloride) is a quinine derivative that inhibits growth of pneumococci but not of viridans streptococci. For testing, a filter paper disk impregnated with the drug is applied to the surface of a blood agar plate streaked with a lawn of a pure culture.

QUELLUNG REACTION. The most useful method for the identification of *S. pneumoniae* is the Neufeld quellung or capsular precipitation reaction. It is easy to perform, rapid, and not only identifies an organism as a pneumococcus but also specifies its type. It can be used directly for the identification of pneumococci in sputum, spinal fluid, exudates, or culture. The test is performed by mixing on a slide a loopful of emulsified sputum (or other clinical material) with a loopful of antipneumococcal serum and methylene blue. The preparation is examined immediately under the oil immersion lens. In a positive reaction, which occurs when pneumococci are brought into contact with homologous anticapsular serum, the capsule becomes more refractile and greatly swollen in appearance.

Unfortunately, there is at **present no** generally available source of diagnostic sera for the typing of pneumococci in the United States. Pools of antisera reacting with the first 33 types of pneumococci are available commercially, and a highly concentrated antiserum, onmiserum, which reacts with all 82 pneumococcal capsular types is provided by the Statens Seruminstitut in Copenhagen, Denmark. Also available from the Copenhagen source are antisera reacting with each of the 82 pneumococcal serotypes.

ANIMAL INOCULATION. If no organisms can be seen in the gram stain of a sputum specimen from a patient suspected of having pneumococcal pneumonia, the sputum should be injected intraperitoneally into a white mouse. The mouse is exquisitely sensitive to most of the capsular types of pneumococci and succumbs to fatal infection 16 to 48 hours after infection. A single colony-forming unit of some types is a lethal dose. The mouse usually effectively eliminates other organisms that may be present in the sputum, and pneumococci may be isolated in pure culture from the heart blood. Several types of pneumococci, however, of which type 14 is the most commonly encountered, are less virulent for the mouse and do not produce fatal infections within four days.

Genetic Variation The possession of a capsule by the pneumococcus provides an easily recognized marker for genetic studies. When cultured on the surface of solid media, encapsulated organisms form characteristic glistening colonies that are mucoid or smooth and contain S organisms. If such organisms are cultured in the presence of homologous antiserum, they produce rough, granular colonies composed of nonencapsulated rough or R cells. In such a culture the antiserum selects for R mutants present in any pneumococcal culture. Conversely, when broth cultures of R pneumococci are inoculated into mice, the R organisms are replaced by S pneumococci of the same serologic type as that from which the R strain was derived. In the animal, the less virulent organisms are destroyed by the host, and the more virulent encapsulated forms survive and are specifically selected. The exquisite sensitivity of the mouse to most pneumococcal capsular types permits detection of small numbers of S organisms that arise from back-mutations and that would be undetectable unless cultured in a selective environment. The conventional method of maintaining the maximum virulence of a culture by several passages through a mouse is based on this principle.

A second type of genetic variation that occurs in *S. pneumoniae* is transformation. This phenomenon was first observed in 1928 by Griffith and further studied by Avery, MacLeod, and McCarty in classic experiments that demonstrated conclusively the genetic role of DNA. In Griffith's original experiment, it was observed that mice injected with unencapsulated avirulent type 2 *S. pneumoniae*, together with heat-killed cells from a virulent encapsulated type 3 strain, frequently succumbed to the infection. From these infected animals living

organisms of the virulent encapsulated type 3 could be isolated. The active principle in the heat-killed organisms responsible for transforming the avirulent organisms to virulent ones was later identified by Avery's group as DNA. The transformation in pneumococci of a number of additional characteristics other than capsule type has also been demonstrated, as has been the transformation of genetic markers between pneumococci and streptococci. The study of transformation in the pneumococcus continues to be an intriguing area of interest for the molecular geneticist, who is currently examining binding and uptake of DNA by the cell and its integration into the chromosome. The pneumococcus system provides an accessible model for the study of genetic recombination (Chap. 8). The recent isolation of pneumococcal bacteriophages should also prove useful for studies on the mechanism of DNA uptake.

Antigenic Structure

Capsular Antigens Pneumococci may be separated immunologically into 82 types on the basis of their polysaccharide capsule. These polysaccharides are high-molecular-weight gels whose sugar composition varies with the immunologic type (Chap. 6). The structure of types 3, 6, and 8 has been fully characterized, and the biosynthesis pathway of type 3 has been defined. Type 3 polysaccharide consists of repeating units of cellobiuronic acid (D-glucuronic acid linked to D-glucose by a β-1,4 linkage; Fig. 28-2). Some of the pneumococcal types cross-react with other types of pneumococci, with *Klebsiella*, *Rhizobium*, enterobacteria, fungi, and with group A human erythrocytes. The range of substances eliciting cross-reactions with certain pneumococci is indicative of the wide distribution in nature

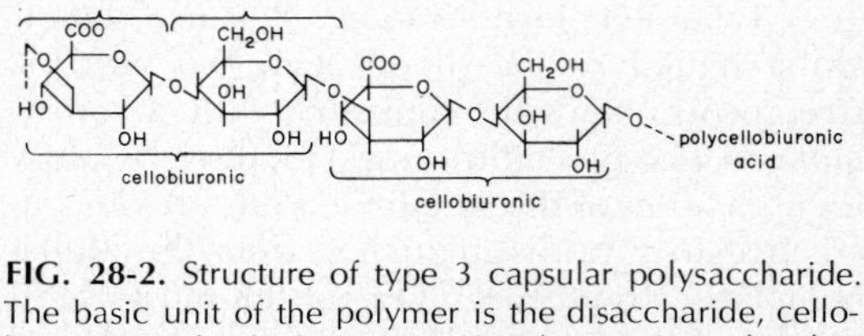

FIG. 28-2. Structure of type 3 capsular polysaccharide. The basic unit of the polymer is the disaccharide, cellobiuronic acid, which consists of D-glucuronic acid and D-glucose connected by a β-1,4 glycosidic bond.

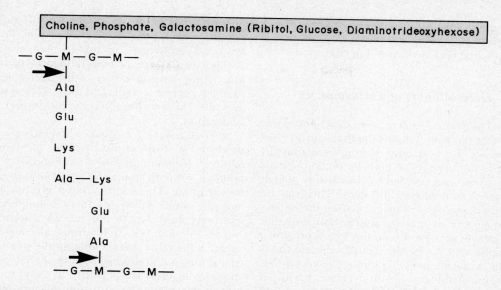

FIG. 28—3. Schematic diagram of proposed cell wall structure of *S. pneumoniae*. The basic element is the N-acetylgluco-samine-N-acetylmuramic acid backbone of a typical peptidoglycan which has two kinds of substituents attached to it: (1) the usual tetrapeptide (2 alanine, 1 glutamic acid, 1 lysine), which are further cross-linked, and (2) chains of a tei-choic acid polymer. The arrow indicates site of attach of autolysin. (Adapted from Mossner and Tomasz: J Biol Chem 245:287, 1970)

of polysaccharides similar to those of the pneu-mococci.

The type 12 pneumococcus interacts with concanavallin A, the binding apparently oc-curring through kojibiosyl residues (0-α-D-glucopyranosyl-(1→2)-D-glucose) in the pneu-mococcus polysaccharide.

As will be discussed on page 450, the poly-saccharide capsule is essential to the pathoge-nicity of the pneumococcus, and antibodies that protect man or animals against infection are directed against this capsular material.

Somatic Antigens A species-specific car-bohydrate, the C polysaccharide, is a major structural component of the cell wall of all pneumococci. This C antigen is a teichoic acid polymer rich in choline, galactosamine, and phosphate, and it probably also contains ribitol, glucose, and diaminotrideoxyhexose. Although the structure of the pneumococcal teichoic acid has not been established, a tentative model has been proposed to illustrate the basic features of the pneumococcal cell wall (Fig. 28-3). The basic element of the wall is a peptidoglycan backbone with two different substituents, tetra-peptides and chains of teichoic acid polymer. Cross-linking of the polysaccharide backbone

occurs via the tetrapeptide substituents and teichoic acid chains. In deoxycholate-induced lysis, one of the major enzymes involved is an autolysin (N-acetylmuramyl-L-alanine amidase) that cleaves the amide bond between alanine and muramic acid. Walls prepared from pneu-mococci in which the cell wall choline has been completely replaced by ethanolamine are totally resistant to the action of this enzyme, emphasizing the existence of a key role for cho-line in the pneumococcus.

Another major antigenic component of the pneumococcus is the F or Forssman antigen, a determinant that cross-reacts with the Forss-man series of mammalian cell surface antigens. The F antigen is a lipoteichoic acid and, like the C antigen, contains choline as a constituent of its teichoic acid. Unlike the C antigen, how-ever, it occurs in the cell membrane and is strongly bound to fatty acids.

Type-specific protein antigens, analogous to the M proteins of *S. pyogenes* but immunologi-cally distinct, are present in pneumococci. No correlation has been shown between the pres-ence of a specific type of M protein and type of organism based on capsular polysaccharide. Antibodies to the pneumococcal M protein do not inhibit phagocytosis and are therefore not protective. The transformation of pneumococci from one M protein type to another can be accomplished both in vitro and in vivo.

Determinants of Pathogenicity

The pneumococcus is an excellent example of an extracellular parasite that damages the tissues of the host only as long as it remains outside the phagocytic cell. Protection against phagocytosis is provided by the capsule, which exerts an antiphagocytic effect. This can be readily demonstrated by comparing the behavior in mice of an encapsulated S strain with that of a nonencapsulated R strain. The S organism is highly virulent for the mouse, whereas the R strain is avirulent and rapidly phagocytosed. Removal of the capsule by treatment with an enzyme specific for the polysaccharide renders the organism nonpathogenic and readily susceptible to phagocytosis. Antibodies against the capsular polysaccharide combine specifically with it, rendering the organism susceptible to phagocytosis.

Many aspects of the pathogenesis of pneumococcal infection remain ill defined. The capsular polysaccharide, although relatively nontoxic, is present in a soluble form in the body fluids of infected animals and man. High levels in the serum or urine are associated with severe infections accompanied by bacteremia, empyema, and a high mortality rate. Excessive amounts of free polysaccharide neutralize antibody and make it inaccessible to the invading organisms. Another observation, the explanation for which remains obscure, is the relationship between certain serotypes and the more severe forms of pneumococcal infection. Recent findings suggest that a correlation exists between the more virulent serotypes and reactivity with the Fc portion of the immunoglobulin. The capsular polysaccharide probably plays a role in this nonspecific binding similar to that of protein A of *Staphylococcus aureus*. The importance of this role remains to be clarified.

Pneumococci produce a hemolysin, pneumolysin 0, with properties similar to those of streptolysin 0. It is an SH-activated cholesterol-sensitive cytolytic toxin that disrupts cell membranes. In addition to its hemolytic activity, it is dermatoxic and lethal. The role of pneumolysin in the pathogenesis of human pneumococcal infections is unknown. Pneumococcal septicemia in rabbits, however, is accompanied by a spherocytic hemolytic anemia. Prior immunization with the material protects against a challenge dose. This system provides an excellent model for further investigation.

Neuraminidase, a glycosidic enzyme, is produced by fresh clinical isolates of S. *pneumoniae*. Neuraminidases are produced by a number of pathogenic bacteria and by the myxoviruses. Their action is on glycoprotein and glycolipid substrates in cell membranes and body fluid, where they cleave a terminal N-acetyl-neuraminic acid from an adjacent sugar. Although a specific role for the pneumococcal enzyme in disease has not been demonstrated, the organism's ability to grow in the human nasopharynx and in the mucous secretions within the bronchial tree requires special metabolic capacities. Neuraminidase is only one of these factors contributing to the invasiveness of the organism.

The basic question that remains unanswered and that, if answered, might prevent morbidity and mortality from pneumococcal infections is the identification of the factor or factors responsible for lethality. At present pneumococci are believed to produce disease solely through their capacity to multiply in the tissues. The possibility remains, however, that a toxin is elaborated under in vivo conditions of growth and that new techniques will be required for its demonstration. Complex multifaceted alterations occur in the metabolism of the host following infection, but it is as yet unknown whether any of the observed biochemical alterations are responsible for the lethal action of the organism.

Clinical Infection

Epidemiology Pneumococcal pneumonia is the most common form of acute bacterial pneumonia: one case occurs annually for every 500 persons in the United States. The organisms are carried in the nasopharynx of healthy contact carriers, who constitute the major reservoir for pneumococcal infections. Multiple infections within family units, however, indicate that infections also result from contact with another case. The carrier rate, ranging from about 5 to 60 percent, varies with the season of the year, as does the frequency rate of the various types. Pneumococcal infections are usually more numerous during the winter months when frequent viral infections of the upper respiratory tract predispose to infection and spread of the organisms.

Since serologic typing was important for effective treatment with type-specific antisera before the advent of modern chemotherapy, retrospective studies have provided an excellent insight into the epidemiology of the pneumococcal carrier state. Seventy-five percent of all cases of pneumococcal pneumonia in the adult are caused by nine types: types 1, 3, 4, 5, 7, 8, 12, 14, and 19. During the past 40 years the predominance of pneumococcal capsular types has changed. A shift has been observed away from the predominance of types 1, 2, and 3 infections previously observed to a more balanced distribution, with types 8 and 4 now more common. In pneumonias of infants and children the most frequent type is type 14. Except for type 3, which is a common inhabitant of the normal pharynx, pneumococci of the higher numbered types are usually associated with the carrier state rather than the more virulent lower-numbered types.

The incidence of pneumococcal infections is highest in the 30 to 50 age group, where occurrence is often conditioned by underlying chronic obstructive pulmonary disease.

Pathogenesis Pneumococcal pneumonia is rarely a primary infection and results only when the normal defense barriers of the respiratory tract are disturbed. Chilling, anesthesia, and morphine and alcoholic intoxication commonly predispose to pneumococcal disease. By slowing epiglottal reflex these factors facilitate aspiration of infected secretions from the upper respiratory tract. Viral infections of the upper respiratory tract are a major contributory cause of pneumococcal pneumonia and often precede its abrupt onset. Pneumococci present in the nasopharynx proliferate in the viral-modified environment and are carried down into the alveoli by the thin bronchial secretions. A number of additional clinical conditions also predispose to acute pneumococcal pneumonia: cardiac failure, noxious gases, pulmonary stasis resulting from prolonged bed rest. In all of these cases fluid accumulates in the alveoli, providing an excellent culture medium for the organism.

THE PNEUMOCOCCAL LESION. Invasion of alveolar tissue by pneumococci results in an outpouring of edema fluid that facilitates rapid multiplication and spread of the organisms to other alveoli. Polymorphonuclear leukocytes and red blood cells accumulate in the infected alveoli, leading to complete consolidation of the lobe or segment. Crowding of leukocytes in the alveoli promotes phagocytosis and destruction of the invading organisms. Macrophages participate in the final stages of resolution, and in most of the less serious cases, recovery is complete and the lung parenchyma is restored to its normal state. Effective present-day antibiotic therapy, however, frequently alters or halts the classic inflammatory response so that the distinguishing histologic features of the spreading pneumonic lesion are obscured.

In the adult, pneumococcal pneumonia characteristically involves one or more complete lobes. In infants, young children, and the aged, however, the lesions may be more patchy in their distribution and localized around the bronchi.

From the primary lesion in the lung, pneumococci may invade the pleural cavity and pericardium with the formation of extensive purulent foci (empyema). In fulminating infections bacteremia is also common and may lead to infections of the meninges, heart valves, or joints.

PHAGOCYTIC DEFENSE. The phagocytic cells in the lungs provide the major line of defense against pneumococcal infections (Chap. 18). In the early stages of the developing lesion before antibody levels are sufficiently high to be beneficial in controlling the infection, phagocytosis of encapsulated bacteria occurs by the antibody-independent mechanism of surface phagocytosis. This type of phagocytosis results when leukocytes trap the organisms against tissue surfaces, against the surfaces of adjacent leukocytes, or against interstices of fibrin clots. In the normal adult natural host resistance is high, and even without any form of treatment 7 of every 10 patients with pneumococcal pneumonia will recover.

Clinical Manifestations Classical pneumococcal pneumonia strikes suddenly with a single violent shaking chill and fever that ranges between 102 and 106F (38.8 and 41.1C). The patient usually presents a history of a mild upper respiratory infection preceding the acute onset by a few days. Severe pleuritic pain is often present, and a cough developing during the course of the disease is productive of rusty mucopurulent sputum. In untreated cases recovery may be as dramatic as the onset, with fever terminating abruptly by crisis 5 to 10 days after onset. In other cases fever subsides more gradually by lysis. A dramatic crisis often occurs within 24 hours in patients receiving effective antibiotic therapy.

The classic presentation of acute pneumococcal pneumonia is unmistakable. Atypical cases often occur, however, in which a diagnosis is less obvious. This is especially true in the case of the alcoholic, the elderly, or the debilitated patient in whom symptoms may be less dramatic or overshadowed by symptoms of severe prostration, confusion, or delirium.

Extrapulmonary Disease. The most common complication of pneumococcal pneumonia is pleurisy with effusion. If bacteria gain access to the effusion the leukocyte response is greatly increased, and empyema results. Empyema, meningitis, pericarditis, and endocarditis are serious complications associated with an increased risk of death.

Meningitis. The pneumococcus is the most common cause of bacterial meningitis in adults and of recurrent meningitis in all age groups. It is usually preceded by pulmonary infection or by symptomatic primary infection of the upper respiratory tract and contiguous structures, ie, sinusitis, mastoiditis, or otitis. Alcoholism, head trauma, sickle cell disease, multiple myeloma, and general debility predispose to pneumococcal meningitis.

Prognosis.   The case fatality rate of untreated pneumococcal pneumonia is about 30 percent. With specific therapy the overall fatality rate is about 5 percent. However, in adults with bacteremic pneumococcal disease, there remains a high case fatality rate (approximately 25 percent) despite antibiotic treatment and shift in prevalent capsular types. Prognosis is influenced adversely by increasing age, an extrapulmonary site of infection, the presence of cirrhosis or diabetes mellitus, immunodeficiency diseases, and infection with certain capsular types, especially type 3. The case fatality rate in type 3 bacteremic pneumococcal pneumonia is over 50 percent, even with antibiotic therapy.

Immunity Spontaneous recovery from pneumococcal pneumonia is dependent on the production of type-specific antibodies which are first demonstrable in the serum 5 to 6 days after onset. Agglutination by type-specific antibody of the organisms in edema-filled alveoli immobilizes the organisms and halts spread of the lesion. Also, by combination with the antiphagocytic capsular polysaccharide, phagocytosis is accelerated.

The bactericidal power of the blood of normal individuals varies with the type of pneumococcus and with the age of the individual. Blood of newborn babies has the same killing power as that of their mothers, but this power is lost within three to five weeks. After that it is observed in an increasing number of persons as they become older until the age of 55 years, when the bactericidal capacity decreases.

Recurrent attacks of pneumococcal infection are usually caused by pneumococci of a different serologic type. Also, persistence of pneumococci in cultures of sputum and throat swabs of patients with pneumococcal pneumonia may be attributed to new types of pneumococci that are acquired during the course of infection. Multiple types are more frequently encountered in patients with chronic respiratory tract infections in whom pneumococci persist longer than in uncomplicated cases. Persistence is not related to the patient's inability to develop antibodies to specific pneumococcal types or to the appearance of drug-resistant organisms.

The immune status of an individual may be determined by the detection in the patient's serum of type-specific antibodies to the polysaccharide capsule. A variety of different serologic tests are useful for this purpose (p. 453). Circulating antibody may also be detected by the intradermal injection of a small amount of the purified homologous polysaccharide. If circulating antibody is present, an immediate wheal and erythema reaction appears within 15 to 30 minutes at the site of the injection. This reaction, known as the Francis test, is attributed to the reaction of polysaccharide and homologous antibody at the local site. Prior to the advent of modern chemotherapy it was widely used to determine the effective dose of type-specific antiserum to be used for treatment.

Laboratory Diagnosis Although a diagnosis of classic acute lobar pneumonia can usually be made on the basis of physical examination and roentgenographic findings, atypical cases, nonpulmonary infections, and pneumonia caused by other organisms are more difficult to diagnose. Also, a number of noninfectious diseases, such as pulmonary infarction, congestive heart failure, and atelectasis may simulate pneumonia and require specific laboratory studies for their differential diagnosis.

The proper collection of sputum is the physician's responsibility and demands that the specimens be mucus expectorated from the lungs rather than samples of saliva. When pneumococcal pneumonia is suspected, blood should be drawn by venipuncture prior to the administration of antibiotics. The pneumococcus is a delicate organism and does not survive for long periods on dry swabs or in physiologic saline. For culture, swabs should be placed immediately in sterile nutrient broth for transport to the laboratory.

A direct examination should be made of sputum smears stained by the gram method to determine the probable etiology of the infection. If positive for gram-positive lancet-shaped diplococci, a presumptive diagnosis of pneumococcal pneumonia may be made. Cultural identification, however, is required to distinguish the pneumococcus definitely from certain other gram-positive cocci. If typing sera are available, the most simple, rapid, and accurate method for the identification of pneumococci by direct examination is the quellung reaction (p. 447).

Specimens for culture should be planted immediately on (1) an enriched medium, such as brain-heart infusion or trypticase soy agar and broth containing 5 percent blood, and (2) in thioglycolate broth. For blood cultures 5 to 15 ml of blood should be inoculated into trypticase soy broth and thioglycolate broth maintaining a ratio of approximately 1:10 between blood and medium. Subcultures should be made by streaking the surface of a blood agar plate. Pour plates with samples of blood provide valuable information on the magnitude of the bacteremia and prognosis of the infection. For culture of body fluids blood agar plates

should be streaked, and 0.5 to 1 ml of the specimen should be inoculated into blood broth. Presumptive identification of pneumococci is based on the appearance of alpha-hemolytic colonies containing organisms that are bile soluble, optochin sensitive, ferment inulin, and give a positive quellung reaction (see p. 447).

Serologic Diagnosis. *Detection of Pneumococcal Antibodies.* A number of techniques have been employed for the demonstration of an immunologic response to pneumococcal infection, including agglutination, quantitative precipitation, mouse protection tests, and bactericidal tests with whole blood. The complement-fixation test cannot be used, since human antibodies to pneumococcal capsular polysaccharides do not fix complement. More recently, indirect hemagglutination, indirect fluorescent antibody, and radioimmunoassay techniques have been employed. The latter test, employing as antigens pneumococcal polysaccharides labeled intrinsically with ^{14}C, has been especially useful in the detection not only of an immunologic response to infection but also of a response following the administration of pneumococcal vaccines. The method is exquisitely sensitive, being capable of detecting specific capsular antibody in nanogram amounts, and requires very small amounts of serum for the assay procedure.

Detection of Capsular Polysaccharide. Capsular polysaccharide appears in the serum and body fluids of patients with pneumococcal infection. The presence of large quantities of the soluble polysaccharide is associated with severe infection accompanied by bacteremia, empyema, and a high mortality rate. In some patients, especially those with slowly resolving infection, capsular polysaccharide may be detected in the urine for several months. First observed by Dochez and Avery over 50 years ago, the phenomenon has been reinvestigated with the more sensitive immunologic methods now available. Counter-immunoelectrophoresis has been utilized to demonstrate specific bacterial antigens in the blood, urine, and spinal fluid of patients and to establish a diagnosis of pneumococcal infection. The pneumococcal capsular antigen present in serum or pleural or cerebrospinal fluids is similar both physically and immunologically to purified pneumococcal polysaccharide (PPP). The polysaccharide in urine, however, is a smaller molecule and has only partial immunologic identity with the PPP. Unanswered at the present time is whether the polysaccharide found in the sera and body fluids of patients with severe infections simply reflects the large amounts produced in these individuals or whether the polysaccharide per se has a deleterious effect on the host or host defense mechanisms. Also unknown is the mechanism by which polysaccharide is ultimately eliminated from the body, since there is no evidence that mammalian cells can degrade pneumococcal polysaccharides.

Treatment   Penicillin G is the recommended drug for all types of pneumococcal infection. Antimicrobial therapy should be started immediately after specimens are obtained for culture and should not be withheld until culture results are available. The choice of drug in the treatment of bacterial pneumonia is based on the results of gram-stained smears of sputum and is usually directed against the pneumococcus. Delay in the administration of specific antipneumococcal therapy probably accounts for the high death rate that is still observed in patients with bacteremic pneumococcal infection. Penicillin G is the drug of choice in the treatment of pneumococcal pneumonia. It is given intramuscularly in a dosage of 600,000 to 1.2 million units per day. Oral penicillin may also be used effectively, but its absorption from the gastrointestinal tract is less predictable, especially in acutely ill patients. In the presence of shock, aqueous penicillin should be given intravenously. Broad-spectrum antibiotics, such as the tetracyclines and cephalosporins, as well as erythromycin, are useful for patients who are highly allergic to penicillin. Treatment should be continued for at least a week to prevent relapse of infection.

Response to penicillin therapy is usually very dramatic, and bacteremia, if present, will clear in a few hours. Failure to respond to penicillin therapy cannot be attributed to penicillin-resistant strain of pneumococcus, since resistant strains are only rarely encountered in clinical practice. Initial response to treatment, followed by relapse, is usually due to the presence of a mixed infection.

Empyema and purulent pericarditis are treated by repeated aspiration of pus and injection of penicillin through a thoracentesis needle or thoracotomy tube. Treatment is facilitated by the use of two enzymes isolated from filtrates of S. pyogenes, streptokinase and streptodornase. Streptokinase lyses the fibrin contained in purulent exudates, and streptodornase depolymerizes the DNA. Long-standing purulent exudates are thus liquefied and can be aspirated.

Prevention   In the United States the case fatality rate of 20 to 30 percent in pneumococcal bacteremia has remained essentially unchanged by two decades of antibiotic therapy. Attempts to reduce this rate have focused on the development of a pneumococcal vaccine for use in certain high-risk groups. Although pilot studies with polyvalent vaccines containing the 12 or 14 types most frequently associated with bacteremic pneumonia have demonstrated the effectiveness of such an approach, the sheer magnitude of proper surveillance has prevented complete acceptance of a massive immunization program. Major problems are anticipated in the selection of pneumococcal types most likely to cause disease, in identifying and vaccinating high-risk groups, and in subsequent surveillance of the population to determine both the effectiveness of the vaccine and its effect on the ecology of the pneumococcus.

Immunization of the general population with pneumococcal polysaccharide is not justified because of the low incidence of the disease under ordinary circumstances. In certain high-risk groups, however, especially the elderly and those with underlying systemic diseases, immunization with polysaccharide vaccine may be indicated. Also, in areas where pneumococcal pneumonia is still highly endemic and epidemics occasionally occur, as in the gold and diamond mines of South Africa, immunoprophylaxis would be useful.

FURTHER READING

Books and Reviews

Finland M: Excursions into epidemiology: selected studies during the past four decades at Boston City Hospital. J Infect Dis 128:76, 1973

Kass EH, Green GM, Goldstein E: Mechanisms of antibacterial action in the respiratory tract. Bacteriol Rev 30: 488, 1966

Selected Papers

Austrian R: Random gleanings from a life with the pneumococcus. J Infect Dis 131:474, 1975

Briles EB, Tomasz A: Pneumococcal Forssman antigen. A choline-containing lipoteichoic acid. J Biol Chem 248:6394, 1973

Heidelberger M, Nimmich W: Additional immunochemical relationships of capsular polysaccharides of klebsiella and pneumococci. J Immunol 109:1337, 1972

Kaiser AB, Schaffner W: Prospectives: the prevention of bacteremic pneumococcal pneumonia. JAMA 230:404, 1974

McDonnell M, Ronda-Lain C, Tomasz A: "Diplophage": a bacteriophage of *Diplococcus pneumoniae*. Virology 63:577, 1975

Mosser JL, Tomasz A: Choline-containing teichoic acid as a structural component of pneumococcal cell wall and its role in sensitivity to lysis by an autolytic enzyme. J Biol Chem 245:287, 1970

Mufson MA, Kruss DM, Wasil RE, Metzgar WI: Capsular types and outcome of bacteremic pneumococcal disease in the antibiotic era. Arch Intern Med 134:505, 1974

Page MI, Lunn JS: Pneumococcal serotypes associated with acute pneumonia. Am J Epidemiol 98:255, 1973

Seto H, Tomasz A: Early stages in DNA binding and uptake during genetic transformation of pneumococci. Proc Natl Acad Sci USA 71:1493, 1974

Stephens CG, Reed WP, Kronvall G, Williams RC Jr: Reactions between certain strains of pneumococci and Fc of IgG. J Immunol 112:1955, 1974

Winkelstein JA, Shin HS: The role of immunoglobulin in the interaction of pneumococci and the properdin pathway: evidence for its specificity and lack of requirement for the Fc portion of the molecule. J Immunol 112:1635, 1974

29
Neisseria

TABLE 29-1 CHARACTERISTICS DIFFERENTIATING THE SPECIES OF GENUS NEISSERIA

	N. gonorrhoeae	N. meningitidis	N. sicca	N. subflava	N. flavescens	N. mucosa	N. lactamicus
Acid from:							
Glucose	+	+	+	+	−	+	+
Maltose	−	+	+	+	−	+	+
Sucrose	−	−	+	±	−	+	−
Lactose	−	−	−	−	−	−	+
Polysaccharide produced from 5% sucrose	0	0	+	±	+	+	0
Reduction of:							
Nitrate	−	−	−	−	−	+	−
Nitrite	−	±	+	+	+	+	+
Pigment	−	−	±	+	+	−	−
Extra CO_2 for growth	+	+	−	−	−	−	−

Two species of the genus *Neisseria* are of major medical importance: *N. meningitidis* and *N. gonorrhoeae*. The organisms are genetically very closely related, but the clinical manifestations of the diseases they produce are quite different. Discovered in 1885 by Neisser, for whom the genus is named, *N. gonorrhoeae* is the etiologic agent of gonorrhea, the most prevalent of the classical venereal diseases. The sixth and seventh decades of the twentieth century find a worldwide epidemic of gonorrhea in progress.

N. meningitidis is the causative agent of meningococcal meningitis. This disease also has the potential for occurring in epidemic form. Because of the tendency of this illness to be recognized in clusters, there is a great deal of concern when a patient with meningococcal infection is identified. Within the last decade the identification and purification of capsular antigens of two of the types of *N. meningitidis* have resulted in the preparation and commercial availability of vaccines for use in epidemic situations.

Man is the only known reservoir of the members of the genus *Neisseria*, which includes, in addition to *N. meningitidis* and *N. gonorrhoeae*, nonpathogenic organisms that inhabit the upper respiratory tract and other mucosal surfaces of the body. In these positions as resident flora, the other *Neisseria* can be confused with *N. gonorrhoeae* or *N. meningitidis*. Unusual situations occur in which certain of the other species may be responsible for invasive disease in the human host. Species within the genus are shown in Table 29-1.

The genus *Neisseria* is one of four genera included in the family Neisseriaceae. Other genera in the family include *Branhamella*, *Moraxella*, and *Acinetobacter*. The taxonomic classification and an outline of distinguishing characteristics of the four genera of the family Neisseriaceae are given in Table 29-2.

GENUS NEISSERIA

Morphology

Neisseria are gram-negative cocci, 0.6 to 1.0 μm in diameter. The organisms are usually seen in pairs with adjacent sides flattened. Fresh isolates of most *N. meningitidis* serogroups are encapsulated. *N. gonorrhoeae* does not produce a capsule, but pili are present on virulent organisms. *Neisseria* are not motile.

The *Neisseria* are structurally like other gram-negative bacteria. The ultrastructure of the cytoplasm and the cell wall of the meningococcus and the gonococcus are similar. The cell envelope is composed of three major elements: the cytoplasmic membrane, the rigid peptidoglycan layer, and the outer membrane which contains lipopolysaccharide, phospholipid, and proteins which are immunologically significant.

TABLE 29-2 DIFFERENTIAL PROPERTIES OF THE GENERA OF THE FAMILY NEISSERIACEAE

Genus	Morphology	Fermentation of Glucose	Oxidase	Penicillin	G & C Moles %
Neisseria°	Gram-negative cocci	+	+	Sensitive	47–52
Branhamella†	Gram-negative cocci	–	+	Sensitive	40–45
Moraxella‡	Short gram-negative rods	–	+	Sensitive	40–46
Acinetobacter§	Short gram-negative rods	±	–	Sensitive	39–47

°Species: N. gonorrhoeae, N. meningitidis, N. sicca, N. subflava (includes perflava), N. flavescens, N. mucosa, N. lactamicus (species incertae sedis)
†Single species in genus: B. catarrhalis (previously N. catarrhalis)
‡Species: M. lacunata, M. bovis, M. nonliquefaciens, M. phenylpyruvica, M. osloensis
§Single species in genus: A. calcoaceticus. Includes two groups:
(1) Ferments glucose; includes organisms known formerly as Herellea vaginicola, Bacterium anitratum, Achromobacter anitratum, Acinetobacter anitratum
(2) Does not ferment glucose; includes organisms known formerly as Mima polymorpha, Acinetobacter lwoffi, Achromobacter hemolyticus var alcaligenes

Physiology

Neisseria are aerobic or facultatively anaerobic organisms. Most strains of *N. meningitidis* and *N. gonorrhoeae* utilize glucose, but the acid produced arises primarily from an oxidative pathway rather than by fermentation, explaining the weak reaction that is usually observed. All *Neisseria* produce catalase and cytochrome oxidase.

Members of the genus are very susceptible to adverse environmental conditions, such as drying, chilling, exposure to unfavorable pH or to sunlight. They should be handled in the laboratory with minimal delay.

Cultural Characteristics

N. meningitidis and *N. gonorrhoeae* are fastidious organisms with complex nutritional growth requirements. Free iron is required for growth, and starch, cholesterol, or albumin should be added to media to neutralize the inhibitory effects of fatty acids.

Cultures derived from normally sterile sites, such as the cerebrospinal fluid, blood, or synovial fluid, can be inoculated on nonselective media, such as chocolate agar. Growth of primary isolates is enhanced by incubation in the presence of 2 to 8 percent CO_2. Some of the apparently beneficial effects of the CO_2 atmosphere may be a result of the increased moisture present in the incubator or candle jar used for culture.

The Thayer-Martin selective medium permits recognition of *N. meningitidis* and *N. gonorrhoeae* from materials contaminated with other bacterial flora. This medium contains chocolate agar modified by the addition of vancomycin to inhibit gram-positive bacteria, colistimethate for inhibition of gram-negative enteric flora, and nystatin for the inhibition of yeast. Most nonpathogenic *Neisseria* species fail to grow in this medium, but only rarely are either meningococci or gonococci inhibited.

Laboratory Identification

A number of biochemical reactions are useful in the differentiation of *N. meningitidis* and *N. gonorrhoeae* from other species that are present in clinical material (Table 29-1). Colonies of *Neisseria* species may be recognized by use of the oxidase test that employs the indicator dye tetramethyl-*p*-phenylenediamine dihydrochloride. When exposed to this dye, colonies turn dark purple within seconds. Since all *Neisseria* are oxidase positive, however, the finding of oxidase-positive gram-negative diplococci in a clinical specimen requires additional tests for confimation and identification of species. Organisms are rapidly killed by the oxidase reagent, therefore, subculture to chocolate agar of the unused portion of the colony should be made immediately.

The distinction between *N. gonorrhoeae* and *N. meningitidis* is usually based upon sugar fermentations. *N. meningitidis* produces acid from both glucose and maltose, whereas *N. gonorrhoeae* produces acid from glucose only. These differential tests of pure cultures can be complicated by some of the growth characteristics of these organisms. For example, the production of acid from carbohydrate sources may be masked by the alkaline products of enzymatic peptone degradation. Supplementary methods of identification are available and may need to be utilized.

A valuable but not fully appreciated differential diagnostic test is based on the synthesis from sucrose of an iodine-reacting polysaccharide by *Neisseria* species other than *N. gonorrhoeae*, *N. meningitidis*, and *N. lactamicus*. The test is simply done by incubating a streaked culture on 5 percent sucrose agar and then treating the culture with modified Gram's iodine. A positive test shows a darkening of the colonies to a red-blue or blue-black color.

Other techniques that are not yet available in service laboratories may become practical as the methodology is standardized. One such test is that of determining the nutritional profile of the organism in question. Chemically defined agar media have been developed that support the growth of *N. meningitidis*, *N. gonorrhoeae*, and *N. lactamicus*. The nutritional profile of each species is distinct and serves to differentiate and identify it. Gas-liquid chromatography is a second such test. The method provides a rapid and accurate means of determining the composition of bacteria and identifying their metabolic products.

In summary, the identification of isolates as *Neisseria* species is based upon the growth of gram-negative, oxidase-positive, catalase-positive diplococci that produce characteristic colonies on blood or chocolate agar plates. The differential utilization of carbohydrates forms the basis for initial speciation. Further immunoserologic diagnosis of *N. meningitidis* can be made on the basis of the identifiable surface antigens, as discussed on page 461.

NEISSERIA MENINGITIDIS

Antigenic Structure

Eight groups of *N. meningitidis*, designated A, B, C, D, X, Y, Z, and Z', have been identified on the basis of agglutination reactions. Organisms in groups A, B, and C are responsible for the great majority of clinically recognized disease. The group A capsular antigen consists of N-acetyl-O-acetyl mannosamine phosphate. The B and C antigens consist of polymers of N-acetyl neuraminic acid (sialic acid). The C antigen is acetyl neuraminic acid but differs immunologically from the B antigen even after removal of the O-acetyl groups. The capsular antigens of the other meningococcal groups have not been characterized. Identification and purification of the group A, B, and C polysaccharide antigens have resulted in the production and testing of these materials as vaccines.

Antigenic similarities to meningococci have been found in unrelated bacteria. Most *Escherichia coli* isolated from the cerebrospinal fluids of newborn infants with meningitis have a K1 capsular polysaccharide antigen that is immunologically identical to that of the group B meningococcus and correlates with the apparent invasiveness of the organism in the neonate. This antigen is easily degraded in the host and is a very poor immunogen in man and animals.

Further distinction of organisms within the B group has been accomplished by a bactericidal technique that identifies at least 10 distinct serotypes of group B organisms. Similarly a bactericidal serotyping technique has been used epidemiologically to examine epidemics of group C meningococcal disease. Cross-reactivity of the bactericidal antibodies with some strains of *N. gonorrhoeae* is observed. At the present time techniques are available for the identification of an epidemic strain of meningococcus, but their role in immunity and vaccine production remains unclear.

In addition to the capsular polysaccharide antigens are the somatic antigens, one of which is a nucleoprotein fraction, and one of which is a somatic carbohydrate antigen. These have not been chemically defined and appear to be common to *Neisseria* within a specific serogroup. These antigens probably account at least in part for the cross-reactivity observed in agglutination testing.

Determinants of Pathogenicity

The capsular polysaccharides contribute to the invasive properties of the meningococci by inhibiting phagocytosis. In the presence of specific antibody, organisms are readily ingested and destroyed by the phagocytic leukocytes. There is no evidence to indicate that intracellular meningococcal organisms that are visible on gram stain can multiply within host cells.

The endotoxins of the meningococcus are basically similar to those of other gram-negative bacteria and are responsible for the extensive vascular damage that is a varying component of the disease they produce.

Clinical Infection

History The first recognition of disease caused by *N. meningitidis* occurred in 1805, with the description of an epidemic of meningitis in Geneva, Switzerland. One year later an outbreak in Medfield, Massachusetts, marked the first recognized outbreak in North America. The causative organism, however, was not identified until 1887, when Weichselbaum described the gram-negative diplococcus in the spinal fluid of patients.

Epidemiology Meningococcal disease is worldwide in distribution and varies from sporadic cases observed in the community to epidemics of infection. In 1973 cases occurred in every state of the United States. Although the reported number of cases of disease in the United States from 1948 to 1973 has been less than 3 cases per 100,000 of the population, in 1945 an outbreak of group A meningococcal disease occurred with a reported case rate of 14 cases per 100,000 of the population (Fig. 29-1). The potential of a meningococcal epidemic is illustrated by the urban epidemic which began in Sao Paulo, Brazil, in June 1971. The disease has continued through the subsequent three years with an attack rate of 65 per 100,000 per month. In February and March of 1974 the predominant strain of *N. meningitidis* changed from serogroup C to serogroup A. Thirteen thousand persons suspected of having meningococcal disease were admitted to the hospitals in Sao Paulo in July and August of 1974.

The adult nasopharyngeal carrier is important in the transmission of meningococci and provides a reservoir of infection from which the organisms are introduced into a household. The median duration of carriage in a nonepidemic setting is 10 months. The carrier rate is higher in members of the household of a patient with meningococcal disease. In community epidemic situations, carriage rates of 15 percent have been observed in households with identified disease as compared with 3.6 percent in households without disease. An investigation of an extended family with several infected children revealed a 44 percent carriage rate, whereas a rate of 3 percent was found in samples of unrelated populations in the same geographic area.

The peak occurrence of disease is in children from 6 to 24 months of age. A lower peak in incidence occurs in the 10- to-20-year age group and is related primarily to outbreaks of disease in the military population.

Meningococcal disease in military populations is associated with nasopharyngeal carriage rates as high as 90 percent. The intimate contact provided by army barracks increases exposure of susceptible recruits from a variety of geographic areas to carriers harboring the organism.

It is of practical importance to emphasize that susceptible intimate household contacts are those at greatest risk of acquiring meningococcal disease. This should focus attention on young children within the family setting of recognized cases and place the fear of acquisition of disease in proper perspective.

Immunity Antibodies, as measured by a bactericidal assay, are present in the blood of very young infants. These antibodies, detectable at birth and for the subsequent few months of life, are presumably transplacentally acquired. The lowest antibody titer is present in infants between 6 and 24 months of age which correlates well with the peak of incidence of sporadic meningococcal disease.

The presence in serum of humoral antibodies of the IgG, IgM, and IgA classes correlates with resistance to infection. Recruits who subse-

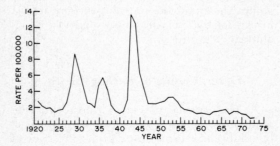

FIG. 29-1 Meningococcal infections. Reported cases per 100,000 population by year, United States, 1920-1973. (From Morbidity and Mortality. CDC Weekly Report for Year Ending December 29, 1973. vol 22 [53]:44, 1973)

quently developed meningococcal disease during basic training were proven to be serosusceptible at their time of entry into the army camp. Also, carriers have been shown to develop antibody titers within two weeks of acquisition of the carrier state. Immunity to the meningococcus is initiated and broadened by this carriage of different strains of the organism, which occurs irregularly throughout life.

Pathogenesis and Clinical Manifestations

Meningococci enter the body via the upper respiratory tract and establish themselves in the membranes of the nasopharynx. Nasopharyngeal acquisition of the organism precedes hematogenous dissemination by an indeterminate time. The incubation period is a matter of days and is usually less than one week. Dissemination of meningococci via the bloodstream results in metastatic lesions in various areas of the body, such as the skin, meninges, joints, eyes, and lungs. The clinical manifestations vary depending on the site of localization.

The spectrum of illness includes a mild febrile disease which may be accompanied by pharyngitis but is without other specific manifestations of meningococcal infection. Systemic disease characterized by fever and prostration is more readily identified. Infrequently an erythematous macular rash is observed, which usually is superseded by the appearance of a petechial eruption rapidly developing into large areas of ecchymosis. This vasculitic purpura is initiated by emboli of meningococci and is considered the hallmark of meningococcal disease. It is characteristic of the more severe fulminant disease. Meningococcemia may be accompanied by meningitis, arthritis, pericarditis, and involvement of virtually any organ system. Disseminated intravascular coagulation and gram-negative shock may be present. Hemorrhage into adrenal tissue with the resultant hypoadrenergic state is referred to as the "Waterhouse-Friderichsen syndrome." The patient may survive meningococcal disease with no detectable sequelae or with direct residua of the infection that are evident for the remainder of his life. Such sequelae include eighth nerve deafness and central nervous system damage and may include necrosis of large areas of skin or tissue secondary to vascular thrombosis. These lesions may require skin grafting or amputation of necrotic digits or an even larger portion of an extremity.

The characteristic petechial eruption usually permits an accurate presumptive diagnosis and allows appropriate initial therapy of the illness. Septicemia with the gonococcus, other pyogenic organisms, or *Rickettsia rickettsiae* in the geographic area of occurrence of Rocky Mountain spotted fever may present problems in differential diagnosis.

Laboratory Diagnosis Meningococcal infection is specifically diagnosed by the identification of *Neisseria meningitidis* in materials obtained from the patient. If inflammatory exudates, such as spinal fluid, are available, a rapid presumptive diagnosis may be made by finding the characteristic gram-negative diplococci in stained smears. The organisms may also be occasionally demonstrated in gram stains of petechial lesions. In cases of overwhelming septicemia the meningococci have been demonstrated in buffy coat smears from peripheral blood or, rarely, in a drop of blood obtained from an ear lobe or even a fingertip for routine differential white blood count.

The materials submitted to the laboratory for culture vary with the illness of the patient. Blood, cerebrospinal fluid, material from petechial skin lesions, synovial fluid, and a nasopharyngeal or throat swab may yield positive cultures. Thayer-Martin selective medium is used for the culture of materials expected to yield a mixture of organisms. Specimens of blood, spinal fluid, or other normally sterile materials are inoculated into blood culture bottles of trypticase soy broth with increased CO_2 and on the surface of a chocolate agar plate.

The immunofluorescent technique may be used for detecting meningococci in smears of cerebrospinal fluid sediments, and it is especially valuable for detecting organisms that have been rendered nonviable as a result of prior chemotherapy. The meningococcal polysaccharide antigens can be precipitated by the use of group-specific polysaccharide antisera. Countercurrent immunoelectrophoresis has been used for the rapid identification of meningococcal polysaccharide in the blood, spinal fluid, and synovial fluid.

Methods are also available for demonstrating the serologic response of a patient with meningococcal infection. A passive hemagglutination inhibition assay detects the presence of antibodies in the patient's serum, a radioactive antigen binding test being the most sensitive assay at the present time. Unfortunately, however, these tests do not become positive until several days after symptoms of disease appear.

Treatment   Penicillin remains the drug of choice for therapy of meningococcal infections. *Neisseria meningitidis* is exquisitely sensitive to penicillin, with minimal inhibitory concentrations usually in the range of 0.3 μg/ml. Therapy is administered with high-dosage aqueous penicillin G using the intravenous route. In penicillin-sensitive individuals, chloramphenicol is an effective alternative form of therapy. In addition to the essential specific antimicrobial therapy, supportive measures for possible complications, such as gram-negative shock or disseminated intravascular coagulation, are important aspects of the care of such patients.

Prevention   PROPHYLAXIS.   Antimicrobial prophylaxis of exposed individuals remains a controversial issue. Prior to the emergence of resistance to sulfonamide therapy, this drug was used efficiently to eradicate the organisms from the nasopharynx of individuals. It has been an interesting puzzle to microbiologists and clinicians that similar use of penicillin, to which the organism is sensitive, fails to eradicate the carrier state. When prophylaxis seems advisable, a choice may be made between two chemotherapeutic agents, rifampin and minocycline, both of which are efficacious in the eradication of the carrier state. Treatment with rifampin for a short period eliminates *N. meningitidis* from the nasopharynx, but during subsequent weeks rifampin-resistant strains may recolonize the nasopharynx. Minocycline also eradicates the carrier state, but a recently recognized side effect of the drug, vestibular dysfunction with resultant disturbance of equilibrium, is now limiting its use. The combined use of the two drugs probably has the greatest efficacy but is a practical impossibility because of the high incidence of side effects in patients receiving the combination.

Decisions concerning the use of such prophylaxis should be made with a complete awareness of the individuals at greatest risk. These usually include (1) children, primarily those less than six years of age who live in the same household or who have a household type of intimate contact with an index case, and (2) recruits in the setting of an army camp. If rifampin or minocycline prophylaxis is given, this does not obviate the need for close observation of contact persons. Meningococcal meningitis has been reported in a patient who received rifampin prophylaxis. Similarly the utilization of penicillin at the prophylactic dosage does not appear to prevent meningococcal disease.

Within the hospital setting it is usually unnecessary to utilize such prophylactic therapy for personnel exposed to meningococcal disease. The occurrence of secondary disease among this group is exceedingly rare. In this setting the recognition of disease and prompt therapy of the patient with appropriate antimicrobials tend to decrease the spread of illness. Physicians who have intimate contact with an untreated patient may take prophylaxis depending upon the individual situation.

IMMUNIZATION.   Group A and group C meningococcal vaccines are licensed and available. The vaccines consist of purified type-specific meningococcal polysaccharide. A single dose of 50 μg is administered, which produces 90 percent serologic response in adults and older children. The data supporting the use of such vaccines have been acquired largely from immunization of over 350,000 Army and Navy personnel. The vaccine produces a significant reduction in meningococcal disease caused by the specific serotype of the vaccine. The carrier state also is significantly lower in vaccinated individuals than in unvaccinated controls. It has been established from these clinical trials that the achieved levels of antibody are protective for this group of individuals.

In contrast, the antibody response of infants during their first year of life is less than optimal. Levels of serum antibody achieved in response to a single dose of vaccine are not considered to be protective. Licensed vaccine is therefore limited to use in military populations where epidemic disease is likely. Vaccine also will be available by specific requests during other epidemic situations for attempted control of an outbreak of infection. At present it cannot be recommended for routine use in children, as its efficacy has not been established.

The development of type-specific vaccines for groups A and C meningococci constitutes a significant contribution to preventive medicine. The group B organisms continue to pose a problem because the polysaccharide is a very poor immunogen. The theoretical possibility that immunization with the group A and/or group C polysaccharides will prevent disease with organisms within these serogroups but will allow other serogroups of organisms to emerge as epidemiologically significant awaits the test of experience with the present vaccines.

NEISSERIA GONORRHOEAE

Antigenic Structure

The antigenic composition of *N. gonorrhoeae* is complex and poorly defined. There are currently no recognized groups or types within the species, although variation between strains does exist. Two major classes of antigens associated with the surface layers have been detected: the pili protein antigen and a polysaccharide antigen that is found in the lipopolysaccharide of the cell wall. Neither of these, however, has been well characterized.

The gonococcus shares a number of antigens with *N. meningitidis*, other *Neisseria*, *Branhamella*, and *Staphylococcus*. Antigonococcal conjugates for use in the fluorescent antibody procedure for the detection of gonococci in exudates must be absorbed with meningococci and staphylococci to eliminate cross-reactivity.

Determinants of Pathogenicity

Current concepts of virulence factors of gonococci are derived primarily from observations that have been made by use of the four major colonial types. The colony forms, designated T1, T2, T3, and T4, reflect differences in the surface antigens of the organisms in the colony. Differences in colony form may be distinguished by direct microscopic examination. Types 1 and 2 are small and dense; types 3 and 4 are appreciably larger and more granular. Types 1 and 2 are predominant in primary isolates, but nonselective subculture leads to the rapid emergence of types 3 or 4. Continued propagation of types 1 and 2 can be effected, however, if individual type 1 or 2 colonies are selected by direct microscopic examination for subculture.

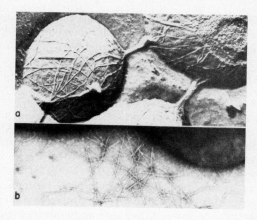

FIG. 29-2. Gonococci and gonococcal pili. A. Freeze-fracture, freeze-etch preparation of gonococci with pili on surface. ×80,000. B. Negatively stained gonococcus with pili radiating from surface. Uranyl acetate. ×70,500. (From Buchanan, Swanson, Holmes, Kraus, Gotschlich: J Clin Invest 52:2896, 1973)

Colony types 1 and 2 are virulent for humans, and colony types 3 and 4 are avirulent. Three properties of the organisms of types 1 and 2 colonies contribute to their ability to produce disease:

(1) The cells of types 1 and 2 are piliated, whereas type 3 cocci contain few or no pili. (Fig. 29-2; Chap. 3). Gonococcal pili from many strains are serologically identical and are composed of helical aggregations of tubelike structures. They are approximately 70 A in diameter and 2 μm in length; each subunit has a molecular weight of about 23,000. Pili confer to cell walls an enhanced ability to adhere to host cells and to each other. This stickiness may be demonstrated in vitro where organisms from colony types 1 and 2 adhere to cultured human amnion cells more avidly than do type 4 organisms. The same phenomenon also may occur in the human urethra, permitting attachment in spite of the flow of urine.

(2) Organisms from the virulent colony types are relatively resistant to phagocytosis by polymorphonuclear leukocytes. Although gonococci of all colony types are readily destroyed following phagocytosis, ingestion of piliated gonococci by macrophages is very inefficient compared with that of nonpiliated strains.

(3) Small spherical structures found on the cell surface are often seen in association with pili. They occur less frequently in colony type

4 organisms and may be associated in some currently unknown way with the damage done to the host during gonococcal infection.

Clinical Infection

The term gonorrhea meaning "flow of seed" was introduced by Galen in 130 AD. Although anicent writings refer to medical conditions characterized by a urethral discharge, it was not until the thirteenth century that physicians were definitely applying the term to a venereally transmitted disease similar to gonorrhea as we know it. Syphilis and gonorrhea often were acquired simultaneously, and descriptions of the two diseases were intermingled. In 1767, the great physician, John Hunter, acquired both syphilis and gonorrhea during an autoinoculation experiment using urethral exudate of a patient erroneously thought to have only gonorrhea. Hunter ascribed his subsequent syphilitic symptoms to gonorrhea, and the confusion of the two diseases became complete. They were not effectively differentiated until the middle of the nineteenth century.

Epidemiology Gonorrhea is the most common of the classical venereal diseases.

Most areas of the world are now affected by the current pandemic. Since the beginning of the twentieth century, when rates of gonorrhea first were recorded, increases and decreases in incidence have been associated with major social changes and with disruptions caused by warfare. Prior to the present period the highest rates in the United States occurred during and just after World War II. As shown in Figure 29-3, the rate decreased through the late 1940s and early 1950s and was followed by a period of quiescence until the early 1960s, when the current pandemic rapidly spread. In the United States, over 900,000 cases were reported to the Center for Disease Control during 1974, an increase of almost 10 percent over the number reported in 1973. Even this does not represent the true incidence, since underreporting is common.

Yearly, seasonal peaks of incidence of gonorrhea occur from July through September, both in the southern and in the northern areas of the United States. The prevalence of gonorrhea in the United States is markedly affected by age. In both males and females the disease is most common in persons 20 to 24 years of age and is only slightly less common among the 15-to-19 and the 25-to-30-year olds. The yearly increases in incidence of gonorrhea have been

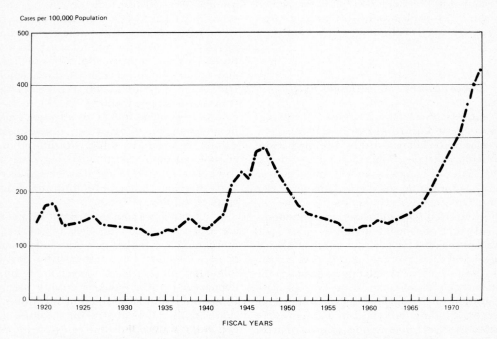

FIG. 29-3. Reported cases of gonorrhea in the United States per 100,000 population.

due primarily to increases among persons 15 to 30 years old. Most cases are casually acquired; prostitution is not at present a major factor in its spread in most areas of the United States. There is a general trend toward increased prevalence in nonwhite individuals, persons of low socioeconomic groups, and urban dwellers.

Pathogenesis Autopsy material of persons who have died of intercurrent disease during the acute phase of gonorrhea have provided information on the histopathology of acute gonorrhea. The primary infection usually begins at the columnar epithelium of the urethra and periurethral ducts and glands of either sex. Cervical, conjunctival, and rectal mucosa also may serve as the portal of entry. Within less than 1 hour following contact with the mucosal surface, the infection is established, and the bacteria are anchored by pili to surface urethral cells. Penetration occurs through intercellular spaces, and organisms reach the subepithelial connective tissue by the third day. The resulting inflammatory response consists of a dense infiltration of polymorphonuclear leukocytes. Obstruction of ducts and glands by this exudate results in retention cysts and abscesses. Spread to other areas often occurs by direct extension through lymphatic vessels and less commonly by blood vessels.

In vitro perfusion of human fallopian tubes has provided a suitable model for study by electron microscopy of the disease process. Initial contact between the organism and the host is at the microvilli. Gonococcal pili extend over the membrane of the epithelial cells as the attached cocci penetrate the mucosal lining of the fallopian tube. Foci of infection develop in the subepithelial connective tissue, resulting in disorganization of collagen connective tissue and local extension of disease. Destruction of epithelial cells by gonococci depletes the mucosal lining, thereby permitting more rapid penetration by other gonococci.

Clinical Manifestations DISEASE IN THE MALE. When compared with many other infectious diseases, gonorrhea is not highly contagious. An unprotected male has approximately a 22 percent chance of acquiring gonorrhea from intercourse with an infected female, and the risk is considerably reduced by use of a condom. Acute gonorrhea in the male has an incubation period of two to eight days, with most cases occurring within four days of infection. The patient presents with burning on urination and a yellow purulent urethral discharge that signifies acute anterior urethritis. The patient may be febrile and have a leukocytosis, but systemic signs are generally lacking. The infection may be asymptomatic in approximately 10 percent of cases, although the patient retains the capacity to transmit disease. Treatment with appropriate antimicrobial agents in adequate doses leads to rapid resolution of clinical disease. In the preantibiotic era most males had resolution of disease within a month. However, approximately 1 percent of males develop complications, the most common being urethral strictures, epididymitis or prostatitis. Less common are septicemia, peritonitis, and meningitis. Another frequent sequela of gonorrhea in the male is the subsequent development of nongonococcal urethritis (nonspecific urethritis) (Chap. 59).

DISEASE IN THE FEMALE. Screening of asymptomatic women has shown prevalence rates of gonorrhea between 1 and 8 percent. Lower rates of infection are observed from such groups as private obstetric practices, and higher rates from such groups as manpower training programs, neighborhood clinics, and venereal disease clinics. The risk to a female from intercourse with an infected male is not definitely known but is probably higher than for the male. The question of whether the use of oral contraceptives alters the susceptibility of a woman to gonorrhea, apart from influencing sexual activity, has not been definitely answered.

Between 20 and 80 percent of women with gonorrhea are asymptomatic, depending upon the population studied. Signs of disease in those who are symptomatic include burning or frequency of urination, vaginal discharge, fever, and abdominal pain. The major complication of gonorrhea in women is the development of pelvic inflammatory disease (PID) by gonococcal infection of the fallopian tubes. This disease affects approximately 10 percent of women with gonorrhea and has two important consequences: (1) Gonococcal PID is a major cause of sterility because of the scars from the infection that block the passage of ova down the fallopian tubes. (2) Scar formation also blocks the normal flow of fluid through the fallopian tubes. In areas where fluid accumulates, infection by other bacteria, often anaerobic, may develop. This leads to chronic PID, a very debilitating and painful disease without satisfactory forms of therapy. Other complications occasionally encountered are infectious perihepatitis and generalized peritonitis.

Approximately 50 percent of females with gonorrhea have concomitant rectal colonization, and proctitis occasionally develops. In 10 percent of women, the rectal site is the only area colonized. Fewer heterosexual males have rectal colonization, but in male homosexuals it is very common.

The other major site of extragenital colonization in both males and females is the pharynx. In about 5 percent of persons who practice fellatio it is the only site of infection. Pharyngeal gonococcal infection is most often asymptomatic, but in some instances it is associated with clinically apparent pharyngitis.

DISSEMINATED GONOCOCCAL DISEASE.   The gonococcal arthritis–dermatitis syndrome is the most common manifestation of disseminated gonococcal disease and is the result of gonococcal bacteremia. Male and female patients in whom this syndrome occurs usually have had asymptomatic genitourinary infection. Although more reported cases have been in women, males with asymptomatic gonorrhea are equally at risk. The incidence of gonococcal bacteremia is approximately 1 percent of all persons with gonorrhea.

The acute form of the gonococcal dermatitis syndrome is heralded by fever, chills, malaise, intermittent bacteremia, polyarticular arthritis or tenosynovitis, and the development of typical skin lesions. The small distal joints are the predominant sites of involvement, and there is usually a paucity of synovial effusion. Joint fluid, if obtained, is most often sterile. The characteristic skin lesions are few in number, occur on the distal dorsal surfaces of the wrists, elbows, and ankles, and usually begin as small petechial or papular lesions. Suppuration, bulbous formation, and central necrosis also are common.

If therapy is not received during this stage, which usually lasts about three days, the patient may progress to the septic joint form of disease. Blood cultures rarely yield *N. gonorrhoeae*, symptoms of septicemia such as fever and chills cease, and the disease becomes more prominent in a single joint. Overt arthritis, with increased quantity and pressure of synovial fluid, develops. The synovial fluid is characteristic of pyarthrosis, with decreased sugar, poor mucin clot formation, and a pronounced granulocytic response.

Other rare forms of gonococcal disease that may follow bacteremic spread include subacute bacterial endocarditis and meningitis. The organisms responsible for disseminated gonococcal infection are usually highly sensitive to penicillin.

DISEASE IN CHILDREN.   Although gonorrhea is most commonly acquired during sexual contact between adults, a significant number of cases each year occur in infants and children. Gonorrhea in this age group may be a result of sexual abuse, but in infancy it usually results from contamination during passage through an infected birth canal.

In the perinatal period, infection of the eye is the most common manifestation of gonorrhea. Prior to the use of silver nitrate for ophthalmic prophylaxis, gonococcal ophthalmia was the cause of blindness in approximately half of the children admitted to schools for the blind. The disease is now a rare cause of blindness, but gonococcal ophthalmia neonatorum continues to occur. Prevention of disease may be based upon the diagnosis and treatment of the mother prior to birth or prophylactic treatment of the eyes of the newborn after birth. Following birth, all states require prophylactic care of the eyes of the newborn; 1 percent silver nitrate is the most satisfactory agent. Failure of silver nitrate prophylaxis, however, does occur and is more common in premature infants or after prolonged rupture of membranes. Silver nitrate instillation is inadequate treatment for established infection, and some of the failures may be due to the presence of active disease by the time of birth.

Neonatal gonococcal arthritis is a highly destructive form of infectious arthritis. The organism usually is acquired from the infected mother at the time of birth. Infection of any mucous membrane may enable dissemination to occur.

Gonorrheal vulvovaginitis is a disease usually seen in girls 2 to 8 years of age. The alkaline pH of the prepubescent vagina is cited as one factor favoring the establishment of gonococcal disease in this age group. The disease usually is self-limited, but it occasionally progresses to invasion of the fallopian tubes or peritonitis. The source of disease is often uncertain.

peritonitis. The source of disease is often uncertain. Although sexual abuse usually is suspected, it appears that the disease may occasionally also be transmitted through contact with fomites which have been contaminated by other family members.

Laboratory Diagnosis MICROSCOPIC EXAMINATION. Gram stain of purulent materials, including urethral discharge from an infected male, conjunctival discharge, and purulent synovial fluid, will reveal many polymorphonuclear leukocytes and intracellular gram-negative diplococci. Gram stains of cervical materials from the female are often misleading because of morphologically similar saprophytic organisms. Examination of scrapings from skin lesions also may yield organisms on gram stain or by fluorescent antibody staining.

CULTURE. A definitive diagnosis is established by isolating the gonococcus in the laboratory. The materials submitted include urethral exudate and endocervical secretions. The pharynx and rectum also may be colonized in infected individuals and may provide cultural evidence of infection. Blood cultures often are positive in disseminated disease, and, in the presence of pyarthrosis, synovial fluid usually yields the gonococcus. In the neonate, cultures of gastric aspirate and the conjunctivae are also helpful. The laboratory processing and identification of materials are discussed on page 458 of this chapter.

Persons suspected of having either meningococcal or gonococcal infection should have complete identification of the isolates. *N. meningitidis* has been recovered from all the sites in which *N. gonorrhoeae* is commonly found.

SEROLOGIC TESTS. In infected males, there is a significant immunologic response to gonococcal infection that may be measured by several systems: (1) Humoral antibody of the IgG classes usually can be detected by the time the patient has clinically apparent disease. Few patients have detectable specific IgM antibodies in the early period of disease. (2) Local secretory IgA in the urethral secretions of infected males can be detected early. (3) In patients with uncomplicated gonococcal urethritis, cell-mediated immunity is activated. Lymphocyte blastogenesis may be induced by gonococcal antigens in some patients with their first infec-

tion and in most patients who have had multiple infections.

Because of the difficulty in obtaining an adequate endocervical culture from women and because a single endocervical culture from women with asymptomatic gonorrhea fails to provide a diagnosis in 20 percent of cases, a serologic method for the diagnosis of gonorrhea would be useful. Two methods for detecting antigonococcal antibody that show promise of clinical usefulness are the immunofluorescent antibody technique (IFA) and the antipilus antibody determination. In clinical studies the IFA technique has accurately diagnosed approximately 80 percent of women with asymptomatic gonorrhea and has given very few false positive reactions. The antipilus antibody technique is the first serologic test using a single defined antigen. It is based upon the finding that pili from many strains of *N. gonorrhoeae* may be antigenically similar. The test appears to be more reliable than any other available and correctly identifies approximately 90 percent of women with asymptomatic endocervical infection. Experience with these tests remains limited.

Treatment Standards for the treatment of all forms of gonorrhea are regularly published by the Center for Disease Control. As modifications of these recommendations are needed they are published in the weekly issue of the *Morbidity and Mortality Report* and should be consulted by physicians treating any patient with gonorrhea. The current recommended regimen of choice for uncomplicated gonococcal infections in men and women is aqueous procaine penicillin G intramuscularly together with probenecid by mouth just before the injection. Alternative regimens are ampicillin by mouth together with probenecid. For the patient who is allergic to the penicillins or to probenecid, tetracycline by mouth or spectinomycin intramuscularly may be used.

Control Each case of gonorrhea should be reported to the local public health department. In some instances, contact tracing by the private physician may supplement public health efforts to control disease.

A number of factors contribute to the difficulties encountered in the control of gonorrhea: (1) Gonococcal infection has a very short incubation period, making it possible for secondary and tertiary cases to transmit disease before recognition and treatment of the primary case. (2) The disease is frequently asymptomatic, and the diagnosis is made only with appropriate cultures. (3) Social acceptance of sexual activity with multiple partners provides the opportunity for wide and rapid dissemination of gonorrhea and other venereal diseases. (4) During the past decade gonococcal isolates have undergone a progressive increase in the mean minimal inhibitory concentrations for penicillin. This has made the use of single injection therapy of disease increasingly difficult.

FURTHER READING

Neisseriaceae

Review

Henriksen SD: Moraxella, Actinobacter, and the mimae. Bacteriol Rev 37:522, 1973

Neisseria meningitidis

Selected Papers

Artenstein MS, Gold R, Zimmerly JG, et al: Prevention of meningococcal disease by group C polysaccharide vaccine. N Engl J Med 282:417, 1970

Frasch CE, Chapman SS: Classification of Neisseria meningitidis group B into distinct serotypes. I. Serological typing by a microbactericidal method. Infect Immun 5: 98, 1972

Frasch CE, Chapman SS: Classification of Neisseria meningitidis group B into distinct serotypes. III. Application of a new bactericidal inhibition technique to distribution of serotypes among cases and carriers. J Infect Dis 127:149, 1973

Gold R, Winklehake JL, Mars RS, Artenstein MS: Identification of an epidemic strain of group C Neisseria meningitidis by bactericidal serotyping. J Infect Dis 124: 593, 1971

Gotschlich EC, Liu TY, Artenstein MS: Human immunity to the meningococcus. III. Preparation and immunochemical properties of the group A, group B, and group C meningococcal polysaccharides. J Exp Med 129: 1349, 1969

Gotschlich EC, Rey M, Triau R, Sparks KO: Quantitative determination of the human immune response to immunization with meningococcal vaccines. J Clin Immunol 51:89, 1972

Greenfield S, Feldman HA: Familial carriers and meningococcal meningitis. N Engl J Med 277:497, 1967

Greenfield S, Sheehe PR, Feldman HA: Meningococcal

carriage in a population of "normal" families. J Infect Dis 123:67, 1971

Morbidity and Mortality Weekly Report. 23:275, 349, 1974

Munford RS, Sussuarana de Vasuncelos ZJ, Phillips CJ, et al: Eradication of carriage of Neisseria meningitidis in families: A study in Brazil. J Infect Dis 129:644, 1974

Munford, RS, Taunay A de E, Marais JS, Frager TW, Feldman RA: Spread of meningococcal infection with households. Lancet 1:1275, 1974

Tramont EC, Sadoff JC, Artenstein MS: Cross reactivity of Neisseria gonorrhoeae and Neisseria meningitidis and the nature of antigens involved in the bactericidal reaction. J Infect Dis 130:240, 1974

Weidmer CE, Dunkel TB, Pettyjohn FS, Smith CO, Leibovitz A: Effectiveness of rifampin in eradicating the meningococcal carrier state in a relatively closed population. Emergence of resistant strains. J Infect Dis 124:172, 1971

Wyle FA, Artenstein MS, Brandt BL, et al: Immunologic response of man to group B meningococcal polysaccharide vaccines. J Infect Dis 126:514, 1972

Neisseria gonorrhoeae

Selected Papers

Cooperman MB: Gonococcus arthritis in infancy. Am J Dis Child 33:923, 1927

Danielsson D, Thyresson N, Falk V, Barr J: Serological investigation of the immature response in various types of gonococcal infection. Acta Derm Venereol 52:467, 1972

Handsfield HH, Lipman JO, Harnisch JP, Tronca E, Holmes KK: Asymptomatic gonorrhea in men. Diagnosis, natural course, prevalence and significance. N Engl J Med 290:117, 1974

Holmes KK, Counts GW, Beaty HN: Disseminated gonococcal infection. Ann Intern Med 79:979, 1971

Kellogg DS, Thayer JD: Virulence of gonococci. Ann Rev Med 20:323, 1969

Krook G, Juhlin I: Problems in diagnosis, treatment and control of gonorrheal infections. IV. The correlation between the doses of penicillin, concentration in blood, IC_{50} values of gonococci, and results of treatment. Acta Derm Venereol 45:242, 1965

Morbidity and Mortality Weekly Report. 23:40, Oct 5, 1974

Swanson J, Zeligs B: Studies on gonococcus infection. VI. Electron microscopic study on in vitro phagocytosis of gonococci by human leukocytes. Infect Immun 10:645, 1974

Ward ME, Watt PJ, Robertson JN: The human fallopian tube: A laboratory model for gonococcal infection. J Infect Dis 129:650, 1974

Wiesner PJ, Tronca E, Bonin P, Pedersen AHB, Holmes KK: Clinical spectrum of pharyngeal gonococcus infection. N Engl J Med 288:181, 1973

30
Haemophilus

Members of the genus *Haemophilus* are strict parasites. They are found in various types of lesions and secretions of vertebrates and on normal mucous membranes. Some species are pathogenic. The genus is a relatively homogeneous one, containing small gram-negative nonmotile bacilli characterized by a requirement for growth factors present in blood. Thus, the name *haemo* (Gr, blood) *philos* (Gr, loving).

Historical and Clinical Perspective *Haemophilus influenzae* causes acute bacterial meningitis in infants and young children, causes several other serious pediatric diseases, and is associated with chronic pulmonary disease in adults. This prototype strain of the genus was first isolated by Pfeiffer during the 1892 influenza epidemic. The frequency of the organism in the nasopharynx of patients led to the erroneous conclusion that it was responsible for the influenza, thus the designation, "the influenza bacillus." *H. influenzae* was apparently only a secondary cause of pulmonary infections during epidemics of true viral influenza. This type of interaction was demonstrated for the influenza virus of swine and a closely related bacterium, *H. suis*, in the important experiments by Shope in the 1930s.

The basic concepts for the epidemiology, pathogenesis, and immunity in *H. influenzae* disease are based on data provided by the classic studies of Dr. Margaret Pittman during the 1930s and 1940s. She demonstrated the two major colony types of the organism, the small granular (R or rough) colony produced by non-encapsulated organisms from the respiratory tract, and the mucoid iridescent (S or smooth) colonies of encapsulated bacteria from sites of invasive disease. These latter strains were considered virulent and were further characterized serologically, being grouped into six types (a–f) on the basis of unique capsular materials.

Subsequent studies have shown that rough or unencapsulated *H. influenzae* are associated commonly with chronic respiratory disease, principally in adults but also in immunocompromised patients. Encapsulated *H. influenzae*, on the other hand, cause invasive diseases, including meningitis, pyarthrosis, cellulitis, pneumonia, pericarditis, and acute epiglottitis. The classic descriptions for meningitis and epiglottitis were written by Alexander in 1942. She emphasized the importance of the type b organism as the cause of most invasive disease and of the clinical implications for immunity to the type b polysaccharide capsular substance.

Organisms of Medical Importance *H. influenzae* type b is the most common cause of acute bacterial meningitis in infancy and childhood, being responsible for 10,000 to 20,000 cases annually in the United States alone. There is also increasing awareness of the importance of unencapsulated *H. influenzae* in pulmonary disease, as emphasized in the monograph by the late J. Robert May (Turk and May 1967).

Other species of *Haemophilus* commonly

TABLE 30-1   PRACTICAL DIFFERENTIATION OF HAEMOPHILUS SPECIES

	Site of Isolation						
Species	Blood or CSF	Wound or Pus	Sputum or Ear	Eye	Chancroid	Urine	Animal
H. influenzae (encapsulated)	+	+	−	−	−	−	−
H. influenzae (nontypable)	−	−	+	−	−	±	−
H. aegyptius	−	−	−	+	−	−	−
H. haemolyticus	−	−	+	−	−	−	−
H. ducreyi	−	−	−	−	+	−	−
H. aphrophilus	+	+	−	−	−	−	−
H. parainfluenzae	±	−	+	−	−	−	+
H. parahaemolyticus	±	−	+	−	−	−	+
H. paraphrophilus	±	−	+	−	−	±	−
H. suis	−	−	−	−	−	−	+
H. gallinarum	−	−	−	−	−	−	+

±*Indicates an uncommon or unconfirmed association*

encountered in clinical and/or laboratory bacteriology are indicated in Table 30-1. These may also be known by eponyms: the influenza bacillus of Pfeiffer *(H. influenzae)*, the tropical Koch-Weeks bacillus *(H. aegyptius)*, the organism isolated from chancroid by Ducrey *(H. ducreyi)*, and the swine bacillus of Shope *(H. suis)*. The names for other species are self-explanatory either from the source of isolation or from growth characteristics.

HAEMOPHILUS INFLUENZAE

Morphology and Physiology

Microscopic Morphology Rapidly proliferating organisms, as seen in cerebrospinal fluid, joint fluid, or on primary growth on enriched media, are small and uniform coccobacillary forms, usually 0.2 to 0.3 by 0.5 to 0.8 μm (Fig. 30-1). Faint refractile capsules may be present and are readily demonstrated by specific quellung reactions with type-specific antisera. The organism is gram-negative but may appear gram-variable unless the staining procedure is very carefully carried out. Unencapsulated organisms from sputum or ear aspirates are often more elongated and may exhibit bipolar staining with the gram stain, leading to an erroneous diagnosis of S. *pneumoniae*. Rough colonies demonstrate this microscopic pleomorphic appearance routinely and often contain long threads and filaments (Fig. 30-2). Electron microscopic examination of *H. influ-*

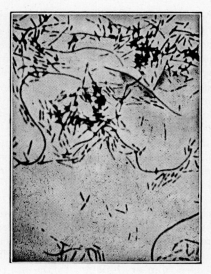

FIG. 30-2. Unencapsulated *H. influenzae* from rough colony.

enzae reveals a cell wall 200 A thick, with an ultrastructure similar to that of other gram-negative organisms. The polysaccharide capsule lies outside the cell wall, although a thin layer of capsule may be strongly bonded to the cell wall.

Cultural Characteristics For the laboratory cultivation of *Haemophilus*, enriched agar media, such as chocolate, Levinthal, and Fildes, have been recommended. Growth on blood agar is sparse, and fresh human or sheep blood plates should not be used because they contain heat-labile inhibitors. Such blood can be used, however, in the preparation of chocolate agar plates where defibrinated blood is added to the agar base and heated at 80C until the color is chocolate brown. *Haemophilus* may also grow as satellites around other organisms, eg, hemolytic staphylococci that are also present in the clinical specimen. Such colonies are larger than those growing at a distance because of increased levels of the V factor made available by the staphylococcus. *Haemophilus* can also grow in broth that is adequately enriched and aerated. Optimum growth occurs at 37C and pH 7.4 to 7.8 but will occur over a temperature range of 25 to 40C and at pH 6.6 to 7.8. Incubation under 10 percent CO_2 enhances or is necessary for the growth of some strains.

Growth on semisolid agar is apparent 18 to 24 hours after inoculation. A majority of clinical

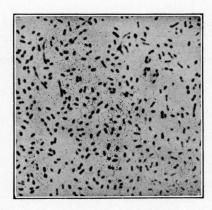

FIG. 30-1. Primary growth of *H. influenzae* on chocolate agar.

isolates are from respiratory specimens, and, thus, colonies are usually very small and dew-like and develop a coarse or rough appearance. These colonies are usually 0.5 to 1.5 mm in diameter. *H. influenzae* from invasive disease (usually type b from blood, CSF, or wound) produces the mucoid, glistening colonies described by Pittman. These may reach 3 or 4 mm in diameter on enriched medium, and they develop a central umbilication in the second 24 hours. Smooth colonies often spontaneously convert to rough colonies due to loss of encapsulation (p. 473).

Nutritional Requirements   Species of *Haemophilus* require one or both of two growth factors (Table 30-2). The V factor is necessary for growth of all except two species. This factor is released from erythrocytes by the mild heat used in the preparation of chocolate agar but is destroyed by excessive heat. Since substitution in defined media is possible of the nicotinamide adenine nucleotides (di or tri), the V factor is considered synonymous with these coenzymes. The two species which will grow in the absence of V factor require increased levels of CO_2; one of these organisms is itself hemolytic. The X factor is heat stable, is derived from erythrocytes, and is hemin or hematin but not hemoglobin per se. This cofactor is apparently an iron complex playing an essential role in respiratory metabolism, as it is not required during anaerobic growth. The species designated *para-* do not require this cofactor, a property employed during laboratory differentiation using X and V disks.

Haemophilus is aerobic but facultatively anaerobic. In the absence of oxygen, nitrate is used as an electron acceptor. Indole is produced from tryptophan by many strains of *H. influenzae*, and in isolates from clinical specimens can often be recognized by its characteristic odor. Like *S. pneumoniae* the organism is bile soluble.

Differentiation from other species is based primarily on growth requirements and source of culture (Table 30-2). Sugar fermentation patterns are usually not helpful in practical identification. Some species that are currently included in the genus, at least as species incertae, require medium enrichment using serum or elevated osmolality. The growth requirements for *H. suis*, *H. gallinarium*, and *H. ducreyi*, and additional authoritative details, will be found in the eighth edition of *Bergey's Manual of Determinative Bacteriology*.

Resistance   *H. influenzae* is very susceptible to the common disinfectants and to desiccation. An exposure to 55C for 30 minutes is lethal. Cultures of the organism are difficult to maintain in the laboratory because of their tendency to autolyze. Proper maintenance of viable virulent organisms requires frequent transfers on chocolate agar. Preservation is best accomplished by lyophilization.

Genetics   The studies of Pittman referred to above established the relationship between colony type, antigenic structure, and virulence of *H. influenzae*. Smooth to rough transitions in form, as observed when clinical isolates from invasive disease are subcultured on artificial media, reflect loss of specific capsular poly-

TABLE 30-2   DIFFERENTIAL PROPERTIES OF SPECIES OF HAEMOPHILUS[*]

Species	V Factor Requirement	X Factor Requirement	Increased CO_2 Requirement	Hemolysis
H. influenzae	+	+	−	−
H. aegyptius	+	+	−	−
H. haemolyticus	+	+	−	+
H. ducreyi	−	+	+	sl.
H. aphrophilus	−	+	+	−
H. parainfluenzae	+	−	−	−
H. parahaemolyticus	+	−	−	+
H. paraphrophilus	+	−	+	−
H. suis	+	+	−	−
H. gallinarium	+	+	+	−

[*]See also Zinneman and Biberstein: In Buchanan and Gibbons (eds): Bergey's Manual of Determinative Bacteriology, 8th ed. Baltimore, Williams & Wilkins, 1974, p 364.

saccharide synthesis by mutation. The spontaneous mutation rate for this property is relatively high and may be increased by suboptimal culture conditions or by the presence of type-specific antisera. Such S → R transitions may occur in vivo, as evidenced by unencapsulated organisms in the upper respiratory tract of patients recovering from *H. influenzae* type b meningitis.

The elaboration of a type-specific polysaccharide capsule by *H. influenzae* provides a convenient marker for genetic studies dealing with the transfer of DNA from one organism to another. Transformations and transductions mediated by DNA from species of *Haemophilus* have been extensively studied and the enzymology and genetics of their restriction and modification systems characterized. In *H. influenzae,* strain-specific restriction endonucleases recognize DNA from other strains as foreign. Protection against restriction is provided by a modification methylase that methylates a limited number of adenine or cytosine residues in the recognized nucleotide sequence. Each of the serologic types of *H. inflenzae* carries different DNA restriction and modification systems. These systems are powerful tools for the molecular biologist who has successfully used *Haemophilus*-derived enzymes to analyze the structure and function of viral genomes (p. 166). At the present time, however, it is not known what role if any is played in vivo by genetic exchange among the large reservoir of primarily nontypable *H. influenzae* and other organisms that are found in the nasopharynx as a part of the normal flora.

Antigenic Structure

Capsular Serotypes The major antigenic determinant of encapsulated *H. influenzae* is the capsular polysaccharide. This polysaccharide confers type specificity on the organism and is the basis of the grouping of the organism into six serotypes, types a, b, c, d, e, and f. The unique chemical specificity of each type is shown in Table 30-3. Of the six capsular types type b is the only one that contains a pentose as the sugar component of its polysaccharide. The other types contain either a hexose or hexosamine moiety. Whether this difference contributes to its greater pathogenic potential for

infants is unknown. In vivo growth of the organism promotes active synthesis and release of the capsular material, and specific antibody and in vitro conditions suppress capsule synthesis. The loss of encapsulation during culture is synonymous with conversion from smooth to rough colonies and the loss of virulence. The medical importance of immunity directed against the capsular antigen is discussed on page 475.

Serologic Capsular Reactions Encapsulated *H. influenzae* may be typed by the quellung (capsular swelling) reaction (p. 447), using antisera prepared against the type-specific polysaccharides a, b, c, d, e, and f. Typing may be done directly on fresh specimens from infected patients or on primary isolates. Agglutination and fluorescent antibody techniques may also be employed but must be interpreted very carefully. Because cell wall (somatic) or group specificity antibodies may contaminate type-specific sera and because of the low potency of diagnostic reagents, organisms should be serotyped by more than one method. The serotype of free capsular polysaccharide antigen which is liberated in vitro (or in vivo) may be identified serologically by use of the precipitin test, agar gel diffusion, or by adsorption to solid particles, such as erythrocytes (hemagglutination) or latex particles (flocculation). Since type b organisms cause over 95 percent of invasive disease, detection of the ribose phosphate polysaccharide of type b is especially important. The detection of type b capsular antigen in body fluids from infected patients may allow rapid and specific diagnosis (p. 476).

A modification of the capsular antigen precipitation test has been useful as a screening technique and for the identification of bacteria

TABLE 30-3 CAPSULAR POLYSACCHARIDES OF H. INFLUENZAE

Type	Sugar	PO_4	Acetyl
a	Glucose	+	−
b	Ribose (ribitol)	+	−
c	Galactose	+	−
d	Hexose	−	−
e	Hexosamine	−	+
f	Galactosamine	+	+

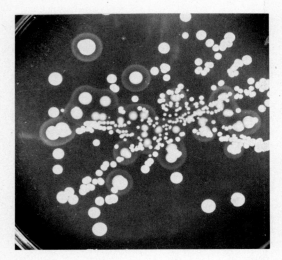

FIG. 30-3. Halo of specific immune precipitin surrounding *H. influenzae* type b colonies on agar containing type b antiserum. (Courtesy of Richard M. Michaels)

cross-reacting with type b capsular polysaccharide. The technique, as illustrated in Figure 30-3, depends upon the formation in agar medium containing antisera of an immunoprecipitin halo around a bacterial colony from which the soluble antigen diffuses. Using this screening technique a number of organisms in other genera have been shown to have antigens cross-reactive with the type b polysaccharide of *H. influenzae*. Cross-reactions are known to occur between *H. influenzae* type b and strains of pneumococci, streptococci, *Escherichia coli*, *Staphylococcus*, *Lactobacillus* species, *Bacillus* species, and others. Cross-reactivity between *E. coli* and *H. influenzae* type b has been attributed to shared specificities of acidic polysaccharides or K antigens, while in gram-positive species the cross-reacting antigens are cell wall polyribitol phosphate teichoic acids.

Noncapsular Antigens Somatic antigens have been identified in all strains, but their location in the bacterial cell and their chemical composition have not been well documented. Some of these antigens are common to untypable and to all encapsulated types of *H. influenzae*; while others appear to be more specific for certain types and strains within a type. Antisera prepared against these somatic antigens have proved useful in agglutination and immunofluorescence tests (FA) for the confirmation of nontypable rough isolates of *H. influenzae* from

such specimens as sputum or ear exudates. Further studies with the somatic antigens and their characterization are indicated in order to clarify the role of nontypable organisms in such conditions as otitis media.

Clinical Infection

Pathogenesis RESPIRATORY PORTAL OF ENTRY. Infection with *H. influenzae* occurs following the inhalation of infected droplets from clinically active cases, convalescent patients, and carriers. Nonhuman reservoirs for *H. influenzae* are not known. The natural history of infections in children is poorly understood, but clinical experience suggests that the organisms initially colonize the nasopharynx. Both rough and smooth variants of *H. influenzae* are carried in the human respiratory tract with low frequency and are associated with sinus, middle ear, and tracheobronchial disease. The organisms are established in the tracheobronchial tree, perhaps in synergy with a virus, as shown for *H. suis* by Shope, or perhaps by paralysis of normal cilia clearance functions, as demonstrated by Denny. However, the relevance of viral synergy, toxic bacterial products, and local immunity to the production of clinical respiratory tract disease has yet to be proved. The strains usually associated with chronic respiratory disease are nonencapsulated and probably do not invade tissue. The presence of encapsulated *H. influenzae* (especially type b) in sputum or ear aspirates may indicate tissue invasion.

BLOODSTREAM INVASION. It has been postulated for many years that *H. influenzae* meningitis, pyarthrosis, or other pyogenic diseases follow respiratory colonization. Epidemiologic culture data indicate concomitant respiratory infection in many patients or family members of patients with invasive disease. Moreover, by careful choice and manipulation of animal models, experimental empyema and meningitis can be produced following respiratory inoculation. Although the precise mechanisms by which invasion from the respiratory tract occurs are still unknown, viral synergy may play an important role. Acquisition of virulence by previously avirulent organisms may occur by in vivo encapsulation, as occurs following genetic exchange between two capsular types. The polysaccharide capsule then would prevent phagocytosis and bacterial killing. Host factors also undoubtedly play a critical role, as evidenced by increased incidence of invasive disease in individuals who are nonimmune and/or genetically susceptible.

Specific Immunity The importance of immunity in defense against *Haemophilus* disease was suggested in 1931 by Wright and Fothergill, who showed that the age-specific frequency of *H. influenzae* meningitis decreases in proportion to increasing antibacterial activity in blood. Invasive disease was shown to occur during the age of relative humoral immunodeficiency, 3 months to 3 years. This fundamental observation on age-specific disease susceptibility in the absence of antibody is one argument supporting an important role for specific anticapsular immunity in protection against meningitis and other *H. influenzae* diseases. Other important findings supporting a role for anticapsular immunity include (1) the high susceptibility of patients with inborn or other humoral immunodeficiencies and its reversal by passively administered specific antibody in gamma globulin, (2) the fact that convalescent immune responses are usually protective and correlate quantitatively with anticapsular antibody levels, (3) preferential virulence of the type b encapsulated organisms, and, most important, (4) the quantitative correlation of the protective activity of antiserum with anticapsular antibody and its specific absorption with purified capsular polysaccharide.

Principles of anticapsular immunity have been utilized in the study of animal models for pyogenic infections, eg, the susceptibility of young rabbits or weanling rats, and also in the development of purified type-specific substances for vaccination against human disease. Antibody against the type b polysaccharide, whether naturally occurring or vaccine induced, should prevent tissue invasion by the virulent type b organism. Recent experimental results suggest that immunity induced by exposure to cross-reactive antigens of nonpathogenic bacteria may also be effective in protection.

Clinical Manifestations *H. influenzae* causes a number of infections of the upper respiratory tract, such as pharyngitis, otitis media, and sinusitis. These infections are important especially in chronic pulmonary disease. Moreover, respiratory foci probably serve as areas for invasion of the bloodstream and spread to other parts of the body.

MENINGITIS. The most serious of the diseases produced by *H. influenzae* is an acute bacterial meningitis. *H. influenzae* meningitis occurs rarely in infants under the age of 3 months and is uncommon in children over the age of 6 years. Cases have been reported, however, in both neonates and adults. The distribution of disease is equal in males and females and in races, except for the increased susceptibility in association with sickle cell anemia. Patients with humoral immunodeficiency are especially susceptible. The incicence of disease is approximately 5 per 100,000 population and is reported to be increasing in recent years. Overt symptoms, cerebrospinal fluid pleiocytosis, and positive cultures are often preceded by several days of respiratory symptoms, during which invasion presumably occurs. Clinical and laboratory findings are typical of a pyogenic infection. Therapy can prevent mortality in 90 to 97 percent of cases, but residual central nervous system deficits are demonstrable in one-third of patients.

ACUTE BACTERIAL EPIGLOTTITIS. This disease, rarely caused by organisms other than *H. influenzae* type b, has an acute onset and is rapidly progressive. It occurs in children who are older than meningitis patients and even occasionally in adults. The infected epiglottis has microabscesses, and the marked edema may cause complete airway obstruction, requiring emergency tracheotomy. Severe septicemia is often present in this too often fatal illness.

OTHER INFECTIONS. *H. influenzae* type b is also a common cause of childhood pyarthrosis and is associated with superficial cellulitis and, rarely, pericarditis. Pneumonia with empyema due to encapsulated *H. influenzae* occurs occasionally in the very young or in debilitated adults. These diseases are uncommon, however, and the epidemiologic and pathogenic relationships are even less well defined than for other clinical entities.

Laboratory Diagnosis *H. influenzae* organisms may often be identified by direct examination of gram-stained clinical specimens, including cerebrospinal fluids, arthrocentesis, thoracocentesis, middle ear aspirates, and sputum specimens. However, the organism's variable size, coccobacillary shape, and tendency to remain gram-positive if not carefully decolorized may be confusing. A specific quellung reaction is helpful except for unencapsulated organisms from the respiratory tract. The specimen should be cultured promptly on chocolate agar or other suitable media and incubated in the presence of 10 percent CO_2 (p. 471).

Detection of specific polysaccharide antigen in body fluids is also a valuable diagnostic aid and has been successfully used for diagnosis (and prognosis) of meningitis since it was first introduced by Alexander in 1942. The presence of specific antigen in serum or CSF provides a presumptive diagnosis of *H. influenzae* infection even in the absence of a positive culture. Countercurrent immunoelectrophoresis (CIE) and other rapid and semiquantitative techniques for the detection of bacterial antigens have also been used (Fig. 30-4). Using CIE, rapid diagnosis can be made in 90 percent of confirmed *H. influenzae* type b meningitis and in a majority of other infections caused by this organism.

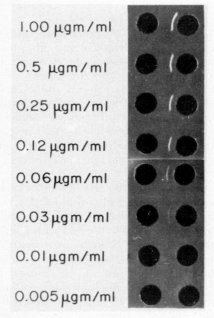

1.00 µgm/ml

0.5 µgm/ml

0.25 µgm/ml

0.12 µgm/ml

0.06 µgm/ml

0.03 µgm/ml

0.01 µgm/ml

0.005 µgm/ml

FIG. 30-4. Countercurrent immunoelectrophoresis of purified *H. influenzae* type b antigen (µg dry weight/ml, in [−] well on left) and rabbit antiserum against *H. influenzae* type b ([+] right wells). (Courtesy of Donald Coonrod)

Treatment and Prophylaxis The antibiotic of choice for therapy in any *Haemophilus* infection should be determined by in vitro evidence of sensitivity. While most *H. influenzae* are sensitive to ampicillin, chloramphenicol, tetracyclines, sulfonamides, and cotrimoxazole, and while therapy with one or combinations of these has been shown to be effective, the sensitivity of the organism and a therapeutic result cannot be assumed. More than thirty ampicillin-resistant *H. influenzae* isolates have been reported in the United States since December 1973. L forms of *H. influenzae*, resistant to penicillin, may arise during therapy with penicillins, and some *H. influenzae* strains produce penicillinase. The current recommendation for initial treatment of *H. influenzae* meningitis and other invasive diseases caused by this organism is chloramphenicol with ampicillin or penicillin G.

Antibiotics are not indicated for routine contacts of patients with *Haemophilus influenzae* disease. Since secondary cases in siblings of meningitis or epiglottitis patients are known, these family contacts should probably be cultured and observed carefully.

A type-specific capsular polysaccharide (PRP) vaccine has been developed and is currently under investigation. Preliminary results with this vaccine appear very promising. The PRP vaccine is nontoxic and immunogenic for adults, but infants respond with low antibody titers. In animal systems antibody formed in response to purified type b polysaccharide is protective. If future and more extensive studies show that general protection is provided, it may be possible to reduce the incidence and sequelae of invasive disease caused by this organism.

OTHER HAEMOPHILUS SPECIES

Haemophilus aegyptius (Koch-Weeks Bacillus)

This organism is closely related to *H. influenzae* but may be differentiated serologically. Unlike *H. influenzae*, *H. aegyptius* does not produce indole. It is sensitive to drying, requiring that specimens be carefully handled and cultured immediately. Unencapsulated *H. aegyptius* is infectious for man and causes a purulent conjunctivitis, especially in children. Associated pathogenic factors and immune responses have not been defined. The conjunctivitis usually responds to locally applied sulfonamides.

Haemophilus ducreyi (Chancroid Bacillus)

This organism is the cause of a venereal disease. It is an obligate parasite, transmitted by direct contact, and very sensitive to drying. In temperate climates *H. ducreyi* may be responsible for up to 10 percent of venereal disease in civilian populations, but in troops invading tropical countries the frequency of chancroid has been second only to gonorrhea.

H. ducreyi is demonstrable in smears from pustular skin lesions or bubo aspirates. The microscopic appearance is described as resembling a school of red fish, but organisms in fresh smears may appear gram-positive. The pleomorphic organisms may be seen intracellularly or extracellularly. *H. ducreyi* grows on meat infusion or blood-enriched medium with increased CO_2, but primary isolation may be very difficult. Serologic diagnosis is also possible, since isolates share antigenic patterns.

Clinical chancroid usually follows a one to two week incubation period. One to five lesions occur, which are flat, measure 2 to 20 mm, and are centrally umbilicate. The erythema is out of proportion to any induration, ie, it is a soft or nonsyphilitic chancre. Lesions are limited to the skin except for associated lymphadenitis (buboes). Response to sulfonamides and/or tetracycline was satisfactory until the war in Vietnam, when refractory cases appeared. Aminoglycoside antibiotics may be necessary for such cases.

Haemophilus aphrophilus

A finite number of *H. aphrophilus* infections have been reported. Most strains are cultured from the blood of patients with a damaged endocardium, congenital heart disease, secondary brain abscess, or otherwise compromised defenses. This organism may also rarely cause sinusitis, pneumonia, or abscesses elsewhere. *H. aphrophilus* is a very fastidious and microaerophilic organism and is killed rapidly on drying. It requires increased CO_2 for growth, thus the name, *aphros* (Gr, foam). Sutter and Feingold have reviewed detailed fermentation and other reactions differentiating *H. aphrophilus* from similar species. Its relationship to the HB* group organism *Actinobacillus actinomycetemcomitans* is not established sufficiently to require reclassification. However, the antibiotic sensitivity pattern is atypical for *Haemophilus*, most strains being resistant to ampicillin and requiring therapy with chloramphenicol, gentamicin, or tetracycline.

FURTHER READING

Books and Reviews

Robbins JB, Schneerson R, Argaman M, Handzel Z: *Haemophilus influenzae* type b: Disease and immunity in humans. Ann Int Med 78:259, 1973

Sell SHW, Karzon DT (eds): *Haemophilus influenzae.* Proceedings of a conference on Antigen-Antibody Systems, Epidemiology and Immunoprophylaxis. Nashville, Vanderbilt Univ Press, 1973

Turk DC, May RF: *Haemophilus influenzae:* Its Clinical Importance. London, English Univ Press. 1967

Selected Papers

Alexander HE, Ellis C, Leidy G: Treatment of type-specific *Haemophilus influenzae* infections in infancy and childhood. J Pediatr 20:673, 1942

Anderson P, Johnston RB, Smith DH: Human serum activities against *Haemophilus influenzae* type b. J Clin Invest 51:31, 1972

Bradshaw M, Schneerson R, Parke JC, Robbins JB: Bacterial antigens cross reactive with the capsular polysaccharide of *Haemophilus influenzae* type b. Lancet 1:1095, 1971

Deacon WE, Albritton DC, Edmundson WF, Olansky S: Study of Ducrey's bacillus and recognition of a gram-positive smooth phase. Proc Soc Exp Biol Med 86:261, 1954

Degré M, Solberg LA: Synergistic effect in viral-bacterial infection. Acta Pathol Microbiol Scand (B) 79:129, 1971

Denny F: Effect of a toxin produced by *Haemophilus influenzae* on ciliated epithelium. J Infect Dis 129:93, 1974

Edwards EA, Huehl PM, Pechinpaugh RO: Diagnosis of bacterial meningitis by counter-immunoelectrophoresis. J Lab Clin Med 80:449, 1972

Fothergill LD, Wright J: Influenzal meningitis: The relationship of age incidence to the bactericidal power of blood against the causal organism. J Immunol 24:273, 1933

Nelson JD: Should ampicillin be abandoned for treatment of *Haemophilus influenzae* disease? JAMA 229:332, 1974

Pittman M: Variation and type specificity in the bacterial

Hemophilic bacilli of uncertain status.

species *Haemophilus influenzae.* J Bacteriol 59:413, 1950

Robbins JB, Parke JC, Schneerson R, Whisnant JK: Quantitative measurement of "natural" and immunization-induced *Haemophilus influenzae* type b capsular polysaccharide antibodies. Pediatr Res 7:103, 1973

Shope RE: The influenzae of swine and man. Harvey Lect 36:183, 1935

Sutter VL, Finegold SM: *Haemophilus aphrophilus* infections: Clinical and bacteriological studies. Ann NY Acad Sci 174:468, 1970

Williams JD, Andrews J: Sensitivity of *Haeomphilus influenzae* to antibiotics. Br Med J 1:134, 1974

Zamenhof S, Leidy G, Fitzgerald PL, Alexander HE, Chargaff E: Polyribosephosphate, the type-specific substance of *Haemophilus influenzae* type b. J Biol Chem 203:695, 1953

31
Bordetella

The clinical syndrome of whooping cough or pertussis has been traced to a classic description given in the latter part of the sixteenth century. It is an acute bacterial disease localized to the respiratory tract and characterized by paroxysmal coughing. Systemic reactions may include neurologic manifestations with permanent central nervous system sequelae. The severity of the illness prompted early investigative work, and the causative organism, *Bordetella pertussis*, was first isolated in 1906 by Bordet and Gengou. Subsequently, similar illness has also been attributed to *Bordetella parapertussis* and *Bordetella bronchiseptica* on a few occasions. The standardization of vaccine and its widespread use within the United States and other countries has been associated with a dramatic decline in the incidence of disease and its attendant morbidity and mortality. Unfortunately, investigative interest in the organism and the pathogenesis of the clinical disease waned concomitantly.

Morphology

The three members of the genus *Bordetella* are *B. pertussis*, *B. parapertussis*, and *B. bronchiseptica*. The organisms are small, gram-negative coccobacilli, 0.2 to 0.3 μm by 0.5 to 1.0 μm, appearing singly, in pairs, and in small clusters. Upon primary isolation cells are uniform in size, but in subcultures they become quite pleomorphic, and filamentous and thick bacillary forms are common. Bipolar metachromatic staining may be demonstrated with toluidine blue. The only motile member of the genus is *B. bronchiseptica*, which possesses lateral flagella. Capsules are produced but can be demonstrated only by special stains and not by capsular swelling.

Physiology

Bordetella organisms are strict aerobes, with a metabolism that is respiratory, never fermentative. They do not produce H_2S, indole, or acetylmethylcarbinol. Differential characteristics of the three species are summarized in Table 31-1.

Unlike *Haemophilus* species, *Bordetella* organisms have no specific growth requirement for hemin (X factor) and coenzyme I (V factor). Primary isolation does require, however, the addition of charcoal, ion-exchange resins, or 15 to 20 percent blood to neutralize the toxic effect of such substances as unsaturated fatty acids, colloidal sulfur, sulfides, or peroxides. Modified Bordet-Gengou medium (potato—glycerol—blood agar) is recommended for this purpose. Colonies of *B. pertussis* on this medium are smooth, convex, glistening, almost transparent, and pearl-like in appearance. All three species produce a zone of hemolysis which varies with cultural conditions.

B. pertussis freshly isolated from patients in the catarrhal stage of pertussis are smooth colony-forming organisms (phase I). Adaptation to other media, such as blood or chocolate agar, results in transition to the avirulent rough colony-producing form (phase IV). The term "cul-

TABLE 31-1 DIFFERENTIAL CHARACTERISTICS OF SPECIES OF GENUS BORDETELLA

	B. pertussis	B. parapertussis	B. bronchiseptica
Motility	−	−	+
Reduces nitrate	−	−	+
Utilizes citrate	−	+	+
Produces urease	−	+	+
Growth on peptone agar	−	+	+
Browning of peptone agar	−	+	−
Growth on Bordet-Gengou agar	3 – 4 days	1 – 2 days	1 – 2 days
Litmus milk alkaline	−, (12 – 14)°	1 – 4 days	1 – 4 days
G + C content moles % Tm	61	61	66

Modified from Buchanan and Gibbons (eds): Bergey's Manual of Determinative Bacteriology, 8th ed. 1974, p 283. Courtesy Williams & Wilkins
+ = all strains positive; − = all strains negative
°Modulated phase II to IV organisms (+) in 12 to 14 days

tural modulation" has been used to describe a change in phenotype of the organism that occurs in almost all members of a population as a result of changes in environment. The changes are reversible, and a single colony will undergo the transition to phase IV. This cultural modulation from phase I through intermediate forms (phases II and III) to rough colony-forming organisms (phase IV) alters the antigenicity of the organism. In addition, the bacteria lose or alter other properties, including the dermonecrosis and histamine-sensitizing factors, the heat-labile toxin, and the protective factor.

Antigenic Structure

Protection against infection with *B. pertussis* in the experimental mouse and in human illness is an immunologic response to an antigen of the bacterium. The nature of the protective antigen of *B. pertussis* is unknown. However, extensive serologic investigations have described distinct antigens of the genus *Bordetella*. There is a single heat-stable surface 0 antigen common to smooth strains of *B. pertussis*, *B. parapertussis*, and *B. bronchiseptica* and to rough strains of *B. pertussis* and *B. bronchiseptica*. This 0 antigen is a protein easily extractable from cells and is found in the supernatant fluids of cell cultures. This antigen is not responsible for protection against infection.

The antigenic differences among species and among strains of each of the species are determined by the heat-labile or capsular antigens of Kauffmann. (The serotype is often indicated by numbers, eg, *B. pertussis* 1. 2. 4.) Eldering postulated the existence of 14 K antigens designated as "factors" on the basis of agglutinin absorption tests (Table 31-2). This scheme explained most of the observed serologic relationships. Factor 7 is common to all strains of the three species of *Bordetella* organisms. Factor 14 is specific for *B. parapertussis*, and factor 12 is specific for *B. bronchiseptica*.

Factors 1 through 6 are found only in strains of *B. pertussis*. The serotypes per se of *B. pertussis* are not significant determinants of the severity of disease or of protection against infection. However, these antigens are essential in vaccine production, as they provide a method of assaying for the alterations in antigenicity which occur with cultural modulation of the strains. Factor 1 antigen is present in all strains of *B. pertussis*, and it has been suggested that the agglutinating antigen (agglutinogen) of the organism is primarily factor 1. Persons sustaining natural infection or immunization with *B. pertussis* vaccine form agglutinins. These antibodies offer a practical means of assessment of experience with antigen and an indirect measure of immunity, since studies have demonstrated that protection from disease correlates well with agglutinin titers of 1:320 or greater. In addition, specific antisera produced against the individual antigens provide a method of surveillance during an epidemic when strains of common antigenic patterns will predominate.

Other antigenic components of *Bordetella* organisms are discussed in the following section.

Determinants of Pathogenicity

B. pertussis is a pathogenic organism with unique properties. The multiple cellular components of this bacterium have been studied in relationship to its biologic activities in hopes of elucidating the pathogenesis of disease. These components include the O and K

TABLE 31-2 SUMMARY OF HEAT-LABILE K ANTIGENS* OF BORDETELLA

Species	Common Antigen	Species-specific Antigen	Other Antigens Present
B. pertussis	7	1	2- 6
B. parapertussis	7	14	8-10
B. bronchiseptica	7	12	8-11

Adapted from Eldering et al: J Bacteriol 74:135, 1957
*Antigens often referred to as "factors"

antigens, discussed above, heat-labile toxin (HLT), lipopolysaccharide (endotoxin), histamine-sensitizing factor (HSF), lymphocytosis-promoting factor (LPF), protective factor, and hemagglutinin.

Heat-labile toxin (HLT) is considered to be a protein contained within the bacterial cell which can be released by cell lysis and is destroyed when heated to 56C for 15 minutes. It is dermonecrotic, and intravenous or intraperitoneal injection of HLT into mice causes death within 48 hours. It does not sensitize the mice to histamine. HLT is antigenic in mice but does not protect against brain infection in the mouse. HLT is distinct from protective factor. HLT apparently does not stimulate antibody production in man, and its role in the pathogenesis of human illness is unknown.

The lipopolysaccharide or endotoxin of the cell wall is heat stable and similar to endotoxins prepared from other gram-negative bacteria. This material does not induce formation of antibodies with protective activity.

The histamine-sensitizing factor (HSF) and lymphocytosis-promoting factor (LPF) of *B. pertussis* have fascinated workers because these are properties unique to *B. pertussis*. Preparation of purified materials either by saline extraction and starch block electrophoresis or by density gradient centrifugation has produced homogeneous material which is thermostable. This material contains HSF and LPF, hemagglutinin, and protective antigen. It is not established whether these activities are all part of a complex molecule or are closely related separate substances. When injected into mice, this purified material results in decreased body weight and late death of the animals in three to four days.

HSF is located in the cell wall, is thermolabile at 80C for 30 minutes, and is antigenic. It produces a primary sensitization to histamine in the experimental mouse. Minute amounts of HSF induce a dose-dependent response which is reproducible and uniform under standard conditions. It is suggested that HSF directly blocks the action of catecholamines, as current experimental work has shown that beta adrenergic blocking agents can simulate this effect in mice. Although the importance of HSF in the pathogenesis of human illness remains to be delineated, it is tempting to consider its importance in such physiologic and pharmacologic

events of clinical pertussis as the paroxysmal cough and the CNS toxicity.

The purified preparation of HSF and LPF also contains hemagglutinating activity. The purified material visualized by electron microscopy consists of large filamentous molecules which will adsorb onto RBC membranes, thereby causing agglutination.

The striking lymphocytosis observed in association with clinical pertussis has been duplicated in the mouse and offers a means of studying this phenomenon. It has been proposed that lymphocytic migration from small vessels is hindered by adsorption of the LPF onto lymphocyte surfaces. The lymphocytosis is then created by the resulting entrapment of cells within the vascular and lymphatic compartment rather than by an increase in newly formed cells. LPF is also being considered as the factor which slows weight gain and causes late death in mice.

Clinical Infection

Epidemiology Several features of the epidemiology have intrigued students of this disease for a number of years. Pertussis has not usually been a disease with marked seasonal variations in incidence, in contrast to several other childhood infections. The disease is worldwide in its distribution, and in the United States the number of reported cases has declined from approximately 120,000 in 1950 to 1,759 in 1973 (Fig. 31-1). Reported deaths declined from approximately 1,100 in 1950 to 12 in 1970. Most deaths occur in infants under 1 year of age, and the decline in case fatality over the past several decades has been associated with a gradual increase in the age of patients sustaining infection.

The illness is highly communicable, as evidenced by attack rates of 90 percent in unimmunized household contacts of persons with pertussis. Man is the only known source of *B. pertussis*, and excretion of organisms is limited almost entirely to persons with active infection. Asymptomatic carriers are unusual, and prolonged presence of organisms during convalescence is extremely rare.

Pathogenesis Following aspiration of infected droplets, the organisms proliferate

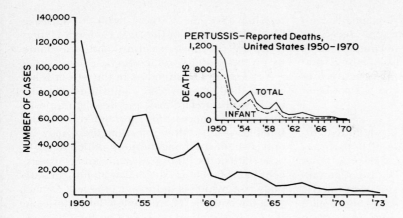

FIG. 31-1. Pertussis. Reported cases by year, United States, 1950-1973. (Adapted from CDC Morbidity and Mortality 22 (53):45, 1973)

within the respiratory tract. Symptoms almost always begin within 10 days after exposure to pertussis, although the incubation period can vary from 5 to 21 days. The clinical illness is divided into three separate stages for descriptive purposes. The catarrhal or prodromal stage lasts from one to two weeks. During this period, the child exhibits only mild symptoms of an uncomplicated upper respiratory infection, including sneezing, a watery nasal discharge, frequent cough, and occasionally conjunctivitis. Physical examination does not reveal any serious objective findings. The second stage usually lasts from one to six weeks and is characterized by progression to a paroxysmal cough. A characteristic paryoxysm is one in which 5 to 20 forcible hacking coughs are produced in 15 to 20 seconds and is often terminated with the production of mucus or associated vomiting. There is no time for breathing between coughs, and the paroxysm may be sufficiently prolonged to induce anoxia. The final inspiratory breath which takes place through the narrowed glottis produces the characteristic whoop. These early stages of illness are frequently associated with leukocytosis of 12,000 to 200,000 per cu mm, and with a lymphocytosis of 60 percent.

The observed limitation of *B. pertussis* invasion to the superficial layers of the upper respiratory tract in a susceptible host remains unexplained. An even greater puzzle for immunologists is the obvious protection from respiratory invasion provided by parenteral administration of inactivated *B. pertussis* vaccine. Recent work demonstrates that production of antibodies in various immunoglobulin classes in the respiratory tract and a titer rise in serum IgA occurs in the mouse after intranasal inoculation with live organisms. This helps to define the host response during actual infection but leaves unanswered the question of how vaccine-induced immunity is achieved. The contribution of cell-mediated immunity to the host response is yet to be defined.

The third stage of illness is that of convalescence and coughing and may persist for as long as several months after the initial onset of illness. The persistence of the paroxysmal cough long after viable pertussis organisms have disappeared from the respiratory tract is unexplained. An understanding of the pathogenesis of the cough is of potential therapeutic importance, since the clinical course of the disease is not appreciably altered by administration of specific antimicrobial agents.

Clinical Manifestations The clinical syndrome of pertussis is readily defined in the presence of the paroxysmal cough and associated whoop, but the illness is of variable severity, and the milder respiratory syndromes caused by *B. pertussis* are impossible to distinguish on clinical grounds alone. As many as 20 percent of pertussis infections have been estimated to be atypical illnesses and those patients are infectious for others.

The morbidity and mortality associated with the disease have resulted primarily from compromise of the central nervous system during the acute illness and from secondary bacterial infection usually involving ears, sinuses, or the lower respiratory tract. The neuropathology of infants dying with pertussis and central nervous system involvement is nonspecific and indistinguishable from changes produced by anoxia. Central nervous system compromise is clearly not a result of actual invasion by *B. pertussis*, but the role of the multiple reactive substances produced by the bacteria has not been determined.

Laboratory Diagnosis The definitive diagnosis depends upon isolation of *B. pertussis* (or less commonly, *B. parapertussis* or *B. bronchiseptica*) from the patient. The isolation rate of the organism from the respiratory tract is greatest during the catarrhal stage, and organisms are not usually detectable for longer than the first four weeks of illness. An appropriate specimen from patients for cultivation is either a nasopharyngeal swab or a cough plate.

Isolation of *B. pertussis* from clinical specimens is dependent upon careful transport and efficient processing of the materials obtained for culture. If the specimen will not be planted for one to two hours, the swab should be placed in 0.25 to 0.50 ml of casamino acid solution with a pH of 7.2 to prevent drying of the swab. When the specimen will be shipped to another laboratory or holding time exceeds two hours, other organisms may overgrow the *B. pertussis*. Swabs should therefore be placed in modified Stuart's medium (SBL) or Mishulow's charcoal agar. These media are better able to maintain the viability of organisms and to support growth under the conditions of transport. Modified Bordet-Gengou agar is recommended for primary isolation of the organism. The addition of 0.25 to 0.5 unit/ml of penicillin to a second plate is useful in inhibiting the growth of the gram-positive flora of the respiratory tract without affecting growth of *B. pertussis* organisms.

In addition to the biochemical reactions listed in Table 31-1, serologic identification of *B. pertussis* will confirm the isolation. A slide agglutination test can be performed with a standard inoculum or organisms and specific antiserum which is available commercially.

Fluorescent antibody (FA) staining has been used to identify *B. pertussis* upon direct smears of nasopharyngeal swabs and for identification of organisms growing on Bordet-Gengou plates. The FA technique with standardized antiserum is useful in experienced hands. The FA procedure does not substitute for cultural isolation but does offer the advantage of rapid identification of organisms. The Analytical Bac-

teriology Section of the Center for Disease Control and many of the state bacterial laboratories are prepared to culture and/or examine by FA techniques for *B. pertussis*.

Assessment of antibodies in the serum is accomplished by measuring agglutinins. The test is not well standardized, and the agglutinin titers are not necessarily correlated with the immune status. After infection there may be only a slight rise in agglutinins, which tends to occur late in the illness. An acute and convalescent pair of sera are needed to define an antibody rise, which is indicative of recent contact with the antigen. There are few laboratories in the United States prepared to perform tests of *B. pertussis* agglutinin titers.

Treatment Erythromycin is currently the drug of choice for therapy of pertussis infection. The organism is sensitive to this drug in vitro, and administration eliminates the organism from the nasopharynx and therefore shortens the period of communicability. There is some evidence to suggest that if erythromycin is administered early during the catarrhal stage the paroxysmal manifestations may be shortened. Tetracycline and chloramphenicol are considered adequate alternative antimicrobial agents. Secondary bacterial infection may necessitate additional appropriate therapy directed at the responsible pathogen. Supportive measures, such as careful suction to remove tenacious secretions, hydration, nutrition, and electrolyte balance, are of great importance. Oxygen therapy with increased humidity appears to be beneficial. Some persons feel that the administration of human pertussis immune serum globulin is a useful adjunct to therapy, but the efficacy of this treatment has not been established.

Prevention It has been recommended that contacts of an infected individual who is under four years of age and previously immunized against pertussis should receive a booster dose of vaccine. They should also receive erythromycin, since immunity conferred by vaccine is not absolute. Unimmunized contacts should receive chemoprophylaxis with erythromycin for approximately 10 days after the contact with the patient has ceased. Human pertussis immune serum globulin may be administered to exposed infants under the age of 2 years who have not been immunized, but protection afforded by this measure is not reliable. The best protective measures for young infants are adequate immunization and avoidance of contact with pertussis.

Active Immunization. Protection of the young infant against pertussis is important because the greatest number of severe complications and highest morbidity occur in this age group. Passive protection is not afforded by the quantity of antibody that traverses the placenta. Routine primary immunization is begun at about two months of age unless pertussis is prevalent in the community, in which case immunization should be begun earlier. A total of 12 protective units of pertussis vaccine is recommended, and this is divided into three equal doses given four to eight weeks apart. The vaccine is usually given in a combined preparation containing adsorbed diphtheria and tetanus toxoids and pertussis vaccine (DTP). These are depot antigens and appear to be more immunogenic and less reactive than a similar plain antigen product without adjuvant. A booster injection is given 12 to 18 months after primary immunization or prior to school entry.

Immunization has been successful in the prevention of disease, and widespread usage of vaccine has been associated with the continued decline of reported cases of pertussis. Neither natural disease nor immunization afford lifetime immunity. Susceptibility to illness has been shown to increase with the number of years after disease or immunization, and outbreaks of illness have occurred in recent years which frequently involve adults and older children. Persons at risk include hospital personnel who may be exposed to patients excreting *B. pertussis*.

The effectiveness of the vaccine in young children has not encouraged the development of purified immunogens. The factor(s) that produce toxicity or contribute to postvaccination encephalopathy have not been defined, and thus it is impossible to test vaccines for this activity. The mouse weight gain test has been employed in the United States as the most accurate animal assessment of potential toxicity of vaccine for humans. Vaccine-associated encephalopathy is estimated to occur once in 5 to 10 million injections in the United States. The estimated incidence of CNS complications of natural disease has ranged from 1.5 percent to 14 percent in hospitalized cases. One-third of these individuals recover, one-third have varying neurologic sequelae, and one-third die or have severe deficits. The risks of immunization appear to be far less than those associated with the natural disease. Further research is essential to understand the nature of the host's pharmacologic reactions and mechanisms of immunity against this infection localized to the respiratory tract.

FURTHER READING

Books and Reviews

Lapin JH: Whooping Cough. Springfield, Ill, Thomas, 1943
Munoz J: Symposium on relationship of structure of microorganisms to their immunochemical properties. I. Immunological and other biological activities of *Bordetella pertussis* antigens. Bacteriol Rev 27:325, 1963
Pittman M: *Bordetella pertussis* — bacterial and host factors in the pathogenesis and prevention of whooping cough. In Mudd S (ed): Infectious Agents and Host Reactions. Philadelphia, Saunders, 1970, Chap 11
Rowatt E: The growth of *Bordetella pertussis:* A review. J Gen Microbiol 17:297, 1957

Selected Papers

Bass JW, Klenk EL, Kothermei JB, et al: Antimicrobial treatment of pertussis. J Pediatr, 75:768, 1969
Eldering G, Kendrick P: *Bacillus para-pertussis.* A species resembling both *Bacillus pertussis* and *Bacillus bronchisepticus* but identical with neither. J Bacteriol 35:561, 1938
Miller JJ, Silverberg RJ, Saito TM, Humber JB: An agglutinative reaction for *Hemophilus pertussis.* II. Its relation to clinical immunity. J Pediatr 22:644, 1943
Morse I, Bray KK: The occurrence and properties of leukocytosis and the lymphocytosis-stimulating material in the supernatant fluids of *Bordetella pertussis* cultures. J Exp Med 129:523, 1969
Ross R, Munoz J, Cameron C: Histamine sensitizing factor, mouse protective antigens, and other antigens of some members of the genus *Bordetella.* J Bacteriol 99:57, 1969
Sato Y, Arai H, Suzuki K: Leukocytosis promoting factor of *Bordetella pertussis.* II. Biological properties. Infect Immun 7:992, 1973

32
Listeria and Erysipelothrix

TABLE 32-1   PRIMARY CLINICAL MANIFESTATIONS OF HUMAN LISTERIOSIS

	Cases
Meningitis, meningoencephalitis, or encephalitis	469
Septicemia: neonates	51
others	59
Pregnant women: prepartum flulike symptoms	5
abortion	12
postpartum, of infected infant	17
Endocarditis	7
Abscess	5
Pneumonia	5
Conjunctivitis	2
Infectious mononucleosis	2
Pharyngitis	2
Cutaneous papules and pustules	1
Persistent headache	1
Fever	2
No disease; routine culture	1
Total	641

From Killinger and Schubert: Proceedings of the Third International Symposium on Listeriosis, Bilthoven, The Netherlands, 1966

Only two organisms in the genera *Listeria* and *Erysipelothrix* are of medical importance, *Listeria monocytogenes* and *Erysipelothrix rhusiopathiae*. *L. monocytogenes* is widely distributed in nature and in a variety of animal reservoirs. In man it produces infection with protean manifestations. Meningitis is most frequent, but the most unique of its many clinical forms is infection of the genital tract of the gravid female and infection of the offspring either before birth or during delivery (Table 32-1). Listeriosis has been recognized in recent years with increased frequency.

E. rhusiopathiae is the cause of erysipeloid in man, an acute self-limited infection of the skin occurring primarily in occupational groups which handle animals and animal products.

Listeria and *Erysipelothrix* organisms resemble corynebacteria morphologically, and until the Eighth Edition of *Bergey's Manual* they were classified with these organisms in the family Corynebacteriaceae. Other properties, however, are more similar to those of the Lactobacillaceae, the group with which they are tentatively associated in Part 16 of Bergey's scheme. *Listeria* and *Erysipelothrix* do not contain arabinogalactan in their cell walls, as do the coryneform organisms but instead contain the sugar rhamnose (Chap. 33). A marked difference also exists in the G + C content of the DNA of the various organisms (Table 32-2).

LISTERIA MONOCYTOGENES

Morphology and Physiology

The *Listeria* are small gram-positive coccobacilli that have a tendency to occur in short chains of three to five organisms. In stained preparations they assume a typical diphtheroid palisade arrangement, a property that resulted previously in their incorrect classification with the corynebacteria. *L. monocytogenes* is 0.4 to 0.5 by 0.5 to 2.0 μm in size. In preparations from rough cultures, elongated rods and filaments 5 to 100 μm in length are observed. It is motile by means of peritrichous flagella; four flagella are produced at 20 to 25C, but fewer flagella are formed at 37C.

L. monocytogenes grows well on sheep blood

TABLE 32-2   DISTINGUISHING PROPERTIES OF CERTAIN NONSPORULATING GRAM-POSITIVE BACTERIA

	Listeria monocytogenes	Erysipelothrix rhusiopathiae	Streptococcus pyogenes	Streptococcus faecalis	Corynebacterium sp.	Lactobacillus sp.
Morphology	Rod	Rod	Coccus	Coccus	Rod	Rod
β-Hemolysis	+	−	+	−	±	−
Catalase	+	−	−	−	+	−
Motility	+	−	−	−	−	−
Acid from:						
Glucose	+	+	+	+	±	+
Mannitol	−	−	−	+	±	±
Keratoconjunctivitis	+	−	−	−	−	−
G + C content*	38	36	34−38	33−38	57−60	34−50

Adapted from Buchner and Schneierson: Am J Med 45:904, 1968
°Guanine and cytosine content of DNA (moles percent).

agar medium and tryptose agar. On blood agar a narrow zone of β hemolysis surrounds the colony. On the clear tryptose agar, colonies are recognized by their characteristic blue-green color as seen with oblique light. The amount of hemolysis varies; some strains are strongly hemolytic, while other hemolyze very weakly. The optimal temperature for growth is 37C, but growth occurs at all temperatures down to 2.5C.

L. monocytogenes is aerobic to microaerophilic, but growth is improved when cultures are incubated under reduced oxygen and a 5 to 10 percent concentration of CO_2. Catalase is produced, a property that is useful in the organism's differentiation from streptococci. L. monocytogenes ferments a number of sugars with the formation of acid only (Table 32-2). All strains hydrolyze Tweens, and some produce a phosphomonoesterase that causes opacity in egg yolk media.

Laboratory Identification

The identification of L. monocytogenes is based on the typical diphtheroidlike appearance of the organisms and motility in semisolid agar. Useful biochemical properties for the differentiation of Listeria are listed in Table 32-2.

Animal Inoculation Animal pathogenicity testing is useful in differentiating L. monocytogenes from gram-positive organisms possessing similar morphologic properties, eg, corynebacteria, Erysipelothrix, and streptococci. The instillation of L. monocytogenes into the conjunctival sac of a young rabbit produces a purulent keratoconjunctivitis within 24 to 36 hours (Anton test). The inoculation of the marginal ear vein of the rabbit produces a marked monocytosis. Intraperitoneal injection of mice also results in necrotic foci in the liver and death of the animal.

Antigenic Structure

Strains of L. monocytogenes have been separated into four major serologic groups and a number of serotypes on the basis of their O and H antigens. Variation has been observed in the frequency of types observed in various parts of the world. At present, type 1b accounts for more than half of the cases. Serotype 2 listeria are rarely encountered, and type 3 is uncommon in the United States.

Determinants of Pathogenicity

L. monocytogenes produces a hemolysin that appears to play an important role in the pathogenesis of the infection. It is similar in many ways to the oxygen-labile cytolytic toxins of a number of other bacterial species. The hemolysin is elaborated into the culture medium during growth of the organism; it is nondialyzable, heat labile, and antigenic. It is sensitive to oxidative inactivation and can be reactivated by reducing substances, such as cysteine.

Listeria hemolysin may function during listeric infection by disrupting membranes, especially those of the phagocytic vacuole and the lysosomes. Hydrolytic enzymes of lysosomes are solubilized, and peritoneal monocytes are degranulated. When injected intravenously hemolysin is lethal for the mouse. Electrocardiograms show serious alterations in heart rate and rhythm indicative of damage to cardiac tissue. The lethal effect following hemolysin treatment probably results from toxic injury to contractile and pacemaker myocardial tissue.

The precise nature of the lipolytic soluble antigen(s) of L. monocytogenes is unclear. A correlation exists in Listeria among hemolysin production, lipolytic activity, and virulence. All avirulent and most nonhemolysin-producing strains show either diminished or no lipolytic activity. The lipolytic antigen and the hemolytic antigen appear to be two distinct antigens rather than a single antigen with both hemolytic and lipolytic activity.

Clinical Infection

Epidemiology L. monocytogenes is worldwide in its distribution. It has been isolated from human beings with disease, from healthy carriers, and from a wide range of other mammals, birds, fish, ticks, and crustacea. There also is a high incidence in plants and soil samples and in the feces of animals. The basic question of whether L. monocytogenes is primarily soil borne or originates from animals excreting the organisms in their feces has not been resolved.

It is currently believed, however, that *L. monocytogenes* is a saprophytic organism that lives in a plant–soil environment and can thus be contracted by humans and animals from many sources via many possible routes. The oral route of infection is probably common.

Pathogenesis In human beings, listeriosis is characterized by widely disseminated abscesses or granulomas. Lesions are present in the liver, spleen, adrenals, respiratory tract, intestinal tract, central nervous system, and skin. The fetus may be infected transplacentally through the umbilical vein with production of septicemia. This is the only proved example of human-to-human transmission of listeriosis. Infection also may be acquired during delivery through contact with infective secretions. Listeriosis of the newborn, contracted intrapartum, usually is localized in the central nervous system; in prepartum infection, listeria from the infected placenta are widely disseminated, resulting in granulomatous foci in many organs.

Listeric infection occurs in some patients as a complication of chronic primary disorders, such as neoplasm, alcoholism, cardiovascular disease, and diabetes. Corticosteroids appear to enhance the susceptibility of patients to infections with listeria and to increase the mortality rate.

Clinical Manifestations Genital tract infection in the gravid female with infection of the offspring is the most characteristic of infections caused by *L. monocytogenes*. In the newborn who is infected at the time of delivery, symptoms begin one to four weeks after birth and are similar to early symptoms observed in any other bacterial meningitis.

Prepartum listeriosis, however, results in abortion, premature delivery, stillbirth, or death within a short period after birth. Cardiorespiratory distress, vomiting, and diarrhea are common, and meningitis, hepatosplenomegaly, and maculopapular skin lesions on the legs and trunk are frequently observed. Usually the mother has no symptomatic illness or only a history of a very benign and self-limited illness resembling influenza during the last trimester of pregnancy.

Meningitis in the adult is the most commonly recognized form of listeriosis. Early in the disease the cells in the cerebrospinal fluid will be mostly granulocytes, but later there may be a predominance of mononuclear cells.

In the adult, febrile pharyngitis with cervical and generalized lymphadenopathy can be caused by *Listeria*. The similarity of these clinical manifestations to those of infectious mononucleosis may make differentiation difficult. There is no reliable evidence at this time, however, that *L. monocytogenes* causes either infectious mononucleosis or repeated abortion.

Disseminated listeriosis in the adult results in pneumonia, empyema, and infective endocarditis. Generalized infection is observed most frequently in patients with carcinoma or other debilitating diseases. Its development in these patients may be augmented by corticosteroid therapy.

Immunity Antigenic stimulation by *L. monocytogenes* results in the synthesis of humoral antibodies that can ,be detected by agglutination, immunofluorescence, and other serologic procedures. *L. monocytogenes*, however, is an intracellular organism. In infections with which it is associated, cellular immunity is of greater importance, and resistance is mediated by thymus-derived lymphocytes and activated macrophages.

Laboratory Diagnosis The diagnosis of listeriosis is based on the isolation of *L. monocytogenes* from the appropriate clinical materials depending upon the syndrome. Such materials would include cervical and vaginal secretions, lochia, cord blood, meconium, blood, and cerebrospinal fluid. The direct examination of gram stains of these materials is extremely useful and will alert the laboratory to the possibility of a *L. monocytogenes* infection.

Specimens should be routinely stored at 4C for at least four weeks and possibly up to six months; subcultures should be made during this period. Useful procedures for the differentiation of *L. monocytogenes* from diphtheroids and other organisms with which it may be confused are listed in Table 32-2. Cultures identified as *L. monocytogenes* should be sent to the Center for Disease Control for complete serologic identification.

The serologic diagnosis of listeriosis is unreliable because *L. monocytogenes* cross-reacts with a number of other gram-positive organisms.

Treatment   The fatality rate in untreated cases of meningitis is 70 to 90 percent; it is much lower in treated cases. The prognosis is still poor in listeriosis of the newborn. Penicillin is the drug of choice, but erythromycin and the tetracyclines also are very effective.

Prevention   Effective control of *Listeria* infections is hampered by difficulties in recognition of human and animal infection. In the newborn, listeriosis is preventable by early recognition and prompt treatment of the mother. Prevention should center on elimination of animal reservoirs and pasteurization of milk; contact with infected animals or animal products should be avoided.

ERYSIPELOTHRIX RHUSIOPATHIAE

E. rhusiopathiae is a nonsporogenous, nonmotile, nonencapsulated gram-positive rod. In smooth colonies organisms are short, slender, straight or slightly curved, 0.2 to 0.4 μm by 0.5 to 2.5 μm in size. In rough colonies long filamentous structures and chains are present.

E. rhusiopathiae is microaerophilic when first isolated and grows in a band a few millimeters below the surface of a semisolid tube of agar. Heart infusion agar containing rabbit blood and incubation in the presence of 5 percent CO_2 are suitable for primary isolation. On blood agar plates alpha hemolysis is produced, although a slight but definite clearing occurs around the colonies upon prolonged incubation. Black colonies are produced on tellurite medium. Properties useful in the identification and differentiation of *Erysipelothrix* from *Listeria* and corynebacteria are listed in Table 32-2.

E. rhusiopathiae is widespread in its distribution. It occurs in the surface slime of fresh and salt-water fish and causes disease in swine, horses, sheep, and other animals. Man acquires the infection by contact with animals or animal products. The disease is more prevalent in the male, especially abattoir employees, butchers, and those handling fish, animal hides, and bones. Most infections are related to skin injury.

The disease in man is characterized by a nonsuppurative violaceous lesion at the site of inoculation, which is usually on the hand or fingers. The lesions burn and itch, but usually there is no pain, no systemic symptoms, and no lymphangitis. The disease remains localized and lasts only a few days; resolution is rapid. Erysipelothrix infections rarely are disseminated. Following bacteremia, however, infective endocarditis, septic arthritis, and death may ensue.

A laboratory diagnosis can be made by culture of the organism from aspirated or biopsied material taken from the margin of the lesion.

Penicillin is the drug of choice. Erythromycin may be used in patients sensitive to penicillin.

FURTHER READING

Books and Reviews

Gray ML, Killinger AH: *Listeria monocytogenes* and listeria infections. Bacteriol Rev 30:309, 1966

Grieco MH, Sheldon C: *Erysipelothrix rhusiopathiae*. Ann NY Acad Sci 174:523, 1970

Hoeprich PD: Listeriosis. In Hoeprich PD (ed.): Infectious Diseases. Hagerstown, Md, Harper and Row, 1972, Chap 46

Killinger AH: *Listeria monocytogenes*. In Lennette EH, Spaulding EH; Truant JP (eds.): Manual of Clinical Microbiology, 2nd ed. Washington, DC, Am Soc Microbiol, 1974, Chap 13

Proceedings of the Third International Symposium on Listeriosis, Bilthoven, The Netherlands. July 13-16, 1966

Seebiger HPR: Listeriosis. New York, Hafner, 1961

Selected Papers

McCallum RE, Sword CP: Mechanisms of pathogenesis in *Listeria monocytogenes* infection. Infect Immun 5:863, 872, 1972

Moore RM, Zehmer RB: Listeriosis in the United States — 1971. J Infect Dis 127:610, 1973

Outteridge PM, Osebold JW, Zee YC: Activity of macrophage and neutrophil cellular fractions from normal and immune sheep against *Listeria monocytogenes*. Infect Immun 5:814, 1972

Ratzan KR, Musher DM, Keusch GT, Weinstein L: Correlation of increased metabolic activity, resistance to infection, enhanced phagocytosis, and inhibition of bacterial growth by macrophages from Listeria- and BCG-infected mice. Infect Immun 5:499, 1972

Srivastava KK, Siddique IH: Quantitative chemical composition of peptidoglycan of *Listeria monocytogenes*. Infect Immun 7:700, 1973

Stuart MR, Pease PE: A numerical study on the relationships of Listeria and Erysipelothrix. J Gen Microbiol 73:551, 1972

Sword CP, Kingdon GC: *Listeria monocytogenes* toxin. In Kadis S, Montie TC, Ajl SJ (eds.): Microbial Toxins. New York, Academic Press, 1971, pp. 357-377

Watson BB, Lavizzo JC: Extracellular antigens from *Listeria monocytogenes*. Infect Immun 7:753, 1973

Weis J, Seeliger HPR: Incidence of *Listeria monocytogenes* in nature. Appl Microbiol 30:29, 1975

33
Corynebacterium

CORYNEBACTERIUM DIPHTHERIAE

Diphtheria is the prototype of a toxigenic disease. It is an acute infection caused by *Corynebacterium diphtheriae* lysogenic for a bacteriophage carrying the gene for diphtheria toxin. The primary lesion that usually occurs in the throat or nasopharynx is characterized by the presence of a spreading grayish pseudomembranous growth. As the organisms multiply at this site they elaborate a potent exotoxin that is transported by the blood to remote tissues of the body causing hemorrhagic and necrotic damage in various organs.

The history of diphtheria is a fascinating account of the successful study and conquest of an infectious disease. It is an account that emphasizes the importance of basic research in providing practical solutions to clinical problems. Diphtheria was first established as a specific clinical entity in 1826 following the publication of a classic monograph by Pierre Bretonneau, but its bacterial etiology was not fully established until 1888. Klebs had earlier described the characteristic bacilli in pseudomembranes from diphtheritic throats, and Löffler had isolated the organism in pure culture, but complete understanding of the pathogenesis of the infection was provided only with the discovery by Roux and Yersin of a soluble exotoxin in the filtrates of cultures. This finding opened the door to immunologic studies that resulted in the discovery of antitoxin and toxoid, the two biologicals that have been so successfully employed in passive and active immunization against the disease.

Corynebacterium diphtheriae is the only major human pathogen of the corynebacteria group of organisms, a group that also contains a number of harmless, poorly described saprophytes frequently found on the surface of mucous membranes. The corynebacteria are taxonomically related to the mycobacteria and nocardia because of similarities in their cell wall components, and they exhibit cross-reactivity with them. Mureins of the three genera contain *meso*-α,ε-diaminopimelic acid, and arabinose and galactose are major sugars of their wall polysaccharide. Cornyebacteria also contain considerable amounts of mycolic acids in the lipids associated with their outer envelope. Mycolic acids found in the corynebacteria are similar to the large saturated, α-branched, β-hydroxy fatty acids of the mycobacteria but contain fewer carbon atoms.

Morphology

C. diphtheriae is a slender, gram-positive, rod-shaped organism that is not acid-fast and does not form spores. Cells range in length from 1.5 to 5 μm and in width from 0.5 to 1 μm. They characteristically appear in stained smears in palisades, or as individual cells lying at sharp angles to each other in V and L formation. These Chinese character formations are caused by the snapping movement involved when two corynebacterial cells divide. When grown on nutritionally complete media at a maximum rate, diphtheria bacilli are uniform in shape. When grown, however, on suboptimal media, such as Löffler's coagulated serum or Pai's coagulated egg medium, the cells are pleomorphic and stain irregularly with methylene blue or toluidine blue. Club-shaped swellings and beaded and barred forms are common. The metachromatic (Babes-Ernst) granules that are responsible for the beaded appearance represent accumulations of polymerized polyphosphates.

Physiology

Cultural Characteristics Although *C. diphtheriae* is a facultatively aerobic organism, it grows best under aerobic conditions. Complex media are used both for the primary isolation and characterization of colonies and for the commercial production of toxin. Most strains grow as a waxy pellicle on the surface of liquid media. On Löffler's coagulated serum medium, which is useful for the primary isolation of the organism, minute, grayish white, glistening colonies appear after 12 to 24 hours' incubation at 37C. Since this medium is nutritionally inadequate for the diphtheria bacillus, unbalanced cell wall synthesis causes the organisms to become pleomorphic and to assume their easily recognizable morphology. Löffler's medium is also useful because it does not support the growth of streptococci and pneumococci that may be present in the clinical specimen.

The incorporation of tellurite salts into the medium reduces the number of contaminants and gives to the colonies a characteristic gray or black color, which aids in the differentiation of *C. diphtheriae* into the three major colonial types: gravis, mitis, and intermedius. Colonies of gravis strains are large, flat, gray to black with a dull surface, mitis organisms produce medium-sized colonies that are smaller, blacker, glossy, and more convex, and colonies of intermedius strains are very small and either smooth or rough. The tellurite ion passes through the cell membrane into the cytoplasm where it is reduced to the metal tellurium and is precipitated inside the cell. No constant relationship exists between the severity of the disease and the three colony types.

Resistance *C. diphtheriae* is more resistant to the action of light, desiccation, and freezing than are most nonsporebearing bacilli. Organisms have been isolated from dried fragments of pseudomembranes after 14 weeks. The organisms are, however, killed by boiling for 1 minute or by exposure to a temperature of 58C for 10 minutes. They are readily destroyed by most of the routinely employed disinfectants.

Antigenic Structure

All diphtheria toxins are immunologically identical. The organism *C. diphtheriae*, however, is an antigenically heterogeneous species. Agglutination tests with whole cell suspensions show a large number of serologic types. The three major colonial types, gravis, mitis, and intermedius, reflect differences in the cell surface of the organisms and constitute the major biotypes of the organism. Within each of these cultural types is a more or less separate group of agglutinating serotypes. Additional differences in cell surface components have also been detected by the more sensitive tests of bacteriophage typing and bacteriocin production. The antigens responsible for the type specificity of *C. diphtheriae* strains are heat-labile proteins, the K antigens, localized in the superficial layers of the wall. These antigens play an important role in antibacterial immunity and hypersensitivity separate from antitoxic immunity. The occurrence of different antigenic types of *C. diphtheriae* probably explains the occurrence of diphtheria in immunized individuals who show a detectable level of circulating antitoxin. The K antigens on the surface, together with the glycolipid cord factor (see below), are major determinants of invasiveness and virulence in diphtheria bacilli.

The heat-stable O antigen of *C. diphtheriae* is a group antigen common to the corynebacteria parasitic for man and animals. It is a polysaccharide containing arabinogalactans and is the antigen responsible for the cross-reactivity with mycobacteria and nocardia. Corynebacterial cells and their subcellular components are excellent antigens. When administered to animals with immunizing agents they also function as adjuvants (Chap. 13).

Determinants of Pathogenicity

Invasiveness Since both toxigenic and nontoxigenic strains of *C. diphtheriae* are capable of colonizing mucous membranes, factors other than toxin contribute to the organism's invasiveness and ability to establish and maintain itself in the human host. The precise relationship of these traits to the pathogenesis of the disease is ill defined at the present time. In addition to the surface K antigens, the organisms contain a cord factor that is considered to be a necessary adjunct of virulence. The cord factor, a toxic glycolipid, is a 6-6' diester of trehalose containing the mycolic acids characteristic of *C. diphtheriae*, corynemycolic acid ($C_{32}H_{62}O_3$) and corynemycolenic acid ($C_{32}H_{64}O_3$). The pharmacologic activity of the cord factor of *C. diphtheriae* is similar to that of the cord factor isolated from *M. tuberculosis*. It is lethal for the mouse, causing a disruption of mitochondria and reduction of respiration and phosphorylation.

Additional factors that are also thought to play a role in the invasiveness of *C. diphtheriae* include neuraminidase and N-acetylneuraminate lyase. For bacteria inhabiting the mucous membranes, these enzymes could provide a readily available source of energy by degrading the N-acetylneuraminic acid residues cleaved from its mucinous environment.

Exotoxin An understanding of the biochemical base of any pathologic process is necessary for a complete understanding of the intracellular events responsible for the fundamental expression of the disease. Most naturally occurring diseases are too complex at the cellular level to dissect successfully and define definitively the primary biochemical lesion. In diphtheria, however, the exotoxin produced by *C. diphtheriae* is the major biochemical determinant in the pathogenesis of the infection and accounts for essentially all of the pathologic effects. The study of the molecular biology of its production and mode of action has provided a model system for the use of modern tools and concepts in the study of a disease process.

LYSOGENY AND *TOX* GENE. Toxin is produced only by those strains of *C. diphtheriae* lysogenic for a bacteriophage carrying the *tox* gene. Nontoxigenic strains, however, may be converted to the lysogenic, toxigenic state by treatment with a suitable *tox* corynebacteriophage. The integration of prophage into host genome is a stable relationship, and toxigenicity is not lost in truly lysogenic strains. Although most of the studies have been conducted with the β phage the *tox* gene has been detected in a variety of corynebacteriophages that differ both genetically and serologically. The *tox* gene is expressed early during vegetative replication of the phage. It appears to be made on the cytoplasmic membrane and to serve no essential viral function. Toxin is released before any phage particles appear and ceases to be formed when the cells undergo lysis.

The yield of toxin by a toxigenic strain is markedly influenced by environmental and cultural conditions, especially the inorganic iron content of the medium. Toxin production is enhanced by any condition that prevents viral maturation or lengthens the period between phage induction and cell lysis, a condition favored by low levels of iron. The successful use for many years of the Park and Williams strain 8 for the commercial production of toxin is linked to its ability to grow in media containing very low levels of iron. Under such conditions toxin may account for approximately 5 percent of the total bacterial protein. Structural changes in the low-iron phenotype of this organism have been revealed by electron micrography and chemical analyses. Cells are usually longer than their high-iron conterpart because of delay in division and have a more simple cell wall. The effect of these changes on permeability of the cell and the facilitated release of exotoxin has been suggested, but at the present time it is still unclear how the effect of iron on toxin production is mediated. One of the most attractive

mechanisms advanced is a regulatory process in which an iron-containing protein functions as the repressor of the *tox* gene.

PROPERTIES.   Diphtheria toxin is produced and released extracellularly as a single polypeptide chain with a molecular weight of about 62,000. It consists of two fragments, A and B, with molecular weights of 24,000 and 38,000, respectively. Both of these fragments are required for a toxic effect in animals and in tissue culture cells. As the native toxin molecule is released from the host bacterium, it is nontoxic because the active site on the A fragment is masked. Activation, however, may be accomplished by proteases present in the bacterial culture medium or experimentally by mild treatment with trypsin in the presence of sulfhydryl reducing agents. All of the enzymatic activity of the toxin molecule resides in fragment A. This fragment alone, however, is unable to enter the cell without the hydrophobic fragment B. Fragment B apparently provides a mechanism for the attachment of fragment A to sensitive sites on the cell membrane and for its transport into the cell.

Both A and B moieties of the toxin contain a number of antigenic determinants. Antitoxin consists of a mixture of antibodies specific for different parts of the toxin molecule. In native toxin or toxoid most of the antigenic determinants in fragment A are deeply buried and are not available either to stimulate antibody production or to participate in the precipitation of antibody. Also, although anti-A antibody inhibits the enzymic activity of toxin, it does not protect animals or cells against the lethal action of toxin. Antibodies directed against fragment B, however, neutralize toxin with great efficiency, supporting the theory that antitoxin acts by preventing the attachment of toxin to cells and that fragment B is required for the initial attachment.

Animals vary widely in their susceptibility to diphtheria toxin. It is lethal for man, rabbits, guinea pigs, and birds in doses as low as 160 nanograms per kilogram of body weight. Rats and mice are highly resistant because their cells apparently lack binding sites for fragment B. In the human a single gene located on chromosome 5 is responsible for sensitivity to the toxin. The exquisite sensitivity of rabbits and guinea pigs to diphtheria toxin has provided excellent experimental models for the study of the mode of action of the toxin and for its biologic standardization.

MODE OF ACTION. Diphtheria toxin inhibits protein synthesis in eukaryotic cells under conditions where no inhibition in other metabolic functions and no evidence of membrane damage are observed. Nicotinamide adenine dinucleotide (NAD) is an absolute requirement for this inhibition of protein synthesis, which can be demonstrated both in tissue culture cells and in cell-free systems. Toxin inactivates the peptidyl-tRNA elongation factor, EF-2, the factor required in protein synthesis for the translocation of polypeptidyl-transfer RNA from the so-called acceptor site to the donor site on the eukaryotic ribosome (Chap. 7). The inactivation is accomplished by its ADP-ribosylation with the adenosine diphosphate ribose (ADPR) moiety of NAD. The reaction catalyzed by the diphtheria toxin is as follows:

$$\text{EF-2} + \text{NAD} \underset{\text{toxin}}{\rightleftharpoons} \text{ADPR—EF-2} +$$
$$\text{nicotinamide} + \text{H}^+$$

Whereas the reaction is reversible, its equilibrium at physiologic pH lies far to the right. No eukaryotic protein other than EF-2 is capable of accepting ADPR from NAD in the presence of diphtheria toxin. Also, toxin has no effect on polypeptide chain elongation in procaryotic systems or in mitochondria, where a different protein, EF-G, replaces the EF-2 factor. As discussed above, all of the enzymatic activity of the toxin resides in the fragment A moiety that has a single binding site for NAD. This activity remains masked in the intact molecule until the induction of conformational changes that expose the active enzyme site.

Clinical Infection

Epidemiology Diphtheria occurs throughout the world, often in epidemic form, but is now relatively uncommon in the United States and Western Europe. The marked decrease in incidence is attributable to successful programs for the active immunization of preschool children. Even though the annual number of cases is small, the problem has been a serious one in certain population clusters where most of the cases are confined. The highest annual attack rates are in the South in the 1 to 9-year age group. The attack rate for unimmunized children is 70 times higher than that of children having received three or more injections of toxoid. Because of the low immunization status of adults, diphtheria occurs in the older age groups at about the same low frequency as in the past, with adults 15 years of age and older now accounting for approximately 25 percent of all cases in the United States. Severe complications are also more prevalent in the elderly. During the last 10 years a number of widely scattered epidemics of diphtheria have occurred in the United States, providing an opportunity for epidemiologic analysis of the diphtheria problem in this country and the evaluation of current measures for its control. The persons affected were of the lower socioeconomic groups, most of whom lived in crowded slum areas with limited access to health care facilities.

Man is the only natural host of *C. diphtheriae* and is therefore the only significant reservoir of infection. The organisms inhabit the upper respiratory tract and, from this locus, are transmitted from person to person via droplet infection. Discharges from extrarespiratory sites, such as skin ulcers, also provide a source of pharyngeal disease. Diphtheria may occur during any month of the year, but crowding and close interpersonal contact during the winter months result in a higher frequency, especially in the South, from September through January. Asymptomatic carriers and persons in the incubation stage of the disease are the major source of most infections.

Immunity The immune status of the individual is the major factor determining whether or not clinical disease will follow invasion and infection of the body by toxin-producing diphtheria bacilli. In diphtheria immunity against the clinical disease depends primarily upon the presence of antitoxin in the circulation. Antitoxin is a true antibody formed in response to either clinical or subclinical infection or as a result of artificial active immunization (p. 498). The antitoxin may be transferred to other persons either naturally, by transplacental passage in utero, or artificially, by transfusion.

The immunization of infants and preschool children with diphtheria toxoid has materially reduced the incidence of diphtheria in children and, as a result, has decreased the carrier rate and opportunity for natural reinforcement of immunity to diphtheria by subclinical infection. As a result an increasing number of adults are without protective antitoxic immunity to diphtheria. Also, a much lower percentage of newborns are immune during the first months of life. The immune status of an individual may be assessed by the determination of serum antitoxin levels or by the Schick test.

SCHICK TEST. This test is performed by injecting into the skin of the forearm 0.1 ml of highly purified toxin (diluted to contain 0.02 MLD). As defined by Ehrlich, the MLD (minimal lethal dose) is the smallest amount of toxin that will kill a guinea pig weighing 250 g within four days after subcutaneous injection. When administering a Schick test a control should always be performed on the other forearm in order to detect pseudoreactions. For the control a similar amount of the same material that has been heated to 60C for 30 minutes in order to destroy the toxic activity is used. A positive reaction is characterized by a local inflammatory reaction that reaches a maximal intensity within four to seven days and fades gradually, leaving an area of brownish pigmentation. A positive Schick reaction indicates the absence of immunity to diphtheria. A negative Schick reaction signifies that the antitoxin level of the blood is greater than 0.03 units per milliliter and that the individual is immune under ordinary conditions of exposure. Allergic reactions are sometimes observed in adults and older children, especially in areas where diphtheria is endemic. These reactions are probably the result of previous infections with corynebacteria or artificial immunization with toxoid. If such individuals are immune, they will give a pseudoreaction characterized by the development of erythema at the site of injection of both the test and control arms. The reaction reaches its maximum intensity within 24 to 36 hours and then fades and disappears completely within the next 72 hours. If, however, the individual is allergic but has no antitoxin or a low level of antitoxin in his blood, he will give a combined reaction. The reaction in the control arm subsides by the fifth or sixth day, whereas that in the test arm reaches its maximum on the fifth day and persists for several days.

Pathogenesis Following exposure of a susceptible individual to *C. diphtheriae* there is a short incubation period of one to four days up to one week, during which time the organism establishes itself on the superficial epithelial cells of the upper respiratory tract. The initial lesion usually occurs on the tonsils and oropharynx and, from this site, may spread to the nasopharynx, larynx, and trachea. Infections of the mucous membranes of the conjunctiva and genitalia are rare. In the tropics, where hygienic conditions are poor, diphtherial skin lesions are relatively common due to the secondary infection of open sores. The organisms grow rapidly in the local lesion, producing an exotoxin that causes necrosis of cells in the area. An inflammatory reaction results, accompanied by the outpouring of a fibrinous exudate. At first patchy in appearance, as the local exudative lesions coalesce, a very tough adherent pseudomembrane forms. It is grayish to black in color and contains, in addition to the fibrin, necrotic epithelial cells, lymphocytes, polymorphonuclear leukocytes, erythrocytes, and *C. diphtheriae*. The pseudomembrane adheres very tenaciously to the underlying tissues, and if attempts are made to forcibly remove it a raw bleeding surface is exposed.

Clinical Manifestations The clinical manifestations vary depending on the virulence of the organism, host resistance, and the anatomic location of the lesion. In the nonimmune individual there is an abrupt onset characterized by moderate fever, chills, malaise, and a mild sore throat. The cervical lymph nodes become edematous and tender, especially when there is involvement of the nasopharynx. Swelling may be so pronounced that the classic bull neck appearance results. Extension from the nasopharynx to the larynx and trachea results in a very severe form of the disease in which mechanical obstruction of the airway by the membrane and accompanying edema introduce the risk of suffocation. Death ensues unless the airway is restored by tracheotomy or intubation.

The growth of *C. diphtheriae* is restricted to the mucosal epithelium, and, rarely if ever, do the organisms invade the deeper tissues and produce lesions in other parts of the body. The reasons for this high degree of tissue specificity are unknown. The absorption of the toxin into the general circulation, however, results in systemic manifestations and lesions in a number of organs. The most serious complications are usually associated with nasopharyngeal diphtheria and involve the heart and nervous system. Cardiac abnormalities which appear after the second week of the disease are seen in approximately 20 percent of diphtheria patients and are responsible for more than half of the case fatalities. The exotoxin causes fatty myocardial degeneration, resulting in cardiac dysfunction and circulatory collapse. The myocardial damage is reversible, and if the patient survives recovery is usually complete.

When neurologic symptoms occur, their appearance is late, usually in the third to fifth week of the disease. Involvement of the cranial nerves characteristically leads to paralysis of the soft palate. As a result difficulty is encountered in swallowing, and fluids are regurgitated through the nose. The most common manifestation of peripheral nerve involvement is a polyneuritis of the lower extremities, varying in severity from a mild weakness to paralysis of certain muscle groups. Recovery from both cranial and peripheral nerve dysfunction is usually complete.

Although diphtheria is usually a disease of the upper respiratory tract, primary or secondary lesions may occur in other parts of the body. In tropical areas cutaneous diphtheria is relatively common, especially as a secondary infection of septic skin lesions. Diphtheria has been considered rare in temperate zones, but an increased number of outbreaks in the United States and Canada, primarily in indigent and derelict groups, are now being reported. In skin diphtheria, lesions usually appear at the site of minor abrasions as chronic, spreading, nonhealing ulcers covered by a grayish membrane. The etiology of cutaneous diphtheria is complex. In addition to *C. diphtheriae,* either *Streptococcus pyogenes* or *Staphylococcus aureus* is usually present in the lesion, which fails to heal until proper diphtheria therapy is instituted. Mitis strains are usually associated with such infections, and such sequelae as polyneuritis, although infrequent, may occur.

Laboratory Diagnosis   Isolation of the organism and proof of toxigenicity is necessary for the microbiologic diagnosis of diphtheria. Since the early administration of antitoxin is of paramount importance in the outcome of the infection, the clinician should institute therapy immediately on the basis of clinical findings without waiting for the laboratory report. Streptococcal pharyngitis and Vincent's infection may be confused with diphtheria and should

always be considered when making a laboratory diagnosis. Swabs containing material from the lesions should be transported promptly to the laboratory and personnel alerted to the presumptive diagnosis of diphtheria. A Löffler's slant, a tellurite plate, and a blood agar plate should be inoculated immediately, and a smear stained with gentian violet should be examined in order to rule out infection with Vincent's fusospirochetal group of organisms. No attempt should be made to identify *C. diphtheriae* directly from smears of clinical material. Löffler's slants should be examined after 16 to 24 hours by staining with methylene blue and looking for the typical pleomorphic forms. Blood agar plates should be examined for β-hemolytic streptococci and any characteristic grayish colonies on tellurite medium should be transferred to Löffler slants. Confirmatory fermentation reactions may be carried out, and the isolate on Löffler's medium should be tested for pathogenicity either by the in vivo virulence test or in vitro gel diffusion technique.

IN VIVO TEST.   Animal inoculation is recommended for laboratories that seldom isolate *C. diphtheriae.* Either guinea pigs or rabbits may be used; one animal is sufficient for both test and control. The test is performed by injecting intracutaneously into the shaved animal 0.2 ml of a 48-hour infusion broth culture of the test organism. Five hours later 500 units of diphtheria antitoxin is injected intraperitoneally into the guinea pig (or into the ear vein of the rabbit), and after 30 minutes a second 0.2 ml sample is injected intracutaneously into the control area opposite the test site. Preliminary readings are made at 24 and 48 hours. If a toxigenic strain is present, a necrotic area appears at 48 to 72 hours at the site of the test injection. At the control site only a pinkish nodule develops, which does not proceed to ulceration because of the prior administration of antitoxin.

IN VITRO TEST.   The gel diffusion test for determining pathogenicity is more rapid than the in vivo method, but unless plates are carefully prepared false negative results may be obtained. In the test antitoxin-soaked strips of filter paper are placed on the surface of a serum agar medium, and the plate is inoculated heavily by streaking a line of inoculum perpendicular to the strip. The plates should be read daily for three days. If the organism is toxigenic a white line of toxin–antitoxin precipitate appears, extending out at a 45 degree angle from the intersection of the line of inoculum and the front of antitoxin diffusing from the filter paper.

Treatment   Diphtheria antitoxin in adequate amounts is the only specific and effective treatment for diphtheria. It should be administered immediately as soon as a presumptive diagnosis of diphtheria is made clinically without waiting for a laboratory confirmation. In severe cases the prognosis depends to a great extent upon how early in the course of the infection antitoxin therapy is initiated. The toxin binds rapidly and irreversibly to susceptible tissue cells and, once bound, cannot be displaced by antitoxin. The role of antitoxin is to prevent any further binding to undamaged cells of free toxin circulating in the blood. This it does by binding to determinants on the toxin molecule at the C-terminal 17,000 dalton end, thereby preventing attachment of fragment B to the tissue cell (p. 494).

Diphtheria antitoxin should be administered in a single dose by the intramuscular or intravenous route. The subcutaneous route should not be used, since absorption is slow and adequate blood levels are not reached until 72 hours after injection. The amount of antitoxin given is dependent upon the severity of the infection, but there is a general lack of agreement among clinicians as to what constitutes adequate therapy. One conservative scheme specifies 10,000 to 20,000 units intramuscularly for mild cases and 50,000 to 100,000 units by the intravenous route for severe cases.*

Since commercial diphtheria antitoxin is usually produced in horses, the patient should be tested for hypersensitivity to horse serum before therapy is started to avoid the possible occurrence of anaphylaxis. The test utilizes a 1:10 dilution of horse serum and may be ophthalmic, in which one drop of the serum is instilled into the conjunctiva of one eye, or an intracutaneous skin test utilizing 0.1 ml of the diluted antitoxin. If the patient is hypersensitive to horse serum the conjunctiva will de-

velop redness in 15 to 30 minutes. In the skin test a wheal with pseudopodia surrounded by an area of erythema appears at the site of the injection. If a positive reaction is obtained by either method, desensitization with small subcutaneous doses of antitoxin should be carried out. A syringe filled with epinephrine should be available at the bedside before antitoxin is administered by any route. Although anaphylaxis is rare, allergic reactions are frequent, and complications occur in about 10 percent of patients.

Diphtheria bacilli are susceptible to penicillin, erythromycin, and the tetracyclines, but antimicrobials cannot be substituted for antitoxin in the treatment of the patient. They are useful, however, in the prevention of secondary infections and in the treatment of chronic carriers. Without chemotherapy, from 1 to 15 percent of persons who recover from diphtheria become carriers, harboring *C. diphtheriae* for weeks or months following infection. Carriage of the organisms is greater following nasal infection. The current recommended treatment of carriers is either erythromycin or penicillin for six days followed by reculture two weeks after completion of therapy to assure eradication of the organisms.

Prevention   Active immunization is the key to the control and prevention of clinical diphtheria. For this purpose toxoid is administered either as fluid toxoid or as alum-precipitated toxoid, both of which are excellent immunizing agents. Toxoid is prepared by treating diphtheria toxin with 0.3 percent formalin at a temperature of 37C until the product is completely nontoxic. The addition of alum to the fluid toxoid precipitates the toxin, which if resuspended yields a partially purified preparation with increased antigenic efficiency because of the local stimulatory effect of the alum.

The primary course of immunization should be started in infancy between the second and third months of life. It usually consists of two doses of alum-precipitated toxoid combined with tetanus toxoid and pertussis vaccine given one month apart. A booster dose should be given one year later and a second booster at the time the child enters school. Young children rarely exhibit either local or general hypersensitivity reactions to the toxoid, but in older children and adults one must be aware of the

*Diphtheria antitoxin is standardized in units by comparing its ability to neutralize toxin with that of the official standard unit of antitoxin, maintained in vacuo at the State Serum Institute in Copenhagen. In terms of protective units the standard unit of antitoxin will neutralize 100 MLD of toxin.

possibility of a sensitivity reaction. This may be detected by the prior administration of a Moloney test, in which 0.1 ml of a 1:10 dilution of fluid toxoid is given intracutaneously. The development of a local reaction indicates sensitivity to the proteins of *C. diphtheriae,* to other corynebacteria, or to the toxin itself. Approximately 50 percent of individuals over the age of 15 give positive reactions to the test and, if administered the full immunizing doses of toxoid, would develop severe local and general reactions. Such reactors present a problem in the immunization of adult population groups, and the toxoid should be administered very cautiously in multiple, small, suitably diluted doses. By repeating the Moloney test each week for three weeks Schick-positive, Moloney-positive reactors can be converted to Schick negative. A highly purified toxoid preparation is now available for use in adults to circumvent the undesirable systemic effects attributable to antibacterial hypersensitivity.

Since immunity developed following the original immunization wanes, the United States Public Health Service now recommends that everyone receive a booster of tetanus-diphtheria toxoid at 10-year intervals. Immunization with diphtheria toxoid does not prevent nasopharyngeal carriage of *C. diphtheriae* and may not be uniformly effective in preventing clinical disease. Epidemiologic analysis, however, does indicate quite conclusively that both the attack rate and the case fatality rate are significantly lower in individuals who have received the full immunization series, and when disease does occur, it is usually mild. Severe complications are more often seen in the elderly who also are farther away from their basic series of inoculation.

Passive immunization by the use of 1,000 to 3,000 units of antitoxin may be employed for the protection of nonimmunized individuals heavily exposed to virulent organisms. Since such protection is of short duration and introduces the risk of inducing sensitization or of eliciting an anaphylactic reaction in an individual previously sensitized to the foreign protein, its use should be limited to high-risk situations. Active immunization with toxoid should be given concomitantly with the antitoxin.

An outbreak of diphtheria in a closed community, such as a school, should prompt careful surveillance of all exposed individuals so that antitoxin may be administered at the first sign of illness. Exposed individuals should be Schick tested, and toxoid should be administered to all Shick-positive reactors.

OTHER CORYNEBACTERIA

As currently constituted, the genus *Corynebacterium* includes three major groups: (1) human and animal parasites and pathogens, (2) plant pathogenic corynebacteria, and (3) nonpathogenic corynebacteria. Anaerobic diphtheroids, such as *C. acnes* and *C. parvum,* are now excluded from the genes *Corynebacterium* and reclassified in the genus *Propionibacterium* (p. 639). The tendency in the past to classify many organisms as corynebacteria solely on the basis of morphology has resulted in the placing of a number of unrelated or distantly related organisms in the genus. The taxonomy and classification of this group of organisms is still unsatisfactory and presents many unresolved problems.

Species currently accepted as human and animal parasites and pathogens are listed in Table 33-1. Except for *C. diphtheriae, C. pseudotuberculosis* is the only species producing an exotoxin. This exotoxin is, however, antigenically distinct from that of *C. diphtheriae. C. pseudotuberculosis* is closely related to *C. diphtheriae,* is susceptible to some of the bacteriophages used in typing the diphtheria bacillus, and when lysogenized with a *tox*+ phage, synthesizes diphtheria toxin. *C. pseudotuberculosis* causes ulcerative lymphangitis, abscesses, and other chronic purulent infections in sheep, horses, cows, and occasionally in man. *C. ulcerans,* an organism intermediate between *C. diphtheriae* and *C. pseudotuberculosis,* has been isolated from the nasopharynx of healthy individuals and from patients with a diphtherialike disease.

Not included in Table 33-1 are *C. pyogenes* and *C. haemolyticum.* These organisms represent a well-defined group and are a common cause of pyogenic infections in domestic animals. Unlike the other corynebacteria, however, they lack arabinose in their cell wall and share a cell wall polysaccharide antigen with Lancefield group G streptococci. They do not produce an exotoxin and may be distinguished from *C. diphtheriae* on the basis of cultural and

TABLE 33-1 CORYNEBACTERIA PARASITIC AND PATHOGENIC
FOR MAN AND ANIMALS

Species	Hemolysis	Sucrose Fermentation	Nitrate Reduction	Urease	Other Properties
C. diphtheriae	+	−	+	−	Human pathogen; specific exotoxin
C. pseudodiphtheriticum	−	−	+	+	Nonpathogenic; nasopharyngeal mucosa of man; no acid from any carbohydrate
C. xerosis	−	+	+	−	Nonpathogenic; skin and mucous membranes of man
C. pseudotuberculosis	+	v*	v*	v*	Primarily animal pathogen; specific exotoxin
C. renale	−	−	−	+	Animal pathogen
C. kutscheri	−	+	−	+	Parasite of mice and rats
C. equi	−	−	+	−	Primarily animal pathogen
C. bovis	−	−	−	+	Parasite on cow's udder; may cause mastitis

*Variable reaction.

biochemical properties. Unlike *C. diphtheriae*, *C. pyogenes* and *C. haemolyticum* grow poorly on tellurite media, show weakly positive catalase activity, and ferment lactose.

The two nonpathogenic species most often cultured from clinical materials are *C. pseudodiphtheriticum* and *C. xerosis*. *C. pseudodiphtheriticum* is found in the nasopharynx of man. It is a short, rather regular rod that stains evenly except for a transverse medial unstained septum; metachromatic granules and club forms are usually absent. *C. xerosis* inhabits the skin and mucous membranes of man, especially the conjunctiva. Differentiating properties are listed Table 33-1.

Erythrasma An organism possibly related to *C. xerosis* has been isolated from the lesions of the skin disease, erythrasma, previously believed to be caused by a fungus. The disease is characterized by the presence of scaly plaques which fluoresce coral red under Wood's light at 365 nm. The causative agent *C. minutissimum*, is nutritionally exacting and, when grown aerobically on a solid medium containing tissue culture medium base and 20 percent bovine fetal serum, produces colonies that display a coral red to orange fluorescence similar to that of the skin lesions. Colonies grown on blood agar do not possess this characteristic fluorescence. A large number of lipophilic corynebacteria have also been isolated from the skin. These strains have not been well characterized, but all of them require lipid for growth. Except for this property they resemble *C. xerosis*.

Traditionally, with the exception of *C. diphtheriae*, corynebacteria have been considered unimportant as disease producers for man. There has been, however, an increased awareness that in the proper setting, such as in an altered host, diphtheroids may assume the role of opportunistic invaders. A number of cases of endocarditis following cardiac surgery, meningitis, and osteomyelitis have been attributed a diphtheroid etiology. Because of the presence of such organisms as common contaminants of clinical material, their recognition and acceptance as the cause of infection has been made with reservation.

CORYNEBACTERIUM VAGINALE (HAEMOPHILUS VAGINALE)

The taxonomic position of this organism is unresolved. In the Eighth Edition of *Bergey's Manual* it is listed as species incertae sedis, *Haemophilus vaginalis*, but with the editorial comment, "This species does not belong in the genus *Haemophilus*." Morphologically the organism appears as small bacilli and coccobacilli, 0.3 to 0.6 by 1 to 2 μm, often showing club formation and metachromatic granules. It is gram-variable, with retention of gram stain being more pronounced in young cultures 8 to 12 hours old. On optimal media it stains

uniformly gram-positive. It is a facultative anaerobe and requires an enriched medium for
growth, but unlike *Haemophilus* species, it
does not require either hemin or nicotinamide
adenine nucleotides.

Interest in *C. vaginale* has centered on its
role as a cause of nonspecific vaginitis and urethritis. Masses of bacteria may be found on the
surface of epithelial cells in the discharge.
These cells observed in wet mounts are referred to as "clue cells" and are considered
characteristic of *C. vaginale* infection.

FURTHER READING

Books and Reviews

Barksdale L: *Corynebacterium diphtheriae* and its relatives. Bacteriol Rev 34:378, 1970

Barksdale L, Arden SB: Persisting bacteriophage infections, lysogeny, and phage conversions. Annu Rev Microbiol 28:265, 1974

Collier RJ: Diphtheria toxin: Mode of action and structure.
Bacteriol Rev 39:54, 1975

Gill DM, Pappenheimer AM Jr, Uchida T: Diphtheria toxin, protein synthesis, and the cell. Fed Proc 32:1508,
1973

Honjo T, Hayaishi O: Enzymatic ADP-ribosylation of proteins and regulation of cellular activity. In Horecker BL,
Stadtman ER (eds): Current Topics in Cellular Regulation. New York, Academic Press, 1973, vol 7, pp 87-
127

Selected Papers

Bezjak V, Farsey SJ: *Corynebacterium diphtheriae* in skin
lesions in Ugandan children. Bull WHO 43:643, 1970

Brooks GF, Bennett JV, Feldman RA: Diphtheria in the
United States, 1959-1970. J Infect Dis 129:172, 1974

Collier RJ, Kandel J: Structure and activity of diphtheria
toxin. I. Thiol-dependent dissociation of a fraction of
toxin into enzymatically active and inactive fragments. J
Biol Chem 246:1496, 1971

Creagan RP: Genetic analysis of the cell surface: association of human chromosome 5 with sensitivity to diphtheria toxin in mouse-human somatic cell hybrids. Proc
Natl Acad Sci USA 72:2237, 1975

Drazin R, Kandel J, Collier RJ: Structure and activity of
diphtheria toxin. II. Attack by trypsin at a specific site
within the intact toxin molecule. J Biol Chem 246:1504,
1971

Gibson LF, Colman G: Diphthericin types, bacteriophage
types and serotypes of *Corynebacterium diphtheriae*
strains isolated in Australia. J Hyg (Camb) 71:679, 1973

Gill DM, Dinius LL: Observations on the structure of diphtheria toxin. J Biol Chem 246:1485, 1971

Gill DM, Pappenheimer AM Jr: Structure-activity relationships in diphtheria toxin. J Biol Chem 246:1492, 1971

Honjo T, Nishizuka Y, Kato-I, Hayaishi O: Adenosine diphosphate ribosylation of aminoacyl transferase II and
inhibition of protein synthesis by diphtheria toxin. J Biol
Chem 246:4251, 1971

Kandel J, Collier J, Chung DW: Interaction of fragment A
from diphtheria toxin with nicotinamide adenine dinucleotide. J Biol Chem 249:2088, 1974

McCloskey RV, Saragea A, Maximescu P: Phage typing in
diphtheria outbreaks in the southwestern United States,
1968-1971. J Infect Dis 126:196, 1972

McCloskey RV, Eller JJ, Green M. Mauney CV, Richards
SEM: The 1970 epidemic of diphtheria in San Antonio.
Ann Intern Med 75:495, 1971

McLaughlin JV, Bickham ST, Wiggins GL, et al: Antibiotic
susceptibility patterns of recent isolates of *Corynebacterium diphtheriae*. Appl Microbiol 21:844, 1971

Miller LW, Bickham S, Jones WL, Heather CD, Morris RH:
Diphtheria carriers and the effect of erythromycin therapy. Antimicrob Agents Chemother 6:166:1974

Singer RA: Temperature-sensitive mutants of toxinogenic
corynebacteriophage beta. I. Genetics. Virology 55:
347, 1973

Uchida T, Gill DM, Pappenheimer AM Jr: Mutation in the
structural gene for diphtheria toxin carried by temperate phage β. Nature [New Biol] 233:8, 1971

Uchida T, Pappenheimer AM Jr, Harper AA: Diphtheria
toxin and related proteins. III. Reconstitution of hybrid
"diphtheria toxin" from nontoxic mutant proteins. J Biol
Chem 248:3851, 1973

34
Mycobacteriaceae

The most distinctive property of the Mycobacteriaceae is their characteristic staining. They stain with difficulty, but once stained they are resistant to decolorization with acid alcohol. For this reason they are often referred to as acid-fast bacilli. The family contains a wide range of nutritional types, including saprophytic species that are present in the soil as well as parasitic organisms that have not been cultured in vitro. The pathogenic members of the family cause some of the most important of human infections, including leprosy and tuberculosis. Most species of birds, mammals, and cold-blooded animals are susceptible to their own specific pathogenic species, although there is considerable cross-infection between animals and man.

The Mycobacteriaceae contain a single genus, *Mycobacterium*, whose properties characterize the family. In the Bergey classification scheme they are grouped with the Actinomycetes and related organisms in Part 17. Also included in this group are the corynebacteria and nocardias that have a number of features in common with the mycobacteria. Arabinose and galactose are present in the cell walls of the three genera; they possess a common cell wall antigen, and they contain mycolic acid.

MYCOBACTERIUM LEPRAE

Leprosy is an ancient disease. It was known in India as an old disease when mentioned in the Vedas of 1400 BC. Not all the skin lesions called "leprosy" in the Old Testament of the Bible were leprosy, but almost certainly some of them were.

The lepra cell, which is a modified monocyte, was recognized in 1840 by Danielssen, and in 1847 his son-in-law, Hansen, discovered the bacilli in the lepra cell. Neisser confirmed the observation of Hansen.

M. leprae of man and *M. lepraemurium* of rats are the causes of human and rat leprosy, respectively. These two antigenically independent species have both achieved a status of complete parasitism and cannot be grown on artificial media.

In some parts of the tropics, leprosy occurs in an active or progressive form in 1 percent of the population. There are approximately 20 million persons with leprosy in the world at the present time. In the United States in 1967 there were approximately 2,000 cases of leprosy known to the United States Public Health Service. This disease is endemic in some parts of Louisiana, Texas, Florida, and California and all parts of Hawaii and Puerto Rico.

A total of 166 cases of leprosy have been followed for a number of years at the leprosy clinic in San Francisco. Among 198 family contacts of patients with lepromatous leprosy 16 developed clinical leprosy within a 7 year period. This represents an attack rate of 80.8 per 1,000 contacts examined.

Morphology and Physiology

When stained by the Ziehl-Neelsen method, leprosy bacilli are found predominantly in modified mononuclear or epithelioid structures called "lepra cells." Large numbers of bacilli are packed in the cells in an arrangement that suggests packets of cigars. The individual rods vary in length from 1 to 7 μm and in width from 0.2 to 1.4 μm. The rods are usually straight or slightly curved and, when stained, may appear solid red or show granules and beads that are slightly larger than the average diameter of the cell. *M. leprae* is acid-fast, gram-positive, and nonsporogenous.

In lepromatous patients who receive chemotherapy for six months there is a decrease in the presence of solid staining rods from 53 percent to 3 percent. These observations have been confirmed by the use of an experimental mouse model in which *M. leprae* from patients are introduced into the foot pads of mice.

A study of thin sections of *M. leprae* in lepromatous nodules shows that this organism's structure resembles that of *M. tuberculosis*, with a three-layered cell wall and a complex intracytoplasmic membrane system that connects with the plasma membrane. Surrounding the individual bacilli is an ill-defined structure of low density, but it is not certain whether it is a product of the cell or of the host. All well-controlled attempts to cultivate *M. leprae* have met with failure, including the attempt to grow the organism in cultures of various types of human cells.

M. leprae obtained from lepromatous skin nodules contain a phenolase that converts 3,4-dihydroxyphenylalanine (dopa) to a colored product having an absorption peak at 540 nm. Phenolase activity has never been detected in other mycobacteria or nocardias.

Antigenic Structure

Patients with leprosy may give positive skin tests with lepromin prepared from leprous nodules but react equally well to PPD or to tuberculin made from the acid-fast saprophyte, M. phlei. In complement-fixation tests using as antigen cultured strains of acid-fast bacilli from lepromatous lesions, M. tuberculosis, and M. phlei, the same percentage of positive reactions was obtained with all antigens. It was observed, however, that the more active cases gave the highest percentage of positive complement-fixation reactions, while the less active cases had the highest percentage of positive skin tests.

Rabbits immunized with leprosy bacilli separated from the tissues of lepromatous nodules by differential centrifugation develop antibody to specific antigens of the leprosy bacilli, with only a little cross-reaction with the human tissue. The cross-reacting antibodies, detected by the agar gel technique, can be removed by absorption. Using specific antisera, lepromatous antigens have been demonstrated in the sera of two patients. The sera of other patients with lepromatous leprosy, however, gave a very faint reaction with leprosy antigen but very strong reactions with antigens from human tubercle bacilli. This confirms the presence of cross-reacting antibodies responsible for the complement-fixation reaction to human and M. phlei antigens.

Patients with lepromatous leprosy frequently have much higher hemagglutinin titers to soluble tuberculin antigen than are found in patients with active tuberculosis, even though their skin tests are negative to both lepromin and to PPD made from the human tubercle bacillus.

Active cases of leprosy have a high percentage of biologically false positive Wassermann and Kahn reactions.

Lepromin Test   It was hoped when this test was introduced that it would be as specific in leprosy as the tuberculin test is in tuberculosis. Lepromin is made by grinding lepromatous nodules in physiologic saline to a final concentration of 1 g per 20 ml. The supernate, after filtration, is sterilized by autoclaving at 120C for 15 minutes and preserved by the addition of 0.5 percent phenol. Good preparations contain many more leprae bacilli than tissue fragments. The test dose is 0.1 ml of lepromin injected intracutaneously. Two types of reactions occur: (1) the early reaction that resembles the tuberculin reaction and which appears in 24 to 48 hours and (2) the late reaction that begins between the seventh and tenth days as a small papule and gradually increases in size by the twenty-fifth to thirtieth day. In the more severe reactions the center of the nodule becomes necrotic and sloughs out. The late lepromin reactions are caused by the intact leprosy bacilli in the lepromin, and if they are removed by filtration or broken up by sonic vibration or by chemical treatment, the tuberculinlike reaction is intensified and the late lepromin reactions reduced or eliminated.

The negative lepromin reaction in the acute lepromatous stage of the disease can be explained by assuming that the patient is in the preallergic stage analogous to the preallergic stage in tuberculosis, in which the bacilli multiply in mononuclear cells before the tuberculin reaction becomes positive.

Positive lepromin tests can be elicited in patients with tuberculosis in areas of the world where there is no leprosy, and positive lepromin tests can be induced in normal, healthy children by vaccination with BCG, which is an attenuated bovine tubercle bacillus. A delayed leprominlike test has been elicited by injecting the whole dead bacilli of human, avian, or Battey types of Mycobacterium.

Pathogenesis

Experimental Disease in Animals   Shepard succeeded in 1960 in infecting the foot pads of mice with strains of human leprosy bacilli. These infections could be passed from mouse to mouse without alteration in morphology or virulence. All attempts, however, to cultivate human leprosy bacilli in tissue cultures of human cells have failed.

The generation time for M. leprae in the mouse foot pad model is 20 to 30 days. The reduced temperature of the foot pad is the secret of the successful inoculation. The preferred site for initial growth of M. leprae in man and mice is peripheral sites of heat loss that average about 30C. The intravenous injection of *M. leprae* into mice results in lesions in the nose and the front feet. The bacilli that are shed from the nose of man have been growing at that site at a temperature of about 30C. The optimum temperature for *M. marinum* also is about 30C, although it will grow on artificial media at lower temperatures.

The distribution of the lesions in leprosy has always been a mystery. The skin usually shows the most obvious lesions, especially the skin of the ears, nose, and face. The peripheral nerves, however, both the large and small branches, show a haphazard asymmetrical type of lesion. In contrast to tuberculosis, the internal organs are not infected. The lesions may be present in the nose, pharynx, and mouth but do not extend into the lungs, liver, spleen, or brain. It is obvious that the bacilli have to pass through the bloodstream to reach the deeper layers of the skin and the peripheral nerves. In 1959, Brand called attention to this distribution of lesions and suggested that growth of *M. leprae* was conditioned by temperature and that the internal organs were too hot for multiplication of the organism. Shepard's study of the temperature requirement for growth of *M. leprae* in the foot pad of the mouse confirms Brand's theory.

The armadillo has been proposed as a new animal model for leprosy. The armadillo can be infected with leprosy bacilli and gives larger yields of more concentrated bacilli than can be obtained from the foot pad of the mouse.

Experimental Disease in Man Man is highly resistant to experimental infection. A number of attempts have been made to infect human beings experimentally but with negative results. In one series reported, of 145 recorded attempts to infect man, only 1 was successful.

The most convincing experiment occurred during World War II when two American marines were tattooed in June 1943, in Melbourne, Australia, and early in 1946 they both developed leprosy which began in the areas that had been tattooed.

Clinical Infection

Transmission The clinical evidence for the transmission of leprosy is quite conclusive. There are many examples of Europeans developing leprosy after a single contact with South Sea Island prostitutes. It must be emphasized, however, that man actually is very resistant to the development of leprosy even when exposed over a period of years.

The incubation period is difficult to determine. It appears to vary from a minimum of a few months to a maximum of 30 years, with an average of 2 to 7 years. Black refers to a 15-year-old girl in whom he demonstrated leprosy bacilli in smears from an apparently normal ear lobe two years before the patient developed cutaneous and neural leprosy of the forearms and legs. In India 25 of 254 contacts had leprosy bacilli in their skin, and 4 of these subsequently developed clinical leprosy.

Evidence also has been presented that leprosy may be transmitted by the bites of some arthropods, such as head lice and mosquitoes.

Types of Diseases Ridley and Jopling classified clinical leprosy into a five-group system; two subgroups were subsequently added. The main five subgroups are shown in Figure 34-1.

The major portion of the exposed population have subclinical infections. The mildest form of clinical leprosy is the tuberculoid, while the dramatic disease, the lepromatous, is the least frequent (Fig. 34-2). The prognosis is poor in the lepromatous type of leprosy, where the lepromin test is negative and bacilli are present in the large mononuclear cells in great abundance. Such patients have a defect in their cellular immunity. A preliminary report has shown that a transfer of white blood cells or a prepared transfer factor produced dramatic improvement in a few cases of lepromatous leprosy. The patient shown in Figure 34-2 made a dramatic recovery after 12 months of treatment with promacetin (Fig. 34-3).

Laboratory Diagnosis The diagnosis may be suspected from the symptoms and from the type and distribution of the lesions plus a history of living in an endemic area. Diagnosis is made by the demonstration of acid-fast bacilli in smears of skin, in nasal scrapings, and in tissue sections. The bacilli are very difficult and often impossible to detect in tissue from the typical tuberculoid leprosy. The administration of corticoid hormones, however, increases the size of the lesions, promotes the growth of *M. leprae* in the local lesions, and thus makes the diagnosis easier.

Treatment Experimental chemotherapy in the disease produced in the mouse foot pad

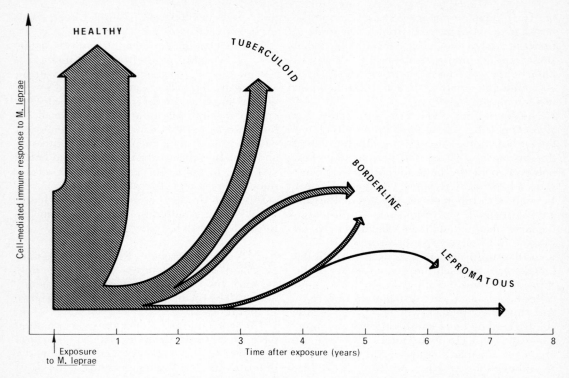

FIG. 34-1. A schematic representation of the hypothesis of how the development of subclinical infection and various types of leprosy are related to time of onset of cell-mediated immune response to *M. leprae* antigens after the initial exposure. The thickness of the lines indicates the proportion of individuals from the exposed population that is likely to fall into each category. The indicated incubation periods, 2 to 3 years in tuberculoid and 6 to 7 years in lepromatous leprosy, probably represent the shortest incubation periods. They are often considerably longer. (From Godal, Myrvang, Stanford, and Samuel: Recent advances in the immunology of leprosy. Bull Inst Pasteur 72:273, 1974)

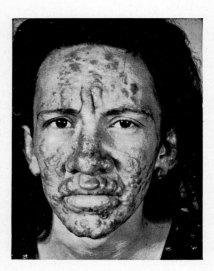

FIG. 34-2. Leprosy before treatment. (From Johansen et al: Public Health Rep 65:204, 1950)

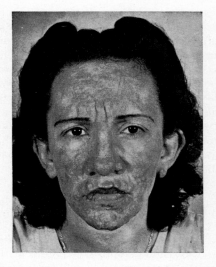

FIG. 34-3. Leprosy after 12-month treatment with pro-macetin. (From Johansen et al: Public Health Rep 65: 204, 1950)

was reviewed by Shepard in 1973. The most widely used drug is 4',4'-diaminodiphenyl-sulfone (DDS) or dapsone, but some organisms develop resistance to DDS. The next most effective drug is clofazimine (B663) which can be used if resistance to dapsone occurs. Shepard's studies showed that rifampin was much more rapidly bactericidal than was DDS or B663.

The toxic reaction in patients with lepromatous leprosy receiving DDS resembles erythema nodosum. Cortisone reduces the severity of symptoms but has other undesirable effects.

Prevention There is now reason for optimism in the prevention of leprosy and perhaps the eventual elimination of the disease from the world. Man is the only host and the *M. leprae* organisms cannot multiply in the soil or spontaneously in animals.

The elimination of the disease in endemic areas would begin with the early detection and rigid isolation of all acute lepromatous and nonspecific or indeterminate types of cases. The diagnosed cases should be isolated in (1) leper colonies or (2) leprosy villages. This should be followed by (1) prophylactic chemotherapy for individuals in close contact with the patient and (2) active immunization with BCG of the remaining children in the village.

BCG vaccination of children who are tuberculin-negative and lepromin-negative results in a conversion both to tuberculin and to lepromin. In a controlled study in Uganda it was shown that BCG vaccination gave 78 percent protection against leprosy for over four years. BCG vaccination of mice infected in the foot pad with *M. leprae* also caused a marked reduction in the multiplication of leprosy bacilli.

BCG vaccination promises to be useful in the prevention of leprosy. It may prove more effective than sulfone chemoprophylaxis in the handling of all contacts of new cases of leprosy.

RAT LEPROSY

This disease, caused by *M. lepraemurium*, was discovered among rats in Odessa in 1903. Since then it has been found in many parts of the world. Rat leprosy occurs spontaneously among house rats and is characterized by subcutaneous indurations, swelling of lymph nodes, emaciation, and sometimes ulceration and loss of hair. The disease is chronic,

and rats often live for six months to one year after becoming infected. The characteristic lesion is a thickened area under the skin of the abdomen or flank which resembles adipose tissue except that it is less shiny and more nodular and gray than fat. The resemblance to fat is so close, however, that it is often overlooked by those unfamiliar with the condition. Acid-fast bacilli resembling *M. leprae* are found in large numbers in the mononuclear cells of the subcutaneous tissues, and in the lymph nodes and nodules in the liver and lungs.

Rats can be infected by direct inoculation of infected tissues, but the disease probably is transmitted naturally from rat to rat by fleas.

Although the disease is not identical to leprosy, the resemblance is sufficiently great to suggest that rats are a potential source of human leprosy. The distribution of the disease in various parts of the world, however, does not correspond with the distribution of human leprosy.

The natural host for both *M. leprae* and *M. lepraemurium* is the monocyte. *M. lepraemurium* can be maintained for months in tissue cultures of monocytes. *M. lepraemurium* grows in these cells and can be subcultured repeatedly. The average generation time is seven days (Fig. 34-4).

Solid staining forms of *M. lepraemurium* will grow in cultured macrophages, while the bead-

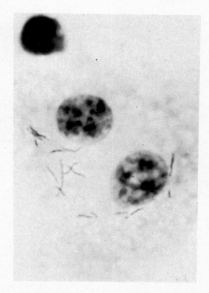

FIG. 34-4. Macrophage with *M. lepraemurium* in a 20-day-old culture showing elongation of the organisms. ×2,000. (From Chang et al: J Bacteriol 93:1119, 1967)

ed and granular ones will not. It has been assumed that the solid staining forms of *M. lepraemurium* are alive.

The studies of Chang and Anderson, however, on the cultivation of *M. lepraemurium* demonstrated that there are two causes for beaded or absent staining: (1) death of the organism and (2) a change that immediately precedes rapid growth and division.

The rat leprosy bacilli have been cultured in rat fibroblasts. Specific antigens elaborated by the bacilli in culture have been purified and studied with the gel diffusion method, using antisera produced by rats infected with the organisms and antisera induced in rabbits by injecting bacilli freed from experimental lesions in rats. There appear to be one or more specific antigens characteristic of *M. lepraemurium* with very little cross-reaction with *M. tuberculosis*.

FURTHER READING

Books and Reviews

Badger LF: Epidemiology. In Cochrane RG (ed): Leprosy in Theory and Practice. Bristol, England, John Wright and Sons Ltd. 1959

Trautman JR, Enna CD: Leprosy. In Tice F (ed): Practice of Medicine. Hagerstown, Md, Harper & Row, 1970, vol 3, Chap 33

Selected Papers

Brown JAK, Stone MM, Sutherland L: BCG vaccination of children against leprosy in Uganda: Results at the end of the second follow-up. Br Med J 1:24, 1968

Bullock WE, Fields TP, Brandriss MW: An evaluation of transfer factor in immunotherapy with lepromatous lepers. N Engl J Med 287:1053, 1972

Chang YT, Anderson RN: Morphological changes of *Mycobacterium lepraemurium* grown in cultures of mouse peritoneal macrophages. J Bacteriol 99:867, 1969.

Dwyer JM, Bullock WE, Fields JP: Disturbance of blood T and B lymphocytes ratio in lepromatous leprosy. N Engl J Med 288:1036, 1973

Editorial: Leprosy: Disordered cellular immunity. JAMA 228:79, 1974

Fasal P, Fasal E, Levy L: Leprosy prophylaxis. JAMA 199:906, 1967

Godal T, Myrvang B, Stanford JL, Samuel DR: Recent advances in the immunology of leprosy with special reference to new approaches in immunoprophylaxis. Bull Inst Pasteur 72:273, 1974

Kircheimer WF, Storrs EF, Binford CH: Attempt to establish the armadillo *(Dasypos novemcinctus linn)* as a model for the study of leprosy. Int J Lepr 40:229, 1972

Kircheimer WF: Leprosy. Am J Med Technol 40:474, 1974

Kircheimer WF, Sanchez RM: Survival of *Mycobacterium leprae* in cutaneous inoculation sites of armadillos. Lepr India 41(1):5, 1975

Levine M: Hemagglutination of tuberculin sensitized sheep cells in Hansen's disease (leprosy). Proc Soc Exp Biol Med 76:171, 1951

Lim SD, Fusaro R, Good RA: Leprosy. VI. The treatment of leprosy patients with intravenous infusion of leukocytes from normal persons. Clin Immunol Immunopathol 1:122, 1972

Mansfield RE: An improved method for fluorochrome staining of mycobacteria in tissues and smears. Am J Clin Path 53:394, 1970

Morbidity and Mortality Weekly Report. Leprosy—In the United States and Puerto Rico, 19:17, 1970.

Prabhakaran J, Kircheimer WF: Use of 3,4-dihydroxy-phenylalanine oxidation in the identification of *Mycobacterium leprae*. J Bacteriol 92:1267, 1966

Rees RJW, Garbutt EW: Studies on *Mycobacterium lepraemurium* in tissue cultures. Brit J Exp Path 43:221, 1962

Ridley OS, Jopling WH: Classification of leprosy according to immunity. A five-group system. Int J Lepr 34:255, 1966

Shankara Manja K, Narayanan E, Kasturi G, Kircheimer WF, Balasubrahmanyan M: Non-cultivable mycobacteria in some field collected arthropods. Lepr India 45(4):231, 1973

Shepard CC: Experimental chemotherapy in leprosy then and now. Int J Lepr 41:307, 1973

Shepard CC, McRae DH: *Mycobacterium leprae* in mice: Minimal infectious dose, relation between staining quality and infectivity, and effect of cortisone. J Bacteriol 89:365, 1965

Shepard CC: Minimal effective doses in mice of clofazimine (B663) and ethioamide against *Mycobacterium leprae*. Proc Soc Exp Biol Med 132:120, 1969

Storrs E, Walsh GP, Burchfield HP: Leprosy in the armadillo: New model for biomedical research. Science 183:851, 1974

Turk JL, Walters MFT: Cell mediated immunity in patients with leprosy. Lancet 2:243, 1969

35
Mycobacterium Tuberculosis

The occurrence of obvious tuberculosis in bones of some of the Egyptian mummies suggests that tuberculosis is an ancient disease. Although it is no longer the most common cause of death in countries with a high standard of living, it remains the number one killer in the world as a whole. The causative agent of tuberculosis, *Mycobacterium tuberculosis*, was isolated by Robert Koch in 1882. Koch found the bacillus constantly associated with the clinical disease, isolated it in pure culture, reproduced the disease in guinea pigs and rabbits with the culture, and recovered the bacillus in pure culture from the experimentally infected animals. These rigid requirements, Koch's postulates, must be fulfilled before a particular microorganism can be accepted as the cause of a specific infectious disease.

Morphology

Tubercle bacilli are slender, straight, or slightly curved rods with rounded ends. They vary in width from 0.2 to 0.5 μm and in length from 1 to 4μm. True branching is seen occasionally in old cultures and sometimes in smears from caseous lymph nodes. Branching forms may be produced at will under certain specific cultural conditions.

The bacilli are acid-fast, nonmotile, and nonsporogenous and have no capsules (Fig. 35-1). Electron micrographs of thin sections show that

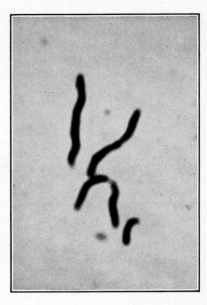

FIG. 35-2. Tubercle bacilli stained uniformly by the Ziehl-Neelsen method. ×3,600. (From Yegian and Kurung: Am Rev Tuberc 56:36, 1947)

the rather thick wall is composed of three layers enclosing a plasma membrane that is also three layers in thickness.

Tubercle bacilli from either cultures or secretions may be stained by the Ziehl-Neelsen method. With this stain the bacilli are seen as brilliant red rods against a deep, sky-blue background (Fig. 35-2).

The cell wall is unlike that of gram-positive or gram-negative cells and contains high con-

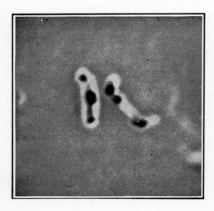

FIG. 35-1. Tubercle bacilli. The protoplasm of the bacillus has been stained by the Ziehl-Neelsen method and the unstained cell wall outlined by the addition of nigrosin. ×3,600. (From Yegian and Vanderlinde: J Bacteriol 54: 777, 1947)

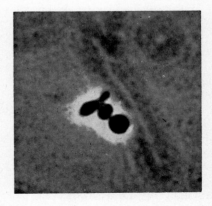

FIG. 35-3. Spheroplast formation by lysozyme treatment. (From Thacore and Willett: Proc Soc Exp Biol Med 114: 43, 1963)

centrations of lipids. It is the physical structure, however, that gives the organism its acid-fastness and gram-positiveness and not the mycolic acids and other lipids. Spheroplast formation in tubercle bacilli grown in the presence of lysozyme has been demonstrated (Fig. 35-3). Cells also can be induced to produce an L-type growth.

Much's Granules Some specimens of pus from tuberculus abscesses, serous exudates, lymph nodes, or sputum contain no acid-fast organisms but produce tuberculosis when inoculated into susceptible animals. In 1908 Much demonstrated gram-positive granules in short chains or irregular clumps in these materials. Later studies by Kahn and Brieger have demonstrated that these non-acid-fast forms are indeed alive.

Physiology

Tubercle bacilli will not grow on the usual type of media but do grow slowly on inspissated serum, coagulated egg, or potato medium. After 10 to 20 days at 37C, small, dry, scaly colonies with corrugated surfaces are produced. The bovine strains grow more slowly and less luxuriantly than do bacilli of human origin. On glycerin broth, prepared by adding 5 percent glycerin to beef or veal infusion peptone broth, growth of the human and bovine strains is confined to the surface of the medium. A thin, gray, almost transparent, veil-like film grows over the entire surface of the broth. This film gradually thickens into a white or slightly yellowish, wrinkled membrane that covers the entire surface of the culture fluid. The generation time of tubercle bacilli on the Proskauer-Beck basal synthetic medium is 20.5 to 24 hours but can be shortened to 13.2 to 15.7 hours by adding beef serum to the basal medium. The addition of 5 percent glycerin inhibits the growth of the vole bacillus, has little or no effect on the bovine bacillus, but accelerates appreciably the growth of the human and avian strains. Tubercle bacilli will grow over a pH range of 6.0 to 7.6. The optimal pH for the maintenance of virulence is pH 6.8. The optimal temperature for the isolation of avian strains is 40C, human and bovine strains 37C, and bacilli from cold-blooded animals 25C.

After a number of generations in the laboratory, however, temperature requirements of the organisms are less exacting.

Tubercle bacilli are obligate aerobes and will not grow in the absence of oxygen. Even a moderate reduction in the oxygen tension results in an appreciable decrease in the metabolism of the bacilli.

The addition to broth media of a long-chain fatty acid derivative, known commercially as Tween 80, alters the surface conditions so that tubercle bacilli multiply much more rapidly, giving a smooth, homogeneous type of growth throughout the culture medium. On hydrolysis free oleic acid, which is toxic for the organism, is liberated, but this effect may be neutralized by adding small amounts of bovine albumin to the medium. Since homogeneous suspensions of organisms grown on other types of media are prepared with great difficulty, the advantages of this medium (Dubos medium) are obvious.

After primary isolation, tubercle bacilli grow readily on synthetic media containing glycerol, asparagine, citrate, and inorganic salts. While growing on synthetic media, the tubercle bacillus synthesizes all of the known B-complex vitamins. The addition of vitamins to synthetic media does not increase appreciably either the rate or the quantity of growth.

Resistance Tubercle bacilli may remain viable in culture media for two to eight months. Organisms from cultures are killed in 2 hours when exposed to direct sunlight, but bacilli contained in sputum require an exposure of 20 to 30 hours. When protected from direct sunlight, they live in putrefying sputum for weeks and in dried sputum for as long as six to eight months. Droplets of dried sputum adhering to dust particles in the air may be infectious for 8 to 10 days. Tubercle bacilli are resistant to the usual chemical disinfectants. A 5 percent solution of phenol requires 24 hours to disinfect sputum.

Tubercle bacilli possess no greater resistance to moist heat than do other bacteria. Pasteurization temperatures are, therefore, efficacious in eliminating them from milk and milk products.

Variability Tubercle bacilli were dissociated by Petroff in the Trudeau Laboratory in 1927. The standard nomenclature employed since 1936 uses S to designate a smooth colony

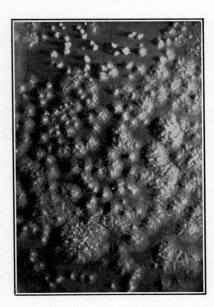

FIG. 35-4. Rough colonies of the human virulent strain H37Rv. (Grown by William Steenken; photographed by Joseph Kurung)

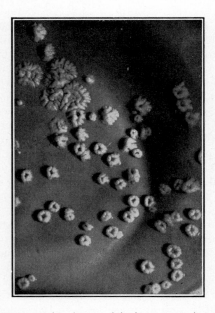

FIG. 35-5. Rough colonies of the human avirulent strain H37Ra. Note the large, flatter, intermediate colonies. (Grown by William Steenken; photographed by Joseph Kurung)

and R to designate a rough one. With few exceptions the virulent organisms produce R colonies (Fig. 35-4), but there are also R colonies which are avirulent (Fig. 35-5).

Antigenic Structure

The acid-fast bacteria may be separated into mammalian, avian, cold-blooded, and saprophytic types by agglutination, agglutinin adsorption, and complement fixation. The avian bacilli have specific antigens by which they can be separated into subtypes and also have an antigen in common with both human and bovine organisms.

Antibodies in the sera of patients with tuberculosis can be detected by a number of techniques and are present in most patients with active tuberculosis. Some severely ill patients are negative, and some healthy individuals with positive tuberculin tests have antituberculous antibodies. There is no reliable serologic test for clinically active tuberculosis.

Antibodies have been demonstrated in the spinal fluid of 97.1 percent of the patients with tuberculosis meningitis by use of a modified hemagglutinin test and concentrated protein from spinal fluid.

All attempts to transfer immunity from one animal to another of the same species have failed. There are many reasons for believing that immunity is not mediated by the classical types of humoral antibodies. In contrast to these negative findings, Lurie's classic studies have demonstrated that monocytes from immunized rabbits retain their ability to destroy tubercle bacilli when transferred to the anterior chamber of the eyes of the normal rabbits.

The detailed studies of Fong, Chin, and Elberg have shown that polymorphonuclear leukocytes do not transfer resistance. Lymphocytes transfer hypersensitivity but not resistance, while histocytes transfer immunity that is still detectable after a second transfer to a normal animal.

Hypersensitivity to tuberculoprotein can be transferred from animal to animal and from tuberculin-sensitive individuals to previously tuberculin-negative ones by the injection of white blood cells. This phenomenon was discovered by Chase and confirmed by a number of other investigators. Cortisone can suppress completely the tuberculin skin test without interfering with the passive transfer of hypersensitivity to a normal animal. The specific alteration required for passive transfer develops very rapidly, and white cells from the peritoneum of guinea pigs can effect the transfer 24 hours after infection. The sensitivity transferred by the white cells of ordinary stock guinea pigs persists for only a few weeks in contrast to that of man. The unknown substance in disrupted human cells that can transfer tuberculin sensitivity is referred to as transfer factor.

Cells from the peritoneal exudate of guinea pigs with positive tuberculin reactions are inhibited from migrating out of capillary tubes onto glass. The factor inhibiting migration is the sensitivity of the cell itself to tuberculin.

Bacteriophage Typing Freshly isolated strains of human tubercle bacilli can be separated into types A, B, C, and an intermediate between A and B. Type A is found most frequently in Japan, Hong Kong, and Rhodesia. Types A and B occur with equal frequency in Britain. Type A and intermediate type A-B are found in Madras, and type C occurs predominantly in the United States. By bacteriophage typing, Stead and Bates demonstrated that a soldier who acquired an infection with type A in the Far East transmitted this type to two civilians after returning to this country.

Determinants of Pathogenicity

The acid-fast bacilli produce neither exotoxins nor endotoxins. No single structure, antigen, or mechanism has been advanced that can explain the virulence of the organism. Virulent strains of human and bovine bacilli grow in strands or cords (Fig. 35-6), while avirulent dissociates of the same strain show no particular arrangment of the organisms (Fig. 35-7). A cord factor can be obtained from virulent organisms that has some toxicity for mice when given in very large doses. This factor is found primarily in the wax C fraction and inhibits various dehydrogenases in the animal.

The violent toxic symptoms induced in spontaneously infected human beings and in experimentally infected animals by the injection of minute amounts of tuberculin are manifestations of allergy to tuberculoprotein and not reactions to endotoxin.

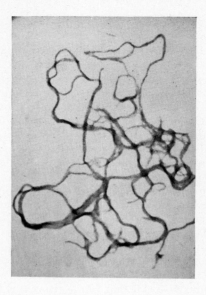

FIG. 35-6. Cord growth of virulent H37Rv. (From Yegian and Kurung: Am Rev Tuberc 65:181, 1952)

Catalase is produced by both virulent and saprophytic strains of mycobacteria, but the ability to synthesize catalase seems to be one of the factors necessary for virulence. There is a reasonably good correlation between the loss of ability to synthesize catalase and the loss of virulence in strains that have become resistant to isoniazid.

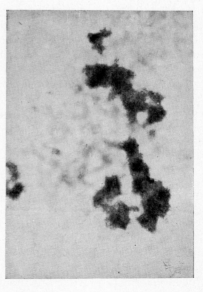

FIG. 35-7. Absence of cord growth with avirulent H37Ra. (From Yegian and Kurung: Am Rev Tuberc 65:181, 1952)

Tuberculin

Between 1891 and 1901 Koch prepared a series of tuberculins, and subsequently more than 50 kinds of tuberculin were investigated, of which only 2 have survived the test ot time. These are Koch's original preparation known as Old Tuberculin (OT) and Seibert's purified protein derivative (PPD).

The purified protein derivative of tuberculin contains a mixture of tuberculoproteins having molecular weights of 2,000 and 9,000, in contrast to the native antigenic tuberculoprotein studied by Seibert that had a molecular weight of 32,000.

PPD is a dry powder that is dry diluted with lactose and made into tablets in the proper proportions so that solutions can be made that will contain 0.00002, 0.0001, or 0.005 mg in the injection dose of 0.1 ml. Some errors may occur in making the dry dilutions of 0.00002 and 0.0001 mg. Hence it is more accurate and more economincal to use a tablet of 0.005 mg diluted in buffered saline to make the 0.0001 mg and 0.00002 mg strengths.

False positive tuberculin reactions will not develop in individuals who are skin tested over a period of months or years with 0.0001 or 0.005 mg of PPD, provided the individual has never been infected with either a tubercle bacillus or one of the other classified or unclassified mycobacteria. However, individuals who give small reactions or even zero reactions to the 0.0001 mg dose but who are positive to the 0.005 mg dose often get a booster effect from the 0.0001 mg dose. This reaction is not evident in two to four days but appears after one week, reaches its maximum at one month, and persists for six to twelve months.

It has been demonstrated, however, that positive skin tests to 5 TU doses of tuberculin can be passively transferred in routine transfusions with fresh blood from donors with positive skin tests.

Tuberculin Tests   Koch originally injected his tuberculin subcutaneously, and positive results were estimated from the severity of the constitutional symptoms and the degree of febrile reaction. The temperature after 6 to 12 hours often exceeded 104F (40C). This method is useful in veterinary practice but should not be used on patients because the generalized tuberculin reaction may reactivate a smolder-ing tuberculous infection. To avoid this danger, von Pirquet introduced the scratch test, in which two drops of undiluted tuberculin were deposited on the skin, after which the superficial layers of the skin were scratched with a needle and the tuberculin allowed to dry. Degrees of sensitivity could not be measured by this method. In 1908 Mantoux introduced the intracutaneous skin test that made quantitative measurements possible. By this method 0.1 ml of a particular dilution of OT or PPD is injected into the superficial layers of the skin and the area of induration read 48 to 72 hours later. Indurations measuring less than 5 mm are read as doubtful or negative. Reactions of 1 to 3 cm are frequently seen in highly allergic patients, and a vesicle often forms in the center of the inflamed area. Actual ulceration of the skin may occur beneath the vesicle, but only rarely does a febrile or constitutional reaction follow the most severe cutaneous reaction. Most false negative tests result from injecting the tuberculin into the deeper layers of the skin, where it drains away from the local area through the lymphatics. Patients critically ill with tuberculosis or other diseases, especially patients with tuberculous effusions of the pleura, pericardium, meninges, or peritoneum, may fail to react to tuberculin or react only to the strong doses, such as 1 mg of OT or second strength PPD (0.005).

Several multiple puncture methods have been introduced that are modifications of von Pirquet's scratch test procedure. In the Heaf test a special tuberculin of intermediate concentration is spread on a small area of the skin, and the tuberculin is introduced into the superficial layer of the skin by small needle points that are activated by a spring gun. The Tine test may be the practical answer for the busy physician in office or clinic practice, but doubtful reactions should be confirmed by the Mantoux test.

Doses of Tuberculin   The doses of tuberculin employed in a particular study are sometimes recorded as 0.1 ml of a specific dilution, as milligrams of OT or PPD, or in tuberculin units (TU). Comparable doses of OT, PPD, and TU are given in Table 35-1. Both PPD and OT contain a mixture of tuberculoproteins that vary in their ability to elicit reactions.

It has been shown that children under six months of age who have not been exposed to

TABLE 35-1 COMPARABLE DOSES OF OT AND PPD

Dilution of OT	Tuberculin Injected (mg)*	PPD Injected (mg)†	Tuberculin Units (TU)	Strength
1:100,000	0.001		0.1	
1:10,000	0.01	0.00002	1.0	First
1:2,000	0.05	0.0001	5.0	Intermediate
1:1,000	0.1		10.0	
1:100	1.0	0.005	100.0	Second

From Smith: Am Rev Respir Dis 99:820, 1969
*Based on 1 ml of concentrated OT = 1,000 mg
†Based on milligrams of protein

tuberculosis give negative reactions to 0.005 mg of PPD. When, however, 2 to 10 times more concentrated PPD is given to the young children, false positive reactions are obtained. BCG vaccination is usually administered only to individuals who have a negative reaction to 100 TU. After vaccination with the BCG used in this country, some individuals react to 5 to 10 TU, but many do not react to less than 200 TU. Nevertheless, the reaction to the strong dose of tuberculin is considered specific, since the subjects failed to react to the same large dose before vaccination. The degree of allergy, following BCG vaccination, does not necessarily indicate the degree of immunity.

Some individuals, particularly Blacks and patients having skin, eye, or glandular infections, are exquisitely sensitive to tuberculin. They may give positive reactions to 0.01 TU and often give large reactions with necrotic centers when injected with 1 TU. Patients suspected of having tuberculosis of the eye or skin should be given an initial dose of 0.01 TU and the dose increased, if the reaction is negative as indicated in the table. Other patients, even those with extensive disease, will not be harmed by an initial dose of 5 TU.

Only since the introduction of iodinated isotopic PPD have we learned about the rapid disappearance of tuberculin from the site of injection. Approximately 50 percent of the intracutaneous Mantoux dose disappears in 1 hour, 75 percent in 5 hours, and 96 percent in 24 hours. The facility with which the major part of the dose injected disappears through the lymphatics gives a good physiologic basis for the varied results obtained with a standard dose of tuberculin when the capillaries are artificially or naturally constricted or dilated. There are clinical observations to show that some tuberculin does remain fixed to the cells in the skin for weeks and months when a subreacting dose is given to a sensitized individual and when a large dose is given to a person who has not yet developed the allergy characteristic of tuberculosis. It is known that individuals receiving corticoid hormones may not react to tuberculin but will react several weeks later at that site when the corticoid has been discontinued.

In practical clinical work with patients, a conclusive negative tuberculin test may be of more value than a positive test, since a positive merely proves previous infection and not that the patient's present symptoms are from active tubercular disease. On the other hand, there is both clinical and experimental work showing that patients in good physical condition who give negative tuberculin tests to 1: 100 OT, or 0.005 mg of PPD (100 TU) have not been infected and are not now suffering from infection with either human or other classified or unclassified *Mycobacterium* organisms. There are about 1 percent who are exceptions to this rule.

Any severe illness may depress or eliminate the tuberculin reaction, but measles is a unique example of a relatively mild illness that may depress the tuberculin test for months. This depression is attributable to a specific effect of the measles virus on the human lymphocytes that renders them insusceptible to the stimulating effect of PPD.

Stability of Tuberculin Reaction Fifty years ago, when almost everyone over 20 years of age had a positive tuberculin test, it was assumed that tuberculin sensitivity, when once acquired, would persist for the remainder of the individual's life. This is true even now when the tubercle bacilli persist in lesions that are microscopically but not macroscopically active. If the tubercle bacilli are completely eliminated, the tuberculin reaction should slowly decrease and finally disappear. This occurs in man and in animals and persons who have been vaccinated with BCG but not superinfected with tubercle bacilli. There are individual examples of physicians who have had clinical tuberculosis, with a high degree of allergy to tuberculin, whose allergy slowly declined until the 100 TU dose was required to obtain even a slight tuberculin reaction.

Spontaneous disappearance of tuberculin sensitivity to the atypical mycobacteria occurs with even greater frequency than to infection with *M. tuberculosis.* Indirect evidence presented in the studies of Grzybowski and Allen in Ontario, Canada, show that a marked reduction in reactions to human tuberculin occurred between 1923 and 1959.

False Positive and False Negative Tuberculin Tests Both false positive and false negative tuberculin tests do occur, although the latter are much more frequent than the former. False positives may occur (1) when a platinum needle, sterilized by flaming has not cooled, (2) from a small hematoma, (3) from a slight skin infection at the site of the injection, (4) from tuberculin contaminated with bacteria. In a series of 448 medical students, 61, or 3.6 percent, had false positive skin tests to the 5 TU dose. The positive tests were shown to be false when the same students failed to give a positive reaction to 20 times as much human or avian PPD.

False negative tuberculin reactions are most frequently caused by (1) old deteriorated tuberculin, (2) injection of the tuberculin into the deeper layers of the skin, (3) the leak out of tuberculin after injection, (4) the physiologic condition of the skin, and (5) the presence of multiple tests.

When multiple skin tests are performed simultaneously the average size of the reaction may be materially reduced regardless of whether the sensitized white cells were passively transferred or actively induced with tubercle bacilli in animals or man.

Booster Effect of Tuberculin Test The first evidence for the booster effect of a tuberculin test was reported in 1938. Of 137 agricultural students who were negative to 10 TU of PPD made from the human tubercle bacillus but positive to 10 TU of PPD made from the avian tubercle bacillus, 46 were found to give good reactions to 10 TU of human PPD when the test was repeated six months later. The researchers concluded that "the original injection of avian tuberculin increased an already existing sensitivity in these individuals so they reacted upon a second injection of human PPD" (McCarter et al: *Am J Med Sci* 195:479, 1938).

The isoniazid prophylactic studies of Ferebee from 1957 to 1961 revealed the extent of the booster effect of a single 5 TU dose of tuberculin even when there was little or no reaction to the tuberculin. Tuberculin-negative individuals who received the placebo and not the isoniazid were retested after one year. It was found that the percentage of converters whose tuberculin reaction had increased to 8 mm or more varied from a low of 15.8 percent in a Georgia group to 21.1 percent in a Massachusetts group and 25.3 percent in a Wisconsin group.

An example of the difficulties that may arise from the booster effect is found in the report on tuberculin conversion on the USS *Long Beach.* A microepidemic had occurred on this ship, and all sailors with pulmonary infections had been removed. Skin tests were performed on all remaining sailors and on new sailors. Those with positive tuberculin reactions were given isoniazid, and those with a negative tuberculin reaction to 5 TU of PPD were observed and retested over the next year. A yearly conversion rate of 0.25 percent was anticipated, but a conversion rate of 9 percent was actually found. Most of the converters had not been in contact with the original open case, and none of them had any evidence of clinical disease. It appears that these were pseudoconversions from the previous tuberculin test. Ferebee had found that the conversion rate for the booster effect of the tuberculin test at age 20 was exactly 9 percent. The age of Navy recruits is in the 20-year range.

Diagnostic Significance of Positive Tuberculin Test It has been known for many years that patients acutely ill with tuberculosis or other diseases may fail to give a positive tuberculin reaction to 1 TU or 5 TU and occasionally even to 250 TU. It was assumed that this resulted from some type of hyposensitization, some exhaustion reaction, or a physiologic inability of the skin to react. This phenomenon is not infrequently seen in patients with miliary tuberculosis and generalized primary infections.

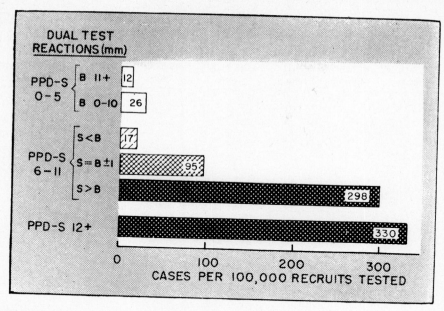

FIG. 35-8. Tuberculosis morbidity among 624,860 white US Navy recruits according to their reactions to 0.001 mg PPD-S and PPD-B. (From Palmer and Edwards: JAMA 205:167, 1968)

Less than 1 percent of patients with tuberculosis who are in good physical condition will fail to give a positive skin reaction to 1, 5, or 250 TU doses of tuberculin. The older the patients and the poorer their general physical conditions, the larger will be the number with false negative reactions. At the Durham Veterans Administration Hospital 6.1 percent did not react to the 5 TU dose, at an Ohio State Sanitorium 8.7 percent failed to react, 10 percent did not react at the St. Alban's Naval Hospital, 17.6 percent did not react at the Mayo Clinic, and 31 percent failed to react at Duke Hospital.

The Public Health Service found in their tuberculin surveys on healthy individuals that the 5 TU dose of PPD-S would detect most, if not all, individuals who had been infected with tubercle bacilli. The experience of physicians at the hospitals listed above indicates, however, that sick patients and especially elderly sick patients have their allergy suppressed so they may give a zero or less than 5 mm reaction to the 5 TU dose of PPD-S.

The dual test method of Palmer and Edwards using 5 TU doses of PPD-S and PPD-B (Fig. 35-8) has been used by Smith and Johnston in studies on 264 medical students and students of nursing (Table 35-2). Thirty-seven of these students gave definitely larger reactions to the 5

TU of PPD-S, indicating that they had been infected with the human tubercle bacillus. Four students gave a zero reaction to the 5 TU dose of PPD-S but an average size reaction of 9.5 mm to the 5 TU dose of PPD-B. On retesting these students with 250 TU doses of PPD-S and PPD-A, they gave an average of 11 mm reaction to PPD-S and 20 mm reaction to PPD-A, suggesting that they had been infected with one of the other species of mycobacteria.

If this group had been tested repeatedly with 5 TU doses of PPD-S, their allergy could have been boosted to such an extent that they would have given a greater than 5 mm reaction to PPD-S. They would have been labeled as tuberculin converted and treated unnecessarily with isoniazid. The 71 students who were negative to both 5 TU and 250 TU doses of PPD-S and PPD-A cannot be boosted to a false positive test with tuberculin. This was first demonstrated by Seibert many years ago when she made the original PPD-S.

At the Mayo Clinic it was reported in 1972 that 13.3 percent of patients subsequently proved to have tuberculosis failed to react to the 5 TU dose. Among 100 newly admitted patients to a Veterans Hospital in California over a 10-year period 10 percent failed to react to the

TABLE 35-2   Reactions of Medical Students and Students of Nursing to 5 TU [0.0001 MG] AND 100 TU [0.005 MG]

Students	PPD-S* (5 TU) mm†	PPD-B* (5 TU) mm	PPD-Y* (5 TU) mm	PPD-Scot* (5 TU) mm	PPD-F* (5 TU) mm	OT (1:100) mm	PPD-S* (100 TU) mm	PPD-A* (100 TU) mm
Medical 41	0	0	0	0	—	0	0	0
Nurses 30	0	0	0	0	—	0	0	0
Medical 44	0	0	0	0	—	5.7	5.3	11.3
Nurses 24	0	0	0	0	—	—	7.6	26.0
Medical 29	0	—	—	—	0	—	5.3	12.6
Medical 8	0	—	—	—	6.6	—	2.7	12.5
Medical 39	0	0	0	10.7	—	8.3	7.1	13.1
Nurses 8	0	0	0	10.3	—	—	14.7	18.5
Medical 4	0	9.5	0	0	—	13.3	11	20
Medical 4	39	12	19	17.5	—	—	—	—
Medical 33	17	9.7	11.1	14.7	—	—	—	—

From Smith and Johnston: Am Rev Respir Dis 90:902, 1964
*PPD-S = human PPD; PPD-B = Battey PPD; PPD-Y = photochromogen PPD; PPD-Scot = scotochromogen PPD; PPD-F = M. fortuitum; PPD-A = M. avium
†Of induration

5 TU dose although the new NCDC PPD-5 TU solution was used.

Clinical and Epidemiologic Significance of Positive or Negative Tuberculin Reaction   There are three groups of individuals based on their tuberculin reactions.

(1) Individuals negative to 5 TU but positive to 250 TU of PPD-S may be infected with one of the other classified or unclassified mycobacteria, which in some instances can be identified by retesting with 5 TU doses of PPD made from the other mycobacteria.

(2) Individuals positive to 250 TU, regardless of the infecting organism, have an immunity to reinfection with human tubercle bacilli that is almost as great as the immunity conferred by BCG vaccination and much greater than that conferred by a naturally acquired 15+ mm reaction to 5 TU of PPD-S. For example, nurses who are negative to 5 TU of PPD-S but positive to 250 TU of PPD-S can be safely assigned to the care of tuberculosis patients without having BCG vaccine. This is in sharp contrast to group 3.

(3) Individuals who are negative to both 5 TU and 250 TU PPD-S can be assumed to have escaped infection with both human and other classified and unclassified mycobacteria. Individuals in this group are easily infected when exposed to patients with tuberculosis and should be given BCG if their occupation or place of residence will expose them to individuals who may have active tuberculosis.

Experimental Disease in Laboratory Animals

Monkeys and anthropoid apes are very susceptible to experimental infections with the human and bovine strains of tubercle bacilli but comparatively resistant to the avian type. The primates acquire tuberculosis spontaneously from casual contact with man.

The guinea pig, the mouse, and the rabbit are the most useful animals for laboratory studies. Only a few bacilli are required to infect guinea pigs. Since they are equally susceptible to the human and bovine strains, guinea pig inoculation is an ideal diagnostic method for the detection of small numbers of organisms in contaminated material (p. 522).

The host–parasite relationship in experimental airborne tuberculosis in guinea pigs has been studied by Donald W. Smith and his associates. By using minute doses of tubercle bacilli and studying the very early days of the infection the roles of (1) the quantity of tubercle bacillus antigen, (2) the sensitized lymphocytes, and (3) the stimulated monocytes have been elucidated for normal guinea pigs and guinea pigs previously immunized with BCG vaccine.

Clinical Infection

Man is very susceptible to tuberculous infection but remarkably resistant to tuberculous disease. In certain epidemics in schoolchildren initiated by an open case of tuberculosis in a teacher or fellow student, as many as 50 to 70 percent of the students became infected, as measured by the tuberculin reaction, although only a few developed clinical infection during the period of observation.

Epidemiology

Forty years ago the death rate from tuberculosis was exceedingly high in infants, adoles-

cents, and young adults and relatively low in late middle age and in old age. With improved standards of living and the adoption of the control measures recommended by the National Tuberculosis Association, a high percentage of the open carriers of tubercle bacilli have been discovered, isolated in sanatoria, and treated. This has resulted in a sharp reduction of death in infancy, adolescence, and the early years of adult life.

Forty years ago the death rate for females was always higher than than that of males in all age groups and all races. This is no longer true. The highest death rates are now in nonwhite and white males after the age of 30 and in nonwhite and white females after the age of 60 (Fig. 35-9). There is considerable variation in the new case rate by states. The number of newly reported cases of tuberculosis each year has not declined proportionally to the decrease in deaths, and the influence of puberty on the activation of clinical disease is still apparent.

SMALL EPIDEMICS OF TUBERCULOSIS. Large epidemics of tuberculosis were precipitated when tubercle bacilli were introduced for the first time in groups of races who had never been exposed to the infection. Indeed, the Alaskan Indians and Eskimos are only now emerging from a major epidemic that has persisted on a high level for about 100 years.

The great success in protecting infants,

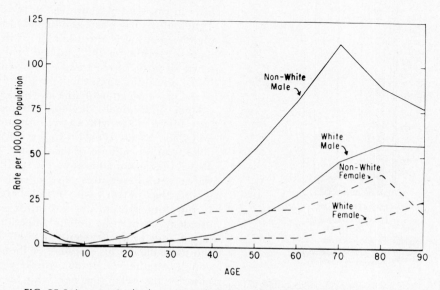

FIG. 35-9. Increase in death rate in males after 30 and females after 60 years of age.

schoolchildren, and young adults from infection with tubercle bacilli has resulted in a concentration of large numbers of highly susceptible individuals. Small epidemics usually arise from infections caused by a single individual. One schoolteacher in Denmark infected 70 to 105 tuberculin-negative students. After infection, 41 of the 105 developed primary infections, demonstrated by x-ray and by the isolation of tubercle bacilli from gastric lavage. Fifteen of the students developed postprimary (reinfection) progressive type of tuberculosis over the next 12 years. A summary of the epidemic is shown in Figure 35-10. A severe school epidemic that developed in the Whitesboro School District in New York State was traced to one bus driver. Among 228 children who rode his bus for less than 40 days, 66, or 28.9 percent, reacted to tuberculin and 42, or 18.4 percent, developed active pulmonary infections. In a group of 30 who rode the bus for more than 40 days, 56.7 percent developed positive tuberculin tests and 30 percent active pulmonary tuberculosis.

The most recent and dramatic example of a good spreader was reported from a school in Nova Scotia in 1969. An effective tuberculosis control program in the district Clair reduced the new cases of clinical tuberculosis to an average of 4 cases per year. Yearly tuberculin testing in the high school had shown that only 42, or 7.3 percent, of the 574 students were tuberculin positive.

One of the tuberculin-negative students visited her grandmother, from whom she apparently received the infection and, several months later, developed a cough. Subsequently she took a 10-hour bus trip with the bus driver and 48 other girls, all of whom were known to have negative tuberculins. She apparently infected everyone except the bus driver. In the course of the epidemic 234 other tuberculin-negative students, or 43.9 percent, were infected. There were 33 new cases of clinical tuberculosis among the students.

With the increase of tuberculin-negative individuals in the population each good spreader can infect many more susceptibles than they could when the positive rate of tuberculin reactors was high.

A Veterans Hospital patient studied by Riley and his associates contaminated the air in his room so thoroughly that it infected 15 guinea pigs in the room to which the air was evacuated. This patient also had tubercular laryngitis, and Riley calculated that he was more infectious than the average child with measles.

Transmission For practical purposes man may be regarded as the sole carrier of tuberculosis in the United States at the present time. Tuberculosis has been eliminated almost completely from herds of cattle as a result of large-scale tuberculin testing followed by the slaughter of all positive reactors. Any residual foci of infection can be controlled completely by universal pasteurization of milk and milk products.

Some individuals develop chronic pulmonary tuberculosis with cavity formation in the lungs and tubercle bacilli in the sputum without obvious symptoms of the disease. Individuals who have stainable tubercle bacilli in their saliva can disseminate the organisms more readily than persons who have tubercle bacilli in purulent sputum but not in the saliva. Individuals with tuberculous infections of the larynx and tubercle bacilli in their saliva are the most dangerous because of their constant cough. Another dangerous spreader of the disease is the schoolteacher who has tubercle bacilli in her sputum and saliva only when she

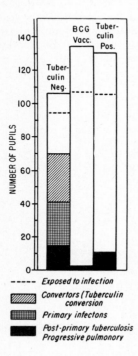

FIG. 35-10. A 12-year follow-up on children infected by one teacher. (From Hyge: Dan Med Bull 4:13, 1957)

has a virus cold. Such a teacher caused the epidemic referred to in Figure 35-10. Lincoln has collected a large series of microepidemics or out-breaks of tuberculosis among tuberculin-negative groups. She refers to one itinerant juggler with far advanced tuberculosis, who in one month infected 54 individuals in one small village.

Puffer's study of tuberculous and nontuberculous families in Tennessee presents evidence that some families are more susceptible to tuberculosis than others and that these susceptible families are gradually being reduced in number.

Jewish people have no increased resistance to tuberculous infection but have a definite resistance to tuberculous disease.

The difference between the White race and the Black is shown best by the studies of Roth, in which he compared the attack rate of White and Black soldiers in the United States Army between 1922 and 1936. The food, clothing, housing, medical care, and other environmental factors were identical. The morbidity rate was 210 per 100,000 for the White soldiers and 256 for Black soldiers, but the mortality rate was 24 per 100,000 for the Whites and 99 for the Blacks. The death rate of the Black was approximately four times as great as that of the White before the introduction of the new antibiotics, but with drug therapy there is now no significant difference.

Pathogenesis   Tubercle bacilli gain entrance to the body by inhalation, ingestion, or directly through the skin. Inhalation is the most frequent method of infection and invasion through the skin the most unusual. The local manifestations of a primary infection vary with the route of invasion. With inhalation, the primary lesion develops in the lungs, and the tracheobronchial lymph nodes are infected most extensively. With ingestion, the primary lesion may be in the mouth or tonsils, with an enlargement of the lymph nodes of the neck producing a condition called "cervical adenitis" or "scrofula." If the organisms penetrate the intestinal mucosa, the primary lesion occurs in the wall of the intestine and is accompanied by mesenteric adenitis with or without peritonitis. When entrance is by way of the skin, an ulceration develops at the point of invasion, accompanied by an extensive involvement of the regional lymph nodes.

When first introduced, tubercle bacilli multiply unchecked. The infecting organisms may be held temporarily and mechanically in the regional lymph nodes, but in a period of days they reach the thoracic ducts and the general circulation. Eventually all parts of the body are infected by a generalized dissemination before the conditions of hypersensitivity and relative resistance can be developed. The tuberculin test becomes positive between the fourth and the twelfth week following infection, and after this the bacilli spread slowly, if at all, through the lymphatics.

Most of the bacilli scattered throughout the body during the early part of the primary infection do not find locations suitable for development and disappear, but some remain in microscopic foci and may give rise 1 to 10 years later to infections of the bones, joints, lungs, and other organs. Of particular importance are those that reach the brain. Some of these develop into tuberculomas, which become encapsulated and heal or calcify, while others rupture into the meninges and initiate a tuberculous meningitis, followed by a bloodstream invasion referred to as "miliary tuberculosis." Miliary tuberculosis also may result from the rupture of a caseous lymph node into a vein or into one of the large lymph vessels without the development of an associated meningitis.

In countries with a high standard of living and a good tuberculosis control program the incidence of tuberculous infection in children has decreased rapidly during the past 40 years. In many instances primary infections have been postponed to adult life and often present very difficult diagnostic problems.

REINFECTION TUBERCULOSIS.   This is almost exclusively a disease of the lungs. Most pathologists believe that reinfection develops from the extension of infection to the lungs from a caseous focus resulting from a primary infection in the lymphatic system. Our experimental studies and clinical experience are in accord with this view.

Recently Stead has reviewed this subject and concluded that exogenous reinfection is relatively rare. He has presented evidence that foci develop in the upper parts of the lung as the result of the primary bloodstream dissemination. These foci may progress directly to disease or may remain quiescent for 10 to 20 or more years before becoming active. The age of

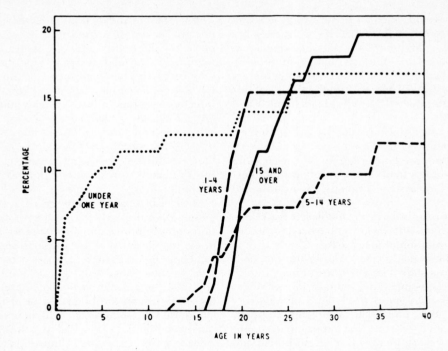

FIG. 35-11. Influence of age at time of infection on age when disease develops. (From Zeidberg, Dillon, and Gass: Am Rev Tuberc 70:1009, 1954)

the patient at the time of the initial infection appears to determine the rapidity with which clinical disease appears (Fig. 35-11).

CONGENITAL TUBERCULOSIS. This form of the disease is quite unusual. Most cases of childhood tuberculosis, even in infants of only a few weeks of age, are acquired in the home.

SILICOTUBERCULOSIS. The inhalation of inorganic dust containing free silica injures the lungs and predisposes the individual to the development of pulmonary tuberculosis. The mortality rate from tuberculosis of workmen exposed to silica dust may be as high as 190 per 100,000 as compared with 65 for the unexposed workers. Experimental silicosis in guinea pigs has been studied to determine the influence of an associated infection with tubercle bacilli. The presence of silica lowers the resistance of the tissues so much that even the relatively avirulent R$_1$ strain regularly produces progressive fatal infection in the silicotic animals.

Dust from organic materials and inorganic dusts other than those containing silica do not predispose the individual to the development of tuberculosis.

Laboratory Diagnosis

A relatively rich medium is required for primary isolation of *M. tuberculosis*. Contaminated sputum or other materials should be treated with a solution containing sodium hydroxide (2 percent) and sodium citrate (0.05 M) to which is added 0.5 g of N-acetyl-L-cysteine for each 100 ml of solution.

The specimen and the decontaminating solution are mixed in equal volumes in a 50 ml centrifuge tube, shaken for 5 to 30 seconds, and allowed to stand at room temperature for 15 minutes. Phosphate buffer is then added to make a 50 ml volume, and the specimen is centrifuged for 30 minutes, after which the supernate is discarded and 1 ml of bovine albumin is added to the sediment. The specimen is diluted 10 times with sterile physiologic saline and planted on Löwenstein-Jensen medium and Middlebrook's 7H10 agar. This method of decontamination and culture increases the number of positive cultures of *M. tuberculosis* and also the positive cultures of other species of mycobacteria and *Nocardia*.

Treatment

Success in the treatment of tuberculosis depends primarily upon measures that conserve and support the patient's innate and acquired resistance to the disease. Rest, both mental and physical, good food, fresh air, and pleasant surroundings, preferably in a sanatorium, give the patient the best possible chances for recovery. Tuberculous patients have a high requirement for ascorbic acid (vitamin C) and possibly also for vitamins A and D. Supplementing the diet with these vitamins is often advantageous.

The precipitous decline in the death rate since 1945 is attributable primarily to the combination of new drugs and improved thoracic surgery. The discovery that the simultaneous administration of two drugs postponed for months or years the emergence of drug-resistant strains has been an important factor in this success. The death rate from progressive primary tuberculosis in children, principally miliary tuberculosis and tuberculous meningitis, was reduced from 21.5 percent in 1946 to 1.5 percent in 1954.

Cortisone, meticortin, and corticotropin reduce or even abolish the tuberculin reaction and at the same time alleviate the symptoms of tuberculosis. Unfortunately, the ultimate effect is to disseminate the disease in animals and in man. Fortunately, the harmful effect of the hormones can be neutralized by the simultaneous administration of antituberculous drugs.

Streptomycin was the first antibiotic introduced that was effective clinically on tubercle bacilli. With its use, however, resistant strains developed in a few months unless a second specific antibiotic was given simultaneously. Para-aminosalicylic acid (PAS) given simultaneously with streptomycin or isonicotinic acid hydrazide (INH) delays the appearance of resistant strains for one year or more.

At the present time six additional antituberculosis drugs are available. The last one, ethambutol, was approved by the Council on Drugs of the AMA in 1969. A seventh drug, rifampin, is proving effective.

Prevention

Theoretically tuberculosis could be prevented and eventually eradicated if every active case were diagnosed, isolated, and treated. The application of these procedures is the cause of the declining incidence and death from tuberculosis in Western countries. The new drugs have speeded up the process but did not initiate it, nor can they alone eliminate tuberculosis.

Tuberculin testing of schoolchildren has become a refined technique of finding isolated spreaders of tubercle bacilli in the community.

Isoniazid Prophylaxis There are two relatively effective methods for preventing clinical tuberculosis, isoniazid prophylaxis and BCG vaccination. These methods should be considered as complementary and not competitive. BCG vaccination is useless after the individuals have been infected with tubercle bacilli, and isoniazid prophylaxis affords no protection, after it is stopped, to the individuals who have not been infected.

The effectiveness of isoniazid was studied in a large group of individuals with positive tuberculin reactions. Isoniazid was given in doses of 100 mg three times each day for one full year; an equal number of individuals were given a placebo. Ferebee summarized the results after a seven-year follow-up. The best protection against clinical disease was seen in recent converters, in whom the protection was 68 percent. In those with a 10^+ mm skin reaction to 5 TU of PPD, protection was obtained in 60 percent. Individuals with 5 to 9 mm skin reactions had only 40 percent protection, and those with 0 to 4 mm skin reactions showed no evidence of protection when compared with the controls.

Comstock and his associates protected about 60 percent of a group of 7,333 Eskimos in Alaska with INH prophylaxis. The 20-year study of INH prophylaxis in the children of Houston, Texas, was even more dramatic.

The attempts by Khoury and his associates, however, to use isoniazid prophylaxis in a slum area of the District of Columbia was an acknowledged failure. There was poor cooperation for skin testing, x-rays, and taking isoniazid. This was in sharp contrast to the good cooperation shown by the Eskimos of Comstock and the middle-class families of Ferebee.

BCG Prophylaxis   After years of investigation Calmette and Guérin obtained a bovine strain of the tubercle bacillus with a low and relatively fixed degree of virulence. This organism, known as the Bacillus of Calmette and Guérin, or BCG, has been used to vaccinate approximately 10,000,000 individuals. This vaccine is harmless when properly prepared and administered but gives a relative rather than an absolute immunity.

The vaccine should be administered only to those individuals who have a negative tuberculin reaction to 0.005 mg of PPD or 1 mg of OT. If a positive reaction to the larger dose of tuberculin does not develop by the end of the third month, the procedure may be repeated. Positive tuberculin reactions usually are obtained in 92 to 100 percent of the individuals receiving the vaccine, and the state of hypersensitivity persists for three to four years or longer. The accidental vaccination of a tuberculin-positive individual results in the rapid development, at the site of inoculation, of a superficial ulceration that persists for a few weeks but does not injure the patient.

The vaccine may be administered by the intracutaneous method of Wallgren or the transcutaneous or multiple puncture method of Rosenthal.

Four large-scale vaccination trials have been completed. They were the 20-year study of BCG and placebos in the North American Indian by Aronson and his associates, the 19-year study of infants in the slums of Chicago by Rosenthal and his co-workers, the 5-year study of schoolchildren in Puerto Rico and Georgia by the US Public Health Service, and the 10-year study of British schoolchildren in England. BCG afforded about 80 percent protection in the Aronson, Rosenthal, and British studies, but only 36 percent in Puerto Rico and apparently no protection in the Georgia studies.

The British children were subjected to the most elaborate and meticulous follow-up studies and revealed an 83 percent protection after 5 years and a 79 percent protection after 9 to 10 years following a single BCG vaccination. In many ways the British study has been the most conclusive study of all. The investigators kept the original positive reaction to 3 TU and to 250 TU separate but studied simultaneously with the BCG vaccinated and the controls. The breakdown rate in these asymptomatic x-ray-negative children was four times as great as in the BCG-vaccinated group (Table 35-3).

The only obvious difference in the four studies was the method of selecting the subjects for vaccination. In the Aronson, Rosenthal, and British studies only individuals who were negative to 100 TU (1 to 100 OT or second strength PPD) were selected for study and control, but in the US Public Health study individuals who were negative and gave 5 mm or less reaction to 5 TU (0.0001 mg PPD) were included in the study and control group. This method

TABLE 35-3   BCG AND CONTROLS IN BRITISH STUDY

Immunology Status	Number of Children	Number Starting in 3 Months	Annual Incidence per 100,000
A. Negative, not vaccinated	13,200	64	194
B. Negative, not vaccinated	6,400	33	206
Total	19,600	97	198
A. Negative, BCG vaccinated	14,100	13	37
B. Negative, BCG vaccinated	6,400	5	31
Total	20,500	18	35
A. Positive to 3 TU	15,800	69	175
B. Positive to 3 TU	8,600	37	172
Total	24,400	106	174
A. Positive to 100 TU	6,500	12	74
B. Positive to 100 TU	3,500	6	69
Total	10,000	18	72
Total of 3 TU + 100 TU	34,400	124	144

From Br Med J 1:413, 1956

of selection introduced a minimum of 31.4 percent of immunes in the Puerto Rico group and a minimum of 52.7 percent immunes in the Georgia group. In fairness to these excellent investigators of the US Public Health Service, one should realize that it was not known at the time of the actual vaccinations that these low-grade tuberculin reactors would be almost as immune as those who were vaccinated with BCG. Palmer and Long found that the other classified mycobacteria gave from 50 to 80 percent as much protection in guinea pigs as did BCG.

BCG vaccination can be recommended for special groups in which the morbidity rates are high and the factors favoring rapid transmission of the organisms temporarily uncontrollable. Such groups include the Indians, the inhabitants of certain slum areas in the large cities, Naval recruits and other military personnel who are confined to crowded quarters and who are exposed to uncontrolled infection, and nurses, medical students, and hospital attendants whose professional duties necessitate almost constant exposure to infection.

FURTHER READING

Books and Reviews

Dannenberg AM Jr: Cellular hypersensitivity and cellular immunity. Bacteriol Rev 32:85, 1968

Lawrence HS: Delayed sensitivity and homograft sensitivity. Annu Rev Med 11:207, 1960

Lester W: Chemotherapy of tuberculosis. Clin Notes Respir Dis 9:3, 1970

Luri MB: Resistance to Tuberculosis: Experimental Studies in Native and Acquired Defensive Mechanisms. Cambridge, Harvard Univ Press, 1964

Mackaness GB, Bladen RY: In Mudd S (ed): Cellular Immunity in Infectious Agents and Host Reactions. Philadelphia, Saunders, 1970, p 22

Rich AR: The Pathogenesis of Tuberculosis. Springfield, Ill, Thomas, 1951

Selected Papers

Barclay WR, et al: Protection of monkeys against tuberculosis by aerosol vaccination with Bacillus Calmette-Guérin. Am Rev Resp Dis 107:351, 1973

Bates, JH, Mitchison, DA: Geographic distribution of bacteriophage types of *Mycobacterium tuberculosis*. Am Rev Respir Dis 100:189, 1969

Carr DT: The tuberculin test. Am Rev Respir Dis 105:855, 1972

Chase MW: The cellular transfer of cutaneous hypersensitivity to tuberculins. Proc Soc Exp Biol Med 59:134, 1945

Ching-Tsai: The diagnosis of tuberculous meningitis by immunologic reaction of cerebrospinal fluid. Am Rev Respir Dis 100:565, 1969

Chusid EL, Shah R, Siltzbach LE: Tuberculin tests during the course of sarcoidosis in 350 patients. Am Rev Respir Dis 104:13, 1971

Comstock GW, Ferebee SH, Hammes LM: A controlled trial of communitywide isionazid prophylaxis in Alaska. Am Rev Respir Dis 95:935, 1967

Council on Drugs. Evaluation of a new antituberculous agent—ethambutol hydrochloride (Myambutol). JAMA 208:2463, 1969

David JR, Al-Askari S, Lawrence HS, Thomas L: Delayed hypersensitivity in vitro. J Immunol 93:264, 274, 279, 1964

Doster B, Murray FJ, Newman R, Woolpert SF: Ethambutol in the initial treatment of pulmonary tuberculosis. Am Rev Respir Dis 107:177, 1973

Duboczy BO, White FC: Further studies with the direct latex agglutination test in tuberculosis. Am Rev Respir Dis 100:364, 1969

Edwards LB, Livesay VT, Acquaviva FA, Palmer CE: Height, weight, tuberculous infection and tuberculous disease. Arch Environ Health 22:106, 1971

Edwards PQ: The tuberculin test. Am Rev Respir Dis 106: 282, 1972

Ferebee SH: Isoniazid prophylaxis for the few or for the many? Bull Natl Tuberc Respir Dis Assoc 54:2, 1968

Galindo B, Myrvik QN: Migratory response of granulomatous alveolar cells from BCG-sensitized rabbits. J Immunol 105:227, 1970

Guld J, Waaler H, Sundaksan TK, Kaufmann PC, TenDam HG: The duration of BCG-induced tuberculin sensitivity in children, and its irrelevance for revaccination. Bull WHO 39:829, 1968

Hardy MA, Schmidek HH: Epidemiology of tuberculosis aboard a ship. JAMA 203:175, 1968

Hsu HK: Isoniazid in the prevention and treatment of tuberculosis—a 20-year study of the effectiveness in children. JAMA 229:528, 1974

Hyde L: Clinical significance of the tuberculin test. Am Rev Respir Dis 105:453, 1972

Kent DC, Schwartz R: Active pulmonary tuberculosis with negative tuberculin skin tests. Am Rev Respir Dis 95: 411, 1967

Khoury SA, Theodore E, Platts VJ: Isoniazid therapy in a slum area. Am Rev Respir Dis 99:345, 1969

Lincoln EM: Epidemics of tuberculosis. Arch Environ Health 14:473, 1967

Magnus K, Edwards LB: The effect of repeated tuberculin testing on postvaccination allergy. Lancet 2:643, 1955

McCarter J, Getz HR, Stiehm RH: A comparison of intracutaneous reactions in man to purified protein derivatives of several species of acid-fast bacteria. Am J Med Sci 195:479, 1938

Mohr JA, Killebrew L, Muchmore HG: Transfer of delayed hypersensitivity by blood transfusions in man. JAMA 207:517, 1969

Moulding T: Chemoprophylaxis of tuberculosis: When is the benefit worth the risk and cost? Ann Intern Med 74: 761, 1971

Murohashi R, Kondo E, Yoshida K: The role of lipids in acid-fastness in mycobacteria. Am Rev Respir Dis 99: 794, 1969

Newman R, Doster B, Murray FJ, Ferebee S: Rifampin in initial treatment of pulmonary tuberculosis. Am Rev Respir Dis 103:461, 1971

Ochs CW: Tuberculin conversion. JAMA 200:1019, 1967

Oort J, Turk JL: The fate of (I[131]) labeled antigens in the skin of normal guinea pigs and those with delayed type hypersensitivity. Immunology 6:148, 1963

Palmer CE, Long MW: Effects of infection with atypical mycobacteria on vaccination and tuberculosis. Am Rev Respir Dis 94:553, 1966

Palmer ED, Edwards LB: Identifying the tuberculous infected. JAMA 205:167, 1968

Pepys J: The relationship of nonspecific and specific factors in a tuberculin reaction. Am Rev Tuberc 71:49, 1955

Pope H, Smith DT: Synthesis of B-complex vitamins by tubercle bacilli when grown on synthetic media. Am Rev Tuberc 54:559, 1946

Rado TA, Bates JH, Engel HWB, et al: World Health Organization studies on bacteriophage typing of mycobacteria. Am Rev Respir Dis 111:459, 1975

Ribi E, Anacker RL, Barkley WR, et al: Efficiency of mycobacterial cell walls as a vaccine against airborne tuberculosis in the Rhesus monkey. J Infect Dis 123:527, 1971

Ribi E: Currents in tuberculosis research. J Infect Dis 123: 562, 1971

Rideout VK, Hiltz TE: Epidemic in a high school in Nova Scotia. Can J Public Health 60:22, 1969

Riley RL, Mills CC, O'Grady F, et al: Infectiousness of air from a tuberculosis ward. Am Rev Respir Dis 85:511, 1962

Smith DT: Progressive primary tuberculosis in the adult and its differention from lymphomas and mycotic infections. N Engl J Med 241:198, 1949

Smith DT, Johnston WW: Single and multiple infections with atypical and typical mycobacteria. Am Rev Respir Dis 90:899, 1964

Smith DT: The tuberculin unit. Am Rev Respir Dis 99:820, 1969

Smith DT: The diagnostic and prognostic value of the second strength dose of PPD (5 micrograms). Am Rev Respir Dis 101:317, 1970

Smith DT: The problem of the "boost" effect in tuberculin testing. Am Rev Respir Dis 106:118, 1972

Smith DT, Abernathy RS, Smith GB Jr, Bondurant S: The apical localization of reinfection pulmonary tuberculosis. Am Rev Respir Dis 70:547, 557, 570, 1954

Smith DT: The antigenicity and allergenicity of tuberculin and the anamnestic effect of a tuberculin test. Arch Environ Health 14:569, 1967

Smith DT: Diagnostic and prognostic significance of the quantitative tuberculin test: the influence of subclinical infection with atypical mycobacteria. Ann Intern Med 67:919, 1967

Stead WW: Pathogenesis of first episode of chronic pulmonary tuberculosis in man: recrudescence of residuals of primary infection on exogenous reinfection. Am Rev Respir Dis 95:729, 1967

Stead WW, Bates JH: Evidence of "silent" bacillemia in primary tuberculosis. Ann Intern Med 74:559, 1971

Turkey JW, DuFour EH, Seibert F: Lack of sensitization following reported skin tests with standard tuberculin (PPD-S). Am Rev Tuberc 62:77, 1950

Valentine FT, Lawrence HS: Lymphocyte stimulation: transfer of cellular hypersensitivity to antigen in vitro. Science 165:1014, 1969

Vall-Spihosa A, Lester TW: Rifampin: Characteristics and role in the chemotherapy of tuberculosis. Ann Intern Med 74:758, 1971

36
Other Mycobacterium Species

TABLE 36-1 Differential Properties of Clinically Significant Species of Mycobacteria*

| Property | M. tuber-culosis | M. afri-canum | M. bovis | Group I | | Group II | | |
				M. kan-sasii	M. mari-num	M. scro-fulaceum	M. gordonae	M. fla-vescens
Speed of growth	S	S	S	S	S	S	S	S
Niacin production	+	+	−	−	−	−	−	−
Nitrate reduction	+	±	−	+	−	−	−	+
Catalase, > 45 mm foam	−	−	−	+	−	+	+	+
Catalase, 68C/20 min	−	−	−	+	±	+	+	+
Pigment, dark	−	−	−	−	−	+	+	+
Pigment, light	−	−	−	+	+	−§	−§	−
Tween 80 hydrolysis (5 day)	−	−	−	+	+	−	+	+
Tellurite reduction (3 day)	−	−	−	−	−	−	−	−
NaCl tolerance	−	−	−	−	−	−	−	+
Arylsulfatase (3 day)	−	−	−	−	−	−	−	−
MacConkey agar	−	−	−	−	−	−	−	−
Strains tested	239	4	61	144	65	94	130	25
Clinical significance	+	+	+	+	+	+	−	−

Data provided by George P. Kubica
Key: + = more than 75 percent of strains positive; − = more than 75 percent of strains negative; ± = high degree of variability (40 to 60 percent with positive reactions)
†Comprised of 2 distinct subspecies: M. chelonei subsp chelonei (contains the now unrecognized M. borstelense) does not grow on 5 percent NaCl; M. chelonei subsp abscessus does grow on NaCl
‡Pigment increases with age and independent of light exposure
§Pigment may intensify with prolonged light exposure

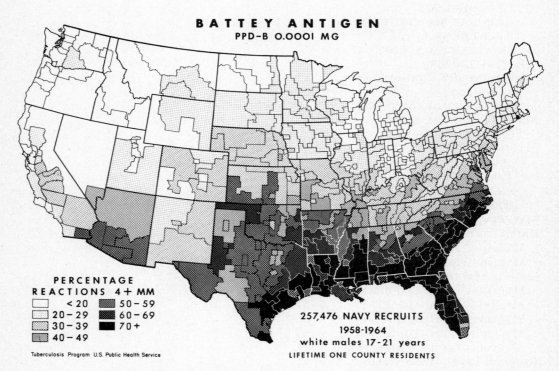

BATTEY ANTIGEN
PPD-B 0.0001 MG

PERCENTAGE
REACTIONS 4 + MM
< 20   50 − 59
20 − 29   60 − 69
30 − 39   70 +
40 − 49

Tuberculosis Program U.S. Public Health Service

257,476 NAVY RECRUITS
1958-1964
white males 17-21 years
LIFETIME ONE COUNTY RESIDENTS

FIG. 36-1. Geographic variations in the frequency of reactors to the Battey antigen (Batteyin) among U.S. Navy recruits. (From Palmer and Edwards: Tuberkuloza 18:193, 1966)

TABLE 36-1 CONT.

Group III						Group IV				
M. xenopi	*M. avium*	*M. intracellulare*	*M. gastri*	*M. terrae complex*	*M. triviale*	*M. fortuitum*	*M. chelonei§*	*M. vaccae*	*M. smegmatis*	*M. phlei*
S	S	S	S	S	S	F	F	F	F	F
–	–	–	–	–	–	–	–	–	–	–
–	–	–	–	+	+	+	–	+	+	+
–	–	–	–	+	+	+	+	+	+	+
+	+	+	–	+	+	+	+	±	+	+
+‡	–	–	–	–	–	–	–	±	–	+
–	–§	–‡	–	–	–	–	–	+	–	–
–	–	–	+	+	+	–	–	+	+	+
–	+	+	–	–	–	±	±	+	+	+
–	–	–	–	–	+	+	+†	+	+	+
±	–	–	–	–	–	+	+	–	–	–
–	–	±	–	–	–	+	+	–	–	–
10	114	240	16	90	27	61	35	10	29	26
+	+	+	–	–	–	+	+	–	–	–

For many years it has been known that *Mycobacterium bovis* frequently and *Mycobacterium avium* occasionally produce disease in man that is indistinguishable clinically from that caused by *Mycobacterium tuberculosis*. In recent years there has been a dramatic decrease in infections caused by the bovine species but an increase or an increased recognition of disease caused by the avian organism. During the past 20 years it has become evident that a number of newly recognized species of mycobacteria, often erroneously designated "atypical," produce disease in man much more frequently than the well-known bovine or avian organisms. These mycobacteria are unique in that they have no known regular animal host but apparently occur in the soil. The species vary in frequency depending upon locale, soil, and other climatic and environmental factors. They appear to be endemic in certain geographic areas. At the present time there is no evidence that this group of mycobacteria can be transmitted directly from man to man. They can and do, however, produce severe and even fatal disease in man. Careful morphologic, cultural, metabolic, and animal studies have permitted the classification presented in Table 36-1.

These mycobacteria are ubiquitous and have been found in practically every part of the world except Alaska. However, their frequency varies greatly in different parts of the world and even in different parts of the same country (Figs. 36-1 and 36-2).

Mycobacterium bovis

Mycobacterium bovis was differentiated from *M. tuberculosis* by Theobald Smith in 1896. The rods often are shorter and plumper than the human tubercle bacillus, and primary isolation is somewhat more difficult. Since growth is inhibited by glycerol, the colonies are smaller than the human species on glycerol agar.

M. bovis produces spontaneous tuberculosis in a wide range of animals, including man. Experimentally it is highly pathogenic for rabbits and guinea pigs, slightly pathogenic for dogs, horses, rats, and mice, and not pathogenic for fowl. Fifty years ago most dairy herds were heavily infected with bovine tubercle bacilli, and in the absence of pasteurization the raw milk produced disease in man, particularly extrapulmonary lesions, such as those of glands and bone and joint disease in children. Although somewhat less virulent for man than the human species, progressive fatal pulmonary disease did occur. Tuberculin testing of cows, however, with the slaughter of the positive reactors, has reduced the incidence of infection in cows to less than 3 percent in the United States. Bovine infections of man have been eliminated where pasteurized milk is consumed. There is still a minimal amount of spread from cows to swine.

Hopefully, bovine tuberculosis eventually will be eliminated as a cause of disease in man and animals. It is still necessary, however, to

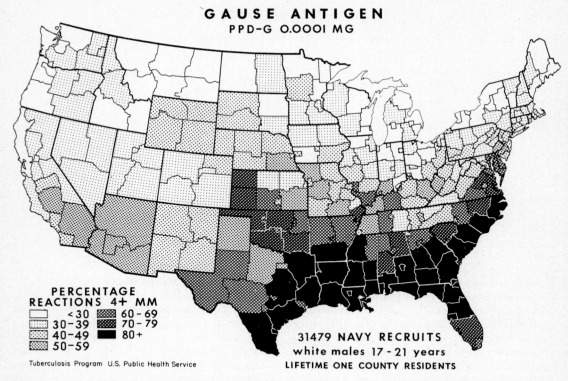

GAUSE ANTIGEN
PPD-G 0.0001 MG

PERCENTAGE
REACTIONS 4+ MM

<30	60-69
30-39	70-79
40-49	80+
50-59	

Tuberculosis Program U.S. Public Health Service

31479 NAVY RECRUITS
white males 17 - 21 years
LIFETIME ONE COUNTY RESIDENTS

FIG. 36-2. Geographic variations in the frequency of reactors to the Gause scotochromogen (Scrofulin) *(Mycobacterium scrofulaceum)*. (From Palmer and Edwards: Tuberkuloza 18:193, 1966)

include it in the differential diagnosis, since as late as 1970 Karlson and Carr found 6 cases among 2,086 individuals with culture-proven clinical tuberculosis.

Mycobacterium paratuberculosis

M. paratuberculosis produces a disease in cattle and sheep first described by Johne and Frothingham in 1895. The infection is confined to the mucosa and submucosa of the ileum, cecum, and upper colon. The lesions are proliferative and granulomatous and contain enormous numbers of acid-fast monocytic cells. The lesions do not caseate or ulcerate. The disease causes diarrhea and prevents the proper absorption of food. The incubation period is long, the progress of the disease is slow, and it is invariably fatal.

Mycobacterium paratuberculosis is a small, acid-fast rod, 1 to 2 μm long and 0.5 μm wide. All attempts at cultivation of the bacillus failed until Twort incorporated heat-killed tubercle bacilli or timothy bacilli *(M. smegmatis)* in the

egg-glycine medium. A growth-promoting factor, isolated from *M. phlei* by Francis and his associates in 1953, was named mycobactin. This factor subsequently was identified as sideramine, a metal-chelating growth factor.

Since *M. paratuberculosis* shares some antigens with *M. avium*, avian tuberculin can be used as a skin test in cows suspected of having Johne's disease. A tuberculin made from cultures of *M. paratuberculosis* reacts in cows infected with *M. avium*. The degree of allergy is not very high in Johne's disease, which is consistent with the lack of caseation in the lesions. The skin test becomes negative in the terminal stages of the disease, while a positive complement-fixation test appears early in the process and usually is present until death.

Mycobacterium Microti (The Vole Bacillus)

This organism was isolated in 1937 by Wells from the field mouse or vole. *M. microti* is somewhat longer and thinner than other mammalian species in culture. Irregular S-shaped, hook-shaped, semicircular, and circular forms have been seen in tissues of infected voles. Growth is slow on all types of media, often requiring as long as four to five weeks for the appearance of minute colonies. Primary growth does not occur on media containing glycerol, nor is subculture growth enhanced by glycerol. The growth is definitely slower than that of the human and bovine species.

M. microti is the cause of general tuberculosis in voles. Localized but not systemic infections are induced in guinea pigs, rabbits, and calves. Vaccines prepared from the vole bacillus were included in pilot studies with BCG to test the effectiveness of BCG vaccination in humans. The percentage of protection after 7.5 to 10 years was practically the same as that from BCG.

Mycobacterium ulcerans

This pathogenic species was isolated in Australia in 1948. In preparations from culture the organisms are 0.2 by 1.5 to 3 μm, but they are somewhat larger in tissue preparations and are frequently beaded. *M. ulcerans* will not grow at 37C and grows very slowly on primary isolation even at 30 and 33C. After nine weeks' incubation, primary colonies are 2 to 3 mm in diameter, round, smooth, low convex, opaque, and white to pale cream in color. *M. ulcerans* is antigenically distinct from other known mycobacteria by both complement fixation and skin test.

Skin ulcers produced in man by *M. ulcerans* are characterized by indolent extensions from areas of inconspicuous induration to involve large new areas. Rats and mice can be infected with cultures, but guinea pigs, rabbits, fowl, and lizards are resistant.

A toxin is produced by *M. ulcerans* that causes inflammation and necrosis when injected into the skin of guinea pigs. This is the only known toxin produced by a *Mycobacterium* species.

Mycobacterium marinum

This organism was isolated in 1926 by Aronson from tuberculous lesions of salt water

fish. The bacilli may be short, thick and uniformly staining when present in clumps in the tissue, but long, thin, beaded, and barred rods may be seen scattered throughout the tissue.

In 1949–50, Linell and Norden studied an epidemic of skin infections in 80 patients in the town of Orebro, Sweden. The lesions were usually located on the outside of the elbows (Fig. 36-3), although they were also present on other parts of the body (Fig. 36-4). The infection began as a small papule that increased in size to that of a bean, ulcerated, and discharged pus that contained acid-fast organisms. The lesion healed spontaneously but sometimes required two years for healing. Epidemics of the same type have occurred in Seattle and in Colorado.

Linell and Norden isolated the causative organism from the lesions of the patients and from the water of a swimming pool and finally proved the pathogenicity of the organism for man by inoculating themselves and reproducing the disease. When grown on Löwenstein-Jensen medium at 31C, the organism produces soft, grayish white colonies with slightly yellow streaks. After exposure to daylight at room temperature, colonies first develop an intense

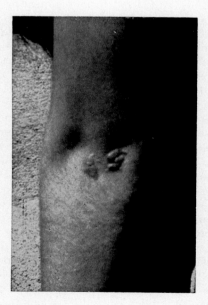

FIG. 36-3. Granulomatous lesion of the elbow of six months' duration showing granulations and some satellite lesions. (Photograph by Mary S. Romer. Courtesy of Norma Johannis, Colorado State Department of Health)

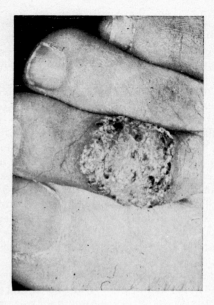

FIG. 36-4. Verrucous lesion of the toe suggesting tuberculous verrucosa cutis. (Photographed by James A. Philpott, Jr. Courtesy of Norma Johannis, Colorado State Department of Health)

orange yellow to orange pigment and finally turn red.

Mice are most susceptible to experimental infections, with local lesions appearing after intraperitoneal infection in the scrotum, tail, paws, and lungs. M. marinum has a wide range of pathogenicity for poikilothermic species of animals. M. ulcerans and M. marinum can be differentiated by inoculation of minute doses into the foot pads of mice.

Epidemics are readily recognized, but the single sporadic infection is usually misdiagnosed. The epidemics in Washington and Colorado followed swimming in fresh water lakes, but one in Alabama followed swimming in a salt water bay.

The prognosis is variable. The lesions of some patients heal while the cultures are growing, or more often while antibiotic sensitivity tests are being run. Others heal following treatment with the proper antibiotic. We have seen one patient, however, with granulomatous lesions of a knee and leg that persisted for 12 years although he was treated with all of the known antibiotics, including rifampin. This patient was finally cured by Cahn and Smith by a complicated procedure in which hyposensitization with avian PPD was followed by potassium iodide by mouth and, finally, stimulating doses of x-ray to increase the circulation in the lesion. The iodides were continued with the x-ray stimulation.

Mycobacterium kansasii

This organism is usually longer and wider than tubercle bacilli and characteristically shows alternate stained and unstained bands, especially in young liquid cultures containing oleic acid and Tween. They usually are arranged in curving strands and are acid-fast. M. kansasii contains mycoside A. This is a specific glycolipid containing 2-0-methyl fucose, 2-0-methyl rhamnose, and 2:4-di-0-methyl rhamnose.

After two weeks of incubation in the dark on glycerol egg slants, colonies appear which are raised, with irregular surface and margins, and are ivory or off-white in color. If grown in lighted incubators, the colonies are lemon yellow and become orange or red-orange with age.

At room temperature growth occurs in three weeks and at 31 to 37C in one or two weeks. No growth occurs at 45C. Biochemical properties of the organism are shown in Table 36-1.

Antigenic Structure M. kansasii shares common antigens with human and other mycobacteria but has at least one antigen that is not present in M. tuberculosis. M. kansasii organisms absorb the agglutinin from the sera of rabbits immunized to either the human or the M. kansasii organism, while human tubercle bacilli absorb agglutinins specific for the human but not the agglutinins to M. kansasii.

Patients infected with M. kansasii who have reactions of the same size to both human PPD and kansasii PPD probably have had a subclinical infection with the human bacillus as well as a clinical infection with M. kansasii.

M. kansasii must be differentiated from M. marinum, which is also photochromogenic, as shown in Table 36-1. The two species can be distinguished by nitrate reduction and catalase production > 45 minutes. M. simiae is also a photochromogen, and M. szulgai is a photochrome when grown at 25C but a scotochrome at 37C.

Pathogenesis M. kansasii produces pulmonary and extrapulmonary disease in man that is almost indistinguishable from that produced by *M. tuberculosis*. Progressive disease can be produced in hamsters when large doses (10^6 to 10^7) of viable organisms are injected intravenously or intraperitoneally. It is relatively nonpathogenic for guinea pigs, rabbits, or fowl, but large doses of organisms (4 mg moist weight) injected into guinea pigs produce a high degree of specific sensitivity to PPD prepared from *M. kansasii*. A double infection with *M. tuberculosis* and *M. kansasii* results in a marked reinforcement of both tuberculin and kansasiin but not the batteyin or fortuitin reactions.

Clinical Infection EPIDEMIOLOGY. There is no evidence that this organism spreads directly from man to man or that children become infected when a sputum-positive member remains in a family for months to years. The infection is, however, much more prevalent in some geographic areas. Seven percent of patients admitted to Suburban Cook County Tuberculosis Hospital – Sanitorium were infected with *M. kansasii*, and no infection has been observed in the children of these patients. *M. kansasii* is the most frequent cause of atypical tuberculosis in the Houston – Dallas area of Texas. Oklahoma also is an area of high infection with *M. kansasii*. Children there develop positive skin tests much sooner to PPDs made from *M. kansasii* than to PPDs from *M. tuberculosis* or from the Battey or scotochrome types. A positive skin rate of 50 percent by age 17 does not increase very much after that age.

CLINICAL MANIFESTATIONS. Primary infections are more frequent than reinfections with *M. kansasii* but are less frequently detected. Lymph node enlargement, especially in the neck, is probably the most frequent clinical form of the disease. In a study of 28 children in Texas with cervical adenitis, 6 were caused by *M. tuberculosis*, 8 by *M. kansasii*, 2 by scotochromogens, and 2 by nonphotochromogens (Battey type). A few children have hilar lymph node disease without adenitis. The onset is usually insidious but may be abrupt, with pleural pain, fever, and hemorrhages. Cavities are often present. Symptomatology of reinfection with pulmonary disease is indistinguishable from that shown by infection with *M. tuberculosis*.

Subclinical infections with *M. kansasii*, as shown by positive skin tests, indicate that the disease in the United States is more localized than infections with *M. scrofulaceum* or *M. intracellulare*. *M. kansasii* infections are found more frequently in areas around Chicago, Dallas and Houston, Texas, and in some parts of California. It usually is not found in the East, Southeast, and other southern areas. Thirteen cases, however, have been found in North Carolina, all of which came from 1 of the 100 counties of the state.

TREATMENT. Experimental studies in mice indicate that rifampin alone will cure *M. kansasii* infections. The addition of streptomycin enhanced the response, but further improvement was not obtained by the addition of isoniazid.

Of 35 patients treated with multiple antibiotics and followed for 10 years, only 4 had relapses.

Mycobacterium scrofulaceum

The scotochromogens are organisms that produce, in a dark incubator, yellow and orange colonies that become more reddish when grown in the light. They are almost as slow-growing as human tubercle bacilli. The colonies are smooth and soft but become dome shaped as growth continues.

When grown in a medium containing Tween 80, *M. scrofulaceum*, the pathogenic scotochromogen from human infections, has no crossbars and resembles *M. tuberculosis*. However, in medium containing free oleic acid (but not Tween 80), the crossbars may develop. Another slow-growing species of scotochromogen is the tap water organism (*M. gordonae*) which is rarely pathogenic. This species, in contrast to *M. scrofulaceum*, does hydrolyze Tween. For differential biochemical reactions see Table 36-1.

Pathogenesis Some strains of scotochrome mycobacteria are pathogenic. They are frequently found as the sole etiologic agent in cervical adenitis in young children. First reported in Canada in 1956, these organisms are now being isolated from cervical lymph nodes in various parts of the world. Skin tests of 29,540 Navy recruits with standardized scoto-

chrome PPD° gave a reaction rate of 48.7 percent. Another scotochrome PPD† gave a 5 mm
or more reaction in approximately 50 percent of
the medical students tested.

If scotochrome mycobacteria are able to invade and grow in guinea pig tissue, a positive
skin reaction would be expected in normal
animals because of their constant exposure to
saprophytic species. No direct testing of normal
stock guinea pigs has been done, but several
hundred guinea pigs sensitized with other
mycobacteria, such as avian, human, photochrome, and Battey, have been tested with a
battery of PPDs. Under these conditions, all of
the observed reactions to the scotochrome were
of the cross-reaction type, with no instance of as
large a reaction as previously observed when
the scotochrome was used to sensitize the
guinea pigs. These observations suggest that
certain strains of scotochromes have a high
degree of invasiveness but a low degree of
pathogenicity for man, while they have neither
for the guinea pig.

Guinea pigs sensitized to scotochrome° gave
appreciable cross-reaction with avian and Battey but very little cross-reaction with human or
photochrome (Fig. 36-5). Guinea pigs sensitized to R₁ human tubercle bacilli gave large
homologous reactions, with very small cross-
reactions to photochromes, larger reactions to
scotochromes, and the largest cross-reactions to
avian and Battey.

M. flavescens is the third scotochrome included in Table 36-1. It can be differentiated
from M. scrofulaceum and M. gordonae by its
ability to reduce nitrogen and tolerate NaCl.

In 1973 a new pathogen was isolated from
five cases involving middle-aged men and
women with pulmonary cavities. This organism
appears to be a photochrome when grown at
25C but a scotochrome when grown at 37C. It
has been named M. szulgai. Patients infected
with this organism responded well to triple-
drug therapy.

Laboratory Diagnosis The great majority
of scotochromes isolated are saprophytes.
However, in the absence of other pathogenic
organisms, when isolated from a lymph node,
spinal fluid, blood, or surgically excised pulmonary tissue, the pathogenicity of the strain
may be assumed for purposes of therapy.

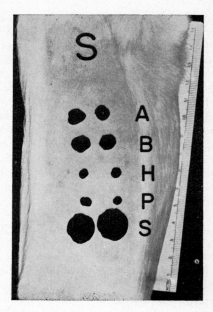

FIG. 36-5. Tuberculin reactions in a guinea pig sensitized with 4 mg of a scotochrome culture. The homologous PPD is largest. There are good cross-reactions with
avialin and Batteyin but poor cross-reactions with
tuberculin and kansasiin. (From Smith and Johnston: Am
Rev Respir Dis 90:899, 1964)

Treatment Most of the antibiotics that
are effective against M. tuberculosis may be
somewhat effective against M. scrofulaceum.

Mycobacterium gordonae

Mycobacterium gordonae is a slow-growing scotochromogen that is frequently isolated
from sputum of patients who do not have mycobacterial infections. The frequency with which
it appears in gastric washings is much greater
than that in sputum, but this discrepancy is due
to its presence in unsterilized tap water used in
gastric lavage. It is also found in soil and natural waters.

The rate of growth and the color and appearance of the colonies is the same as that of M.
scrofulaceum (Table 36-1).

Mycobacterium avium

This organism was isolated from birds in
1891. The acid-fast rods are short and resemble
the bovine species more closely than the human bacillus. Avian bacilli grow on the usual

media employed for the isolation of the human tubercle bacillus and at the same rate or a little faster than the human species. The optimal temperature is 40C, although the organism will grow at temperatures between 30C and 44C.

Avian bacilli are strongly catalase-positive but niacin-negative. With minor exceptions, the virulence of the strains can be predicted from the colonial types: Rough and smooth colonies are virulent, while the opaque colonies are not virulent (Fig. 36-6).

Mycobacteria of the avian-Battey complex have been divided into serologic groups by agglutination with absorbed sera. Serotypes I and II are the most prevalent types in chickens, other birds, and man. Serotypes III to VIII rarely occur in birds but are found in cattle, swine, and man.

Avian bacilli produce spontaneous disease in domestic fowls and other birds and can spread from these sources to cows, swine, and man. Avian infection is usually asymptomatic in cows and sheep but produces a specific allergy that is more reactive to tuberculin made from *M. paratuberculosis* and the avian bacillus than to tuberculin made from the human and bovine

bacilli. Swine may have an asymptomatic infection, but caseous lesions in the lymph nodes are the most common form of clinical disease and occasionally may be fatal.

The incidence of human infections is difficult to assess. There are probably many more avian infections than suggested by the literature.

Treatment Avian strains are usually highly resistant to the usual antituberculous drugs. However, all strains isolated from patients should be assayed for susceptibility.

Mycobacterium intracellulare

Strains of *M. intracellulare* (Battey type of group III) have undoubtedly been isolated from patients with pulmonary disease for the past 75 years, but since they are soft in consistency, grow slowly at room temperature, and are not pathogenic for guinea pigs, they were discarded as contaminants. Our current knowledge of this group began at the Battey State Hospital for Tuberculosis at Rome, Georgia, in 1950. About 1 percent of all hospital admissions from 1950 to 1955 had a peculiar type of *Mycobacterium* in their sputum: Some were mixed infections with typical human tubercle bacilli, but 65 patients showed only the newly recognized organism that was consistently present in repeated cultures. This organism can easily be misdiagnosed. It grows luxuriantly in the cytoplasm of mammalian cells without producing necrosis, is strongly acid-fast, grows readily on all kinds of ordinary laboratory media, and is not pathogenic for guinea pigs, rabbits, or fowl. It shows profuse branching when observed in hanging drop slides (Fig. 36-7).

Pathogenicity is variable. Some isolates kill mice but not guinea pigs. Most virulent avian strains grow better at 44C than at 37C, while most Battey strains grow better at 37C than at 44C. Stock strains of avirulent variants of avian strains may adapt to good growth at 37C, and they are then indistinguishable by the usual tests from avirulent Battey strains. It should be kept in mind, however, that the isolation of Battey strains in pure culture from lymph nodes, biopsies, and necropsies in man may be the sole explanation of the disease.

On a solid medium the colonies are characteristically thin, translucent, and radially lobed, in contrast to the dark, heavily corded colonies of *M. tuberculosis*. *M. intracellulare* provides a

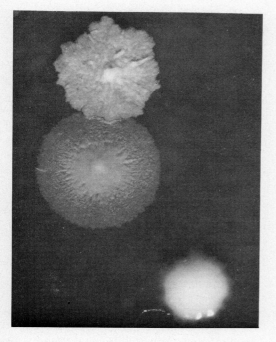

FIG. 36-6. Rough, transparent, and opaque colonies of *M. avium*, serotype 2, on oleic acid-albumin agar. Original magnification, ×15. (From Schaefer et al: Am Rev Respir Dis 102:499, 1970)

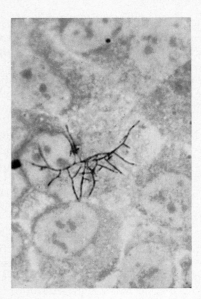

FIG. 36-7. Battey strain from human pulmonary disease after 3 days' growth in HeLa cells. Note branching. ×1,200. (From Brosbe, Sugihara, and Smith: J Bacteriol 84:1282, 1962)

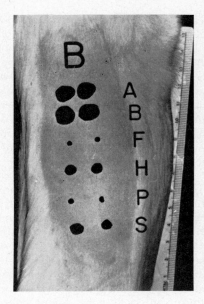

FIG. 36-8. Tuberculin reaction in a guinea pig sensitized to 4 mg of Battey-Boone nonphotochromogen (*M. intracellulare*). Note the large reaction to Batteyin (B) and equally large reaction to avialin (A), less to scrofulin, and still less to tuberculin (H), kansasiin (P), and fortuitin (F). (From Smith and Johnston: Am Rev Respir Dis 90:899, 1964)

negative niacin test, hydrolysis of Tween 80, and nitrate reduction; catalase is positive at 68C, and tellurite is reduced in three days.

Johnston and Smith sensitized guinea pigs with the Battey-Boone strain of *Mycobacterium* and obtained large reactions to the homologous PPD-B and almost equally large reactions to PPD-A, less extensive cross-reactions with scrofulin, and progressively less with tuberculin, kansasiin, and fortuitin (Fig. 36-8). Double infections with Battey-Boone and human bacilli showed equally large reactions with avian, batteyin, tuberculin, and scrofulin, but much smaller reactions with kansasiin and fortuitin.

The study of Meissner and associates in 1974 of a numerical analysis of slowly growing mycobacteria indicates that *M. intracellulare* should be merged with *M. avium* with more specific designations being made by serologic type.

Clinical Infection EPIDEMIOLOGY. The soil has always been considered a likely source of endemic infections with various mycobacteria. Battey type nonphotochromogens have been isolated from bronchial secretions and saliva of healthy individuals, suggesting that the source is dusty air.

CLINICAL MANIFESTATIONS. Skin tests suggest that infection with the Battey-Boone type of *Mycobacterium* is more frequent than that with *M. tuberculosis* but less frequent than that with *M. scrofulaceum*. The Battey type organisms are less frequently found as a cause of adenitis but are more frequently present in pulmonary disease. The symptoms and x-ray findings are indistinguishable from those of patients with *M. tuberculosis* infections.

Except for *M. tuberculosis*, *M. intracellulare* is the most common cause of pulmonary infections in North Carolina, Georgia, and Florida.

TREATMENT. Rifampin with streptomycin is recommended for the treatment of *M. intracellulare* infections.

Mycobacterium xenopi

This organism was first isolated from a skin lesion on the back of a South African toad, *Xenopus laevis*. Although isolated from a cold-blooded animal, its optimal temperature for growth is 42C. The colonies are usually yellowish in color when grown in a dark incubator. A bacteriophage typing scheme for *M. xenopi* is available.

M. xenopi has been isolated in England from the sputum of patients. It also has been isolated from granulomatous lesions in swine. For biochemical reactions, see Table 36-1.

In contrast to the other group III organisms, *M. xenopi* is usually susceptible to the antibiotics used for the treatment of infections with *M. tuberculosis*.

Rapid-Growing Mycobacteria

In this group of rapid-growing mycobacteria are two definite pathogens that do not produce pigment, *M. fortuitum* and *M. chelonei*. The rapid-growing, pigmented members of this ubiquitous group are saprophytes that produce brilliant red, yellow, or orange colonies.

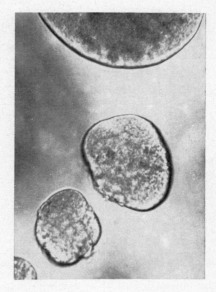

FIG. 36-9. Colonies of strain 444 of *M. fortuitum* on Bennett's agar at 6 days. ×680. (From Gordon and Mihm: J Gen Microbiol 21:736, 1959)

Mycobacterium fortuitum This organism was isolated from abscesses in man in 1938. It was later shown, however, that the organism isolated in 1932 from lymph glands in cows was identical with *M. fortuitum*. *M. fortuitum* has been isolated from cold-blooded animals and from the soil.

After 72 hours' cultivation on glycerol agar, *M. fortuitum* appears as acid-fast rods 1 to 3 μm long, although some coccoid forms and some long, beaded, and occasionally swollen nonacid-fast bacilli are seen. In pus, long and filamentous forms appear, and sometimes there is definite branching. When growing on corn meal-glycerol agar, filamentous colonies are produced, and numerous branching organisms are seen. After two to three days on glycerol agar at 28C soft, waxy, butyrous colonies may be seen (Fig. 36-9).

This is the most rapidly growing of all the pathogenic species of mycobacteria and must be distinguished from the other saprophytic, rapidly growing species. *M. fortuitum* produces an enzyme that releases free phenolphthalein, which can then be detected by treatment with alkali. It appears to be the only pathogenic mycobacterium that can grow in one week on an agar medium where $NaNO_2$ is the sole source of nitrogen.

M. fortuitum is highly pathogenic for mice. Following intravenous inoculation, characteristic abscesses and granulomatous formations appear in the internal organs. Rabbits and guinea pigs cannot be infected. *M. fortuitum* gives a specific reaction to the PPD-F with very slight cross-reactions with human, avian, Battey, and photochrome tuberculins. In Edwards' study of 3,415 Navy recruits, only 7.7 percent gave skin reactions of more than 2 mm to 5 TU or PPD-F, with an average of 4.8 mm (Table 36-2). This was the lowest reaction to any of the specific PPDs but probably represents true primary infections, since the cross-reactions to fortuitum are so slight.

In a study of 82 medical students by Smith and Johnston with PPD-F, 14.6 percent gave positive reactions of 5 mm or more of induration. There was very little cross-reaction with PPDs from other mycobacteria when guinea pigs were infected with *M. fortuitum*.

The pulmonary cases cannot be distinguished by x-ray from typical tuberculosis. This organism can also produce superficial ulceration, which must be differentiated from that caused by *M. ulcerans* and *M. marinum*.

The organism can be cultured from sputum. There is little doubt that many strains of *M. fortuitum* have been incorrectly diagnosed as *M. tuberculosis* when the cultures are not inspected for three to four weeks after they are plated. At that time *M. fortuitum* presents a colorless, sometimes rough looking growth that

TABLE 36-2   FREQUENCY AND MEAN SIZE OF REACTIONS AMONG NAVY
RECRUITS TO 0.0001 MG OF PPD ANTIGENS PREPARED FROM
VARIOUS STRAINS OF MYCOBACTERIA

| PPD Antigen | Prepared From | Number Tested | Reactions of 2 mm or More | |
			Percentage	Mean Size (mm)
PPD-S	M. tuberculosis	212,462	8.6	10.3
PPD-F	M. fortuitum	3,415	7.7	4.8
PPD-240	Unclassified; (Group III)	3,729	12.0	5.8
PPD-Y	M. kansasii	13,913	13.1	6.2
PPD-63	Unclassified; (Group III)	9,473	17.5	7.0
PPD-sm	M. smegmatis	14,239	18.3	5.7
PPD-ph	M. phlei	15,229	23.1	6.4
PPD-216	Unclassified; (Group II)	10,060	28.4	9.0
PPD-A	M. avium	10,769	30.5	6.7
PPD-B	Unclassified; (Battey type)	212,462	35.1	7.7
PPD-269	Unclassified; (Group III)	8,402	39.0	7.2
PPD-G	Unclassified; (Group III)	29,540	48.7	10.3

(Modified from Edwards: Ann NY Acad Sci 106:36, 1963)

may be almost identical to that seen with the human tubercle bacillus (Fig. 36-10). In older cultures a very faint color may be seen that is also seen with the human tubercle bacillus. The secret to the isolation of *M. fortuitum* is the inspection of cultures at 4 to 14 days and selection of the colorless, rapid growers for specific study. Other characteristics are rapid growth on ordinary media at room temperature as well as at 37C, surface growth on broth, and uniform resistance to INH, PAS, and streptomycin.

No effective treatment of infections with this organism has been described.

Mycobacterium chelonei   The species previously designated as *M. abscessus* and *M. borstelense* have been merged in the new species, *M. chelonei*. Subspecies *chelonei* fails to grow in 5 percent NaCl, whereas subspecies *abscessus* does grow in NaCl. Other characteristics can be found in Table 36-1.

These rapidly growing species have been isolated from patients with chronic pulmonary disease. *M. chelonei* has also been cultured from an abscess in the thyroid gland of a 4-year-old child. Subtotal resection of the thyroid followed by treatment with ethionamide resulted in a cure. *M. chelonei* is susceptible in vitro to erythromycin.

Other Mycobacteria

Mycobacterium terrae   This is a slow-growing, nonphotochromogenic organism that

has not been isolated from clinical infections. It appears in the older literature as the "radish" group. It is niacin-negative and tellurite-negative but shows nitrate reduction, catalase activity, and hydrolysis of Tween 80.

Mycobacterium gastri   *Mycobacterium gastri* is a common contaminant that is often isolated from gastric juice and may be mistaken for *M. intracellulare*. It is very inert biochemically but shows hydrolysis of Tween at both 5 and 10 days. It is negative to all other biochemical tests.

Mycobacterium triviale   This group III mycobacterium usually is classified as a nonpathogenic organism, although it has been isolated from the synovial fluid of infants. Its biochemical reactions are given in Table 36-1.

Mycobacterium phlei   This organism is a rapid-growing saprophytic species first described in 1898 as the timothy grass bacillus. Growth which appears in two to four days on glycerol agar may be soft, smooth, butyrous, deep yellow to orange, waxy, and coarsely wrinkled, suggesting the presence of both smooth and rough type colonies. Growth occurs from 28C to 52C, and the organism survives 60C for four hours. This organism is believed to be distributed widely in soil, in dust, and on plants but is rarely isolated in clinical laboratories. It is not pathogenic for any animal species tested, including man.

Edwards found in her studies that PPD pre-

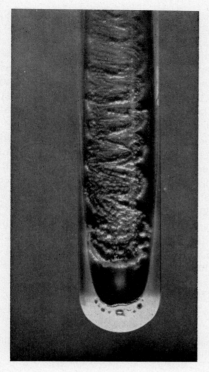

FIG. 36-10 Culture of *M. fortuitum*. Note the rough type of growth which is easily mistaken for the human *M. tuberculosis*. This is the strain used for the production of fortuitin.

pared from *M. phlei* gave an average reaction of 6.4 mm in 23.1 percent of 14,239 Navy recruits. These reactions may, however, have been cross-reactions from other mycobacterial infections.

Mycobacterium smegmatis This organism, isolated in 1889 from human smegma, is referred to as the "smegma bacillus." Growth which appears after 2 to 3 days on glycerol agar is first white, rough, and finely wrinkled; after 14 days it is waxy and creamy yellow to orange. Smooth forms also are present. It grows best between 28C and 45C and does not survive 60C for four hours. It is almost constantly present in smegma and is also distributed widely in soil, dust, and water.

Edwards found that PPD made from *M. smegmatis* gave an average reaction of 5.7 mm in 18.3 percent of 14,239 Navy recruits. These may, however, have been cross-reactions from infections with other mycobacterial species.

Multiple Infections with Mycobacterium Species

It is a mathematical certainty that some patients and perhaps even more normal individuals will have primary infections with two or more mycobacteria. In the past, when practically every young adult had been infected with a human tubercle bacillus, infections with the other less virulent species of mycobacteria had little effect on the size of the tuberculin reaction, which would be greatest to the more virulent human bacillus. If such infections preceded infection with *M. tuberculosis*, they might have had an immunizing effect against clinical disease with *M. tuberculosis*. Experimental work has shown that *M. kansasii* gives in animals almost as good immunity as does BCG. Avian and Battey strains give significant immunity, while scotochromes give lesser, although definitely measurable, immunity.

The importance of infections with atypical mycobacteria in protection from clinical tuberculosis was demonstrated by the study of Naval recruits by Palmer and Edwards. These investigators gave simultaneously 5 TU doses of PPD-S from the human tubercle bacillus and 5 TU of PPD-B from the Battey bacillus. When the PPD-B reaction was 2+ mm greater than the PPD-S reaction the morbidity rate due to *M. tuberculosis* was only 17 per 100,000. When the reactions were 10 mm or over and within 2 mm of each other the morbidity rate was 95 per 100,000. When, however, the PPD-S was definitely greater than the PPD-B the Battey reaction was obviously a cross-reaction and not a double infection, and the morbidity rate was 289 per 100,000.

In our studies on medical students it is apparent that some students have had only a single infection, all the other reactions being definitely cross-reactions. In these instances the reaction to the homologous type is the largest. The experiments with guinea pigs suggest that a double infection will give two large reactions, one to each of the infecting organisms, and a third or fourth may be almost as large because of a double cross-reaction.

Sarcoidosis

This clinical syndrome is characterized by involvement of skin, glands, bones, lungs, and other internal organs and is difficult to differentiate from some forms of tuberculosis.

The etiologic agent is unknown, but the pathologic reaction is characterized by a granulomatous reaction without caseation.

The tuberculin test is usually negative even to 250 TU doses.

When properly prepared suspensions of sarcoid tissue from lymph nodes or spleen are injected intracutaneously, a nodular lesion appears in about two months which on biopsy shows the characteristic lesions of sarcoid disease. This is known as the Kveim test. It is positive in about 85 percent of active cases and positive in about 3 percent of individuals with other diseases.

All attempts to isolate the active agent by culture or animal inoculation have failed. The active agent cannot be demonstrated with certainty by stains of pathologic specimens. This suggests that the active agent is dead when the disease is fully developed. But the nonviable products must be present in large amounts to explain the activity of the Kveim test. This concept is supported by the serologic studies of Chapman and his associates. In 1966, Chapman and Speight reported that 79.7 percent of sera from 280 patients with sarcoidosis had antibodies to two or three of the antigens isolated from atypical mycobacteria.

In 1950 Smith and Scott were using their modification of the Middlebrook-Dubos hemagglutinin test to study patients with tuberculosis. Eleven cases of sarcoid were encountered among the controls. Seven of the eleven sarcoid patients had hemagglutinin tests as high as any of the active cases of tuberculosis.

In the same year, Levine, in Hawaii, used the Smith and Scott modification of the Middlebrook-Dubos test in testing for antibodies in lepers. He found that the lepromatous lepers had higher hemagglutinin tests than did sputum-positive patients with tuberculosis.

In lepromatous leprosy we have an example of high antibody titers in the presence of depressed skin test to lepromin and tuberculin. The excess amount of antigen in lepromatous leprosy is obvious from the massive numbers of leprosy bacilli in monocytes in the lesions.

In sarcoidosis the tuberculin-type test is suppressed. The excess amount of antigen can be assumed from the behavior of the Kveim test and from Chapman's demonstration of excess antibodies in the serum.

Direct evidence that some, or all, of the atypical mycobacteria can induce the sarcoid reaction in man is difficult to obtain. In 1970, Greenberg, Jenkins and associates demonstrated inclusions which could have been bacilli in epithelioid cells of five sarcoid patients.

In 1970, Vaner and Schwartz demonstrated acid-fast rods in 30 consecutive cases of sarcoidosis. This was followed by the report, in 1971, of Richter and associates who detected mycobacteria by fluorescent microscopy in sarcoidosis. The student is warned that, at the present time, the evidence that the atypical mycobacteria are the cause of sarcoidosis is circumstantial only.

The most comprehensive review of the sarcoid problem was published by Mitchell and Scadding in 1974. The best review on treatment was by Johns, Zachary, and Ball in 1974.

FURTHER READING

Books and Reviews

Feldman WH: Avian tuberculous infections. Baltimore, Williams & Wilkins, 1938

Linell F, Norden A: *Mycobacterium balnei,* a new acid-fast bacillus occurring in swimming pools. Acta Tuberc Scand (Suppl): 33:1-84, 1954

Richter J, Barták, F, Halova RR: Detection of mycobacteria by fluorescent microscopy in sarcoidosis. In Levinsky L, Macholda F (eds): Fifth International Conference on Sarcoidosis. June 16-21, 1969. Prague, University Karlova, 1971, p. 375

Runyon EH: Manual of Clinical Microbiology. Bethesda, Md, American Society of Microbiology, 1970, p 112

Selected Papers

Adams RM, Remington JS, Steinberg J, Seibert JS: Tropical fish aquariums: a source of *Mycobacterium marinum* infection resembling sporotrichosis. JAMA 211:457, 1970

Aronson JD: Spontaneous tuberculosis in snakes. J Infect Dis 44:215, 1929

Awe RJ, Gangapharam PRJ, Jenkins DE: Clinical significance of *M. fortuitum* infections in pulmonary disease. Am Rev Respir Dis 107:1087, 1973

Bailey RK, Wyles S, Dingley M, Hesse F, Kent GW: The isolation of high catalase *Mycobacterium kansasii* from tap water. Am Rev Respir Dis 101:430, 1970

Black BG, Chapman JS: Cervical adenitis in children due to human and unclassified mycobacteria. Pediatrics 33: 887, 1964

Brown J, Berman DJ, Torrie JH: Quantitative studies of mycobacteria sensitins in cattle. Am Rev Respir Dis 105:95, 1971

Cahn BJ, Smith DT: Sporotrichoid *Mycobacterium marinum* infections. Cutis 9:485, 1972

Carpenter RL, Patnode RA, Goldsmith JB: Comparative study of skin-test reactions to various mycobacterial antigens in Choctaw County, Oklahoma. Am Rev Resp Dis 95:6, 1967

Chaparas SD, Sheagren JH, Demeo A, Hendrick S: Correlation of human skin reactivity with lymphocyte transformation induced by mycobacterial antigens and histoplasmins. Am Rev Respir Dis 101:67, 1970

Chapman JS, Speight M: Further studies of mycobacterial antibodies in sera of sarcoid patients. Acta Med Scand (Suppl) 425:61, 1964

Chapman JS, Speight M: Tolerance of atypical mycobacteria: the effect of metal ions in various concentrations. Am Rev Respir Dis 103:372, 1971

Conner DH, Lunn HF: Buruli ulceration: a clinicopathologic study of 38 Ugandans with *Mycobacterium ulcerans.* Arch Pathol 81:183, 1966

Dechairo DC, Kittredge D, Meyers A, Corrales T: Septic arthritis due to *Mycobacterium triviale.* Am Rev Respir Dis 108:1224, 1973

Edwards LB, Acguaviva FA, Livesay VT, Cross FW, Palmer CE: An atlas of sensitivity to tuberculin PPD-B and histoplasmin in the United States. Am Rev Respir Dis 99:1, 1969

Edwards LB, Palmer CE: Isolation of "atypical" mycobacteria from healthy persons. Am Rev Respir Dis 80:747, 1959

Feldman RA, Long MW, David HL: *Mycobacterium marinum:* a leisure time pathogen. J Infect Dis 129:618, 1974

Fields BT Jr, Bishop MC, Brosbe EA, Bates JH: Pulmonary disease caused by *Mycobacterium xenopi* and *Histoplasma capsulatum.* Am Rev Respir Dis 99:590, 1969

Froman S, Scammon L: Enhancement of virulence for chickens of Battey-type mycobacteria by preincubation at 42°C. Am Rev Respir Dis 90:804, 1964

Gonzales EP, Crosby RN, Walker SH: *Mycobacterium aquae* in a hydrocephalic child. Pediatrics 48:974, 1971

Gracey DR, Byrd RB: Scotochromogens and pulmonary disease. Am Rev Respir Dis 101:959, 1970

Greenberg SD, Györkey F, Weo TC, Jenkens DE, Györkey P: The ultrastructure of the pulmonary granuloma in "sarcoidosis." Am Rev Respir Dis 102:648, 1970

Gruff H, Henning HG: Pulmonary mycobacteriosis due to rapidly growing acid-fast bacillus, *Mycobacterium chelonei.* Am Rev Respir Dis 105:618, 1972

Gunnels JJ, Bates JN: Characterization and mycobacterial typing of *Mycobacterium xenopi.* Am Rev Respir Dis 105:388, 1972

Gutman LT, Handwerger S, Zwadyk P, Abramowsky CR: Thyroiditis due to *M. chelonei.* Am Rev Respir Dis 110:807, 1974

Hand WL, Sanford JP: *Mycobacterium fortuitum*—a human pathogen. Ann Intern Med 73:971, 1970

Hatler BG, Young WG Jr, Sealy WC, Gentry WH, Cox CB: Surgical management of pulmonary tuberculosis due to atypical mycobacteria. J Thorac Cardiovasc Surg 59:366, 1970

Jarnagin JL, Richards WK, Muhm RL, Ellis EM: The isolation of *Mycobacterium xenopi* from granulomatous lesions in swine. Am Rev Respir Dis 104:763, 1971

Johanson WG Jr, Nicholson DP: Pulmonary disease due to *Mycobacterium kansasii.* Am Rev Respir Dis 90:73, 1969

Johns CJ, Zachary JB, Ball WC Jr: A ten year study of corticosteroid treatment in pulmonary sarcoidosis. Johns Hopkins Med J 134:271, 1974

Johnston WW, Smith DT, Vandiviere H Mac III: Simultaneous or sequential infection with different mycobacteria. Arch Environ Health 11:37, 1965

Karlson AG, Carr DT: Tuberculosis caused by *Mycobacterium bovis.* Ann Intern Med 73:979, 1970

Krieg RD, Hockmeyer WT, Connor DH: Toxins of *Mycobacterium ulcerans.* Arch Dermatol 110:783, 1974

Kubica GP: Differential identification of mycobacteria. VII. Key features for identification of clinically significant mycobacteria. Am Rev Respir Dis 107:9, 1973

Levine M: Hemagglutination of tuberculin sensitized sheep cells in Hansen's disease. Proc Soc Exp Biol Med 76:171, 1951

Lincoln EM, Gilbert LA: Disease in children other than *Mycobacterium tuberculosis.* Am Rev Respir Dis 105:683, 1972

Marks J, Schwabacher H: Infection due to *Mycobacterium xenopi.* Br Med J 1:32, 1965

McClatchy JK, Waggoner RF, Lester W: In vitro susceptibility of mycobacteria to rifampin. Am Rev Respir Dis 100:234, 1969

McCool JA: Anonymous mycobacteria (group II scotochromogens) as a cause of cervical lymphadenitis in children. NC Med J 26:152, 1965

Meissner G, Schroder KH, Amadio GE, ANZ W: A cooperative numerical analysis of slowly growing mycobacteria. J Gen Microbiol 83:207, 1974

Mitchell DN, Scadding JG: Sarcoidosis. Am Rev Respir Dis 110:774, 1974

Molavi A, Weinstein L: In vitro activity of erythromycin against atypical mycobacterium. J Infect Dis 123:216, 1971

Mollohan CS, Romer MS: Public health significance of swimming pool granuloma. Am J Public Health 51:883, 1961

Morbidity and Mortality Weekly Report. *Mycobacterium marinum* from salt water in Alabama. 18:359, 1969

Palmer CE, Long MW: Effects of infection with atypical mycobacteria on BCG vaccination and tuberculosis. Am Rev Respir Dis 94:553, 1966

Palmer CE, Long MW, Edwards LB: Identifying the tuberculous infected. JAMA 205:167, 1968

Raucher C, Kerby G, Ruth, WF: A ten-year clinical experience with *Mycobacterium kansasii.* Chest 66:17, 1974

Richter PE: Pulmonary disease related to *Mycobacterium xenopi.* Med J Aust 1:1246, 1969

Runyon EH: *Mycobacterium intracellulare.* Am Rev Respir Dis 95:861, 1967

Runyon EH: Identification of mycobacterial pathogens utilizing colony characteristics. Am J Clin Path 54:578, 1970

Runyon EH: Whence mycobacteria and mycobacterioses? Ann Intern Med 75:467, 1971

Saito H, Tasaka H: Comparison of the pathogenicity for mice of *Mycobacterium fortuitum* and *Mycobacterium abscessus.* J Bacteriol 99:851, 1969

Salyer KE, Votter TP, Dorman GW: Cervical adenitis in children with atypical mycobacteria. Plast Reconstr Surg 47:47, 1971

Schaefer WB: Serologic identification of the atypical mycobacteria and its value in epidemiologic studies. Am Rev Respir Dis 96:115, 1967

Schaefer WB, Davis CL, Cohn ML: Pathogenicity of transparent, opaque, and rough variants of *Mycobacterium avium* in chickens and mice. Am Rev Respir Dis 102:499, 1970

Schaefer WB, Wolinsky E, Jenkins PA, Marks J: *Mycobacterium szulgai*. A new pathogen. Am Rev Respir Dis 108:1320, 1973

Shronts JS, Rynearson K, Wolinsky F: Rifampin alone and combined with other drugs in *M. kansasii* and *M. intracellulare* infections in mice. Am Rev Respir Dis 104: 728, 1971

Silcox VA, David HL: Differential identification of *M. kansasii* and *M. marinum*. Appl Microbiol 21:327, 1971

Smith DT, Scott NA: Clinical interpretation of Middlebrook and Dubos hemagglutinin test. Am Rev Tuberc 62:121, 1950

Vaner J, Schwarz J: Demonstration of acid-fast rods in sarcoidosis. Am Rev Respir Dis 101:395, 1970

Warring FC Jr: Mycobacteria in a New England hospital. Am Rev Respir Dis 96:115, 1967

Wayne LG, Runyon EH, Kubica GP: Mycobacteria: a guide to nomenclature usage. Am Rev Respir Dis 100: 732, 1969

Wheeler CW, Hanks JH: Utilization of external growth factors by intracellular microbes: *Mycobacterium paratuberculosis* and wood pigeon mycobacteria. J Bacteriol 89:889, 1965

Yoder WD, Schaefer WB: Comparison of seroagglutination tests in chickens for identification of *M. avium* and *M. intracellulare*. Am Rev Respir Dis 103:173, 1971

37
Actinomycetes

Standing midway between the true bacteria and the more complex molds are a number of pathogenic microorganisms that have been placed in the order Actinomycetales. Colonies of these organisms have some gross resemblances to the hyphomycetes, usually being dry, tough, and wrinkled, and sometimes covered with a down of aerial mycelium. These mold-like organisms are characterized by a delicate mycelium from 0.5 to 2.0 μm, usually less than 1.0 μm in diameter, and hence within bacterial dimensions. The mycelium is septate and shows a marked tendency to branch. The component parts of the mycelium often stain unevenly but do not contain recognizable nuclei.

In the Actinomycetaceae the mycelial filaments fragment into bacillary and coccoid forms, and under special conditions some members of the group grow in diphtheroid forms. Those organisms that are anaerobic or microaerophilic, non-acid-fast, obligate parasites are placed in the genera *Actinomyces* and *Arachnia*.

In the Nocardiaceae mycelium may be extensive or rudimentary. The organisms are aerobic, partially acid-fast or non-acid-fast, and saprophytic but facultative parasites.

The Streptomycetaceae form aerial hyphae that segment into spores. This is one of the distinguishing morphologic features of the organisms within the family.

Many schemes for the classification of this group have been proposed, but differences of opinion still exist among investigators, particularly in respect to the phylogenetic relations among these organisms. Some regard them as degraded fungi, others see them as a primary stock from which both bacteria and fungi have developed, and still others prefer to call them "higher bacteria." There is, however, a general agreement that the actinomycetes belong in an intermediate position between bacteria and fungi. The actinomyces are similar to corynebacteria in microscopic morphology, while the nocardias are similar to the mycobacteria in that some species are acid-fast. Cummins reports that the nocardias, mycobacteria, and corynebacteria have arabinose and galactose as cell wall sugars and a common cell wall antigen.

ANAEROBIC ACTINOMYCETES

The genus *Actinomyces* includes several species of importance to medical microbiologists: *A. israelii, A. bovis,* and *A. naeslundii. Arachnia propionica,* the only organism in the genus *Arachnia,* will be included in this discussion because of its similarity to *A. israelii* and *A. naeslundii.* It differs from the *Actinomyces* in its cell wall composition and high production of propionic acid from glucose. All cause a chronic suppurative or granulomatous infection characterized by the formation of abscesses, multiple draining sinuses, and the appearance of tangled mycelial masses, or granules, in the discharges and in tissue sections. *A. bovis,* however, affects cattle, not man.

Morphology

Microscopic Appearance   In tissues the organisms are found in organized colonies or granules composed of densely packed and tangled filaments, 1 μm or less in diameter (Fig. 37-1). The ends of the filaments, at the periphery of the granule, are encased in a

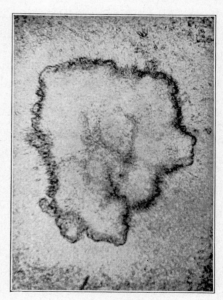

FIG. 37-1. *Actinomyces israelii.* Granule in pus. ×350. (From Conant et al: Manual of Clinical Mycology, 3rd ed. 1971. Courtesy of W. B. Saunders Co)

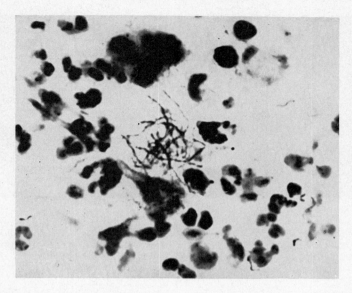

FIG. 37-2. *Actinomyces israelii.* Gram stain of crushed granule showing gram-positive branching hyphae. ×1300 (From Conant et al: Manual of Clinical Mycology, 4rd ed. 1971. Courtesy of W. B. Saunders Co)

sheath of material and resemble clubs. An examination of sectioned granules of A. *bovis* by light and phase microscopy and ultrathin sections by electron microscopy reveals hyphae tips that are quite distinct within the material that is apparently secreted by the fungus. The granule itself is a mycelial mass cemented by a polysaccharide-protein complex and contains about 50 percent calcium phosphate.

In sections of tissue stained with hematoxylin and eosin, the filaments take the hematoxylin stain, and the sheaths or clubs, if present, are stained with eosin. When granules from sputum or pus are crushed between slides and stained by Gram's method, the preparation reveals gram-positive branching filaments, short diphtheroid forms, and coccoid elements (Fig. 37-2).

Cultural Characteristics

Actinomyces species are catalase-negative, anaerobic, microaerophilic organisms. They may be cultured directly from uncontaminated materials in thioglycolate broth, anaerobic chopped-meat medium, or in deep-shake cultures of beef infusion-glucose agar at 37C. In the latter medium, lobulated colonies, pinpoint to large in size, appear in four to five days.

They are found at varying depths below the surface of the agar but often form a band 1 to 1.5 cm from the surface of the medium (Fig. 37-3).

For identification of an isolate, colonies are picked from the above media, emulsified in sterile water if necessary, and streaked onto the

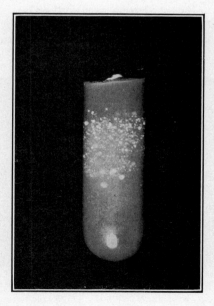

FIG. 37-3. *Actinomyces israelii.* Culture in shake tube of beef infusion glucose agar (pH 7.6).

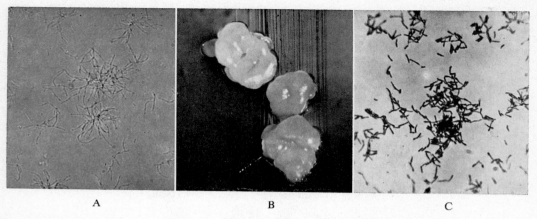

FIG. 37-4. A. *Actinomyces israelii.* Spidery colony on BHI agar plate, 24 hours. ×500. B. *Actinomyces israelii.* Molar tooth colony on BHI agar plate, 15 days. C. *Actinomyces israelii.* Gram stain of smear from rough colony showing diphtheroid forms. ×1200. (Courtesy of Mycology Unit, Center for Disease Control, Atlanta, Ga)

surface of brain-heart infusion agar plates that are incubated at 37C under 95 percent nitrogen and 5 percent CO_2. The appearance of microcolonies at 24 hours, macrocolonies at five to seven days, and a negative catalase test identify the isolate as a species of *Actinomyces* or *Arachnia* (Figs. 37-4 to 37-6).

Laboratory Identification

Pus, collected from closed lesions by aspiration with a sterile needle and syringe, should be examined for granules. If granules are present they should be crushed and stained by Gram's method to demonstrate gram-positive, branching filaments. The granule may be cultured by washing several times in sterile distilled water, crushing the granule with a glass rod in a test tube, and streaking the resulting emulsion over an agar surface. Several media, eg, beef extract-starch-blood agar, brain-heart infusion agar, or synthetic maintenance medium, may be used for the isolation. *Arachnia propionica* differs from *Actinomyces* in that it contains diaminopimelic acid in its cell wall

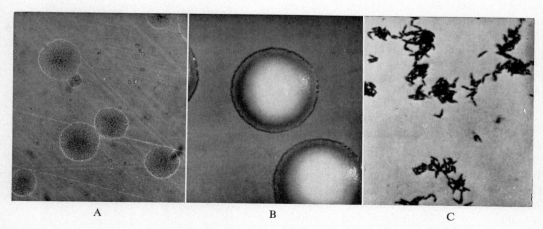

FIG. 37-5. A. *Actinomyces bovis.* Entire colony on BHI agar plate, 24 hours. ×100. B. *Actinomyces bovis.* Smooth colony on BHI agar plate, 10 days. C. *Actinomyces bovis.* Gram stain of smear from smooth colony showing diphtheroid forms. ×1000. (Courtesy of Mycology Unit, Center for Disease Control, Atlanta, Ga)

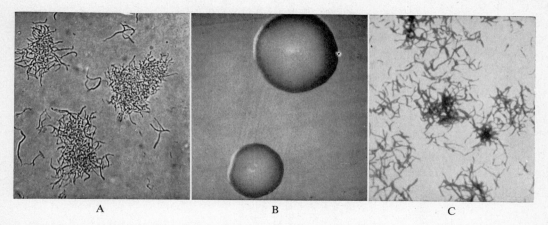

FIG. 37-6. A. **Actinomyces naeslundii.** Dense tangled mycelial colony on BHI agar plate, 24 hours. ×475. B. *Actinomyces naeslundii.* Smooth colony on BHI agar plate, 7 days. C. *Actinomyces naeslundii.* Gram stain smear from smooth colony showing branching diphtheroid forms. ×900. (Courtesy of Mycology Unit, Center for Disease Control, Atlanta, Ga)

(actinomyces do not) and that its major fermentation products from glucose are CO_2, acetic acid, and propionic acid.

Table 37-1 summarizes the cultural and physiologic properties helpful in the identification of *Actinomyces* and *Arachnia*.

Antigenic Structure

Antigenically related components exist in the cytoplasmic fractions of *A. israelii* and *Mycobacterium* species, but cell wall fractions show specificity. Cytoplasmic components of *Nocardia* species are antigenically related to *A. israelii*, whereas certain cell wall fractions are species- and type-specific. Agar-gel diffusion tests show *A. israelii* and *A. bovis* to be antigenically distinct, whereas *A. naeslundii* shows antigenic relationship to both of these species. A comparison of fluorescent antibody (FA) and agar-gel diffusion techniques for distinguishing *A. israelii* from *A. naeslundii* shows the FA test to be more specific. Also, FA conjugates show that two serotypes of *A. israelii* exist. Identification solely on the basis of serologic techniques, however, cannot be accomplished. They are of limited value but do complement the cultural techniques.

Clinical Infection

Epidemiology The worldwide occurrence of actinomycosis is illustrated best by Cope's statement that ". . . wherever there is a microscope and a laboratory, the fungus has been found to be the cause of disease."[*] The disease has been observed in a 28-day-old infant and in a patient 75 years of age. The disease occurs primarily, however, in patients between the ages of 15 and 35. All races are equally susceptible.

Pathogenesis The fungi are normal inhabitants of the oral cavity and are found around carious teeth and in tonsillar crypts. At one time actinomycosis was a fairly common disease in agricultural workers, suggesting that the infection was acquired from some exogenous source. However, in view of our present knowledge, the higher incidence may have been due to poor oral hygiene. Actinomycosis is an endogenous infection. Reports of foreign bodies in the lesions, such as particles of straw in cervicofacial infections, would seem to indicate that the fungus lives in nature and can be introduced into the body as a contaminant. In general, when foreign bodies are found in such lesions they probably represent the means by which the fungus was inoculated deeper into the tissue from its natural oral habitat. There have been no reports of man-to-man or animal-to-man transmission. Indeed, it is difficult to infect laboratory animals directly with granules

[*]*Cope VZ: Actinmycosis. London, Oxford Univ Press, 1938, p 26.*

TABLE 37-1 DIFFERENTIAL CHARACTERISTICS OF ACTINOMYCES ISRAELII, A. BOVIS, A. NAESLUNDII, AND ARACHNIA PROPIONICA

Characteristic	A. israelii	A. bovis	A. naeslundii	A. propionica
Isolated from	Man	Cattle	Man	Man
Metabolism	Obligate anaerobe	Obligate anaerobe	Facultative aerobe	Facultative aerobe
Microscopic colonies (2–4 days)	Mycelial and spidery (Fig. 37-4A)	Smooth, round, dewdrop (Fig. 37-5A)	Dense, tangled mycelial center, hyphal fringe (Fig. 37-6A)	Mycelial and spidery
Macroscopic colonies (5–7 days)	Raised, rough, molar-tooth appearance (Fig. 37-4B)	Convex, smooth, entire (Fig. 37-5B)	Convex and smooth, lobulated and rough (Fig. 37-6B)	Raised, rough molar-tooth appearance
Microscopic	Gram-positive branching diphtheroids (Fig. 37-4C)	Gram-positive branching diphtheroids (Fig. 37-5C)	Gram-positive branching diphtheroids (Fig. 37-6C)	Gram-positive branching diphtheroids
Gelatin liquefaction	–	–	–	–
$NO_3 \rightarrow NO_2$	V	–	+	+
Starch hydrolyzed	V	+	V	+
Sugar fermentations				
Glucose	A	A	A	A
Xylose	A	–	–	–
Mannitol	V	–	–	A
Raffinose	–	–	A	A
Mannose	A	–	A	A

A-acid production; V-variable reaction

from lesions or with pure cultures. The pathogenesis of actinomycosis is not completely understood.

The possible role of associated organisms, such as *Bacterium actinomycetemcomitans*, anaerobic diphtheroids, or anaerobic streptococci, in the pathogenesis of actinomycosis has been investigated. In a bacteriologic study of specimens from 650 patients with closed lesions, *A. israelii* was never found in pure culture. Such results apparently indicate that a symbiotic relationship may be the cause of the varied results obtained in the treatment of this disease.

Clinical Manifestations Actinomycosis usually is differentiated into cervicofacial, thoracic, and abdominal types of infection.

Cervicofacial actinomycosis is the most common form of the disease. The jaws and tissues of the face and neck are affected, and the disease is characterized by swelling and hardness, with the formation of multiple abscesses which eventually break down to form draining sinuses. The sanguinopurulent drainage from the sinuses usually contains macroscopic granules. The infection is first noted in the lower jaw, particularly in the region of infected teeth or following tooth extractions or other operative procedures in the mouth. The disease progresses by a slow and direct extension of the infection through the tissues. Pain is minimal unless there is a secondary infection. If the disease is localized, the patient's general health usually is good.

Thoracic actinomycosis is an infection of the lungs and thoracic cage. Until extension through the thoracic skin results in multiple draining sinuses, the diagnosis often is not suspected. Infection usually is confined to the hilar region and the base of the lungs. Direct extension through the tissues to the lung surface and pleura may result in an inflammatory process, with pleural thickening, empyema, and osteomyelitis of the ribs. Hematogenous spread from a primary lung infection can result in the formation of foci in tissues, such as the liver, kidneys, and brain.

Abdominal actinomycosis originates in the region of the cecum and may simulate acute or subacute appendicitis. Infection by an *Actinomyces* should be suspected when an appendectomy wound fails to heal and irregular tender masses appear in the abdomen. Later in the disease, evidence of destruction of vertebral bodies or of the formation of a psoas abscess should suggest infection. Infection extends to the abdominal skin, and sinuses from which granules may be obtained are formed. Generalized infection can occur, especially by extension through the diaphragm to the pleural cavity.

Treatment Actinomycosis responds to the sulfonamides, penicillin, chlortetracycline, oxytetracycline, isoniazid, and stilbamidine. Prolonged and vigorous treatment with penicillin, however, is the treatment of choice.

AEROBIC ACTINOMYCETES

The aerobic actinomycetes include *Nocardia*, *Streptomyces*, and *Actinomadura*. Not only does the separation of the aerobic actinomycetes from mycobacteria and corynebacteria present a problem, but the grouping into genera has encountered differences of opinion. Some investigators assert that they should be grouped as *Nocardia*, others as *Streptomyces*, and another opinion in *Bergey's* Eighth Edition, under genera incertae sedis, states that the genus *Actinomadura* should be used because of differences in cell wall composition.

Morphology

Microscopically the growth consists of delicate, branching hyphae, 1 μm or less in diameter when examined in undisturbed preparations, such as cell cultures. The hyphae fragment readily into bacillary and coccoid forms and in stained smears are gram positive and partially acid-fast. Study of the fine structure of *Nocardia* reveals a cell wall, a triple-layered cell membrane, a nuclear region, polyribosomes, and mesosomes.

Pathogenic species of *Nocardia*, *Streptomyces*, and *Actinomadura* present such rudimentary morphology that it is difficult or impossible to separate species on a morphologic basis. Therefore, biochemical and physiologic characteristics are used for their identification.

The formation of aerial hyphae with their segmentation into spores has been one of the distinguishing morphologic features of *Actino-*

TABLE 37-2 COMPARISON OF PATHOGENIC AEROBIC ACTINOMYCETES

Species	Granule	Cell Wall	Growth at 40-45C	Fragmentation of Mycelium	Acid-fast	Casein	Decomposition of Tyrosine	Xanthine	Utilizes Paraffin	Liquefy Gelatin	Urease
Nocardia asteroides	No granule formed in systemic nocardiosis; Cause mycetoma?	IV	+	+	+	-	-	-	+	+	+
Nocardia brasiliensis	Small; white to yellowish; soft; with or without clubs. No granule formed in systemic disease	IV	-	+	+	+	+	-	+	+	+
Nocardia caviae	Small; white to yellowish; soft; with or without clubs	IV	-	+	+	-	-	+	+	+	+
Actinomadura madurae	Large (1-10 mm); white to yellowish; soft; lobulated; large clubs at periphery	III	-	-	-	+	+	-	-	+	-
Actinomadura pelletierii	Large (0.3-0.5 mm); red; firm; smooth border	III	-	-	-	+	+	-	-	+	-
Streptomyces somaliensis	Large (1-2 mm); yellow to brownish; hard; round; smooth border	I	-	-	-	+	+	-	-	+	-
Streptomyces paraguayensis	Large (0.5 mm); black; firm; clubs at periphery	I	-	-	-	+	+	+*	-	-	+

*Six weeks

madura and *Streptomyces* and separates these genera from *Nocardia*. Table 37-2 illustrates the morphologic, physiologic, and biochemical differences of the aerobic actinomycetes.

Cultural Characteristics

Nocardia is readily cultured on all common laboratory media, as are all species of *Actinomadura* and *Streptomyces*. From closed lesions, subcutaneous abscesses, and spinal fluid, cultures may be made directly on Sabouraud's agar and brain-heart infusion blood agar for incubation at room temperature and 37C, respectively. Sputum and exudates from draining sinuses must be streaked carefully on agar plates of the above media for adequate separation of resulting colonies. Antibiotics should not be used in these media for the purpose of curtailing bacterial contaminants, since species are susceptible in vitro to most of the antibacterial agents. *N. asteroides* grows at 40 to 50C and, therefore, cultures from contaminated materials can be incubated at these temperatures in order to inhibit contamination.

N. asteroides on Sabouraud's agar appears glabrous and somewhat granular, varying in color from yellow to deep orange. An occasional isolate will produce a chalky white surface and will have an earthy odor resembling a *Streptomyces* (Fig. 37-7).

N. brasiliensis has a similar type of growth on Sabouraud's agar and must be differentiated by other criteria (Table 37-2).

All species of *Actinomadura* and *Streptomyces* develop slow-growing, variously pigmented (cream to yellow and orange, pink to coral and brick red, or gray to black), glabrous, wrinkled, or granular colonies, some of which resemble colonies of acid-fast bacteria (Fig. 37-8). Pigmentation of a single strain may vary from transfer to transfer on Sabouraud's agar but remains fairly constant on Czapek's agar. Some strains produce an aerial, chalky white mycelium that may be lost on subculture, subsequent colonies remaining smooth and glabrous. Some colonies may be membranous and difficult to remove from the agar surface, whereas others are soft and granular and easily removed. Some species may have the characteristic earthy odor. In liquid media they usually produce surface pellicles, with the medium remaining clear.

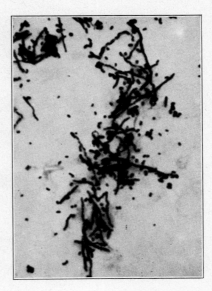

FIG. 37-7. *Nocardia asteroides.* Culture on Sabouraud's glucose agar at room temperature for 12 days.

Laboratory Identification

Nocardia In clinical materials, such as sputum, spinal fluid, or other exudates from systemic nocardiosis, no organized granules are present, and only grampositive, branching, or bacillary elements are seen (Fig. 37-9). Granules are not observed in tissues from systemic infections. Hematoxylin and eosin-stained sections reveal only an acute inflammatory response, but no organisms are seen. In gram-stained sections, however, *Nocardia asteroides* appears as gram-positive, delicate, branching, bacillary forms, 1 μm in diameter, scattered throughout areas of necrosis (Fig. 37-10). When associated with mycetoma, *Nocardia* species do produce a granule (Fig. 37-11).

Actinomadura and Streptomyces In tissues or exudates from the localized subcutaneous lesion small white to yellow, red or black granules may be seen (Fig. 37-12). Such granules are composed of a delicate, branching mycelium that may or may not have clubs on the hyphae at the periphery. In sectioned tissues the size of the granule, pigmentation, morphology, and staining reaction with hematoxylin and eosin are characteristic for the species identification of *Actinomadura*

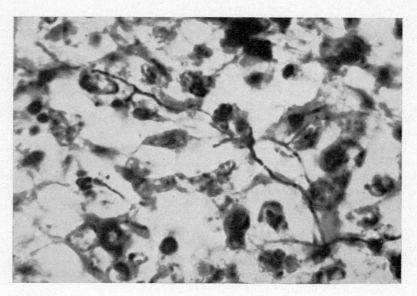

FIG. 37-8. *Nocardia brasiliensis.* Culture on Sabouraud's glucose agar at room temperature for 15 days.

madurae, Streptomyces somaliensis, and *Actinomadura pelletierii.*

Antigenic Structure

Because *Nocardia* is acid-fast and is culturally and morphologically similar to *Mycobacterium tuberculosis,* several studies have been initiated to determine whether they also are antigenically similar. Antigens common to both organisms can be demonstrated by complement-fixation, agglutination, and precipitation tests. The question of cross-allergic reac-

tions was investigated by Drake and Henrici, who showed that animals injected with *N. asteroides* reacted to skin tests with a polysaccharide, a protein, and a crude extract of powdered defatted organisms but did not react to tuberculin. Likewise, tuberculous animals with a

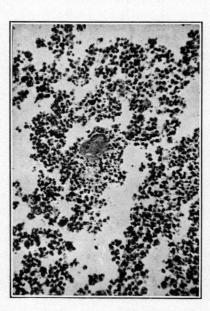

FIG. 37-10. *Nocardia asteroides.* Gram-stained section of brain abscess showing gram-positive, branching filaments. (From Conant et al: Manual of Clinical Mycology, 3rd ed. 1971. Courtesy of W.B. Saunders Co.)

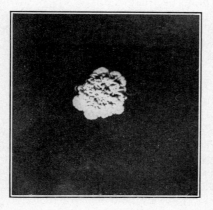

FIG. 37-9. *Nocardia asteroides.* Gram stain of sputum smear. ×1524.

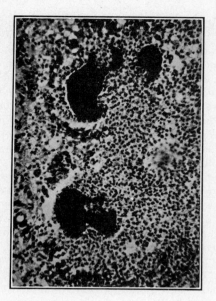

FIG. 37-11. *Nocardia brasiliensis.* Small granule in subcutaneous tissue. ×147.

high degree of allergy did not react to the allergens of *N. asteroides.* A slight tuberculin sensitivity has been demonstrated in guinea pigs inoculated with killed *N. asteroides* in water-in-oil emulsion. Small reactions to the international standard tuberculin, PPD-S, also have been obtained in rabbits sensitized with a PPD made from *N. asteroides.* Since the animals gave larger reactions to the homologous PPD the reaction was considered specific.

A PPD (purified protein derivative) and a sensitin have been prepared from *Nocardia* species. Guinea pigs sensitized with heat-killed oil suspensions of these organisms give larger delayed skin test reactions to the homologous PPD than to the heterologous PPDs or to human-type tuberculin. Sensitin of *N. asteroides* at a 0.2 γ per 0.1 ml dose does not give reactions in the skin of patients infected with *N. brasiliensis, A. madurae,* and tuberculosis or in healthy controls. When the dose is raised to 2.0 γ per 0.1 ml, however, cross-reactions occur in tuberculous patients. Polysaccharides from *N. asteroides* and *N. brasiliensis* have been prepared which are species-specific in agar-gel

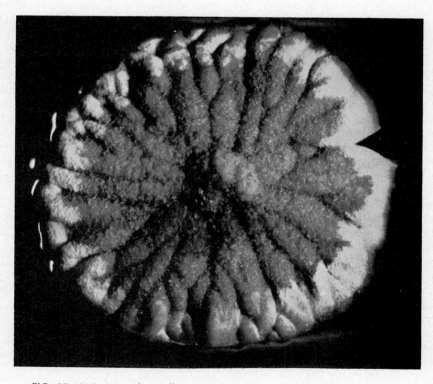

FIG. 37-12. *Actinomadura pelletierii.* Red granules in subcutaneous tissue. ×147.

diffusion studies. An immunochemical study has been made of the polysaccharide from *N. brasiliensis*. A polypeptide skin test antigen obtained from *N. asteroides* is strain specific.

Polysaccharides from a number of strains of *Nocardia* and *Streptomyces* have been used in precipitin tests to show antigenic similarities between *N. asteroides* and *N. brasiliensis*, between *A. madurae* and *A. pelletierii*, and between *S. paraguayensis* and *Streptomyces* species. *S. somaliensis* antigen reacted only in its homologous serum.

Clinical Infection

Epidemiology   Aerobic actinomycosis occurs throughout the world. The mycetomas, however, are more common in tropical and subtropical areas. The causative organisms have been isolated from soil, and there are no reports of man-to-man or animal-to-man transmission. Nocardiosis occurs in all age groups with no preference for race, whereas the mycetomas occur in the middle-aged group, and men are involved three to five times as often as women. *Nocardia* is an opportunistic pathogen. Nocardiosis is very prevalent as a secondary infection in patients with chronic debilitating primary illness who are receiving corticosteroids.

Clinical Manifestations   ACTINOMYCOTIC MYCETOMA.   The majority of infections caused by aerobic actinomycetes are subcutaneous, suppurative tumefactions, or mycetomas. Actinomycotic mycetoma develops as a unilateral infection of the extremities and follows an injury that introduces the causative organism into the tissues. A nodule, pustule, or indurated mass accompanied by moderate pain may appear in a few days to several months after exposure. Other pustules or nodules appear, which upon rupture discharge a serous or serosanguineous exudate. The infection of tissues may take months or years. Multiple abscesses throughout the infected area break down to form numerous fistulas from which typical actinomycotic granules are discharged. The bones of the foot may show decalcification and small punched-out areas. The infection may spread by the lumphatics to involve the leg but does not metastasize.

NOCARDIOSIS.   Systemic nocardiosis is not uncommon. The infection usually is pulmonary in origin and simulates tuberculosis clinically, by x-ray, and by the presence of delicate acid-fast filaments in the sputum. X-rays show hilar involvement, infiltration, and often cavities, and the lesions may simulate unresolved pneumonia or even metastatic tumors. Weight loss, fever, malaise, a productive cough, and hemoptysis are the usual symptoms. Physical examination of the chest shows the percussion note to be impaired and breath sounds diminished.

Metastasis to the brain is frequent, presenting symptoms of brain abscess or brain tumor. When the brain is involved, pulmonary symptoms may disappear. In severe cases metastasis to all organs may result, but involvement of the bone is rare.

Treatment   The importance of an early diagnosis and prompt specific treatment is essential. Sulfadiazine is the drug of choice in the treatment of systemic nocardiosis. If the patient is sensitive to this drug, other choices among the sulfonamides will be necessary.

In the treatment of actinomycotic mycetomas chemotherapy with the sulfonamides is effective when surgical intervention allows drainage of the deeply affected tissues. On the basis of in vitro testing, *N. brasiliensis* is partially inhibited by a 1:50,000 and completely inhibited by a 1:10,000 dilution of DDS (4,4-diaminodiphenylsulfone). Aerobic actinomycetes are inhibited by sulfamethoxypyridazine as follows: *N. asteroides* is inhibited by 256 μg, *N. brasiliensis* by 4 to 16 μg, *A. madurae* by 4 to 32 μg, *A. pelletierii* by 8 to 16 μg, and *S. somaliensis* by 64 to 256 μg per ml. Long-standing infection with scar tissue formation and fibrosis of extensive tissue areas is amenable only to amputation.

FURTHER READING

Books and Reviews

Al-Doory Y: A bibliography of actinomycosis. Mycopathol Mycol Appl 44:1, 1971

Georg LK, Coleman RM: Comparative pathogenicity of various *Actinomyces* species. In Prauser H (ed) Jena International Symposium on Taxonomy, Sept 1968, p 35-45, 1970

Kurup PV, Randhawa HS, Gupta HP: Nocardiosis: a review. Mycopathol Mycol Appl 40:193, 1970

Lynch JB: Mycetoma in the Sudan. Ann R Coll Surg Engl 35:319, 1964

Pine L: Classification and phylogenetic relationship of microaerophilic actinomycetes. Int J Syst Bacteriol 20:445, 1970

Vanbreuseghem R: Early diagnosis, treatment and epidemiology of mycetoma. Rev Med Vet Mycol 6:49, 1967

Selected Papers

Adar R, Antebi E, David R, Mozes M: Abdominal actinomycosis. Isr J Med Sci 8:148, 1972

Affronti LF: Purified protein derivatives (PPD) and other antigens prepared from atypical acid-fast organisms and *Nocardia asteroides*. Am Rev Tuberc Pulmon Dis 79:284, 1959

Ajello L, Bascom WC: A Mexican case of mycetoma caused by *Streptomyces somaliensis*. Dermatol Int 7:17, 1968

Aron R, Gordon W: Pulmonary nocardiosis, case report and evaluation of current therapy. S Afr Med J 46:29, 1972

Bach MC, Monaco AP, Finland M: Pulmonary nocardiosis. Therapy with minocycline and with erythromycin plus ampicillin. JAMA 224:1378, 1973

Berd D: *Nocardia asteroides*. A taxonomic study with correlations. Am Rev Respir Dis 108:909, 1973

Berd D: *Nocardia brasiliensis* infection in the United States. A report of nine cases with a review of the literature. Am J Clin Pathol 60:254, 1973

Bergeron J, Mullens JF, Ajello L: Mycetoma caused by *Nocardia pelletierii* in the United States. Arch Dermatol 99:564, 1969

Bojalil LF, Zamora A: Precipitin and skin tests in the diagnosis of mycetoma due to *Nocardia brasiliensis*. Proc Soc Exp Biol Med 113:40, 1963

Brewer NS, Spencer RJ, Nichols DR: Primary anorectal actinomycosis. JAMA 228:1397, 1974

Brock DW, Georg LK: Determination and analysis of *Actinomyces israelii* serotypes by fluorescent-antibody procedures. J Bacteriol 97:581, 1969

Brock DW, George LK, Brown JM, Hicklin MD: Actinomycosis caused by *Arachnia propionica*: Report of 11 cases. Am J Clin Pathol 59:66, 1973

Cameron HM, Gatei D, Bremmer AD: The deep mycoses in Kenya: A histopathological study. 1. Mycetoma. East Afri Med Jour 50:382, 1973

Causey WA: *Nocardia caviae*: A report of 13 new isolations with clinical correlation. Appl Microbiol 28:193, 1974

Causey WA, Sieger B: Systemic nocardiosis caused by *Nocardia brasiliensis*. Am Rev Respir Dis 109:134, 1974

Causey WA, Howell P, Brinker J: Systemic *Nocardia caviae* infection. Chest 65:360, 1974

Cohen ML, Weiss EB: Successful treatment of *Pneumocystis carinii* and *Nocardia asteroides* in a renal transplant patient. Am J Med, 50:269, 1971

Coleman RM, Georg LK: Comparative pathogenicity of *Actinomyces naeslundii* and *Actinomyces israelii*. Appl Microbiol 18:427, 1969

Coleman RM, Georg LK, Rozzell AR: *Actinomyces naeslundii* as an agent of human actinomycosis. Appl Microbiol 18:420, 1969

Cross RM, Binford CH: Infections by fungi that are commonly primary pathogens. Is *Nocardia asteroides* an opportunist? Lab Invest 11 (part 2):1103, 1962

Eastridge CE, Prather JR, Hughes FA Jr, Young JM, McCaughan JJ Jr: Actinomycosis: a 24 year experience. South Med J 65:839, 1972

Georg LK, Coleman RM, Brown JM: Evaluation of an agar gel precipitin test for the serodiagnosis of actinomycosis. J Immunol 100:1288, 1968

Georg LK, Robertstad GW, Brinkman SA: Identification of species of *Actinomyces*. J Bacteriol 88:477, 1964

Georg LK, Ajello L, McDurmont C, Hasty TS: The identification of *Nocardia asteroides* and *Nocardia brasiliensis*. Am Rev Respir Dis 84:337, 1961

Gordon RE: Some criteria for the recognition of *Nocardia madurae* (Vincent) Blanchard. J Gen Microbiol 45:355, 1966

Lambert FW Jr, Brown JM, Georg LK: Identification of *Actinomyces israelii* and *Actinomyces naeslundii* by fluorescent-antibody and agar-gel diffusion techniques. J Bacteriol 94:1287, 1967

Magana M: Brief case summaries: Tuberculosis verrucosa cutis and mycetoma. Int J Dermatol 11:82, 1972

Mariat F: Sur la distribution geographique et la réparation des agents de mycetomes. Bull Soc Pathol Exot 56:35, 1963

Mishra SK, Sandhu RS, Randhawa HS, Damodaran VH, Abraham S: Effect of cortisone administration on experimental nocardiosis. Infect Immun 7:123, 1973

Murray IG, Mahgoub ES: Treatment of nocardiosis. Lancet 2:362, 1970

Norman JE deB: Cervicofacial actinomycosis. Oral Surg 29:735, 1970

Orfanakis MG, Wilcox HG, Smith CB: In vitro studies of the combined effect of ampicillin and sulfonamides on *Nocardia asteroides* and results of therapy in four patients. Antimicrob Agents Chemother 1:215, 1972

Pier AC, Fichtner AE: Serologic typing of *Nocardia asteroides* by immunodiffusion. Am Rev Respir Dis 103:698, 1971

Pine L, Georg LK: Reclassification of *Actinomyces propionicus*. Int J Syst Bacteriol 19:267, 1969

Presant CA, Wiernik PH, Serpick AA: Factors affecting survival in nocardiosis. Am Rev Respir Dis 108:1444, 1973

Roberts GD, Brewer NS, Hermans PE: Diagnosis of nocardiosis by blood culture. Mayo Clin Proc 49:293, 1974

Saltzman HA, Chick EW, Conant NF: Nocardiosis as a complication of other diseases. Lab Invest 11(part 2):1110, 1962

Slack JM, Gerencser MA: Two new serological groups of *Actinomyces*. J Bacteriol 103:266, 1970

Viroslav J, Williams TW Jr: Nocardial infection of the pulmonary and central nervous system: Successful treatment with medical therapy. South Med J 64:1381, 1971

Zaias N, Taplin D, Rebell G: Mycetoma. Arch Dermatol 99:215, 1969

38

Enterobacteriaceae: General Characteristics

The family Enterobacteriaceae is composed of a large number of closely related bacterial species that inhabit the large bowel of man and animals, soil, water, and decaying matter. Because of their normal habitat in man they have often been referred to as the enteric bacilli or enterics. Included in this group of organisms are some of the most important intestinal pathogens of man, eg, the agents of typhoid fever and bacillary dysentery. Most enterics, however, do not cause disease when confined to the intestinal tract of a normal host, but given an altered host or an opportunity to invade other body sites, many have the capability of producing disease in any tissue. In fact the organisms of this family are responsible for the majority of nosocomial (hospital-acquired) infections and cause urinary tract and wound infections, pneumonia, meningitis, and septicemia. The medical and economic importance of such infections becomes apparent when one considers that an estimated 2 million patients per year (5 to 10 percent of the total hospital population) acquire infections while hospitalized. The seriousness of the problem is further complicated by the fact that most enterics isolated from nosocomial infections are resistant to multiple antimicrobial agents.

The enterobacteria have also played a very important role in the field of molecular biology. Most of the information contained in Chapters 7, 8, and 9 concerning microbial genetics and regulatory mechanisms has been derived from experimentation with these organisms. Because of this intense study and the need for accurate information on the epidemiology of enteric infections, the speciation and characterization of the family has been carried out to a higher degree than with other microorganisms.

Taxonomy of the Enterobacteriaceae The family Enterobacteriaceae is divided into tribes consisting of closely related species. Table 38-1 presents the classification of the family according to Ewing. This classification scheme, however, is not universally accepted, as evidenced by the scheme from the Eighth Edition of *Bergey's Manual of Determinative Bacteriology* (Table 38-2). Most experts in the field expect that additional changes will take place in the near future. Readers interested in the relative merits of the classification schemes are urged to read the references on this subject listed at the end of this chapter. For the sake of

TABLE 38-1 CLASSIFICATION OF ENTEROBACTERIACEAE ACCORDING TO EWING

Family: Enterobacteriaceae	
Tribe I	Eschericheae
Genus I	*Escherichia*
Genus II	*Shigella*
Tribe II	Edwardsielleae
Genus I	*Edwardsiella*
Tribe III	Salmonelleae
Genus I	*Salmonella*
Genus II	*Arizona*
Genus III	*Citrobacter*
Tribe IV	Klebsielleae
Genus I	*Klebsiella*
Genus II	*Enterobacter*
Genus III	*Serratia*
Tribe V	Proteeae
Genus I	*Proteus*
Genus II	*Providencia*
Tribe VI	Erwinieae
Genus I	*Erwinia*
Genus II	*Pectobacterium*

Adapted from Ewing: Differentiation of Enterobacteriaceae by Biochemical Reactions, Revised. Atlanta, Ga. DHEW Publication No (CDC) 74-8270, 1973

consistency, future references to nomenclature in this section will use the Ewing scheme, since it is the method used in the United States by most clinical journals and the Center for Disease Control at the time of this writing.

One major taxonomic change on which there

TABLE 38-2 CLASSIFICATION OF ENTEROBACTERIACEAE ACCORDING TO BERGEY'S MANUAL

Family: Enterobacteriaceae	
Group I	Eschericheae
Genus I	*Escherichia*
Genus II	*Edwardsiella*
Genus III	*Citrobacter*
Genus IV	*Salmonella*
Genus V	*Shigella*
Group II	Klebsielleae
Genus VI	*Klebsiella*
Genus VII	*Enterobacter*
Genus VIII	*Hafnia*
Genus IX	*Serratia*
Group III	Proteeae
Genus X	*Proteus*
Group IV	Yersinieae
Genus XI	*Yersinia*
Group V	Erwinieae
Genus XII	*Erwinia*

Adapted from Buchanan and Gibbons (eds): Bergey's Manual of Determinative Bacteriology, 8th ed. 1974, Part 8, pp 290-304. Courtesy of The Williams and Wilkins Co.

is general agreement is the inclusion of the genus *Yersinia* in the family Enterobacteriaceae on the basis of biochemical and serologic reactions. However, because of the epidemiologic differences and historical importance of one species, *Yersinia pestis*, the cause of black plague, these organisms will be discussed in Chapter 43. Other taxonomic changes in the enterics will be discussed in later chapters.

Morphology

The Enterobacteriaceae are small (0.5 μm by 3.0 μm), gram-negative, nonsporeforming rods. They may be motile or nonmotile. When motile, movement is by means of peritrichous flagella, a property that aids in differentiating the enterics from the polar flagellated bacteria of the families Pseudomonadaceae and Vibrionaceae, which can be isolated from similar sources. Two genera, *Shigella* and *Klebsiella*, are characteristically nonmotile. Enteric bacilli may possess a well-defined capsule, as in the genus *Klebsiella*, may have a loose, ill-defined coating referred to as a "slime layer," as seen in some *Escherichia*, or may be lacking either structure.

Cell Wall Ultrastructure   Enterobacteriaceae possess complex cell walls composed of mureins, lipoproteins, phospholipids, proteins, and lipopolysaccharides arranged in several layers (Fig. 38-1). The murein-lipoprotein layer constitutes approximately 20 percent of the total cell wall and is responsible for cellular rigidity. This structure resembles a net consisting of chains of N-acetyl glucosamine covalently linked via a β1, 4-glycosidic bond to N-acetyl muramic acid. Rows of these polysaccharide chains are cross-linked by short peptide linkages between meso-diaminopimelic acid and D-alanine. Figure 38-2 depicts this murein net as well as the linkage of the lipoprotein to the murein layer via the ϵ-amino group of a C-terminal lysine and the carboxyl group of a *meso*-diaminopimelic acid group.

The remaining 80 percent of the cell wall is joined to the lipoprotein at the lipid end of the molecule, perhaps forming a lipid bilayer (Fig. 38-1). This portion of the cell wall can be removed by various treatments, such as boiling in 4 percent dodecylsulfate. A major constituent of this portion of the cell wall is the lipopolysaccharide. This molecule contains the specific polysaccharide side-chains that determine the antigenicity of various enteric bacilli (p. 561) and is the portion of the cell responsible for endotoxic activity (p. 561).

Physiology

Biochemical Properties   Enterobacteriaceae are facultative organisms that are biochemically diverse and complex. Under anaerobic or low oxygen conditions they attack carbohydrates fermentatively, but given sufficient oxygen they utilize the tricarboxylic acid cycle for energy production. Various species differ in

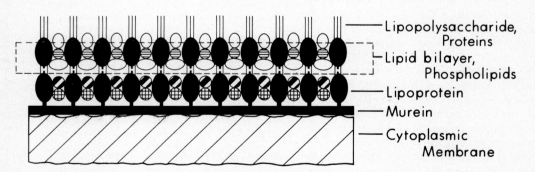

FIG. 38-1. Section through the *Escherichia coli* cell envelope. For the wall, hypothetical subunits are drawn to represent the major building blocks. It is proposed that the pattern of distribution of the lipoprotein molecules over the murein is representative of the arrangement of the subunits. Other major components of the wall, although suggested in this model, do not necessarily have to be in a one-to-one relationship to the number of lipoprotein molecules. The lipid at the N-terminal end of the lipoprotein is drawn in such a way that it is interacting with the lipid A of lipopolysaccharide in a lipid bilayer, of which both components besides phospholipids could be a part. (From Braun: J Infect Dis 128 (Suppl):S10, 1973)

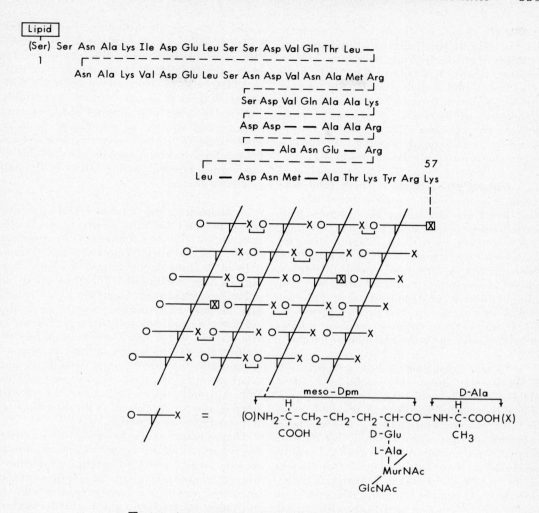

☒ Attachment sites of Lipoprotein replacing D-alanine

FIG. 38-2. Proposed model for the murein net on which only one lipoprotein molecule is drawn. Underlying murein net: The parallel heavy lines symbolize the polysaccharide chains. They are cross-linked by the T-like peptide side-chains. Nothing is known about the conformation of the peptide side-chains. Here they are drawn to allow a long-range covalent fixation of the murein, which is a necessity for *Escherichia coli* and other gram-negative bacteria. Since *E. coli* is cross-linked only to the variable extent of 15 to 30 percent, some links between *meso*-Dpm(o) and D-Ala(x) were left open. Despite the lack of some cross-linking peptide bonds, the conformation of the peptide side-chain is considered to be the same for all. Attachment site of the lipoprotein: to account for the fact that, on the average, one lipoprotein is covalently linked to every tenth to twelfth disaccharide unit of the murein, four attachment sites are indicated in the murein net. For purposes of simplification, only the sequence of one lipoprotein molecule is drawn. The lipoprotein is linked by the ε-amino group of its C-terminal lysine to the carboxyl group of meso-diaminopimelic acid of the murein and replaces there the D-alanine. The sequence is presented in a way that emphasizes its repetitive design. (From Braun: J Infect Dis 128(Suppl):S11, 1973)

the carbohydrates they ferment. These differences, together with the variations in end product production and substrate utilization, form the basis for speciation within this family. The important biochemical reactions of the various genera are discussed in the chapters dealing with the individual organisms and in the section on Laboratory Diagnosis (p. 563). By definition, however, all enterics ferment glucose with the production of acid and reduce nitrates to nitrites but do not produce indol phenol oxidase or liquefy alginate. Most enterics ferment glucose by the mixed acid pathway, but the tribe Klebsielleae is distinguished by its ability to utilize the butanediol fermentative pathway (Chap. 39). Gas formation, in the form of hydrogen and carbon dioxide, during glucose fermentation varies with the species and represents a useful tool in preliminary identification of the organism. For example, all *Shigella* and *Salmonella typhi*, important enteropathogens, characteristically do not produce gas.

Cultural Characteristics   On nondifferential or selective media, such as blood agar or brain-heart infusion agar, the Enterobacteriaceae usually cannot be differentiated but appear as smooth, gray, moist colonies. Hemolysis, which may or may not occur, is usually of the beta type. A variety of special differential and selective media are utilized in the isolation and preliminary characterization of different groups of enterics (p. 563). When grown in broth culture the enterics produce diffuse growth which reflects their facultative nature.

Genetic Interaction   To the geneticist the enterobacteria are a very useful tool. Most of the information concerning genetic mapping and gene transfer has been delineated using the Enterobacteriaceae (Chaps. 7 and 8). These experiments have demonstrated that genetic information can be transferred among distantly related as well as closely related enterobacteria. The transfer of this genetic material, either through transduction, lysogenic conversion, or conjugation, gives rise to hybirds with altered biochemical and/or structural properties. Such hybrids are not merely products of laboratory experimentation but can be isolated in natural settings, particularly the hospital environment. Changes in structural and biochemical properties cause difficulty in proper laboratory speciation, necessitating detailed microbiologic identification procedures. Changes in antimicrobial susceptibility also can occur when a resistant organism possessing the resistance transfer factor (RTF) acts as a male cell and transfers the genes coding for resistance to a female cell via conjugation (Chaps. 8 and 10). Although such hybrids do occur, it is fortunate that the majority of enteric isolates conform to normal identification and sensitivity patterns.

Bacteriocins (Colicins)   A number of Enterobacteriaceae harbor extrachromosomal ele-ments that code for the production of bactericidal substances known as colicins (Chap. 8). Different colicins attack different molecular sites, such as DNA, RNA, or protein synthesis, or ATP formation. They do not act indiscriminately but only attack certain susceptible strains. This selectivity in action has been used with certain species of enterobacteria as an epidemiologic tool and is referred to as colicin typing. Such testing is usually not available in the normal hospital setting but only through reference centers.

Resistance   The enteric bacilli produce no spores and are thus relatively easily destroyed by low concentrations of common germicides and disinfectants. Phenol, formaldehyde, β-glutaraldehyde, and halogen compounds are bactericidal for this group of organisms. Quaternary ammonium compounds may be only bacteriostatic depending on the particular formulation and situation. The use of chlorine in water has been helpful in controlling the dissemination of these organisms, particularly the agents of typhoid fever and other intestinal diseases. The enterics tolerate bile salts and bacteriostatic dyes to a varying degree, a fact that is useful in the development of primary isolation media.

These organisms also are relatively sensitive to drying but can survive for extended periods of time when provided adequate moisture. Moisture-laden respiratory care equipment and anesthesia equipment have served as sources of enteric infections in the hospital environment. Enterics tolerate cold for extended periods of time. They have been isolated from snow and ice after several months, thus providing a mechanism for the contamination of water supplies during the spring thaws. Contaminated ice machines also are sources of infection. Control of enterics in foods can be achieved by pasteurization, thorough cooking, and proper refrigeration.

Antigenic Structure

With certain species of enterobacteria, antigenic characteristics play an important role in epidemiology and classification. This is particularly true with the intestinal pathogens of the genera *Salmonella*, *Shigella*, and certain *Escherichia*. Three major components of the bacterial cell, the O antigen, the H antigen, and the K antigen, are useful in the serologic typing of the Enterobacteriaceae (Fig. 38-3). In addition most Enterobacteriaceae share a common antigen that is detectable by hemagglutination and appears to be associated with the cell wall. This antigen may prove to be useful in further taxonomic and possibly epidemiologic studies.

Capsular Antigens The K or capsular antigens are polysaccharides. In some genera, such as *Klebsiella*, they may exist as true capsules and can be typed by a quellung reaction similar to that used with the pneumococci. In other genera, the K antigen may block the reaction of the O antigen with its homologous antiserum. This effect may be overcome by heating, which alters the K antigen. The best known K antigen is the Vi antigen of *Salmonella typhi*, which may play a role in the pathogenesis of typhoid fever.

Flagellar Antigens The H or flagellar antigens are proteins. Antigenic variation in flagella is thought to be due to the difference in amino acid sequence of the particular flagellar type. With two genera, *Salmonella* and *Arizona*, the flagella for a particular bacterium may exist in one of two phases: phase one (specific), which is not shared by many organisms, or phase two (nonspecific), which is found in many organisms. The Kauffman-White scheme of classification uses the variation in phase type and differences in flagellar antigen to aid in the serologic speciation of these genera.

Somatic Antigens The lipopolysaccharide (LPS) of the cell wall is composed of three distinct regions. The O-specific or cell wall antigen is contained in region I and is a polymer

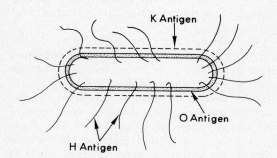

FIG. 38-3. Location of the structural antigens of Enterobacteriaceae.

of repeating oligosaccharide units of three or four monosaccharides. Table 6 in Chapter 6 depicts some of the O-specific units of the genus *Salmonella*. Within certain genera, such as *Escherichia*, *Salmonella*, and *Shigella*, the diversity of these O antigens allows for serologic subgrouping and provides a useful epidemiologic tool. Attached to the O antigen is region II, consisting of a core polysaccharide that appears to be constant within a particular genus of enterobacteria but differs between genera. The lipid A moiety or region III is attached to the core polysaccharide and is believed to be the toxic portion of the molecule. Lipid A also serves to join the LPS to the murein-lipoprotein layer of the cell wall. Figure 38-4 depicts the inner core of *Salmonella* and its attachment to the lipid A. Further discussion of the lipopolysaccharide molecule of the Enterobacteriaceae and other gram-negative organisms can be found in Chapter 6.

Determinants of Pathogenicity

Endotoxin The lipopolysaccharide portion of the cell wall has been referred to as endotoxin. As noted previously, the toxicity appears to reside in the lipid A portion. These toxins can be extracted from the bacterial cell wall by a number of agents, such as phenol-water, trichloracetic acid, or ethylene-diamine-tetraacetate. Upon injection into animals these toxins produce a variety of effects, such as fever, fatal shock, leukocytic alterations, regression of tumors, cytotoxicity, alterations in host response to infection, Sanarelli-Shwartzman reaction, and various metabolic changes. The role of endotoxin in such diseases as urinary tract or wound infection remains unclear. However, when the enteric bacilli enter the bloodstream, endotoxic shock plays an important role. Approximately 30 percent of patients with enteric bacteremia will develop shock, with a mortality of 40 to 90 percent. The cause of this shock is apparently endotoxin, since experiments with animals injected with endotoxin or enteric organisms produce some of the reactions seen in man. The exact mechanism and nature of this syndrome have not been determined. Basically the chief defect in endotoxic shock is an inadequacy of blood supply to vital organs, causing cellular hypoxia and metabolic failure. Survival is directly proportional to the

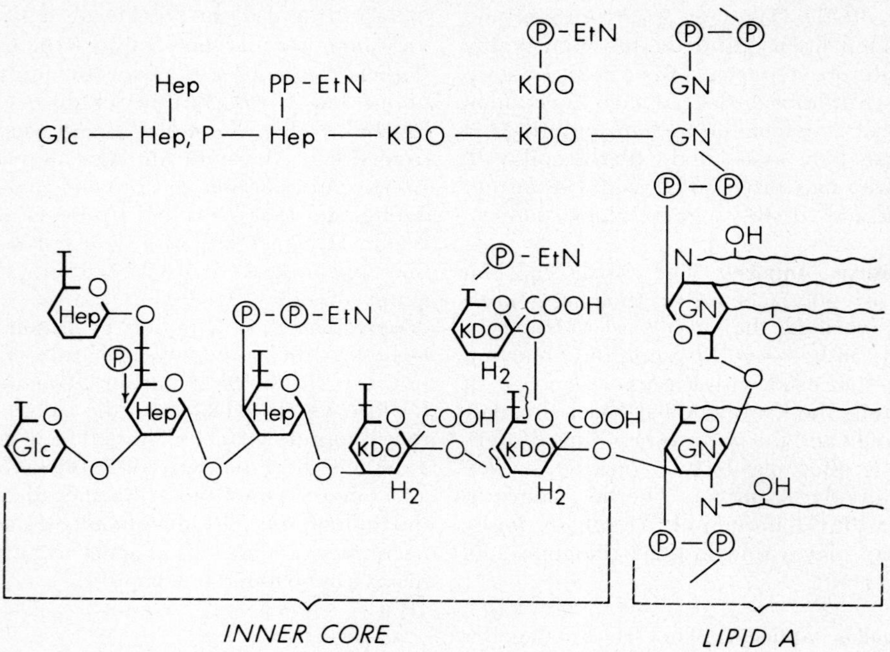

FIG. 38-4. Structure of the inner core and lipid A of a *Salmonella* Rc lipopolysaccharide. Hep = heptose; KDO = 2-keto-3-deoxyoctonate; GIN = glucosamine; P = phosphate; EtN = ethanolamine; ~ = fatty acids. (Adapted from Luderitz et al: J Infect Dis 128(Suppl):S17, 1973)

length of time needed to recognize the development of bacteremia and adequately treat the infection as well as the shock syndrome.

Enterotoxins Enterotoxins are bacterial substances that exert their toxic effect in the intestinal tract, causing a transudation of fluid into the ileum. Enteropathogenic *Escherichia coli* and *Shigella dysenteriae* type 1 are two types of enterobacteria that produce such toxins (Chaps. 39 and 40). The discovery of these toxins has been late in coming because of the lack of an experimental animal. The discovery of *Vibrio cholerae* enterotoxin (Chap. 41), using ileal loops in rabbits, provided the necessary animal model for testing enterobacterial enterotoxin production. Subsequent studies have demonstrated that the response of infant rabbits, rabbit skin, and certain tissue cultures to some types of the enterotoxin is associated with at least two separate transferable plasmids. The enterotoxin fractions of *Shigella dysenteriae* type I may correspond to the neurotoxin described in earlier literature. Preliminary experiments have demonstrated that neurotoxin preparations do have enterotoxic activity. Enterotoxin production in other *Shigella* species has not yet been described, nor has an enterotoxin been isolated from the enteropathogens of the genus *Salmonella*.

Other Factors Members of the genus *Shigella* have been shown to penetrate the epithelial lining of the intestinal tract. The nature of this penetration has not been determined, but it appears to be an important feature of shigella infections and even occurs in enterotoxin-producing strains. Whether these organisms produce an enterotoxin that is quickly absorbed by the intestinal lining is at present unknown.

The surface properties of the bacterial cells of certain enterics appear to play an important role in the etiology of their infections. The capsule of *Klebsiella pneumoniae* functions in a similar manner to the pneumococcal capsule and prevents phagocytosis. The Vi antigen of *Salmonella typhi* also may function in some protective manner and prevent intracellular destruction of the organism. Variation in the O antigen of *S. typhimurium* can cause changes in the virulence of the organism. Losses of O-specific side-chains have been associated with the lowering of the LD_{50} in mice.

A number of enterics produce a variety of factors, such as hemolysins or enzymes, but their precise role in disease is unknown. This is especially true when dealing with urinary tract or wound infections.

Clinical Infection

The Enterobacteriaceae can cause urinary tract and wound infections, pneumonia, meningitis, septicemia, and various gastrointestinal disorders. The nature of these diseases and their epidemiology will be discussed in the chapters dealing with individual organisms. It is useful, however, to think of those infections caused by organisms other than *Salmonella*, *Shigella*, and enteropathogenic *E. coli* as opportunistic or secondary infections. That is, these organisms require some alteration in the host by either mechanical, physiologic, or infectious processes before they can cause disease. These opportunistic infections usually occur outside the large intestine. *Salmonella* and *Shigella*, however, are considered to be true enteric pathogens, and their isolation from feces or other body sites of an individual implies either a diseased or a carrier state. *E. coli* is representative of an organism that can be either opportunistic or a true intestinal pathogen.

Regardless of the site of initial infection, one potential danger with the enterobacteria is the development of bacteremia. It is estimated that as many as 100,000 deaths a year may occur in the United States as a result of enteric bacteremia and subsequent development of shock.

Laboratory Diagnosis

Clinical Material, Transport, and Culture Specimens submitted for isolation of the enterobacteria include sputum, tissue, pus, body fluids, rectal swabs, and feces. To prevent overgrowth of these organisms and to obtain an accurate picture of the microbial flora, these specimens should be cultured immediately or placed in an appropriate transport medium, such as Stuart's or Amies'.

The method of handling the specimen in the laboratory depends upon the specimen source. With all nonfecal specimens any enteric could be a pathogen. Therefore, these specimens are planted on a medium that will allow the growth of most enterics but inhibit the growth of gram-positive and possibly other nonenteric gram-negative rods.

With fecal specimens, the laboratory is seeking to isolate only the intestinal pathogens, ie, *Salmonella*, *Shigella*, and in some cases enteropathogenic *E. coli*. Since fecal specimens contain the opportunistic organisms in larger quantities than the pathogens, media that suppress the growth of the opportunists but favor isolation of the pathogens are required.

All of the enteric media, regardless of purpose, contain various acid-base indicators to demonstrate carbohydrate fermentation. Most of the media also contain the carbohydrate, lactose. This is because the majority of the organisms in the genera *Escherichia*, *Enterobacter*, and *Klebsiella*, the enteric organisms present in greatest numbers in fecal material, ferment this carbohydrate while intestinal pathogens usually do not. This provides the laboratory a convenient method of selecting different types of organisms from a specimen. It must be stressed, however, that this is only a preliminary aid, since strain variation within species does occur, underlining the need for additional biochemical tests for accurate identification. Some media also contain iron salts for the detection of H_2S production to aid in the identification of potential *Salmonella* colonies. Table 38-3 lists several of the common enteric isolation media and their uses.

Laboratory Identification Colonies selected from the primary isolation media are

TABLE 38-3 MEDIA USED FOR ISOLATION OF ENTERICS

Differential Media that Permit Most Enterics to Grow
1. MacConkey's agar
2. Eosin-methylene blue agar
3. Desoxycholate agars
More Highly Selective Media Used for Cultivation of Intestinal Pathogens
1. Salmonella-Shigella agar
2. Desoxycholate citrate agar
3. Hektoen-enteric agar
4. Xylose-lysine desoxycholate agar
Enrichment Broths Used to Select for Growth of Intestinal Pathogens
1. Selenite broth
2. G-N broth
3. Tetrathionate broth

speciated by various biochemical tests. The reactions used by Ewing to divide the family into the tribes are presented in Table 38-4. Major reactions of the individual organisms will be covered in the following chapters. The choice of additional tests for speciation varies from laboratory to laboratory. The reader interested in more detailed biochemical reactions should refer to the publications of Ewing and to *Bergey's Manual*.

Serologic tests for the identification of the enterics are used in varying degrees dependent upon the organism. For example, speciation of *Salmonella* and *Shigella* is based on serologic reactions entirely, whereas the genus *Proteus* is speciated on the basis of biochemical reactions. Separation of the enteropathogenic *E. coli* in infants from the other types of *E. coli* is accomplished by serologic determination of the O, H, and K antigens.

Treatment

Table 38-5 lists the various agents useful in the treatment of enterobacterial infections. Despite the discovery of newer antimicrobial agents, adequate treatment of enterobacterial infections remains a major therapeutic problem. Several factors contribute to this problem. One of the most important is that the usual pa-

TABLE 38-5   ANTIMICROBIALS USEFUL IN TREATMENT OF ENTEROBACTERIAL DISEASES*

A. Penicillins
   1. Ampicillin
   2. Carbenicillin
B. Cephalosporins
C. Aminoglycosides
   1. Kanamycin
   2. Gentamicin
   3. Neomycin
   4. Streptomycin
D. Polymyxins
   1. Polymyxin B
   2. Colistin (Polymyxin E)
E. Other Antimicrobials
   1. Chloramphenicol
   2. Tetracyclines
   3. Trimethoprim-sulfamethoxazole
   4. Sulfonamides

See text and Chapters 39–42 for applicability to various species

tient having such infections has been compromised in some manner. In addition, the indiscriminate use of antimicrobials results in the selection of resistant strains of organisms that have the potential of transferring their resistance factors to previously sensitive organisms. A number of reports regarding outbreaks of such resistant forms are found in the literature. The biochemical nature and genetics of the re-

TABLE 38-4   DIFFERENTIATION OF THE TRIBES OF ENTEROBACTERIACEAE BY BIOCHEMICAL METHODS

Test of Substrate	Tribes				
	Escherichiaeae	Edwardsielleae	Salmonelleae	Klebsielleae	Proteeae
Hydrogen sulfide (TSI)	−	+	+	−	+ or −
Urease	−	−	−	− or (+)	+ or −
Indol	+ or −	+	−	−	+ or −
Methyl red	+	+	+	−	+
Voges-Proskauer	−	−	−	+	−
Citrate (Simmons)	−	−	+	+	d
KCN	−	−	− or +	+	+
Phenylalanine deaminase	−	−	−	−	+
Mucate	d	−	d	+ or −	−
Mannitol	+ or −	−	+	+	− or +

From Ewing: Differentiation of Enterobacteriaceae by Biochemical Reactions, Revised. Atlanta, Ga., DHEW Publication No (CDC) 74-8270, 1973.

Note: S. typhi, S. enteritidis *bioserotype paratyphi-A, and some rare bioserotypes fail to utilize citrate. Cultures of* S. enteritidis *bioserotype paratyphi-A and some rare bioserotypes may fail to produce hydrogen sulfide; an occasional strain of almost any serotype of salmonellae may be hydrogen sulfide negative. Some cultures of* P. mirabilis *may yield positive Voges-Proskauer tests. Some strains of* E. agglomerans *deaminate phenylalanine.*

+ = 90% or more positive within 1 or 2 days; − = 90% or more no reactions; (+) = delayed positive (3 or more days); d = different biochemical reactions, +, (+), −; + or − = most cultures positive, some negative; − or + = most strains negative, some positive; − or (+) = most cultures negative, some positive delayed

sistance factors and their transfer are discussed in Chapters 8 and 10. Because of the potential variability in sensitivity of the organisms and harmful side effects of some antimicrobials, careful monitoring of the antimicrobial susceptibility of individual enterobacterial isolates is required.

FURTHER READING

Andersen ES: The ecology of transferable drug resistance in the enterobacteria. Ann Rev Microbiol 22:131, 1968

Boxerbaum B: Antimicrobial drugs for treatment of infections caused by gram-negative bacilli. Med Clin North Am 58:623, 1974

Brachman PS, Eichoff TC (eds): Proceedings of the International Conference on Nosocomial Infections. Atlanta, Georgia, CDC, 1970

Cluff LE, Sanders WE, Robson HG: Bacteremia and bacteremic shock. In Cluff LE, Johnson JE (eds): Clinical Concepts of Infectious Diseases. Baltimore, Williams & Wilkins, 1972, pp 85-99

Cowan ST: Family I Enterobacteriaceae. In Buchanan RE, Gibbons NE (eds): Bergey's Manual of Determinative Bacteriology, 8th ed. Baltimore, Williams & Wilkins, 1974, pp 290-340

Edwards PR, Ewing WH: Identification of Enterobacteriaceae, 3rd ed. Minneapolis, Burgess, 1972

Ewing WH: Differentiation of Enterobacteriaceae by Biochemical Reactions, Revised. Atlanta, Ga, DHEW Publication No (CDC) 74-8270, 1973

Ewing WH, Martin WJ: Enterobacteriaceae. In Lennette EH, Spaulding EH, Truant JP (eds): Manual of Clinical Microbiology, 2nd ed. Washington, DC, American Society for Microbiology, 1974, pp 189-221

Hoeprich PD: Manifestation of infectious diseases. In Hoeprich PD (ed): Infectious Disease. Hagerstown, Md, Harper and Row, 1972, pp 65-69

Kass EH, Wolff SM (eds): Bacterial lipopolysaccharides: Chemistry, biology and clinical significance of endotoxin. J Infect Dis 128 (Suppl): July, 1973, S1-S305

McHenry MC, Hawk WA: Bacteremia caused by gram-negative bacilli. Med Clin North Am 58:623, 1974

Whang HY, Neter E: Production of common enterobacterial antigen by members of family Enterobacteriaceae. Experientia 29:96, 1973

39
Opportunistic Enterobacteriaceae

Clinically it is useful to divide the family Enterobacteriaceae into the intestinal pathogens and the opportunistic pathogens. The opportunists constitute those enterics that can be found as part of the normal bowel flora or as free living forms and which can serve as potential pathogens for nonintestinal tissue. Opportunists include organisms of the genera *Escherichia*, *Edwardsiella*, *Arizona*, and *Citrobacter*, and the tribes Klebsielleae and Proteeae. The genera *Escherichia* and *Arizona* are included in the definition of opportunists despite the association of certain strains with intestinal disease because most isolates of these genera are from extraintestinal sources. All of the opportunistic enteric bacilli are capable of producing similar disease, but the epidemiology, frequency, severity, and treatment of these diseases may vary with the different species. In fact, differences in antimicrobial susceptibility and epidemiology of the same species may be seen in different institutional settings. Discussion of the overall medical importance of these opportunists is found in Chapter 38.

TRIBE KLEBSIELLEAE

The tribe Klebsielleae consists of three genera, *Klebsiella*, *Enterobacter*, and *Serratia*. *Klebsiella* is the second most populous facultative enteric genus found in the bowel of man. *Enterobacter* and *Serratia* also inhabit the intestinal tract but are present in smaller numbers. Some species of *Enterobacter* are more commonly found in water, sewage, and soil.

The Klebsielleae have become the third leading cause of nosocomial infections in the United States and, in some institutions, have replaced *Escherichia coli* as the most frequent isolate. The epidemiology of the individual genera of this tribe has been difficult to assess because of the numerous taxonomic changes that have occurred and the lack of definitive methods of speciation. During the past 10 to 15 years, reliable methods have become available to the clinical laboratories permitting the acquisition of more accurate epidemiologic data. Table 39-1 correlates the present classification scheme of Ewing with some of the former nomenclature used to describe this tribe.

Genus Klebsiella

The most commonly isolated member of the tribe Klebsielleae is *Klebsiella pneumoniae* (Friedländer's bacillus). As its name implies, it can cause pneumonia and was originally thought to be the cause of the classic lobar pneumonia, the true agent of which is *Streptococcus pneumoniae*. Like all other opportunistic enterics *K. pneumoniae* can cause infection of other body sites besides the respiratory tract.

The remaining two species of *Klebsiella*, *K. ozaenae* and *K. rhinoscleromatis*, are causative agents of chronic infections of the nasal mucosa and pharynx and are rare in the United States.

Biochemical and Cultural Characteristics Speciation of the *Klebsiella* can be achieved by the tests shown in Table 39-2. All species

TABLE 39-1 COMPARISON OF PRESENT NOMENCLATURE OF KLEBSIELLEAE WITH OLDER USAGE

Present Taxonomy		Older Synonyms
Genus	*Klebsiella*	
Species	*K. pneumoniae*	Same but includes nonmotile *Aerobacter aerogenes*
	K. ozaenae	Same
	K. rhinoscleromatis	Same
Genus	*Enterobacter*	*Aerobacter*
Species	*E. cloacae*	*Aerobacter cloacae, Aerobacter A, Cloacae A*
	E. aerogenes	*Aerobacter aerogenes, Aerobacter B, Cloacae B*
	E. hafniae	Hafnia group, *E. alvei, Bacterium cadaveria*
	E. agglomerans	*Erwinia herbicola, Escherichia adecarboxylata, Bacterium typhiflavum,* and others
Genus	*Serratia*	
Species	*S. marcescens*	Same
	S. liquefaciens	*Enterobacter liquefaciens*
	S. rubidaea	*Bacterium rubidaeum*

TABLE 39-2   SPECIATION OF GENUS KLEBSIELLA

Test	K. pneumoniae	K. ozaenae	K. rhinoscleromatis
Lactose fermentation	+	±	−
Voges-Proskauer	+	−	−
Methyl red	−	+	+
Citrate (Simmons)	+	±	+
Lysine decarboxylase	+	±	−
Malonate	+	−	+

are characteristically nonmotile, which is useful in separating them from other members of the tribe. With the exception of *K. rhinoscleromatis*, most isolates ferment lactose. The presence of a large capsule causes colonies of *Klebsiella* growing on agar to appear large, moist, and mucoid.

Antigenic Structure *Klebsiella* possess O and K antigens, of which the polysaccharide K antigen has proven to be the most useful for serologic typing. Seventy-two different K antigens have been described. All species of *Klebsiella* share common antigens and thus are able to be typed with the same set of antisera. The majority of *K. ozaenae* strains belong to type 4, whereas most of *K. rhinoscleromatis* strains possess type 3 antigen.

No single serologic type of *K. pneumoniae* is more virulent than other types, nor is one found to be more frequently associated with different infections. Nevertheless, serologic typing provides a very useful tool for determining distribution of these organisms during large outbreaks of disease.

Clinical Infection *K. pneumoniae* can cause a primary pneumonia. Generally, this occurs in middle-aged and older men who have underlying medical problems, such as alcoholism, chronic bronchopulmonary disease, or diabetes mellitus. A thick, nonputrid, bloody sputum occurs in approximately one-fourth to three-fourths of patients with pneumonia caused by *Klebsiella*. Abscess formation and necrosis are more likely to occur with *Klebsiella pneumoniae* than in other bacterial pneumonias. Positive blood cultures occur in about 25 percent of klebsiella pneumonias. Some authors report a mortality rate of 50 percent despite adequate antimicrobial therapy, with mortality correlating closely with the occurrence of bacteremia.

In addition to primary pneumonia, *K. pneumoniae* has been associated with urinary tract and wound infections, septicemia, and meningitis. At some institutions it has become the leading cause of septicemia.

K. ozaenae has been implicated in a chronic atrophic rhinitis characterized by a fetid odor. *K. rhinoscleromatis* produces a granulomatous destruction of the nose and pharynx that is relatively rare in this country, but common in Southeast Europe, India, and Central America.

Treatment The majority of *K. pneumoniae* isolates are resistant to ampicillin and carbenicillin. Cephalosporins are usually effective, a property that is useful in differentiating *Klebsiella* from the organisms of the genus *Enterobacter*. Other antibiotics listed in Chapter 38 also are usually effective against this organism, but strains isolated from nosocomial infections usually are resistant to multiple antimicrobials.

Genus Enterobacter

The clinical importance of the genus *Enterobacter* as a separate entity was not greatly appreciated until the 1960s. Prior to this time, separation of the *Enterobacter* from the *Klebsiella* was not routinely attempted, and many infections were reported as being caused by the *Klebsiella-Aerobacter* group. How many of these diseases were in reality caused by *Enterobacter* is not known. Recent studies indicate that *Enterobacter* infections occur less frequently than those caused by *Klebsiella*. The organisms of this genus, however, are capable of causing infections similar to those caused by other enterobacteria.

Biochemical and Cultural Characteristics The genus *Enterobacter* can be divided into four genera on the basis of the biochemical

TABLE 39-3 SPECIATION OF GENUS ENTEROBACTER

Test	E. cloacae	E. aerogenes	E. hafniae	E. agglomerans
Lysine	−	+	+	−
Ornithine decarboxylase	+	+	+	−
Arginine dihydrolase	+	−	−	−
Adonitol fermentation	±	+	−	±

tests shown in Table 39-3. They are differentiated from *Klebsiella* by the fact that all are motile, and with the exception of *E. agglomerans*, all decarboxylate ornithine. Most isolates of *Enterobacter*, with the exception of *E. hafniae*, ferment lactose rapidly. With *E. hafniae* more biochemical tests will be positive at 25C than at 37C.

Antigenic Structure All *Enterobacter* possess O and H antigens, while only a portion of the strains possess K antigens. The characterization of these antigens for the entire genus has not been completely established to the same extent as with other enteric bacilli.

Clinical Infection *Enterobacter*, like most Enterobacteriaceae, are capable of producing disease in any body tissue but have been most frequently isolated from urinary tract infections. *E. cloacae* accounts for the majority of isolates of this genus, but all species have been isolated from clinical specimens. Two species, *E. agglomerans* (formerly classified as *Erwinia*) and *E. cloacae* were associated with a nationwide epidemic involving contaminated intravenous fluids. These species were isolated from eight hospitals in seven states and were responsible for 150 bacteremias and nine deaths.

Treatment With the exception of ampicillin and cephalosporins, most of the antimicrobials discussed in Chapter 38 are useful in the treatment of *Enterobacter* infections. As with all enterics, resistance patterns vary with individual isolates.

Genus Serratia

The organisms of the genus *Serratia* were at one time thought to be harmless saphrophytes and were used to determine air current patterns in hospitals. These organisms, however, are rapidly emerging as major entities in nosocomial infections. Almost all *Serratia* infections are associated with underlying disease, changing physiologic patterns, immunosuppressive treatment, or mechanical manipulations of the patient.

Biochemical and Cultural Characteristics Organisms of the genus *Serratia* can be differentiated from other enterobacteria by the production of an extracellular DNase. The three species *S. marcescens*, *S. liquefaciens*, and *S. rubidaea* can be differentiated by the decarboxylase and fermentation tests listed in Table 39-4. The majority of *S. rubidaea* form a pink to red pigment, as do some strains of *S. marcescens*. Pigment production by *S. marcescens* is enhanced by incubation at room temperature.

Clinical Infections *S. marcescens* is the most frequent isolate of the genus *Serratia* and has been associated with a number of nosocomial epidemics involving pneumonia, septicemia, urinary tract infections, and wound infections. Urinary tract infections are associated with underlying abnormalities or instrumentation. Pneumonia with this organism has been transmitted by contaminated respiratory care equipment and is similar to pneumonia caused by *Klebsiella* except that necrosis and

TABLE 39-4 SPECIATION OF GENUS SERRATIA

Test	S. marcescens	S. liquefaciens	S. rubidaea
Ornithine decarboxylase	+	+	−
Arabinose fermentation	−	+	+
DNase	+	+	+

abscess formation are less likely to occur. Infection with pigmented *Serratia* may cause sputum to be tinged with red, thus giving the false impression of hemoptysis.

S. *liquefaciens* and S. *rubidaea* are associated with similar infections but are less frequently isolated.

Treatment The majority of S. *marcescens* isolates are resistant to multiple antimicrobials. Although resistant strains of S. *liquefaciens* do occur, this organism tends to be more sensitive than S. *marcescens*, with some strains being sensitive to ampicillin.

TRIBE PROTEEAE

The organisms of the tribe Proteeae are characterized by their motility and ability to deaminate phenylalanine. With the exception of a rare isolate, they do not ferment lactose. Ewing favors the division of the tribe into two genera, *Proteus* and *Providencia*, while other taxonomists classify the *Providencia* as *Proteus inconstans*. Recent investigations on DNA homology, phage and bacteriocin susceptibility, and characterization of enzymes indicates that the taxonomy of the tribe will change in the near future.

The majority of clinical isolates of this tribe are from urine, although other infections occur. Some studies indicate that the Proteeae are responsible for approximately 10 to 15 percent of the nosocomial infections in the United States.

Genus Proteus

The organisms of the genus *Proteus* are found in soil, water, sewage, and decaying animal matter as well as the human intestinal tract. All possess a powerful urease, which distinguishes them from the genus *Providencia*.

Biochemical and Cultural Characteristics
The genus *Proteus* can be divided into four species by the biochemical tests listed in Table 39-5. *P. mirabilis* is the only species that does not produce indol from tryptophan. *P. mirabilis* and *P. vulgaris* are actively motile at 37C, producing a thin translucent sheet of growth on nonselective agars. This phenomenon is referred to as "swarming." On certain enteric isolation media the production of hydrogen sulfide by *P. mirabilis* and *P. vulgaris* may cause the colonies of these organisms to be confused with those of the enteric pathogens of the genus *Salmonella*. All *Proteus* species can tolerate alkaline pH and thus can be isolated on media designed for the selective isolation of the organisms of the genus *Vibrio* (Chap. 41).

Antigenic Structure Several studies have attempted to group *Proteus* strains on the basis of their O, H, and K antigens, but these studies have not been sufficiently correlated to be useful as an epidemiologic tool. The most important use of the *Proteus* antigens is in the diagnosis of rickettsial diseases. Certain *P. vulgaris* strains (OX-19, OX-K, OX-2) share antigens with the Rickettsia. This cross-reactivity allows the *Proteus* to serve as the antigen for the detection of rickettsial antibodies. (Chap. 57).

Clinical Infection *P. mirabilis* accounts for the majority of *Proteus* infections in man, causing community- as well as hospital-acquired urinary tract infections. Wound infections, pneumonia, and septicemia can also occur. The frequency of infection with other *Proteus* species is difficult to assess because of the tendency of various laboratories to lump these organisms into a group called the "indol-positive" *proteus*. Despite this tendency several nosocomial outbreaks with other species, particularly *P. rettgeri*, have been described.

Proteus pneumonias are similar to those of *Klebsiella*. Bacteremias are common in debili-

TABLE 39-5   Speciation of Genus Proteus

Test	P. mirabilis	P. morganii	P. rettgeri	P. vulgaris
Urease	+	+	+	+
Indol	−	+	+	+
H$_2$S	+	−	−	+
Ornithine decarboxylase	+	+	−	−

tated patients and are associated with high mortality rates.

When *Proteus* infects the urinary tract, the hydrolysis of urea to ammonia raises the pH of the urine, resulting in precipitation of calcium and magnesium salts and the formation of calculi. Urease also may be important in the severity of the disease. When urease activity is absent, the number of organisms in the kidneys and the extent of renal damage are less than when the enzyme is present. Evidence indicates that the alkalization of urine by urease causes increased damage to renal epithelium.

Treatment *P. mirabilis* differs from the other *Proteus* species in being sensitive to ampicillin and the cephalosporins. Most isolates of all species are sensitive to aminoglycoside antibiotics and to the combination of trimethroperim and sulfamethoxazole. Resistant forms do occur, particularly in patients with previous antimicrobial therapy.

Genus Providencia

The genus *Providencia* has been associated with a number of nosocomial infections involving urinary tract infections, septicemia, wound infections, and pneumonia. Several institutions report that *P. stuartii* is becoming an increasingly important cause of infections in burn patients. Most of these isolates have been resistant to multiple antimicrobials, even the aminoglycosides. Both *P. alcalifaciens* and *P. stuartii* deaminate phenylalanine but do not produce urease, nor do they possess the ability to decarboxylate amino acids. *P. stuartii* can be differentiated from *P. alcalifaciens* by the ability to ferment inositol. Treatment of infections depends upon the susceptibility pattern of individual isolates, but the limited experience with these organisms indicates that *P. alcalifaciens* are usually more susceptible to antimicrobials than are *P. stuartii* isolates.

TRIBE EDWARDSIELLEAE

Edwardsiella tarda is the only species presently classified in the tribe Edwardsielleae. Formerly it has been classified as the Asakusa group and the Bartholomew group. A number of isolates from animal sources, primarily cold-blooded types, have been reported. In man *Edwardsiella* infections are rare, but the organism has been isolated from wound infections, sepsis, and meningitis. The organism also has been isolated from human feces in cases of gastroenteritis.

E. tarda produces indol, H_2S, lysine and ornithine decarboxylases. Lactose is not fermented, nor can acetate be used as the sole carbon source. The production of H_2S may cause colonies of these organisms to be confused with the enteric pathogens of the genus *Salmonella*.

Most *E. tarda* isolates are sensitive to most antimicrobials used in the treatment of enterobacterial infections.

OPPORTUNISTS OF TRIBE SALMONELLEAE

In addition to the intestinal pathogens of the genus *Salmonella*, the tribe Salmonelleae contains two genera, *Citrobacter* and *Arizona*, that can be isolated from secondary infections. The biochemical differentiation of this tribe is found in Table 39-6.

Genus Citrobacter

The genus *Citrobacter* contains two species, *Citrobacter freundii* and *Citrobacter diversus*, a newly described species. Both organisms have been isolated from urinary tract infections, wounds, blood, sputa, and spinal fluid. The organisms differ in their susceptibility to antimicrobials: *C. diversus* resembles *Klebsiella* in its resistance to ampicillin and carbenicillin, and most *C. freundii* strains resemble *Enterobacter* and are resistant to ampicillin and the cephalosporins.

Genus Arizona

Most organisms of the genus *Arizona* have been isolated from animals, particularly reptiles and birds. One species is described, *Arizona hinshawii*, formerly referred to as *Paracolobacterium arizonae*. Although isolates of this organism from man are rare, diseases such as gastroenteritis, bacteremia, pyelonephritis, osteomyelitis, and otitis media have

TABLE 39-6   DIFFERENTIATION OF THE TRIBE SALMONELLEAE

Biochemical Test	Salmonella species	Citrobacter diversus*	Citrobacter freundii	Arizona hinshawii †
H₂S production	+	−	±	+
Indol production	−	+	−	−
Malonate production	−	+	±	+
Lysine decarboxylase	+	−	−	+
Growth in KCN	−	−	+	−

Previously classified as aberrant E. cloacae, Levinea, *and* Citrobacter koseri
†Previously Paracolobacterium arizonae

been attributed to it. Its importance in human gastroenteritis is difficult to assess, since the majority of strains may ferment lactose, and laboratory technicians have been trained to regard lactose-fermenting organisms as normal fecal flora. It appears, however, that man is an accidental host in most infections with this organism.

Genus *Arizona* shares some biochemical characteristics and a number of antigens with the genus *Salmonella,* causing some taxonomists to consider it a species of *Salmonella.* Most isolates are sensitive to the antimicrobials used in treatment of gram-negative infections.

TRIBE ESCHERICHIEAE

Two closely related genera, *Shigella* and *Escherichia,* comprise the divisions of the tribe Escherichieae. All *Shigella* are intestinal pathogens and as such will be discussed in Chapter 40. The genus *Escherichia* contains a single species, *Escherichia coli,* which is the predominant facultative organism found in the large bowel. Accurate differentiation between the two genera can require many biochemical and serologic tests. In most cases, however, differentiation is achieved easily, since *E. coli* usually is motile, ferments lactose and other carbohydrates, produces lysine decarboxylase, and utilizes acetate as the sole carbon source.

Genus Escherichia

E. coli occupies a unique position among opportunistic enteric bacilli in that certain strains are capable of causing primary intestinal disease as well as extraintestinal infection. In addition, *E. coli* has been the subject of more experimental research than any microorganism, especially in the field of molecular biology.

Biochemical and Cultural Characteristics *E. coli* grows well in most commonly used media. Some strains produce beta hemolysis on blood agar. Most are motile, ferment lactose, and produce gas from the fermentation of glucose. Some strains, especially those formerly classified as Alkalescens-Dispar, are anaerogenic and nonmotile and, thus, can be confused with *Shigella.* Table 39-7 lists the biochemical reactions useful in characterizing *E. coli.*

TABLE 39-7   CHARACTERISTICS OF ESCHERICHIA COLI USING SELECTED BIOCHEMICAL TESTS

Test	Reaction (% Positive)
Indol	96.3
Lysine decarboxylase	82.1
Mucate	91.6
Acetate	93.5
Gas from glucose	92.0
Lactose	95.8
Motility	62.1

Adapted from Ewing: Differentiation of Enterobacteriaceae by Biochemical Reactions, Revised. Atlanta, Ga. DHEW Publication No (CDC) 74-8270, 1973

Antigenic Structure Serologic typing of the O, K, and H antigens of *E. coli* provides a useful epidemiologic tool, especially in infantile diarrhea. Presently at least 150 O, 90 K, and 50 H antigenic types have been described. The K antigens are divided on physical behavior into three main types, L, A, and B. The serologic type of an *E. coli* isolate is given in the form: O type:K type:H type, as in the example *E. coli* 111:58(B4):2.

Clinical Infection *E. coli* is the most common cause of urinary tract infections in man, both hospital and community acquired. It is also the most frequent cause of gram-negative sepsis and has been isolated from cerebrospinal fluid and wounds and from cases of pneumonia. *E. coli* accounts for the majority of cases of meningitis seen in premature infants and neonates but is a less frequent cause of meningitis in older populations.

Enteropathogenic strains of *E. coli* are responsible for an acute diarrhea seen in children under 2 years of age. Ewing and co-workers have reported that 80 percent of the *E. coli* that are enteropathogenic for human infants belong to the 20 serotypes listed in Table 39-8. Epidemics of these enteropathogens have caused hospital nurseries to close down to stem the number of infections.

TABLE 39-8 SEROLOGIC TYPES OF E. COLI ASSOCIATED WITH INFANTILE DIARRHEA

O Antigen	K Antigen	H Antigen
26	60 (B 6)	NM*
26	60 (B 6)	11
55	59 (B 5)	NM
55	59 (B 5)	6
55	59 (B 5)	7
86a	61 (B 7)	34
111a, 111b	58 (B 4)	NM
111a, 111b	58 (B 4)	2
111a, 111b	58 (B 4)	12
111a, 111b	58 (B 4)	21
119	69 (B 14)	6
125a, 125c	70 (B 15)	21
126	71 (B 16)	NM
126	71 (B 16)	27
127a	63 (B 8)	NM
127a	63 (B 8)	9
127a	63 (B 8)	21
128a, 128b	67 (B 12)	2
128a, 128b	67 (B 12)	7
128a, 128c	67 (B 12)	12

NM = Nonmotile
Adapted from Edwards and Ewing: Identification of Enterobacteriaceae, 3rd ed. 1972. Courtesy of Burgess Publishing Co.

Recent evidence demonstrates that *E. coli* can be the causative agent of diarrhea in adults. The frequency of such infections is not clear, but several reports of outbreaks involving a number of people have appeared. The enteropathogenicity of *E. coli* in adults appears to be mediated by either of two mechanisms: (1) production of an enterotoxin and (2) a shigella-like penetration of intestinal mucosa. The toxin causes fluid accumulation in the jejunal and ileal portion of the intestine, while the *E. coli* that cause intestinal mucosa penetration apparently resides primarily in the colon. Regardless of type of disease, invasion of extraintestinal tissue is extremely rare. Death due to dehydration and electrolyte imbalance may occur in the very young and very old.

The enteropathogenic *E. coli* appear to be of low virulence when compared with the intestinal pathogen *Shigella*. Volunteer studies indicate that it may require 10^6 to 10^7 *E. coli* to produce the symptoms produced by about 2×10^2 *Shigella*.

ENTEROTOXINS. Two enterotoxins, one heat labile (LT), the other heat stable (ST), have been isolated from *E. coli*. The relationship of the human enterotoxins to those isolated from animal diseases is not yet known. The ability to produce these enterotoxins is associated with two transferable plasmids, one coding for both enterotoxins, the second coding for the ST only. The LT is similar in many respects to the enterotoxin of *Vibrio cholerae*. Both the LT and cholera enterotoxin stimulate the adenylate cyclase in epithelial cells of the small intestinal mucosa. This stimulation of enzyme activity increases the permeability of the intestinal lining, subsequent fluid loss, and thus diarrhea. The LT and cholera enterotoxin also share immunologic reactivity, are cytopathic for Y-1 adrenal tumor and Chinese hamster ovary cells, and increase capillary permeability of rabbit skin at the site of injection. The LT and cholera enterotoxin may, however, differ in their initial binding sites within the intestinal tract.

Unlike the LT and the cholera enterotoxin, the ST does not stimulate adenyl cyclase activity or antibody production and is not reactive in the rabbit skin test. The ST is a smaller molecule than is the LT and is not immunogenic. When injected into ileal loops of rabbits, the ST will produce its maximal response in 4 hours rather than the 10 hours required for the LT. The suckling mouse is unique in its ability to detect ST and is positive within 4 hours of inoculation.

The discovery of enterotoxins requires that in the absence of known pathogens, the enteropathogenic *E. coli* be considered in the differential diagnosis of diarrhea. Tests for the detection of enterotoxin production, although presently available only at reference centers, may be an important serologic procedure for clinical relevance in large outbreaks.

Treatment *E. coli* isolated from community-acquired infections is usually sensitive to most antimicrobials used to treat gram-negative organisms (Chap. 38). Resistant forms, however, can and do appear, especially in patients with a history of prior antibiotic therapy. The best treatment of diarrhea appears to be management of fluid and electrolyte balance. Although infantile diarrhea has been controlled by a number of antibiotics, the rapid emergence of resistant forms requires close surveillance of sensitivity patterns.

FURTHER READING

Books and Reviews

Coetzee JN: Genetics of the Proteus Group. Annu Rev Microbiol 26:23, 1972

Edwards PR, Ewing WH: Identification of Enterobacteriaceae, 3rd ed. Minneapolis, Burgess, 1972

Edwards PR, Fife MA, Ramsey CH: Studies on Arizona group of Enterobacteriaceae. Bacteriol Rev 23:155, 1959

Ewing WH: Differentiation of Enterobacteriaceae by biochemical reactions, Revised. Atlanta, Ga, DHEW Publ No (CDC) 74-8270. 1973

Selected Papers

Adler JL, Burke JP, Martin DF, Finland M: Proteus infections in a general hospital. I. Biochemical characteristics and antibiotic susceptibility of the organism. Ann Intern Med 75:517, 1971

Bennett JV, Scheckler WE, Maki DG, Brachman PS: Current national patterns. United States. Proceedings of the International Conference on Noscomial Infections. CDC. 1970, pp 42-49

DuPont HL, Formal SB, Hornick RB, et al: Pathogenesis of *Escherichia coli* diarrhea. N Engl J Med 285:1, 1972

Edwards LD, Cross A, Levin S, Landau W: Outbreak of a nosocomial infection with a strain of *Proteus rettgeri* resistant to many antimicrobials. Am J Clin Pathol 6:41, 1974

Eickhoff TC, Steinhauer BW, Finland M: The Klebsiella-Enterobacter-Serratia division: Biochemical and serological characteristics and susceptibility to antibiotics. Ann Intern Med 65:1163, 1966

Eickhoff TC, Steinhauer BW, Finland M: The Klebsiella-Enterobacter-Serratia division: Clinical and epidemological characteristics. Ann Intern Med 65:1180, 1966

Fields BN, Uwaydah MM, Kunz LJ, Swartz MN: The so-called "Paracolon" bacteria. A bacteriologic and clinical reappraisal. Am J Med 42:89, 1967

Finland M: Changing ecology of bacterial infection as related to antibacterial therapy. J Infect Dis 122:419, 1970

Grady GF, Keusch GT: Pathogenesis of bacterial diarrheas (Parts 1 and 2). N Engl J Med 285:831, 891, 1971

Gyles C, So M, Falkow F: The enterotoxin plasmid of *Escherichia coli*. J Infect Dis 130:40, 1974

Jones SR, Ragsdale AA, Kutscher E, Sanford JP: Clinical and bacteriological observations on a recently recognized species of Enterobacteriaceae, *Citrobacter diversus*. J Infect Dis 128:563, 1973

Kantor HS: Enterotoxins of *Escherichia coli* and *Vibrio cholerae*: Tools for the molecular biologist. J Infect Dis 131(Suppl):s22, 1975

Maki DG, Hennekens CG, Phillips CW, Shaw WV, Bennett JV: Nosocomial urinary tract infections with *Serratia marcescens*: An epidemiological study. J Infect Dis 128:579, 1973

Malowany MS, Chester B, Allerhand J: Isolation and microbiological differentiation of *Klebsiella rhinoscleromatis* and *Klebsiella ozaenae* in cases of chronic rhinitis. Am J Clin Pathol 58:550, 1972

Meyers BR, Bottone E, Hirschman SZ, Schneierson SS: Infection caused by microorganisms of the genus *Erwinia*. Ann Intern Med 76:9, 1972

Morbidity and Mortality. Special suppl to vol 20:No 9. Nosocomial bacteremias associated with intravenous fluid therapy—USA, 1971

Overturf GD, Wilkins J, Ressler R: Emergence of resistance of *Providencia stuartii* to multiple antibiotics: Speciation and biochemical characteristics of *Providencia*. J Infect Dis 129:353, 1974

Pierce AK, Sanford JP: Aerobic gram-negative bacillary pneumonias. Am Rev Respir Dis 110:647, 1974

Selden R, Lee S, Wang WLL, Bennett JV, Eickhoff TC: Nosocomial *Klebsiella* infections: Intestinal colonization as a reservoir. Ann Intern Med 74:657, 1971

Shore EG, Dean AG, Holik KJ, Davis BR: Enterotoxin producing *Escherichia coli* and diarrheal disease in adult travelers: A prospective study. J Infect Dis 129:577, 1974

Solberg CO, Matsen JM: Infections with Providence bacilli. Am J Med 50:241, 1971

Sonnenwirth AC, Kallus BA: Meningitis due to *Edwardsiella tarda*. Am J Clin Pathol 49:92, 1968

Washington JA II, Birk RJ, Ritts RE Jr: Bacteriologic and epidemiologic characteristics of *Enterobacter hafniae* and *Enterobacter liquefaciens*. J Infect Dis 124:379, 1971

40
Enterobacteriaceae: Salmonella and Shigella, Intestinal Pathogens

For the adult population of well-developed countries, diarrhea generally represents at most an inconvenience. However, among the very young and old and the malnourished in marginal living conditions, diarrhea represents a crippling, even life-threatening entity. Diarrhea also has altered military history by incapacitating large numbers of men, making them unfit for battle.

The causes of diarrhea are many, ranging from the psychologic to the infectious. The infectious processes are caused by protozoan, bacterial, and viral agents. The family Enterobacteriaceae contains two of the most common and important causes of diarrhea, the genera *Salmonella* and *Shigella*. Although these two genera belong to the same family of bacteria and cause a similar clinical syndrome, they differ greatly in their microbiologic, epidemiologic, and pathologic properties.

SHIGELLA

Shigella are primarily human pathogens and have been isolated only occasionally from other animals, principally primates. The genus *Shigella* is classified in the tribe *Escherichieae* together with the genus *Escherichia*. *S. dysenteriae*, *S. flexneri*, *S. boydii*, and *S. sonnei* constitute the four species of the genus. Speciation is based upon serologic and biochemical reactions. All four species can cause bacillary dysentery, but the severity of disease, mortality, and frequency of isolation differ for each species.

Physiology

Biochemical and Cultural Characteristics
All shigella are nonmotile, do not produce H_2S, and, except for certain types of *S. flexneri*,

do not produce gas during carbohydrate fermentation. These factors distinguish them from most salmonella. In contrast to *E. coli* they do not produce lysine decarboxylase, utilize acetate as a carbon source, or ferment lactose rapidly. *S. sonnei* will ferment lactose upon extended incubation. Some of the biochemical tests useful in speciation of the genus are found in Table 40-1. For detailed biochemical information the reader is referred to the publications of Ewing and co-workers.

Resistance to Physical and Chemical Agents
Shigella are less resistant than salmonella and other enterics to a variety of physical and chemical agents. High concentrations of acids are detrimental, necessitating the use of well-buffered media. High concentrations of bile also are inhibitory to some strains, making certain enteric media, such as SS agar (Salmonella–Shigella agar), unsuitable for isolation of shigella from clinical specimens. They tolerate low temperatures if adequate moisture is available.

Antigenic Structure

All shigella possess O antigens, and some possess K antigens. Those strains possessing K antigens appear as smooth colonies when grown on agar. The K antigen is not significant in the serologic typing of shigella but, when present, interferes with the determination of the O antigen type. This interference usually can be removed by boiling the cell suspension. Using the O antigen, the shigella are divided into four groups designated A, B, C, and D, which correspond to the species *S. dysenteriae*, *S. flexneri*, *S. boydii*, and *S. sonnei*, respectively. Each major group or species is also subdivided into types on the basis of the O antigen. These subgroups are designated by Arabic

TABLE 40-1   BIOCHEMICAL TESTS USEFUL IN THE SPECIATION OF SHIGELLA

Test	S. dysenteriae	S. flexneri	S. flexneri 6	S. boydii	S. sonnei
Mannitol	−	+	+	+	+
Ornithine decarboxylase	−	−	−	−	+
Arginine dihydrolase	±	−	±	±	−
Jordan's tartrate	±	−	−	−	+
Indol	+	±	−	±	−

numbers. At the present time there are 10 serologic types of *S. dysenteriae*, 6 of *S. flexneri*, 15
of *S. boydii*, and 1 of *S. sonnei* described.

Determinants of Pathogenicity

Bacillary dysentery follows penetration
of the epithelial cells of the mucous surface of
the terminal ileum and colon by invasive shigella. After multiplication of the bacteria in the
epithelial lining, a local inflammation occurs,
followed by cell death and sloughing of the lining. Noninvasive shigella mutants are incapable of producing disease. Whether or not a toxic
substance is excreted intracellularly by the bacteria is not yet known. *Shigella dysenteriae*
type 1, however, is known to produce an enterotoxin that is cytotoxic for Hela cells. In addition, a second cytoxic fraction with different
physical properties has been discovered in the
crude enterotoxin preparations. It is not known
whether this second cytotoxic molecule represents a subunit of the enterotoxin or is a separate entity. No toxins have yet been isolated
from other *Shigella* species, but the severity of
disease caused by other shigella is much less
than that of the disease caused by *S. dysenteriae* type 1.

The enterotoxic fractions appear to be the
same as the neurotoxin described in earlier literature. Like the *E. coli* LT and *V. cholerae*
enterotoxins, the shigella enterotoxin is heat
labile and causes fluid accumulation in ileal
loops of rabbits. It does not activate the adenyl
cyclase system, however, nor does it increase
vascular permeability in rabbit skin. The role of
enterotoxin in bacillary dysentery is not yet
resolved, since nontoxigenic but invasive *S.
dysenteriae* type 1 mutants can cause disease.
In addition, enterotoxin activity occurs primarily in the small intestine, as compared to the
large bowel involvement of the classic bacillary
dysentery. It may be possible that the cytotoxic
properties of the enterotoxin itself and the cytotoxic fraction combined with the intracellular
penetration by the bacteria are responsible for
the increased severity of disease seen with *S.
dysenteriae* type 1.

Clinical Infection

Epidemiology During 1973, 22,000 cases
of shigellosis were reported to the Center for

Disease Control in Atlanta. Of these the majority (60 to 80 percent) of the isolates were *S. sonnei*. *S. flexneri* is the next most frequent isolate
in the United States, and *S. boydii* and *S. dysenteriae* are isolated only rarely in the United
States.

Since animal hosts are lacking, the spread of
shigella is from man to man and the reservoirs
are carriers who shed the organisms in their
feces. From these carriers the shigella can be
spread via flies, fingers, food, or feces. Shigella
can be isolated from clothing, toilet seats, or
water contaminated by infected individuals.
Outbreaks involving many people occur in
closed groups, such as mental hospitals, prison-
er-of-war camps, or in areas where water supplies have been contaminated.

Pathogenesis All *Shigella* species cause
bacillary dysentery, a diarrhea characterized by
watery feces tinged with blood, mucus, and
groups of polymorphonuclear leukocytes.
Studies in healthy volunteers indicate as few as
200 bacilli are needed to produce disease. The
percentage of affected individuals increases as
the number of infecting organisms increases.
The organism enters the small bowel, multiplies, then proceeds to the terminal ileum and
colon, where it penetrates the epithelial cells
and multiplies. This causes inflammation,
sloughing of cells, and superficial ulceration.
Rarely does the organism penetrate the intestinal wall and spread to other parts of the body.
In previously healthy adults spontaneous cure
can occur within two to seven days. In the very
young and old, and in malnourished individuals,
the disease is longer lasting, and the mortality
due to dehydration and electrolyte imbalance is
higher. Rectal prolapse also can occur but is
rare.

Death is most likely to occur in the pediatric
population and when *S. dysenteriae* is the causative organism. A recent epidemic of *S. dysenteriae* in Central America was associated with a
mortality rate in children of 20 to 25 percent.

Laboratory Diagnosis The best specimen
for diagnosis of shigellosis is a rectal swab of an
ulcer taken by sigmoidoscopic examination.
Feces also can be used, but because the shigella are sensitive to the acids present in fecal
material, the time interval between the collection of the specimen and the inoculation of
media is important. Specimens that cannot be

planted immediately should be placed in transport media or buffered glycerol preparations. Serologic typing of isolates is required for complete epidemiologic determination and identification.

Treatment   Because of the self-limiting nature of the disease in its usual settings in the United States most people do not seek treatment. However, the use of antibiotics decreases the severity and mortality of the disease. Ampicillin, tetracycline, and chloramphenicol have been effective, but since resistant forms are being isolated more frequently, accurate sensitivity testing is required. The organisms isolated during the Central American epidemics were resistant to multiple antimicrobials.

Control   Since man represents the major source of organisms, adequate sanitation together with detection and treatment of carriers are the only effective control methods. Vaccines that only raise humoral antibody levels are not effective, presumably because of the local nature of the infection. Oral vaccines that may alter the immune status of the intestine itself are currently being developed and tested. If at all possible, persons with disease should be kept on enteric isolation until cultures are negative. Carriers should be treated and should not be allowed to handle foods. Proper sewage disposal and water chlorination are important measures required for controlling all gram-negative enteropathogens.

SALMONELLA

In contrast to the genus *Shigella*, the genus *Salmonella* is composed of a more complex and diverse group of organisms. They infect many animal species besides man and are capable of invading extraintestinal tissues, causing enteric fevers, the most severe of which is typhoid fever. The genus *Salmonella* is more reactive biochemically and contains over 1,500 antigenic types.

Taxonomy   The Kauffmann-White antigenic scheme for the genus *Salmonella* gives species status to each antigenic type. Ewing and co-workers have proposed that there are only three species of *Salmonella*: *S. cholerae-suis*, *S. typhi*, and *S. enteritidis*, with the other

TABLE 40-2   COMPARISON OF NOMENCLATURE FOR GENUS SALMONELLA

Kauffmann-White	Ewing
S. typhi	S. typhi
S. cholerae-suis	S. cholerae-suis
S. typhimurium	S. enteritidis sero typhimurium
S. derby	S. enteritidis sero derby

antigenic types being serotypes of *S. enteritidis*. A comparison of the two systems is shown in Table 40-2. Further discussion of these schemes is found on page 579. The Ewing scheme currently is being used by the Center for Disease Control.

Physiology

Biochemical and Cultural Characteristics The salmonellas, with the exception of a rare isolate, do not ferment lactose. Most are motile and produce H_2S and gas from glucose fermentation. *S. typhi*, however, does not produce gas from glucose fermentation, and H_2S production may be very slight. Biochemical tests used to differentiate the genus *Salmonella* from the other genera of the tribe Salmonelleae are described in the preceding chapter (Table 39-6). The characteristics used to speciate the genus *Salmonella* are shown in Table 40-3.

Resistance to Physical and Chemical Agents The salmonellas are capable of tolerating relatively large concentrations of bile, a fact that is used in the designing of media for the isolation of these organisms. The members of this genus are typical of the enterics in their resistance to other physical and chemical agents. One species, *S. cholerae-suis*, is used as the standard test organism for phenolic preparations.

Antigenic Structure

The O and H antigens are the major antigens used to type the salmonella. The O antigens are similar to those of other enterobacteria, but the H antigens of salmonella are diphasic. That is, the H antigens can exist in either of two major phases, phase one or specific phase, and phase two or nonspecific phase.

TABLE 40-3 BIOCHEMICAL SPECIATION OF SALMONELLA

Test	S. typhi	S. cholerae-suis	S. enteritidis*
Citrate	−	−	+
Ornithine decarboxylase	+	−	+
Gas from glucose	−	+	+
Trehalose	−	+	+

Adapted from Ewing: Differentiation of Enterobacteriaceae by Biochemical Reactions, Revised. Atlanta, Ga. DHEW Publ. No. (CDC) 74-8270. 1973
°Commonly isolated bioserotypes

The phase one antigens are shared by only a few organisms and react only with homologous antisera, while the phase two antigens are shared by many organisms and will cross-react with heterologous antisera. The numerous antigenic types of salmonella were organized by Kauffmann and White to form a logical classification system that is immensely important for epidemiologic work. According to this scheme the salmonellas are grouped into major groups based on common O antigens. These groups are designated by capital Arabic letters A through I. Subdivision of the major groups into species or serotypes is then accomplished by the determination of the remaining O and H antigens (both phases one and two). Ewing utilizes the same Kauffmann-White antigenic types in his classification scheme. The only difference between the Ewing and the Kauffmann-White systems is that of taxonomy. The Kauffmann-White method designates each antigenic type as a species, whereas the Ewing system designates the same antigenic type as a serotype of *S. enteritidis*.

Because of the great number of possible serotypes only large reference centers are capable of complete serotyping of salmonella isolates. Of all the 1,500 serologic types of salmonella described, however, 38 percent of the serotypes account for 95 percent of all clinical isolates. This greatly simplifies the number of antisera required to identify clinical isolates. Of 500,000 salmonella, Kelterborn reported that group B was responsible for 47 percent of all isolates. Groups C, C_2, D, and E_2 accounted for 13, 7, 24, and 4.4 percent respectively of the remaining isolates.

The capsular antigens play a minor role in the serologic classification of the salmonella but may have important pathogenic significance. The *S. typhi* capsular antigen, the Vi (for virulence) antigen, may play a role in preventing intracellular destruction of the organism. This antigen may be found in other salmonella or other enterics, such as *Citrobacter* or *Escherichia*.

Determinants of Pathogenicity

Like the invasive shigella, virulent salmonella penetrate the epithelial lining of the small bowel. However, unlike the shigella, the salmonella do not merely reside in the epithelial lining but pass directly through the epithelial cells into the subepithelial tissue. The biochemical mechanism of penetration is not known, but the process appears to be similar to phagocytosis. As the bacteria approach the epithelium, the brush border begins to degenerate and the bacteria enter the cell. They are then surrounded by inverted cytoplasmic membranes similar to phagocytic vacuoles. The salmonella pass through the epithelial cells into the lamina propria. Occasionally epithelial penetration occurs at the intercellular junction. After penetration, the organisms are ingested by macrophages, where they multiply readily and may pass to other body sites. Epithelial destruction occurs in later stages of disease, but the mechanism of this destruction is not known.

The ability of the salmonella to survive intracellularly may be due to surface O antigens or, in the case of *S. typhi*, the presence of the Vi antigen. Studies in human volunteers show that those organisms containing Vi antigen are clearly more virulent than those not possessing the antigen. Non-Vi strains, however, are capable of producing disease in volunteers, albeit at a lower rate.

The exact role endotoxin may play in salmonella infection is unclear. As with all enteric endotoxins, endotoxin from salmonella can

cause a variety of effects when injected parenterally into animals. Presumably salmonella
endotoxin could be responsible for fever and
possibly shock during salmonella bacteremia.
However, when endotoxin-tolerant human
volunteers were infected with *S. typhi*, classical symptoms of typhoid fever were seen. It is
possible that the fever observed in these volunteers was due to the endotoxin of the infecting
S. typhi stimulating endogenous pyrogen release from macrophages and polymorphonuclear leukocytes. The nature of the role of endotoxin in disease is further complicated by its
ability to activate the chemotactic properties of
the complement system. The endotoxic stimulation of the chemotactic activity may cause the
localization of leukocytes in the classic enteric
lesions seen in typhoid fever.

To date no enterotoxic substances have been
isolated from any of the salmonella.

Clinical Infection

Epidemiology Salmonellosis probably
represents the largest single communicable
disease problem in the United States today.
During 1974, 21,980 cases of salmonellosis,
excluding typhoid fever, were reported in the
United States. Since most infections are not
reported, however, the actual rate of infection
has been estimated at about 2 million cases per
year.

Contaminated food and water are the mechanisms of transmission for all salmonella, including *S. typhi;* the only difference is the source of
the infection. In *S. typhi* infection (typhoid
fever) the human carrier is the source, whereas
in the other salmonelloses, animals are most
important. The role of proper sewage disposal
and water treatment in control of these diseases
must not be underestimated. The epidemiology of typhoid fever in a migrant worker camp in
Florida in 1974 serves as an example of the
spread of salmonella via contaminated water.
This outbreak of typhoid fever involved a
probable 225 individuals (no deaths) and was
the largest in the United States since 1939. The
source was a suspected typhoid carrier, and the
means of transmission was drinking water from
a well. A faulty sewage system coupled with a
poor well design led to the contamination of
the well water. A nonfunctioning chlorinator
failed to purify the water and contributed to the
epidemic.

Food-borne salmonellosis is quite common,
and for the nontyphoidal types probably constitutes the major source of infection today. *S.
typhi* also can be spread via food, as evidenced
by the infamous Typhoid Mary incident at the
turn of the century which involved a carrier
who was a cook. Recent large-scale typhoid outbreaks in Aberdeen, Scotland (515 cases), and
Germany (344 cases) involved contaminated
corned beef and potato salad, respectively.

Poultry products represent the largest source
of nontyphoid salmonella in the United States.
Meat products are contaminated during slaughter, and those which are improperly cooked or
refrigerated allow the salmonella to proliferate
to the infective dose. Eggs dried by processes
that do not reach a killing temperature have
contaminated cake mixes and other products.

Dogs and other pets harbor salmonella for
long periods. Pet turtles also are sources of
salmonella, and most states either ban the sale
of turtles or require that they be certified as free
of salmonella.

Clinical Manifestations The actual disease process may present as any of three distinct clinical entities: a gastroenteritis, a septicemia with focal lesions, or an enteric fever,
such as typhoid fever.

Gastroenteritis. Salmonella gastroenteritis, like shigellosis, represents an actual
infection of the bowel and usually occurs about
18 hours after ingestion of the organism. The
disease is characterized by diarrhea, fever, and
abdominal pain that is usually self-limiting and
lasts for two to five days. In extreme cases the
symptoms may last for several weeks. In most
cases affected individuals do not seek medical
attention. Dehydration and electrolyte imbalance constitute the major threat to the very
young and old. While the organism can be
isolated from feces for several weeks, the
occurrence of chronic carriers who shed the
organism after one year is rare. Any species of
salmonella can produce the disease, but the
most common cause is *S. enteritidis* serotype
typhimurium.

Septicemia. Salmonella septicemia is
prolonged and characterized by fever, chills,
anorexia, and anemia. Focal lesions may develop in any tissue, producing osteomyelitis,
pneumonia, pulmonary abscesses, meningitis,
or endocarditis. Gastroenteritis is minor or

even absent, and the organism rarely is isolated from the feces. *S. cholerae-suis* is a frequent isolate from this type of disease.

TYPHOID FEVER AND OTHER ENTERIC FEVERS.

The prototype and most severe enteric fever is typhoid fever, and the causative agent is *S. typhi*. Other salmonella, particularly serotypes paratyphi A and paratyphi B, also can cause enteric fevers, but the symptoms are milder and the mortality rate is lower. Man is the only known host for *S. typhi*, and transmission is via food and water contaminated by diseased individuals or carriers. Volunteer studies show that approximately 25 percent of people will become infected upon ingestion of 10^5 viable organisms. The rate of infection becomes 95 percent when the number of organisms is increased to 10^9.

During the first week of infection the symptoms, consisting of fever, lethargy, malaise, and general aches and pains, can be confused with a variety of other illnesses. Constipation rather than diarrhea is the rule. During this time the organism is penetrating the intestinal wall, infecting the regional lymphatics. Some organisms also are carried by the bloodstream to other parts of the reticuloendothelial system. At both sites they are phagocytosed but not killed. After intracellular multiplication, they reenter the bloodstream, causing a prolonged bacteremia. This occurs during the second week of illness. Infection of the biliary system and other tissue also occurs at this time. The patient is severely ill, with fever sustained at about 104F (40C), and is often delirious. The abdomen is very tender and may have rose-colored spots; diarrhea begins in most patients. At this time the organisms are reinfecting the intestinal tract from the gallbladder and may cause necrosis of Peyer's patches. By the third week, patients are exhausted and still febrile but begin to show improvement if no complications occur. Complications include intestinal perforation, severe bleeding, thrombophlebitis, cholecystitis, pneumonia, or abscess formation. The death rate varies from 2 to 10 percent; the lower mortality usually occurs where adequate supportive therapy is available. Relapse may occur in about 10 percent of untreated patients but, since the introduction of antibiotic therapy, is uncommon.

About 3 percent of typhoid patients develop into chronic carriers who serve as sources of future infections. These patients appear to have escarified gallbladders in which the organisms reside. Some studies indicate that these individuals may be deficient in IgM and it is because of this deficiency that they are unable to eliminate the organism.

Infection occurs with equal frequency in both sexes, but women are three to four times more likely to become carriers than men.

Laboratory Diagnosis Isolation of salmonella constitutes a positive laboratory diagnosis of salmonellosis. During the acute stages of gastroenteritis the number of salmonella in feces is large, and the stool represents the specimen of choice. Although the salmonella are not as sensitive to acid conditions as are the shigella, it is still appropriate to buffer the feces if there will be a delay in placing the material in proper cultural media.

Blood cultures represent the best specimen for the detection of septicemia and enteric fevers in the first two weeks of illness. Positive blood cultures will occur in 95 percent of patients with typhoid fever during this time and will decrease to 25 percent or less by the fourth week. Bone marrow cultures may be positive for *S. typhi* after the blood becomes negative. Positive stools are found in only about 25 percent of typhoid patients during the first week but are found in about 85 percent of patients by the third week. Urine may be positive in about 25 percent of patients with typhoid fever. Any other appropriate specimen, such as sputum in the case of pulmonary abscesses, may yield salmonella.

Determination of serum agglutinins (Widal test) also can pinpoint salmonella infections. These serologic tests must be interpreted carefully, however, since cross-reactions with non-salmonella can be obtained.

Treatment Dixon and others have demonstrated that antibiotic treatment of uncomplicated gastroenteritis only serves to prolong the carrier state and may help to promote drug resistance in the salmonella. Treatment should center around supportive therapy and prevention of dehydration and electrolyte imbalance.

In cases of enteric fever or septicemia, ampicillin or chloramphenicol is the drug of choice. In 1972, however, an epidemic in Mexico was caused by a chloramphenicol-resistant strain of *S. typhi*, and ampicillin resistance also occurred in some isolates. The combination of trimethroprim-sulfamethoxazole proved effective in the treatment of these infections. About 50 cases involving these strains were imported into the United States.

Ampicillin, not chloramphenicol, is the drug of choice in treatment of chronic *S. typhi* carriers without gallbladder disease. Cholecystectomy alone produces an 85 percent cure rate of the chronic carrier state and remains the therapy of choice when gallstones or gallbladder disease is present.

Control   Prevention of salmonellosis requires that water standards be kept and that all food should be properly cooked and/or refrigerated. Temperatures below 40F (4.4C) halt salmonella proliferation on foods, while those above 140F (60C) kill the organisms. Efforts also are being made to control salmonella in foods by regulations on slaughterhouses and the use of antibiotics in feeds.

Detection and treatment of carriers, particularly *S. typhi*, constitute a major control mechanism. Utilization of enteric isolation procedures is helpful in preventing spread of these organisms in health care facilities.

Various vaccines have been tried to control typhoid fever. While some encouraging results have been obtained by use of the K vaccine (containing Vi antigen) in children living in endemic areas, no vaccine has proved to be entirely successful in preventing disease, especially when the number of ingested organisms is large.

FURTHER READING

Books and Reviews

Craig JP: The enterotoxic enteropathies. In Smith H, Pearce JP (eds): Symposium 22: Microbiol Pathogenicity in Man and Animals. Cambridge, Cambridge Univ Press, 1972, pp. 129-155

Edwards PR, Ewing WH: Identification of Enterobacteriaceae, 3rd ed. Minneapolis, Burgess, 1972

Hook EW, Johnson WD: Typhoid fever. In Hoeprich PD (ed): Infectious Diseases. Hagerstown, Md, Harper & Row, 1972

Selected Papers

Aberdeen's typhoid bacillus. Lancet 1:645, 1973

Baker EF, Anderson HW, Allard J: Epidemiological aspects of turtle-associated salmonellosis. Arch Environ Health 24:1, 1972

Dixon IMS: Effect of antibiotic treatment on duration of excretion of *Salmonella typhimurium* by children. Br Med J 2:1343, 1965

Ewing WH: Differentiation of Enterobacteriaceae by Biochemical Reactions, Revised. Atlanta, Ga. DHEW Publ No (CDC) 74-8270, 1973

Ewing WH: The nomenclature of Salmonella, its usage, and definitions for the three species. Can J Microbiol 11:1629, 1972

Ewing WH, et al: Biochemical reactions of Shigella. Atlanta, Ga. DHEW Publ No (HSM) 72-8081, 1971

Feldman RE, Baine WB, Nitzkin JL, Saslow MS, Pollard RA Jr: Epidemiology of *Salmonella typhi* infection in migrant labor camp in Dade County, Florida. J Infect Dis 130:334, 1974

Formal SB, Gemske P, Giannella RA, Austin S: Mechanisms of Shigella pathogenesis. Am J Clin Nutr 25:1427, 1972

Grady GF, Keusch GT: Pathogenesis of bacterial diarrheas. Parts 1 and 2. N Engl J Med 285:831, 891, 1971

Hornick RB, Greisman SE, Woodward TE, et al: Typhoid fever: Pathogenesis and immunologic control. N Engl J Med 283:686, 1970

Levine MM, DuPont HL, Formal SB, et al: Pathogenesis of *Shigella dysenteriae* (Shiga) dysentery. J Infect Dis 127:261, 1973

Martin WJ, Ewing WH: Prevalence of serotypes of salmonella. Appl Microbiol 17:111, 1969

Morbidity and Mortality Weekly Report. Follow-up on chloramphenicol-resistant *Salmonella typhi* — Mexico. 22:159, 1973

41
Vibrionaceae

The Eighth Edition of *Bergey's Manual of Determinative Bacteriology* has established a new taxonomic family, the Vibrionaceae. Included in this family are three genera that are of clinical importance, the genus *Vibrio*, the genus *Aeromonas*, and the genus *Plesiomonas*. The majority of clinical infections caused by *Vibrio* species are enteric in nature, ranging from the dread Asiatic cholera to isolated sporadic cases of diarrhea. In contrast, the *Aeromonas* and *Plesiomonas* have been isolated from a variety of other sources, such as blood, spinal fluid, and urine, as well as feces.

All members of this family are gram-negative, facultative organisms and do not have exacting nutritional requirements. Since they can grow on media used for the isolation of the Enterobacteriaceae and may be isolated from similar sources, they can be mistaken for enterobacteria (Chap. 38). In contrast to the enterobacteria, however, all members of the Vibrionaceae are oxidase positive, and when motile, movement is by means of polar rather than peritrichous flagella. Metabolism is both respiratory and fermentative. Additional characteristics for identification may be found in the sections dealing with the individual organisms.

VIBRIO

The genus *Vibrio* contains some of the most important intestinal pathogens of man, including the cause of epidemic asiatic cholera, *Vibrio cholerae*. Another intestinal pathogen, *Vibrio parahaemolyticus*, is the leading cause of diarrhea in Japan and is being isolated more frequently in other parts of the world as laboratories become more familiar with its characteristics. Other vibrios, known variously as "non-

agglutinable vibrios" and "noncholera vibrios," can cause diarrhea in man and occasionally have been associated with limited epidemics.

Taxonomy

Vibrio cholerae Recent advances in taxonomic procedures employing such approaches as numerical taxonomy and DNA base ratio and homology have resulted in a number of taxonomic changes that temporarily may cause confusion among the microbiologist, clinician, and epidemiologist. The major change is the inclusion of the eltor and the nonagglutinable vibrios of medical importance into the species epithet, *Vibrio cholerae*. The species is then further subdivided into biotypes and serotypes. Table 41-1 depicts some of the biochemical properties that distinguish the various biotypes. Additional differential tests are listed in the Eighth Edition of *Bergey's Manual*. One test of major epidemiologic importance reflects the fact that only the biotypes cholerae and eltor, the organisms producing a more devastating disease and widespread epidemics, are capable of agglutinating in the antiserum of O type 1 (p. 586). The inability of the other biotypes to agglutinate in this antisera is responsible for the designation "nonagglutinable vibrios."

Other Vibrios According to the Eighth Edition of *Bergey's Manual* the two species, V. *parahaemolyticus* and V. *alginolyticus*, have been incorporated into a single species V. *parahaemolyticus*. The two former species epithets are used as biotypes of the new species. The microaerophilic vibrios formerly designated V. *fetus* are included in the new genus *Campylo-*

TABLE 41-1   DISTINGUISHING FEATURES OF THE BIOTYPES OF V. CHOLERAE

Test	Cholerae	Eltor	Proteus	Albensis
Agglutination by 0:1 antiserum	+	+	−	−
Tube hemolysis	−	d	+	−
NO$_3$ → NO$_2$	+	+	−	+
Fermentation of sucrose	+	+	+	+
Fermentation of mannose	+	+	+	−
Voges-Proskauer at 22C	−	+	d	+

d = delayed reaction
Adapted from Buchanan and Gibbons (eds): Bergey's Manual of Determinative Bacteriology, 8th ed. 1974. Courtesy of Williams and Wilkins Co

bacter (Chap. 48). The other species in the genus are not clinically important.

Vibrio cholerae

No infection except plague arouses such panic as cholera. The disease is endemic in the Bengal region of India and Bangladesh. From this region it has spread in a wave of pandemics. Since 1817 there have been seven pandemics, the most recent occurring from the early 1960s to the early 1970s and involving the countries of Africa, Western Europe, the Philippines, and other areas of Southeast Asia. This pandemic provided the impetus for research efforts that have been successful in the elucidation of the pathogenic processes of the disease as well as providing significant advancements in treatment. In addition, the work on cholera has provided useful methods and approaches for research into other causes of diarrhea (Chap. 38).

Morphology The cholera vibrios are short (0.5 by 1.5 to 3.0 μm), gram-negative rods that upon initial isolation appear to be comma shaped. In fact, Koch initially named his isolates the "Kommabacillus." Upon serial transfer in the laboratory the organisms revert to straight forms. Motility is by means of a single thick polar flagellum, which in electron micrographs reveals an inner core and an outer sheath. Biotype albensis occasionally may produce lophotrichous forms. Spheroplasts are readily formed in unfavorable environments.

Physiology *Vibrio cholerae* is a facultatively anaerobic organism with an optimum temperature of 18 to 37C. Its metabolism is both respiratory and fermentative, and fermentation is by the mixed acid pathway with no gas production (Chap. 4).

BIOCHEMICAL AND CULTURAL CHARACTERISTICS. Cholera vibrios will grow on simple media providing a utilizable carbohydrate, inorganic nitrogen, sulfur, phosphorus, minerals, and adequate buffering. They grow best at pH 7.0 but can tolerate alkaline conditions to pH 9.5, a property used in the design of isolation media. They are extremely sensitive to an acid pH; a pH of 6.0 or less will sterilize cultures. When grown on meat extract agar, fresh isolates of the organism develop a translucent colonial growth with an iridescent green to red-bronze color when viewed at low magnification with oblique lighting. Older cultures, especially those transferred on laboratory media for a period of time, become opaque and corrugated (rugose variant) or rough. Growth does not occur or is very sparse on common enteric media, such as eosin-methylene blue, Salmonella-Shigella, or brilliant green agars. However, most strains will grow on MacConkey's agar. A variety of media have been developed to aid in primary isolation of the cholera vibrios from clinical specimens. These include tellurite-taurocholate gelatin agar (TTGA) and thiosulfate citrate bile salts (TCBS) agar. Use of these media is discussed on page 588.

Laboratory Diagnosis Although prompt recognition of *V. cholerae* is important and serologic procedures are of prime importance, laboratories in this country are more likely to rely upon biochemical tests for initial identification. Some of the biochemical tests that distinguish *Vibrio cholerae* from related forms are shown in Table 41-2. A variety of tests, such as the string test and darkfield motility test, are useful in the hands of experienced field workers but may cause confusion and misinterpretation in the hands of less experienced laboratory personnel. Historically, the eltor biotypes have been characterized by a positive tube hemolysin test. Technical difficulties with the test procedure, however, and the isolation of hemolysin-negative strains from the seventh pandemic

TABLE 41-2 BIOCHEMICAL PROPERTIES OF VIBRIO CHOLERAE

Test	Reaction
Indophenol oxidase	+
Indol	+
0/129 sensitive	+
Lecithinase	+
Growth without added NaCl	+
Lysine decarboxylase (Moeller's medium)	+
Ornithine decarboxylase "	+
Arginine dihydrolase "	−
Citrate utilization	Varies
Growth at 5C	−
Sucrose fermentation	+
Reaction on triple sugar iron (TSI)	A/A No gas

Adapted from Buchanan and Gibbons (eds): Bergey's Manual of Determinative Bacteriology, 8th ed. 1974. Courtesy of Williams and Wilkins Co

have lessened the importance of this test in differentiating the eltor from the cholerae biotype. The tests currently of value in distinguishing these two biotypes are listed in Table 41-3. As with most *Vibrio*, the cholera vibrios are sensitive to 0/129 (2,4 diamine-6,7-diisopropyl pteridine), a trait which aids in their separation from other oxidase-positive, gram-negative rods.

TABLE 41-3   BIOCHEMICAL DIFFERENTIATION OF SEROTYPE 0:1 VIBRIO CHOLERAE

Test	Biotype	
	Cholerae	Eltor
Voges-Proskauer test at 22C	−	+
Chicken erythrocyte agglutination	−	+
Polymyxin B sensitivity 50 IU	+	−
Group IV cholera phage sensitivity	+	−

Antigenic Structure   The O or somatic antigens constitute the antigens of major importance in the serologic grouping of the cholera vibrios. All cholera vibrios appear to share the same H antigen. The majority of strains are classified into six antigenic O groups. Serogroup O type 1(0:1) contains the biotypes cholerae and eltor. Three antigenic factors, A, B, and C, are used to subdivide the 0:1 into the serotypes ogawa, inaba, and hikojima. Table 41-4 depicts the combinations of A, B, C antigens found in the serotypes 0:1. The biotypes, eltor and cholerae, of serogroup 0:1 are causative agents of classic cholera, and the isolation of this serogroup from feces has important significance both to the individual patient and to the community at large (p. 587). The other serogroups are associated with milder forms of disease with apparently limited epidemic potential.

TABLE 41-4   ANTIGENIC DETERMINATES OF SEROGROUP 0:1

Serotype	O factors
Ogawa	AB
Inaba	AC
Hikojima	ABC

Conversion among the serotypes ogawa, inaba, and hikojima can occur both in experimental animals and in natural infection. Serologic conversion appears to be related to the appearance of agglutinating antibody in the serum.

Immunochemical studies on the lipopolysaccharide from an inaba strain reveal an absence of KDO (2-keto-3-deoxyoctonate) in the inner core polysaccharide, showing a fundamental difference between the families Vibrionaceae and Enterobacteriaceae. Further studies are required before the nature of the lipopolysaccharide can be determined.

Determinants of Pathogenicity   The important clinical features of cholera are the result of host reaction to an extracellular enterotoxin. De and Chatterje were the first to describe the experimental model using ligated intestinal loops of rabbits, which led to the discovery of the enterotoxin and opened the way for research into the pathogenesis of other gastrointestinal diseases. Purification and subsequent characterization of the enterotoxin have revealed that the enterotoxin (choleragen) is a protein of about 84,000 daltons with little or no carbohydrate or lipid. Spontaneous conversion into toxoid (choleragenoid) can occur. The enterotoxin appears to consist of two peptides of 56,000 and 28,000 daltons, while the toxoid consists of a single peptide of 56,000 daltons. Recent experimental evidence shows that the 28,000-dalton peptide may represent an aggregate of smaller fragments that can be integrated into the formation of toxoid.

The enterotoxins produced by the various serotypes and biotypes appear to be homogeneous, in contrast to *E. coli* enterotoxin (Chap. 39). Like the LT of *E. coli*, however, it stimulates the adenyl cyclase system of cells in the small intestine to produce cyclic AMP, which in turn results in the loss of fluid and electrolytes. The effect of toxin appears to be a stimulation of existing enzymes rather than synthesis of new enzymes. The mechanism by which cyclic AMP causes such fluid loss has not yet been determined. The enterotoxin is active in a number of other test systems, such as rabbit skin permeability, tissue culture cytotoxicity, fat cell lipase stimulation, and mouse foot edema. The mechanism of action of enterotoxin in these systems also seems to be a result of cyclic AMP stimulation. These various tests have proven to be useful in the elucidation of enterotoxin mode of action and have provided insight into the physiology of enterotoxin stimulation.

Clinical Infection EPIDEMIOLOGY. Organisms of the serotype 0:1 (biotypes cholerae and eltor) are capable of causing widespread disease involving large numbers of people. A 1947 epidemic in Egypt involved 33,000 cases with 20,000 deaths. The most recent pandemic has spread to 60 countries and affected 171,329 persons.

The human carrier serves as the source of new cases of cholera. He sheds large numbers of organisms in his feces, which contaminate water and food supplies. Two types of carriers exist, the convalescent and the chronic carrier. The convalescent carrier or individual recovering from the disease is usually under 50 years of age and sheds the organism for several months to one year after his illness. The chronic carrier, on the other hand, is usually over 50 years of age and more difficult to detect. The chronic carrier appears to carry the organisms in the gallbladder and only sheds them intermittently. The shedding occurs during natural purging that may result from noncholera intestinal infection. The purging action apparently lowers the natural antagonism of the large bowel for the vibrios and allows them to survive passage to the outside. Detection of such carriers requires careful epidemiologic follow-up on the index cases because most chronic carriers are members of the household of the index case. Daily rectal cultures or induced purging may be required to detect the carrier. The carrier rate in endemic regions can vary from 1 in 300 to 20 percent.

The spread of the organism from the endemic areas to new areas is greatly facilitated by the freedom of modern international travel and the presence of carriers. During an East Pakistan (Bangladesh) epidemic involving both eltor and cholerae biotypes, Bart and co-workers found that the clinical case rate to infection rate was 1:36 for the eltor and 1:4 for the cholerae biotype. In addition to revealing a higher potential for disease with the cholerae biotype, this study demonstrates how the disease can spread via nonsymptomatic carriers.

The role of animals, however, in the spread of cholera has been minimized. It was recently reported that serotype 0:1 organisms were found in domesticated animals during periods of human infection. It has been suggested that in the absence of human carriers intermittent excretion of vibrios from cows and chickens may serve as a source of new infections. In addition, contaminated shellfish have served as sources of new cases.

PATHOGENESIS AND CLINICAL MANIFESTATIONS. Classic Asiatic cholera is one of the most devastating diseases known to man. The incubation period may be hours or days, with a mean of two to three days. The onset is abrupt, with vomiting and diarrhea. Fluid loss in severe cases approaches 15 to 20 liters per day. The voided fluid is watery, without traces of odor or enteric organisms, and contains no protein but is high in sodium, potassium, bicarbonate, and chloride. Hypovolemic shock and metabolic acidosis are consequences of this fluid loss. By the time the patient reaches the hospital his eyes and cheeks are sunken, skin turgor is diminished, and his hands have a washerwoman appearance. Usually the voice is low and hoarse. The untreated case fatality rate is over 60 percent, and higher attack rates are seen in children. There are also significant differences in the incidence of hospitalized cases compared with milder forms of the disease with respect to the biotype of the infecting agent—a higher disease rate is associated with the cholerae biotype.

The nonagglutinable vibrios can cause isolated as well as focal outbreaks of diarrhea. However, the volume of fluid loss does not approach that of classic cholera, and the disease is usually self-limiting.

The organisms remain in the intestinal tract in both types of disease, and the epithelial lining of the intestine appears to remain intact. Earlier studies that described desquamated or sloughed intestinal epithelium probably resulted from a delay in postmortem examination of victims residing in tropical climates.

LABORATORY DIAGNOSIS. The laboratory diagnosis of cholera depends upon the isolation and identification of *V. cholerae*. Immunologic studies using acute and convalescent sera are useful in retrospective epidemiologic studies. Since *V. cholerae* are susceptible to desiccation and acidic conditions, vomitus, stool, and rectal swabs should be cultured quickly or placed in a suitable transport medium. The Amies' and Cary-Blair modifications of Stuart's transport medium make excellent holding media for the preservation of the sample, as does feces-soaked blotter paper stored in airtight plastic bags.

Upon arrival in the laboratory, the specimen should be placed on a nonselective medium, a selective medium, and an enrichment broth. Nutrient agar or taurocholate gelatin agar (TCGA) are excellent nonselective media and are useful for visualization of the iridescent qualities of V. cholerae colonies illuminated with transmitted oblique lighting. V. cholerae colonies are also surrounded by cloudy zones of hydrolyzed gelatin on TCGA. Thiosulfate citrate bile salts medium (TCBS) is excellent for the isolation of V. cholerae. Yellow colonies (sucrose fermenting) which are oxidase positive should be subjected to identification procedures. However, suspected V. cholerae colonies growing on TCBS should be subcultured to a nonselective medium before serologic procedures are performed. This eliminates the dangers of misinterpretation that can occur using TCBS. Alkaline peptone (pH 8.5) broth incubated six to eight hours is a good enrichment broth for isolation of V. cholerae. Overnight incubation of the broth is also acceptable if the six-to-eight-hour incubation cannot be accomplished. Subcultures of the broth are made to the same media as the initial stool culture.

During recent cholera outbreaks in Calcutta and the Philippines, direct fluorescent antibody procedures on stools provided over 90 percent correlation with cultural methods in patients with acute diarrhea. Such procedures, however, were not useful in the detection of carrier states.

TREATMENT. Recent advances in the treatment of cholera have resulted in a marked drop in mortality rate to less than 1 percent. Prompt replacement of fluid and electrolyte losses causes a rapid response and reversal of the patient's condition within a matter of hours. Initial shock symptoms are treated with intravenous fluids that provide 133 mEq of sodium, 98 mEq of chloride, 13 mEq of potassium, and 48 mEq of bicarbonate per liter of pyrogen-free water. After initial recovery, fluid and electrolyte balance can be maintained with an oral solution of glucose and electrolytes. The oral therapy thus eliminates the need for large volumes of pyrogen-free solutions and is a direct result of research that showed that the absorptive powers of the colon remain intact during

the disease. Oral therapy also can be administered by paramedical personnel, a significant advantage in the rural areas of undeveloped countries. Tetracycline, although not directly affecting the enterotoxin, lowers the number of infecting organisms and thereby reduces the fluid loss by almost 60 percent. Also, because of its concentration in the bile, tetracycline aids in eliminating the carrier state.

PREVENTION AND CONTROL. The primary defense in the control of cholera is the maintenance of adequate sewage treatment and water purification systems, together with the prompt detection and treatment of cases and carriers. In countries with adequate sanitation, cholera is limited to imported cases. Paradoxically, the single case of cholera in the United States since 1911 occurred in a Texas man who did not leave this country or knowingly have contact with any carrier. Extensive epidemiologic studies failed to reveal a source of this infection. No other cases were found at the time of the initial infection, nor have any subsequent cases occurred. The fact that this infection did not spread to others is attributed to astute primary clinical observation, laboratory confirmation, and prompt action by local authorities.

Travelers to countries with known cholera are cautioned against eating uncooked vegetables, unpeeled fruits, and raw seafood and drinking unbottled beverages. Swimming should be done at beaches not contaminated with human sewage.

The present pandemic has illustrated that the current vaccines do not afford significant protection against disease, especially if large numbers of organisms are ingested. Trial toxoid vaccines were discontinued when a formalinized preparation partially reverted to toxin and caused reactions at the inoculation site. Some degree of protection appeared to be afforded to the volunteers in this study. Further work on the characterization of the toxin-toxoid are required before clinical effectiveness is attained. Currently, efforts are being made to develop an oral toxoid-attenuated organism vaccine. At present United States travelers to foreign countries are not required to have valid cholera vaccine certification.

The role of quarantine measures has been questioned, especially in view of the failure of such measures to control the spread of the current pandemic. The usefulness of tetracycline prophylaxis is also limited and not recommended. In endemic areas the major control measure remains the prompt detection and treatment of asymptomatic carriers.

Vibrio parahaemolyticus

Vibro parahaemolyticus is a marine organism that inhabits estuaries throughout the world. Its role in human disease was not recognized until 1951. Since that time efforts, primarily by the Japanese, have revealed that biotype parahaemolyticus is a major cause of gastroenteritis involving seafood. In addition, both biotypes parahaemolyticus and alginolyticus have been isolated from infections of the extremities, eyes, and ears of individuals in contact with the marine environment.

Morphology and Physiology *V. parahaemolyticus* resembles the other vibrio species in its structural and staining characteristics. The metabolism of the organism is both fermentative and respiratory, with no gas produced during fermentation.

CULTURAL CHARACTERISTICS. *V. parahaemolyticus* resembles *V. cholerae* in its simple nutritional requirements and preference for an alkaline environment. Optimum growth occurs between pH 7.6 and 9.0. This permits the use of the same selective media as used for the isolation of *V. cholerae.* Unlike the cholera vibrios, however, members of this species are halophilic (salt-loving) and require at least 2 percent NaCl for growth. Biotype alginolyticus can even tolerate 11 percent NaCl, a property

useful in its differentiation from biotype parahaemolyticus. Salt requirements can be satisfied by the addition to the medium of two or three drops of a sterile 20 to 30 percent solution of NaCl. When provided with the appropriate conditions for growth, the generation time of this species is 9 to 15 minutes, a property of considerable importance in the epidemiology of gastroenteritis (p. 590).

BIOCHEMICAL CHARACTERISTICS. On TCBS (thiosulfate citrate bile salts) medium, biotype parahaemolyticus produces a large green (nonsucrose-fermenting), smooth colony, while biotype alginolyticus (not a cause of diarrhea) will appear yellow because of its fermentation of sucrose. Typical colonies giving oxidase-positive reactions should be inoculated into the media listed in Table 41-5 for identification.

Antigenic Structure The O and K antigens are useful for the serologic typing of *V. parahaemolyticus.* Currently there are 11 O types and 57 K types recognized. No particular serotype appears to be more prevalent or more virulent than any other serotype.

Determinants of Pathogenicity When injected into the ileal loops of rabbits, cultures of biotype parahaemolyticus cause an outpouring of fluid similar to that seen in cholera or in *E. coli* gastroenteritis. There is little or no change in the lining of the intestine. To date no enterotoxin has been isolated. However, over 95 percent of gastroenteritis isolates give a positive Kanagawa hemolysis test, whereas isolates from other infections or from the environment

TABLE 41-5 CHARACTERISTICS OF MARINE VIBRIOS

Test or Medium*	Biotype parahaemolyticus	Biotype alginolyticus	Other Marine Vibrios
Triple sugar iron agar	Alkaline/acid	Acid/acid	Either acid/acid or alkaline/acid
Voges-Proskauer	Negative	Positive	Varies
Sucrose fermentation	Negative	Positive	Varies
Peptone (NoNaCl)	0†	0	0
Peptone (3–7% NaCl)	Growth	Growth	Growth
Peptone (11% NaCl)	No growth	Growth	No growth
Lysine decarboxylase	100	100	50
Arginine dihydrolase	0	0	50
Ornithine decarboxylase	80-90	50	10
Cholera red test	96	90	10

*Unless stated otherwise, all media are supplemented with 3% NaCl
†Numbers refer to percentage of strains giving positive reactions

do not. The Kanagawa hemolysis test detects the presence of a heat-stable hemolysin that lyses human or rabbit erythrocytes but not horse erythrocytes. Human volunteer studies indicate that Kanagawa-negative strains are incapable of producing symptoms regardless of infecting dose, whereas 10^5 to 10^7 Kanagawa-positive organisms will produce classic symptoms within 12 hours. The precise relationship of the hemolysin to the enteropathogenic symptoms is not known.

Clinical Infection EPIDEMIOLOGY. Gastroenteritis follows the ingestion of contaminated seafood. In Japan V. *parahaemolyticus* causes over 50 percent of diarrhea during the summer. Its presence in other parts of the world is becoming more apparent as laboratories and clinicians become aware of this organism. In the United States in the period 1969-1972, there have been 13 outbreaks involving approximately 1,200 individuals. Two of these outbreaks were caused by raw seafood inadequately refrigerated. Seafood cooked for an inadequate time followed by inadequate refrigeration, and cooked seafood cross-contaminated with raw seafood accounted for the other 11 outbreaks. In Japan the disease is most commonly associated with the eating of suski, a vinegared riceball topped with fish. When suski is eaten in shops, the disease rarely occurs, but when it is delivered to the home, the same preparation can cause diarrhea. The delay in transit coupled with the rapid generation time of the organism apparently permits the number of ingested bacteria to reach a minimal infective dose.

CLINICAL MANIFESTATIONS. Gastroenteritis ranges from a self-limiting diarrhea to a choleralike illness. Diarrhea is explosive and watery with no blood or mucus, although shigellalike disease has been reported in India, Japan, and Australia. Headache and fever may be present. Symptoms may persist for as long as 10 days, but the median is 72 hours, and a few individuals require hospitalization. In contrast to V. *cholerae* there is a fatty infiltration and cloudy swelling in livers of patients infected with V. *parahaemolyticus*. Localized infections may be produced by both biotypes.

LABORATORY DIAGNOSIS. Feces and rectal swabs should be cultured quickly or placed into a suitable transport medium (Cary-Blair or Amies'). Specimens should be inoculated into TCBS and alkaline peptone broth (pH 8.5) supplemented with 3 percent NaCl. After overnight incubation alkaline peptone broth is subcultured to TCBS, and final identification is made as discussed on page 589. Sucrose-positive organisms that are oxidase positive should be checked to rule out the possibility of V. *cholerae*. Positively identified isolates of biotype parahaemolyticus should be reported to local health authorities for investigation of possible outbreaks of diarrhea.

Such persons as boat workers, seafood cooks, or swimmers who develop localized infections after contact with a marine environment should submit appropriate specimens for isolation and identification of both biotypes of V. *parahaemolyticus*. Close cooperation between the laboratory and clinical personnel is required to ensure that proper isolation procedures are followed.

TREATMENT.   Since the gastroenteritis produced by this organism usually is self-limiting, most cases are not treated. In severe cases, however, fluid and electrolyte replacement should be given and antibiotics administered. The organisms are usually sensitive to chloramphenicol, kanamycin, tetracycline, and the cephalothins.

CONTROL.   The ubiquitous nature of V. *parahaemolyticus* prevents its removal from the environment. Control measures are aimed at keeping the number of organisms present in seafood below the minimal infective dose. Refrigeration of seafood eaten raw is absolutely essential. Cooked seafood that is served chilled, such as crab or shrimp, must not come in contact with the organism and also should be refrigerated. An outbreak involving crabs resulted when cooked crabs were returned to their original containers and stored in a basement until the following day. Similarly, shrimp cooked and stored at ambient temperature resulted in a major outbreak in Louisiana.

AEROMONAS

The genus *Aeromonas* contains several species, all of which are found free-living in

TABLE 41-6 BIOCHEMICAL CHARACTERISTICS OF AEROMONAS HYDROPHILIA AND PLESIOMONAS SHIGELLOIDES

Tests or Substrates	A. hydrophilia*	P. shigelloides*
Indol phenol oxidase	100	98
H₂S	0	0
Glucose fermentation	100	100
Lactose fermentation	9	65
Mannitol fermentation	99	0
Inositol	0	100
Lysine decarboxylase	0	96
Ornithine decarboxylase	0	50
Arginine dihydrolase	75	93
Simmons' citrate	52	0
Voges-Proskauer	33	0

Numbers indicate percentage of strains giving positive reactions.
Adapted from Ewing and Hugh: Aeromonas. In Lennette, Spaulding, and Truant (eds): Manual of Clinical Microbiology, 2nd ed. 1974. Courtesy of American Society for Microbiology

water. Most are pathogens for cold-blooded animals and have not been incriminated in human disease. One species, however, *Aeromonas hydrophilia*, is a well-documented pathogen of man, causing septicemia, osteomyelitis, and wound infections. It has also been isolated from cases of diarrhea and from the urine of asymptomatic individuals. Most infections are seen in persons with debilitating diseases, particularly neoplasms.

Aeromonas hydrophilia grows quite readily on media used for the Enterobacteriaceae and is often misidentified as an enteric bacillus. In contrast to the enteric bacilli, *Aeromonas hydrophilia* is oxidase positive and possesses a single polar flagellum. The distinguishing biochemical reactions are listed in Table 41-6. Most isolates are sensitive to gentamicin, tetracycline, and chloramphenicol and are resistant to ampicillin and cephalothins.

PLESIOMONAS

Plesimonas shigelloides is classified by some taxonomists as an *Aeromonas* and in some medical literature is referred to as *Aeromonas shigelloides*. In man this organism has been isolated from the blood and spinal fluid and has been incriminated in gastroenteritis. Like *Aeromonas hydrophilia* this organism can be confused with the Enterobacteriaceae. Its biochemical characteristics are listed in Table 41-6.

FURTHER READING

Books and Reviews

Craig JP: The enterotoxic enteropathies. In Smith H, Pearce JH (eds): Microbial Pathogenicity in Man and Animals. London, Cambridge Univ Press, 1972, pp. 129-155

Ewing WH, Hugh R: Aeromonas. In Lennette EH, Spaulding EH, Truant JP (eds): Manual of Clinical Microbiology, 2nd ed. Washington, DC, American Society for Microbiology, 1974, pp. 230-237

Feeley JC, Balows A: Vibrio. In Lennette EH, Spaulding EH, Truant JP (eds): Manual of Clinical Microbiology, 2nd ed. Washington, DC, American Society for Microbiology, 1974, pp 238-245

Finkelstein RA: Cholera. CRC Crit Rev Microbiol 2:533, 1973

Sanyal SC, Sen PC: Human volunteer studies on pathogenicity of *Vibrio parahaemolyticus*. International Symposium on *Vibrio parahaemolyticus*. Tokyo, Japan, Saukon Publishing Co, 1973, pp 227-230

Schubert RHW: Aeromonas. In Buchanan RE, Gibbons NE (eds): Bergey's Manual of Determinative Bacteriology, 8th ed. Baltimore, Williams & Wilkins, 1974, pp 345-449

Shewan JM, Veron M: Vibrio. In Buchanan RE, Gibbons NE (eds): Bergey's Manual of Determinative Bacteriology, 8th ed. Baltimore, Williams & Wilkins, 1974, pp 340-345

Selected Papers

Carpenter CJ: Cholera and other enterotoxin-related diseases. J Infect Dis 125:551, 1972

Feeley JC, Oseasohn RO (eds): Workshop on the immunology of cholera. Williamsburg, Va. J Infect Dis 121 (Suppl): May 1970, pp S1-S150

Gangarosa EJ, Barker WH: Cholera implications for the United States. JAMA 227:170, 1974

MacKenzie DJM. Cholera: Whither prevention? Med Clin North Am 51:625, 1967

McCormak WM, Islam S, Fahimuddin, Mosley WH: A community study of inapparent cholera infections. Am J Epidemiol 89:658, 1969

Morbidity and Mortality Weekly Report. *Vibrio parahaemolyticus* gastroenteritis — United States, 1969-1972. 22:231, 1973

Smith MR: *Vibrio parahaemolyticus.* Clin Med 78:22, 1971

Von Graevenitz A, Mensch AH: The genus *Aeromonas* in human bactriology. N Engl J Med 278:245, 1968

Weissman JB, DeWitt WE, Thompson J, et al: A case of cholera in Texas, 1973. Am J Epidemiol 100:487, 1975

Zen-Yoji H, LeClair RA, Ohta K, Montague TS: Comparison of *Vibrio parahaemolyticus* cultures isolated in the United States with those isolated in Japan. J Infect Dis 127:237, 1973

42
Pseudomonas

The genus *Pseudomonas* is composed of a large number of nonfermentative, aerobic, gram-negative rods that inhabit the soil and water. In their natural habitat these widely distributed organisms play an important role in the decomposition of organic matter. Several species are major plant pathogens, while others can infect animals. A few are pathogenic for both plants and animals. While most *Pseudomonas* species do not infect man, some are important opportunistic pathogens that infect individuals with impaired host defenses. Such human infections usually are severe, difficult to treat, and are hospital acquired (nosocomial).

PSEUDOMONAS AERUGINOSA

The *Pseudomonas* species most frequently associated with human disease is *P. aeruginosa*. In some hospitals this organism causes 10 to 20 percent of the nosocomial infections. It has replaced *Staphylococcus aureus* as the major pathogen of cystic fibrosis patients and is frequently isolated from individuals with neoplastic disease or severe burns.

Morphology and Ultrastructure

P. aeruginosa is a gram-negative rod, 0.5 to 1.0 by 3.0 to 4.0 μm. It usually possesses a single polar flagellum, but occasionally two or three flagella may be produced. When grown in the absence of sucrose, an extracellular polysaccharide slime layer, similar to a capsule, is produced.

The cell wall structure of *P. aeruginosa* is similar to that of the Enterobacteriaceae (Chap. 38 and Fig. 38-1). The inner core of *P. aeruginosa* lipopolysaccharide (LPS) contains KDO (2-keto-3-deoxyoctonic acid), as do the enteric bacilli, but the side-chains of the *P. aeruginosa* LPS contain amino sugars rather than the neutral sugars found in the enterobacteria LPS. Also, lipid A of *P. aeruginosa* LPS lacks β-hydroxymyristic acid.

Strains isolated from clinical specimens frequently possess pili that may promote attachment to cell surfaces and may play a role in resistance to phagocytosis.

Physiology

Biochemical and Cultural Characteristics *P. aeruginosa* is an extremely adaptable organism that can utilize over 80 different organic compounds for growth, and ammonia can serve as a nitrogen source. *P. aeruginosa* will grow on media used for the isolation of the enterobacteria, and its ability to tolerate alkaline conditions also permits it to grow on vibrio isolation media. Although an aerobic organism, *P. aeruginosa* can utilize nitrate as an electron acceptor and grow anaerobically. A temperature of 35C is optimal for growth, but growth can occur at 42C. Clinical isolates grown on blood agar are frequently beta hemolytic.

P. aeruginosa is the only *Pseudomonas* species that produces the chloroform-soluble pigment, pyocyanin, although a number of strains of this species do not produce this phenazine pigment. The use of specialized media (Pseudomonas P agar) enhances pigment production. In addition to pyocyanin a number of water-soluble fluorescent pigments also may be produced. These pigments can be detected in the tissue of burn patients as well as in culture by the use of a Wood's light. A few strains also produce a red pigment.

Energy from carbohydrates is derived by oxidative rather than fermentative metabolism. Since the acid produced by the oxidative pathway is less than that produced by other organisms using a fermentative pathway, carbohydrate utilization by *P. aeruginosa* as well as by other nonfermentative bacteria must be tested for in the O-F medium of Hugh and Leifson. The carbohydrate reactions listed in Table 42-1 are based upon reactions in this basal medium. Also listed in Table 42-1 are useful biochemical reactions for the identification of *P. aeruginosa* and other medically important *Pseudomonas* species.

Resistance *P. aeruginosa* is more resistant to chemical disinfection than are other vegetative bacteria. When adequate moisture is provided, it can survive in a variety of places, such as respiratory care equipment, cold-water humidifiers, instruments, bedpans, floors, baths, and water faucets. Most of the commonly used antibiotics and antimicrobials are ineffective against *Pseudomonas* (p. 000). It has been isolated from certain types of quaternary am-

TABLE 42-1 SOME CHARACTERISTICS OF PSEUDOMONAS SPECIES ENCOUNTERED IN CLINICAL SPECIMENS*

Test or Substrate	P. aeruginosa	P. cepacia	P. maltophilia	P. mallei	P. pseudomallei	P. putida	P. stutzeri	P. alcaligenes	P. fluorescens
Indo phenol oxidase	100	90	0	67	100	100	100	100	100
Glucose oxidation	100	100	56	100	100	100	100	0	100
Maltose oxidation	0	100	100	0	96	35	100	0	70
Lactose oxidation	0	100	0	17	100	28	0	0	26
Mannitol oxidation	81	100	0	0	100	19	89	0	94
2-Ketogluconate	100	12	0	0	0	74	2	—	70
Nitrate to gas	94	0	0	0	85	0	100	0	2
Pyocyanin production	58	0	0	0	0	0	0	0	0
Lysine decarboxylase	0	93	20	0	0	0	0	0	0
Ornithine decarboxylase	0	29	0	0	0	0	0	0	0
Arginine dihydrolase	96	0	0	83	100	97	0	8	98
Growth at 42C	100	71	10	0	100	0	100	0	70

Adapted from Hugh and Gilardi: In Lennette, Spaulding, and Truant (eds): Manual of Clinical Microbiology, 2nd ed. 1974. Courtesy of American Society for Microbiology
*Numbers equal percentage of strains yielding positive reactions

monium compounds and from hexachlorophene soaps. Phenolics and beta glutaraldehyde are usually effective disinfectants against it. Boiling water kills the organisms, as does complete desiccation.

Genetics Gene transfer between strains of *P. aeruginosa* can occur through conjugation and transduction (Chap. 8). Resistance to at least one antibiotic, carbenicillin, can be genetically transferred via an R factor. Strain differences can be detected by serologic typing, phage typing, and pyocin (bacteriocin) typing.

Antigenic Structure

The O, or somatic, antigen of *P. aeruginosa* has been used to group various strains for epidemiologic purposes. Several antigenic schema using the O antigen are currently in use. These include the schema of Verder and Evans, Habs, Lanyi, and of Fischer. In spite of the number of schema proposed, serologic typing of the O antigen provides a less cumbersome and less variable system of epidemiologic characterization than does pyocin or phage typing. Bacteriophage and pyocin typing, however, may be necessary for complete characterization of *Pseudomonas* strains isolated during an epidemic. At present, an international study group is attempting to establish a serotyping method based upon specific somatic antigens.

The slime layer of *Pseudomonas* is also im-

munogenic and may play a role in protecting the bacterial cell from phagocytosis. Active and passive immunization against this slime material can protect mice from the toxic and lethal effects of challenge in live bacteria.

Determinants of Pathogenicity

The mechanism by which *P. aeruginosa* produces disease in man is not understood. A number of enzymes and toxins, in addition to slime and endotoxin, cause pathologic effects in animals, but their role in human disease has not been determined.

At least two types of proteases are produced by *P. aeruginosa*. They may be responsible for the hemorrhagic skin lesions observed in some infections, and in *P. aeruginosa* eye infections they may cause the destruction of corneal tissue. No lethal effect, however, appears to be associated with them.

Two hemolysins, one of which is a phospholipase and the other a glycolipid, are produced. They have no lethal activity, but in *P. aeruginosa* pneumonia the phospholipase may contribute to the invasiveness of the organism by destroying the pulmonary surfactant and attacking the pulmonary tissue to produce atelectasis and necrosis.

At least three exotoxins, A, B, and C, which are lethal for mice and dogs and which cause hypotensive shock in monkeys, have been identified. Exotoxin A has been isolated and partially characterized, and it appears to be a protein. It does not, however, affect phagocytic capabilities, nor does it cause necrosis of the skin. The production of these lethal toxins in vivo is unpredictable, and their role in human disease has not been determined. In addition to the enzymes and exotoxins, the pigment pyocyanin may contribute to the overall disease process through its effect on the oxygen uptake of tissue cells, including leukocytes. An enterotoxin has been recently discovered and may be responsible for diarrhea associated with *P. aeruginosa* intestinal infection.

Clinical Infection

Epidemiology   *P. aeruginosa* infections occur in individuals with altered host defenses. These include burn patients, persons with malignant or metabolic disease, or those who have had prior instrumentation or manipulation. The frequency of urinary tract infections is higher in individuals with advanced age. Prolonged treatment with immunosuppressive or antimicrobial drugs and radiation therapy also predispose individuals to *Pseudomonas* infections.

The ubiquitous nature of *P. aeruginosa* enhances its spread. It is not only present in soil and water but is found in approximately 10 percent of normal stools and on the skin of some normal individuals. Almost any site in the hospital environment may harbor the organism, especially if moisture is present. Contaminated respiratory equipment, catheters, instruments, intravenous fluids, and even soap are vehicles for its spread. Transmission from patient to patient via hospital personnel is more significant in spreading the organism throughout a hospital unit than is airborne spread. A nationwide epidemiologic surveillance of community hospital infection reveals that *P. aeruginosa* is responsible for 10 percent of nosocomial infections seen, 11 percent of all blood isolates, and about 4 percent of nosocomial epidemics. In specialized units, such as burn or cancer centers, *P. aeruginosa* may cause 30 percent of all infections.

Pathogenesis and Clinical Manifestations
P. aeruginosa can infect almost any tissue or body site. Localized lesions occur at site of burns or wounds, in corneal tissue, the urinary tract, or lungs. Bacterial endocarditis and gastroenteritis also can be caused by *P. aeruginosa*. Infection of corneal tissue may result in loss of the eye. From a localized infection the organisms may spread via the hematogenous route, producing a septicemia and focal lesions in other tissues. With septicemia the mortality rate may reach 80 percent. In *Pseudomonas* pneumonias, patients present with toxicity, confusion, and progressive cyanosis. Empyema is common. X-rays reveal infiltrates in the lower lobes that are nodular and may necrose, with abscess formation. The mortality is high in *Pseudomonas* pneumonia. The major body defense against *Pseudomonas* infection appear to be a functioning phagocytic system. In patients with leukemia, mortality is highest when patients become severely leukopenic. In patients with cystic fibrosis, the organisms are frequently encapsulated, which may prevent their phagocytosis.

Laboratory Diagnosis   A diagnosis is made by isolation of the organism. *P. aeruginosa* will grow on almost any of the laboratory media in use today. Isolation from properly collected and transported clinical specimens does not require any unusual procedures. Properties useful in the identification of the organism are listed in Table 42-1.

Treatment   Most antimicrobial agents are ineffective for the treatment of *P. aeruginosa* infections. A majority of the strains are susceptible to gentamicin, tobramycin, and colistin, but resistant forms develop, especially during long-term treatment. Approximately 50 percent of *P. aeruginosa* are sensitive to carbenicillin. Gentamicin and carbenicillin appear to act synergistically in vivo, and combination therapy with these two drugs is recommended in life-threatening situations. The antibiotics should not be mixed prior to injection, since in vitro inactivation occurs. Sulfamylon applied topically limits the bacterial density in burns and prevents spread of the organisms to other body sites.

A heptavalent vaccine has been developed (Pseudogen) that has proved effective in burn patients in decreasing the incidence of pseudomonas bacteremia and the resulting high mortality. When Pseudogen was administered concurrently with hyperimmune gamma globulin, no deaths were seen in 186 vaccinated individuals. Maximum tolerable levels of vaccine must be given before effects are observed. Little or no benefit has been obtained by use of the vaccine in cystic fibrosis patients, and the role of vaccine in cancer patients has not been completely evaluated. Granulocyte transfusions may prove useful in the treatment of granulocytopenic individuals.

Control The spread of *P. aeruginosa* is enhanced by failure to observe proper isolation procedures, handwashing techniques, disinfection, and guidelines for care of catheters and respiratory equipment. Hospital surveillance and access to strain typing are useful measures in locating sources of infections and preventing their spread.

OTHER PSEUDOMONAS SPECIES

A number of other *Pseudomonas* species are isolated from clinical specimens and the hospital environment. When these organisms are isolated, however, careful evaluation of the clinical setting must be made, since these organisms may represent contaminants rather than etiologic agents of disease. Most of them are common inhabitants of the soil, but *P. mallei* appears to be a specialized animal pathogen. Characteristics that are useful for the laboratory identification of these organisms are listed in Table 42-1.

Pseudomonas cepacia The organism was formerly classified as EO-1, *P. multivorans*, and *P. kingii*. It is frequently isolated from the hospital environment and clinical specimens. It has been associated with endocarditis, septicemia, wound infections, and urinary tract infections. Most patients in whom *P. cepacia* has been associated with disease were debilitated or had had prior instrumentation or manipulation. One hospital infection involving pressure transducers contaminated with *P. cepacia* has occurred in the United States. Bacterial endocarditis in a heroin addict has been documented. A number of isolates are resistant to most antibiotics, including gentamicin. However, most are sensitive to chloramphenicol or the combination sulfamethoxazole and trimethroprim.

Pseudomonas maltophilia This pseudomonad is frequently isolated from the oropharynx and sputum of normal adults as well as from many sites in the environment. The significance of laboratory isolation of this organism requires close clinical evaluation. Documented cases, however, of *P. maltophilia* infection of wounds, the urinary tract, and the blood have occurred. Antimicrobial susceptibility varies, but most isolates are susceptible to chloramphenicol, colistin, tetracycline, and sulfisoxazole.

Pseudomonas mallei This organism is the cause of glanders, a disease in horses and donkeys. Man is infected by direct contact through skin abrasions and inhalation. Since equine glanders has been eliminated in the United States and Canada, the disease is rarely seen in this country.

Pseudomonas pseudomallei This organism is a common inhabitant of the soil in Southeast Asia. It causes melioidosis, a glanders-like disease in man. The organism gains entrance into the body by inhalation or through abraded skin. In the body it may not cause any immediate problems but follows the course of a benign pulmonary disease. It may mimic tuberculosis or fungal diseases. Melioidosis can also present as an acute fulminating septicemia that is rapidly fatal. Reactivation of quiescent disease may occur after years, giving the disease the nickname "Vietnamese time bomb." The organism can be isolated from sputum, urine, pus, or blood. Most strains are sensitive to tetracycline, chloramphenicol, and sulfadiazine. Prompt treatment lowers the mortality rate of the fulminating form.

Other Species *P. stutzeri, P. putida, P. alcaligenes,* and *P. acidovorans* are isolated from clinical material but frequently are not the etiologic agents of disease. Rarely, however, they may be significant causes of wound, pleural, and urinary tract infections. *P. fluorescens* is frequently isolated from the hospital environment or blood products. Since this organism grows poorly at 37C, however, the symptoms seen in man, such as fever, may be caused by endotoxin rather than by an infectious process.

Further Reading

Books and Reviews

Artenstein MS, Sanford JP (eds): Symposium on *Pseudomonas aeruginosa*. J. Infect Dis 130(Suppl): Nov 1974, pp S1-S166

Doudoroff M, Palleroni NJ: Pseudomonas. In Buchanan RE, Gibbons NE (eds): Bergey's Manual of Determinative Bacteriology, 8th ed. Baltimore, Williams & Wilkins, 1974, pp 217-241

Howe C, Sampath A, Spotnitz M: The pseudomallei group: A review. J Infect Dis 124:598, 1971

Hugh R, Gilardi GL: Pseudomonas. In Lennette EH, Spaulding EH, Truant JP (eds): Manual of Clinical Microbiology, 2nd ed. Washington, DC, American Society for Microbiology, 1974, pp 250-269

Selected Papers

Boxenbaum B: Antimicrobial drugs for the treatment of infections caused by aerobic gram-negative bacilli. Med Clin North Am 58:519, 1974

Gilardi GL: Characterizatiom of nonfermentative nonfastidious gram-negative bacteria encountered in medical bacteriology. J Appl Bacteriol 34:623, 1971

Gilardi GL: Infrequently encountered *Pseudomonas* species causing infection in humans. Ann Intern Med 77: 211, 1972

Morbidity and Mortality Weekly Report. Nosocomial *Pseudomonas cepacia* bacteremia caused by contaminated pressure transducers. 23:423, 1974

Pedersen MM, Manso E, Pickett MJ: Nonfermentative bacilli associated with man. III. Pathogenicity and antibiotic susceptibility. Am J Clin Pathol 54:178, 1970

Pierce AK, Sanford JP: Aerobic gram-negative bacillary pneumonias. Am Rev Respir Dis 110:647, 1974

43
Yersinia

The three species in the genus *Yersinia* are primarily animal pathogens but also produce human disease. *Y. pestis* is the cause of plague, and *Y. pseudotuberculosis* and *Y. enterocolitica* usually are associated in man with gastrointestinal disease and involvement of the mesenteric lymphatics. Previously classified in the genus *Pasteurella*, numerical classification has shown a clear-cut relationship to members of the Enterobacteriaceae, in which family they are now placed.

YERSINIA PESTIS

Occasional fragments of early writing suggest that plague was present in the West in the pre-Christian era, but the extent of the disease is unknown. The first documented pandemic occurred during the reign of Emperor Justinian in 542 A.D. It probably began in Egypt or Ethiopia, spread widely, and lasted 60 years. Approximately 100 million persons died of the infection, and towns were completely decimated.

The second pandemic, known as the "Black Death," started in the fourteenth century. The disease originated in Central Asia and became rampant throughout Europe, the Near East, India, and China. Both rats and infectious droplets from pneumonic victims played a prominent role in transmission of the disease. In Europe alone, 25 million persons died, one-fourth of the entire population. Following the second pandemic the disease became endemic among urban rat populations in many affected areas, and periodic smaller epidemic continued to occur through the seventeenth century. From that time until 1894 a general decline of the disease occurred, the reasons for which are incompletely understood.

In 1855, warfare facilitated spread of a Burmese focus of disease, and slow migration brought infected persons to Canton and Hong Kong in 1894. Modern transportation enabled rapid spread of the disease and precipitated the current and third pandemic. Virtually the entire world was affected, including for the first time the United States. During the third pandemic, foci of plague were firmly established among wild commensal rodents in large areas. These foci currently give rise to sporadic cases of plague, which have a potential for dissemination even in countries with high standards of public health. The third pandemic, however, appears to be approaching quiescence.

Morphology

The causative agent, *Yersinia pestis,* is a gram-negative, nonmotile coccobacillus (Fig. 43-1). It shows marked bipolar staining, especially in tissue impressions, aspirates of buboes, and pus stained with Wayson's stain. The cells have a safety-pin appearance, with the polar bodies staining blue and the remainder light blue to reddish. Freshly isolated virulent organisms are encapsulated.

Physiology

Yersinia are facultative anaerobes. They are anaerogenic and usually do not ferment lactose. They are oxidase negative and do not produce catalase.

Cultural Characteristics *Y. pestis* can grow over a wide temperature range, from 0 to 43C, the optimal temperature for growth being 28C. It can grow on ordinary laboratory media even from small inocula. On nutrient agar plates, small mucoid colonies appear in one to

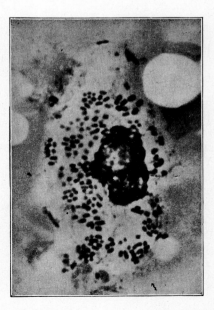

FIG. 43-1. *Pasteurella pestis* in monocyte from mouse lung. Giemsa stain. ×1,500. (From Meyer: J Immunol 64: 139, 1950)

two days. On desoxycholate agar very small red colonies may be seen on the second day of incubation. No hemolysis is produced on blood agar.

Strain Identification Three biotypes have been identified on the basis of their ability to reduce nitrates to nitrites and to ferment glycerol. These biotypes have been designated orientalis, mediaevalis, and antigua, and are characterized by differences in their geographic distribution. Orientalis is the usual biotype of western North America. *Y. pestis* strains are also characterized by quantitative differences in their antigens, as described below.

Antigenic Structure

At least 20 different antigens have been detected in *Y. pestis* by gel diffusion and biochemical analysis; 15 of these are shared with *Y. pseudotuberculosis*. Most of these antigens have received an alphabetical designation. Fraction 1 antigen, murine toxin, and D antigen are unique to *Y. pestis*. M and N antigens are found only in *Y. pseudotuberculosis*. Quantitative differences occur in the content of the F-1 antigen and the murine toxin, which vary independently from one isolate to another. Variations also exist in the protein patterns of isolates from various areas and may be of use epidemiologically in the future.

Determinants of Virulence

The availability of a number of mutants of *Y. pestis* has provided information on properties of the organism that contribute to its virulence. Five determinants of virulence have been defined: (1) V and W antigens, (2) fraction 1 antigen (envelope antigen), (3) pesticin, coagulase, and fibrinolysin formation, (4) ability to absorb certain pigments, and (5) purine synthesis. The importance of each of these factors separately is difficult to assess. The V and W antigens appear to confer on *Y. pestis* the ability for small numbers of bacilli to establish infection in animals. Once infection is established, the envelope antigen (F-1), pesticin, coagulase, and fibrinolysin contribute to the disease process.

(1) V and W antigens are always produced together and consist of a protein and a lipo-protein fraction. These antigens enable the organism to resist phagocytosis by the polymorphonuclear leukocyte. They are selectively produced during periods of stasis of bacterial growth. Factors which promote bacterial growth, such as the proper ionic conditions, repress V and W formation. The Mg^{++} concentration and essential absence of Ca^{++} in mammalian intracellular fluid permit stimulation of V and W production following phagocytosis.

(2) Fraction 1 antigen (F-1) is a soluble antigen contained within the bacterial envelope. It consists of two immunologically identical complexes: a protein complexed with polysaccharides (fraction 1A), which contains N-acetyl-glucosamine and hexuronic acid, and a protein alone (fraction 1B). Fraction 1 apparently consists of a series of serologically identical molecular aggregates. Maximal production occurs at 37C, and none is produced at very low temperatures. It is essential for virulence in the guinea pig, but not in the mouse. Its role in human infections is unknown. It is highly immunogenic, however, and may constitute as much as 7 percent of the dry weight of the organism. Antibody to fraction 1 appears to be protective in both human and experimental animals.

(3) Pesticin I, coagulase, and fibrinolysin production are always correlated. Pesticin I is a bacteriocin produced by *Y. pestis* that inhibits the growth of *Y. pseudotuberculosis* as well as some strains of *E. coli* and *Y. enterocolitica*. The production of coagulase and fibrinolysin is apparently a function of bacteriocinogenic conversion. Strains of *Y. pestis* lacking these antigens are fully infectious for the mouse or guinea pig, but lethality is attenuated.

(4) An interesting relationship exists in *Y. pestis* between pigmentation and virulence. In virulent strains an unidentified surface component is present that results in the absorption of hemin and basic aromatic dyes to form colored colonies. In mice, avirulent nonpigmented organisms may be restored to their original expression of virulence by providing an excess of free serum iron. Also, the in vivo virulence of pigmented *Y. pestis* is enhanced by an injection of Fe^{++} sufficient to saturate serum transferrin. This observation, however, is not unique to *Y. pestis* but also occurs following experimental infection with *Pasteurella multocida*, *Y. pseudotuberculosis*, and many other organisms.

(5) Loss of the ability to complete the synthesis de novo of purine ribotides is correlated

in *Y. pestis* with a loss of virulence. This is also observed with other members of the Enterobacteriaceae.

Two additional factors that may be associated with the expression of virulence of *Y. pestis* are murine toxin and endotoxin. Although the LD_{50} of murine toxin for rats and mice is less than 1 microgram, it is relatively atoxic for other animals, hence the name "murine toxin." It is a protein which in highly purified preparations inhibits the respiration of muscle mitochondria of sensitive animals by preventing reduction of coenzyme Q. The effect is most pronounced on the peripheral vascular system, resulting in shock and fatty degeneration and necrosis of the liver.

The role of *Y. pestis* endotoxin is ill defined. Endotoxin shock is produced in sensitive animals. A biphasic febrile response, induced tolerance, and both localized and generalized Shwartzman reactions are produced by the lipopolysaccharide of the cell wall.

Clinical Infection

Epidemiology   At the present time over 90 percent of the total world incidence of plague occurs in Southeast Asia, especially in South Vietnam, Burma, Nepal, and Indonesia. Another major active focus is in Brazil. Outbreaks in the present pandemic, however, have been less extensive than in the past (Fig. 43-2).

Plague was introduced into the United States from China in 1900, when the first human case of the disease was reported from San Francisco. Within the next decade, studies showed the presence of infected wild rodents, especially ground squirrels, in wide areas south of San Francisco. In 1907-1908 a major epidemic occurred in San Francisco, with 167 cases. Permanent foci of plague now exist that involve at least 57 wild rodent species and their fleas. These extend as far east as Kansas, Oklahoma, and Texas, and to approximal areas of Canada and Mexico. The disease does not have natural foci in North America east of these areas. During the current pandemic, infected fleas are the major mechanism for transmission.

Plague is perpetuated by three cycles: (1) natural foci among commensal rodents with transmission by fleas (sylvatic plague, wild plague), (2) urban rat plague which is transmitted by the rat flea (domestic plague, urban plague), and (3) human plague which may be acquired by contact with either of the former cycles and which may be transmitted by pneu-

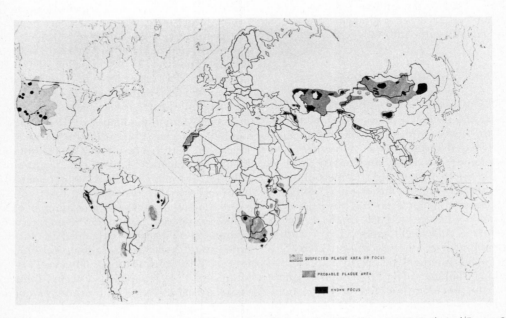

FIG. 43-2. Locations of known and probable foci and areas of plague in 1969. (From WHO Technical Report Series 447:6, 1970)

monic spread or, rarely, by the bite of a human flea (Fig. 43-3).

SYLVATIC PLAGUE. This is the only form prevalent in the United States. Wild rodent plague, in the area west of the 100th meridian, is one of the largest world reservoirs. A major factor in the restriction of plague to the western United States is the presence of dense colonies of rodents, such as prairie dogs, in the western areas.

Flea-related Factors. In nature the flea is essential for the perpetuation of plague. At least four flea-related factors influence the epidemic potential of plague. (1) Fleas vary greatly in their vector efficiency. Most wild rodent fleas are relatively inefficient in the transmission of disease to humans. The oriental rat flea, however, *Xenopsylla cheopis*, is highly efficient and has been the classic vector in urban rat-borne epidemics. (2) The restricted feeding habits of most wild rodents limit their threat to humans. However, the spread of infection within rodent populations, especially between

different species that commingle, is facilitated by the transfer of fleas from one rodent host to another. Humans occasionally have been infected when wild rodent deaths during an epizootic left hungry fleas in search of a new host. Dog and cat fleas are very poor vectors and have not been associated with plague outbreaks. (3) Some infective wild rodent fleas survive in burrows for long periods of time even after the rodent hosts have died. Survival of fleas for as long as 15 months has been shown. (4) The development of DDT-resistant fleas in some areas may influence the epidemic potential of plague. This has occurred in some instances concomitant with widespread DDT spraying during malaria control programs.

Transmission of plague by fleas may occur in several ways. The most efficient method involves ingestion of the organism by the flea during a blood meal from a bacteremic host. In the flea stomach, the infected blood is coagulated by coagulase which is produced by *Y. pestis* in the presence of an enzyme of the flea stomach. Bacteria are thus trapped in a matrix of fibrin which fixes them to the spines of the

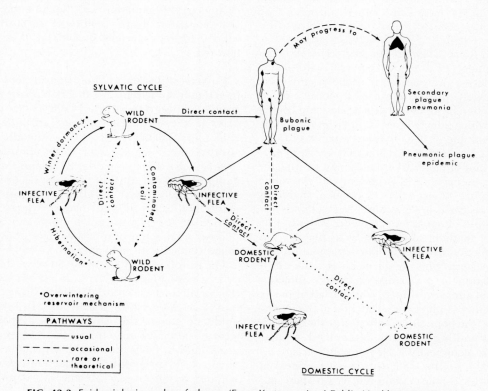

FIG. 43-3. Epidemiologic cycles of plague. (From Kartman: Am J Public Health 56:1554, 1966)

flea's proventriculus. As the bacteria multiply, the proventriculus is occluded, causing blocking. The time between ingestion and blocking is the extrinsic incubation time, and usually for *X. cheopis* this is about two weeks. During subsequent attempts to obtain a blood meal, regurgitation of infected material results in infection of the new host. The hungry flea also becomes less fastidious about his host and will readily attack man. Hot, dry weather adversely affects all stages in the life cycle of the flea, explaining the subsidence of many epidemics at the beginning of a hot and dry season. Blocking is enhanced at temperatures below 26C. Above 27C the fibrinolytic factor of *Y. pestis* and the trypsinlike activity of the flea stomach enzyme are activated, destroying the fibrin meshwork needed for blocking. Decreased blocking results in decreased vector efficiency.

Mechanical transmission via contaminated mouth parts of the flea is also important in the transmission of plague, especially in wild plague. The fleas of many wild rodents do not become blocked or may be poor vectors even when blocked. Mechanical transmission by such fleas which are highly prevalent may be the primary means by which enzootics and epizootics occur.

Wild Rodent-related Factors. The essential components of a natural focus for wild plague include the presence of *Y. pestis* organisms of sufficient virulence to cause infection, a dense population of rodents that may develop bacteremia when infected, and a high index and infestation rate of fleas that are capable of transmitting the infection. Over 200 species of rodents and other small animals may be infected during an enzootic. Ten rodent and two rabbit genera are of especial importance, including squirrels, field mice, prairie dogs, chipmunks, and voles. Populations of wild rodents vary widely in their susceptibility to plague. The introduction of disease into a population may cause catastrophic death of almost the entire population or may cause extensive infection without apparent illness. This variation in susceptibility to plague is a function of the experience of the population with former outbreaks of plague and is genetically determined. Animals that are genetically highly susceptible are unlikely to survive the disease to manifest an immune response. Inherently resistant animals, however, may survive and demonstrate serologic evidence of exposure.

Reservoirs of Infection. The maintenance of plague foci is enhanced by a commingling of rodents or other mammals of differing susceptibility. The relatively resistant species act as a reservoir of the infection. Although they do not succumb, they develop bacteremia that serves to perpetuate the infected fleas. The relatively susceptible species augment the level of infectivity of the local flea population, and deaths among this species may bring them into contact with humans or domestic animals.

The hibernating habits of some wild rodents also facilitate survival of plague during the winter months. Animals are much more resistant to plague during hibernation; an infected animal may survive through the winter and transmit disease again in the spring.

Attenuated *Y. pestis* organisms have been isolated from natural foci. These organisms may produce infection without causing death and provide another mechanism for perpetuation of the disease. It is not known at present whether these attenuated strains reacquire virulence. Perpetuation of the infection is also facilitated by the ability of *Y. pestis* to survive for long periods in the soil of animal burrows.

Human Infection. The transmission of infection from wild plague foci to humans is an accidental occurrence. From 1908 to 1968, 120 cases in the United States were attributed to wild sources. Disease is usually sporadic and always bubonic in character. Cases often occur in areas of extensive mortality among the rodent populations. Most of the cases occur from June through August, and the victims are primarily children and adult males. A large proportion of the victims are hunters and other persons who come into professional or avocational contact with wild animals.

The American Indians of the Southwest comprise a particularly high-risk group, especially the Navajos, whose cultural patterns bring them into close contact with prairie dogs. In 1965 an epidemic among the Navajos was associated with an extensive epizootic of the local prairie dog colonies. Dogs associated with these outbreaks developed antibody to fraction 1 antigen without serious disease. Domestic dogs and cats bring infected wild rodents and their fleas into the area of human habitations, increasing the danger of infection among domestic rodents.

URBAN PLAGUE. Urban plague has been the principal cause of the massive epidemics of plague in recent history. The characteristics of this form of plague are quite distinct from those of wild plague, although there has been extensive interaction between the two forms. Urban plague is characterized by an accompanying epizootic of plague among the rodents, particularly the black rat that lives in close proximity to human habitations. An epizootic occurs when there is a sufficiently dense population of susceptible domestic rats, a high index of parasitism with fleas capable of transmitting disease (the flea index), adequate climatic conditions, and introduction of disease. Centers for commerce, especially seaports, have been frequent sites of explosive disease. During the eras of epidemic human plague, the natural history of the epidemic included a gradual onset of fatal disease among the domestic rodents. As the infected fleas moved from the dead or dying rodents to other living rodents, the rate of death among the rodents increased. Human cases could be expected when approximately 10 percent of the rats were infected. Human cases usually began as bubonic disease, and usually there was only one or a few cases per family. The disease was seasonal, and the onset of adverse climatic conditions would curtail an epidemic. The disease was also cyclical, with severe disease following seasons of no disease or mild disease.

Initial epizootics characteristically caused the death of essentially the entire population of domestic rodents. Subsequent generations of rodents, however, were relatively more resistant to plague and, after several such epizootics, developed herd resistance and did not die of the disease, with the result that the severity of subsequent epidemics gradually declined. This probably accounts in large part for the fact that epidemic urban plague during the current pandemic has been declining for several decades. Repopulation of an urban area by a susceptible species of rodent, however, may again lead to extensive epizootic and epidemic disease, as occurred in Bombay in 1948 following an influx of susceptile bandicoots.

RURAL PLAGUE. Urban plague has been commonly disseminated to rural areas through lines of commerce. Grain shipments in Vietnam have probably played a role in the establishment of new foci. In rural areas, the disease first affects domestic rats, from which it is then spread to commensal wild rodents, thereby establishing a focus of wild plague. In contrast to urban plague, rural plague causes small numbers of sporadic human cases. There is little tendency for rural plague to disappear, since the constant influx of susceptible rodents from wild sources precludes the development of effective herd immunity.

INTERHUMAN TRANSMISSION. Pneumonic plague is the clinical form of the disease with the greatest potential for rapid dissemination. It occurs following close contact with a victim of bubonic plague who has developed secondary lung involvement and exhales the organism in droplets. This form of disease may be widespread and rapid in onset and is the only form of plague that is directly contagious. Epidemiologic characteristics of pneumonic plague show that familial spread is most common, and disease is most frequent in areas of overcrowding. Cold weather with high humidity fosters the disease. Although most epidemics are predominantly either bubonic or pneumonic in clinical presentation, recent epidemics in Vietnam have been mixed. Factors that determine whether an epidemic will be predominantly bubonic or pneumonic are not well understood.

Pathogenesis and Clinical Manifestations

The various clinical forms of plague overlap but may be grouped as predominantly bubonic, septicemic, or pneumonic.

Bubonic plague is essentially the only form of disease that occurs in man following infection from a wild focus. The bubo represents the infected regional lymph node which drains the area of skin through which the organism was introduced. The groin is the region most commonly affected, with axillary and cervical nodes affected less frequently. Buboes in more than one site are extremely rare. The incubation period of bubonic plague is usually less than a week, and the bubo may be preceded by prodromata of chills, fever, malaise, confusion, nausea, and pains in the limbs and back. Onset of disease is usually sudden. Patients may experience pain at the site of the future bubo before it is palpable. The lesion itself is tender, the node is enlarged and may suppurate, and erythema of the surrounding tissues is common. The bubo of plague cannot be distinguished clinically from other causes of acute lymphadenitis. Bacteremia is usually present even in mild cases; approximately one-half of early blood cultures will yield the organism. The level of bacteremia is usually low, and organisms are seldom seen on direct observation of stained buffy coat smears.

Pulmonary involvement is common in all severe cases of plague and is often the immediate cause of death. Hemorrhagic and edematous effusions predominate, probably associated with emboli that may be septic and originate from the bubo. Endotoxin-mediated effects are observed. Another primary manifestation of bubonic plague is congestion of the vessels of the conjunctivae. The three clinical findings that traditionally have been most useful in the diagnosis of plague are a rapid rise in temperature, regional buboes, and conjunctivitis. In very mild plague, the only clinical finding may be vesiculation at the site of inoculation. Slightly more active disease, with local buboes but without systemic signs of disease, is termed "pestis minor."

At the opposite extreme is septicemic plague. In this form of disease, the patient experiences a very high level of bacteremia early in the course of disease before local buboes evolve. The mortality rate, treated and untreated, is high, with rapid peripheral vascular collapse. A prominent finding in this, as well as in other forms of plague, is disseminated intravascular coagulation with a generalized Shwartzman phenomenon. Purpuric lesions with intravascular thrombi occur in all areas of the body. This manifestation of disease is more common in children than in adults.

Plague meningitis is an infrequent complication. Clinical evidence suggests that it is most common in persons who experience an attenuated form of infection such as that which occurs in the partially immune or following inadequate treatment. The clinical findings are those of an acute bacterial meningitis.

Pneumonic plague usually arises from septic embolization to the lungs. Patients also may acquire the pneumonic form following pharyngeal plague and direct extension into the lung from the cervical or tonsillar buboes. Inhalation of organisms in droplet nuclei dispersed by another person with plague also provides a mechanism for direct inoculation of the lung parenchyma. This was probably the etiology of the highly fatal, fulminant epidemics in China in the late 1890s. The average length of time in untreated patients with pneumonic plague from the first appearance of symptoms to death is less than two days. The disease is highly contagious. Marked central nervous system abnormalities, including convulsions, incoordination, stupor, and delirium, usually accompany the disease.

Laboratory Diagnosis Clinical materials containing *Y. pestis* are extremely hazardous. Suspicious cultures or specimens should be sent immediately to a laboratory with facilities for making a rapid definitive identification. Aspirates from buboes, pus from the area of the flea bite, sputum, throat swabs, or blood should be carefully collected and placed in Cary-Blair transport media for transfer to the laboratory.

Serologic Diagnosis. Antibodies to the F-1 antigen (p. 601) may be detected by use of the agglutination test or the complement-fixation test. The complement-fixation test also may be used for detecting the F-1 antigen in either tissue extracts or the organism itself. Complement-fixing antibodies decrease rapidly following recovery from plague. The passive hemagglutination test which uses tanned erythrocytes coated with F-1 antigen or murine toxin is also a sensitive indicator of antigen or antibody. This antibody may persist for several years following recovery from plague and is a sensitive test for identifying a quiescent plague focus. This antibody, however, is often not apparent during the first week of the infection, and a rise in titer may not be apparent until two weeks after onset of clinical disease.

Precipitin tests are useful in the detection of F-1 antigen in dried and decomposed carcasses of animals. An immunofluorescent test using F-1 antibody is a rapid and generally accurate method of identifying *Y. pestis*, although cross-reaction with *Y. pseudotuberculosis* may occur in a small percentage of cases.

Treatment Streptomycin is bactericidal and highly effective for most strains. Resistant organisms have been observed in the Far East but not in the United States. Alternative treatment is tetracycline or chloramphenicol. Kanamycin appears to be equally as effective as streptomycin and to show no cross-resistance. Penicillin is inadequate, and the sulfonamides are not uniformly effective. Sulfamethoxazole-trimethoprim has been used successfully in the treatment of a small number of patients, but further evaluation is necessary.

Prevention An effective vaccine for immunization against plague is available. In spite of widespread plague among Vietnamese civilians, by the end of 1969 only 8 cases had occurred in United States military personnel. Two types of vaccine are available: live attenuated vaccine and a vaccine of killed virulent organisms. Considerable experience has been gained in the past with the use of live attenuated vaccines, but these are no longer used in the United States. A vaccine of killed virulent organisms is employed, the efficacy of which appears to be directly proportional to the content of F-1 antigen. Immunization is recommended for persons traveling to Vietnam, Laos, and Cambodia and for persons at risk from contact with plague-infected rodents. The primary series consists of three doses of vaccine given four or more weeks apart and a booster each six months thereafter. Severe reactions to the vaccine have not been common, although immediate and generalized urticaria and anaphylaxis may occur. There is no evidence that vaccine protects against pneumonic plague.

Control Plague is one of the internationally quarantinable diseases, and reporting of cases is mandatory. Public health authorities may institute enforced quarantine and/or disinfection of persons, ships, and aircraft arriving with known or suspected infected persons or animals. Efforts to prevent plague have been directed toward preventing transportation of rats, especially by ships and airplanes. Current methods of shipping and docking make the classic importation of shipboard rats into Western countries unlikely, but the possibility of spreading diseased rats by container shipping may still exist.

Control of urban plague has proceeded along the principles of flea control, which should precede rat control, rodent extermination, treatment and/or quarantine of cases, quarantine of contacts of pneumonic plague, restriction of movement in highly infected areas, thorough garbage disposal, and application of good personal hygiene.

YERSINIA PSEUDOTUBERCULOSIS AND YERSINIA ENTEROCOLITICA

The term "yersiniosis" denotes infection with *Yersinia* species other than *Y. pestis*, namely, *Y. pseudotuberculosis* and *Y. enterocolitica*. These are zoonotic diseases, in which human infection appears to be acquired accidentally from disease cycles of wild and domestic animals.

Morphology and Physiology

Unlike the plague bacillus, *Y. pseudotuberculosis* and *Y. enterocolitica* are motile. The flagella are parapolar or peritrichous in location and are produced during growth at 22C but not at 37C. A microscopically visible capsule is not produced.

Both species may be isolated from clinical material by culture on blood agar and the usual media used for the enteric bacilli. They are characterized by urease production, an acid slant and butt on TSI agar, and no hydrogen sulfide production. Growth requirements and metabolic pathways are similar to those of the other Enterobacteriaceae.

Differentiation of *Y. enterocolitica* from *Y. pseudotuberculosis* is based on biochemical differences between the species, as shown in Table 43-1. The results of many of these tests are markedly affected by temperature, a property that should be noted in the interpretation of results.

Antigenic Structure

Yersinia pseudotuberculosis The V and W antigens of *Y. pestis* are also present in *Y. pseudotuberculosis*. *Y. pseudotuberculosis*, however, does not produce coagulase, fibrinolysin, pesticin I, or murine toxin. Fraction 1 is usually absent from *Y. pseudotuberculosis*, but a few strains produce a similar antigen. Pig-

TABLE 43-1   DISTINGUISHING PROPERTIES OF
YERSINIA SPECIES

	Yersinia pseudotuberculosis	Yersinia enterocolitica	Yersinia pestis
Oxidase	−	−	−
β-Galactosidase	+	+(d)	+
Indole	−	−(d)	−
Rhamnose fermentation	+	−	−
Melibiose fermentation	+	−	−
Cellobiose fermentation	−	+	−
Sucrose fermentation	−	+(d)	−
Ornithine decarboxylation	−	+(d)	−
Salicin fermentation	+	−(d)	+
Aesculin hydrolysis	+	−(d)	+
Urease	+	+	−
Motility at 25C	+	+	−

From Nilehn: Acta Pathol Microbiol Scand (B) (Suppl) 206:20, 1969
The signs, + and −, denote the behavior of the majority of strains within a species;
(d) indicates the occurrence of different biochemical types (rare exceptions omitted).

mentation of *Y. pseudotuberculosis* is less pronounced than in *Y. pestis*, but as in *Y. pestis*, virulence is greatly enhanced by the presence of free iron compounds. A potential determinant of virulence that is common to both organisms is an exotoxin that is similar to the plague murine toxin and an endotoxin. Pesticin I of *Y. pestis* inhibits some strain of *Y. pseudotuberculosis*.

The O-antigen specificity is conferred by 3,6-dideoxyhexoses, some of which also are present in the cell walls of *Salmonella* groups B and D and are responsible for the cross-reactions in agglutination tests. There are at least five serologic types of *Y. pseudotuberculosis*, each of which is characterized by type-specific O and H antigens. Serotyping can be done either by slide agglutination or by passive hemagglutination tests.

Yersinia enterocolitica *Y. enterocolitica* bears little antigenic relationship to other *Yersinia* but cross-reacts with *Brucella*.

Most species of *Brucella* show complete cross-reaction with *Y. enterocolitica* type 9. Differentiation between the two organisms, however, can be made by means of a quantitative Rose-Bengal plate. For diagnostic purposes, it should be kept in mind that a positive brucella agglutination titer may represent a *Y. enterocolitica* type 9 infection. The antigenic determinant responsible for this cross-reactivity is probably lipopolysaccharide of the cell wall. There is also antigenic similarity between some *Y. enterocolitica* strains and *Vibrio cholerae* serotype inaba.

Strains of *Y. enterocolitica* have been separated into five recognized biotypes on the basis of cultural and biochemical characteristics. Phage typing and serotyping according to O and H antigens have proved useful. Twenty-seven serotypes have been identified on the basis of their O and H antigens.

Clinical Infection

Epidemiology The yersinioses have been recognized in wild and domestic mammals, birds, invertebrates, and amphibians. Clinically apparent disease in human beings with both species has occurred in all areas of the world, but the majority of cases have come from Northern Europe, especially France, Germany, and the Scandinavian countries.

Sources of infection in human beings are poorly defined. Direct contamination of food or water by infected animals may account for cases in which identical strains have been obtained from a person and his pet or a domestic animal, frequently a pig, in a *Y. enterocolitica*-related disease. Most reports are of individual cases or small family outbreaks. Secondary cases are common, and a high attack rate also appears to be common. A single school outbreak of *Y. enterocolitica* enteritis in Japan involved 20 percent of the entire student body. Person-to-person spread within related families and between personnel on hospital wards has demonstrated the potential for rapid transmission under appropriate conditions.

Contamination of water supplies by *Y. enterocolitica* has been demonstrated. Survival of both organisms in various types of water is shortest in the spring and summer and longest in the fall and winter, a finding probably attributable to the ability of the organisms to grow at the lower temperature. The majority of human infections occur during the winter and early spring. The incidence of infection with both organisms is the same for males and females. *Y. enterocolitica* is primarily a disease of the very young, including infants, while *Y. pseudotuberculosis* more commonly affects persons 10 to 20 years of age.

In the United States *Y. pseudotuberculosis* has been identified in six species of domestic mammals and several wild mammals, including deer, rabbits, and rodents. Wild birds also are reservoirs of *Y. pseudotuberculosis*. Fecal-oral spread of both *Y. enterocolitica* and *Y. pseudotuberculosis* appears to be the major natural method of transmission.

The relative clinical importance of *Y. enterocolitica* and *Y. pseudotuberculosis* as causes of gastrointestinal disease in the United States is unknown. Surveys of routine stool cultures suggest that rarely are the organisms found in normal persons. In Japan, however, a convalescent carrier rate of 10 percent was found one month following a school outbreak. In some areas of the world these *Yersinia* species are considered to be as common a cause of serious gastrointestinal disease as is shigellosis. It is expected that as physicians and laboratories in the United States become more familiar with these organisms, their importance will be clarified.

Pathogenesis The primary lesion results from invasion of the wall of the small intestine, usually in the area of the ileum. Ulcers of the intestinal mucosa at the site of lymphoid tissue may develop and lead to extensive loss of blood and fluid, strongly resembling the intestinal findings in typhoid fever. The mesenteric nodes usually are the most extensively involved structures. Enlarged nodes may become confluent. Histopathologic differentiation of these lesions from gastrointestinal infection with *Francisella tularensis*, *Salmonella* species, and cat-scratch fever occasionally may be difficult.

Although usually restricted to the gastrointestinal tract, invasion of the portal system leading to liver involvement and generalized septicemia, with colonization in other parts of the body, may occur.

Clinical Manifestations A short prodromal period of approximately one day precedes symptoms of gastrointestinal disease. The majority of naturally acquired human cases present primarily with gastrointestinal symptoms, including diarrhea and mesenteric lymphatic involvement. Systemic symptoms usually accompany the focal gastrointestinal complaints and consist of headache which may be severe, malaise, and fever associated with convulsions. Both organisms produce severe abdominal pain which, together with enlarged mesenteric nodes, has resulted in many instances in exploratory surgery in the expectation of appendicitis. In one series reported, only 3.8 percent of patients who underwent surgery for a clinical diagnosis of appendicitis yielded *Y. enterocolitica* in culture. The uncomplicated case of gastroenteritis caused by either *Y. enterocolitica* or *Y. pseudotuberculosis* is not clinically distinguishable from that caused by *Salmonella* or *Shigella*.

Complications consisting of septicemia and hepatic abscesses may occur in a small number of patients, most of whom have preexisting liver disease, are diabetics, or are receiving corticosteroids. An arthritis-erythema nodosum syndrome also has been reported extensively by Scandinavian physicians but has not been observed in the United States or Canada. Patients with this syndrome are predominantly female in the 15-to-45-year age group. The arthritis usually is preceded by abdominal pain and diarrhea and often affects multiple large joints sequentially.

Laboratory Diagnosis A definitive diagnosis can be made only by culture of the organism. The organisms can be isolated from mesenteric lymph nodes, feces, blood (in generalized septicemia), effusions from serous cavities, and tissue specimens. For selective enrichment and holding, the specimen should be placed in isotonic saline with or without potassium tellurite and promptly refrigerated.

Treatment   The susceptibility of *Y. enterocolitica* and *Y. pseudotuberculosis* to ampicillin, tetracycline, and other commonly used antibiotics is variable, necessitating the sensitivity testing of each isolate. Most strains are sensitive to the aminoglycosides and to sulfamethoxazole-trimethoprim. Other forms of supportive care, such as maintenance of fluid and electrolyte balance, are essential in the care of the severely ill patient.

FURTHER READING

Books and Reviews

Ahvonen P: Human yersiniosis. I and II. Ann Clin Res 40: 30, 39, 1972

Brubaker RR: The genus *Yersinia:* Biochemistry and genetics of virulence. Curr Top Microbiol Immunol 57:111, 1972

Chen TH: The immunoserology of plague. In Kwapinski JBG (ed): Research in Immunochemistry and Immunobiology. Baltimore, Univ Park Press, 1972, vol 1, p 233

International Symposium on Pseudotuberculosis. Symposium Series Immunobiol, Standard Vol 9. Basel and New York, Karger, 1968

Mair NS: The laboratory diagnosis of infection with *Pasteurella pseudotuberculosis.* In Dyke SC (ed): Recent Advances in Clinical Pathology, Series 5. Boston, Little, Brown, 1968, p 35

Pollitzer R: Plague. WHO Monograph Series, No 22. Geneva, Switzerland, World Health Organization, 1954

Trends in research on plague immunization. J Infect Dis 129:(Suppl) May 1974 S1-S120

Selected Papers

Butler T: A clinical study of bubonic plague. Am J Med 53: 268, 1972

Cavanaugh DC: Specific effect of temperature upon transmission of the plague bacillus by the oriental rat flea, *Xenopsylla cheopis.* Am J Trop Med Hyg 20:264, 1971

Gordon JE, Knies PT: Flea versus rat control in human plague. Am J Med Sci 213:362, 1947

Gutman LT, Ottesen EA, Quan TT, Noce PS, Katz SL: An inter-familial outbreak of *Yersinia enterocolitica* enteritis. N Engl J Med 288:1372, 1973

Hubbert WT: Yersiniosis in mammals and birds in the United States. Case reports and review. Am J Trop Med Hyg 21:458, 1972

Hudson BW, Quan SF, Goldenberg MI: Serum antibody responses in a population of *Microtus californicus* and associated rodent species during and after *P. pestis* epizootics in the San Francisco Bay area. Zoonoses Res 3: 15, 1964

Kartman L, Goldenberg MI, Hubbert WT: Recent observations on the epidemiology of plague in the United States. Am J Public Health 56:1554, 1966

Kartman L: Historical and ecological observations on plague in the United States. Trop Geogr Med 22:257, 1970

Knapp W, Thal E: A simplified antigenic scheme for *Yersinia enterocolitica* ("Pasteurella X") based on biochemical characteristics. Zentralbl Bakteriol [Orig A] 223:88, 1973

Legters LJ, Cottingham AJ, Hunter DH: Clinical and epidemiologic notes on defined outbreak of plague in Viet Nam. Am J Trop Med Hyg 19:639, 1970

Mair NS: Yersiniosis in wildlife and its public health implications. J Wildl Dis 9:64, 1973

Nilehn B: Studies on *Yersinia enterocolitica.* Acta Pathol Microbiol Scand (B) (Suppl) 206:1, 1969

Reed WP, Palmer DL, Williams RC, Kisch AL: Bubonic plague in the Southwestern United States. Medicine 49: 465, 1970

Surgalla MJ, Beesley EC, Albizo JM: Practical applications of new laboratory methods of plague investigations. Bull WHO 42:993, 1970

Toivanen P, Toivanen A, Olkkonen L, Aantaa S: Hospital outbreak of *Yersinia enterocolitica* infection. Lancet 1: 801, 1973

44
Francisella

Tularemia is a major zoonotic disease indigenous to many areas of the United States. It is caused by *Francisella tularensis*, which is transmitted to man by insect vectors or by the handling or ingestion of infected animals. Human disease, often referred to as "deerfly fever" or "rabbit fever," is characterized by a focal ulcer at the site of entry of the organisms and enlargement of the regional lymph nodes.

Most of the early work on the etiology and epidemiology of tularemia was carried out by epidemiologists in the United States. The organism was first isolated in 1911 by McCoy and Chapin from ground squirrels in Tulare County, California, hence the name tularemia. These workers found animals in the area to be infected with a plaguelike organism that caused disease and produced lesions resembling those of plague. Human cases were recognized under circumstances that implicated rabbits as the source of infection. Extensive studies by Francis and his colleagues of the United States Public Health Service resulted in a classic description of the human disease, definition of the zoonotic nature of the disease, implication of several vectors and means of transmission, and bacteriologic description of the organism.

The disease was subsequently recognized in Europe and the Far East. Widespread enzootic disease with associated human cases has occurred in Russia and Scandinavia. In some of these areas endemic disease has had serious economic consequences.

Previously classified as *Bacterium tularense* and *Pasteurella tularensis*, the organism is currently classified in the genus *Francisella*, which is a genus of uncertain affiliation. *F. novicida*, isolated from water, is the only other member of the genus and is not known to infect man.

FRANCISELLA TULARENSIS

Morphology

F. tularensis is a small, poorly staining, gram-negative coccobacillus, approximately 0.5 by 0.2 μm in size. It is nonmotile, nonencapsulated, and displays bipolar staining. Young cultures may be relatively uniform in appearance, but older cultures are characterized by extreme pleomorphism (Fig. 44-1).

Physiology

Cultural Characteristics *F. tularensis* is an obligate aerobe but is catalase negative. Growth occurs over a temperature range of 24 to 39C, with an optimal of 35 to 37C. It survives best at low temperatures. The genus is characterized by a growth requirement for cysteine or cystine. No growth is obtained on ordinary culture media, but slow growth is obtained on semisolid media, such as gelatinized egg yolk and media containing cysteine, glucose, and defibrinated rabbit blood or serum. Growth from small inocula is greatly enhanced by the addition of a low-molecular-weight cellular component that has not been completely characterized. This substance forms complexes with iron and copper ions and may be partially replaced by iron salts and sideramines. On blood media, colonies of *F. tularensis* may produce greening directly under the colony but no true hemolysis. Colonies are nonpigmented.

Biochemical Properties *F. tularensis* ferments glucose, maltose, and mannose with acid and no gas. H_2S is produced on media containing cysteine.

Determinants of Pathogenicity

A general correlation exists between a smooth colonial morphology, high degree of virulence for experimental animals, acriflavin reaction, acid agglutination, and staining with crystal violet. Fresh isolates of the organism produce smooth colonies, but repeated passage on artificial media results in a change from the smooth to the rough form and loss of a surface antigen that is a major determinant of pathogenicity.

In addition to changes in virulence that accompany colonial variation, inherent differences exist among the wild strains of *F. tularensis*. Strains with high virulence for men are most often associated with tickborne tularemia of rabbits, exhibit citrulline ureidase activity, and ferment glycerol. These strains are the major type in the United States. Strains of

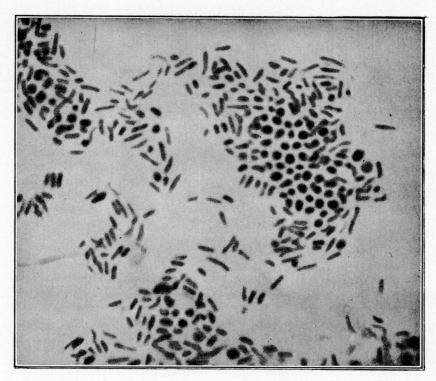

FIG. 44-1. *Francisella tularensis.* From culture on glucose cystine agar, showing coccoid and bacillary forms in the same field. Approx ×5,000. (From Army Medical Museum. Courtesy of Edward Francis, USPHS)

lesser virulence for man are associated with waterborne disease of rodents, seldom ferment glycerol, and do not exhibit citrulline ureidase activity. These strains also are found in the United States but are the predominant type in Europe, Russia, and the Far East. In some areas both types are present. Factors conferring virulence to the organism are poorly understood. No exotoxin has been identified.

Antigenic Structure

Different immunologic types of *F. tularensis* have not been detected. Three major antigens have been obtained from all strains tested: (1) a polysaccharide antigen that produces an immediate wheal and erythematous skin reaction in patients recovering from tularemia, (2) cell wall and envelope antigens that apparently contain the immunizing antigen and are responsible for endotoxic activity, and (3) a protein antigen that is responsible for a delayed type of hypersensitivity reaction in patients with the disease. A common protein antigen is shared by *F. tularensis* and members of the genus *Brucella.*

Clinical Infection

Epidemiology Tularemia is a reportable disease in the United States. Since 1939 when 2,291 cases were reported, there has been a steady decline in the annual number of reported cases (Fig. 44-2). In 1974, there were 144 cases of tularemia. The majority of the cases are from rural areas and are predominantly adult males. Women and children commonly acquire the infection by skinning a rabbit. Seasonal peaks occur during the winter and summer months (Fig. 44-3).

Tularemia is enzootic in all areas of the continental United States as well as most other areas of the world that are north of the equator, except for the British Isles. Rodents and rabbits

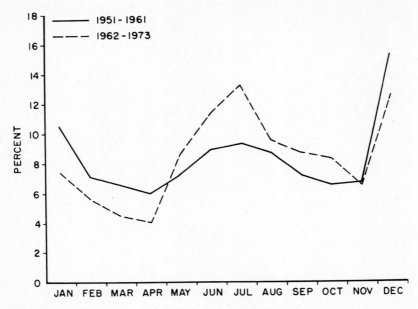

FIG. 44-2. Reported cases of tularemia in the United States, 1950 to 1973. (From Boyce: J Infect Dis 131:197 1975)

are the major reservoirs of infection. Other wild and domestic mammals suceptible to tularemia include the deer, fox, mink, racoon, opposum, beaver, mouse, rat, mole, dog, cat, sheep, and horse. Many species of birds also are probably naturally infected.

Two strains of tularemia may be recognized in the United States. Type A, which accounts for approximately 80 percent of recognized human cases in North America, is highly virulent for man and usually tickborne and rabbit associated. A second natural complex of virulent tularemia, type B, occurs among sheep keds and may be transmitted to man by mosquitoes and/or ticks. Type B is less virulent for man and usually is associated with disease of water-dwelling rodents, such as muskrats, and with associated contamination of streams. The source of the disease in the muskrats and beavers may be an epizootic of tularemia in a neighboring highly susceptible rodent population, leading to a rodent die-off in the area adjacent to the water, contamination of water, and disease of the larger rodents. Apparent disease from tularemia among rodent species ranges from asymptomatic disease to bacteremia with survival to the rapid death of the entire colony.

F. tularensis has been recovered from over 54 arthropod species, half of which are known

to have transmitted the disease to man. Although ticks, especially *Dermacentor andersoni, Dermacentor variabilis,* and *Amblyomma americanum,* are the most common arthropod vectors, other bloodsucking arthropods may be involved, including deerflies, mites, blackflies, mosquitoes, and occasionally lice. *F. tularensis* may be transmitted directly from an infected female tick to her offspring, an example of transovarial passage of infection.

There are many methods by which man may become infected with *F. tularensis* other than by contact with infected animals or through the bite of an arthropod vector. These include ingestion of inadequately cooked infected meat, usually rabbit, leading to primary cervical or gastrointestinal tularemia, which presents without a lesion of the skin. Ingestion of contaminated water, and inhalation of contaminated aerosols may lead to disease. Two exampleas of this latter mode of transmission are (1) laboratory-acquired infections, which are common and from which a great deal has been learned concerning the natural history of the disease, and (2) inhalation of dust that has been contaminated with infected vole feces during an epizootic. Other methods for acquiring the disease include direct inoculation into the skin from an infected animal bite or scratch and,

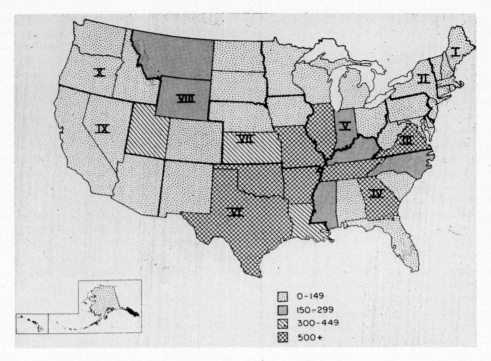

FIG. 44-3. Seasonal distribution of tularemia in the United States, 1951 to 1973. Presented as the percentage of annual number of reported cases of tularemia that occurred during each month. (From Boyce: J Infect Dis 131:197, 1975)

very rarely, direct spread from an infected person. This is known to have occurred only in the case of a pathologist who accidentally contaminated himself while handling infected material. Under normal circumstances person-to-person transfer does not occur. Congenital infection has been reported.

Tularemia in human beings is usually a sporadic disease, but it may be epidemic in circumstances that favor the arthropod vector, such as the deerfly, and when water or food supplies are contaminated. Regional differences in the ecology of the reservoirs of tularemia markedly affect its epidemiologic characteristics, which must be determined for each area if a clinical or veterinary problem exists. No other disease is so varied in its reservoirs, vectors, and ecology.

Pathogenesis *F. tularensis* is a facultative intracellular parasite. Macrophages of the fixed reticuloendothelial system and circulating mononuclear phagocytes ingest and harbor the organism. Peripheral polymorphonuclear leukocytes, however, phagocytose *F. tularensis* only in the presence of immune serum. Infect-

ed tissue is characterized by invasion of macrophages, necrosis, and granuloma formation.

In the original description of tularemia, Francis recognized at least four clinical forms, glandular, ulceroglandular, oculoglandular, and typhoidal. Tularemic meningitis, gastrointestinal disease, bacterial endocarditis, and pneumonia were subsequently described. These variations in presentation depend largely upon the method by which the person has acquired the infection, the virulence of the organism, and the individual degree of resistance to tularemia.

Most infections in the United States are acquired from the bite of a contaminated arthropod, usually a tick, deerfly, or mosquito, and lead to an ulceroglandular form of disease. Ulceration at the site of inoculation and regional lymphadenitis are similar following the arthropod bite or direct inoculation, such as occurs during the dressing of an infected rabbit. At the site of inoculation, a single punched-out ulcer, develops within one to three days. Lymphangitic spread from the ulcer to the draining nodes may be apparent as induration and erythema. Painful and swollen regional nodes may be the first sign of disease that the patient notices.

Clinical Manifestations Systemic signs of disease that occur suddenly early in the course of illness include back pain, anorexia, headache, chills and fever, sweating, and prostration. Nonproductive cough, nausea, vomiting, and abdominal pain also are common. Over 10 percent of patients develop a rash that may be macular, papular, or blotchy, is painless, is not pruritic, and lasts a week. In the Scandinavian countries, a third of the patients with tularemia develop erythema nodosum, but this is rare in other parts of the world.

In untreated cases the primary ulcer often suppurates and heals with scarring in four to seven weeks. Lymphadenopathy is often of long duration, and convalescence usually extends from three to six months. Suppuration sometimes continues for years, and relapses are frequent. Before specific therapy became available, the mortality rate was about 10 percent, but it is now less than 1 percent. In areas of the world where less virulent disease is prevalent, such as Russia and Japan, low mortality rates have always prevailed.

Oculoglandular disease accounts for less than 5 percent of the cases and is similar to ulceroglandular except that the conjunctival sac is the primary site of inoculation. Infection commonly occurs during the skinning of rabbits. In the early stages a papule may be found in the conjunctiva. The histopathology is a granulomatous conjuntivitis that may suppurate. Involved lymph nodes are the preauricular, parotid, submaxillary, and cervical. Although blindness is uncommon, the disease often is accompanied by severe systemic signs of disease which may be fatal.

The two forms of the disease which do not present with a primary ulcer are glandular and typhoidal tularemia. Glandular disease may resemble sporotrichosis. Typhoidal disease is characterized by general and severe systemic signs and must be differentiated from typhoid fever, brucellosis, tuberculosis, and other generalized bacterial diseases. Blood and sputum cultures most frequently yield *F. tularensis*. Hepatosplenomegaly is common, and the mortality rate is particularly high. Diagnosis is more difficult because there is no history of contact with an appropriate vector or source.

Pulmonary disease commonly accompanies tularemia and may be the dominant feature. Roentgenographic findings, which are not specific for tularemia, include bronchopneumonia, pleural effusion, hilar adenopathy, nodular infiltrations, and peribronchial thickening. The etiology of these changes probably includes hematogenous spread to the lung parenchyma, extension from involved hilar lymph nodes and, occasionally, inhalation of bacteria. Most of the 42 cases of laboratory-acquired tularemia included in Overholt's report were assumed to have resulted from inhaled infected particles. Persons with tularemic pulmonary involvement, however, seldom disseminate disease to other persons, and secondary spread is extremely rare. Other rare forms of tularemia have included meningitis following septicemia, gastrointestinal disease following ingestion of infected food, and congenital infection.

Immunity Agglutinating antibody is usually found in the serum by the second to third week of primary illness and may persist for years. The agglutinating and precipitating antibodies to *F. tularensis* probably confer little protective immunity to virulent strains, since persons and animals with high titers of these antibodies have subsequently acquired the disease. The major factor in acquired resistance appears to be a cellular immune mechanism involving an activated macrophage population. Evidence for this comes from several observations: (1) Resistance of experimental animals to tularemia is conferred by immunization with viable, attenuated strains of organisms but not with killed organisms. (2) The presence of circulating antibody, either passively or actively acquired, does not necessarily enhance the ability to resist challenge. (3) Peritoneal macrophages from immune animals have shown enhanced destruction of *F. tularensis* and prolonged cell viability after phagocytosis as compared with cells from nonimmune animals. This phenomenon is little influenced by specific antibody. (4) Protective immunity to *F. tularensis* may be conferred by the transfer of macrophages from immune animals.

SKIN TEST. The preceding findings are consistent with the concept that *F. tularensis* is a facultative intracellular parasite of the reticuloendothelial system and that development of protective immunity is coincident with the development of cell-mediated immunity. A skin test using phenolized and diluted vaccine gives a delayed reaction within seven days of the onset of disease in approximately 90 percent of persons with known tularemia. This skin test has been useful in epidemiologic studies on the prevalence of tularemia in endemic areas and in hazardous occupations. A reactive status persists for many years after infection or vaccination, long after circulating antibody has greatly decreased. The tularemia skin test does not elicit a response in persons previously infected with *Brucella* species without *F. tularensis* infection. The skin test also is more sensitive than most serologic tests, being reactive both earlier and longer. In one study, only 72 percent of persons with delayed hypersensitivity had demonstrable circulating antibody.

Laboratory Diagnosis Diagnosis of tularemia by recovery of *F. tularensis* is uncommon because of the requirement for special media and frequent overgrowth by other organisms. Overgrowth may be partially controlled by the use of selective inhibitors, such as penicillin G and cycloheximide. Another obstacle in the recovery of *F. tularensis* from clinical specimens is the reluctance of many laboratories to attempt isolation because of the high rate of laboratory-acquired disease. This is especially true when animal inoculation is used. Even in laboratories well equipped to attempt isolation, however, the proportion of isolates to suspected cases is low when compared with most bacterial diseases. In patients with pulmonary foci of disease, pharyngeal secretions and morning gastric aspirates may yield an isolate, as may the primary ulcer and regional node.

Fluorescent antibody identification of *F. tularensis* organisms or antigen in tissues of naturally infected animals has shown good correlation with histopathologic findings and may be useful in situations where the organisms are nonviable, as in highly decomposed tissue. Under such circumstances, a thermostable antigen may be extracted from organisms or infected tissue and identified by a precipitin reaction with appropriate antibody.

The agglutination test is the most commonly used serologic method for the diagnosis of tularemia. It usually becomes positive by the second week of disease, at which time the titer rises sharply to a maximum of over 1:1,280 in

four to eight weeks, and persists for a variable time. The skin test is usually reactive before the agglutination test.

The antibody response to infection or to vaccination with attenuated or killed *F. tularensis* includes production of agglutinins that cross-react with *Brucella abortus* and *Brucella melitensis*. The agglutinating titer to *Brucella* that is stimulated by *F. tularensis* is usually two to four dilutions lower than to *F. tularensis*. *Brucella* fails to absorb antifrancisella agglutinins. Similarly, agglutinating antibody to *Brucella* cross-reacts with *F. tularensis*, but the titer to *Brucella* is not ablated by absorption with *F. tularensis*. Cross-reaction with fluorescent antibody appears to be less common than with agglutination.

Treatment Streptomycin is the recommended treatment for tularemia. Bactericidal concentrations are readily achieved, and there is little clinical tendency to relapse. By contrast, clinical studies with both chloramphenicol and tetracyclines have demonstrated recurrent disease, and failure of these drugs to erradicate subcutaneous deposits of bacteria has been shown in volunteers. Treatment during early infection is more likely to result in eradication of bacteria than is treatment of chronic tularemia. Strains naturally resistant to streptomycin, chloramphenicol, or tetracycline are exceedingly rare. Penicillin is inefficacious.

Prevention Prevention involves avoidance of animals likely to be infected, especially rabbits, protection from biting arthropods, and provision of clean water supplies. The natural foci of disease appear to be stable and are not likely to be eradicated. Rabbits sick with tularemia are more easily caught by dogs or cats and may therefore be brought into contact with human beings. Persons at risk include rabbit hunters, all persons who handle wet skins of potentially infected animals, such as muskrats and beavers, sheepshearers, and persons in endemic areas whose field work brings them into contact with rodents. Precautionary measures may include wearing clothing with secure ankles and wrists to protect against attachment of ticks.

At high risk are all laboratory personnel handling cultures of *F. tularensis* and infected laboratory animals. Persons likely to be exposed in this way, including the animal handlers, should consider receiving live vaccine.

VACCINATION.   Attenuated live tularemia vaccine is available through the United States Army Biological Laboratories and Center for Disease Control. Experimental and clinical experience with the use of this vaccine has been acquired in Russia, Japan, and the United States. The tularemia vaccine and the vaccine of bacillus Calmette-Guérin for tuberculosis are the only currently used live bacterial vaccines. Use of the tularemia vaccine should be restricted to persons whose risk of exposure is high, such as sheepherders, sheepshearers, trappers, and laboratory personnel.

The vaccine usually is administered by scarification, producing a papular-vesicular lesion at the site of the take, similar to that in smallpox vaccination. Reactions to vaccine have not been severe, but regional lymphadenitis does occur. Vaccinated persons promptly develop cutaneous delayed hypersensitivity. Most vaccinees show an antibody response that reaches a peak within one month for half of the vaccinees and in the remainder within two months. The dose of *F. tularensis* in vaccinated persons is several logarithms higher than it is for non-immune persons, which is estimated to be 10 to 50 virulent organisms. When clinical disease does occur in previously vaccinated individuals, it is modified.

FURTHER READING

Books and Reviews

Reilly JR: Tularemia. In Davis JW (ed): Infectious Diseases of Wild Mammals. Ames, Iowa, Iowa State Univ Press, 1970, p 175

Selected Papers

Bell TF: Ecology of tularemia in North America. J Jinsen Med 11:34, 1965

Buchanan TM, Brooks GF, Brachman PS: The tularemia skin test: 325 skin tests in 210 persons: Serologic correlation and review of the literature. Ann Intern Med 74: 336, 1971

Claflin JL, Larson CL: Infection-immunity in tularemia: Specificity of cellular immunity. Infect Immun 5:311, 1972

Dahlstrand S, Ringertz O, Zetterberg B: Airborne tularemia in Sweden. Scand J Infect Dis 3:7, 1971

Francis E: Symptoms, diagnosis and pathology of tularemia. JAMA 91:1155, 1928

Jellison WL, Owen CR, Bell JF: Tularemia and animal populations: ecology and epizoology. Wildl Dis 17:22 1961

Overholt EL, Tigertt WD, Kadull PJ, et al: An analysis of 42 cases of laboratory acquired tularemia. Treatment with broad spectrum antibiotics. Am J Med 30:785, 1961

Young LS, Bicknell DS, Archer BG, et al: Tularemia epidemic: Vermont, 1968. Forty-seven cases linked to contact with muskrats. N Engl J Med 280:1253, 1969

45
Pasteurella, Actinobacillus, Streptobacillus

PASTEURELLA

Organisms of the genus *Pasteurella* have a wide host spectrum and cause epidemic and septicemic diseases of domestic animals and birds. Man also may be infected. The genus comprises an extremely heterogeneous group of organisms, but only four species are currently recognized: *P. multocida, P. pneumotropica, P. haemolytica,* and *P. ureae. P. multocida,* the major human pathogen of the genus, derives its name from its wide range of hosts, ie, *many killing,* and now includes as minor biotypes those organisms previously classified as different species because of their isolation from different animal hosts.

Pasteurella multocida

Morphology and Physiology *Pasteurella* are small, nonmotile, ovoid or rod-shaped organisms, approximately 1.4 by 0.4 μm in size. They are gram-negative and show bipolar staining, especially in preparations from infected tissue. Virulent *P. multocida* organisms are encapsulated.

Media containing blood or hematin should be used for culture. *P. multocida* is nonhemolytic but may produce a brownish discoloration of the medium in areas of confluent growth. The optimum temperature for growth is 37C, with growth occurring between 25 and 40C.

Pasteurella are facultatively anaerobic. They are catalase positive and usually oxidase positive. Their metabolism is fermentative, and acid is produced by most strains from glucose, mannitol, and sucrose. Distinguishing properties of *P. multocida* are shown in Table 45-1.

Colonial Morphology and Pathogenicity Four principal colonial variations occur: mucoid, smooth (iridescent), smooth (noniridescent), and rough. Most mucoid colonies are serotype A. There is a close relationship among colony morphology, acriflavin reaction, and hemagglutination. Flocculation with acriflavin is associated with rough or noniridescent colonies that fail to hemagglutinate and are deficient in capsular material. Cells that remain suspended in acriflavin contain capsular material that is typable by indirect hemagglutination and are mucoid or smooth (iridescent).

TABLE 45-1 PROPERTIES OF THE SPECIES OF GENUS PASTEURELLA

Characteristic	P. multo- cida	P. pneumo- tropica	P. haemo- lytica	P. ureae
Hemolysis on blood agar	−	−	+	−
Growth on MacConkey's agar	−	−	+	+
Indole	+	+	−	−
Urease	−	+	−	+
Mannitol	+	−	+	+

− = 90 percent or more strains negative; + = 90 percent or more strains positive

Encapsulated organisms are usually pathogenic for mice, but other, ill-defined factors, including the somatic antigens, play an important role in pathogenicity.

Virulence is greatly enhanced in vivo by the provision of free iron in the form of ferric ammonium citrate, hematin, lysed mouse erythrocytes, and purified hemoglobins. Conversely, one serum component that participates in the bacteriostasis of *P. multocida* includes transferrin. Interference with the iron metabolism of the organism is believed to be significant in host resistance to infection.

Antigenic Structure Five major antigenic types of *P. multocida* have been identified and designated A to E on the basis of their capsular or surface polysaccharides. Typing by use of standard agglutination procedures is usually complicated by the presence of common somatic antigens and in mucoid strains by capsular hyaluronic acid. The typing of *P. multocida* based on O antigens has been described for capsular types A and D. *P. multocida* strains may be characterized by both somatic O antigen and capsular components, and serotypes are assigned formulas such as 1:A, 2:A, 1:B where the numeral designates the somatic type and the letter designates the capsular type. There is a broad relationship between serologic type and host distribution when both capsular and somatic type are identified. The cell walls of both *P. multocida* and *P. haemolytica* contain significant endotoxin activity. No exotoxin has been demonstrated.

Clinical Infection EPIDEMIOLOGY. The *Pasteurella* species are present as normal flora in many domestic animals. *P. multocida* occupies an ecologic niche in the nasopharynx of the cat similar to that of the alpha-hemolytic streptococcus in man. It survives poorly in soil and water and is transmitted most commonly by direct contact, usually a bite. The tonsils of dogs are a site commonly colonized with *P. multocida*. The organism is more common in young male dogs, and the rate of colonization is higher in the cold seasons. Rates of colonization for the dog vary, but the majority of cats harbor *P. multocida*, as do many other domestic animals. Colonized animals are generally asymptomatic, and the disease apparently occurs during stressful situations, such as the shipping of cattle, when highly virulent organisms may be recovered from diseased animals. *P. multocida* is responsible for outbreaks of cholera of domestic or wild fowl, hemorrhagic septicemia of cattle, and primary and secondary pneumonias.

P. multocida types A and D are widely distributed in nature, and the majority of respiratory tract disease in man is due to type A. Types B and C have been recovered primarily from cattle, bison, and buffaloes. Organisms recovered from human disease following dog or cat bite or scratch are usually nontypable, rough, and lack pathogenicity for mice.

PATHOGENESIS AND CLINICAL MANIFESTATIONS. Human disease caused by *P. multocida*, or by other members of the genus which are rarely pathogenic for man, may be of three types: (1) infection via bites or scratches, (2) superinfection of a chronically diseased lung, and (3) other foci of disease which are secondary to septicemia.

Animal bites are common and frequently require medical attention. *P. multocida* can be recovered from approximately one-half of infected animal bites. In addition, half of the wounds that initially are colonized with *P. multocida* develop frank infection. Wounds that have been sutured are particularly prone to develop infection with *P. multocida*. Complications of bites infected with *P. multocida* are common. Cat bites may progress to pyarthrosis, necrotizing synovitis, and osteomyelitis of the underlying bone, presumably due to the depth of the bite and associated trauma of adjacent tissue. Regional lymphadenitis, with severe local pain, swelling, and discoloration, follows the often sudden onset of signs of infection.

Septicemia occurs primarily in persons with underlying disease which impairs reticuloendothelial function, such as cirrhosis of the liver and rheumatoid arthritis, but also has been reported in apparently normal persons.

The second most common form of infection with *P. multocida* is infection of the lung in patients with preexisting chronic pulmonary disease. These patients are usually middle-aged or older. Lower respiratory tract diseases associated with recovery of *P. multocida* are bronchiectasis, bronchogenic carcinoma, chronic bronchitis, emphysema, pulmonary abscess, and pneumonia, including sinusitis, mastoiditis, and chronic otitis media. *P. multocida* also has been recovered from upper respiratory tract infections. Disease with *P. multocida* in these settings of previous chronic disease may present with asymptomatic colonization, insidious progression to apparent pulmonary disease, or an acute or fulminant onset.

Other sites of infection with *P. multocida* are unusual and represent either hematogenous dissemination during bacteremia or local extension. Examples are meningitis, chorioamnionitis with premature delivery, cerebellar abscess, and infectious endocarditis.

LABORATORY DIAGNOSIS. Identification of the causative agent requires culture of appropriate specimens from the patient, depending on the area of involvement. Early morning sputa, bronchial washing, or nasal swabs from respiratory tract infections, purulent exudate from animal bites, spinal fluid, and repeated blood cultures are appropriate for this purpose.

TREATMENT. Among the gram-negative rods the *Pasteurella* species are unusual in their uniform sensitivity to penicillin. The mean inhibitory concentrations of tetracycline, ampicillin, and benzyl penicillin are less than 0.5 μg/ml. As with other pyogenic infections, localized abscesses must be drained. Following an animal bite, the wound should be meticulously cleaned and suturing avoided. Initiation of treatment with penicillin or tetracycline at the time of the bite is recommended.

PREVENTION. A number of vaccines and antisera preparations have been used in attempts to control veterinary disease due to these organisms. These have lacked efficacy, however, and are no longer used. More precise knowledge concerning the antigenic structure of strains causing particular veterinary diseases may make possible the production of more efficacious products.

ACTINOBACILLUS

Species in the genus *Actinobacillus* cause acute septicemia or granulomatous lesions in cattle and sheep. One ill-defined species now associated with this genus as species incertae sedis is *A. actinomycetemcomitans*, a human pathogen. This is a small, nonmotile, nonencapsulated, gram-negative coccobacillus. It grows best on serum or blood agar in an atmosphere of 10 percent carbon dioxide. Growth is optimal at 37C. Colonies on agar are about 1 mm in diameter after two to three days, are starlike, and are adherent to the agar. Growth in broth is granular.

Most clinical isolates of *A. actinomycetemcomitans* have been from infected blood and bone. Although some isolates have been obtained from lesions also infected with *Actinomyces* species, from which the organism's name is derived, most isolates have been obtained in the absence of *Actinomyces*. The organism is a normal inhabitant of the human mouth. The apparent etiology of some cases of human disease is related to impaired host defenses in such diseases as malignant lymphoma and leukemias. A number of cases of subacute bacterial endocarditis due to *A. actinomycetemcomitans* also have been described.

STREPTOBACILLUS

The primary human pathogen of this genus is *Streptobacillus moniliformis*, the cause of one type of rat-bite fever and of a milkborne disease known as "Haverhill fever."

S. moniliformis is a nonencapsulated, nonmotile, gram-negative bacillus, 0.3 to 0.7 μm by 1 to 5 μm in length. The organism frequently occurs in chains and filaments 10 to 150 μm long. It is often pleomorphic and may produce a series of bulbous swellings. It is a facultative anaerobe and requires CO_2 and moisture for primary isolation (Fig. 45-1). The most distinguishing characteristic of the organism is the spontaneous development of L-phase variants during in vitro culture (Fig. 45-2). The designa-

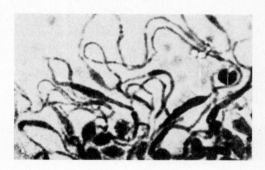

FIG. 45-1. Edge of a colony of *Streptobacillus moniliformis*. ×3000. (From Sharp: The Role of Mycoplasmas and L forms of Bacteria in Disease. 1970. Courtesy of Charles C Thomas)

tion "L-phase" was first used by Klieneberger-Nobel to refer to the pleuropneumonialike organism associated with *S. moniliformis* in cultures. It is now known that most bacteria and fungi are capable of similar changes, but this organism remains the prototype of this phenomenon.

Human disease caused by this organism is uncommon and is related to poor living conditions. Only 70 cases had been reported in the United States through 1965. *S. moniliformis* is a common inhabitant of the nasopharynx of wild and laboratory rats. Although the disease usually is acquired by the bite of a rat or other rodent, it also may be transmitted by means of milk, water, and food.

The disease begins one to five days following the introduction of the organism. The onset is abrupt, with chills, fever, vomiting, headache, and severe pains in the joints. A maculopapular rash develops within the first 48 hours, and one or more joints become swollen and painful.

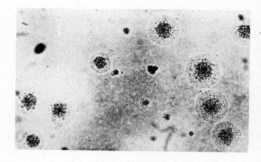

FIG. 45-2. L-form colony of *Streptobacillus moniliformis* produced spontaneously. ×100. (From Sharp: The Role of Mycoplasmas and L Forms of Bacteria in Disease. 1970. Courtesy of Charles C Thomas)

Acute arthritis is a characteristic and persistent symptom.

Diagnosis is made by isolation of the organism from the blood or from joint fluids and pus. Agglutinins appear in the patient's serum within 10 days and reach a maximum in three or four weeks. A titer of 1:80 is considered diagnostic, and a fourfold rise in titer is significant. Pencillin and streptomycin have been successfully used in treatment.

FURTHER READING

Books and Reviews

Carter GR: Pasteurellosis *(Pasteurella multocida).* Vet Rev Annot 6:105, 1960

Carter GR: Pasteurellosis: *Pasteurella multocida* and *Pasteurella hemolytica.* In Brandly CA (ed): Advances in Veterinary Sciences. New York, Academic Press, 1967, vol 11, p 321

Selected Papers

Holloway WJ, Scott EG, Adams YB: *Pasteurella multocida* infection in man. Am J Clin Pathol 51:705, 1969

Holmes MA, Brandon G: *Pasteurella multocida* infections in 16 persons in Oregon. Public Health Rep 80:1107, 1965

Hubbert WT, Rosen MN: I. *Pasteurella multocida* infection due to animal bite. II. *Pasteurella multocida* infection in man unrelated to animal bite. Am J Public Health 60:1103, 1109, 1970

Lee MLH, Buhr AJ: Dog bites and local infection with *Pasteurella septica.* Br Med J 1:169, 1960

Manioka S, Murata M: Serological studies on *Pasteurella multocida.* I and II. Cornell Vet 51:498, 507, 1961

Murata M, Horiuchi T, Namioka S: Studies on the pathogenicity of *Pasteurella multocida* for mice and chickens on the basis of O-groups. Cornell Vet 54:294, 1964

Smith JE: Studies on *Pasteurella septica.* I. The occurrence in the nose and tonsils of dogs. J Comp Pathol 65:239, 1955

Tindall JP, Harrison CM: *Pasteurella multocida* infections following animal injuries, especially cat bites. Arch Dermatol 105:412, 1972

46
Brucella

Malaise, anorexia, fever, and profound muscular weakness characterized a debilitating illness first recognized by Marston in 1861 and called "gastric remittent fever." The responsible organism, *Micrococcus melitensis*, was isolated in 1887 by Sir David Bruce. The organism derived its species name from Melita (honey), the Roman name for the Isle of Malta where the disease was recognized. The classic description of the clinical illness by Hughes in 1897 altered its designation to the more frequently used term, "undulant fever." The subsequent rapid acquisition of knowledge of brucellosis was a direct result of the morbidity sustained by the armed forces of Great Britain which used Malta as a major military site in the first part of the twentieth century. The thousands of days of illness per year were such a liability that physicians were brought together by the Mediterranean Fever Commission to initiate investigation of this disease.

Recognition of infections with other members of the genus *Brucella* occurred independently. Nocard, in 1862, first recognized the presence of bacteria between the fetal membranes and the wall of the uterus of the pregnant cow, but it remained for Bang, a Danish veterinarian, to isolate the organism, *B. abortus*. In a report of his findings in 1897, Bang linked the organism to infectious abortions in animals. The third member of the genus was identified in 1914, when Traum isolated *B. suis* from a premature pig.

The relationship of these three organisms was unknown until Alice Evans, working for the Diary Division of the Bureau of Animal Industry, noted the close bacteriologic and serologic relationships between *M. melitensis* and *B. abortus*. As a result of her observations the genus *Brucella* was recognized and named in honor of Sir David Bruce.

Brucellae are mammalian parasites and pathogens with a relatively wide host range. They are facultatively intracellular. Six species are currently recognized, *B. melitensis*, *B. abortus*, *B. suis*, *B. neotomae*, *B. ovis*, and *B. canis*.

Morphology and Physiology

Brucella are small, nonmotile rods, usually coccobacillary but with a size range of 0.5 to 0.7 by 0.6 to 1.5 μm. Organisms occur singly

TABLE 46-1 DIFFERENTIAL CHARACTERISTICS OF SPECIES AND BIOTYPES IN GENUS BRUCELLA

| Species | Biotypes | CO_2 Required | H_2S Produced | Growth on Dye Media* | | | Agglutination in Monospecific Sera | |
				Basic Fuchsin 1:100,000	Thionine 1:25,000	Thionine 1:100,000	Abortus	Melitensis
B. melitensis	1	–	–	+	–	+	–	+
	2	–	–	+	–	+	+	–
	3	–	–	+	–	+	+	+
B. abortus	1	±	+	+	–	–	+	–
	2	+	+	–	–	–	+	–
	3	±	+	+	+	+	+	–
	4	±	+	+	–	–	–	+
	5	–	–	+	–	+	–	+
	6	–	±	+	–	+	–	+
	7	–	±	+	–	+	+	–
	8	+	–	+	–	+	+	+
	9	±	+	+	–	+	–	+
B. suis	1	–	+	–	+	+	+	–
	2	–	–	–	–	+	+	–
	3	–	–	+	+	+	+	–
	4	–	–	+	+	+	+	+
B. neotomae		–	+	–	–	+	+	–
B. ovis		+	–	+	+	+	–	–
B. canis		–	–	–	+	+	–	–

Modified from WHO Technical Report Series No 464:1971, p 71
*Species differentiation is obtained on albimi or tryptose agar with graded concentrations of dyes. Interpretation should be controlled with the reference strains of each species

or in groups, and capsules, if present, are small. They are gram-negative but frequently take the counterstain poorly and require a minimum of three minutes for good definition.

The brucellae are strict aerobes. They grow slowly and require complex media for primary isolation. Such media as serum-dextrose agar or trypticase agar are satisfactory for this use (p. 628). Colonies of *Brucella* are spheroidal in shape and 2 to 7 mm in diameter. The colonial morphology may be altered by the conditions of growth, but usually colonies are moist, translucent, and slightly opalescent.

The members of this genus comprise a closely knit genetic group as defined by DNA hybridization studies. The differentiation of the three most common *Brucella* species is based upon quantitative differences in several physiologic tests (Table 46-1). The need for increased CO_2 for growth is characteristic of *B. abortus*. The ability to produce H_2S for a period of four to five days is more typical of *B. abortus* or *B. suis*. *B. melitensis* usually grows in the presence of both basic fuchsin and thionin, whereas thionin inhibits *B. abortus* and basic fuchsin inhibits *B. suis*.

Within each of these three species of *Brucella*, a number of strains or biotypes have been recognized based on these and additional biochemical properties. Antigenic differences between the species permit serologic confirmation of identification by agglutination with monospecific antisera.

Antigenic Structure

B. abortus, *B. melitensis*, and *B. suis* occur in the smooth phase in nature. Serial propagation in the laboratory results in a change in antigenicity of the organism with visible alterations in colonial morphology and a reduction in virulence for laboratory animals. For these reasons, propagation of the organisms in the laboratory prior to identification or for use as antigens in serologic testing requires rigorous monitoring of the cultures. The present hypothesis of the antigenic structure of these three species recognizes two antigenic determinants, A (Abortus) and M (Melitensis), present on the lipopolysaccharide-protein complex. The quantity of each antigen present and their spatial distribution would allow for the antigenic variation observed between the species.

Quantitative agglutination–absorption tests differentiate between the smooth phase antigens of the three species. Monospecific antisera are produced by absorption of heterologous antiserum. *B. melitensis* absorption leaves serum reactive only with *B. abortus* and *B. suis*. *B. abortus* and *B. suis* are indistinguishable by agglutination tests. Absorption of a second aliquot with *B. abortus* leaves serum specific for *B. melitensis*. There is some antigenic cross-reaction of the brucellae with other organisms, such as *Yersinia enterocolitica*, *Francisella tularensis*, and *Vibrio cholerae*.

Determinants of Pathogenicity

Recognition of brucella organisms within macrophages and documentation of their multiplication within cells have intrigued investigators, and attempts have been made to define these interactions. The predilection of *B. abortus* for fetal bovine tissues was quantitated by Smith and co-workers who extracted the organisms from tissues and calculated that of the total organisms present (ca 0.3 to 1.4 times 10^{-4}), 60 to 85 percent were present in fetal cotyledons, 1 to 25 percent were present in the chorion, and 2 to 8 percent were present in fetal fluids (allantoic and amniotic). They also described the presence of erythritol, a four-carbon polyhydric alcohol ($OHCH_2CHOHCHOHCH_2OH$), in these same tissues of the pregnant cow, sheep, and goat but not in the human placenta. Erythritol seems to be a fetal product measurable in amniotic and allantoic fluids from normal bovine fetuses. This alcohol functions efficiently as a carbohydrate source in a basal medium for *B. abortus*. It also enhances the intracellular growth of the organisms in an in vitro system employing phagocytes and *B. abortus*. There is, therefore, a significant correlation of the organotropism in cattle, sheep, and goats with the presence of erythritol. The absence of such tissue localization in human disease correlates with the absence of large amounts of erythritol in these organs. The similar intracellular localization of the bacteria in human illness, however, indicates that other factors contributory to the pathogenesis of brucellosis have not yet been elucidated.

Clinical Infection

Epidemiology *Brucella* organisms are distributed throughout the world, and the epidemiology is intricately related to animal infections. Human infection is a direct result of contact with infected animals, and for this reason it is necessary to consider animal disease.

INFECTION IN ANIMALS. The pathogenesis of infection in the various animal species is similar. Under natural conditions goats harbor *B. melitensis*, cattle harbor *B. abortus*, swine harbor *B. suis*, and sheep harbor *B. melitensis* or, less frequently, *B. abortus*. Infrequently dogs may be reservoirs of any of the three species mentioned if they come in contact with infected animals, but more recently *B. canis* has been identified as a significant pathogen for dogs particularly in kennels of beagles. Other animals which may be infected with brucellae include buffalo and the Bactrian camel (*B. abortus*), as well as reindeer and caribou (*B. suis*). In very unusual situations other farm animals, such as horses and poultry, may become infected with brucella, but these do not constitute a large reservoir or significant source of human infections. Infection of the animal occurs through the gastrointestinal tract, skin, and mucous membranes, including the conjunctivae. Animal food substances may come in contact with *Brucella*-infected materials, and their ingestion by the animal results in infection. *B. ovis*, *B. suis*, and *B. canis* are also transmitted with some frequency from an infected male to a female at the time of breeding. Infection of lymph nodes nearest the portal of entry is followed by bacteremia, which in the pregnant or lactating animal can lead to massive multiplication of the organism in the uterus and mammary glands. Brucellae localize in chorionic epithelial cells and cause necrosis of placental cotyledons. The animal fetus may become infected or may be aborted because of asphyxia alone.

Animals usually recover spontaneously but excrete the bacteria for varying intervals of time in vaginal secretions, urine, and milk, all of which are infectious. *B. melitensis* is excreted for months in the milk of infected goats, as originally demonstrated by Zammit on the Isle of Malta. Sheep tend to excrete the organisms for a shorter interval of time. The organisms are extremely long-lived under the proper environmental conditions. Survival is altered by pH and temperature, and exposure to sunlight will kill the organisms after a few hours. *B. melitensis* has been shown to survive in damp soil for as long as 72 days, in milk for 17 days, and in seawater for 25 days. It is clear that potential communicability can represent a threat to an entire herd of animals and persons in contact with the animals and infected materials.

Pathogenesis Man acquires the organisms through contact with infected materials. Within the United States, 90 percent of brucellosis in man is caused by contact with infected materials rather than by ingestion of contaminated fresh milk and milk products. Seventy-one percent of reported cases of brucellosis in 1972 were abattoir-related illness. The occurrence of disease principally in males between the ages of 20 and 50 years reflects this occupational hazard. Other occupations at risk include veterinarians, livestock producers, farmers, dairymen, and laboratory personnel working with the organism.

Organisms can enter through abraded skin, from which site they gain access to lymphatics and lymph nodes. There is often local lymphadenopathy and subsequent bloodstream invasion secondary to the bacterial multiplication and dissemination from the primary node. The subsequent localization of the organisms occurs particularly in the reticuloendothelial system. They have been observed inside the phagocytes, including mononuclear cells and macrophages. Intracellular organisms are protected from antibody and antibiotics. In infected tissues there is a granulomatous response, which in some situations may go on to abscess formation and even caseation. Sites, such as the spleen, are particularly heavily involved, and the bone marrow frequently has detectable granulomas. The liver tends to be less involved but has been a good source of positive biopsy materials.

Clinical Manifestations The incubation period of disease may be as short as three days but is sometimes several months in duration. More commonly, there is a time period of approximately three weeks after known exposure to organisms before the onset of symptoms. Weakness is seen in the vast majority of patients and is the most outstanding complaint. Fatigue, especially that occurring late in the day, results in the inability to perform normal activities. Chills, sweats, and anorexia are seen in approximately three-fourths of the patients with acute illness, and over one-half of the patients report generalized muscle aching, headache, and backache. These nonspecific symptoms may be accompanied by associated mental depression and increased nervousness.

The findings on physical examination are minimal in contrast to the multiple complaints. Over 90 percent of patients have fever, but only 10 to 20 percent have palpable splenomegaly or lymphadenopathy. The fever tends to be intermittent with characteristic diurnal variation. Disease may begin either insidiously or with a rather abrupt onset. The majority of patients with infection by *B. abortus* have a self-limited disease. *B. melitensis* is the most invasive species in man, and illness due to *B. melitensis* or *B. suis* may be more severe or chronic. Chronic brucellosis is difficult to diagnose or define but is usually nonbacteremic and occurs without demonstrable localized foci of infection.

Complications resulting from brucella infections are usually attributable to the granulomatous lesions which have occurred in various organs and tissues. Analysis of a large series of patients by Spink showed that at least 10 percent of patients were suffering from debilitating neuropsychiatric disorders. The complaints may be nonspecific, or there may be localized specific dysfunction. The second most common complication is *Brucella* infection of a bone or joint. The vertebral column is involved most frequently, and the invasion of the intervertebral disk and adjacent vertebral bodies constitutes osteomyelitis. In addition, a few cases of endocarditis due to *Brucella* have been recorded. The viscera, such as the spleen, liver, and bone marrow, may have evidence of infection for a significant period of time. The liver may be enlarged or tender, but only on rare occasions is there jaundice, hepatic failure, or subsequent cirrhosis.

Immunity Following natural infection in both man and animals there is an initial IgM antibody response followed by an IgG antibody response. In human brucellosis, IgM antibody makes up the majority of agglutinating antibody, whereas IgG antibody fixes complement. This pattern of response is different in other species of animals.

Laboratory Diagnosis Analysis of the clinical illness described above reveals that the findings in this group of patients are nonspecific when considered individually. Therefore evaluation of patients with these symptoms often includes a number of tests dictated by the differential diagnosis. At least one blood culture should be obtained from every patient suspected of having brucellosis. Other materials can also be examined, including the CSF in the presence of CNS symptoms, bone marrow, and tissues (eg, lymph nodes and liver). The intracellular localization of brucella organisms, particularly within reticuloendothelial cells, may be responsible for the positive cultures obtained from bone marrow aspirates at a time when blood cultures are negative from the same patient. Isolation of brucella organisms makes the definitive diagnosis. Isolation of organisms from tissues of infected animals may also be important.

CULTURE. In vitro growth of brucella organisms from patient specimens requires careful and informed laboratory processing of materials. For primary culture, direct inoculation of materials onto solid media is recommended in order to facilitate the recognition and isolation of the developing colonies and to limit the establishment of nonsmooth mutant organisms. Such media as serum-dextrose agar, serum-potato infusion agar, trypticase agar, brucella agar with serum, and 5 percent sheep blood agar have been found satisfactory for this use. Duplicate plates should be incubated under atmospheric conditions and in the presence of 10 percent CO_2, since this is often an essential requirement for growth of *B. abortus* on primary isolation. The commonly used method for attempted isolation from blood and body fluids employs the Casteñada bottle containing both a solid and a liquid medium. All cultures should be kept for 21 to 35 days before discarding as negative. Transfers or subcultures should be made from the original flask every four to five days to fresh medium. These subsequent subcultures should also be observed for 21 to 35 days. The conventional cultural methods employed in most hospital and laboratory situations are adequate to identify the positive cultures encountered from patients or in animal surveillance studies. The Food and Agriculture Organization of the United

Nations (FAO) and World Health Organization (WHO) Brucellosis Reference Centers will perform the metabolic testing which may be necessary for identification of atypical cultures of epidemiologic significance.

Laboratories processing materials, such as animal tissue or milk, which may be heavily contaminated with other microorganisms employ either animal inoculation or the use of selective media containing antibiotics to inhibit bacteria other than brucella.

SEROLOGIC DIAGNOSIS.   The serologic diagnosis of infection accomplished by the standard tube agglutination test is very sensitive and yields the highest degree of reproducibility. The success of the agglutination test depends largely upon the selection and standardization of the antigen. A single antigen will accurately diagnose disease with any one of the three commonly encountered species of *Brucella*. Cross-reactivity of the serum agglutinins to *Brucella* with *F. tularensis, V. cholerae,* and organisms of the genus *Yersinia* demonstrates the slight cross-antigenicity of these organisms. The homologous titer is considerably higher than the heterologous titer, affording help in evaluating the presence of agglutinins. The recently developed card agglutintion test recognizes greater than 90 percent of patients with positive tube agglutination tests. This test can be performed and interpreted in four minutes and may become a useful screening test, as it is superior to the slide agglutination test. Sera should also be examined by the standard tube agglutination test, particularly during the first week of illness.

It has been long observed that there is a prozone phenomenon in the measurement of agglutinating antibodies to brucella organisms. This phenomenon is apparently due to the presence of blocking antibodies. During the acute phase of illness when IgM agglutinating antibodies predominate, it is easy to detect the agglutination reaction. As IgG antibodies are formed during the course of the infection some of them bind with antigen and thus prevent its agglutination by the large IgM molecule. A modified Coombs (antiglobulin) test has been used to increase the efficiency of serologic diagnosis. With the use of antiglobulin to bind the incomplete antibody and antigen, agglutination can again be detected.

Extensive data gathered by Spink and co-workers indicate a relatively high incidence of brucella agglutinins in the serum of normal individuals. The titer varies with the geographic location and exposure to the organisms but is usually less than 1:100. More recent comparative serologic studies by Buchanan indicate that a single titer of greater than 1:160 by the standard tube agglutination test is presumptive evidence of infection with brucella organisms. A fourfold rise in agglutinins is seen in the first three months of infection in more than 90 percent of patients with cultures positive for brucellosis. To date, there is no evidence that antibiotic therapy alters the appearance or persistence of antibodies to the brucella organisms.

Other serologic determinations include specific indirect immunofluorescence, complement fixation, and the 2-mercaptoethanol (2-ME) agglutination test. Immunofluorescence requires preparation of materials and interpretation by experienced personnel and is less practical for rapid diagnosis than is the card agglutination test. Complement fixation requires rigid adherence to the standardization of the test conditions and reagents but has the advantage of indicating active or recent infection. The 2ME test has been more reliably utilized to demonstrate IgG (2 ME-resistant) agglutinin, suggestive of active disease in a symptomatic patient. The absence of such agglutinins mitigates against active disease, which may be helpful in evaluation for chronic brucellosis.

SKIN TEST.   The brucella skin test has been investigated and utilized because it is a measurement of sensitization to the antigens of the organism and may remain positive after the agglutination test becomes negative. The most commonly used antigens are those producing a delayed type of dermal reaction, and one of the more standardized products is brucellergen, a nucleoprotein fraction of brucella cells. Brucellergen is commercially available for clinical use. A positive intradermal test indicates contact with the brucella antigen at an undetermined point in time. Since the application of the intradermal test can result in a rise in serum agglutinins, serologic studies should be done prior to application of intradermal skin tests.

Treatment Tetracycline remains the drug of choice for therapy of the illness and is usually continued for a minimum of three weeks. Streptomycin has been used in combination with tetracycline, and recent analysis of a large series of patients indicates that antibiotic combinations including streptomycin produced a significantly lower relapse rate than combinations without streptomycin. Although many other antimicrobial agents have been effective in vitro, none have shown greater therapeutic efficacy in patients. The intracellular position of many of these organisms contributes to the continued recovery of bacteria from the blood despite antibiotic therapy. Intracellular killing of brucella organisms is essential for the final eradication of the bacteria and is dependent upon the normal bactericidal mechanisms of the phagocyte. Antibiotic therapy has not been completely satisfactory, and clinical or bacteriologic relapses occur in 0.9 percent to 30 percent of patients.

Prevention CONTROL OF ANIMAL DISEASE. There has been a decline in the reported cases of brucellosis in the United States from 3,510 in 1950 to 213 in 1970. The continued decline of recognized illness is a result of controls exerted on the animal reservoirs of infection. Regulations governing the pasteurization of milk were effective in reducing the infection of milk and dairy products. In addition to this, the United States Livestock Sanitary Association (now the United States Animal Health Association) and the Bureau of Animal Industry of the United States Department of Agriculture formulated the State Federal Cooperative Brucellosis Eradication Program. Their recommendations were reinforced by the 1953 USPHS Milk Ordinance and Code. The majority of states are now certified Brucellosis-free or Modified-certified for cattle, but only a few have achieved validated Brucellosis-free status for swine. This is reflected in the data collected through extensive study of 1,644 abattoir-associated cases of brucellosis occurring in the United States from 1960 to 1972, which revealed that 90 percent of these patients were exposed to infected hogs. Iowa, Virginia, California, and Illinois account for 88 percent of the reported hog-associated illnesses. Specific recommendations have been made to help control such abattoir-related infections.

An effective vaccine is available for animal immunization. In animals immunized during the first six to eight months of life, abortion is prevented, organisms are not excreted in the milk, and the animal has a permanent immunity against natural infection. In such animals there is only a transitory rise in complement-fixing antibodies, and the animal is serologically negative six months to one year after immunization. The strains employed for this purpose are the attenuated *B. abortus* strain 19 for cattle and the *B. melitensis* strain Rev I for sheep and goats.

PROPHYLAXIS IN MAN. Prevention of human brucellosis is primarily dependent upon control of the animal sources of infection. Modifications of milk and dairy product processing as well as animal surveillance and animal immunization have greatly reduced the dangers of this disease within the United States. The population at risk consists almost exclusively of those persons in contact with animals or their contaminated materials. Available vaccines are suitable only for animals. The disease remains one of economic importance in many countries of the world where control of infected animal herds has not been readily accomplished.

FURTHER READING

Books and Reviews

Alton CG, Jones LM: Laboratory Techniques in Brucellosis

Buchanan, RE and Gibbons NE: Bergey's Manual of Determinative Bacteriology, 8th ed, Williams & Wilkins, 1974

Spink WM: The Nature of brucellosis. Minneapolis, Univer Minnesota Press, 1956

WHO Technical Report Series No 464. Joint FAO/WHO Expert Committee on Brucellosis. 5th report, 1971

Selected Papers

Buchanan TM, Faber LC, Feldman RA: Brucellosis in the United States, 1960-72. An abattoir-associated disease. Part I. Clinical features and therapy. Medicine 53:403, 1974.

Buchanan TM, Sulzer CR, Frix MK, Feldman RA: Brucellosis in the United States, 1960-72. An abattoir-associated disease. Part II. Diagnostic aspects. Medicine 53: 415, 1974

Buchanan TM, Hendricks SL, Patton CM, Feldman RA: Brucellosis in the United States, 1960-72. An abattoir-associated disease. Part III. Epidemiology and evidence for acquired immunity. Medicine 53:427, 1974

Busch LA, Parker RL: Brucellosis in the United States. J Infect Dis 125:289, 1972

Elberg SS: Immunity to brucella infection. Medicine 52: 339, 1973

Smith H, Keppie J, Pearce JH, Fuller R, Williams AE: The chemical basis of the virulence of *Br. abortus*. 1. Isolation of *Br. abortus* from bovine foetal tissue. Br J Exp Pathol 42:631, 1961

Smith H, Keppie J, Pearce JH, Fuller R, Williams AE: Isolation of *Br. abortus* from bovine foetal tissue. Br J Exp Pathol 42:631, 1961

Smith H, Keppie J, Pierce JH, Fuller R, Williams AE: Erythritol. A constituent of bovine foetal fluids which stimulate the growth of *Br. abortus* in bovine phagocytes. Br J Exp Pathol 43:31, 1962

Smith H, Keppie J, Pearce JH, Fuller R, Williams AE: III. Foetal erythritol a cause of the localization of *Br. abortus* in pregnant cows. Br J Exp Pathol 43:530, 1962

47
Bacillus

The genus *Bacillus* includes members of the family Bacillaceae that are aerobic or facultative anaerobic rod-shaped organisms. Species in the genus are widely distributed in nature and often are encountered as contaminants of laboratory cultures. The only major pathogen of significance in the genus is *Bacillus anthracis,* the cause of anthrax. Other species have been studied extensively and have been especially useful in model studies on mechanisms of differentiation in procaryotic cells (Chap. 5).

BACILLUS ANTHRACIS

Anthrax is primarily a disease of herbivorous animals, particularly sheep and cattle and to a lesser extent horses, hogs, and goats. It is caused by *Bacillus anthracis,* a gram-positive, aerobic, spore-forming bacillus that was isolated by Robert Koch in 1877. Man accidentally encounters this disease in an agricultural setting, with the development of a local skin infection that may become generalized. The disease also may be acquired in an industrial setting from the processing of hides or animal hair, with resultant inhalation anthrax that produces a virulent type of pneumonia. Rarely the disease may be acquired by ingestion. Widespread immunization of animals has remarkably diminished outbreaks of this disease in herds, with the result that it is now a very rare illness for man.

Morphology and Physiology

The anthrax bacillus is a straight rod, 5 to 10 μm long and 1 to 3 μm wide. When examined in smears from the blood or tissues of an infected animal the organisms usually are found singly or in pairs. Their ends appear square, and the corners are often so sharp that the bacilli in the chains are in contact at these points, leaving an oval opening between the organisms. Unlike most members of the genus, *B. anthracis* is nonmotile. Bacilli are encapsulated during growth in the infected animal, but capsules cannot be demonstrated in vitro unless the organisms are cultured on bicarbonate media in the presence of 5 percent CO_2. Spores are formed in culture, in the soil, and in tissues and exudates of dead animals but not in the blood or tissues of living animals.

Cultural Characteristics The organisms grow well on most common laboratory media, but for demonstration of characteristic colonial morphology, specimens should be inoculated on 5 percent blood agar plates, prepared with blood free of antibiotics. Maximal growth of the organism is obtained at pH 7.0 to 7.4 under aerobic conditions, but sparse growth occurs in the absence of oxygen. The optimal temperature for maximal growth is 37C, but growth does not cease until temperatures as low as 12C and as high as 45C are reached. By continued cultivation, the organism may become adapted to either a low or high temperature and eventually attain luxuriant growth. The bacilli grow readily on simple laboratory media, producing in 24 hours large, raised, opaque, grayish white, plumose colonies 2 to 3 mm in diameter and possessing an irregular, fringelike edge. Tangled masses of long, hairlike curls can be seen with a colony microscope. The colony is membranous in consistency and emulsifies with difficulty. No hemolysis is produced. A selective medium, referred to as PLET, has been described that permits growth of *B. anthracis* while inhibiting common contaminants, enteric organisms, and even closely related spore-formers, such as *B. cereus.* Although PLET medium is useful for monitoring purposes, it is recommended that for culture of clinical materials, nonselective media be employed.

Laboratory Identification Biochemical properties useful in the identification of *B. anthracis* are listed in Table 47-1. Neither morphology nor the usual cultural characteristics will differentiate *B. anthracis* from nonmotile strains of *B. cereus,* the organism most easily mistaken for *B. anthracis.* Virulent strains of *B. anthracis,* however, are the only organisms that produce rough colonies when grown in the absence of increased CO_2 and mucoid colonies when grown on sodium bicarbonate medium in an atmosphere of 5 percent CO_2.

The string-of-pearls reaction also clearly separates virulent and avirulent *B. anthracis* from *B. cereus* and other aerobic sporeformers. The string-of-pearls reaction is most dramatic. It can be demonstrated following a three-to-six hour incubation of *B. anthracis* on the surface of a solid medium containing 0.05 to 0.5 units of penicillin G per milliliter. The cells become large and spherical and occur in chains on the

TABLE 47–1   DIFFERENTIAL CHARACTERISTICS OF BACILLUS ANTHRACIS
AND BACILLUS CEREUS

Characteristic	B. anthracis	B. cereus
Blood agar colony	Rough, flat, usually many comma-shaped outgrowths	Rough, flat, none or few comma-shaped outgrowths
Hemolysis	None or very weak	Usually beta hemolytic
Tenacity°	Positive	Negative
Bicarbonate medium (CO_2)	White, round, raised, glistening, mucoid	Flat, dull
Fluorescent–antibody test	Positive	Negative
Gamma phage	Susceptible	Resistant
Animal pathogenicity	Positive	Negative
Litmus milk	Not reduced or slowly reduced and peptonized	Usually reduced in 2 to 3 days
Methylene blue	Not reduced or slightly reduced in 24 hours	Usually reduced in 24 hours
Motility	Negative	Usually positive

Adapted from Lennette, Spaulding, and Traunt (eds).: Manual of Clinical Microbiology, 2nd ed. 1974. Courtesy of American Society for Microbiology
°*Refers to appearance of colony when pushed gently; resembles beaten egg whites*

surface of agar, resembling a string of pearls. Another useful test for differentiating *B. anthracis* and *B. cereus* is based on the susceptibility of *B. anthracis* to a variant bacteriophage, gamma phage; no lysis of *B. cereus* occurs. Confirmation of the identity of an isolate may be obtained by the inoculation of a mouse with a suspension of organisms from an agar plate. Death from anthrax infection usually occurs within two to five days, and organisms can be recovered from the heart blood.

Resistance   Because of its ability to produce spores, the anthrax bacillus is extremely resistant to adverse chemical and physical environments. A temperature of 120C for 15 minutes is usually adequate for inactivating the spore. The vegetative cell is comparable in resistance to other nonspore-forming bacteria and is destroyed by a temperature of 54C in 30 minutes. Spores remain viable for years in contaminated pastures and remain a source of infection for long periods.

Antigenic Structure

Three antigens of *B. anthracis* have been partially characterized: (1) the capsular polypeptide, (2) a polysaccharide somatic antigen, and (3) a complex protein toxin. Unlike most bacterial capsules, the capsule of *B. anthracis* is a polypeptide of high molecular weight consisting exclusively of D-glutamic acid. There appears to be a single antigenic capsular type.

The somatic polysaccharide antigen is a component of the cell wall and contains equimolar amounts of D-glucosamine and D-galactose. Antibodies to this antigen are not protective.

Anthrax toxin is a complex toxin consisting of three components: protective antigen (PA), lethal factor (LF), and edema factor (EF). All of the components appear to be nondialyzable proteins or lipoproteins, highly thermolabile and displaying evidence of molecular heterogeneity. The components are serologically active and distinct. They are also immunogenic. Some biologic activity can be demonstrated upon injection of either protective factor or lethal factor alone, but maximal biologic activity occurs only when the various components are combined.

Determinants of Pathogenicity

Only strains of *B. anthracis* that produce both a capsule and a toxin are fully virulent. The glutamyl polypeptide capsule interferes with phagocytosis and appears to be a major factor in the organism's pathogenesis, especially during the early stages of infection. Antibodies against the capsular antigen are produced, but they are not protective against the disease. The signs and symptoms of anthrax are attributable to a toxin that builds up gradually in the infected animal to become maximal at the time of death. The pathophysiology of the bacillary disease and the toxemia from sterile toxin are very similar. In both cases and in all animal hosts tested, respiratory failure and anoxia result from action of the toxin on the central nervous system.

The complex toxin derived from the thoracic and peritoneal exudates of infected animals consists of the three components, PA, LF, and EF. Maximum toxicity occurs only when all components are present. A combination of PA and LF are required for lethality; EF and LF combined have no biologic activity. Although toxoiding of the toxin and of its components has been demonstrated, data in this area are limited.

Clinical Infection

Epidemiology Spontaneous disease occurs in herbivorous animals that acquire the infection by ingestion of spores that probably enter the body through microscopic cuts or abrasions of the oral or intestinal mucosa. When a pasture has been contaminated with anthrax spores, it may remain a source of infection for 20 to 30 years. Although it is impossible to determine the precise time of infection in a case of spontaneous anthrax, it is certain that the duration of the disease is only a few days. The infected animal remains asymptomatic until a few hours before death. Mortality in herbivorous animals is usually about 80 percent. Sporadic cases continue to occur in the United States; in 1968 a total of 165 cases of anthrax occurred on 34 farms in California. Many species of animals acquire the natural disease, and epizootics continue to occur in wildlife sanctuaries in Africa.

The most common form of human anthrax is industrial anthrax, which results from contact with animal products, such as wool, hide, goat hair, skin, and bones imported from Africa, the Middle East, and Asia. Less commonly, anthrax is acquired in an agricultural setting from working with infected animals. One of the most recent episodes of anthrax in this country resulted from imported bongo drums covered with animal hide containing the spores. Cutaneous anthrax also has resulted from contact with finished products, such as shaving brushes made with animal bristles, ivory keys on a piano, and wool products.

Pathogenesis Man becomes infected by one of three mechanisms. The organisms can gain access through small abrasions or cuts and multiply locally, with a fairly dramatic inflammatory response. They also may gain access by inhalation, where they multiply in the lung and are swept to the draining hilar lymph nodes, where marked hemorrhagic necrosis may occur. A rare method of infection is ingestion of infected meat, with resultant invasion of the gastrointestinal mucosa and ulceration. From all three surface areas, invasion of the bloodstream may occur with profound toxemia. Metastatic infections, such as meningitis, may complicate the primary process.

Clinical Manifestation Anthrax presents in one of three ways, depending on the mode of infection. Cutaneous anthrax begins two to five days after infection as a small papule that develops within a few days into a vesicle filled with dark bluish black fluid. Rupture of the vesicle reveals a black eschar at the base, with a very prominent inflammatory ring of reaction around the eschar, sometimes called a "malignant pustule." The lesion is classically found on the hands, forearms, or head. It is rarely found on the trunk or lower extremities. The pulmonary infection is known as "woolsorters disease" and occurs in patients who handle raw wool, hides, or horse hair and acquire the disease by the inhalation of spores. The patient's symptoms are typically those of a respiratory infection with fever, malaise, myalgia, and unproductive cough. Within several days, however, it rapidly becomes a very severe infection with marked respiratory distress and cyanosis. With the sudden worsening of the illness, death usually supervenes within 24 hours. Infection of the gastrointestinal tract, which occurs rarely, is associated with nausea, vomiting, and diarrhea. Occasionally there is loss of blood either through hematemesis or in the stools. This is associated with profound prostration, with eventual development of shock and death. From all three of these surface infections there may be invasion of the bloodstream and localization in the meninges, with a resultant fatal meningitis.

Anthrax infection in man provides permanent immunity, and second attacks are extremely rare.

Laboratory Diagnosis Specimens for culture should be obtained either from a malignant pustule, from the sputum, or from a blood culture. A gram stain and fluorescent antibody stain are useful in making a presumptive diagnosis. The organism will grow readily on most laboratory media. However the greatest problems are the frequency with which nonpathogenic species of bacilli, such as *B. cereus,* are confused with *B. anthracis* and the fact that most laboratory personnel have never seen *B. anthracis.*

Acute and convalescent sera should be obtained, since antibodies to the organism can be demonstrated by agar-gel diffusion, complement fixation, and hemagglutination procedures. These procedures are available at the Communicable Disease Center, and acute and convalescent sera of suspect cases may be submitted to the CDC.

Treatment   *B. anthracis* is quite susceptible to penicillin and when used early in the course of the illness is curative. The major difficulty is the lack of clinical suspicion of anthrax because of its rarity. Cutaneous anthrax may therefore be diagnosed as another illness, with prescription of an antibiotic appropriate to that illness. With pulmonary anthrax the diagnosis usually is made at postmortem, as is the case with gastrointestinal anthrax. If the diagnosis of pulmonary anthrax is made in sufficient time, large intravenous doses of penicillin should be instituted as quickly as possible. In patients allergic to penicillin, tetracycline may be used. If a skin lesion is mistakenly identified as a staphylococcal infection, incision and drainage may be attempted. This can lead to disastrous results because of widespread dissemination of the organism.

Prevention   Animals   with   known   or suspected anthrax should be handled with care and their carcasses buried deeply to prevent the spread of spores to new pastures. Wool, horse hair, and hides coming from areas where epidemic anthrax is present should be gas sterilized. A vaccine is available for outbreaks of human anthrax in an industrial setting.

IMMUNIZATION.   Active   immunization   is the only known method of preventing anthrax in herbivorous animals in areas where the pasture land is already contaminated with spores. Pasteur's famous attenuated living anthrax vaccine was effective but difficult to maintain at a desired level of virulence, and it has been su-

perseded by a living spore vaccine made from a nonencapsulated strain *of B. anthracis.* In a comparison of this vaccine with an alum-precipitated protective antigen vaccine, it was shown that the living vaccine gave good protection but caused some local disease in the animals. The protection afforded by the protective antigen was 100 percent after one month but dropped to 52 percent in three and one-half months. The use of both materials simultaneously provides a marked increase in level of resistance and is the recommended procedure for animal immunization when available. The widespread use of a living spore vaccine in South Africa has reduced the incidence of anthrax in the cattle of this area by over 99 percent. The alum-precipitated protective antigen has been used in industrial plants to protect workers in high-risk situations. This antigen appears to be quite effective, and no harmful side effects are produced.

OTHER AEROBIC SPORE-FORMING BACILLI

Gram-positive aerobic, spore-forming bacilli are ubiquitous in nature, commonly found in soil and water. In the Eighth Edition of *Bergey's Manual* 48 different species of *Bacillus* have been recognized. Within the genus there is great diversity in the properties of the organisms included. Variations occur in metabolic type and in nutritional requirements for growth. Vegetative cell walls of the different species vary in structure, composition, and susceptibility to lytic enzymes. One of the most reliable diagnostic properties of the genus is spore formation. Among the members of the genus are several species that produce antibiotics, but only one, polymyxin made by *B. polymyxa,* is of clinical use.

Several species, such as *B. thuringiensis,* produce disease in insects, some of which have been used in insect control. There is no evidence to suggest that they cause human infection. One species, *B. cereus,* produces a toxin and has a limited ability to produce disease in animals; it has been implicated in outbreaks of human food poisoning. *B. subtilis* is present in the air, dust, brackish water, and infusion of vegetable matter. It is a common laboratory contaminant and may appear in clinical specimens as a secondary contaminant of wounds.

FURTHER READING

Books and Reviews

Bonventre PF, Johnson CE: *Bacillus cereus* toxin. In Montie TC, Kadis S, Ajl SJ (eds): Microbial Toxins. New York, Academic Press, 1970, vol 3, pp 415-435

Brachman PS: Anthrax. In Hoeprich PD (ed): Infectious Diseases. Hagerstown, Md, Harper & Row, 1972

Lincoln RE, Fish DC: Anthrax toxin. In Montie TC, Kadis S, Ajl SJ (eds): Microbial Toxins. New York, Academic Press, 1970, vol 3, pp 361-413

Selected Papers

Brachman PS: Anthrax. Ann NY Acad Sci, 174:577, 1970

Burdon KL, Wende RD: On the differentiation of anthrax bacilli from *Bacillus cereus*. J Infect Dis 107:224, 1960

Ellar DJ, Lundgren DB: Ordered substructure in the cell wall of *Bacillus cereus*. J Bacteriol 94:1778, 1967

Fish DC, Mahlandt BG, Dobbs JP, Lincoln RF: Purification and properties of in vitro-produced anthrax toxin components. J Bacteriol 95:907, 1968

Fitz-James PC, Young IE: Comparison of species and varieties of the genus *Bacillus*. J Bacteriol 78:743, 755, 765, 1959

Gold H: Treatment of anthrax. Fed Proc 26:1563, 1967

Gordon MA, Moody MD, Barton AM, Boyd FM: Industrial air sampling for anthrax bacteria. Arch Indust Hyg Occup Med 10:16, 1954

Jones WI Jr, Klein F, Walker JS, et al: Growth of anthrax bacilli in resistant, susceptible, and immunized hosts. J. Bacteriol 94:600, 1967

Klein F, DeArmon IA Jr, Lincoln RE, Mahlandt BG, Fernelius AL: Immunity against *Bacillus anthracis* from protective antigen live vaccine. J Immunol 88:15, 1962

Morbidity and Mortality Weekly Reports. Animal Anthrax in California, 17:279, 1968

Nungester WJ: Proceedings of the conference on progress in the understanding of anthrax. Fed Proc 26:1491, 1967

Weinstein L, Colburn CG: *Bacillus subtilis* meningitis and bacteremia. Arch Intern Med 86:585, 1950

48

Introduction to the Anaerobic Bacteria: Non-spore-forming Anaerobes

Recognition of the anaerobic nature of certain species of microorganisms is credited to Pasteur, who, in 1863, noted that motility of certain bacteria was lost upon exposure to air. A number of bacteria which would only grow in gaseous environments having substantially reduced oxygen tensions were isolated prior to 1900. Greater attention was given to the gram-positive, spore-forming, anaerobic bacilli (*Clostridum*) because of their recognized association with important human disease, such as gas gangrene, tetanus, and botulism. Study of non-spore-forming anaerobic bacteria lagged because of their sensitivity to oxygen, fastidious growth requirements, and their occurrence in complex mixtures of anaerobic and facultative species. Provision of anaerobic environments for culture was technically difficult, and broth rather than surface growth on solid media was primarily used. These technical problems made it almost impossible to obtain pure cultures for study.

TABLE 48-1   GENUS IDENTIFICATION OF MEDICALLY SIGNIFICANT ANAEROBIC BACTERIA

I. Rods
  A. Form spores (sometimes difficult to demonstrate) .... *Clostridium**
  B. Do not form spores
    1. Gram-positive cells present (Kopeloff's modification of Gram's stain)
      a. Propionic and acetic acids as the major volatile acid products ..... *Propionibacterium** and *Arachnia**
      b. Acetic and lactic acids (1+ to 1) .... *Bifidobacterium**
      c. Lactic acid sole major product .... *Lactobacillus**
      d. Moderate acetic, major succinic,† ±formic and/or lactic .... *Actinomyces**
      e. Other: butyric and others, acetic and formic, or no major acids .... *Eubacterium** and *Lachnospira*
    2. Only gram-negative cells present (Kopeloff's modification of Gram's stain)
      a. Peritrichous flagella or nonmotile
        i. Produce butyric acid (without much isobutyric and isovaleric acid) .... *Fusobacterium**
        ii. Produce only lactic acid .... *Leptotrichia buccalis*
        iii. Not as above (i, ii) .... *Bacteroides**
      b. Polar flagella.
        i. Fermentative
          a. Produce butyric acid .... *Butyrivibrio*
          b. Produce succinic acid
            1. Spiral-shaped cells .... *Succinivibrio*
            2. Ovoid cells .... *Succinimonas*
        ii. Nonfermentative
          a. Microaerophilic .... *Campylobacter**,‡
          b. Obligately anaerobic .... *Vibrio succinogenes**
      c. Tufts of flagella on concave side of crescent-shaped cells .... *Selenomonas*
      d. Spiral-shaped cells with axial filaments............................ *Treponema** and *Borrelia**
II. Cocci
  A. Gram positive
    1. Occur in packets .... *Sarcina*
    2. Pairs and chains
      a. Require fermentable carbohydrate
        i. Produce butyric acid .... *Coprococcus*
        ii. Do not produce butyric acid .... *Ruminococcus*
      b. Do not require fermentable carbohydrate
        i. Produce lactic acid as sole major fermentation product .... *Streptococcus**
        ii. Not as above (i) .... *Peptostreptococcus** and *Peptococcus**
  B. Gram negative
    1. Produce propionic and acetic acids .... *Veillonella**
    2. Produce butyric and other acids
      a. Ferment carbohydrate and produce budding cells .... *Gemmiger*
      b. Do not ferment carbohydrate .... *Acidaminococcus**
    3. Large cells and produce complex mixture of fermentation acids .... *Megasphaera*

Modified from Holdeman and Moore: Anaerobic Bacteriology Manual, 3rd ed. 1975. Courtesy of Virginia Polytechnic Institute and State University.
*Medically significant: Inclusion of certain genera is on the basis of their isolation from clinical specimens with pathogenicity unproven
†Amount of succinic acid depends on amount of CO_2 present
‡Will grow in 10 percent oxygen but not aerobically or anaerobically

The inadequacies of techniques formerly employed in the culture of anaerobes are reflected in the high percentage of infected specimens submitted for culture in which no organisms could be isolated. With improved anaerobic technology, however, a high incidence of anaerobic organisms in clinical specimens has been demonstrated. The higher isolation rate not only may reflect an improvement in techniques but also may indicate an increased incidence of anaerobic infections. Many anaerobic organisms previously considered to be harmless commensals of our indigenous flora are now recognized as opportunistic pathogens that may produce disease when the host's resistance is lowered. Tissue damage due to surgery and administration of antibiotics, corticosteroids, cytotoxic agents, and other immunosuppressive drugs may modify host defenses and alter the normal flora so that the endogenous anaerobes are able to initiate disease. Modern hospital care has thus apparently created within the population a higher proportion of individuals susceptible to anaerobic infections.

The anaerobic bacteria are widespread in nature. They constitute the predominant part of our normal indigenous flora, and outnumber facultatively anaerobic bacteria of the gut by a factor of 1,000:1 and of the skin, mouth, and upper respiratory tract by 5:1 to 10:1. Recognition of the high incidence of anaerobes in and on our bodies as normal flora is recent, and consequently their contributions to health and disease are just beginning to receive widespread attention. With but few exceptions it has been traditionally taught that the clostridia are the only anaerobes of medical significance. Even now, in spite of substantial laboratory and clinical data, there exists some resistance to re-education and acceptance of a pathogenic role for the non-spore-forming anaerobic bacteria.

The anaerobic bacteria include many different types, both gram-positive and gram-negative. In the Eighth Edition of *Bergey's Manual* they are classified in different parts on the basis of their gram stain reaction, cellular morphology, and intolerance to oxygen. Although DNA homology and other techniques have increased our understanding of relatedness among anaerobes, a need exists for further work on classification and simplification of the procedures required for cultivation and identification. At present there are many anaerobic bacteria that cannot be identified. The student should be

aware that the same organism may have a variety of names coined over the years and that reference to authoritative manuals on anaerobic bacteriology are helpful in reading some of the older literature.

Anaerobic bacteria may be conveniently divided into: (1) the spore-forming clostridia and (2) the non-spore-forming anaerobic bacteria, on the basis of differences in the types of diseases produced and the characteristics of growth. The pathogenic exotoxin-producing clostridia will be covered separately in Chapters 49, 50, and 51 because of the specific disease entities that they produce. It is important to remember, however, that both toxigenic and nonpathogenic clostridia usually are present in infections in combination with the non-spore-forming anaerobes and require similar techniques for isolation and culture. Cultural characteristics and anaerobic methodology common to the study of most anaerobic bacteria are covered in this chapter. The non-spore-forming anaerobes are grouped for discussion within this chapter with emphasis only on genera and species with a recognized relationship to human infection (Table 48-1). Additional information on anaerobic organisms will be found in Chapters 37, 52, 53, 54, 55, and 56 on the *Actinomyces, Treponema, Borrelia, Leptospira, Spirillum, Campylobacter,* and Dental Microbiology.

CLINICAL AND LABORATORY REQUIREMENTS FOR CULTURE AND IDENTIFICATION OF ANAEROBIC BACTERIA

Clinical Requirements Culture of anaerobic bacteria differs from that of many aerobic or facultative pathogens because the medically significant anaerobes also constitute a major part of our normal endogenous flora. Thus, isolation of anaerobic bacteria may be clinically meaningless unless the specimen is derived from a site that is normally sterile. The locations of normal body flora must be appreciated and these sites avoided in collecting specimens to allow correct interpretation of culture results (Table 48-2). For this reason the following

TABLE 48-2 INCIDENCE OF ANAEROBIC BACTERIA AS NORMAL FLORA IN HUMANS

Anatomic Site	Cocci		Bacilli								
			Gram positive						Gram negative		
	Gram Positive	Gram Negative	Clos-tridium	Actino-myces	Bifido-bacterium	Eubac-terium	Lacto-bacillus†	Propioni-bacterium	Bacter-oides	Fuso-bacterium	Campylo-bacter
Skin	1	0	0	0	0	U	0	2	0	0	0
Upper respiratory tract*	1	1	0	1	0	±	0	1	1	1	1
Mouth	2	2	±	1	1	1	1	±	2	2	1
Intestine	2	1	2	±	2	2	1	±	2	1	±
External genitalia	1	0	0	0	0	U	0	U	1	1	0
Urethra	±	±	±	0	0	U	±	±	1	1	±
Vagina	1	1	±	0	2	U	2	0	1	±	1

Modified from Sutter, Vargo, and Finegold: Wadsworth Anaerobic Bacteriology Manual, 2nd ed. 1975. Courtesy of University of California

* = includes nasal passages, nasopharynx, oropharynx, and tonsils
† = includes anaerobic, microaerophilic, and facultative strains
U = unknown
0 = not found or rare
± = irregular
1 = usually present
2 = usually present in large numbers

641

TABLE 48-3   Clinical Clues of Possible Anaerobic Infection

1. Clinical setting suggestive of anaerobic infection, ie, pulmonary infection associated with aspiration, infection following bowel surgery, postabortal sepsis.
2. Foul-smelling discharge
3. Location of infection in proximity to a mucosal surface
4. Necrotic tissue, gangrene, pseudomembrane formation
5. Gas in tissues or discharges
6. Clinical signs of infection with negative routine (aerobic) cultures
7. Infection associated with malignancy or other process
8. Infection related to the use of aminoglycosides (oral, parenteral, or topical)
9. Septic thrombophlebitis
10. Bacteremic picture with jaundice
11. Infection following human or other bites
12. Black discoloration of exudates containing blood (infection may involve *Bacteroides melaninogenicus*)
13. Presence of sulfur granules in discharges (actinomycosis)
14. Classical clinical features of gas gangrene

Modified from Finegold and Rosenblatt: Medicine 52:318, 1973

specimens are unacceptable for anaerobic culture: expectorated sputum, throat swabs, nasotracheal or bronchoscopy aspirates, gastrointestinal contents, feces, vaginal secretions, midstream or clean catch urine, and skin or superficial wound swabs. Appropriate specimens include normally sterile body fluids (ie, pleural, joint, bile, peritoneal fluid), surgical specimens from normally sterile sites, abscess contents, blood cultures, and deep wound and transtracheal aspirates. Certain clinical clues are very helpful for the clinician in recognizing

infections most likely to involve anaerobic bacteria (Table 48-3), as well as knowledge of the types of infections from which anaerobes are commonly isolated (Table 48-4).

Culture of anaerobic bacteria generally requires more time than is required for facultative organisms, since many anaerobes grow very slowly and usually must be isolated from complex mixtures containing both anaerobic and facultative species. A direct gram stain of the specimen read by a trained individual can be a significant aid to the clinician in the choice of initial antibiotic therapy.

Communication between clinician and microbiologist is important in the proper interpretation of anaerobic cultures. A complete understanding of the potential pathogenicity of most anaerobic bacteria is lacking. Certain non-spore-forming anaerobes, such as *Bacteroides fragilis* subspecies *fragilis*, subspecies *thetaiotaomicron*, and subspecies *vulgatus*, *B. melaninogenicus*, *Fusobacterium nucleatum*, *F. necrophorum*, and species of *Peptostreptococcus* and *Peptococcus*, consistently are found in infected material and are generally accepted as potentially pathogenic. Less is known regarding many other anaerobic bacteria isolated from infections, and interpretation of their presence in clinical material depends on numerous factors. For example, *Propionibacterium acnes* usually is considered a contaminant, since it is part of the normal flora of the skin. It may in rare circumstances, however, assume the role of a pathogen. Also, in mixed infections the bacteria essential to the infection are difficult to

TABLE 48-4   Infections in which Anaerobic Bacteria are Commonly Isolated or are Predominant Pathogens

Brain abscess	Peritonitis
Otogenic meningitis, extradural or subdural empyema	Appendicitis
	Subphrenic abscess
Chronic otitis media	Other intraabdominal abscess
Dental infections	Wound infections following
Pneumonia secondary to obstructive process	bowel surgery or trauma
	Puerperal sepsis
Aspiration pneumonia	Postabortal sepsis
Lung abscess	Endometritis
Bronchiectasis	Tubo-ovarian abscess
Thoracic empyema	Other gynecologic infections
Breast abscess	Perirectal abscess
Pylephlebitis	Gas-forming cellulitis
Liver abscess	Gas gangrene

Modified from Finegold and Rosenblatt: Medicine 52:318, 1973

define, since many of the same organisms are found in settings of overt infections as well as in harmless colonization. Thus even with anaerobic culture techniques sufficiently sensitive to isolate the anaerobes present, in mixed infection specific roles seldom can be assigned.

Laboratory Requirements* The toxic effects of O_2 on anaerobes necessitate the production and maintenance of a reduced O_2 environment for successful cultivation. Until 1966 when the simplified Gaspak† jar system was introduced, most of the methods available were cumbersome, inadequate, and difficult. Currently, there are a number of culture systems available, but certain principles common to all are essential for optimal recovery of anaerobic bacteria from clinical specimens.

(1) Specimens should be collected in a manner to avoid contamination with normal flora.

(2) Collection and transport to the laboratory must avoid undue exposure of the specimen to oxygen and dehydration. Since the oxygen sensitivity of any anaerobes present is unknown at the time of collection, all specimens should be delivered to the laboratory immediately or in minimal time using stoppered transport tubes or vials containing an O_2-free gas (usually CO_2).

(3) An immediate gram stain of the material is extremely valuable to the physician in his selection of initial antibiotic therapy and to the microbiologist in the choice of appropriate media and methods for culture and as a quality control.

(4) Specimens should be cultured as soon as possible, with the aim of minimizing exposure to oxygen. Enriched media must be freshly made or prepared and held in an O_2-free atmosphere (CO_2 or N_2). Anaerobic culture should include both direct streaking of

---

More detailed information on recommended anaerobic methods, media, controls, isolation, and identification methods are given in the following reference sources: Laboratory Methods in Anaerobic Bacteriology *(CDC Laboratory Manual),* Anaerobic Bacteriology Manual *(VPI Anaerobe Laboratory),* Wadsworth Anaerobic Bacteriology Manual, Manual of Clinical Microbiology, The Pathogenic Anaerobic Bacteria, *articles by Aranki and Freter, and* Bergey's Manual of Determinative Bacteriology, *8th ed.*
†Gaspak (Baltimore Biological Laboratories).

plates and inoculation of enrichment broth. Plates should also be inoculated for aerobic and/or CO_2 incubation.

(5) A properly functioning anaerobic culture system must be utilized. Catalysts used to remove residual oxygen must be active.

(6) Incubation should be continued for a sufficient time to permit isolation of slow-growing organisms. Ideally, plates should be checked at 18 to 24 hours for fast-growing anaerobes *(Clostridium)* and daily thereafter up to five to seven days in order to isolate very slow-growing bacteria, such as actinomycetes.

ANAEROBIC CULTURE SYSTEMS. At present three primary types of anaerobic culture systems are in use: the anaerobic jar, the roll tube, and the anaerobic glove box.

Anaerobic Jar Method. This method employs vented or unvented jars or bags for holding culture plates or tubes. These containers have a leakproof closure and contain a catalyst, palladium, which reacts with residual oxygen in the presence of hydrogen to form water. They are filled with an anaerobic gas mixture provided either by a Gaspak H_2 and CO_2 gas generator envelope, which generates the proper volume of gas when water is added to the packet, or by a mechanical evacuation-replacement system consisting of a vacuum source, manometer, and a gas cylinder (mixture containing 10 percent H_2, 5 to 10 percent CO_2, and N_2). These systems function properly only if the catalyst is kept active. Inoculated media are placed within these jars and incubated in a standard incubator.

Roll Tube Method. This system uses enriched media that has been prepared, sterilized, and stored under O_2-free gas in order to maintain a low oxidation-reduction potential and prevent oxidative changes. The media is kept anaerobic during inoculation either by needle injection through the oxygen impermeable stopper without introducing any air or, more commonly, by passing a gentle stream of O_2-free gas into the tube via a sterile cannula when the stopper is removed. Thus, each tube has its own anaerobic atmosphere and can be incubated in a standard incubator and observed at any time for growth.

Anaerobic Glove Box Method. This method consists of a closed chamber usually made of flexible clear plastic and fitted with gloves for manipulations within the enclosed space. An entry lock which can be evacuated and filled with O_2-free gas is used to pass material in and out of the chamber, which is filled with 10 percent H_2, 5 to 10 percent CO_2, and N_2. Any oxygen introduced into the system is removed by palladium catalyst. The glove box contains all the necessary equipment for bacteriologic work, including incubators, so that standard methods of inoculation, incubation, and isolation can be accomplished completely within an anaerobic environment.

All of these anaerobic systems, however, have certain advantages and disadvantages, and at present there is no really optimal system. Although the roll tube and anaerobic glove box systems yield a higher number of isolates of the more oxygen-sensitive species, the anaerobic bacteria associated with clinical infections appear to be less oxygen sensitive than do other anaerobic members of the normal flora and may not require the more sensitive techniques.

PRIMARY CULTURE. Good anaerobic technology should always include the primary streaking of clinical material on solid media. Since many anaerobic infections are polymicrobic, containing either a mixture of anaerobic species or of anaerobic plus facultatively anaerobic species, introduction of a mixed bacterial inoculum into liquid media will result in growth of the least fastidious, most rapidly growing bacteria at the expense of other strains that may be present in high proportions in the original material. Thus, an organism such as *Escherichia coli*, which is commonly found in association with anaerobic organisms, may outgrow and mask the presence of anaerobic bacteria in a broth culture. Use of solid media circumvents this.

In general the anaerobes are nutritionally very fastidious and require an enriched medium for growth. Growth factor requirements may be met by the addition of yeast extract, blood, vitamin K, hemin, and a fermentable carbohydrate to the base medium. Cooked chopped meat medium containing carbohydrate is probably the best liquid medium for initial culture because it is enriched and a low oxidation-reduction potential is provided by re-ducing substances present in the tissue. Unless the culture is placed in an anaerobic environment for incubation, it should be overlayed with a seal of vaspar (paraffin and Vaseline) to protect the liquid from exposure to oxygen. Thioglycolate prepared and stored under aerobic conditions and without supplementation is inadequate for initial growth of many anaerobic bacteria. For effective use it should either be stored under anaerobic conditions or boiled 10 minutes prior to use, and it should be supplemented with the materials listed above, with serum (inactivated rabbit, bovine, or other) substituted for blood.

Since anaerobic infections often contain a mixture of different species, careful streaking on initial plating media or roll tubes is essential for isolation. In addition to nonselective media, use of antibiotic-containing selective media aids in the isolation of anaerobes from heavily mixed populations. A dissecting microscope is useful in recognizing different colony types sufficiently early so that culture information will have greater clinical value.

IDENTIFICATION. Once the laboratory has determined that an isolate is present in pure culture and will not grow on the surface of blood agar plates exposed to air, a number of identification schemes are available. Although a few species included among the anaerobes will either grow sparsely under aerobic conditions or will grow in a microaerophilic environment with added carbon dioxide, especially after subculture, growth is always more luxuriant under anaerobic conditions. A commonly used scheme of classification and identification to the genus level (VPI *Anaerobic Bacteriology Manual*) is based on gram-stain reaction morphology, motility, and gas-liquid chromatography of volatile fatty acids, nonvolatile acids, and alcohols produced as end products of metabolism (Table 48-1). Species determination is based on gas-liquid chromatography, sugar fermentation, and various biochemical reactions.

SEROLOGIC TECHNIQUES. Immunofluorescence appears promising as a useful technique for the rapid identification of bacteroides and fusobacteria directly in clinical material or in pure culture. Fluorescent antibody conjugates have been used for specific staining of *Actinomyces* and *Propionibacterium*.

NON-SPORE-FORMING ANAEROBES OF MEDICAL SIGNIFICANCE

Morphology and Physiology

MORPHOLOGIC TYPES. The anaerobic bacteria include a variety of morphologic types, including gram-positive and gram-negative bacilli and cocci, comma-shaped organisms, and spirochetes (Table 48-1) Although the clostridia generally stain boldly with the gram stain, many of the non-spore-forming anaerobic bacteria stain poorly, are pale in appearance, and are gram-variable. Better definition may be obtained by the use of Kopeloff's modification of the gram stain. Observation of certain of the anaerobes, including *Campylobacter*, *Treponema*, and *Borrelia*, may require phase contrast or darkfield microscopy.

As a group, anaerobic bacteria are more pleomorphic in appearance than are most aerobic or facultatively anaerobic bacteria, a property that may be useful in their recognition from clinical material. Since pleomorphism, however, is quite variable depending on the chemical environment of infected material or of artificial culture, it cannot be utilized as an absolute requirement for the presence of anaerobes. For example, *Bacteroides fragilis*, a clinically significant organism, demonstrates characteristic vacuolization and pleomorphism on culture in thioglycolate media or certain other media containing fermentable carbohydrate, but it may not always appear pleomorphic in direct smears from clinical material or in other media (Fig. 48-1).

Colonial morphology of most anaerobes on solid and liquid media is not sufficiently unique to aid appreciably in their identification. Characteristics helpful in some instances include production of turbid, granular, or flocculent growth in liquid culture and the size, shape, color, and consistency of colonies on solid media. Hemolysis does not aid in the identification of the organisms to the same extent that it does with certain aerobic or facultatively anaerobic bacteria. Colonial morphology, like cellular morphology, is extremely dependent on the cultural environment.

ANAEROBIOSIS. The basis for oxygen intolerance among anaerobic bacteria remains un-

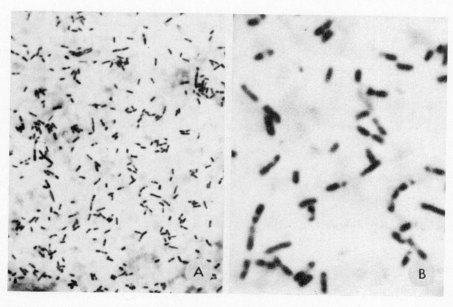

FIG 48-1. *Bacteroides fragilis* subspecies *fragilis* from supplemented thioglycolate. Pleomorphism, which may be considerably more or less apparent than shown here, is highly dependent on the cultural environment and on strain differences. A. ×1000. B. ×1000 enlarged 3 times to demonstrate vacuoles present within cells.

solved at present. Various factors play a role, but no single mechanism has received complete acceptance. Among the proposals are (1) O_2 has a direct toxic effect, (2) O_2 is indirectly toxic by specific mediators such as H_2O_2 or free radicals, (3) an appropriate low oxidation-reduction potential which appears to be required for many anaerobic bacteria is unachievable in the presence of normal O_2 tensions, (4) essential SH-containing enzymes are oxidized and therefore inactivated by O_2, and (5) O_2 inhibits metabolism by reaction with flavoproteins and DPNH oxidases, thereby critically lowering the reducing power of the cell.

One of the more popular theories advanced to explain the toxicity of O_2 for anaerobic bacteria is based on their lack of the enzyme, catalase, and the accumulation of toxic levels of H_2O_2. Although undoubtedly important, experimentation has not substantiated the hypothesis that the absence of catalase is the sole mechanism of oxygen toxicity. Certain species of anaerobes demonstrate low levels of catalase activity, and certain aerobes are devoid of the activity. More recently, it has been proposed that absence of the enzyme, superoxide dismutase, may be a major contributing factor in the inability of anaerobes to survive in oxygen. Since, however, relatively few anaerobic bacteria have been assayed for this enzyme, a primary role cannot be assigned. Indeed, a single mechanism may not be applicable to all anaerobes, and different mechanisms may also apply under different environmental conditions. Anaerobes are not equally intolerant of O_2. Maximum growth occurs at a PO_2 equal to or less than 0.5 percent for strict anaerobes and equal to or less than 3 percent for moderate anaerobes. A few anaerobes demonstrate variable growth at a PO_2 up to 8 percent.

Determinants of Pathogenicity

Since the pathogenic potential among non-spore-forming anaerobic bacteria has only recently been recognized, information on the mechanisms of pathogenicity is limited. No toxins are produced by the non-spore-forming anaerobes that are comparable to the potent toxins of certain clostridia. Endotoxins containing heptone and 2-keto-3-deoxyoctonate (KDO) in the lipopolysaccharide portion have been obtained from certain members of the group, including species of *Fusobacterium*, *Bacteroides*, and *Veillonella*. Endotoxic activity has been detected in 29 strains of the bacteroides and fusobacteria tested. The demonstration of enhanced coagulation (decreased clotting time) in mice injected with whole bacteria, lipopolysaccharide, or lipid A from strains of bacteroides and fusobacteria may be related to thromboembolic disease associated with clinical bacteroides infections.

Except for endotoxin, few bacterial products have been shown to play a role in disease production. *Bacteroides melaninogenicus* produces an enzyme, collagenase, which is capable of hydrolyzing native collagen and appears to play a unique role in the production of experimental infections. A heparinase also is produced by certain bacteroides, thus suggesting an alternate hypothesis to endotoxin for the development of thrombophlebitis and septic pulmonary emboli during bacteroides infections. *Fusobacterium necrophorum* strains produce hemolysins and lipases, which are referred to as toxins but which are much less potent than the toxins of *Clostridium*. A leukocidin toxin has been obtained from strains of *F. necrophorum* isolated from sheep with foot abscess. The toxin is released from the organism during growth and is distinct from endotoxin. It is a macromolecule inactivated slowly at 100C, in contrast to the hemolysin and lipase, which are inactivated by heating at 56C for 30 minutes. Tissue damage in the host is apparently related to inhibition of leukocyte migration and damage to leukocytes, which then release irritant substances. A neuraminidase has been detected in *Fusobacterium polymorphum* (probably a strain of *F. nucleatum*) that may play a role in pathogenicity.

Clinical Infection

Diseases of Animals Extensive studies have centered on two naturally occurring anaerobic infections in domestic animals: liver abscesses in cattle and foot infections of sheep. Although primarily motivated by the economic impact, these studies are significant because of the insight they provide into the complex interrelationships that exist between bacteria within a symbiotic mixture. Ovine interdigital dermatitis and the more serious infective bulbar necrosis are caused by *F. necrophorum* and *Cory-*

nebacterium pyogenes acting as a synergistic mixture. Benign footrot and virulent footrot result when *Bacteroides nodosus (F. nodosus)* is added to the foregoing mixture of bacteria. In cattle, liver abscesses occur when animals are fed diets high in carbohydrate prior to slaughter. *Fusobacterium necrophorum*, which is normally present in the intestine and rumen, escapes into the hepatic portal system when the integrity of the wall of the rumen or intestine is compromised as a result of changes in the rumen microflora and irritating fermentation products produced with the altered diet.

EXPERIMENTAL ANIMAL INFECTIONS. In the past demonstration of infectivity of nonspore-forming anaerobic bacteria for laboratory animals was often unsuccessful. This may have been because of technical difficulties encountered in culturing sufficiently high concentrations of viable organisms for injection. A small number of well-documented early studies, however, increased awareness of the role of anaerobic bacteria in clinical infection and pioneered work on the polymicrobial nature of many anaerobic infections and the combined pathologic activities of organisms in synergistic mixtures.

Early studies demonstrated that aspiration pneumonia and lung abscess were produced by intratracheal inoculation of pyorrhea exudate from human beings into laboratory animals; these findings were correlated with human infections. It was suggested that a fusospirochetal mixture of oral anaerobic bacteria — spirochetes, fusiform bacilli, streptococci, and usually also vibrios — was often the cause of pneumonia and lung abscess that followed aspiration of oral material containing these bacteria. Subsequent studies using guinea pigs, mice, and rabbits examined the potential pathogenicity of anaerobic bacteria and their etiologic role in appendicitis peritonitis, genital infections, soft tissue infections, periodontal disease, skin necrosis, and intrahepatic and intraabdominal abscesses. The findings confirm the potential pathogenicity of certain anaerobic bacteria in synergistic mixtures. Fewer anaerobic species produce infection in pure culture than when included in mixtures with other organisms. Also, clinically similar infections can be produced by a variety of different anaerobic species, suggesting that the pathogenesis of these infections has a greater biochemical than bacterial specificity. An exception is the specific requirement for *B. melaninogenicus* in the experimental production of fusospirochetal

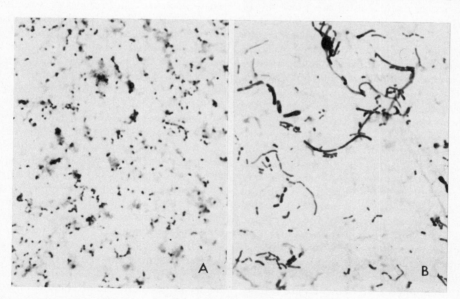

FIG. 48-2. A. *Bacteroides melaninogenicus* from supplemented thioglycolate, 24 hours. The organism often appears as small coccobacilli as shown here. ×1000. B. *Bacteroides melaninogenicus* from chopped meat medium with carbohydrate, 24 hours. ×1000. The same strain is shown in A and B to demonstrate variation in morphology dependent on the culture medium. Pleomorphism is also observed within a single culture, as demonstrated in B.

infection in guinea pigs following inoculation of a mixture of oral bacteria (Fig. 48-2).

Diseases of Man   A number of distinguishing properties characterize anaerobic infections. Most important perhaps is that most of the anaerobic bacteria that cause infection are members of our normal indigenous flora. Mucocutaneous surfaces of the skin and the upper respiratory tract, the gastrointestinal, and the genitourinary tracts are populated with a varied and great abundance of anaerobic organisms (Table 48-2). Thus, except for the clostridia of tetanus, gas gangrene, and botulism that may derive from soil or other exogenous sources, the source of most of the disease-producing anaerobes is endogenous. Therefore, anaerobic infection usually is neither communicable nor transmissible. Although many of these areas of the body would appear to be extremely deleterious aerobic environments for anaerobic organisms, the microenvironment is the crucial determinant. Requirements for low oxidation-reduction potential and oxygen tension are met by the reduced state of the surrounding chemical milieu, such as plaque on the teeth and in gingival margins, organic compounds in hair follicles or sweat glands, and the presence of facultative bacteria that use up the available oxygen and contribute enzymes or growth factors required by the anaerobes' growth. The existence of the anaerobes is thus not on a smooth flat surface exposed to ambient oxygen but rather in microcrevices and pits in the surface from which atmospheric oxygen is excluded physically and chemically. Alterations in the host's defenses may then allow these opportunistic bacteria to invade tissues or spread to other sites.

Another distinguishing characteristic of anaerobic infections is their polymicrobic nature. Although infections do occur with a single species, mixed infection either with a variety of anaerobic species or a combination of facultative and anaerobic species is most common. The propensity for multiple species infections originates in the requirement for growth factors, protective enzymes such as catalase or superoxide dismutase, virulence factors, and a reduced environment, all of which are provided by other anaerobic or facultative bacteria. Deficiencies in individual bacteria may also be compensated for in a compromised host through immunosuppresion, trauma, and various other factors.

Diseases caused by the non-spore-forming anaerobic bacteria usually are characterized by tissue necrosis, abscess formation, and an indolent or chronic course. Acute episodes, such as gram-negative septicemia involving *B. fragilis*, do occur, but normally these infections tend to develop and persist over extended periods of time. Infections often have a putrid odor, a characteristic of anaerobic infection, not infection with *E. coli* as previously was thought. The presence of gas usually is also an indication of anaerobic infection, although gas may occur with certain facultative bacteria.

PATHOGENESIS.   The pathogenesis of infection with non-spore-forming anaerobes is incompletely understood. A number of settings, however, predispose to invasion by endogenous flora.

A change from the normal host–parasite relationship in which there is no apparent harm to the host occurs most often in settings that produce a lowered oxidation–reduction potential in tissues normally well oxygenated and resistant to invasion by anaerobes. Reduction of the normal potential of tissue (approximately +120 mv), and thus predisposition to anaerobic infection, may stem from growth of facultative bacteria in a wound, an impaired blood supply, and tissue necrosis. These may be associated with vascular disease, injection of such vasoconstrictive agents as epinephrine, shock, cold, edema, trauma, surgery, presence of foreign bodies, malignancy, and gas-forming aerobic or facultative bacteria. Conditions appropriate for the initiation of anaerobic infections are thus found in the compromised host in whom the natural balance between tissue resistance and endogenous flora is disturbed by the settings listed previously, by such diseases as diabetes mellitus, or by treatment with immunosuppressive drugs, steroids, cytotoxic agents, or antibiotics.

Once introduced into the affected site, anaerobic bacteria multiply, further reduce the oxidation–reduction potential, and thereby extend tissue damage. The production of toxins, enzymes, and other virulence factors is obviously significant, but their specific role in the overall disease process remains to be clarified. Pathogenicity is not equal among species or strains of anaerobes. For example, certain organisms, such as *B. fragilis* subspecies *fragilis*, have a high incidence of human infection but are found in the indigenous flora in much lower numbers than are other prevalent endogenous organisms that are rarely associated with infection.

CLINICAL MANIFESTATIONS. The types of infections produced by the non-spore-forming anaerobes are related to their normal endogenous locations on the skin and in the upper respiratory, gastrointestinal, and genitourinary tracts.

Intraabdominal Infections. Infectious complications generally derive from spillage of fecal matter into the peritoneal cavity in such settings as penetrating abdominal trauma, surgery, appendicitis, diverticulitis, inflammatory bowel disease, or cancer. The first clinical manifestation is generally peritonitis, which is followed in survivors by abscess formation and localization of the infection. Infectious complications following disruption of the integrity of the lower bowel and colon are more frequent than of the upper bowel because of the higher concentrations of bacteria, especially anaerobes (10^{11} per gram of feces), in the colon. Ninety to ninety-six percent of abdominal infections are associated with anaerobes. The majority are mixed infections with multiple anaerobic species and facultative bacteria (Table 48-5).

Liver Abscess. Liver abscess often follows inflammation of the portal vein (pylephlebitis) or of the bile duct (cholangitis). Intestinal ma-

lignancy or inflammation, direct extension of perinephric, pancreatic, subdiaphragmatic, and lung abscesses, intestinal perforation, or spread of distant infection via the bloodstream and lymphatics also may precipitate solitary or multiple abscesses within the liver. Although the real incidence of anaerobes in these infections is unknown at present due to inadequate anaerobic culture of specimens, recent series indicate that at least 50 percent of liver abscesses involve anaerobes.

Obstetric and Gynecologic Infections. Anaerobes play a prime role in pelvic abscesses, endometritis, vaginal cuff infections following hysterectomy, postabortal sepsis, ovarian abscesses, and other settings. The normal flora of the vulva, vagina, and cervix can become invasive in certain situations predisposing to infection. Among the most common of these are premature rupture of membranes, prolonged labor, extensive manipulations, and hemorrhage during delivery, spontaneous or induced abortion, surgery, malignancy, gonococcal salpingitis, and intrauterine contraceptive devices. Endometritis may be limited or may spread to produce tubo-ovarian infection, pelvic abscess, peritonitis, and septicemia. Chronic pelvic infections may subsequently develop. Although anaerobes are involved in a high percentage of these infections and only anaerobic species are often isolated, many infections are mixed with facultative organisms

TABLE 48-5 ORGANISMS COMMONLY ISOLATED FROM ANAEROBIC INFECTIONS

Type of Infection	Isolates	
	Anaerobic	Facultative and Aerobic
Intraabdominal	B. fragilis, Clostridium, Peptostreptococcus, Peptococcus	E. coli, Klebsiella, Pseudomonas, Proteus, enterococci
Liver abscess	Bacteroides, Fusobacterium, Clostridium, Peptostreptococcus, Peptococcus	E. coli, Klebsiella, Proteus, Pseudomonas, Enterobacter, Streptococcus, S. aureus
Obstetric and gynecologic	B. fragilis, B. melaninogenicus, other Bacteroides, Fusobacterium, Peptostreptococcus, Peptococcus	E. coli, Proteus, Klebsiella, Enterobacter, Streptococcus, Staphylococcus, Lactobacillus, diphtheroids
Pleuropulmonary	B. melaninogenicus, F. nucleatum, Peptostreptococcus, Peptococcus, microaerophilic streptococci	Staphylococcus, Streptococcus, Pseudomonas, enterobacteria
Upper respiratory tract	B. melaninogenicus, F. nucleatum, Peptostreptococcus, Peptococcus, Propionibacterium, spirochetes	Staphylococcus, Streptococcus, diphtheroids
Soft Tissue	Vary with site of infection	Vary
Bacteremia	Bacteroides, Fusobacterium, Peptostreptococcus, Peptococcus, Clostridium	

(Table 48-5). Serious postabortal or postpartum infectious caused by *Clostridium perfringens* fortunately are rare. *Bacteroides* have largely replaced anaerobic or facultative streptococci in puerperal sepsis. The incidence of postabortal sepsis has markedly decreased since the introduction of legalized abortion.

Pleuropulmonary Infections. Anaerobic bacteria are important causes of pneumonitis (pulmonary infiltrate without cavity formation), lung abscess, necrotizing pneumonia, and empyema. Specimens that are properly collected and cultured under anaerobic conditions yield anaerobes in 71 to 95 percent of these infections. Anaerobes are not important agents in lobar pneumonia or in chronic bronchitis.

As in other anaerobic infections, pleuropulmonary foci yield mixed species of bacteria, usually 3 to 4 species but ranging to over 10 species per specimen. In these settings the common anaerobic isolates are *F. nucleatum*, *B. melaninogenicus*, and gram positive cocci (Fig. 48-3). Of interest is the finding that *B. fragilis* is isolated in approximately 20 percent of these infections, although it is not present in the normal flora of the oral cavity.

Aspiration of mouth flora generally is the inciting cause of these diverse pleuropulmonary infections. Important clinical clues include a putrid odor of discharge or sputum, presence of tissue necrosis, subacute or chronic presentation, and settings that predispose to aspiration, such as alcoholism or general anesthesia. Other common underlying conditions are dental infections or other extrapulmonary anaerobic disease, bronchogenic carcinoma, pulmonary embolus with infarction, and bronchiectasis.

Upper Respiratory Tract Infections. Chronic forms of a wide variety of infections of the upper respiratory tract are associated with anaerobes. These include periodontal disease, various fusospirochetal diseases, actinomycosis, peritonsillar abscesses, otitis media, mastoiditis, and sinusitis. *Bacteriodes melaninogenicus* contributes significantly to the pathogenesis of many of these infections (Table 48-5).

The association of anaerobic bacteria with chronic otitis media, mastoiditis, and sinusitis doubtlessly accounts for the contiguous spread of these organisms into the central nervous system and their high incidence in nontraumatic brain abscesses. Hematogenous spread from anaerobic pleuropulmonary infections or sepsis following dental extractions also are sources of brain abscess.

Soft Tissue Infections. Anaerobic infections of the skin and soft tissues usually evolve from traumatic injury, surgery, or ischemia as-

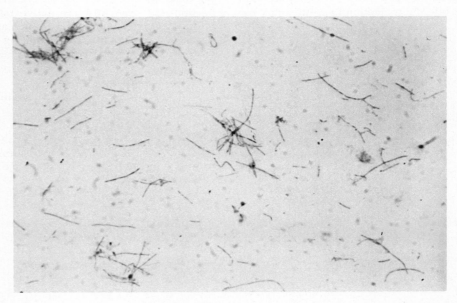

FIG. 48-3. *Fusobacterium nucleatum* from sheep's blood agar plate. This organism may appear as thin bacilli as shown here, often with very tapered ends, or may form long thin filaments. It stains palely gram negative. ×1,000.

sociated with vascular disease or diabetes mellitus. The specific anaerobes involved depend largely on the site of infection or source of the infecting bacteria. For example, human bites that can develop into serious infections usually involve normal flora of the mouth. These diverse anaerobic infections usually produce extensive tissue necrosis with extension along subcutaneous and fascial planes, gas, and a foul odor. Other better characterized infections include (1) progressive bacterial synergistic gangrene, a progressive ulceration of the skin and subcutaneous tissue produced by microaerophilic or anaerobic streptococci and *Staphylococcus aureus* acting synergistically, (2) chronic undermining ulcer of Meleney, an indolent, deep subcutaneous infection producing necrotic ulcers with eroding edges, (3) synergistic necrotizing cellulitis, a rapidly spreading necrotic infection of the skin and connective tissue usually involving a mixed bacterial flora and accompanied by fever, pain, and systemic toxicity, and (4) necrotizing fasciitis, a severe infection often caused by peptostreptococci with wide extension deep into the fascia, systemic toxicity, and a high mortality rate.

Bacteremia. Anaerobic bacteria primarily from abdominal and pelvic infections account for approximately 8 to 11 percent of all bacteremias in a general hospital. Many anaerobic bacteremias involve gram-negative anaerobes that can produce a classical septic shock syndrome. *B. fragilis* is second in incidence only to *E. coli* in gram-negative bacteremia. Anaerobic bacteremias present with sudden fever, chills, and sweating and may be associated with jaundice, septic thrombophlebitis, and suppuration at distant sites from metastases. The current overall mortality in anaerobic bacteremia is 25 to 35 percent, but large differences are found relative to the patient population. Bacteremia stemming from abdominal infections, particularly with underlying diseases, is associated with a higher mortality and poorer prognosis than bacteremia in obstetric patients. *Bacteroides* sepsis is particularly serious during pregnancy. Mortality among neonates is high but the mother is usually spared.

TREATMENT. Therapy for infections involving anaerobic bacteria is limited. Surgical drainage and resection of necrotic tissue are mainstays for closed-space anaerobic infections or mixed infections that are amenable to surgery. Since infections may continue to smolder following surgical intervention, the administration of appropriate antibiotics is important. Parenteral therapy is usually required in order to achieve effective drug levels in necrotic areas. Such chronic infections as lung or liver abscesses must be treated for prolonged periods to prevent relapse.

At present there is no universally accepted method of in vitro antimicrobic susceptibility testing for anaerobes comparable to the disc-diffusion technique (Kirby-Bauer) applicable to facultative bacteria. Agar and broth dilution techniques, however, have demonstrated that many anaerobic species have predictable susceptibility patterns.

Anaerobic bacteria are uniformly resistant to the aminoglycoside antibiotics, making drugs such as gentamicin, kanamycin, neomycin, and streptomycin useless against anaerobes in infection. Although many anaerobes were originally sensitive to tetracycline, increasing resistance has been noted. Approximately two-thirds of clinical isolates of *B. fragilis*, the anaerobe most frequently associated with infection, are now resistant to tetracycline. Most *B. fragilis* strains also are resistant to the usual clinical levels of penicillin G, ampicillin, the synthetic penicillins, and cephalothin. The high association of *B. fragilis* with anaerobic infections of the abdomen and pelvis precludes widespread use of penicillin for these infections. Penicillin G is active, however, against a variety of other anaerobes, including certain other bacteroides, fusobacteria, and anaerobic cocci, and it remains the drug of choice for pleuropulmonary infections.

Chloramphenicol is very active against most anaerobic bacteria, including *B. fragilis*, and is the drug of choice for anaerobic brain abscess. However, the serious side effects of the drug, although infrequent, have generally restricted its use to severe or life-threatening infection. Clindamycin also has an excellent spectrum against anaerobic bacteria and proven clinical effectiveness. Clindamycin should be used only where definite clinical indications exist since pseudomembranous enterocolitis may infrequently accompany its use.

A number of additional drugs are moderately active against anaerobic bacteria at easily achievable clinical levels. A crucial point, however, in using profiles of drug susceptibility is a drug's activity against *B. fragilis* specifically in addition to its overall activity against anaerobes. Drugs with good activity for many anaerobic strains, including 65 to 75 percent of *B. fragilis* strains, are two tetracycline derivatives, doxycycline and minocycline, cefoxitin and carbenicillin. Metronidazole is of interest because of its specificity for anaerobes. It is inactive against aerobic and facultative bacteria, but about 70 percent of all anaerobes are inhibited, including 88 percent of *B. fragilis* strains.

Initial choice of appropriate antibiotic therapy for infections involving anaerobes is important. In anaerobic bacteremias, especially those involving bacteroides or fusobacteria, mortality rates among patients treated with antibiotics active against the infecting anaerobic bacteria are 12 to 16 percent compared to 60 percent mortality among patients receiving inappropriate drugs. Gram stain often aids in the choice of initial therapy, but changes may be necessary when the laboratory obtains the isolates from culture. Since mixed infections containing both anaerobic and facultative species frequently occur, two or even three antibiotics may be required for coverage of known pathogens. Clindamycin is not active against the facultative gram-negative rods, and gentamicin or another antibiotic may be required to cover organisms, such as *E. coli*, especially in pelvic and abdominal infection.

Hyperbaric oxygen theoretically could be an alternate mode of therapy for anaerobic infections, but it has not been evaluated except for clostridial myonecrosis (Chap. 49). The bacteriostatic and bactericidal effects of high oxygen tensions on anaerobic bacteria achievable by hyperbaric oxygenation might be useful clinically as an adjunct to conventional antibiotic and surgical therapy or could serve as an alternate to surgery for inoperable patients.

CLINICAL ISOLATES OF NON-SPORE-FORMING ANAEROBIC BACTERIA

This section presents a brief description of some of the clinically significant, non-spore-forming, anaerobic bacteria. The following anaerobes, listed in decreasing order of incidence, have been isolated from various types of infections: *Bacteroides, Clostridium, Pepto-*

streptococcus and *Peptococcus*, primarily, followed by *Fusobacterium, Eubacterium, Propionibacterium, Lactobacillus,* and *Actinomyces,* and, least frequently, *Bifidobacterium, Veillonella,* and *Acidaminococcus. Treponema,* not included in this list, are covered in Chapter 52.

Anaerobic Gram-negative Bacilli

Bacteroides BACTEROIDES FRAGILIS. This organism is the most frequently isolated anaerobic species from clinical specimens and is involved in serious infections. The species is divided into five subspecies, *fragilis, thetaiotaomicron, vulgatus, distasonis,* and *ovatus.* Subspecies *fragilis* is the most common clinical isolate from infections, yet it is the least numerous of the subspecies in normal fecal flora.

Morphology and Physiology.   Cellular morphology of this gram-negative rod varies widely according to the medium and the gaseous environment. The bacilli may be quite pleomorphic with vacuoles and swellings when grown in some liquid media containing glucose or be fairly regular with rounded ends when grown on blood agar plates (Fig. 48-1). Colonies of *B. fragilis* are low convex, white to gray, semiopaque, glistening, and some strains may be hemolytic. The organisms grow more rapidly than most non-spore-forming anaerobes, and growth is stimulated by bile. *B. fragilis* is a moderate anaerobe growing maximally in $PO_2 < 3$ percent but is capable of surviving prolonged exposures to oxygen, particularly in the presence of blood.

Antigenic Structure.   On the basis of agglutination and gel diffusion assays, strains of bacteroides can be subdivided into serotypes that in general correspond to the five physiologic subspecies groupings. Thermolabile protein and thermostable lipopolysaccharide antigens have been detected which, when further characterized, should provide a basis for serologic classification of the organism into genus, species, and strain.

The antibody response of patients with various infections, including septicemia or abscesses, caused by members of the Bacteroidaceae has been investigated to study the pathologic significance of bacteroides in mixed infections and possibly to devise a method of detecting bacteroides infections that would be clinically useful. Antibodies to bacteroides and fusobacteria have been found in infected patients' sera measured by precipitin and agglutination techniques and are absent in control sera. More sensitive techniques, such as passive hemagglutination, can detect antibodies to *B. fragilis* in healthy individuals. Further work on the serology of the Bacteroidaceae is required to determine whether this can be developed into a useful clinical tool.

Determinants of Pathogenicity. An endotoxin has been isolated from various strains of bacteroides and shown to have endotoxic activity.

Clinical Infection. *B. fragilis* is present in high concentrations in the normal flora of the gastrointestinal tract and in the cervix and is commonly associated with localized infections or septicemias derived from those sites. Although not present in the normal flora of the mouth, *B. fragilis* is isolated from approximately 20 percent of pleuropulmonary disease involving anaerobes. Most strains are resistant to penicillin and ampicillin.

BACTEROIDES MELANINOGENICUS. This organism is subdivided into three subspecies: *asaccharolyticus*, *intermedius*, and *melaninogenicus*, occurring from clinical specimens in the same order. Older synonyms for this organism are *Bacteroides nigrescens* or *Fusiformis melaninogenicus*. These bacteria are small coccobacilli, but usually longer rods also can be observed (Fig. 48-2). Colonies of *B. melaninogenicus* are usually β-hemolytic, and most strains form pigmented colonies on blood agar, becoming tan and then black in four to seven days. Many strains require menadione and hemin for growth. *B. melaninogenicus* is part of the normal flora of the mouth, gastrointestinal tract, and probably the urogenital tract. It is an important agent in oral, pulmonary, obstetric, and gynecologic infections. The organism produces a collagenase which is important in the pathogenesis of certain infections.

BACTEROIDES CORRODENS. This is a somewhat fastidious species that, with improvement in anaerobic techniques, has been isolated more frequently from infection. Although the original description of this organism included both obligately anaerobic and facultative strains, as now defined it refers only to the anaerobic strains. Facultative strains have been placed in a separate genus and species, *Eikenella corrodens*. The obligately anaerobic organisms grow rather slowly and form flattened, translucent colonies that erode or pit the agar. *Bacteroides corrodens* is part of the normal flora of the mouth and may be found in oral and pleuropulmonary infection.

BACTEROIDES ORALIS. Previously considered an uncommon isolate from infections, this organism may play a more significant role in disease than previously recognized. Cellular morphology may be coccobacillary or elongated bacilli. Colonies are yellowish, glistening, and often hemolytic. *Bacteroides oralis* is present in the normal flora of the mouth, gastrointestinal tract, and urogenital tract. Clinical isolations usually are from oral, pulmonary, or genital tract infections.

Fusobacterium FUSOBACTERIUM NUCLEATUM. Previously called *F. fusiforme*, this is the most common of the fusobacteria isolated from infections. The true clinical incidence of fusobacteria, however, is not completely known. In much of the older literature all anaerobic gramnegative rods were termed "bacteroides," and only occasionally were distinctions made, primarily on the basis of thin bacteria with pointed ends. Although not all fusobacteria are thin with pointed ends, *F. nucleatum* characteristically possesses this trait. These organisms may look like scattered wheat straw or may be very long thin filaments (Fig. 48-3). Colonies sometimes are alpha hemolytic and may be convex and translucent, with internal flecking or mottling, or more umbonate, dull, and opaque. *Fusobacterium nucleatum* is present in the normal flora of the mouth and is an important agent in oral infections, lung abscess, and other pleuropulmonary infections.

FUSOBACTERIUM NECROPHORUM. This organism is an important animal pathogen and is found in a variety of human infections. Older synonyms for *F. necrophorum* are *Sphaerophorus necrophorus*, *Bacteroides necrophorus*, and *Sphaerophorus funduliformis*. The organism is very similar in its biochemical reactions to *F. nucleatum* but is more pleomorphic. Bacilli are

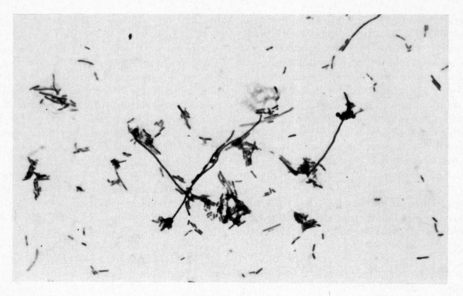

FIG. 48-4. *Fusobacterium necrophorum* from chopped meat medium with carbohydrate. This organism may be highly pleomorphic, appearing as short, long, or filamentous bacilli often with bulbous swellings and round bodies. ×1000.

generally broader, usually with rounded ends, and may be short, long, or filamentous forms often with bulbous swellings and round bodies (Fig 48-4). Colonies may be alpha or beta hemolytic. A lipase and a partially characterized leukocidal toxin are produced. Its normal habitat is probably the gastrointestinal tract, although documentation is incomplete. The organism is found in a variety of human infections, primarily abdominal or pelvic in origin, and is an important agent in liver abscess.

Other fusobacteria, such as *F. mortiferum* and *F. varium*, are also occasionally isolated from clinical material. Although most fusobacteria may be highly pleomorphic, *F. mortiferum* produces especially bizarre forms, as indicated by one of its previous designations, *F. ridiculosum*. Occasional strains of *F. varium* may be resistant to penicillin and to clindamycin.

Anaerobic Gram-positive Bacilli

Eubacterium, Propionibacterium, Lactobacillus, Actinomyces, and Bifidobacterium Of the anaerobic gram-positive bacilli, strains of *Eubacterium* and *Propionibacterium* are isolated most frequently from clinical specimens, fol-

lowed by strains of *Lactobacillus*, *Actinomyces*, and occasionally *Bifidobacterium*. Many of these organisms are slow growing in contrast to *Clostridium*, the spore-forming, anaerobic, gram-positive rods. Strains within the genera *Propionibacterium*, *Lactobacillus*, and *Actinomyces* may show sparse to good growth in a CO_2 incubator or aerobically while other strains are obligately anaerobic. Many gram-positive rods are isolated that cannot be identified by present schemes.

Eubacterium lentum is the most common of the eubacteria isolated from clinical specimens. It is a coccobacillus that often is associated with *B. fragilis* in infection, but little is known of its pathogenic role, if any. It is part of the normal flora of the gastrointestinal tract.

Propionibacterium acnes and *P. granulosum* are normal inhabitants of the gastrointestinal tract and, primarily, of the skin. Consequently they occur most frequently as contaminants, but rarely they appear to be causally associated with infections. They were previously classified as anaerobic members of the genus *Corynebacterium*. *Propionibacterium* may closely resemble *Actinomyces* or *Arachnia propionica* (formerly classified in *Actinomyces* and *Propionibacterium*), since cells are pleomorphic and may be branched and/or diphtheroidal.

Strains of lactobacilli are normal flora in the mouth and gastrointestinal tract and may be the predominant flora in the urogenital tract. A number of species have been isolated from human infection, but *Lactobacillus catenaforme* is especially associated with pleuropulmonary infections.

The *Actinomyces* are covered separately in Chapter 37. Previously their characteristically slow growth resulted in their affiliation with diagnostic mycology laboratories rather than bacteriology laboratories. *Arachnia propionica*, which can also cause actinomycosis, is closely related to *Actinomyces* and to *Propionibacterium*, but because of certain metabolic differences it has been placed in a separate genus.

Bifidobacteria are infrequently involved in infection. *Bifidobacterium eriksonii* has been listed as *Actinomyces eriksonii* in the Eighth Edition of *Bergey's Manual*. Various bifidobacteria are normal flora in the mouth and urogenital tract and occur in high numbers in the gastrointestinal tract.

Anaerobic Gram-positive Cocci

Peptostreptococcus and Peptococcus The most common clinical isolates of *Peptostreptococcus* are *P. anaerobius* and *P. intermedius*; most common isolates of *Peptococcus* are *P. magnus*, *P. asaccharolyticus*, and *P. prevotii*. Since *P. intermedius* produces lactic acid as its major metabolic end product and, after primary anaerobic isolation, often will grow on subculture in air or in a CO_2 incubator, it has been proposed that the organism be reclassified in *Streptococcus* (Table 48-1). *P. magnus* and *P. prevotii*, as listed by the *Anaerobic Bacteriology Manual* of Virginia Polytechnic Institute, are not included in the Eighth Edition of *Bergey's Manual*. The relative importance of cellular morphology (clumps or chains), the presence of catalase, and metabolic patterns in the classification of the *Peptococcus* and *Peptostreptococcus* is controversial. Corresponding to the facultative genera *Staphylococcus* and *Streptococcus*, peptococci generally occur as singles, pairs, and irregular clumps, and peptostreptococci may be in singles, pairs, or chains. Many of the gram-positive anaerobic cocci are similar in colonial appearance and may produce an alpha or beta hemolysis. These species of cocci

are normal flora in the mouth, urogenital tract, and gastrointestinal tract. Both genera are involved in a wide variety of human infection but are particularly important in pleuropulmonary disease, brain abscess, and obstetric and gynecologic infections.

Anaerobic Gram-negative Cocci

Veillonella and Acidaminococcus *Veillonella alcalescens*, *V. parvula*, and *Acidaminococcus fermentans* are isolated from clinical specimens, but little is known of their role, if any, in the pathogenesis of anaerobic infections. *Veillonella* species are small cocci occurring in pairs, short chains, and clumps. It is present in the normal flora of the mouth and the gastrointestinal and urogenital tracts. *Acidaminococcus* cells are larger, and may partially stain gram positive. This genus has been isolated as normal flora from the gastrointestinal and urogenital tracts.

FURTHER READING

Books and Reviews

Balows A, DeHaan RM, Dowell VR Jr, Guze LB (eds.): Anaerobic Bacteria: Role in Disease. Springfield, Ill, Thomas, 1974

Buchanan RE, Gibbons NE (eds.): Bergey's Manual of Determinative Bacteriology, 8th ed. Baltimore, Williams & Wilkins, 1974

Dowell VR Jr, Hawkins TM: Laboratory Methods in Anaerobic Bacteriology. CDC Laboratory Manual. Washington, US Government Printing Office. DHEW Publication No (CDC) 74-8272, 1974

Gorbach SL, Bartlett JG: Anaerobic infections. N Engl J Med, 290:1177, 1237, 1289, 1974

Holdeman LV, Moore WEC: Anaerobic Bacteriology Manual, 3rd ed. Anaerobe Laboratory, Blacksburg, Virginia Polytechnic Institute and State University, 1975

Lennette EH, Spaulding EH, Truant JP (eds.): Manual of Clinical Microbiology, 2nd ed. Washington, American Society for Microbiology, 1974

Miraglia GJ: Pathogenic anaerobic bacteria. CRC Crit Rev Microbiol 3:161, 1974.

Moore WEC, Cato EP, Holdeman LV: Anaerobic bacteria of the gastrointestinal flora and their occurrence in clinical infections. J. Infect Dis 119:641, 1969

Prevot AR: Fredette V (trans): Manual for the Classification and Determination of the Anaerobic Bacteria. Philadelphia, Lea & Febiger, 1965

Sabbaj J, Sutter VL, Finegold SM: Anaerobic pyogenic liver abscess. Ann Intern Med 77:629, 1972

Smith LDS: The Pathogenic Anaerobic Bacteria. Springfield, Ill, Thomas, 1975

Sutter VL, Vargo VL, Finegold SM: Wadsworth Anaerobic

Bacteriology Manual, 2nd ed. Los Angeles, Department of Continuing Education in Health Sciences, University of California, 1975

Selected Papers

Altemeier WA: The pathogenicity of the bacteria of appendicitis peritonitis. Surgery 11:374, 1942

Aranki A, Freter R: Use of anaerobic glove boxes for the cultivation of strictly anaerobic bacteria. Am J Clin Nutr 25:1329, 1972

Bartlett JG, Finegold SM: Anaerobic infections of the lung and pleural space. Am Rev Respir Dis 110:56, 1974

Carter B, Jones CP, Alter RL, Creadick RN, Thomas WL: *Bacteroides* infections in obstetrics and gynecology. Obstet Gynecol 1:491, 1953

Chow AW, Guze LB: Bacteroidaceae bacteremia: clinical experience with 112 patients. Medicine 53:93, 1974

Dowell VR Jr: Comparison of techniques for isolation and identification of anaerobic bacteria. Am J Clin Nutr 25: 1335, 1972

Felner JM, Dowell VR Jr: "Bacteroides" bacteremia. Am J Med 50:787, 1971

Finegold SM, Rosenblatt JE: Practical aspects of anaerobic sepsis. Medicine 52:311, 1973

Finegold SM, Bartlett JG, Chow AN, et al: Management of anaerobic infections. Ann Intern Med 83:375, 1975

Hill GB, Osterhout S, Pratt PC: Liver abscess production by nonsporeforming anaerobic bacteria in a mouse model. Infect Immun 9:599, 1974

Loesche WJ: Oxygen sensitivity of various anaerobic bacteria. Appl Microbiol 18:723, 1969

McCord JM, Keele BB Jr, Fridovich I: An enzyme-based theory of obligate anaerobiosis: the physiological function of superoxide dismutase. Proc Natl Acad Sci USA 68:1024, 1971

McDonald JB, Sutton RM, Knoll ML, Madlener EM, Grainger RM: The pathogenic components of an experimental fusospirochetal infection. J Infect Dis 98:15, 1956

Meleney FL: Bacterial synergism in disease process. Ann Surg 94:961, 1931

Roberts DS: Editorial. Synergistic mechanisms in certain mixed infections. J Infect Dis 120:720, 1969

Smith DT: Experimental aspiratory abscess. Arch Surg 14: 231, 1927

Socransky SS, Gibbons RJ: Required role of *Bacteroides melaninogenicus* in mixed anaerobic infections. J Infect Dis 115:247, 1965

Swenson RM, Michaelson TC, Daly MJ, Spaulding EH: Anaerobic bacterial infections of the female genital tract. Obstet Gynecol 42:538, 1973

Thadepalli H, Gorbach SL, Broido P, Norsen J: A prospective study of infections in penetrating abdominal trauma. Am J Clin Nutr 25:1405, 1972

49
Clostridium Perfringens and Other Clostridia of Wound Infections

CLOSTRIDIUM

The clostridia are gram-positive, anaerobic, spore-forming bacilli. Most species are obligate anaerobes, but a few species are aerotolerant and will grow minimally in air at atmospheric pressure. The pathogenic species produce soluble toxins, some of which are extremely potent. Some species are saccharolytic, producing acid and gas from carbohydrates, and many are proteolytic. The clostridia are widely distributed in nature and are present in soil and in the intestinal tract of man and animals.

The pathogenic clostridia can be divided into three major groups according to the types of diseases they produce. (1) The histotoxic clostridia that will be discussed in this chapter characteristically cause a variety of tissue infections usually subsequent to wounds or other types of traumatic injury. (2) *Clostridium tetani*, the causative agent of tetanus, produces disease through a potent exotoxin that is produced during limited growth within tissue (Chap. 50). (3) *C. botulinum* is the cause of botulism, a food poisoning caused by the ingestion of a powerful exotoxin previously formed by the organism in contaminated food (Chap. 51).

The histotoxic clostridia cause a severe infection of muscle, clostridial myonecrosis. Older and frequently used synonyms for this infection are "gas gangrene" and "clostridial myositis." The term "gas gangrene," however, is misleading, since the presence of gas in the infected tissues may be a late or variable manifestation of the disease, and "clostridial myositis" suggests muscle inflammation rather than the actual pathologic condition, necrosis. The most important histotoxic clostridia are *Clostridium perfringens*, *C. novyi*, and *C. septicum*. Three other organisms of lesser importance also are capable alone of producing clostridial myonecrosis: *C. histolyticum*, *C. sordellii*, and *C. fallax*. All of these histotoxic clostridia produce a variety of toxins of different potencies, and for each species toxins are designated by Greek letters in order of importance or discovery. Thus, the alpha toxins of different species are not identical. None of these histotoxic clostridia are highly invasive pathogens, but they play an opportunistic role that requires a special set of conditions within tissue in order to initiate infection. A spectrum of clinical involvement is seen in clostridial wound infections, ranging from simple contamination of wounds to the most serious type of infection, myonecrosis.

Since the clostridia are so widely distributed in nature, contamination of wounds with these bacteria is very common. Often more than one clostridia is present, including both saprophytic and histotoxic species. An average of 2.6 species of clostridia were isolated from cases of clostridial myonecrosis during World War II, and higher numbers would probably be demonstrated with the improved anaerobic culture techniques currently available. Reported figures for clostridial contamination of wounds in civilian life range up to 39 percent, and contamination during warfare is considerably higher. Only a small proportion of wounds contaminated with *C. perfringens* or other histotoxic clostridia, however, evolve into true clostridial myonecrosis. The incidence of the disease in civilian life is difficult to establish, with considerable variation according to the precipitating incident and geographic location. Its incidence during warfare is from 10 to 100 times greater than during peacetime, occurring in 0.2 to 1 percent of war casualties. An important corollary to the high rate of clostridial contamination of wounds is that the isolation of histotoxic clostridia from wounds or drainage material does not by itself indicate clostridial myonecrosis. Diagnosis of clostridial myonecrosis must be made on clinical grounds, and the bacteriology laboratory contributes to a careful differential diagnosis by demonstrating histotoxic clostridia or other bacteria that are associated with diseases of similar symptomatology.

CLOSTRIDIUM PERFRINGENS

C. perfringens is cultured from 60 to 90 percent of cases of clostridial myonecrosis. There are five types of *C. perfringens*, A to E, separated according to their production of four major lethal toxins (Table 49-1). *C. perfringens* type A is the organism primarily responsible for diseases in man: clostridial myonecrosis, less severe wound infections, and a common form

TABLE 49-1   Toxins and Soluble Antigens of Clostridium perfringens

Type	Group	Disease	Major Lethal Toxins*				Minor Antigens†				
			α	β	ε	ι	δ	θ	κ	λ	μ
A		Gas gangrene in man and animals Food poisoning in man‡	++	−	−	−	−	++	++	−	++
B	1	Lamb dysentery Enterotoxemia of foals	++	++	++	−	−	++	−	++	++
	2	Enterotoxemia of sheep and goats (Iran)	++	++	++	−	−	++	++	−	−
C	1	Enterotoxemia (struck) of sheep	++	++	−	−	++	++	++	−	−
	2	Enterotoxemia of calves and lambs (Colorado)	++	++	−	−	−	++	++	−	−
	3	Enterotoxemia of piglets	++	++	−	−	−	++	+	−	+
	4	Necrotic enteritis (pig-bel) of man (New Guinea)	++	++	−	−	−	++	+	−	++
	5	Necrotic enteritis of man and fowl (Germany)‡	++	++	−	−	−	−	−	−	−
D		Enterotoxemia of sheep, lambs, goats, and cattle	++	−	++	−	−	++	++	+	++
E		Isolated from sheep and cattle; pathogenicity doubtful	++	−	−	++	−	++	++	++	+

Modified from Kadis, Montie, and Ajl (eds): Microbiol Toxins, Vol 2A: Bacterial Protein Toxins. 1971. Courtesy of Academic Press.
+ + = produced by all or most strains; + = produced by less than 50 percent of strains; − = not produced
*Lethal antigens primarily responsible for pathogenicity and type designation
†Lower order of toxicity, some may be involved in pathogenicity
‡Some strains produce heat-resistant spores

of food poisoning. Type A *C. perfringens* has been found in the intestinal tract of almost every animal that has ever been cultured for this organism but is a less common cause of disease in animals than in man. In contrast types B, C, D, and E, which occur only in the intestinal tracts of animals and occasionally man, produce a variety of naturally occurring diseases of domestic animals.

Morphology

Clostridium perfringens usually appears as a short, plump rod, strongly staining gram-positive (Fig. 49-1). The organisms are uniform in appearance, 2 to 4 μm in length and 1 to 1.5 μm in width. The length varies according to the stage of growth and the nutritional and ionic composition of the medium. Rapidly growing organisms may appear almost coccoid or cubical, whereas more elongated cells occur in older cultures. Unlike the other pathogenic clostridia, *C. perfringens* is nonmotile. It does not produce spores in ordinary media, and special media must normally be used to demonstrate sporulation. Capsules may be observed by di-

rect examination of smears from wounds but are not uniformly demonstrable in culture.

Physiology

CULTURAL CHARACTERISTICS.   *C. perfringens* is aerotolerant when compared with many anaerobic bacteria and will survive and even grow in low oxygen tensions, especially when streaked on blood agar plates. Anaerobic culture methods suitable for *C. perfringens* and other clostridia are discussed in Chapter 48. It will grow over a pH range of 5.5 to 8.0 and a temperature range of 20 to 50C. Although it is usually grown at 37C, a temperature of 45C is optimal for many strains. The generation time at this temperature may be as low as 10 minutes. Surface colonies that are produced on blood agar after 24 hours' incubation are circular and smooth and 2 to 4 mm in diameter, but as the colonies increase in size with age, the periphery often loses symmetry and assumes the appearance of a colony of motile bacteria showing swarming. Variation in colonial morphology occurs depending on the degree of encapsulation and smooth to rough transition.

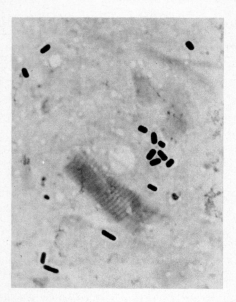

FIG. 49-1. *Clostridium perfringens* directly smeared from infected muscle in clostridial myonecrosis, demonstrating short, plump bacilli which lack spores. A variety of other bacteria including other clostridia may also be present, but polymorphonuclear leukocytes are characteristically absent. Note the disintegrated muscle tissue. ×1000.

LABORATORY IDENTIFICATION. The rapid growth of *C. perfringens* in chopped meat medium at 45C can be utilized to isolate it from mixtures of bacteria. Since *C. perfringens* will outgrow most other organisms during the first four to six hours incubation, blood agar plates streaked after that time and incubated at 37C will have proportionally higher numbers of *C. perfringens*. Although heat treatment (80 to 100C) of mixed cultures is an aid in the isolation of many clostridial species that sporulate well, this method is not recommended for *C. perfringens*. Cultures of clinical isolates of this organism usually contain few spores, and the heat resistance of the spores appears to be inversely related to the toxigenicity of the vegatative forms.

A few easily observable characteristics aid in the identification of *C. perfringens*. In chopped meat glucose media there is abundant growth with gas formation. In vivo toxicity testing may be carried out with supernates from this medium. *C. perfringens* also produces a characteristic pattern of hemolysis on blood agar plates, precipitation in serum or egg yolk media, and stormy fermentation in milk media.

After overnight incubation on rabbit, sheep, ox, or human blood agar, colonies of most strains demonstrate a characteristic target hemolysis resulting from a narrow zone of complete hemolysis due to the theta toxin and a much wider zone of incomplete hemolysis due to the alpha toxin. This double-zone pattern of hemolysis may fade with longer incubation.

A dense opalescence in human serum is produced by growing organisms or by the supernatant fluid from an overnight culture. This reaction, the Nagler reaction, is caused by the alpha toxin (a lecithinase C) and is specifically inhibited by *C. perfringens* antitoxin. A similar and more easily observable reaction occurs with egg yolk agar. This medium can be inoculated directly with wound specimens for screening purposes and is helpful in the identification of pure cultures of *C. perfringens* and other clostridia that produce a lecithinase or a lipase. Presumptive identification of *C. perfringens* can be made by streaking organisms on both sides of an egg yolk agar plate, one-half of which has been covered with *C. perfringens* antitoxin. The inhibition of opalescence on the antitoxin-treated portion, however, is not totally specific for *C. perfringens*. A number of other organisms produce a lecithinase, and although most are not inhibited by the specific antitoxin, the lecithinases of the *C. bifermentans-sordellii* group and *C. paraperfringens* (*barati*) are antigenically similar and are partially inhibited by antitoxin to *C. perfringens* alpha toxin. These organisms can be separated by other tests.

In milk media most strains of *C. perfringens* produce stormy fermentation, in which the fermentation of the lactose in milk produces a large amount of acid, causing the protein (casein) to coagulate. This acid clot is then disrupted and torn apart by the large volume of gas formed from the lactose fermentation. This action in milk media is a useful aid in the identification of *C. perfringens*, but when used alone is not diagnostic, since the reaction also may be produced by a number of other clostridial species, including *C. septicum*. Use of the test requires a pure culture of the organism. Fermentation reactions and other biochemical tests used in the identification of *C. perfringens* are listed in Table 49-2 and are covered in greater detail in the reference manuals listed at the end of this chapter.

TABLE 49-2 CHARACTERISTICS OF FREQUENTLY ENCOUNTERED CLOSTRIDIA

Species	Egg Yolk Agar		Spores	Cooked Meat Medium Digestion	Milk	Gelatin Hydrolysis	Indole	Carbohydrate Fermentation				Principal Fermentation Products
	Lecithinase	Lipase						Glucose	Maltose	Lactose	Sucrose	
Toxigenic, pathogenic for humans												
C. perfringens	+	−	ST	−	CG	+	−	+	+	+	+	A,(P),B
C. novyi A*	+	+	ST	−	C(G)	+	−	+	+	−	−	A,P,B,V
C. novyi B*	+	−	ST	V	C(G)	+	V	+	+	−	−	A,P,B,V
C. septicum	−	−	ST	−	CG	+	−	+	+	+	−	A,B
C. sordellii	+	−	ST	+	CD	+	+	+	+	−	−	A,F,P,IB,IV,IC
C. histolyticum†	−	−	ST	+	CD	+	−	−	−	−	−	A,L
C. tetani	−	−	T	−	−	+	V	−	−	−	−	A,P,B
C. botulinum‡												
Group I*	−	+	ST	+	C(D)	+	−	+	+	−	−	A,P,IB,B,IV, V,IC
Group II*	−	+	ST	−	(C)	+	−	+	+	−	−	A,B
Group III*	V	+	ST	−	C(D)	+	−	+	V	−	−	A,P,B
Nontoxigenic, uncertain pathogenicity for humans												
C. bifermentans	+	−	ST	+	CD	+	+	+	+	−	−	A,F,P,IB,(B), IV,IC
C. ramosum	−	−	T	−	(C)(G)	−	−	+	+	+	+	A,F,L,S
C. sporogenes	−	+	ST	+	CD	+	−	+	+	−	−	A,P,IB,B,IV, V,IC
C. innocuum	−	−	T	−	−	−	−	+	V	−	V	A,(F),B,L
C. paraputrificum	−	−	T	−	C(G)	−	−	+	+	+	+	A,F,B,L
C. subterminale	−	−	ST	+	CD	+	−	−	−	−	−	A,(P),IB,B,IV
C. cadaveris	−	−	T	+	CG	+	+	−	−	−	−	A,(IB),B,IV
C. butyricum	−	−	ST	−	CG	−	−	+	+	+	+	A,F,B
C. tertium†	−	−	T	−	CG	−	−	+	+	+	+	A,B
C. lentoputrescens	−	−	T	−	−	−	+	−	−	−	−	A,B
C. limosum	+	−	ST	+	CD	+	−	−	(	−	−	A
C. cochlearium	−	−	ST	−	−	−	−	−	−	−	−	A,(P),B

+ = positive reaction for 90 to 100 percent of strains; − = negative reaction for 90 to 100 percent of strains; C = curd; D = digestion; G = gas; ST = subterminal; T = terminal; reaction; ( ) = variable;

Fermentation products by gas liquid chromatography: A = acetic; B = butyric; F = formic; IB = isobutyric; IC = isocaproic; IV = isovaleric; L = lactic; P = propionic; S = succinic; V = valeric;

*Toxin neutralization test required for identification

†Growth on aerobically incubated blood agar

‡Group I contains proteolytic strains (types A,B,F,G); Group II, types C and D; Group III, nonproteolytic strains (types B,E,F)

Antigenic Structure

Strains of *C. perfringens* produce at least 12 different soluble substances or toxins, all of which are protein in nature and antigenic (Table 49-1). Of the four major lethal antigens, alpha, beta, epsilon, and iota toxins, the most important is the alpha toxin, which is produced by all five types of *C. perfringens*. All of the toxins are exotoxins.

Many of the other soluble substances or minor antigens are enzymes with defined substrates. These substances are nonlethal and should not be referred to as toxins as has been customary in the past. Examples of these substances are collagenase (kappa antigen), deoxyribonuclease (nu antigen), and hyaluronidase (mu antigen).

In general, serotyping with somatic antigens has not been practical in the further subdivision of *C. perfringens*, although a large number of serologic types exist. One useful application, however, is in epidemiologic studies of outbreaks of food poisoning where a comparison can be made between the serotypes of heat-resistant (100C for 1 hour) *C. perfringens* type A isolated from the feces of patients and the serotype of the incriminated food.

Determinants of Pathogenicity

The toxin of primary importance in the pathogenesis of clostridial myonecrosis is the alpha toxin, which initially was described in terms of its lethal, dermonecrotic, and hemolytic activities. The toxin is a lecithinase C (or phospholipase C) which splits lecithin to phosphorylcholine and a diglyceride. The toxin is activated by Ca^{++} and Mg^{++} ions, and it also hydrolyzes sphingomyelin. Titration of alpha toxin can be performed using in vivo lethality testing and in vitro procedures which are dependent upon its enzymatic action against lecithin-containing substrates, such as egg yolk emulsion, human serum, or erythrocytes of certain animal species. Alpha toxin is an excellent antigen; in vivo protection or therapy of animals is dependent entirely on the alpha antitoxic titer. The in vivo action of alpha toxin is apparently on lecithin-containing lipoprotein complexes in the cell membrane and probably on mitochondria. Disruption or leakage of cell membranes alone can explain the lysis of erythrocytes, destruction of tissue, and edema observed in this disease. Its local activity in the muscle lesion is obvious, but the basis for the generalized toxicity or systemic manifestations and death seen in clostridial myonecrosis is not fully explained. Other substances such as theta, kappa, or mu antigens apparently exert an ancillary role in abetting the local spread of the infection through tissue and providing nutrients for the proliferation of the organism.

Clinical Infections

Wound and Soft Tissue Infections Epidemiology. *C. perfringens* is ubiquitous. Type A strains are commonly found in the intestinal tract of man and animals and are numerous in the soil in both the vegetative and spore forms. The natural habitat of types B through E, which cause a variety of infections in animals, appears to be the intestinal tract of animals and occasionally man, but these types are not permanent inhabitants of the soil, as is type A. Infection may be due to endogenous or exogenous clostridia. In traumatic injuries, either accidental or during warfare, the source of clostridia is usually soil carried into the tissues. The incidence of contamination and infection depends on the concentration of *C. perfringens* in the soil, which varies with the geographic location. Endogenous infections stem from fecal flora present on the skin or on particles of clothing carried into the wound or from clostridia escaping from the bowel when its integrity is disrupted by disease, traumatic injury, or surgery.

One of the essential factors predisposing to clostridial myonecrosis is trauma, associated with deep and lacerating or crush wounds of muscle and vascular damage of major vessels and capillary beds. If ischemia and necrosis are present deep within the muscle, however, the trauma may not be necessarily severe. Such a setting occurs in infections associated with injections of such vasoconstrictive agents as epinephrine. The basis for the requirement of trauma with ischemic or necrotic areas is the anaerobic nature of the clostridia, which require a reduced oxygen tension and oxidation–reduction potential for growth (Chap. 48). Clostridia are unable to initiate infection in healthy tissues in which the oxidation–reduction potential is normal. Even with the high frequency of pathogenic clostridia in wounds, the incidence of gas gangrene remains relatively low because of these growth restrictions.

The principal settings for infections of this type occur during periods of war when massive wounds of muscle contaminated with soil, clothing, and metal fragments are common. Prior to the early 1950s evacuation and medical care of the wounded following injury was delayed, providing optimal conditions for the histotoxic clostridia to initiate infection. More recently, however, rapid evacuation of the wounded and early medical care have drastically reduced the wartime incidence of clostridial myonecrosis. In civilian life, settings that may lead to this disease include automobile and motorcycle accidents, gunshot wounds, compound fractures, industrial accidents, surgical complications, septic abortion, and injections of medications, such as epinephrine. A reduced blood supply stemming from edema, cold, or shock and the presence in the wound of facultative organisms also predispose to clostridial infection.

PATHOGENESIS. When *C. perfringens* is introduced into tissue the primary requirement for initiation of infection is a lowered oxidation–reduction potential. In areas of reduced oxygen tension the pyruvate of muscle is incompletely oxidized, and lactic acid accumulates, causing a drop in pH. The combination of lowered oxidation–reduction potential and pH may activate endogenous proteolytic enzymes, resulting in tissue autolysis. This release of nutrients and the lowered oxidation–reduction potential combine to produce conditions suitable for growth of anaerobic organisms.

Proliferation of the organisms is accompanied by the production of soluble toxins. In true clostridial myonecrosis these toxins diffuse from the initial site of growth and attack healthy muscle and surrounding tissues. These tissues are in turn destroyed by the toxins, thereby permitting spread of the infection into new necrotic areas. The edema fluid and gas accumulated from the metabolism of the organism also increase the pressure within muscle bundles so that circulation is impaired, and the oxidation–reduction potential and pH decrease, providing new areas within muscle suitable for the extension of growth of the clostridia. The disease progresses in this manner, with the organisms moving into new areas be-

hind the destructive action of their toxins. The local infection and its extension into healthy tissues are well understood. The generalized systemic toxicity, however, and the immediate cause of death in clostridial myonecrosis are still unknown, although the alpha toxin is recognized as an essential element in its pathogenesis.

CLINICAL MANIFESTATIONS. Wound infections can be divided into three categories of increasing levels of severity: (1) simple wound contamination, (2) anaerobic cellulitis, and (3) clostridial myonecrosis. Two additional clinical settings, uterine infections and clostridial septicemia, are special types of wound and soft tissue infections with certain unique features. The symptomatology of the three categories, however, may overlap, and an infection may evolve from a cellulitis into true clostridial myonecrosis. The essential clinical features of wound infections are given in Table 49-3.

Simple Wound Contamination. In simple wound contamination one or more histotoxic clostridia may be present without an obvious pathologic process. Either the clostridia present may be nontoxigenic, or the environmental conditions in the wound may be unsuitable for toxin production and the initiation of a progressive infection by toxigenic strains.

Anaerobic Cellulitis. This is a more serious form of wound infection, in which the clostridia infect necrotic tissue already dead as a result of ischemia or direct trauma. The organisms in this case spread through subcutaneous tissue and along fascial planes between muscles but do not invade healthy, intact muscle. Growth of *C. perfringens* within the necrotic tissue is extensive, and gas is normally a prominent feature. Patients, however, are not extremely toxic, and the overall prognosis is considerably better than for clostridial myonecrosis. Careful distinction between this level of infection and true clostridial myonecrosis is necessary in order to avoid the sometimes extreme surgical measures that are unnecessary for anaerobic cellulitis but are required for treatment of clostridial myonecrosis.

Clostridial Myonecrosis (Gas Gangrene). This term should be limited to use in characteristic anaerobic infections of muscle in which

TABLE 49-3   DIFFERENTIATION OF GASSY INFECTIONS OF SOFT TISSUES AND WOUNDS

Criterion	Infected Vascular Gangrene	Anaerobic Cellulitis	Clostridial Myonecrosis	Streptococcal Myonecrosis
Incubation	Over 5 days, usually longer	Almost always over 3 days	Usually under 3 days	3–4 days
Onset	Gradual	Gradual	Acute	Subacute or insidious
Toxemia	None or minimal	None or slight	Very severe	Severe only after some time
Pain	Variable	Absent	Severe	Variable, as a rule fairly severe
Swelling	Often marked	None or slight	Marked	Marked
Skin	Discolored, often black and desiccated	Little change	Tense, often very white	Tense, often with coppery tinge
Exudate	None	None or slight	Variable, may be profuse, serous, and blood stained	Very profuse, seropurulent
Gas	Abundant	Abundant	Rarely pronounced except terminally	Very slight
Smell	Foul	Foul	Variable, may be slight, often sweetish	Very slight, often sour
Muscle	Dead	No change	Marked change	Little change at first except edema

Modified from MacLennan: Bacteriol Rev 26:177, 1962

organisms are invasive and the infection is associated with profound toxemia, extensive local edema, variable amounts of gas, massive tissue damage, and death in untreated cases.

Following injury there is an incubation period usually of 12 to 48 hours before symptoms suddenly appear. The characteristic initial symptom is pain in the affected area which increases in severity as the infection spreads. There is local edema and a thin, blood-stained exudate. The pulse rate rises disproportionately higher than the temperature. If the disease remains untreated, the process advances rapidly with increasing toxemia and extension of the infection. With increased exudation from the area, gas usually becomes obvious, but it is a variable symptom. Changes which occur in skin color, may become black finally. Necrosis of large muscle masses is associated with severe shock and prostration. Infrequently, intravascular hemolysis occurs, producing hemoglobinemia, hemoglobinuria, and renal failure. Death occurs rapidly in untreated cases.

Uterine Infections.   These are a special type of clostridial myonecrosis usually involving the gravid uterus. Prior to legalized abortion many cases followed illegal attempts at mechanically induced abortion by nonmedical practitioners. They may occasionally occur as puerperal infections. The source of *C. perfringens* may be exogenous or endogenous. As in wound infections different levels of clinical involvement occur. In contrast to clostridial myonecrosis from wounds, in uterine myonecrosis septicemia and intravascular hemolysis are common and lead to secondary renal failure. The disease progresses rapidly and has a high mortality.

Clostridial Septicemia.   Invasion of the bloodstream may occur in association with malignancy and may involve a localized myonecrosis in addition to a fulminating clostridial septicemia. There usually is no history of external trauma. The source of the organisms appears to be endogenous and to result from an alteration of the patient's intestinal tract as a consequence of the malignant process. Septicemia also may follow biliary tract or gastrointestinal surgery. *Clostridium septicum* or *C. perfringens* is usually the etiologic agent. Rapid diagnosis and treatment are essential, since in untreated cases death may occur in less than 24 hours after the onset of symptoms.

LABORATORY DIAGNOSIS.   An early diagnosis of clostridial myonecrosis is essential and as previously stated must be made on clinical grounds. Bacteriologic confirmation of the organisms present in the infection is important, however, and valuable information can be gained from a direct smear and gram stain of material from deep within the wound (Fig. 49-1). More than one clostridial species is usually present. Other organisms that are commonly found include *Staphylococcus, Streptococcus, Escherichia, Proteus, Bacillus, Bacteroides,* and other anaerobes. Gram stain and culture aid in differentiating clostridial myonecrosis from rare cases of anaerobic streptococcal myonecrosis or other mixed anaerobic infections (Table 49-3).

TREATMENT.   Simple wound infections with *C. perfringens* can be treated by removal of necrotic tissue and cleansing. They rarely require administration of antibiotics. Anaerobic cellulitis, which is a more serious infection, usually can be treated by opening the wounded area, removing all necrotic tissue, cleansing thoroughly, and administering antibiotics. These infections must be carefully monitored.

Mortality rates of clostridial myonecrosis vary from approximately 15 to 30 percent and are highly dependent on the anatomic location of the infection. Intensive and immediate therapy is indicated. The surgical removal of all infected and necrotic tissue is of prime importance. Intensive antibiotic and antitoxin therapy is partially effective, but if all infected muscles are not excised because of their anatomic location or for other reasons, the results obtained with antibiotic and antitoxic therapy alone are poor. Patients who survive this infection usually require extensive surgery and amputation. Not only is clostridial myonecrosis more common in the areas of the body that have large masses of muscle, such as the buttock, thigh, and shoulder, but also mortality from infections in these sites is higher, and treatment is more difficult because of spread of the infection to the trunk and involvement of areas that cannot be excised.

Although antibiotic therapy alone is ineffective in treating clostridial myonecrosis, there is general agreement on its therapeutic effectiveness as an ancillary agent. Penicillin is the drug of choice, but clindamycin can be substituted in patients with penicillin allergy. Secondary infection with organisms, such as *Escherichia coli,* must be covered with gentamicin or kanamycin. Clindamycin is indicated when *Bacteroides fragilis* is suspected or demonstrated. Although the value of antitoxin, which is available commercially as a polyvalent serum, has been disputed, it is probably a valuable therapeutic adjunct to surgery when used in adequate dosage. In spite of the risk of hypersensitivity reactions, antitoxin therapy is generally employed in a setting of extreme toxemia, particularly with intravascular hemolysis.

Hyperbaric oxygen was introduced in 1961 as an adjunct in the therapy of clostridial myonecrosis. Its effectiveness is supported by clinical use in human beings and by experimental observations in animals, but at present no controlled studies are available on its efficacy in the reduction of mortality in man. The increased survival (approximately 50 percent) of patients with clostridial myonecrosis involving the trunk when treated with hyperbaric oxygen in addition to the standard modes of therapy, however, suggests its effectiveness. The administration of hyperbaric oxygen also appears to have eliminated the necessity for early radical amputation of limbs or excision of tissue in an attempt to check surgically the irreversible spread of infection. Initial surgery can be limited to debridement and removal of frankly necrotic tissue, with hyperbaric oxygen used to halt further spread of the infection and improve oxygenation of marginally viable tissue.

Hyperbaric oxygen usually is administered by giving the patient five to seven intermittent exposures to breathing 100 percent O_2 in a chamber pressurized to 3 atmospheres absolute pressure. The first treatment is given as soon as possible after diagnosis. Further treatments are scheduled to complete a total of three treatments during the first 24 hours with intervals of 6 to 8 hours between treatments, a fourth treatment 6 to 12 hours later, and usually three final treatments at intervals of 6 to 14 hours. Hyperbaric oxygen exerts a direct inhibitory action on the organism and on toxin production. It also exhibits indirect effects by raising the oxidation–reduction potential of the tissues surrounding the infection and preventing spread of the organisms. Preformed alpha toxin is not inactivated by hyperbaric oxygen.

Clostridial septicemia complicating malignancy is amenable to antibiotic therapy with penicillin if initiated early. If localized myonecrosis develops, additional appropriate treatment is required.

PREVENTION.   The most important preventive measure against clostridial myonecrosis is early and adequate wound debridement. The incidence of the disease markedly increases with delay in debridement. Adequate cleansing, removal of necrotic tissue, delay in primary closure of large, ragged wounds, maintenance of drainage, and avoidance of tight packing are all of prime importance in prevention. Administration of prophylactic antibiotic (penicillin) probably reduces the risk of an anaerobic infection particularly if administered shortly after the wound is sustained.

Food Poisoning   This mild form of food poisoning has been recognized with increasing frequency since its association with *C. perfringens* was first demonstrated in 1945. The organisms usually involved are strains of type A that produce heat-resistant spores and minimal amounts of theta toxin, although more typical type A strains also may cause the disease. Eight to twenty-four hours following ingestion of contaminated food, patients develop acute abdominal pain and diarrhea. Nausea may occur, but vomiting is uncommon, as are other signs of infection, such as fever and headache. Symptoms normally last for 12 to 18 hours, and recovery is usually complete except for rare fatalities in elderly or debilitated patients.

The symptoms are attributable to an enterotoxin that is synthesized during sporulation of the organism. Properties of enterotoxin are erythema after intracutaneous injection, fluid accumulation in intestinal loops, and lethality for mice. Clinical symptoms are probably the result of the action of the enterotoxin on the intestinal mucosa. Repeated attacks occur, indicating absence of immunity.

This type of food poisoning usually results from the ingestion of meat dishes such as roasts, poultry, fish, and stews, that are heavily contaminated with *C. perfringens*. Contamination of food may occur at any time, since this organism is so widespread in the environment. Raw meat may be contaminated at slaughter, through handling during preparation, or by exposure to flies and dust. The initial heating or cooking of the food may produce germination of heat-resistant spores, or food may become contaminated after cooking. The clostridia multiply during cooling of the meat or during a storage period and will produce food poisoning if the food is served cool or is inadequately reheated. Symptoms occur only if the organisms multiply to a concentration of 10^6 to 10^7 viable cells per gram of food, such that 10^8 to 10^9 viable bacteria are ingested. A specific diagnosis is made by isolation of *C. perfringens* in higher than normal numbers from the feces of infected patients and, if possible, from samples of the ingested food.

Enteritis Necroticans (Necrotizing Jejunitis, Necrotic Enteritis)   This disease is caused by type C strains of *C. perfringens* and is a more severe disease than *C. perfringens* type A food poisoning. Following an incubation period of less than 24 hours, the onset is sudden, with severe abdominal pain, diarrhea, and in some patients loss of intestinal mucosa with bleeding into the stool. The disease may be fatal, with peripheral circulatory collapse or intestinal obstruction and peritonitis. Although strains causing this disease were originally designated as a new type of *C. perfringens*, type F, they are now considered to be an atypical type C strain producing heat-resistant spores (Table 49-1). In addition to sporadic cases, major outbreaks have been reported from New Guinea, where it is associated with the ingestion of contaminated and inadequately cooked pork (pig feasting), and the disease is called "pig-bel." In New Guinea the disease occurs in four forms, varying in severity and degree of toxicity but having an overall mortality rate of 35 to 40 percent. The beta toxin produced by *C. perfringens* type C is responsible for the symptomatology. The administration of *C. perfringens* type C antitoxin to patients with enteritis necroticans significantly reduces the mortality rate.

OTHER HISTOTOXIC CLOSTRIDIA

Clostridium septicum   *C. septicum* is closely related to *C. chauvoei*, both of which are widely distributed in nature and in the intestinal tract of man and animals. *C. chauvoei* is pathogenic for animals only, but *C. septicum* is pathogenic for man and other animals. Since this organism can escape from the intestinal tract of man and animals and invade tissues shortly after death, the presence of *C. septicum* in pathologic specimens must be interpreted with caution. *C. septicum* is 0.8 μm in diameter and 3 to 5 μm in length. It is motile by means of peritrichous flagella. Colonies on blood agar are surrounded by zones of complete hemolysis, and swarming across the surface of plates may be marked. The major toxin produced by *C. septicum* is alpha toxin, which is lethal, necrotizing, hemolytic, and possibly leukocidic. The organism also produces deoxyribonuclease, hyaluronidase, and an oxygen-labile hemolysin. The percentage of *C. septicum* isolates from cases of clostridial myonecrosis ranges from 5 to 20 percent, according to different reports. Endogenous *C. septicum* from the patient's own intestinal tract may produce septicemia and occasionally localized myonecrosis in patients with underlying carcinoma.

Clostridium novyi *C. novyi* has been differentiated into three major types, A, B, and C, on the basis of the soluble antigens present in toxic filtrates of the organism. These bacteria are found in the soil (especially type A) and in the livers (types A and B) of a variety of apparently healthy animals. Type A *C. novyi* is 4 to 8 μm in length and 1 μm in width, and type B organisms are even larger. These bacteria have oval subterminal spores. They are motile by peritrichous flagella, producing swarming on the surface of blood agar plates.

Type A *C. novyi* rather than type B causes most of the clostridial myonecrosis and other wound infections in man. Both types produce an alpha toxin that is necrotizing and lethal and is the most potent toxic substance in filtrates of *C. novyi* cultures. The alpha toxin apparently increases capillary permeability and produces the intense gelatinous edema in muscle tissue that is characteristic of clostridial myonecrosis caused by *C. novyi*. Beta (type B) and gamma (type A) toxins are lecithinase C enzymes, which are hemolytic, necrotizing, and, in the case of beta toxin, lethal. These toxins produce lecithinase reactions on egg yolk agar plates. Type A also produces a lipase (epsilon antigen) that gives a pearly layer effect (similar to oil on water) on and around colonies on egg yolk agar plates.

The production of the lethal alpha toxin by *C. novyi* appears to be bacteriophage dependent.

Recent studies have demonstrated that curing a toxigenic *C. botulinum* type C of its prophage produces a nontoxigenic strain. Infecting this organism with another specific bacteriophage then can convert the nontoxigenic strain into *C. novyi* type A, which produces the lethal alpha toxin. Continued toxigenicity and interconversion of species of toxigenic *C. botulinum* type C and *C. novyi* type A thus depends upon the presence of specific bacteriophages.

The percentage of clostridial myonecrosis due to *C. novyi* varies in different reported series but was approximately 42 percent during World War II. Since this organism, especially type B, is extremely fastidious and oxygen sensitive, its true occurrence may be greater than reported. Clostridial myonecrosis with *C. novyi* generally is characterized by a high mortality rate and large amounts of edema fluid, with little or no observable gas in the infected tissue.

Clostridium histolyticum *C. histolyticum* has been isolated from the gastrointestinal tract of humans and from the soil. It is an aerotolerant species and produces limited growth on blood agar plates incubated under aerobic conditions, although improved growth is produced in an anaerobic environment. The organism is markedly proteolytic, digesting a variety of native proteins. Several soluble antigens are produced, the most important being the alpha and beta toxins that are lethal and necrotizing. The beta toxin is a collagenase that causes the destruction of collagen fibers and marked disruption of tissues observed in cases of clostridial myonecrosis caused by this organism. The incidence of *C. histolyticum* in cases of clostridial myonecrosis during World War II was between 3 and 6 percent.

Clostridium bifermentans and Clostridium sordellii Although *C. bifermentans* and *C. sordellii* are very similar and for a time were considered a single species, there are sufficient serologic and physiologic differences to justify their separation into different species. *C. sordellii* consists of both pathogenic and nonpathogenic strains and produces urease. *C. bifermentans* is nonpathogenic and urease negative. Both organisms are found in the soil and as part of the normal intestinal flora of man and other animals. Both species produce proteolytic enzymes and a lecithinase that is serologically related to the alpha toxin of *C. perfringens* and is therefore partially inhibited by *C. perfringens* antitoxin. *C. sordellii* also produces a lethal toxin. Clostridial myonecrosis involving *C. sordellii* is characterized by large amounts of edema and thus may resemble infection with *C. novyi*. The incidence of *C. sordellii* in clostridial myonecrosis is about 4 percent.

Clostridium fallax   Although MacLennan considers *C. fallax* capable by itself of causing clostridial myonecrosis, there are few cases on record, and the organism is rarely encountered. *C. fallax* is a strict anaerobe that rapidly loses virulence after isolation and artificial cultivation. Its natural habitat is unknown.

NONPATHOGENIC CLOSTRIDIA

There are a variety of other species of clostridia commonly encountered in soft tissue infections, abscesses, wound infections, anaerobic cellulitis and clostridial myonecrosis. These organisms are usually considered to be nonpathogenic although there are unanswered questions regarding their possible role in the development of infection.

There is a correlation between the incidence in wound infections of the various species of clostridia, both pathogenic and nonpathogenic, and their occurrence in the soil, but the source also may be endogenous organisms on the skin and clothing. Alteration in the integrity of the intestinal wall by disease, surgery, or trauma may also release a variety of endogenous bacteria, including these so-called nonpathogenic clostridial species that may then be isolated from subsequent infections, such as peritonitis and abdominal abscess. It is important to remember that *C. tetani* and *C. botulinum* may also be present in a wound in addition to the histotoxic clostridia and nonpathogenic clostridial species (Chaps. 50 and 51).

Of the clostridia currently labeled nonpathogenic *C. sporogenes* is frequently encountered in wound infection along with *C. bifermentans* and *C. tertium*. Additional organisms which may be isolated from these sources are *C. limosum*, *C. lentoputrescens*, *C. butyricum*, *C. cochlearium*, *C. cadaveris*, (formerly *C. capitovale*), *C. subterminale*, *C. innocuum*, and *C. ramosum* (formerly termed *Bacteroides terebrans* or *B. trichoides*, and *Catenabacterium filamentosum*). Although *C. sporogenes* does not appear to produce toxins, there is some evidence that the organism when associated with frank pathogens, such as *C. perfringens* or *C. novyi*, may play a synergistic role in clostridial myonecrosis. Its presence with either of these organisms is correlated with a high mortality rate.

FURTHER READING

Books and Reviews

Balows A, DeHaan RM, Dowell VR Jr, Guze LB (eds): Anaerobic Bacteria: Role in Disease. Springfield, Ill, Thomas, 1974

Buchanan RE, Gibbons NE (eds): Bergey's Manual of Determinative Bacteriology, 8th ed. Baltimore, Williams & Wilkins, 1974

Dowell VR Jr, Hawkins TM: Laboratory Methods in Anaerobic Bacteriology. CDC Laboratory Manual. Washington, Government Printing Office, DHEW Publication No (CDC) 74-8272, 1974.

Holdeman LV, Moore WEC: Anaerobic Bacteriology Manual, 3rd ed. Anaerobe Laboratory, Blacksburg, Virginia Polytechnic Institute and State University, 1975

Kadis S, Montie TC, Ajl SJ (eds): Microbial Toxins. vol 2A: Bacterial Protein Toxins. New York, Academic Press, 1971

Lennette EH, Spaulding EH, Truant JP (eds): Manual of Clinical Microbiology, 2nd ed. Washington, American Society for Microbiology, 1974

MacLennan JD: The histotoxic clostridial infections of man. Bacteriol Rev 26:177, 1962

Smith LDS: The Pathogenic Anaerobic Bacteria. Springfield, Ill, Thomas, 1975

Sutter VL, Vargo VL, Finegold SM: Wadsworth Anaerobic Bacteriology Manual, 2nd ed. Los Angeles, Department of Continuing Education in Health Sciences, University of California, 1975

Willis AT: Clostridia of Wound Infection. London, Butterworths, 1969

Selected Papers

Alpern RJ, Dowell VR Jr: *Clostridium septicum* infections and malignancy. JAMA 209:385, 1969

Altemeier WA, Fuller WD: Prevention and treatment of gas gangrene. JAMA 217:806, 1971

Eklung MW, Poysky FT, Meyers JA, Pelroy GA: Interspecies conversion of *Clostridium botulinum* type C to *Clostridium novyi* type A by bacteriophage. Science 186:456, 1974

Hauschild AHW, Nolo L, Dorward WJ: The role of enterotoxin in *Clostridium perfringens* type A enteritis. Can J Microbiol 17:987, 1971

Hobbs BC, Smith ME, Oakley CL, Warrock GH, Cruickshank JC: *Clostridium welchii* food poisoning. J Hyg 51:75, 1953

Holland JA, Hill GB, Wolfe WG, et al: Experimental and clinical experience with hyperbaric oxygen in the treatment of clostridial myonecrosis. Surgery 77:75, 1975

Macfarlane MG: On the biochemical mechanism of action of gas gangrene toxins. Symp Soc Gen Microbiol 5: 57, 1955

Macfarlane MG, Knight BCJG: The biochemistry of bacterial toxins. I. The lecithinase activity of *Cl. welchii* toxins. Biochem J 35:884, 1941

Sterne M, Warrack GH: The types of *Clostridium perfringens*. J Pathol 88:279, 1964

50
Clostridium Tetani

Tetanus is a relatively rare disease in well-developed countries. In developing countries where many unimmunized mothers give birth to children with neglected umbilical cord care, neonatal tetanus has a significant impact on overall mortality. In the adult, disease classically follows a puncture wound and is characterized by severe muscle spasms, the most characteristic being that of the jaw, thus the term "trismus" or "lockjaw." Despite many advances in treatment, the mortality rate is quite high, especially in the very young and the very old.

The anaerobic nature of the causative organism, *Clostridium tetani*, was in part responsible for its late isolation and discovery by Kitasato in 1889. The clinical as well as experimental recognition that a small local infection produced by this organism could result in a profound toxemia with neuromuscular manifestations led to the discovery of tetanus toxin and the detection shortly thereafter of its specific antitoxin. Antitoxin proved to be quite effective when administered prophylactically but less so when used therapeutically. However, the discovery that the toxin can be converted to a toxoid that is an excellent immunizing agent provided a remarkably effective method for the prevention of this disease. Widespread use of the toxoid has resulted in a marked reduction in the incidence of tetanus.

Morphology

The tetanus bacillus is quite long and thin when compared with species of other pathogenic clostridia. Individual bacilli range from 2 to 5 μm in width and 3 to 8 μm in length. Young cultures of the organism usually stain gram-positive, but in older cultures and in smears made from wounds the organisms frequently are gram-negative. Under appropriate cultural conditions the organism produces a spore terminally located and of considerably greater diameter than the vegetative cell, giving the characteristic drumstick appearance. The spore does not take the gram stain and appears as a colorless round structure. With prolonged incubation the vegetative cells autolyze, leaving behind either the spore with a portion of the vegetative cell attached or free spores. Most isolates of *C. tetani* possess numerous peritrichous flagella that convey active motility to the organism.

Physiology

C. tetani is an obligate anaerobe, moderately fastidious in respect to its requirement for anaerobiosis. The optimal temperature for growth is 37C, and the optimal pH is 7.4. Nutritional requirements of *C. tetani*, like those of other clostridia, are complex and include a number of amino acids and vitamins. These requirements can be readily met by blood agar or cooked meat broth. Since swarming of the organisms occurs on blood agar plates, the isolation of surface colonies is difficult. The edge of the colony appears as a translucent, finely granular sheet with a delicate filamentous advancing edge. This pronounced motility, especially in the presence of condensed moisture, has been used to advantage in isolating the organism from mixed cultures containing bacteria that are less motile than *C. tetani*. Where isolated colonies can be obtained, faint beta hemolysis is observed. In cooked meat broth a small amount of growth can be detected in 48 hours; no digestion of the meat is noted. The organism does not ferment any carbohydrates. It does not usually liquefy gelatin in 48 hours and produces very little change in litmus milk.

The spore of *C. tetani* conveys to the organism considerable resistance to the various disinfectants and to heat. It is not destroyed by boiling for 20 minutes. For practical purposes, autoclaving at 120C for 15 minutes is the best method for sterilizing contaminated materials.

Laboratory Identification Clinical materials for culture should be transported to the laboratory in vessels containing carbon dioxide. They should be planted immediately both on prereduced solid media and on anaerobic liquid culture media, such as chopped meat medium, and incubated under anaerobic conditions. Sometimes isolation of the organism is difficult because of the presence of other organisms in the specimen. In such cases heating the culture at 80C for 20 minutes after an initial 24-hour incubation period will kill nonspore-forming organisms and permit recovery of *C. tetani*. The rapid motility of the organism may also be useful in its isolation. One-half of a culture plate is inoculated with a culture, the remaining half is left uninoculated and is examined after 24 hours for a thin film of the motile *C. tetani*. Final proof of the isolation of toxin-producing *C. tetani* rests on the in vivo demonstration of toxin production when injected into mice and its neutralization in mice previously inoculated with antitoxin.

Antigenic Structure

Flagella (H), somatic (O), and spore antigens have been demonstrated in *C. tetani*. The spore antigens are different from the H and O antigens of the somatic cell. Strains of the organism have been differentiated into 10 types on the basis of their flagellar antigens. There is a single somatic agglutination group for all strains that permits identification of the organism by use of fluorescein-labeled antisera. Of tremendous practical importance, however, is the production of a single antigenic type of toxin by all strains of *C. tetani* and its neutralization by a single antitoxin.

Determinants of Pathogenicity

Very little is known about the conditions that allow the tetanus bacillus to survive within the human host. When present alone, it rarely produces an invasive cellulitis. Frequently, however, it is found in association with other bacteria that play a more significant role in the local infection and that lower the oxidation-reduction potential at the site of injury.

All of the symptoms in tetanus are attributable to an extremely toxic neurotoxin, tetanospasmin, which is an extracellular protein elaborated by the organism.

Properties of Tetanus Toxin   The purification of toxin is best accomplished by its extraction from cells toward the end of the exponential phase of growth before there is appreciable toxin detectable in the culture medium. The purified active product is a simple protein containing no carbohydrate and with a molecular weight of about 68,000. The toxin exists in two stages, the toxin monomer and a dimer of about twice that molecular weight, which is nontoxic but still antigenic.

Tetanus toxin is one of the most poisonous substances known; only *C. botulinum* toxin and *S. dysenteriae* toxin are comparable in toxicity. There is no simple in vitro test for determining its activity. Toxicity must be assayed by observing its lethal effect on an experimental animal. In quantitating the toxin the most meaningful dose is the LD_{50}, since this level of toxin lies on the steepest part of the dose–response curve. Animals vary in their susceptibility to the toxin. Man and the horse are probably the most susceptible, while birds and cold-blooded animals are usually quite resistant. In mice, pure toxin preparations have a potency of about 30 million MLD/mg protein. Toxin constitutes about 5 to 10 percent of the bacterial weight; however, the physiology of its production and function in the parent organism is unknown.

Although toxin forms nontoxic dimers spontaneously, toxoiding with formaldehyde increases the degree of polymerization and produces a more stable and reliable product. This material is useful in immunization against the disease. Toxoid is nontoxic but retains the single antigenic determinant of tetanus toxin that gives rise to antitoxin antibody.

Mode of Action   The molecular basis for the action of tetanus toxin is unknown. The site of action, however, is the synaptosomes (nipped-off nerve endings) that are high in toxin-fixing capacity. Gangliosides in synaptic membranes are responsible for this binding of tetanus toxin. The gangliosides are water-soluble mucolipids, ceramidyloligosaccharides, containing residues of stearic acid, sphingosine, glucose, galactose, N-acetylgalactosamine, and sialic acid. The fixation of tetanus toxin by the ganglioside is dependent on the number and position of sialic acid residues in the molecule. At present, however, there is no definitive evidence that ganglioside binding has any connection with the mode of action of the toxin.

Physiologic Effects of Toxin   The injection of tetanus toxin into susceptible animals produces two types of neurologic illness. (1) Local injections of small doses of toxin produce local tetanospasm followed by ascending tetanus, the development of increasing muscle spasticity above the site of injection, and eventually generalized tetanic convulsions. (2) Injection of tetanus toxin intravenously or very large doses locally produces descending tetanus characterized by spasticity in the head and neck, spreading to the back and limbs, followed by general tetanic convulsions. There has long been a controversy as to whether tetanus toxin travels to the central nervous system by way of the bloodstream or along the nerves. A number of arguments support the centripetal movement of toxin in nerves. It is probable that the toxin travels within the nerve trunk in the tissue spaces between individual nerve fibers rather than in nerve axons. It is not generally agreed how intravenously injected toxin enters the central nervous system. Since in general tetanus the face muscles, which have very short motor nerves, are first affected, the toxin probably enters the central nervous system along motor nerves as it does in local tetanus. It has been suggested that the toxin may gain entrance to the central nervous system through the floor of the fourth ventricle, an area adjacent to lower cranial motor nerve nuclei, which could account for the early appearance of trismus and involvement of neck muscles.

The modes of action of tetanus toxin and strychnine are similar. Both produce excitation of the central nervous system by specifically blocking synaptic inhibition in the spinal cord, presumably at inhibitory terminals that use glycine as a neurotransmitter. However, tetanus toxin appears to act presynaptically, while strychnine acts postsynaptically. The obliteration of inhibitory reflex responses of nerve fibers by tetanus toxin would permit the uncontrolled spread of impulses initiated anywhere in the central nervous system, resulting in the hyperreflexia of the skeletal muscles. The convulsion pattern is determined by the most powerful muscles at a given joint and in most animals is characterized by tonic extension of the body and of all limbs.

Clinical Infection

Epidemiology Tetanus is a sporadic disease that is seen most frequently in southern, southeastern, and midwestern states. Rising rates of addiction to hard drugs, such as heroin, have led to an increase in clusters of cases in large urban areas. Despite a steady decrease in the incidence rate from 0.3 per hundred thousand population in 1950 to 0.1 per hundred thousand in 1967, there has not been as impressive a decline in the mortality rate.

Pathogenesis The spores of *C. tetani* are ubiquitous. They have been found in 20 to 64 percent of soil samples taken for culture and are present in even higher yields in cultivated lands. They are present in the gastrointestinal tracts of man and animals. If one carefully cultures traumatic wounds, *C. tetani* can also be demonstrated fairly frequently, although it is uncommon for tetanus to develop from these wounds. The most significant feature of the pathogenesis of tetanus is the setting of the wound where the oxidation–reduction potential must be properly poised to permit multiplication of the organism and toxigenesis. Classically the wounds seen in practice are the simple puncture wounds–nail, splinter, or thorn. However, other settings, such as compound fractures, skin-popping by drug addicts, decubitus and varicose ulcers, external otitis, and dental extractions, also provide the proper conditions. The most feared form of tetanus, tetanus neonatorum, is a very significant cause of morbidity and mortality in developing nations. This form of tetanus usually results from cutting of the umbilical cord with unsterile instruments or from improper care of the umbilical stump following delivery. In this country most neonatal cases have followed unattended home deliveries. Tetanus may also follow operative procedures, but with modern hospital facilities this is an extremely rare event.

The lowering of the oxidation–reduction potential is associated with tissue necrosis following traumatic injuries or the injection of necrotizing substances. An important contributing factor is the presence of aerobic bacteria that will grow to the point of removing oxygen and then continue to grow facultatively as anaerobes. This growth will effectively reduce the oxidation–reduction potential to the point where tetanus spores may germinate. Following the germination of the spores, toxin is elaborated and gains entrance to the central nervous system. The infection with *C. tetani* remains localized and inconspicuous with minimal reaction unless other organisms are present. In any collection of cases of tetanus, there is always a small percentage that gives no preceding history of injury.

Clinical Manifestations Following implantation of spores into an appropriate site there is an incubation period of 4 to 10 days. Tetanus may occur rarely in a localized form, developing in muscles adjacent to the site of inoculation. More frequently, however, it is generalized in nature. The earliest manifestation is muscle stiffness, followed by spasm of the masseter muscles, trismus or lockjaw. This is the classic symptom of tetanus. As the disease progresses tetanospasms cause clenching of the jaw, producing a grimace referred to as "risus sardonicus," arching of the back (opisthotonos), flexion of the arms, and extension of the lower extremities. These tetanospasms are relatively brief in duration but may be frequent and exhausting. Respiratory complications, such as aspiration pneumonia and atelectasis, are common. Occasionally the spasms will be of sufficient intensity to produce bone fractures. The disease takes several weeks to run its course, and death may ensue during one of the spasms. Poor prognosis is associated with a short incubation period between injury and seizure, rapid development from muscle spasm to tetanospasms, injury close to the head, extremes of age, and frequency and severity of convulsions. Patients who recover from this disease usually return to a completely normal state after a variable period of stiffness. Except for possible damage to the lungs from pulmonary complications or bone fracture, tetanus leaves no permanent residua.

Immunity There is no evidence that the natural disease confers immunity against subsequent tetanus infection. The tetanus toxin is so toxic that an amount sufficient to cause clinical tetanus is too small to be immunogenic. Recurrent attacks are not uncommon, and for this reason patients who recover from the disease should be actively immunized with toxoid to prevent possible exogenous reinfection or recurrence of infection from spores of *C. tetani* retained within the body. Adequate immunization of pregnant patients is extremely important so that the newborn will have passive immunity at the time of delivery, thereby diminishing the likelihood of tetanus neonatorum. This maternally transmitted immunity will last until active immunization has been started during the first year of life.

Laboratory Diagnosis The diagnosis of tetanus is made on clinical grounds because isolation of the organism can occur in the absence of disease and it is also possible to have tetanus and never isolate the organism. If the local lesion can be detected and gram stained, one can occasionally demonstrate thin gram-positive or gram-negative rods and sometimes spores with varying amounts of the vegetative cell attached. However, most such attempts to demonstrate the organisms directly have been unsuccessful. Material taken from a known wound should be transported to the bacteriology laboratory in transport vessels filled with carbon dioxide and should be cultured under anaerobic conditions.

Treatment The treatment of tetanus varies with the severity of the disease, but in general it is designed to prevent the further elaboration and absorption of toxin. Antitoxin is administered, and because of the immediate and delayed complications resulting from the administration of antitoxin prepared in a horse or sheep, human antitoxin from pooled hyperimmune donors is recommended. In addition, debridement of the wound and removal of any foreign bodies is essential unless the extent or location should preclude such a surgical approach. Large doses of penicillin should be given, and if the patient is allergic to penicillin, tetracycline or clindamycin may be considered. Mild tetanospasm may be controlled with barbiturates and diazepam. With severe tetanospasms, a curarelike agent may be employed to completely paralyze the patient's muscles so that respiratory function may be maintained by positive pressure breathing apparatus. Tracheostomy should be performed after the onset of the first tetanospasm in order to minimize respiratory complications. Good supportive care of the patient should also include careful control of the environment to reduce auditory and visual stimuli to minimize the frequency and severity of tetanospasms.

Prevention Tetanus can be prevented by active or passive immunization. When this is properly applied, the disease is almost completely preventable. During World War II only 12 cases of tetanus occurred in 2,734,819 hospital admissions for wounds and injuries in soldiers who had been previously immunized.

This successful experience resulted in the passage by most state legislatures in this country of laws making admission to primary school contingent upon adequate immunization with tetanus toxoid. This has been the reason for the steady decline in the incidence of this disease.

ACTIVE IMMUNITY.   Routine immunization with tetanus toxoid should begin at one to three months of age, using a combination of tetanus and diphtheria toxoid and pertussis vaccine (DPT). Three doses of DPT should be given at three-week or four-week intervals, with booster doses one and four years later. Immunity to tetanus can be maintained by a single booster dose of toxoid every 10 years. Because young children are very prone to lacerations and puncture wounds, in the past they were exposed repeatedly to booster shots when brought to emergency rooms. In addition, school requirements, camp requirements, and military requirements have led to an inordinate exposure to tetanus toxoid. For this reason patients coming to an emergency room with a history of the basic immunizing series and a history of a booster injection within a four-year period probably do not need to receive a booster injection at the time of injury. Individuals who come to the emergency room with no history of immunization or partial immunization should receive in one arm human immune globulin and in the other arm the first of a series of toxoid injections in order to prevent future tetanus.

PASSIVE IMMUNITY.   Passive immunity may be conferred by the administration of antitoxin. This form of immunity was developed during World War I, when it was recognized that a small dose of tetanus antitoxin prepared in a horse was impressively protective when administered at the time of injury. Because of the risks involved in the use of a foreign serum in a sensitized recipient, human hyperimmune antitetanus globulin is recommended for passive immunization. The prophylactic administration of a single 250-unit dose of antitoxin should be reserved for patients with tetanus-prone wounds who have no record of immunization, who have received only one dose of tetanus

toxoid, or who are not seen until 48 hours after the injury. Penicillin or tetracycline also should be given along with appropriate surgical care. Such persons receiving antitoxin should be given, at the same time, alum-absorbed toxoid administered at a different site and a second dose of toxoid one month later.

FURTHER READING

Books and Reviews

Balos A, DeHaan RM, Dowell VR Jr, Guze LB: Anaerobic Bacteria-Role in Disease. Springfield, Ill, Thomas, 1974.

Smith LD, Holdeman LV: The Pathogenic Anaerobic Bacteria. Springfield, Ill, Thomas, 1968

Van Heyningen WE, Mellanby J: In Kadin S, Montie TC, Ajl Sj (eds): Microbial Toxins. New York, Academic Press, 1971, vol 2A

Willis AT: Clostridia of Wound Infection. London, Butterworths, 1969

Wright GP: Mechanisms of Microbial Pathogenicity. Cambridge, Cambridge Univ Press, 1955

Selected Papers

Brooks GF, Buchanan TM, Bennett JV: Tetanus toxoid immunization of adults: A continuing need. Ann Intern Med 73:603, 1970

Edsall G, Elliott MW, Peebles TC, Levine L, Eldred MC: Excessive use of toxoid boosters. JAMA 202:17, 1967

Johnson DM: Fatal tetanus after prophylaxis with human tetanus globulin. JAMA 207:1519, 1969

MacLennan JD: The serological identification of C. tetani. Br J Exp Pathol 20:371, 1939

Morbidity and Mortality Weekly Report. Tetanus — United States 1968-1969. 19:162, 1970

Murphy SG, Miller KD: Tetanus toxin and antigenic derivatives. I. Purification of the biologically active monomer. J Bacteriol 94:580, 586, 1967

Pascale LR, Wallyn RJ, Goldfein S, Gumbiner SH: Treatment of tetanus by hyperbaric oxygenation. JAMA 189:408, 1964

Smith DT, Pryor WW: Case of tetanus treated with antitoxin and d-tubocurarine. Ann Intern Med 32:728, 1950

Suri JC, Rubbo SD: Immunization against tetanus. J Hyg (Camb) 59:29, 1961

Wessler S, Avioli LA: Tetanus. JAMA 207:123, 1969

Wigley, FM, Wood SH, Waldaman RH: Aerosol immunization of humans with tetanus toxoid. J Immunol 103:1096, 1969

Young LS, LaForce FM, Bennett JV: An evaluation of serologic and antimicrobial therapy in the treatment of tetanus in the United States. J Infect Dis 120:153, 1969

Zacks SI, Sheff MF: Tetanus toxin: Fine structure localization of binding sites in striated muscle. Science 159:643, 1968.

51

Clostridium Botulinum

Botulism is not an infectious disease but is a specific and often fatal type of food poisoning that results from the ingestion of food containing the preformed toxin elaborated by *Clostridium botulinum.* Botulinum toxin is the most potent toxin known. It is a neurotoxin, producing illness characterized by sudden onset and swiftness of course, terminating in profound paralysis and pulmonary arrest.

The disease botulism received its name from the Latin *botulus* (sausage), a term introduced in 1870 to describe a fatal food poisoning syndrome associated with the eating of sausage. Although of historical interest, the name has lost much of its significance, since fish and other animal proteins also transmit the disease, and in the United States plant rather than animal products are more common vehicles.

Morphology and Physiology

Morphology *C. botulinum* is a straight to slightly curved gram-positive rod with rounded ends. Although exhibiting marked variation in size depending on cultural conditions and serologic type, the size falls within the range of 3.4 to 8.6 μm by 0.5 to 1.3 μm. Involution forms on artificial media are frequently observed. *C. botulinum* is motile with peritrichous flagella. It produces heat-resistant spores that are oval, subterminal, and tend to distend the bacillus. These are produced more consistently when the organism is grown on alkaline glucose gelatin media at 20C to 25C; spores usually are not produced at higher temperatures.

Physiology *C. botulinum* is a strict anaerobe, easily cultured in an anaerobic environment on routine media. On blood agar all strains except those of type G are beta hemolytic. The nutritional requirements of the organism are complex, especially those of the nonproteolytic strains.

With the various serologic types of *C. botulinum* (p. 678), there is considerable diversity in the utilization of specific carbohydrates and proteins. All strains, however, ferment glucose and fructose and hydrolyze gelatin. The property of gelatin liquefaction has been an especially useful one in the overall classification of the more than 300 species of clostridia. Primary products of sugar fermentation are acetic and butyric acids, with smaller amounts of other organic acids and alcohols. The action of *C. botulinum* on egg, milk, and other proteins is useful in its classification and has been employed to separate strains into two groups, the strongly proteolytic (ovolytic) organisms and the less proteolytic (nonovolytic) strains. The four major physiologic groups of *C. botulinum* and their relationship to the serologic types are shown in Table 51-1. Considerable diversity in cultural characteristics and colony types is associated with variations in physiologic properties.

Resistance The heat resistance of the spores of *C. botulinum* is greater than that of any other anaerobe. The degree of resistance to various physical and chemical factors depends on the specific strain and serologic type of the organism. Type A is more resistant than types B, C, and D; type E is the least heat-resistant, but variants of this type which are exquisitely heat-resistant have been obtained. In general, the spores may survive several hours at 100C and up to 10 minutes at 120C. The spores are also resistant to irradiation and can survive temperatures of −190C.

TABLE 51-1 RELATIONSHIP BETWEEN PHYSIOLOGIC GROUP AND SEROLOGIC TYPE OF CLOSTRIDIUM BOTULINUM

Group	Serologic Types	Gelatin Liquefaction	Action on Milk	H$_2$S Production
I	A and proteolytic strains of B, C, D, F	+	Digested	+
II	E and nonproteolytic strains of B and F	+	Coagulated with soft curd; not digested	−
III	Nonproteolytic C and D	+	Not changed	−
IV	G	+	Digested slowly	+

Antigenic Structure

The species *C. botulinum* includes a very heterogeneous group of strains which have been divided into seven serologically distinct types, A through G, on the basis of the type of toxin produced. Immunologic differences between these types are constant and clear-cut and of epidemiologic significance.

The antigenic composition of vegetative cells of *C. botulinum* is very complex and has not been completely defined for most of the types. Studies on the ovolytic strains of types A and B have permitted their division into six subgroups on the basis of their heat-labile antigens. These strains of *C. botulinum* share one heat-stable antigen with *Clostridium tetani*, *Clostridium histolyticum*, and *Clostridium sporogenes*. Using the fluorescent antibody technique, cross-reactions have been demonstrated among the ovolytic strains of A, B, and F and between strains of C and D. There are different heat-stable and heat-labile agglutinating antigens among strains of type E. These strains, however, appear to be homogeneous and distinct and do not cross-react with strains of other types. For each of the types, spore antigens appear to be more specific than antigens of the vegetative cells.

Determinants of Pathogenicity

The clinical manifestations of botulism are attributable to the preformed toxin of *C. botulinum* present in the ingested food. Botulinum toxin is the most potent toxin known. One microgram of the purified toxin contains about 200,000 minimal lethal doses (MLD) for a 20 g white mouse.

Extensive work has established the basic requirement for growth and toxigenicity of the various types. The optimal temperature for toxin production varies greatly both within and across types. Best results have been obtained over a temperature range of 30 to 38C, except for *C. botulinum* type E, which grows best at 25 to 28C. Initiation of growth and toxin production occurs only over a narrow pH range of 7.0 to 7.3. *C. botulinum* can be grown on a completely defined synthetic medium, but toxin production is less than that obtained on media containing casein hydrolysate or corn steep liquor.

Although usually classified as an exotoxin because of its high potency and antigenicity, botulinum toxin differs from a classic exotoxin in that it is not released during the life of the organism. Instead, it is produced intracellularly and appears in the medium only upon death and autolysis of the cell. The tremendous size of the toxin molecule as it first appears in the culture medium would also require rupture of the cell membrane for liberation of the toxin. The role played by the toxin in the metabolism of *C. botulinum* is unknown, since the organism may be rendered nontoxigenic without any discernible effect on the growth rate.

The molecules of toxin are believed to be synthesized as progenitor toxins with relatively low specific toxicity or as nontoxic protoxins which are converted to progenitor toxins. Trypsin and other proteolytic enzymes apparently activate progenitor toxin by cleavage of specific arginyl and lysyl bonds. When first isolated crystalline type A toxin was reported to have a molecular weight of 900,000. Subsequent studies, however, have shown that botulinum toxin forms a stable complex with another soluble component of the organism that has hemagglutinating activity and that this complex acts as a homogeneous material during purification. Crystalline toxin has been dissociated into two biologically active fractions: one is toxic, the α component, and the other the β component, is a potent hemagglutinin. The α toxic component is a different protein from the hemagglutinin and has a molecular weight of 1.28×10^5. The hemagglutinin is an aggregate of three molecular species of molecular weight 2.5×10^5, 5×10^5, and 7.5×10^5. In electron micrographs the toxin appears as round or disklike particles, 4 to 4.5 nm, arranged in long strands or tubules, 9 nm in width. The microscopic appearance of the hemagglutinin suggests that it forms a helix with sufficient space within its coil to admit the strands of the toxin. It has been proposed that this is the native structure of the toxin-hemagglutinin complex as it is elaborated by *C. botulinum* into the medium. Dissociated, the toxin is rapidly detoxified and becomes labile even in the cold. The hemagglutinin retains its stability after purification.

Site of Action of Botulinum Toxin   Toxin is absorbed largely from the small intestine and appears in the lymphatics draining the intestine before it is found in the bloodstream.

Much of the ingested toxin may not be absorbed from the small intestine. Some may be completely denatured and destroyed by proteolytic enzymes in the intestine, or it is possible that only the toxin molecules of lower molecular weight are capable of getting into the circulation.

Botulinum intoxication is associated with functional disturbances in the peripheral nervous system. The toxin acts at the myoneural junction to produce complete paralysis of the cholinergic nerve fibers at the point of release of acetylcholine. Botulinum toxin affects both sets of cholinergic transmission points in the autonomic system, the synaptic ganglia and the parasympathetic motor end plates peripherally located in the junction between the nerve and cell fibers. Death occurs from suffocation following paralysis of such respiratory organs as the diaphragm. Although the action of botulinum toxin is primarily on peripheral nerves, clinical manifestations of the disease as well as evidence presented by a number of investigators suggest that the central nervous system may also be involved.

The toxin suppresses the presynaptic release of acetylcholine, but the mechanism of this suppression is unknown. It has been suggested that botulinum toxin in some way antagonizes calcium ion transport through the cell membrane by serotonin. Since the amount of acetylcholine released per nerve impulse is a function of the extracellular concentration of calcium ions, with depletion of calcium ion, the end plate does not release acetylcholine, and the muscle fiber fails to contract. There is at present, however, no direct evidence to support the hypothesis that toxin competes with serotonin or one of its derivatives for a combining site on the nerve cell.

Inactivation of Toxin The susceptibility of toxin to inactivation by various chemical and physical agents is of practical importance because of its role in food poisoning. The resistance of botulinum toxin to various deleterious agents is markedly dependent upon the serologic type of toxin, temperature, pH, and the presence of certain other materials in the medium in which the toxin is tested. In general, thermostability depends upon the substance in which the toxin is dissolved. All toxin types are completely destroyed by boiling for 1 minute or by heating at 75 to 85C for 5 to 10 minutes. At room temperature toxin persists for several days in tap water, an important observation suggesting the possibility of prolonged contamination of water supplies. Toxin is destroyed by direct sunlight within five days unless protected from air, in which case toxin inactivation proceeds at a slower rate. A low pH of 3.5 to 6.8 favors preservation of the toxin, while an alkaline pH favors detoxification. Factors usually found in putrefying canned foods apparently have no effect on the toxin.

Laboratory Detection of Toxin The incrimination of *C. botulinum* as the cause of food poisoning is based on demonstration of the toxin in the food or in serum or gastric contents from the patient. Because of the extreme potency of botulinum toxin, an effective assay for clinical or laboratory use should be rapid, specific, and sensitive. Tests presently available for the detection and assay of toxins, when suitable for low concentrations of toxin, are too slow to be practical. In vitro serologic tests are useful only when the toxin is present in relatively high concentrations and the antiserum is free of hemagglutinating antibodies.

Although too slow to be of use in the diagnosis of a single isolated case of botulism, the in vivo mouse neutralization test is the only test available at present for the detection of small amounts of toxin. A protocol for the performance of this test is shown in Table 51-2. Two mice are injected intraperitoneally with 0.5 ml of each different type of test material. Antitoxin may be mixed with the fluid before inoculation (neutralization test) or inoculated intraperito-

TABLE 51-2 MOUSE NEUTRALIZATION TEST FOR TYPING OF BOTULINUM TOXIN

Cell-free Test Material*	Treatment	Serum
1.2 ml	None	0.3 ml normal
1.2 ml	Heat	0.3 ml normal
1.2 ml	None	0.3 ml antitoxin†
1.2 ml	Trypsin‡	0.3 ml normal
1.2 ml	Trypsin, heat	0.3 ml normal
1.2 ml	Trypsin	0.3 ml antitoxin

From Smith and Holdeman. The Pathogenic Anaerobic Bacteria, 1968. Courtesy of Charles C Thomas
° Food sample extracted by soaking overnight at 4C, centrifuged
‡ Monovalent or polyvalent may be used
† Test material incubated at 37C for 45 minutes with 0.1 percent trypsin, final concentration

neally 30 minutes before the challenge dose of test material is administered (protection test). If all animals die, including those inoculated with heated material, a nonspecific toxic substance is present, and the experiment should be repeated using dilutions of the test material. Survivors are observed for four to five days before discarding.

Clinical Intoxication

C. botulinum is the causative agent of a very lethal type of food poisoning that occurs in several species of animals. In general, food poisoning in a particular animal species is usually associated with certain types of the organism. The reason for this specificity is unknown. Man is susceptible to types A, B, E, and F, birds primarily to A and C, ruminants to C and D, and mink to A, B, C, and E.

Ecology   *C. botulinum* has been isolated from the sediments of lakes and rivers, from virgin and cultivated terrestrial soil, from the intestinal tract of fish, and from the intestinal tract, spleen, and liver of a variety of animals. In general, *C. botulinum* is isolated more frequently from soil containing silt and is easier to culture from manured than from nonmanured land.

The distribution of the various types of *C. botulinum* throughout the world is based on reports of disease in animals and man caused by the different types and upon isolation of the organisms from animals and the soil in various parts of the world. Table 51-3 shows the major geographic areas associated with each type. Although there is a prevalence of certain types of *C. botulinum* food poisoning in various localities, this does not rule out the possibility of spores of other types in the same locality. In the United States types A and B are widely distributed and have been associated with most outbreaks of human botulism. Type A is the predominant type in the Pacific Coast states, in the Rocky Mountains, and in Maine, New York, and Pennsylvania. The strains found in the soil of the Mississippi River Valley, the Great Lakes region, and in New Jersey, Delaware, Maryland, Georgia, and South Carolina are predominantly type B. Type E has in recent years been isolated from several parts of the United States but is especially prevalent in the Great Lakes area.

Disease in Animals   A number of characteristic paralytic diseases of birds and mammals are caused by the ingestion of botulinum toxin in the animals' food. The best known examples include grass or fodder sickness of horses, silage disease in cattle, limberneck in chickens, lamziekte of cattle, and dust sickness in wild birds. Outbreaks of botulism in animals reflect the geographic distribution of the organism, susceptibility of the animal species to the different toxins, and other predisposing factors. Thus, lamziekte in cattle is restricted to areas in which the soil and herbage are markedly deficient in phosphorus. In such areas the cattle are prone to eat putrid bones and carcasses of small animals that have *C. botulinum* in the intestin-

TABLE 51-3   EPIDEMIOLOGY OF THE DIFFERENT TYPES OF C. BOTULINUM

Type	Animals Primarily Affected	Transmission Vehicle	Highest Geographic Incidence
A	Man, chickens (limberneck)	Home-canned vegetables and fruits; meat and fish	Western US, Soviet Ukraine
B	Man, horses, cattle	Prepared meats, especially pork products	France, Norway, Eastern US
C_α	Aquatic wild birds (western duck sickness)	Fly larvae; rotting vegetation of alkaline ponds	Western US and Canada, South America, South Africa, Australia
C_β	Cattle (midland cattle disease), horses (forage poisoning), mink	Carrion	Australia, South Africa, Europe, North America
D	Cattle (lamziekte)	Carrion	South Africa, Australia
E	Man	Uncooked products of fish and marine mammals	Northern Japan, British Columbia, Labrador, Alaska, Great Lakes region, Sweden, Denmark, USSR
F	Man	Homemade liver paste	Denmark

Adapted from Dolman: US Public Health Service, Publ 999-FP-1:5, 1964

al tract. Botulism in sheep results from bone chewing and is associated with periods of drought or with overgrazed ranges. Forage poisoning in cattle and horses occurs in many parts of the world as a result of the ingestion of toxic hay or silage. The toxin in the hay originates from an animal carcass. Carcasses of small animals, especially cats, found in the food or bedding of the animals involved in such outbreaks, have been shown to contain as much as 3,000 MLD of toxin per gram. This toxin diffuses out into the hay or silage.

Type C botulinum toxin is the cause of large epidemics of botulism in aquatic and shore birds. Wild ducks are most frequently involved in these epidemics, which may affect thousands of birds. The disease is the major natural cause of death of ducks in the western United States. Outbreaks have also occurred in domestic ducks, gulls, loons, and sandpipers. Such outbreaks are probably initiated by strong wind action that tears aquatic plants from their mooring on the shore, leaving long rows of uprooted vegetation to decay. Aquatic invertebrates present in the decaying vegetation die because of lack of oxygen, and *C. botulinum* proliferates in their bodies. In searching for food among the masses of decaying vegetation, ducks ingest the toxic bodies of the invertebrates that contain *C. botulinum* organisms. After the duck's death the carcass is invaded by the organisms, and the carcass itself becomes toxic and serves to perpetuate the outbreak. The carcass becomes flyblown, and the fly larvae pick up a considerable amount of toxin both in their exterior slimy coating and by ingestion. The ingestion by ducks of only a few of these fly larvae results in death, and the ducks are invaded postmortem by *C. botulinum* and become flyblown, thus furnishing toxic larvae to poison more ducks. Botulism in pheasants follows a similar pattern.

Carrion eaters, such as the vulture, are almost completely resistant to botulinum toxin. The mechanism of this resistance is unknown, but apparently it cannot be attributed to the presence of antitoxin in the animal's blood.

Disease in Man EPIDEMIOLOGY During the 71 years from 1899 to 1970, 659 outbreaks of botulism have been reported in the United States, involving 1,696 persons and 957 deaths. Since 1935, however, because of improved canning methods in industry and in the home, there has been a gradual decline in the inci-

dence of the disease. Botulism is now considered a comparative rarity but one whose potential is present and which must always be kept in mind.

At the present time most cases of botulism occur in relatively circumscribed outbreaks following the consumption of home-preserved food. Sterilization procedures employed by commercial canneries utilize pressure apparatus in which canned products are held at a temperature of 121.1C for 30 minutes. As a result outbreaks of botulism are rarely associated with canned food. In recent years, however, there have been outbreaks from canned tuna fish and from vichyssoise as well as from smoked fish. The home-canned food most often incriminated as the source of botulism is green beans, which may produce only a slight sharp taste, prompting the housewife to rinse the contents of the jar of beans and serve them in a salad. Foods which are highly acidic, such as tomatoes and citrus fruits, are rarely the source because the organisms will not grow and release toxin at the low pHs encountered, about 4.6. Although the early descriptions of botulism followed the ingestion of contaminated sausage and meat products, botulism of this type is now uncommon. Specialized foods eaten by certain ethnic groups are often responsible for the prevalence of a particular type of botulism poisoning in a given locality. In Japan, izushi (fermented raw fish salad) is often implicated; among the Indians of the northwest Pacific Coast salmon egg cheese or stink eggs are responsible. Among the Alaskan Eskimos muklak is prepared by soaking beluga flippers in seal oil for an extended period before eating. In all of these foods conditions are suitable for growth and toxin production by *C. botulinum*.

Pathogenesis Human botulism results from the ingestion of preformed botulinum toxin in contaminated foods. After ingestion the toxin is absorbed primarily from the upper gastrointestinal tract, but toxin reaching the lower small intestine and colon may be slowly absorbed, perhaps accounting for the delayed onset and prolonged duration of symptoms seen in many patients. The toxin gains access to the peripheral nervous system and, as discussed on page 679, blocks release of acetylcholine.

Several cases have been reported of wound botulism, in which *C. botulism* has contaminated a traumatic wound. The rarity of this form of botulism is probably due to failure of *C. botulinum* spores to germinate readily in tissues. Also, within the setting of the experimental laboratory, the inhalation of aerosolized toxin has resulted in reported cases of clinical botulism.

Clinical Manifestations The incubation period and clinical manifestations are simlar for all types of botulinum toxin. Characteristically, symptoms begin 12 to 36 hours following ingestion of the contaminated food, or they may begin as late as 8 days. Type E botulism appears to have a shorter incubation period than do types A and B. Severe nausea and vomiting are frequently observed with type E intoxication. Weakness, lassitude, and dizziness are often early complaints. There is usually no diarrhea, but constipation is common. The early symptoms of botulism would rarely bring a patient to a physician's attention. Cranial nerve palsy— diplopia (double vision), dysphagia (difficulty in swallowing), and dysphonia (difficulty in speaking)—is usually the presenting symptom. The pupils are dilated; the tongue is very dry and furry. Abdominal distention is especially common in type E intoxication and may lead to a mistaken diagnosis of intestinal obstruction. Fever is rarely observed, and the mental processes remain intact. As the disease progresses, weakness of muscle groups, particularly of the neck, proximal extremities, and respiratory musculature, is often observed, leading ultimately to sudden respiratory paralysis, airway obstruction, and death. The mortality rate is affected by the type of toxin consumed, the distribution of toxin in the food, and the speed with which the disease is diagnosed and antitoxin therapy is initiated. Mortality is about 70 percent for type A toxin, 20 percent for type B, and 30 to 40 percent with type E toxin.

Laboratory Diagnosis The rapid diagnosis and establishment of the type of botulinum toxin affecting the patient is of crucial importance. Unfortunately, however, the disease is difficult to diagnose because, at its onset, the symptoms of botulism are often confused with the symptoms of other diseases and because few physicians are familiar with it. Diagnosis in an isolated case may be extremely difficult, and by the time the nature of the disease is apparent, it is usually too late for therapy. The neurologic diseases most frequently confused with botulism are myasthenia gravis, Guillain-Barré syndrome, and cerebrovascular accidents.

As soon as a diagnosis of botulism is suspected on clinical grounds, a specimen of the patient's blood should be drawn immediately and allowed to clot. Stool and gastric washings specimens should also be obtained if possible. The Center for Disease Control in Atlanta, Georgia, should be called to make arrangements for the laboratory diagnosis.* Collected specimens should be refrigerated until arrangements are made to air express them to Atlanta. Diagnosis is made by the mouse neutralization test described on page 679. If at all possible, the original food specimen should be obtained for similar studies, but all too frequently the original ingested food has been discarded. Since it is imperative to begin specific treatment as quickly as possible, the diagnosis must be made clinically and then confirmed by laboratory methods.

Treatment The efficacy of botulinum antitoxin has been demonstrated. The polyvalent antiserum containing antitoxins to types A, B, and E should be administered as soon as possible after the clinical diagnosis is made. Because the antitoxin is of equine origin, great care should be taken in its administration in order to minimize the risk of anaphylaxis and serum sickness. The patient should be skin-tested for serum sensitivity and, if sensitive to horse serum, should be desensitized before antitoxin is given. The antitoxin can be obtained by calling the Center for Disease Control at the telephone numbers listed on this page. Equally important in the management of these patients is supportive care for the respiratory tract. For this reason it is imperative that they be managed in large medical centers with modern facilities for respiratory monitoring of patients who require ventilatory assistance. In addition to the usual therapeutic approaches, two drugs that have recently been used show promise as a useful adjunct when combined with good medical care, guanidine hydrochloride and germine monoacetate. The use of the drugs in combination is more effective than either drug used alone. Caution is required in their use, however, because of a number of undesirable side effects and potential toxicity.

*Center for Disease Control, Atlanta, Georgia, 30333. Telephones: Day (404)633-3311, Extension 3751 or 3684; Night (404)633-2176 or (404)633-8673.

Prevention Although existing preventive measures for the control of botulism are simple and are effective when properly carried out, the fact that a number of outbreaks still occur each year indicates the need for improved methods of control. The homemaker should be alerted to the necessity of using sterilized containers and pressure cookers in the canning of all foods in order to kill any *C. botulinum* spores that may be on the food. Before any home-canned food is eaten, it should be boiled for one minute or heated at 80C for five minutes to destroy any toxin that might have been produced in the anaerobic environment provided.

The safety record of the canning industry during the past 40 years has been very impressive. Unfortunately, however, minor breaks in technique do occur, and unless rigid controls are constantly monitored there will continue to be sporadic outbreaks. Two deaths resulted from the small outbreak from canned tuna in Michigan in 1963, and the fish canning industry suffered a multimillion dollar loss.

Since botulism is a relatively rare disease, immunization of the entire population is impractical. An effective toxoid is available, however, for laboratory workers in high-risk situations. The recommended schedule for the establishment of active immunity in man is two injections of toxoid, either absorbed on aluminum sulfate or mixed with an equal volume of Freund's adjuvant, given at 0 and at 10 weeks, with a booster injection 52 weeks later.

Economically, botulism in animals is a very important disease, causing the death of many thousands of animals and birds each year. For range cattle, immunization with toxoid is the most practical method for prevention. In addition, lamziekte in cattle may be controlled by keeping the feeding area free of carcasses and by providing a diet adequate in phosphorus. Botulism in sheep can be prevented by supplementing the diet with carbohydrates and protein. Forage poisoning in cattle and horses may be prevented by keeping food and bedding free of carcasses of small animals.

FURTHER READING

Books and Reviews

Balows A, DeHaan RM, Dowell VR Jr, Guze LB: Anaerobic Bacteria—Role in Disease. Springfield, Ill, Thomas, 1974

Boroff DA, DasGupta BR: Botulinum Toxin. In Kaden S, Montie TC, Ajl SJ (eds): Microbial Toxins. New York, Academic Press, 1971, vol 2A

Smith LDS, Holdeman LV: The Pathogenic Anaerobic Bacteria. Springfield, Ill, Thomas, 1968

Selected Papers

Anellis A, Berkowitz D, Swantak W, Strojan C: Radiation sterilization of prototype military foods: Low-temperature irradiation of codfish cake, corned beef, and pork sausage. Appl Microbiol 24:453, 1972

Armstrong, RW, Stenn F, Dowell VR Jr, Ammerman G, Sommers HM: Type E botulism from home-canned gefilte fish. JAMA 210:303, 1969

Boroff DA, Reilly JR: V. Prophylactic immunization of pheasants and ducks against avian botulism. J Bacteriol 77:142, 1959

Boroff DA, Shu-Chen G: Radioimmunoassay for type A toxin of Clostridium botulinum. Appl Microbiol 25:545, 1973

Boroff DA, Nyberg S, Höglund S: Electron microscopy of the toxin and hemagglutinin of type A Clostridium botulinum. Infect Immun 6:1003, 1972

Bott TL, Johnson J Jr, Foster EM, Sugiyama H: Possible origin of high incidence of Clostridium botulinum type E in an inland bay (Green Bay of Lake Michigan). J Bacteriol 95:1542, 1968

Brown GW Jr, King G, Sugiyama H: Penicillin-lysozyme conversion of Clostridium botulinum types A and E into protoplasts and their stabilization as L-form cultures. J Bacteriol 104:1325, 1970

Cardella MA, Duff JT, Wingfield BH, Gottfried C: VI. Purification and detoxification of type D toxin and immunologic response to toxoid. J Bacteriol 79:372, 1960

Craig JM, Pilcher KS: Clostridium botulinum type F isolated from salmon from the Columbia River. Science 153:311, 1966

DasGupta BR, Sugiyama H: Role of a protease in natural activation of Clostridium botulinum neurotoxin. Infect Immun 6:587, 1972

Eklund MW, Poysky FT: Interconversion of type C and D strains of Clostridium botulinum by specific bacteriophages. Appl Microbiol 27:251, 1974

Eklund MW, Poysky FT, Reed SM, Smith CA: Bacteriophage and the toxigenicity of Clostridium botulinum type C. Science 172:480, 1971

Fiock MA, Varinsky A, Duff JT: VII. Purification and detoxication of trypsin-activated type E toxin. J Bacteriol 82:66, 1961

Mandia JW: Serological group II of the proteolytic clostridia. J Immunol 67:49, 1951

Marshall R, Quinn LY: In vitro acetylcholinesterase inhibition by type A botulinum toxin. J Bacteriol 94:812, 1967

Morbidity and Mortality Weekly Report. Surveillance Summary. Botulism—United States, 1899-1967. 17:444, 1968

Ono T, Karashimada T, Iida H: Studies on serum therapy of type E botulism (Part II). J Infect Dis 120:534, 1969

Takagi A, Kawata T, Yamamoto S: Electron microscope studies on ultra thin sections of spores of the clostridium group with special reference to the sporulation and germination process. J Bacteriol 80:37, 1960

Williams-Walls NJ: Type E botulism isolated from fish and crabs. Science 162:375, 1968

52

Introduction to the Spirochetes: Treponema

THE SPIROCHAETACEAE

The family Spirochaetaceae contains slender, helically coiled, flexible organisms with one or more complete turns in the helix. Spirochetes are motile, but motility results from the action of axial fibrils rather than flagella. These are long, flagellalike intracellular organelles that originate at either end of the cell from knoblike structures and extend toward the other end. Axial fibrils are variable in length but overlap one another near the middle of the cell. They are enclosed within the outer envelope. These fibrils determine the spiral shape of the cells and are responsible for the characteristic motility members of this family exhibit. There are five genera in the family Spirochaetaceae, of which only *Treponema*, *Borrelia*, and *Leptospira* species cause major human illnesses. Differentiation among genera of the family Spirochaetaceae is based primarily on morphology (Table 52-1).

The members of the family Spirochaetaceae are 3 to 500 μm long and 0.2 to 0.75 μm wide. Multiplication is by transverse fission. Each cell is composed of a protoplasmic cylinder, axial fibrils, and outer envelope (Fig. 52-1). Cellular motility includes rapid rotation around the long axis, flexation of cells, and locomotion along a helical path. Spirochaetaceae may be aerobic, facultatively anaerobic, or anaerobic. Many are best recognized by darkfield microscopy, since they may be below the resolution of light microscopy.

The three *Treponema* species that are pathogenic for man have not been cultured in vitro. *Treponema pallidum* is the cause of venereal and endemic syphilis and is the type species. *Treponema pertenue* is the cause of yaws, and *Treponema carateum* is the cause of pinta. The differentiation among these pathogenic *Treponema* species is based solely upon differences in the sites of lesions that may be produced in several types of experimental animals (Table 52-2). These distinguishing characteristics are not accepted by all investigators, some of whom consider the three organisms to be minor variants of a single species. There are seven other species of *Treponema*, most of which may be cultivated in vitro. They are seldom major human pathogens but may cause diseases of the oral cavity (Chap 56).

Borrelia species cause relapsing fever in man. No adequate method of speciation of *Borrelia* is available. The organisms currently are identified on the basis of the arthropod vector with which they are associated. Many have been cultured on complex media. Identification is based upon the coarse, uneven coils, the presence of 15 to 30 parallel fibrils, and atypical motion.

Leptospira species cause human and animal leptospirosis and are characterized by their motion, hooking or bending of one or both ends, and the presence of two fibrils. There are two recognized species, *Leptospira interrogans* and *Leptospira biflexa*. *L. interrogans* includes known human and animal pathogens, while *L. biflexa* includes free-living saphrophytes. Serologic characteristics identify complexes by serotype and serogroup, but these complexes have no taxonomic standing.

TABLE 52-1 **PROPERTIES OF GENERA OF THE FAMILY SPIROCHAETACEAE**

Type Species	Characteristics of Genus	Human Disease Produced
Spirochaeta plicatilis	Free-living, regular coils, 2 axial fibrils, anaerobic	None
Cristispira pectinis	Free-living, 2–10 loose coils, ovoid intracellular inclusions, over 100 axial fibrils	None
Treponema pallidum	Tight, regular coils, 3–7 axial fibrils, anaerobic	Syphilis, yaws, pinta, bejel
Borrelia anserina	Coarse, irregular coils, 15–20 axial fibrils, anaerobic	Relapsing fever
Leptospira interrogans	Tight, regular coils, bent or hooked ends, 2 axial fibrils; aerobic	Leptospirosis

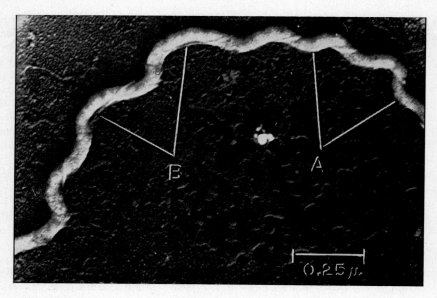

FIG. 52-1. *L. interrogans* (formerly *L. icterohaemorrhagiae*). The protoplasmic cylinder (A) is wound helically around the axial fibrils (B). ×75,000. (From Czekalowski and Eaves: J Pathol 69:129, 1955).

TREPONEMA PALLIDUM

Morphology and Physiology

The name *Treponema* is derived from the Greek words meaning "turning thread." Individual organisms are 5 to 20 μm in length and 0.09 to 0.5 μm in diameter; the ends are finely tapered. Whole cells appear to have a flat wave with one or more planes per cell, giving it the appearance of a helical coil. There are 8 to 14 waves per cell, which are evenly distributed. Its motility is sluggish, with a drifting motion and graceful flexuous movements; it rarely rotates.

The internal structure of *T. pallidum* is in general similar to that of other Spirochaetaceae, with a multilayer cytoplasmic membrane, six flagellalike fibrils which lie between the cell wall and the cytoplasmic membrane, cell wall, and outer envelope. Intracytoplasmic microtubules have been detected, and such structures may be specific for *Treponema* species.

Treponemal organisms have a high content of glycolipid. The axial filaments are composed of amino acids. The composition of the outer

envelope and other cell components is currently under study. No single component of *T. pallidum* has been found to evoke protective antibody.

Virulent strains of *T. pallidum* cannot be grown in vitro, although they will survive for four to seven days at 25C in an anaerobic medium containing albumin, sodium bicarbonate, pyruvate, cysteine, and a bovine serum ultrafiltrate. Virulent strains (eg, the Nichols strain)

TABLE 52-2   TREPONEMAL SPECIES PATHOGENIC FOR HUMAN BEINGS

Organism	Human Disease	Differentiating Characteristics
T. pallidum	Syphilis	Cutaneous lesions in rabbits
	Endemic syphilis	No cutaneous lesions in hamsters or guinea pigs
T. pertenue	Yaws	Cutaneous lesions in rabbits and hamsters, no cutaneous lesions in guinea pigs
T. carateum	Pinta	No cutaneous lesions in rabbits, hamsters, or guinea pigs

are propagated by intratesticular inoculation of rabbits. The division time of organisms in experimental chancres in rabbits is about 30 hours, and division is by transverse fission.

Clinical Infection

History Syphilis was first recognized in Europe at the end of the fifteenth century, when the disease appeared first in the Mediterranean areas and rapidly reached epidemic proportions at this time. One theory is that syphilis is of New World origin and that Columbus's crew acquired syphilis from the West Indies and introduced it into Spain on their return. Alternatively, the disease that had been endemic for centuries in Africa may have been transported to Europe at that time during the migration of armies and civilian populations. The relatively benign African diseases, yaws and bejel, may have been transformed in the susceptible population of Europe into a highly virulent disease with high mortality rates.

Syphilis initially was called the "Italian disease," the "French disease," and the "great pox" as distinguished from smallpox. Its venereal transmission was not recognized until the eighteenth century. Delineation of the characteristics of syphilis was hindered by confusion of its symptoms with those of gonorrhea. In 1767 John Hunter, a great English experimental biologist and physician, inoculated himself with urethral exudate from a patient with gonorrhea. Unfortunately, the patient also had syphilis, and the subsequent symptoms experienced by Hunter convinced two generations of physicians of the unity of gonorrhea and syphilis. The separate nature of gonorrhea and syphilis was demonstrated in 1838 by Ricord, who reported his observations on more than 2,500 human inoculations. Recognition of the stages of syphilis followed, and in 1905 Schaudinn and Hoffman discovered the causative agent. The following year Wassermann introduced the diagnostic blood test that bears his name.

Epidemiology Syphilis is not a highly contagious disease; a person who has had sexual contact with an infected partner has approximately 1 chance in 10 of acquiring disease. The rate of primary and secondary syphilis in the United States in 1974 in civilians was 11.9 per 100,000 population. As is typical of patients with other venereal diseases, persons who acquire syphilis are often promiscuous and have had contact with an average of five other persons during the incubation period. They are also characteristically young. In the United States in 1974 the rate of infectious syphilis for persons aged 15 to 19 years was 19.2 per 100,000; that for the 20- to 24-year-olds was 41.3 per 100,000; for persons over 24 years of age there was a gradual decline in rate which went to 1.5 per 100,000 for persons 50 years of age or older. Since 1958 the overall rate of infectious syphilis has increased, but there has been a progressive decline in the late stages of disease. This presumably is due to the efficacy of early treatment, usually with penicillin, in the prevention of late complications (Fig. 52-2).

An increase in the rate of other venereal diseases also has occurred in the same time period. For example, in one area of the United States, 8 percent of persons with gonorrhea had concomitant syphilis. Since many of these persons with dual diseases are treated in the preprimary stage of syphilis, this infection may never become manifest clinically or serologically.

Psychologic factors are important in the epidemiology of syphilis. Persons who are poorly adjusted, are undergoing major changes in life style, lack societal roots, have not achieved in school or job, and are promiscuous are among those more likely to acquire syphilis. Prostitutes traditionally have been prominent in dissemination of syphilis, but in most developed countries organized prostitution is no longer a major source of disease. Replacing their role in urban areas are casual partners, semiprostitutes who also pursue other occupations, and callgirls. Other persons at high risk of acquiring syphilis include male homosexuals.

TRANSMISSION. *T. pallidum* has the capacity to invade the intact mucous membranes or skin in areas of abrasions. Direct inoculation from contact with an infected person is necessary for infection, since survival of the organism outside the host is very limited. Sexual contact is the common method of transmission and the site of inoculation usually is on the genital organs, the vagina or cervix in females and the penis in males. Other sites include lips, when infected by kissing, and other areas of the skin, when infected through abrasions. Examining

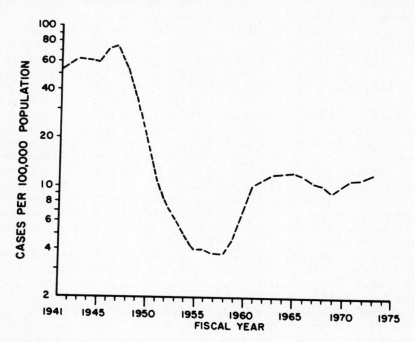

FIG. 52-2. Reported cases of primary and secondary syphilis per 100,000 population in civilians in the United States, 1941–1975. (From Morbid Mortal Week Rep [Annual Suppl] 22:60, 1973).

physicians or pathologists may be infected in this way if appropriate barrier protection is not provided.

Pathogenesis   After invasion, the organism undergoes rapid multiplication and is widely disseminated. Spread through the perivascular lymphatics and then the systemic circulation occurs before the clinical development of the primary lesion. Ten to ninety days later, but usually within three to four weeks, the patient manifests an inflammatory response to the infection at the site of the inoculation. The resulting lesion, the chancre, is characterized by profuse discharge of spirochetes, accumulation of mononuclear leukocytes, lymphocytes, and plasma cells, and swelling of capillary endothelia. The regional lymph nodes are enlarged, and the cellular infiltrate resembles that of the primary lesion. Resolution of the primary lesion is by fibrosis.

Secondary lesions develop when tissues of ectodermal origin, such as skin, mucous membranes, and central nervous system, participate in an inflammatory response. Mucous patches in the mouth are due to local vasculitis. The cellular infiltrate resembles that of the primary lesion, with a predominance of plasma cells.

There is little or no necrosis, and healing is without scarring but may include pigmentary changes.

Tertiary syphilis may involve any organ system and is often asymmetrical. Gummas are lesions typified by extensive necrosis, few giant cells, and paucity of organisms. They commonly occur in internal organs, bone, and skin. The other major form of tertiary lesion is a diffuse chronic inflammation with plasma cells and lymphocytes, but without caseation, that may result in aneurysm of the aorta, paralytic dementia, or tabes dorsalis. Chronic swelling of the capillary endothelium and fibrosis result in the characteristic tissue changes.

Clinical Manifestations   PRIMARY DISEASE. The chancre of primary syphilis is typically a single lesion, nontender, and firm, with a clean surface, raised border, and reddish color. It may be overlooked by women, in whom it is frequently situated on the cervix or vaginal wall. Systemic signs of symptoms are absent, but the draining lymph nodes are frequently enlarged and nontender.

SECONDARY DISEASE.   Two to ten weeks after the primary lesions, the patient may experience secondary disease (Fig. 52-3). Prominent findings include fever, sore throat, generalized lymphadenopathy, headache, and rash. Involvement of the palms and soles is common, in contradistinction to many other dermatologic conditions. On mucous membranes the lesions may appear as white mucous patches. Condylomata lata occur around moist areas, such as the anus and vagina. All secondary lesions of the skin and mucous membranes are highly infectious.

Other signs of this stage of disease may be secondary to the generalized immunologic response. Nephrotic syndrome with immune complex nephritis results from deposition of antigen–antibody complexes within the glomerular basement membrane. Arthritis and arthralgias may have a similar etiology. Involvement of other organ systems also occurs.

Following the last episode of secondary disease, the patient enters the stage of latent disease, the first four years of which are considered early latent, and the subsequent period to be late latent. By definition, persons in the late latent stage of disease have no signs or symptoms of active syphilis but remain seroreactive. If therapy for syphilis is first given during this stage, the patient is unlikely to show regression of nontreponemal antibody determinations. Approximately 60 percent of untreated patients in the late latent stages continue to have an asymptomatic course, while 40 percent develop symptoms of late disease. Progression of disease from late latent to late symptomatic syphilis is usually prevented if appropriate antimicrobial therapy is given at this stage.

TERTIARY DISEASE. *Gummas.* Three to ten years following the last evidence of secondary disease, the patient may develop nonprogressive, localized lesions of the dermal elements or supporting structures of the body, which are called "gummas." Since these lesions are relatively quiescent, the term "benign tertiary syphilis" often is used. Spirochetes are extremely sparse or absent. The gummatous reaction is primarily a pronounced immunologic reaction of the host.

Neurosyphilis. During the early stages of syphilis, approximately one-third of all patients have involvement of the central nervous system, but only half of these, if untreated, develop late neurosyphilis. The interval between primary disease and late neurosyphilis usually is more than five years. Late neurosyphilis may be asymptomatic or, if symptomatic, may present in a variety of ways. Classical presentations include paralytic dementia, tabes dorsalis, amyotropic lateral sclerosis, meningovascular syphilis, seizures, optic atrophy, and gummatous changes of the cord. Neurosyphilis may

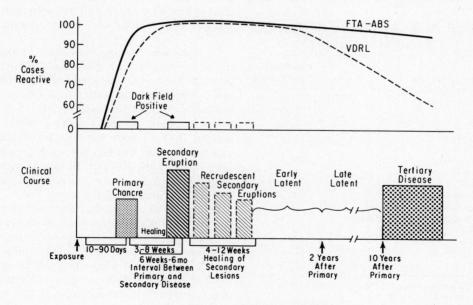

FIG. 52-3. The course of untreated syphilis.

resemble virtually any other neurologic disease.

Cardiovascular Syphilis. Approximatey 10 to 40 years after primary syphillis, the untreated patient may develop signs of cardiovascular involvement. The most commonly involved organs are the great vessels of the heart, where syphilitic aortic and pulmonary arteritis develop. The inflammatory reaction may also cause stenosis, with resulting angina, myocardial insufficiency, and death.

CONGENITAL SYPHILIS.   Congenital syphilis results from transplacental infection of the developing fetus and is often a very severe and mutilating form of the disease. In spite of widespread programs to examine all pregnant women, in 1973 there were 350 reported cases of congenital syphilis in the United States. These trends reflect the general increase in infectious syphilis that has been especially pronounced in young adults.

At the onset of congenital syphilis, *T. pallidum* is liberated directly into the circulation of the fetus, resulting in spirochetemia with widespread dissemination. The mortality rate of untreated congenital syphilis is approximately 25 percent, and an additional 40 percent of children suffer from late stigmata (Table 52-3). Abortion because of congenital syphilis usually occurs during the second trimester of pregnan-

cy, and histopathologic reactions to *T. pallidum* rarely are found in fetal tissue prior to that time. It has been generally thought that the fetus is protected from congenital infection until the sixteenth week of pregnancy, when the Langhans layer of the chorion atrophies. There is also evidence, however, that infection of the fetus may occur earlier but that the typical inflammatory response that results in tissue injury and fetal death does not occur until the fetus becomes immunologically competent. Syphilitic pregnant women who have not been treated may transmit the infection to their fetus at any clinical stage of their disease. In general, the greater the time that has elapsed since the woman's primary or secondary infection, the less likely she is to transmit disease to the fetus. Almost all pregnant women with untreated primary syphilis, 90 percent of women with secondary, and approximately 30 percent of women with latent syphilis may infect their fetuses.

The manifestations of congenital syphilis are highly variable in both signs and intensity. Especially prominent early symptoms include hepatosplenomegaly, jaundice, hemolytic anemia, pneumonia, and multiple long bone involvement. Snuffles, skin lesions, and testicular masses are common.

Late manifestations of congenital syphilis result from both scars of the active disease and the progression of active disease (Table 52-3). Some changes may be prevented by early treatment, but others often progress despite therapy.

Immunity   IMMUNE RESPONSE.   During the initial infection with *T. pallidum*, humoral IgG and IgM antibody is detectable by the time the chancre appears. Thereafter, both IgG and IgM antibodies persist for long periods in the untreated patient. If the patient is adequately treated, IgM antibody declines during the next one to two years, but IgG antibody usually persists through the lifetime of the patient. The stages of syphilis evolve in spite of humoral antibody response.

Inhibition of cell-mediated immunity occurs in early syphilis. Lymphocytes from syphilitic persons show reduced or absent response to treponemal antigens and other antigens to which lymphocytes from nonsyphilitic persons exhibit a lymphoblastic response. Paracortical areas of syphilitic lymph nodes in early stages

TABLE 52-3   STIGMATA OF LATE CONGENITAL SYPHILIS*

Stigmata	Percentage of Total Patients
Frontal boss of Parrott	87
Short maxilla	84
High palatal arch	76
Hutchinson's triad	75
Hutchinson's teeth	63
Interstitial keratitis	9
Eighth nerve deafness	3
Saddle nose	73
Mulberry molars	65
Higouménakis' sign	39
Relative protuberance of mandible	26
Rhagades	7
Saber shin	4
Scaphoid scapulae	0.7
Clutton's joint	0.3

Adapted from Fiumara: Arch Dermatol 102:78, 1970
°An analysis of 271 patients

of disease are correspondingly depleted of lymphocytes. These findings may help to explain the progression of early disease in persons who have achieved an antibody response to their infection.

The inhibition of migration of leukocytes from syphilitic persons by treponemal antigens is further evidence that cell-mediated immunity is activated during the later stages of syphilis. Persons with late secondary syphilis and tertiary syphilis exhibit cell-mediated immunity to treponemal antigen. In addition, there is experimental evidence of nonspecific activation of macrophages several weeks after infection with *T. pallidum.*

NATURAL IMMUNITY. The progressive decline in severity of syphilis between its introduction into Europe during the sixteenth century and the present time indicates that there has occurred a change in the virulence of the organism, the development of relative resistance by affected human populations, or both. Natural humoral or cell-mediated immunity sufficient to protect against disease has not been demonstrated, and the ID_{50} to humans in an experimental situation has been estimated to be as few as 57 organisms.

ACQUIRED IMMUNITY. Persons with untreated syphilis have a relative resistance to reinfection, so that the development of a chancre with second infection is unusual and probably depends upon the challenge inoculum. Following re-exposure untreated persons may develop an increased humoral antibody level.

In persons who have been treated for syphilis, especially if treatment was given during the secondary or earlier stages, the protective effect of prior disease is minor, and active disease following reinfection is common. This applies to persons who maintain a reactive nontreponemal antibody test (serofast) as well as to those who are serononreactive. In summary, although active or prior syphilis modifies the response of the patient to subsequent reinfection, protection is only relative and is unreliable.

Serologic Tests The two types of serologic tests for syphilis are the nontreponemal antigen tests and the treponemal antigen tests (Table 52-4). Although the latter tests indicate

experience with a treponemal infection, they cross-react with antigens other than those of *T. pallidum;* hence no test is specific for syphilis. In the United States yaws and pinta are rare diseases, and, therefore, the treponemal tests generally provide a reliable indication of syphilitic infection.

NONTREPONEMAL TESTS The original test for syphilis, as described by Wassermann, used syphilitic tissue as complement-fixing antigen to detect the presence of antibody (reagin) that is induced by *T. pallidum.* Extracts of other normal tissue, such as beef heart, had similar properties, and purification and standardization of these materials led to the use as antigen of a preparation containing cardiolipin and lecithin in cholesterol.

Two types of tests use cardiolipin–lecithin as antigen: (1) complement-fixation tests, including the Wassermann and Kolmer tests, (2) flocculation tests, including the VDRL (Venereal Disease Research Laboratory), Hinton, and rapid reagin tests. The tests provide similar clinical information and have similar advantages. They are inexpensive to perform and demonstrate rising and falling antibody titers that often correlate with adequacy of therapy and the clinical status of a patient. Disadvantages include a relatively high proportion of biologic acute and chronic false positive reactors and an increasing proportion of false negative reactions in the later stages of untreated syphilis. The technical difficulties include a negative reaction due to the prozone phenomenon when only undiluted serum is tested.

TREPONEMAL TESTS *Treponema pallidum Immobilization (TPI).* This test is based on the capacity of reaginic antibody and complement to immobilize a suspension of living and motile treponemes maintained in rabbit testes. The effect of the test serum on the motility of the spirochetes is determined by darkfield microscopy. The test is difficult and expensive, requires living organisms, and also is positive in the nonveneral treponematoses, bejel, jaws, and pinta. The TPI test is now performed in only a few research laboratories, primarily for comparison with and evaluation of other tests. It also retains a useful clinical role in distinguishing between syphilis and a biologic false positive reaction in patients who have collagen

TABLE 52-4   SEROLOGIC TESTS FOR SYPHILIS

| Antigen | Antigen Source | Tests | Percent Reactivity During | | |
			Primary Stage	Secondary Stage	Tertiary Stage
Nontreponemal Reagin	Extracts of tissue (Cardiolipin – Lecithin – Cholesterol)	Complement fixation (Wassermann, Kolmer)	65	98	60
		Flocculation (VDRL, Hinton, Kahn)	78	97	77
Treponemal	T. pallidum, Reiter strain	RPCF	61	85	72
	T. pallidum	TPI	56	94	92
		FTA-ABS	85	99	95
		IgM-FTA-ABS			

vascular disease with abnormal serum globulins.

Reiter Protein Complement Fixation. Antigen for this test is an extract from a nonvirulent treponeme, the Reiter strain, which may be cultured in vitro. The test detects group antigen; therefore, both false positive and false negative results are not uncommon. Nonvirulent treponemal organisms in the oral cavity may stimulate the production of cross-reacting antibody. Also, the test is frequently nonreactive in late stages of syphilis.

Fluorescent Antibody Tests. The most significant development of the past two decades in the serology of syphilis is the detection of treponemal antibody by fluorescein-labeled antihuman antibody. These tests are used to confirm the validity of a positive reaginic test, to diagnose congenital syphilis, and to diagnose late stages of syphilis. The tests are both sensitive and reliable.

Fluorescent treponemal antibody (FTA) tests use lyophilized Nichols strain organisms as antigen. Antigen is fixed to a slide, and the test serum is applied, allowing reaction of antitreponemal antibody with antigen. The slide is layered with fluorescein isothiocyanate-labeled antihuman gamma globulin, and the presence or absence of antibody is determined by fluorescent microscopy.

The currently used modification of this method is the FTA-ABS (fluorescent treponemal antibody-absorption) test in which test sera are preabsorbed with sorbent* to eliminate

Sorbent originally consisted of a sonicate of Reiter treponemes; other substances may be used.

group antibody. The test is thus rendered relatively specific for disease with virulent treponemal species, usually *T. pallidum.*

The FTA-ABS test is expensive and time-consuming. It is, therefore, recommended not for general screening but for confirmation of positive nontreponemal tests and diagnosis of later stages of syphilis in which the results of nontreponemal tests are frequently falsely negative.

Hemagglutination Tests. A hemagglutination method for serodiagnosis of syphilis has been automated and is both technically easy to perform and inexpensive. It is as sensitive as the FTA-ABS tests, except in primary syphilis, and is highly specific. Further experience with this method will determine its usefulness as a primary test for confirming syphilis. Like the FTA-ABS test, it is unlikely to revert to a nonreactive state following treatment of the patient unless treatment is given very early. The test usually is also reactive in persons with non-syphilitic treponematoses.

IgM-FTA-ABS Test. In the diagnosis of congenital syphilis, it is necessary to differentiate between passive transplacental transfer of maternal antibody to the fetus and production by the fetus of endogenous antitreponemal antibody. Since antibodies of the IgG but not of the IgM class cross the placenta, detection of IgM antibody in the fetal circulation usually indicates antibody production by the fetus due to active fetal infection. The FTA-ABS test will detect immunoglobulin of both the IgG and IgM classes and hence will not distinguish between active infection and passive transfer. This problem stimulated the development of a fluorescent antihuman antibody that is specific for IgM class antitreponemal antibody, the IgM-FTA-ABS test. A reactive test with infant blood is strong evidence of active congenital disease.

FALSE POSITIVE REACTIONS. All of the available serologic tests for syphilis produce occasional reactive results in patients for whom there is no other evidence of syphilitic infection. These reactions are usually called "biologic false positive" (BFP), as distinct from positive reactions due to technical errors. The majority of BFP reactions occur with nontreponemal tests; approximately 1 percent of normal adults will have a BFP reaction by nontreponemal antigen tests. Reaginic antibody is reactive with at least 200 antigens other than those of *T. pallidum*, and although the specific stimulus for this antibody in syphilis as well as other diseases is unknown, it may represent antibody to cellular lipoidal antigens of the host that are liberated during various diseases. For clinical purposes, BFP reactions may be classified as acute, in which the reactivity resolves within six months, or chronic, in which reactivity is persistent.

Acute BFP. Most BFP reactions are detected by nontreponemal tests and occur in patients with other acute illnesses, especially pneumonia, hepatitis, vaccinations, and viral exanthematous disease. The prognosis for the patient's health is not affected by the finding. The titer of antibody usually is low, less than 1:8, and in most instances the FTS-ABS is nonreactive. Approximately two-thirds of patients with BFP reactions have acute reactions, and reactivity subsides in six months or less.

Chronic BFP. Many patients with chronic BFP reactions have or develop systemic disease. Drug addiction, chronic hepatitis, old age, leprosy, and collagen vascular disease are highly associated with chronic BFP reactions. The antibody detected by the VDRL test in chronic BFP reactions is predominantly IgM, whereas in syphilis it is mainly IgG. Patients with chronic BFP reactions and systemic lupus erythematosus commonly also have a reactive FTA-ABS. The TPI test may be helpful in the differential diagnosis in these instances.

Laboratory Diagnosis Efforts to diagnose infectious syphilis suffer from the lack of a method to culture the organism on laboratory media. Three methods are useful in the diagnosis of syphilis: (1) direct visualization of the organism by darkfield microscopy, fluorescent antibody technique, or by special stains of infected tissue, (2) animal inoculation, and (3) demonstration of serologic reactions typical of syphilis.

Patients with a primary chancre as well as with active secondary lesions may be diagnosed by darkfield microscopy. Since this depends upon direct visualization of motile spirochetes, the organisms must be active and viable. Prior use of many antibiotics rapidly destroys the motility of the organisms as do many topical disinfectants. Serous fluid from the base of the lesion should be collected for darkfield examination. Syphilitic lesions of the mouth may harbor indigenous treponemes whose morphologic similarity to pathogenic species can confuse the interpretation of findings. The technique is, however, particularly helpful in making a diagnosis early in the disease prior to the development of seroreactivity. If a darkfield microscope is unavailable, a direct fluorescent antibody stain for *T. pallidum* may be made. Exudate is collected in capillary tubes or slides and stained with specific antibody. Most patients with syphilis that has progressed beyond the primary stage are diagnosed by serologic methods.

Treatment Since *T. pallidum* cannot be grown in vitro, estimates of the sensitivity of strains to antimicrobial agents depend upon the results of treatment of experimental animals, especially rabbits. The minimal inhibitory concentration of penicillin for *T. pallidum* is approximately 0.004 units/ml, making it one of the most sensitive of human pathogens. There is no evidence that the resistance of the organism to penicillin has increased during the past three decades of penicillin use. For these reasons, penicillin has remained the single most widely and successfully used antimicrobial agent for treatment of all stages of syphilis.

Essential requirements for effective therapy include maintenance of at least 0.03 units of penicillin/ml of serum for 7 to 10 days in early syphilis and avoidance of penicillin-free intervals during therapy. Provision of treatment for an individual patient may require frequent injections of short-acting penicillin preparations or the use of long-acting preparations. If the disease is beyond the early stages, the patient should receive adequate doses of penicillin for at least 21 days.

Successful eradication of active disease also has been achieved with erythromycin, tetracyclines, and cephaloridine. However, infected women have delivered syphilitic infants after treatment with these forms of therapy, possibly because of the relatively poor passage of erythromycin and tetracycline into the fetal circulation.

JARISCH-HERXHEIMER REACTION. Two to twelve hours following the treatment of active syphilis with either heavy metals or penicillins, a variable proportion of patients develop an acute focal and systemic reaction usually consisting of headache, malaise, and fever to 38C or above. These symptoms are resolved within a day. The reaction is most commonly observed in the early stages of syphilis and does not affect the course of recovery. In the later stages of syphilis, less than one in four patients develop the reaction. Most reactions in late syphilis are clinically insignificant, but an occasional reaction may produce damage to the central nervous system or the cardiovascular system.

In most patients receiving appropriate therapy during the primary or secondary stages, active disease is totally and permanently arrested. Persistent seroreactivity as measured by FTA-ABS may be avoided if treatment is given during the preprimary stage, but seldom thereafter. Nevertheless, progression to tertiary disease seldom, if ever, occurs. Similarly, therapy during early or late latent syphilis averts the development of symptomatic tertiary disease. Antimicrobial therapy for symptomatic neurosyphilis, optic neuritis, and cardiovascular syphilis may not be followed by significant clinical improvement, and established damage to vital organs may fail to resolve.

Prevention   Methods to control the spread of syphilis have relied extensively on treatment of case contact. Persons with active syphilis are interviewed to identify all sexual contacts that may have occurred during the incubation period. The contacts are examined, and if they are not infectious, they receive treatment appropriate for primary syphilis. Advantage is thus taken of the long incubation period of syphilis by preventing disease in contacts before they themselves can transmit infection.

YAWS (FRAMBESIA)

Yaws is a spirochetal disease of the tropics. It is caused by *T. pertenue*, an organism very closely related to *T. pallidum* (Table 52-2). These two organisms are serologically and morphologically indistinguishable and are differentiated by the type of lesions produced in experimental animals. No serologic test distinguishes human yaws from syphilis.

Yaws is endemic in tropical forest regions of Africa, parts of South America, India, and Indonesia, and many of the Pacific Islands. In these areas it is most commonly acquired in childhood and by direct contact rather than by sexual contact. The disease very rarely occurs congenitally, since most infected children have passed the early stages of disease by the age of sexual maturity.

The course of yaws resembles that of syphilis. The initial lesion is called the "mother yaw" or "framboise" and occurs about a month after the primary infection. It is a painless erythematous papule that heals during the subsequent one or two months. Secondary lesions that resemble the primary lesion occur six weeks to three months later. Recurrent disease may continue to occur for several years. Tertiary lesions are most likely to involve the skin and bones with gummatous ulcerations. Infection of the feet causes a crippling form of disease, called "crab yaws."

Yaws is readily treated with penicillin. Eradication of yaws has accompanied the general improvement in sanitation and standard of living in most areas of the world.

PINTA

Pinta is a disease of tropical areas of Central and South America, caused by *T. carateum*. This organism is serologically and morphologically similar to both *T. pallidum* and *T. pertenue* and is distinguished by failure to produce cutaneous lesions in rabbits, hamsters, or guinea pigs (Table 52-2). Chimpanzees, however, may be experimentally infected.

Human pinta is acquired by person-to-person contact and rarely by sexual intercourse. The primary and secondary lesions are flat, erythematous, and nonulcerating. The healing lesion first becomes hyperpigmented and later, as scarring occurs, will be depigmented. The lesions most commonly occur on the hands, feet, and scalp. Tertiary disease, such as occurs in syphilis, is uncommon in pinta. Treatment with penicillin is highly efficacious.

BEJEL

Bejel is a disease that closely resembles yaws both epidemiologically and in clinical manifestations. It is considered to be a form of endemic syphilis and occurs in areas of the Middle East. Poor hygienic conditions are important in perpetuating these infections, which are decreasing in incidence in most areas. Bejel is transmitted by direct contact, usually during early childhood, and results uniformly in serologic reactions that are indistinguishable from those of syphilis.

FURTHER READING

Books and Reviews

Cannefax G.R., Norins LC, Gillespie EJ: Immunology of sphyilis. Annu Rev Med 18:471, 1967

Clark EG, Danbolt N: The Oslo study of the natural course of untreated syphilis. Med Clin North Am 48:613, 1964

Nabarro D: Congenital Syphilis. London, Edward Arnold, 1954

Newman RB: Laboratory diagnosis of syphilis. In King JW, Falkner WK (eds): Critical Reviews in Clinical Laboratory Sciences, Cleveland, Ohio, CRC Press, 1974, vol 5, p 1

Selected Papers

Alford CA, Polt SS, Cassady GE, Straumfford JV, Remington JS: IgM-fluorescent treponemal antibody in the diagnosis of congenital syphilis. N Engl J Med 280:1086, 1969

Catterall RD: Systemic disease and the biological false positive reaction. Br J Vener Dis 48:1, 1972

Gjestland T: The Oslo study of untreated syphilis — an epidemiologic investigation of the natural course of untreated syphilis based on a restudy of the Boeck-Bruusgaard Material. Acta Derm Venereol [Suppl] 1955

Idsøe O, Guthe T, Willcox RR: Penicillin in the treatment of syphilis. The experience of three decades. Bull WHO (Suppl) 48:1, 1972

Magnuson HJ, Thomas EW, Olansky S, et al: Inoculation syphilis in human volunteers. Medicine 35:33, 1956

Sparling PF: Diagnosis and treatment of syphilis. N Engl J Med 284:642, 1971

53
Borrelia

Spirochetes of the genus *Borrelia* cause relapsing fever in man. This is an acute infection characterized by febrile episodes that subside spontaneously but tend to recur over a period of weeks. The organisms are transmitted by ticks and lice. Other terms used to describe these diseases are "tick fever," "borreliosis," and "famine fever."

Relapsing fever has been known to the western world since the time of Hippocrates. In recent times it has been associated with poverty, crowding, and warfare. Following World War I, louseborne relapsing fever was desseminated through large areas of Europe, carried by louse-infested, dislocated civilians, soldiers, and prisoners. A high mortality rate occurred in these debilitated populations who often were also experiencing epidemic typhus.

Separation of the genus *Borrelia* from other members of the Spirochaetaceae is based on their characteristic morphology as revealed by the electron microscope (Chap. 52). The current classification of *Borrelia* is based on the arthropod vector.

Morphology and Physiology

Borrelia are helical organisms 0.2 to 0.5 μm wide and 3 to 20 μm in length, with 3 to 20 uneven coils. Spirals are coarser and more irregular than those of the treponemes or leptospires and can be seen with light microscopy in preparations stained with Wright or Giemsa stains. Borreliosis is the only disease in which spirochetes may be demonstrated by direct stain in the peripheral blood, and the presence of morphologically typical forms is adequate for diagnosis. In fresh blood the organisms are actively motile; they move in forward and backward waves and in a corkscrewlike motion. Observed variations in morphology depend upon the parasitized host and on the stage of disease.

Borrelia are strict anaerobes. Special culture media containing natural animal proteins are available, but little is known of the nutritional requirements of the organisms. The optimum temperature for growth is 28 to 30C.

In vitro and in vivo culture for diagnostic purposes is difficult and not always successful. If inoculation of experimental animals is attempted, great care should be taken to insure that the animals are free from preexisting borreliosis. Chick embryo cultures have been irregu-

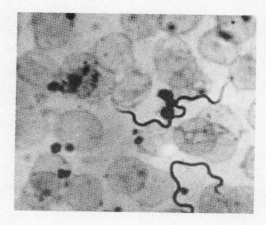

FIG. 53-1. *Borrelia hermii* from *Ornithodoros hermsi* collected at Broune Mountain. Giemsa-stained smear of mouse blood. ×2,300. (From Thompson: JAMA 210: 1045, 1969)

larly successful, as have tissue culture techniques.

Speciation is based upon two considerations: (1) the species responsible for louseborne disease is designated *Borrelia recurrentis*, as opposed to all tickborne strains, and (2) for tickborne strains the close vector-strain relationship has led to the definition of most species by the tick vector. For example, *Borrelia hermsii* is associated with the tick *Ornithodoros hermsi* (Fig. 53-1).

Antigenic Structure

The most striking property of relapsing fever is the capacity of the borrelia to undergo several antigenically distinct variations within a given host during the course of a single infection. Experimental infection of rats with *B. hermsii* has shown the presence of four major serotypes. Antigenic shifts were observed to occur in a regular sequence, were most readily determined by immunofluorescent methods, and stimulated appropriate antibody responses in the host. The organisms disappeared from the peripheral blood coincident with appearance of specific antibody and reappeared after antigenic variation had occurred. The specific antigenic determinant is a polyoside-lipid complex.

In a study of the development of immobilizing antibody in human relapsing fever, most patients were found to develop antibody to both autologous and heterologous strains. A number of other studies have demonstrated that a low level of protection against subsequent relapse strains is afforded by antigenic stimulation with the initial strains of the infection, and there is a frequent lack of cross-protection.

Clinical Infection

Epidemiology Tickborne Disease. The vectors of tickborne borreliosis are ticks of the genus *Ornithodoros*, which comprise the soft ticks.

In the United States, tickborne disease may be transmitted by *Ornithodoros turicatae*, *Ornithodoros parkeri*, and *Ornithodoros hermsi*. Throughout the world, over 15 species of *Ornithodoros* ticks have been found to transmit borreliosis. *Ornithodoros* species feed exclusively on blood, and they often feed at night. They usually have a painless bite and feed for a short time (usually less than an hour) after which they spontaneously leave the host. People are therefore frequently unaware of having received the bite.

When the tick bites a borrelemic host, the borrelia penetrate the tick's celomic cavity. There is a predilection for the coxal and salivary glands and gonads, enabling transovarian passage to occur. The infected tick may survive for years without food in environments of low humidity. The infection is transmitted by ticks both by contamination of the bite with coxal fluid and by the salivary fluid. The life span of the tick is not shortened by carrying borrelia. Many *Ornithodoros* species will feed on a variety of hosts.

B. hermsii and its vector are found primarily at elevations above 3,000 feet and are associated with tree squirrels and chipmunks, which may carry the ticks into cabins where they become established. *O. turicatae* parasitizes goats, sheep, and rodents and is found in caves and animal burrows mainly in Florida and Mexico. *O. parkeri* inhabits the homes of ground squirrels and prairie dogs at lower elevations than *O. hermsi* and is widely distributed geographically. Numerous other small mammals also serve as reservoirs for tickborne *Borrelia*, including rats, mice, rabbits, opposums, and hedgehogs. Birds have not been im-

plicated. Once infected, the tick may harbor the disease for many years. However, tickborne disease is not rapidly spread and, in the United States, is responsible only for sporadic cases.

In the United States relapsing fever is a disease limited to persons who have come into contact with infected ticks. This most commonly results from vocational or avocational exposure, such as vacationing in a tick-infested summer cottage. A recent example was a Boy Scout troop, of which 11 of 42 persons contracted relapsing fever. Most of the infected scouts had slept in a rodent-infested cabin, while the scouts who were younger and did not become infected slept in tents. The spring and summer distribution of disease coincides with the season of maximal tick activity and the avocational invasion of man into tick-infested areas. In the United States foci of tickborne disease occur mainly in the Western states, particularly Oklahoma, California, Washington, Texas, and Kansas, which may reflect the distribution of *Ornithodoros* ticks.

In some areas of Africa, inhabitation of the home by *Ornithodoros moubata* is considered to be good luck and has resulted in introduction of disease.

Louseborne Disease. The human body and head lice, *Pediculus humanus corporis* and *Pediculus humanus capitis*, are the vectors of epidemic relapsing fever caused by *B. recurrentis*. After the louse ingests the borrelia, the organisms pass exclusively into the celomic cavity. Since other organs are not invaded, there occurs neither transovarian transmission nor direct infection during feeding by an intact louse. *Borrelia* escape the louse to infect the host only when the louse is injured, as may occur during scratching. A single louse can, therefore, infect only one person. The infected louse remains infectious for its life span, which is approximately three weeks. Lice may rapidly and widely disseminate disease. Epidemics usually occur in the cold seasons, among the crowded and poor, and in homes with inadequate hygiene. Although *B. recurrentis* is considered to be the louseborne species, tickborne borrelia may also be transmitted by lice. No natural animal reservoir of *B. recurrentis* is known.

Relapsing fever may occasionally be acquired by means other than louse or tick infestation. For example, transplacental transmission has caused congenital disease, and infected blood may be the cause of laboratory accidents leading to infection.

Clinical Manifestations Prior to the development of effective antimicrobial agents, fever induction was used in the therapy of tertiary syphilis. Induced infection with borrelia was often selected for this purpose, and much of our present knowledge concerning prodromata, incubation period, natural history, and complications stem from these experiences.

The symptoms and severity of relapsing fever depend upon the immune status of the host, geographic location, strain of *Borrelia,* and phase of the epidemic. There may also be consistent differences between some characteristics of louseborne disease and tickborne disease, but both forms will be described together (Table 53-1).

The natural history of a course of relapsing fever includes the incubation period, the primary attacks, the afebrile interval, and subsequent attacks. In epidemic, endemic, and therapeutically induced disease, few prodromata have been noted. The incubation period is approximately 6 days, with a range of 2 to 14 days. Late in the incubation period the patient may experience chills. The onset is usually very sudden and accompanied by fever, headache, tachycardia, and muscle pain. The initial attack usually lasts 3 to 7 days, may be longer for louseborne than for tickborne disease, and ends by crisis. The fever is usually continuous.

A macular rash is seen in varying numbers of patients and usually appears near the end of the first paroxysm. Hepatosplenomegaly, jaundice, nausea, and vomiting are common. Bronchitis and bronchopneumonia are frequent in the United States. Meningeal signs with and without encephalitic disease may affect up to 30 percent of some groups of patients, and ocular disease is common.

The crisis is coincidental with the immune response, which causes lysis of the organisms. Occasionally, the crisis is associated with endotoxic shock. Usually, the temperature returns to normal, and the patient is asymptomatic until the subsequent attack. The interval between initial and subsequent attacks is usually shorter with louseborne, 5 to 9 days, than with tickborne disease, which is approximately 14 days.

Data from the period 1921–1941 described the course of untreated tickborne disease as follows: no relapse, 16 percent; 1 relapse, 20 percent; 2 relapses, 27 percent; 3 relapses, 17 percent; 4 or more relapses, 18 percent of cases. A similar distribution of relapses has occurred in some outbreaks of louseborne disease.

Subsequent attacks are usually shorter in duration, less severe, and with increasingly shorter apyrexial periods between attacks but

TABLE 53-1 CLINICAL MANIFESTATIONS IN RELAPSING FEVER

Manifestation	Mean Value or Incidence	
	Tickborne Disease*	Louseborne Disease†
Incubation period	Approx 7 days	—
Duration of primary febrile attack	3.1 days	5.5 days
Duration of afebrile interval	6.8 days	9.25 days
Duration of relapses	2.5	1.9 days
Number of relapses	3	Majority = 1
Maximum temperature (primary attack)	Approx 105F (40.4C)	—
Splenomegaly	41%	77%
Hepatomegaly	17–18%	66%
Jaundice	7%	36%
Rash	28%	8%
Respiratory symptoms	16%	34%
CNS involvement	8–9%	30%

Adapted from Southern and Sanford: Medicine 48:129, 1969
*Based on a review of 1,105 reported cases
†Based on a review of 2,073 reported cases

are otherwise clinically similar to the initial episode. Most physicians fail to diagnose relapsing fever until one or more relapses have occurred.

    Treatment and Prevention Treatment of relapsing fever includes general supportive measures, such as fluid and electrolyte therapy. Evaluation of efficacy of antimicrobial therapy has been inhibited by the lack of information on in vitro sensitivity. The most clinically effective antimicrobial agents appear to be tetracyclines and chloramphenicol. Streptomycin has also been found to modify disease, although it may fail to prevent relapses.

    Prevention of relapsing fever is dependent upon control of exposure to the arthropod vectors. In tickborne borreliosis, this includes wearing protective clothing and careful cleaning of rodent-infested cabins, followed by spraying with appropriate insecticides, such as aldrin, benzenehexachloride, or malathion. Louseborne relapsing fever is controlled by the application of good personal and public standards of hygiene.

FURTHER READING

Books and Reviews

Felsenfeld O: Borrelia, Strains, Vectors, Human and Animal Borreliosis. St. Louis, Mo, Warren H. Green, Inc, 1971

Moulton FR: Relapsing Fever in the Americas. Lancaster, Pa, Science Press Printing Co, 1942

Selected Papers

Bryceson ADM, Parry EHO, Perine PL, et al: Louse-borne relapsing fever. A clinical and laboratory study of 62 cases in Ethiopia and a reconsideration of the literature. Q J Med 39:129, 1970.

Coffey EM, Eveland WC: Experimental relapsing fever initiated by *Borrelia hermsi*. I. Identification of major serotypes in the rat. J Infect Dis 117:23, 29, 1971

Pickett J, Kelly R: Lipid catabolism of relapsing fever borreliae. Infect Immun 9:279, 1974

Southern PM, Sanford JP: Relapsing fever. A clinical and microbiological review. Medicine 48:129, 1969

Thompson RS, Burgdorfer W, Russell R, Francis BJ: Outbreak of tick-borne relapsing fever in Spokane County, Washington, JAMA 210:1045, 1969

Warrell DA, Pope HM, Parry EHO, Perine PL, Bryceson ADM: Cardiorespiratory disturbances associated with infective fever in man: Studies of Ethiopian louse-borne relapsing fever. Clin Sci 39:123, 1970

54
Leptospira

Leptospirosis, an acute illness associated with febrile jaundice and nephritis, was first recognized by Weil in 1886 as a clinical entity distinct from other icteric fevers. Commonly referred to since that time as "Weil's disease," the infection is caused by a leptospira transmitted to man from infected rodents.

By 1948, over 300 cases of human leptospirosis had been reported, most of which were clinically severe and accompanied by jaundice. Recognition of other forms of leptospirosis, however, was exceedingly slow in spite of indications in Europe and other parts of the world that clinically milder and nonicteric forms of leptospirosis were common and that animal reservoirs were not restricted to rodents. In 1938, Meyer described canicola fever in dogs and man. Infection in cattle was reported in 1948, and shortly thereafter human infection by this same strain (serovar[*] *pomona*) was recognized in Georgia.

Evidence of widespread leptospiral disease among cattle, swine, horses, and other livestock led to an appreciation of the economic losses attributable to these infections as well as their threat to human health. By the early 1950s several public health laboratories were capable of evaluating serologic evidence of infection with an increasing number of leptospiral serogroups, and syndromes, such as pretibial fever (Fort Bragg fever), aseptic meningitis, and other mild febrile illnesses, were attributed to leptospiral infection. Commonly used terms for leptospirosis include "swineherds' disease," "Fort Bragg fever," "pretibial fever," "Weil's disease," and "canicola fever."

Morphology

The genus *Leptospira* is characterized by fine coiling of the primary spirals. The name is derived from the Greek word *lepto*, meaning "thin" or "fine" spiral. *Leptospira* are helicoidal organisms, usually 6 to 20 μm in length and 0.1 μm in diameter. The coils are 0.2 to 0.3 μm in overall diameter and 0.5 μm in pitch. In liquid media, one or both ends are usually hooked. In the living state, the organisms are clearly visible by darkfield and much less clearly by phase contrast microscopy.

[*]*The term "serovar" has been adopted in lieu of serotype by the International Committee on Systematic Bacteriology (Leptospira subcommittee), 1973.*

Ultrastructure   *Leptospira* consist of a helicoidal protoplasmic cylinder, two axial filaments, and an outer envelope. The outer envelope is composed of three to five layers and surrounds the whole organism. Located between the outer envelope and the cytoplasmic membrane are two independent axial filaments, each of which is inserted by one end subterminally at opposite ends of the protoplasmic cylinder. The free ends are directed toward the center of the cell where they usually do not overlap. During cellular reproduction septal wall formation occurs at the middle region of the organism, leading to transverse division.

Lipids comprise 18 to 28 percent of the dry weight of the leptospiral cell and are composed of approximately 70 percent phospholipid and 30 percent free fatty acids. The composition of fatty acids is a reflection of those present in the culture medium, since with few exceptions leptospira can neither synthesize fatty acids de novo nor elongate chains.

The major components of the leptospiral cell wall are polysaccharide and peptidoglycan. Alanine, glutamic acid, diaminopimelic acid, glucosamine, and muramic acid are the predominant amino acids and sugars. The diaminopimelic acid content of *Leptospira* serves to differentiate these organisms from treponemes and members of the genus *Spirochaeta*, which instead contain ornithine.

Physiology

Leptospira are aerobic; metabolism is respiratory, with oxygen utilized as the final electron acceptor. They grow well at pH 7.2 to 7.4 in rabbit serum or Tween 80 albumin media. The generation time of pathogenic *Leptospira* cultivated in laboratory media is 12 to 16 hours and 4 to 8 hours in inoculated animals. Long-chain unsaturated fatty acids serve as the major source of carbon and energy and are required by the parasitic strains. *Leptospira* can use inorganic ammonium salts as a source of nitrogen.

Characterization of Species

Two species, *Leptospira interrogans* and *Leptospira biflexa* were proposed by the *Lep-*

tospira subcommittee in 1973. *L. interrogans* includes pathogenic organisms, whereas *L. biflexa* includes the saprophytic or water leptospira that commonly occur in fresh, surface waters. Distinguishing characteristics of the two species, other than their ability to infect animals, include the inhibitory effect of 8-azaguanine, bivalent copper ions, serologic characteristics, and ability to grow at low (5 to 10C) temperatures. The two species also are distinguishable genetically and share no nucleotide sequences as determined by DNA-DNA annealing tests. Each species can be further separated into three genetic groups of strains that have partial DNA homologies.

Antigenic Structure

Each species of *Leptospira* includes a large number of serologically distinct strains as determined by cross-agglutination and agglutinin-absorption tests. The basic taxon is the serovar. Strains that share major agglutinogens are arbitrarily assembled into serogroups. The serogroup is not a recognized taxon and serves primarily serodiagnostic purposes. The serologic relationships do not necessarily correlate with genetic characteristics. Genetic groups may consist of serologically diverse serovars. However, strains with major antigenic affinities (eg, within the same serogroup) usually appear to be genetically homologous.

Among the parasitic leptospiras over 150 serovars are now recognized and classified into approximately 16 serogroups, all of which are characterized by very wide distribution both in variety of animal species affected and in geographic occurrence.

Determinants of Pathogenicity

A number of biologic properties characterize the pathogenic strains of *Leptospira*. (1) Avirulent strains are relatively more sensitive to the leptospiricidal effect of immune serum and complement than are virulent strains. The outer sheath of *Leptospira* is the primary site of action of antibody and complement and has immunogenic properties. The reason for the resistance of virulent *Leptospira* is unknown. (2) Strains of some virulent *Leptospira* produce a soluble hemolysin that appears to be important in the manifestations of leptospirosis in a number of animals species. Previous infection with a hemolytic serotype confers immunity to subsequent hemolytic disease. (3) Some of the

TABLE 54-1 LEPTOSPIRA SEROGROUPS, DISTRIBUTION, AND HOSTS

Serogroup	Distribution	Common Host
Icterohaemorrhagiae	Japan, Germany, England, USA, the world	Rat, mouse, dog, skunk, fox, raccoon
Hebdomadis	Japan, Italy, Eastern Asia, USA	Field mice, dog, cattle, skunk
*Autumnalis**	Japan, Eastern Asia, USA	Field mice, dog, cat, goat
Bataviae	Indonesia, Zaire, Eastern Asia, USA	Rat, cat, fieldmice
Australis	North Queensland, Italy, Malaya, Brazil, USA	Field rat, dog, bandicoot, raccoon, opossum, fox
Pyrogenes	Indonesia, Japan, Italy, Malaya, USA	Dog, nutria
Canicola	Netherlands, Denmark, England, USA, worldwide	Dog, jackal, pig, horse, cattle, sheep
Grippotyphosa	Russia, Germany, Israel, Malaya, Netherlands, USA	Goat, horse, skunk (fieldmice), dog
Pomona	North Queensland, Indonesia, Europe, Asia, South America, USA	Pig, cat, cattle, horse, dog
Sejro	Denmark, Europe, Switzerland	Fieldmice, cattle, dog, horse, pig
Ballum	Denmark, Holland, Yugoslavia, Czechoslovakia, Portugal, Canada, USA, Puerto Rico	House mouse, opossum, pig, skunk
Andamana	Andaman Islands, Finland	Not known
Hyos	Argentina, Queensland, Malaya, France, Italy, Switzerland, USA	Pig, cattle, horse, skunk

Adapted from Schlossbeiger and Brandis: Ann Rev Microbiol 8:133, 1954.
*Identified as the cause of USA pretibial or Fort Bragg fever

clinical manifestations of leptospirosis, such as conjunctival irritation and iritis, are probably caused by cell-mediated sensitivity to leptospiral antigen.

Clinical Infection

Epidemiology Leptospirosis is a zoonotic disease with a wide range of host reservoirs. The predominant natural reservoirs of pathogenic *Leptospira* are wild mammals, although other vertebrates occasionally are infected (Table 54-1). Domestic animals, such as dogs, cattle, swine, sheep, goats, and horses, also may be major sources of human infections. The improved ability of regional laboratories to group *Leptospira* has resulted in the recognition of the large number of serovars endemic in the United States, as well as the extent of infections in a variety of animal species. Nevertheless, it is an infrequently diagnosed human disease. In 1974, 68 cases were reported to the Center for Disease Control.

The major mode of transmission between animals and man is by indirect contact with urine infected with virulent *Leptospira* from an animal with leptospiruria. *Leptospira* from infected soil, food, and water enter the body through a break in the skin and through mucous membranes. Survival of *Leptospira* outside the host is fostered by a temperature of 22C or above, moisture, and a neutral to slightly alkaline environment. *Leptospira* are readily killed by temperatures above 60C, detergents, desiccation, and acidity.

Because of its prevalence in rodents and domestic animals, leptospirosis has been primarily a disease of persons in occupations heavily exposed to animals and animal products, such as sewer workers, swineherders, veterinarians, abattoir workers, and farmers. Also at risk are persons living in rodent-infested housing, such as urban slums, and dog owners. There is a higher incidence in males. At present, the majority of cases occur in the summer and fall in teenagers and young adults. Avocational exposure is now increasingly common.

Common source outbreaks attributed to contaminated ponds or slowly moving streams are numerous; over 14 instances have been reported in the United States since 1939. A high at-

tack rate, summer season, young age group, and the proximity of animals to the water typify most of these outbreaks. In some areas of the world, the runoff during flooding also is highly infectious.

Sporadic disease may be acquired by direct contact with infected animals. Vaccination of domestic animals, which prevents clinical disease, may fail to prevent shedding of *Leptospira*. Pet dogs have been a prominent source of sporadic human cases. The convoluted renal tubules of animal reservoirs harbor viable *Leptospira*, which are passed in the urine. The duration of asymptomatic urinary shedding varies with the animal species; human beings rarely shed *Leptospira* longer than a few months.

Forms of transmission other than direct and indirect contact with contaminated urine are rare. Lactating animals shed *Leptospira* in the milk, but whole milk is leptospirocidal after a few hours, and no known human cases have occurred in this manner. *Leptospira* are not shed in saliva, and animal bites are therefore not a direct source of infection.

Pathogenesis The organism probably invades the human being through small breaks in the skin or intact mucosa. The initial sites of multiplication are unknown. Nonspecific host defenses fail to contain *Leptospira* to any significant extent, and leptospiremia occurs rapidly after infection and continues through the initial acute illness. A local lesion at the site of entry does not develop.

Leptospira usually infect the kidneys. The major renal lesion, common to all forms of leptospirosis and present even in patients with normal renal function, is an interstitial nephritis with associated glomerular swelling and hyperplasia. Late manifestations of this disease may be caused by the host immunologic response to the infection.

Clinical Manifestations The severity of human leptospirosis varies greatly and is determined to a large extent by the infecting strain and by the general health of the host. Severe icteric disease with a high fatality rate occurs in a small proportion of cases and is frequently associated with serogroup *ictohemorrhagiae* serovars. Less severe and anicteric disease is far more prevalent and is commonly caused by serovars of serogroups *australis* and *pyrogenes*;

disease due to those of *canicola, ballum,* and *pomona* is often mild. There is, however, no absolute correlation between severity of disease or clinical syndrome with infecting serogroups.

The incubation period is usually 10 to 12 days but ranges from 3 to 30 days after inoculation. Prominent presenting signs include an abrupt onset of fever, chills, headache, conjunctival suffusion, myalgias, and gastrointestinal complaints. The clinical presentations of leptospirosis often suggest other disease processes, most commonly hepatitis, meningitis, fever of unknown etiology, and encephalitis.

Clinical illness is biphasic, the first leptospiremic stage lasting approximately seven days in most instances. The appearance of humoral antibody coincides with the termination of fever and leptospiremia. A few days after the initial defervescence, a second and shorter febrile period may occur. Routine laboratory studies do not usually aid in the diagnosis.

Infection of the kidneys results in the excretion of organisms in the urine. Renal failure in Weil's disease is not rare and is the cause of death in most fatal cases. With the availability of extracorporeal dialysis, however, the mortality rate is very low, and there is complete return of renal function following recovery.

Certain presentations and complications of leptospirosis require attention. Meningeal irritation is common and probably a frequent cause of undiagnosed aseptic meningitis. Approximately half the patients examined during the second week of illness may have a cerebrospinal fluid lymphocytosis associated with a moderate elevation of cerebrospinal fluid protein. *Leptospira* may be isolated from the cerebrospinal fluid early in the disease. The later onset of symptoms of central nervous system involvement may reflect an untoward antigen–antibody reaction. Permanent neurologic sequelae are exceedingly rare.

An infectious agent from patients with a syndrome named Fort Bragg fever (pretibial fever), first described at Fort Bragg, North Carolina, in 1943, was identified in 1952 as a pathogenic leptospira (serovar *ft. bragg*) in the *Autumnalis* serogroup. Sporadic cases have subsequently been reported from other parts of the United States, including the Pacific Northwest. Clinical characteristics included an unusual symmetrical rash limited to the pretibial areas. The lesions resembled erythema nodosum but were urticarial in a few cases. Fever, headache, a palpable spleen, and leukopenia predominated. A similar syndrome may occur with other *Leptospira* serovars.

IMMUNITY. During the initial immunologic response to leptospirosis, 19 S immunoglobulins comprise the major portion of the antibody produced and are usually detectable within a week after onset of disease. Human convalescent serum contains protective and agglutinating antibodies that persist in a patient's serum for many years.

Laboratory Diagnosis Isolation of *Leptospira* may be accomplished by direct inoculation into laboratory media or by animal inoculation. During the acute phase of disease *Leptospira* can be readily cultured from the blood or cerebrospinal fluid by the use of liquid or semisolid medium. After the first week of disease and for several months therafter, *Leptospira* may be shed intermittently in the urine by a large proportion of patients and may be demonstrated by cultural means. Isolation of *Leptospira* from contaminated specimens may be accomplished by the use of a selective inhibitor, such as 5-fluorouracil, or by intraperitoneal inoculation of young hamsters or guinea pigs. Direct demonstration of *Leptospira* by darkfield microscopy, fluorescent antibody silver impregnation, or staining with aniline dyes is successful in only a small proportion of cases. It is not recommended as a single diagnostic procedure because of the frequently mistaken identification of artifacts as *Leptospira*.

SEROLOGIC TESTS. Antibody may be detected in the patient's serum within a week after the onset of disease. Determination of serovar-specific antibody is technically difficult. The complement-fixation, Patoc I agglutination, hemolytic, hemagglutinating, and indirect immunofluorescent tests show wide cross-reactivity. The most useful strain-specific serologic test is the microscopic agglutination test (agglutination-lysis). This test was the original method for determining antibody response to leptospirosis and remains the reference method. Use of living organisms gives the most specific reaction, with highest titer and fewer cross-reactions. Formalinized antigen also may be used. Results are read by low-power dark-field microscopy. The macroscopic agglutination test, read by direct visualization, is much less specific and sensitive than is the microscopic test. These tests require maintenance of appropriate living or formalinized antigen, are arduous to perform, and are available only in reference laboratories. Since agglutinating antibodies persist for long periods after the acute episode, these tests are useful in determining the past experience of a community with leptospirosis. Various complement-fixation, hemagglutination, hemolytic, and fluorescent antibody tests have been proposed and advantageously used in some laboratories for the diagnosis of human cases. These tests, however, may lack sensitivity in detecting antibodies in animals or for detecting antibodies in retrospect for purposes of serologic survey.

Treatment and Prevention Penicillin, streptomycin, tetracycline, and the macrolide antibiotics are active against *Leptospira* in vitro and in experimentally infected animals. Recovery of human cases is hastened if therapy is initiated during the first two days after onset. When therapy is initiated after the fourth day of illness, the course of the disease usually is not altered.

Vaccines have been effectively used in veterinary medicine and for human beings in endemic areas. Protection is serovar specific.

FURTHER READING

Books and Reviews

Alexander AD: *Leptospira*. In Lennette EH (ed): Manual of Clinical Microbiology, 2nd ed. Washington, DC, American Society of Microbiology, 1974, p 347

Babudieri B: Experimental infections with *Leptospira*. In Handbook of Experimental Pharmacology XVI IIB. New York, Springer Verlag, 1973, pp 23-42

Selected Papers

Auran NE, Johnson RC, Ritzi DM: Isolation of the outer sheath of Leptospira and its immunogenic properties in hamsters. Infect Immun 5:968, 1972

Berman SJ, Tsai CC, Holmes KK, Fresh JW, Watten RH: Sporadic anicteric leptospirosis in South Vietnam. A study in 150 patients. Ann Intern Med 79:167, 1973

Feigin RD, Lobes LA, Anderson D, Pickering L: Human leptospirosis from immunized dogs. Ann Intern Med 79:777, 1973

Haapala DK, Rogul M, Evans LB, Alexander AD: Deoxyribonucleic acid base composition and homology studies of *Leptospira*. J Bacteriol 98:421, 1969

Heath CW, Alexander AD, Calton MM: Leptospirosis in the United States. N Engl J Med 273:857, 915, 1965

Ooi BS, Chen BTM, Tan KK, Oon TK: Human renal leptospirosis. Am J Trop Med Hyg 21:336, 1972

Pertzelan A, Pruzanski W: *Leptospira canicola* infection; report of 81 cases and review of the literature. Am J Trop Med Hyg 12:75, 1963

Tong MJ, Rosenberg EB, Votteri BA, Tsai: Immunological response in leptospirosis. Am J Trop Med Hyg 20:625, 1971

Turner LH: Leptospirosis I, II, and III. Trans R Soc Trop Med Hyg 61:842, 1967; 62:880, 1968; 64:623, 1970

55
Spirillum and Campylobacter

The family Spirillaceae is composed of the two genera, *Spirillum* and *Campylobacter*. Both genera contain organisms that are pathogenic for man. *Spirillum minor* is the cause of one form of rat-bite fever and is the only human pathogen of the genus. *Campylobacter fetus* may cause neonatal septicemia, severe diarrhea, and a variety of other anaerobic infections. Its association with human infections has only recently been appreciated as a result of improvements in anaerobic culture techniques.

The Spirillaceae are rigid, helically curved rods with a variable number of turns. They are motile by means of flagella and move in a corkscrew motion. Most of the organisms in the family are free living in fresh or salt water. Others are saprophytic or parasitic and human or animal pathogens. *Spirillum* species are polytrichous, with flagella at both poles, and they are strict aerobes. *Campylobacter* have a single polar flagellum at one or both poles and are microaerophilic to anaerobic.

SPIRILLUM MINOR

Morphology   *S. minor* is a short, thick organism with tapering ends, 0.2 to 0.5 by 3 to 5 μm in size. It has two or three windings that are thick, regular, and spiral. It is gram-negative but can best be visualized in blood smears with Giemsa or Wright's stain. Silver impregnation methods, such as that of Fontana-Tribondeau, stain the bipolar tufts of flagella. Darkfield illumination of a drop of blood containing the organism is the best method for demonstrating its rapid motility, spiral structure, and flagella.

Laboratory Identification   *S. minor* has not been cultured in artificial media. Proof that the organism produces rat-bite fever has been provided by experimental inoculation of man with blood containing the organism. The diagnosis of rat-bite fever is based upon demonstration of the organisms in infected animals. The primary method is inoculation of white mice and guinea pigs with the patient's blood, exudate from the initial lesion, serum expressed from exanthematous patches, material aspirated from lymph nodes, or ground-up pieces of tissue excised from lesions. Since mice often harbor this organism, it is necessary to ensure that animals are free from spirilla before inoculations are made. Alternatively, diagnosis may be made by examination of blood and exudate from lesions by darkfield illumination and stains. The organism rarely has been detected with certainty in the blood of man but may be found in material from the lesions.

Clinical Infection   Rat-bite fever is an acute infection caused by *S. minor* or *Streptobacillus moniliformis*, both of which are present in the normal oropharyngeal flora of rodents. Differences in clinical manifestations between the two forms, however, permit differentiation of the two diseases. Rat-bite fever caused by *S. minor* is commonly referred to as "Sodoku fever."

Epidemiology.   Rat-bite fever is primarily a bacteremic disease of wild rats that is transmissible to rats, various other animals, and man by the bite of an infected animal. Fleas and other insects are not vectors, and there is no record of transmission of the disease from man to man by contact, excreta, or fomites. Cases attributed to the bites of cats, ferrets, and weasels have been reported.

The infecting organisms are carried into the wound of the bite by the rat's teeth. Spirilla have not been found in the saliva of rats. They may get into the mouth and on the teeth in blood from injured gums, lesions in the mouth, infectious conjunctival exudate that drains through the lacrimal ducts, or exudate from pulmonary lesions. When several persons are bitten by an infected rat, often only the first victim will contract the disease.

Rat-bite fever begins as a wound which may be infected with organisms other than *S. minor*. A variety of cocci, bacilli, and *Actinomycetes* have been found in these conditions.

Clinical Manifestations.   In a case uncomplicated by mixed or secondary infection, the wound of the bite heals promptly. After an incubation period of 5 to 14 days, the site of the wound swells and becomes purplish and painful. A chancrelike indurated ulcer with a black crust may develop at this site and may reach a diameter of 5 to 10 cm. The regional lymphatics are inflamed, and the adjacent lymph nodes become enlarged and tender. The development of the local lesion is accompanied by malaise and headache and a sharp rise of temperature, usually with a chill. After this, periods of fever alternate with afebrile periods. The temperature rises abruptly to 103 to 104F (39.4 to 40C), remains elevated for 24 to 48 hours, and falls rapidly to normal within about 36 hours. The intervening afebrile periods last from three to nine days. In untreated cases this relapsing type of fever may continue for weeks or months, gradually subsiding.

Within the first week of the beginning of the fever, a characteristic purplish maculopapular eruption of the skin of the arms, legs, and trunk, and occasionally on the face and scalp usually appears. The skin lesions do not ulcerate. They fade somewhat during the afebrile periods but reappear, with new patches of eruption, during the paroxysms of fever.

There are few recorded autopsies of cases of rat-bite fever. The local lesion, which is a granuloma without suppuration, shows necrosis of the epithelium and dense round cell infiltration of the corium. Similar round cell infiltration with dilated vessels occurs in the lesions of the skin eruption. In the preantibiotic era, the mortality rate was estimated to be about 10 percent and was usually due to secondary pyogenic infection.

TREATMENT. Penicillin is the drug of choice. Streptomycin also has been used successfully.

CAMPYLOBACTER FETUS

Morphology The genus name *Campylobacter* is derived from the Greek word meaning "curved." Organisms in the genus are gram-negative and are 0.2 to 0.5 μm wide and 1.5 to 5 μm long. They are characteristically comma-shaped when seen in infected tissue but are filamentous or coccoid after in vitro cultivation. They are actively motile, which can best be observed with the phase microscope. The genus is of recent origin and includes three species previously assigned to the genus *Vibrio*: *Campylobacter fetus*, *Campylobacter sputorum*, and *Campylobacter fecalis*. Of these only *C. fetus* is pathogenic for man.

Laboratory Identification For isolation, brucella agar plates and broth containing 10 percent animal blood can be used. Colonies on blood are nonhemolytic. There are three sub-species of *C. fetus*: subspecies *jejuni*, subspecies *fetus*, and subspecies *intestinalis*. Distinctions among the subspecies are based upon differences in temperature tolerance, biochemical properties, and serologic characteristics. In the medical literature a group of organisms has been termed "related vibrios"; most of these are *C. fetus* subspecies *fetus*.

Antigenic Structure The major antigen of *Campylobacter* is the lipopolysaccharide of the cell wall. Colonization or infection in animals results in the formation of IgM, IgA, and IgG classes of antibody with specificity for the lipopolysaccharide. IgA and IgG antibodies that arise following infection are demonstrable in the serum and have opsonizing and immobilizing capacity. Agglutinins are present in the cervicovaginal mucus of animals convalescing from genital infections. A transition in serotype of infecting organism has been observed in cattle with persistent genital infections.

Clinical Infection EPIDEMIOLOGY. The major importance of infections with *Campylobacter* lies in the field of veterinary medicine. Serious economic losses to farmers result from abortions and infertility of infected cattle and sheep. Infection of animals is transmitted venereally and may be harbored asymptomatically for long periods of time in the genitourinary and intestinal tracts. An extensive literature on this subject may be found in veterinary journals.

The mode of transmission to human beings is largely unknown. Because of the prevalence of *Campylobacter* within animal herds, direct transmission from infected animals and indirect transmission from contaminated food or water has been suspected but not proven. Transplacental passage occurs in human beings.

CLINICAL MANIFESTATIONS. Human disease caused by *Campylobacter* usually is recognized only when septicemia occurs, since isolation of the organism from mixed cultures obtained from the primary site is very difficult. Cases of meningitis and arthritis also may be recognized.

Less than 100 cases of human disease with these organisms have been reported. A significant proportion has been in women during the second and third trimester of pregnancy and in premature infants. Most of the other cases have been in older adults with significant underlying disease, such as cirrhosis, leukemia, chronic obstructuve pulmonary disease, and cardiovascular disease. Prominent characteristics of human disease include severe diarrhea and vascular disease, such as arteritis and thrombophlebitis. Sites of involvement and clinical material from which organisms have been recovered include blood, cerebrospinal fluid, joint fluid, abscess cavity, the uterine cervix, bile, and pleural fluid.

Infections with *Campylobacter* species may be more common than is currently recognized. Technical difficulties in their recovery probably greatly decrease the proportion of cases that are documented. Nevertheless, they may be considered in the diagnosis of perinatal morbidity, septicemia, severe diarrhea, and in infections of the compromised host.

LABORATORY DIAGNOSIS.   Diagnosis of *C. fetus* infections can be made only by culture of the organism. The organisms grow on various media, but careful attention must be given to the atmospheric conditions. There is little or no growth under strict anaerobic conditions. *C. fetus* is microaerophilic, and in a semisolid medium, growth occurs only within the first few millimeters below the surface. This is in contrast to some of the other *Campylobacter* that will grow under conditions of strict anaerobiosis.

Antibodies in high titers may be demonstrated in patients with documented infection by use of an indirect hemagglutination test. Experience with this test, however, is still limited.

TREATMENT.   *Campylobacter* usually are sensitive to most antimicrobial agents. Specific sensitivity testing, however, is indicated for optimal treatment of a given case.

FURTHER READING

Spirillum

Babudieri B: Experimental infections by Spirilla. Eichler O (ed): In Handbuch der experimentellen Pharmakologie, New Series, vol 17 IIB, Berlin. New York, Springer Verlag, 1973, p 43

Bayne-Jones S: Rat-bite fever in the United States. International Clinic, 41st ser, 3:235, 1931

Roughgarden JW: Antimicrobial therapy of rat-bite fever. Arch Intern Med 116:39, 1965

Watkins CG: Rat-bite fever. J Pediatr 28:429, 1946

Campylobacter

Bokkenheuser V: *Vibrio fetus* infection in man. 1. Ten cases and some epidemiologic observations. Am J Epidemiol 91:400, 1970

Bokkenheuser V: *Vibrio fetus* infection in man: a serological test. Infect Immun 5:222, 1972

Kahler RL, Sheldon H: *Vibrio fetus* infection in man. N Engl J Med 262:1218, 1960

King EO: The laboratory recognition of *Vibrio fetus* and a closely related *Vibrio* isolated from cases of human vibriosis. Ann N Y Acad Sci 98:700, 1962

Ruben FL, Wolinsky E: Human infection with *Vibrio fetus*. In Day RA (ed): Antimicrobial Agents and Chemotherapy. Ann Arbor, Mich, American Society for Microbiology. 1967, p 143

56

Microbiota of Dental Plaque, Caries, Gingival Disease, Related Systemic Infections

The biology of dental plaque in its specific relation to dental caries and to gingivitis involves a complexity of host–parasite interactions that have eluded bacteriologists and oral biologists since Anton van Leeuwenhoek first described the teeming bacterial forms from his own teeth under a powerful magnifying lens in 1675.

Currently, impressive strides in clinically related biologic research are being made in the study of bacterial mattlike plaque or films that accumulate on the teeth of man and animals. Insidious destruction of the mineralized teeth, of the gingival tissues (gums), and of the bone that surrounds and supports the teeth constitute the most prevalent infectious processes of man. Recent development of experimental animal and human models provides more effective systems for the study of these diseases and the development of new methods of prevention. This also has stimulated broad interest in the biology of dental plaque and in the response of host tissues.

Increased interest in the aerobic and anaerobic oral bacteria of dental plaque and their involvement in bacteremia and valvular heart infections also is being reinforced by an age of artificial heart valves and other vascular prosthetic implants, by immunosuppressive therapy for organ transplants, and by the use of irradiation and cytotoxic drugs in the treatment of neoplastic disease. More sensitive anaerobic culture techniques have expanded the capacity of bacteriologists to study these problems.

These advances and progress in oral disease control have stimulated a dramatic shift in clinical dentistry from overemphasis on dental restorations and extractions to a much stronger emphasis on prevention and control of oral disease.

STREPTOCOCCUS AND LACTOBACILLUS SPECIES ASSOCIATED WITH DENTAL CARIES

Caries is a multifactorial disease that results only when dependent factors coincide, as illustrated in Figure 56-1. (1) Susceptible teeth and tolerance of a cariogenic microflora by the host: Pits and fissures and interproximal spaces tend to entrap food and are more susceptible to decay, as are all exposed surfaces of tooth en-

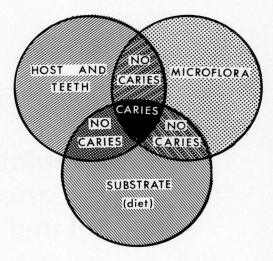

FIG. 56-1. Overlapping circles depicting factors responsible for caries activity. (Courtesy of Dr. P.H. Keyes, National Institute for Dental Research)

amel that have little or no fluoride content. The role of immune host factors in controlling the cariogenic microflora has still to be defined. (2) Dietary sucrose intake: Frequent intake of fermentable carbohydrate in the diet serves as the main energy source for the growth of cariogenic bacteria and as the substrate for the production of acids for demineralization of dental enamel and of an adhesive polysaccharide component of plaque. (3) Cariogenic microflora: The importance of acid-producing microflora adherent to the teeth in the form of a gelatinous mattlike plaque has been established in experimental animal models and strongly implicated in the disease in man (Fig. 56-2).

Cariogenic Streptococci

The taxonomy of streptococci cariogenic for animals and those found on human teeth has not been conclusively defined. Extracellular glucan-forming streptococci designated *Streptococcus mutans* were cultivated from caries lesions in 1924 by Clarke, and since then the role of similar extracellular polysaccharide-producing streptococci in animal caries and their presence in human plaque flora has been well established. Plaque-forming strains similar to *S. mutans* produce, in hamsters, specific transmissible infections that decay the smooth surfaces of their teeth; caries can be transmitted

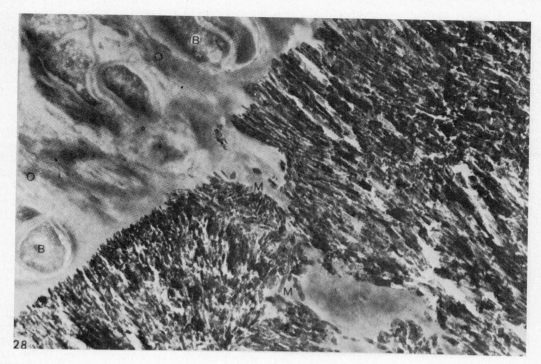

FIG. 56-2. Ultrastructure of a section cut through an early carious lesion in the enamel surface of a human molar covered by dental plaque. Shown are changes in orientation of enamel crystals (M), sectioned plaque bacteria (B), and interbacterial matrix (O). (Courtesy of Drs. R.M. Frank and A. Brandel, Institut Dentaire, Faculté de Medecine, Strasbourg, France)

to germ-free rats by infecting them with a polysaccharide-producing streptococcus from conventional rats, and streptococci of the types most cariogenic for rats and for hamsters can be detected in human dental lesions using immunofluorescence techniques. *S. mutans* has since been found in all parts of the world. Bratthal recognizes five serologic groups of *S. mutans*, including Lancefield group E. The organism, however, has not been sufficiently well characterized to be recognized in the 8th edition of Bergey's Manual.

Microscopic and Cultural Characteristics
Microscopically, gram-positive streptococci similar to *S. mutans* and other streptococci of dental plaque (eg, *Streptococcus mitis, Streptococcus sanguis*) do not differ from other streptococci.

Streptococci in dental plaque and carious lesions can be grown on blood agar or selective mitis-salivarius agar, preferably under anaerobic conditions. Varieties resembling *S. mutans* produce somewhat characteristic colony forms

in 24 hours, 0.5 mm in diameter, highly convex, opaque, with a finely granular surface when viewed with a dissecting microscope by reflected light.

S. mutans produces colonies that are nonhemolytic. It ferments sorbitol and mannitol, produces no ammonia from arginine, and does not grow in 6.5 percent sodium chloride broth. Dextran-forming strains, designated *S. sanguis*, are also common in plaque and produce hard smooth colonies 0.5 mm in diameter on mitis-salivarius agar. They are hemolytic, ferment neither mannitol nor sorbitol, but may split arginine. Strains resembling *S. sanguis* are inhibited by 5 units of bacitracin and by 100 μg of sulfathiazole, while strains similar to *S. mutans* are unaffected.

Metabolic   Products A characteristic common to the streptococci most often implicated in caries is production of capsular polysaccharides from sucrose. These consist mainly of soluble and insoluble dextranase-sensitive polymers of glucose and some levan polymers

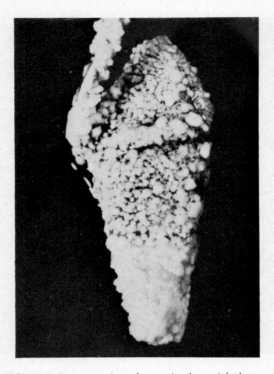

FIG. 56-3. Demonstration of extensive bacterial plaque-like matts or deposits that can form on a tooth incubated in sucrose broth culture of *Streptococcus mutans* for 24 hours, then transferred to fresh broth medium daily for four or more days. (Courtesy of Dr. P.H. Keyes, National Institute of Dental Research)

of fructose formed by enzymes on the cell surface. These cause the bacteria to adhere to walls of the tube or other objects in sucrose broth (Fig. 56-3). This mechanism, plus agglutination of other streptococci by saliva and nonspecific adsorption of salivary components to the enamel surface, contributes to the formation of bacterial plaque matts on teeth. Fermentation end products are not distinctive, mainly lactic acid, with some acetic, formic, and butyric acid. Intracellular glycogen vacuoles are also formed from sucrose, and they contribute to prolonged acid production following a brief sucrose exposure (Fig. 56-4). Acid production and glycogen storage are markedly reduced in plaque deposits on teeth of individuals who are tube-fed.

Oral Lactobacilli

Lactobacilli are members of the family Lactobacillaceae. They are widely distributed in nature, occurring in both parasitic and saprophytic states. When lactose and dextrin diets are consumed they are present in the human oral cavity and human and animal feces. They occur in a wide variety of dairy products.

There is evidence of beneficial effects of these organisms in the flora of the human intestinal tract and the vagina. Interest of early oral researchers was attracted by the acidophilic qualities of oral *Lactobacillus* species, their association with carious lesions, and the effects on their numbers in saliva of increased and decreased sugar intake, which also related to increases and decreases in dental decay. Lactobacilli have produced caries in gnotobiotic animals.

Lactobacillus casei, Lactobacillus fermentum, Bifidobacterium bifidum, and *Lactobacillus acidophilus* are among the main species found in the human oral cavity.

Morphology and Physiology Lactobacilli are gram-positive, nonspore-forming, generally nonmotile rods, varying from short to rather long and slender forms of uniform width, 0.6 to 0.9 μm in diameter, often forming chains.

Colonies are smooth to rough, oval, opaque, creamy white to slightly brown, and catalase negative. Oral strains may require various B-complex vitamins and are microaerophilic and facultative anaerobes. Growth is obtainable in three to four days on blood agar or on Rogosa's and other *Lactobacillus* selective agar media acidified to pH 5.0.

Most oral lactobacilli produce only lactic acid as a fermentation end product and are termed "homofermentative." Species that also produce carbon dioxide and other fermentation products are termed "heterofermentative" (Chap. 3). Although oral lactobacilli grow more slowly than do streptococci, they can reduce the pH of glucose broth to 3.0 in two to four days. A pH approaching 5 or below demineralizes tooth enamel.

Clinical Infection

Dental caries is characterized by a demineralization of the inorganic component of tooth structure and dissolution of the residual organic matrix. It is the main cause of tooth loss before age 25. When the disease is progressive and when it becomes widespread in the dentition, it is termed "rampant caries." There is no

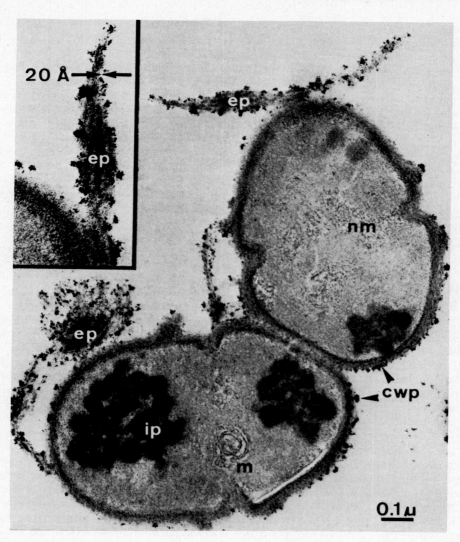

FIG. 56-4. Sucrose-grown cells of streptococci contrasted with osmium black. Heavily electron-dense granules of intra-cellular polysaccharides (ip), mesosomes (m), and nuclear material (nm) are shown in detail. The cell wall has a dense middle layer; its outer surface carries strongly dense osmiophilic particles; labeling sites of polysaccharides (cwp, arrows). In direct continuation with the cell wall there are extracellular polysaccharides (ep). This material consists of very fine protofibrils approximately 20 A thick (inset). ×99,000. Inset, ×165,000. (From Guggenheim and Schroeder: Helv Odontol Acta 11:131, 1967)

disease process analogous to dental caries in any other tissue of the body because of the unique nature of the tooth structure, the avascularity of enamel and the underlying dentin, and because the advanced lesion cannot heal itself.

Localized lesions tend to take the form of pyramidal cavities. The apex of lesions located in occlusal fissures points toward the surface, with the base toward the pulp. On the sides of the teeth the lesion apex is directed toward the pulp. As lesions tend to enlarge and deepen, the pulp eventually becomes exposed and inflamed, frequently leading to irreversible necrosis. Pulp degeneration and/or infection can irritate periodontal tissues at the apex of the root to produce a lesion that may extend into the osseous tissues. Extension of an infection into facial tissues produces the classic picture of a patient with facial cellulitis, showing edema and inflammation, usually with fever and elevated blood leukocyte count. Microorganisms involved in such severe conditions may include pathogenic *Streptococcus pyogenes,* but more often only a mixed streptococcal flora derived originally from the plaque and carious lesions can be detected. Most of these organisms respond to intensive penicillin therapy, but resistant strains of staphylococci, enterics, and anaerobic oral bacteria may be encountered.

Root surface caries, a generalized type of decay associated with advanced gingival disease, occurring on and around root surfaces of the teeth below the crown, is of concern because of difficulty in controlling and restoring such lesions. It may be caused by filamentous bacteria, such as *Actinomyces* species.

CARIES PREVENTION AND CONTROL

Prevention of caries is closely tied to control of bacterial plaque matts on teeth and of gingival disease. Clinical and investigative approaches include (1) influencing patient behavior to improve oral hygiene, to limit sucrose intake, and to bring carious lesions under control with temporary or permanent fillings, (2) the use of fluorides to increase resistance of enamel and investigation of new chemicals to keep bacteria or their products off the teeth, (3) investigation of immunologic prophylaxis.

Plaque control will be considered under plaque disease (p. 717). Efforts to alter patient sucrose intake require careful analysis of diet and detailed directions. Various diet plans are available, such as that of Jay, or contemporary plans may be integrated into total preventive programs.

The use and effectiveness of fluorides to reduce the solubility of the enamel is well established. Water fluoridation is safe and can reduce decay lesions in pits, fissures, and between teeth by 45 to 60 percent and those at the gingival margins by 75 percent. Frequent topical applications have been found to prevent three out of four of the remaining carious lesions.

Other chemicals under investigation range from chlorhexidine, which acts on the tooth surface to prevent bacteria from forming a plaque, to cyanoacrylate and other polymers, used to coat the teeth with a protective film. Dextranase, used to control plaque in experi-

mentally infected rodents, is only partially effective for plaque removal in man. It may prove effective combined with other chemicals, such as certain phosphates, that tend to reduce plaque adherence to enamel.

Of bacteriologic and medical interest is the possibility of a vaccine to control cariogenic bacteria. Most efforts to protect animals have been unsuccessful. Risk of endocarditis would prevent the use of viable streptococcal vaccines. Even the cell wall component is toxic. Protection afforded by antibodies against dextransucrase and other enzymes is being investigated.

Tests for Cariogenic Bacteria

Lactobacillus colony counts of saliva specimens using selective low pH media have been used since the 1930s. Tests in current clinical office use are patterned after Snyder's fermentation test. The test is read daily for three days for degree of acid produced, mainly by lactobacilli and some streptococci. This test has since been miniaturized and the agar content reduced to give a semifluid medium that is more convenient for clinical use, such as Grainger's and Sim's tests. Tests can be performed with saliva or plaque. The latter seems preferable.

The often misleading term "caries activity test" applied to such fermentation tests relates best to their use in longitudinal population studies. In individual use, positive fermentation tests constitute a false positive for caries activity at any time new caries do not develop despite the risk posed by bacteria and diet. Actual caries activity is not readily apparent by visual assessment. Judging development of new caries takes months and is also subject to much error. On the other hand, a set of three tests does give useful immediate information about the acid-producing capacity of the patient's flora that is of value in patient education and dietary control.

FLORA OF BACTERIAL PLAQUE AND GINGIVAL DISEASE

Until recently the filamentous and fusospirochetal organisms were considered to be a normal component of dental plaque matts near the gingival margins or gums. Recent clinical research indicates that these organisms could be considered "normal" only because gingival disease itself was "normal," ie, a condition commonly observable in the adult population. Using highly effective hygienic procedures to free human subjects' teeth of plaque, cumulative changes in microbial populations on tooth surfaces have been followed by direct microscopic examination and cultures over several weeks in human subjects in the total absence of oral hygiene. Cocci and short rods accumulate on the teeth after one to two days, consisting mainly of *Streptococcus* and *Neisseria*, plus some *Veillonella* and *Propionibacterium* species, among others. Filamentous bacteria (*Leptotrichia buccalis* and probably *Bacterionema matruchotii*) and *Fusobacterium* species accumulate in increasing numbers after the second day. Motile oral vibrio forms and spirochetes (*Treponema* and *Borrelia* species) are added in increasing numbers after about one week. This stage usually coincides with the appearance of gingivitis in adults. Restoring effective oral hygiene eradicates gingivitis within a few days.

Pathogenesis of Gingival Disease in Man

Mechanisms involved in destruction of the gingival tissues and underlying bone are complex. Cell wall endotoxins appear to be the most toxic components of plaque bacteria, although they also produce some potentially tissue destructive enzymes. Enzymes liberated by polymorphonuclear leukocytes migrating from inflamed gingivae and enzymes liberated within the inflamed tissues themselves appear to produce most of the tissue destruction observed. Inflammation and the presence of plasma cells, immunoglobulin, and lymphocytes in gingival tissues and various immunologic experiments suggest that the Shwartzman, Arthus, autoimmune, and delayed hypersensitivity reactions may also be involved in gingival disease.

Of concern to clinicians is the extent to which bacteria on teeth may enter the bloodstream. Premedication is required to prevent bacterial endocarditis among high-risk patients, such as those with a history of rheumatic fever.

Anaerobic bacteria far outnumber aerobic species in bacterial matts on teeth. Little interest had been given in the past to their involvement in endocardial infections, mainly because of inadequate culture technology which prevented their detection (Chap. 48). Felner and Dowell reviewed 30 instances of anaerobes in bacterial endocarditis, and one-third were believed to be of oral origin.

A greater risk exists among thousands of patients who have cardiovascular implants or who receive cytotoxic drugs, irradiation therapy, and other immunosuppressive treatments for neoplastic diseases and organ transplants.

Tests Applied to Plaque Control and Prevention

Extensive clinical programs are being used to train patients on a daily basis over a period of a week in the mastery of effective flossing and brushing techniques required for plaque control. Training is incorporated into a combined program of evaluation, diagnosis, and patient education, including use of fermentation tests for dietary control. The bacterial nature of a patient's plaque is demonstrated to him by phase contrast microscopy, and erythrocin dye is used to disclose plaque as an aid to hygiene.

FUSOSPIROCHETAL DISEASE

Fusospirochetal disease is most commonly observed as the painful condition of acute necrotizing ulcerative gingivitis (ANUG) first described by Vincent. The bacterial agents are a symbiotic mixture of indigenous anaerobic species derived from bacterial plaque deposits on the teeth at the gingival margin. A characteristic, thriving flora of active spirochetes, large fusiform bacilli, and vibrio or spiral forms together with other anaerobic species are easily observed by darkfield or phase contrast microscopy.

Fusospirochetal flora can be found in ulcerative or pseudomembranous infections of the throat and oral mucosa, as well as in extensive mixed anaerobic bacterial infections of the oral–facial tissues, submandibular tissues, bronchi, lungs, and in tissues injured by human bites. Infections rarely may spread to other vital organs, including the brain.

Anaerobic infections in the abdominal and female urogenital regions are associated more with anaerobic species common to the intestines and female genitalia, although *Bacteroides*, *Peptostreptococcus*, and sometimes *Fusobacterium* species are common to fusospirochetal infections as well (Chap. 48).

Fusospirochetal flora is also found almost universally with anaerobic filamentous species in well-developed dental plaque at the gingival margins in conditions ranging from mild gingivitis to periodontitis, that is, destruction of the periodontal tissues and bone that surround and support the teeth. These are conditions universally found in adults with inadequate training in preventive oral hygiene. They constitute the most prevalent disease of mankind and cause the greatest loss of teeth among adults. However, the fusospirochetal flora does not appear to be invasive in gingivitis or periodontitis in the absence of pseudomembraneous or ulcerative lesions.

Morphology and Physiology   The fusiform bacilli are slender or stout, straight or slightly curved rods with sharply pointed ends. They vary from 3 to 10 μm in length and 0.3 to 0.8 μm in thickness. They usually consist of a mixture of delicate, curved, pointed, gram-negative *Fusobacterium* species and larger forms of cigar-shaped bacilli, *Leptotrichia buccalis*.

Spirochetes with open wavy undulations, *Treponema buccale* and *Treponema vincentii*, are abundant. Fine, tightly coiled *Treponema macrodentium* and *Treponema denticola* and *Treponema orale* are seen. All are gram-negative. Comma and spiral bacterial forms are gram-negative *Campylobacter* and *Selenomonas* species.

The fusospirochetal flora is difficult to see in dried smears stained by Gram's method. Simple staining with 0.1 percent crystal violet for 30 seconds provides more distinct staining of the larger forms present. Silver stains can be used to demonstrate the more delicate oral *Treponema* species, but these organisms are easily detected and differentiated in wet preparations examined by darkfield (Fig. 56-5) or phase contrast microscopy.

Cultivation.   *Fusobacterium* species and *Bacteroides* species can be cultivated on fresh

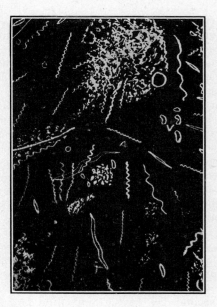

FIG. 56-5. Fusospirochetal symbiotic organisms found in a patient with chronic bronchiectasis. (From Smith: Oral Spirochetes and Related Organisms, 1932. Courtesy of William and Wilkins Co)

blood agar plates incubated anaerobically or in prereduced cooked meat or brain-heart infusion medium supplemented with hemin and vitamin K, as can most other moderate anaerobes likely to be present. Methods for cultivating oral *Treponema* and *Borrelia* spirochetes in media enriched with serum and other supplements have been described in the VPI *Outline of Clinical Methods in Anaerobic Bacteriology*.

Laboratory Identification   For diagnostic purposes cultivation of fusospirochetal flora from surface lesions is unnecessary, since the flora is easily recognized by microscopic examination. Cultivation of the fusospirochetal flora from surface lesions for antibiotic testing is also usually unnecessary because the infections appear to respond uniformly to penicillin or erythromycin. In abscesses and pulmonary infections, anaerobic species of *Bacteroides* or *Peptostreptococcus* may be resistant to some antibiotics and perpetuate the infections. Therefore, efforts should be made to carefully collect exudates from pulmonary infections and other deep infections of the oral–facial tissues for cultivation and testing of any resistant anaerobic species.

Determinants of Pathogenicity The organisms involved do not elaborate potent exotoxins or high levels of tissue-destructive enzymes. Some *Bacteroides* species found in dental plaque produce small amounts of collagenase and several other enzymes that may act in vivo. However, the abundance of gram-negative species that comprise fusospirochetal flora suggests that gram-negative endotoxic cell wall components may be more important in the disease process.

Antigenic Structure and Immune Response Fusiform bacilli have been separated into four distinct serologic groups by agglutination reactions.

Response to antigenic components of bacteria may be important in the disease process. Transformation tests performed with lymphocytes of patients with necrotic ulcerative gingivitis show a marked response to *Fusobacterium* species but not to *Proteus* or *Lactobacillus* species. Patients' sera were devoid of circulating antibodies to these species. However, periodontally diseased patients have been found to give immediate skin test reactions to certain *Actinomyces* found in dental plaque.

Clinical Infection PHARYNGEAL INFECTIONS. Acute necrotic ulcerative gingivitis occurs in young adults under conditions of stress, poor nutrition, and lack of oral hygiene. During World War I this painful condition was known as "trench mouth." This is the most common form of fusospirochetal disease.

As a pseudomembranous, ulcerative disease of the tonsils, pharynx, tongue, or oral mucosa, fusospirochetal disease is termed "Vincent's angina" or "Vincent's stomatitis." This is the most frequent form seen by physicians. Severe forms are often accompanied by foul odor, pain, lymphadenopathy, difficulty in eating and drinking, and lethargy. Body temperature may be elevated 1 to 2 degrees F. The onset is sudden, within 24 to 48 hours. Necrosis and ulceration of the interdental papilla characterize ANUG. Ulcers of the mucosa resemble syphilitic lesions. Malaise and higher temperatures may be a sign of primary stomatitis.

Pharyngeal infections are sufficiently severe at times to be confused with diphtheria. Although cultures for diphtheria bacilli will not detect fusospirochetal flora, the fusospirochetal organisms are easily and rapidly recognized by direct wet smear examination using phase contrast or darkfield microscopy.

In ulcerative gingivitis, electron microscopic studies of biopsy tissues reveal four zones of infection. A bacterial zone is seen at the lesion surface overlying a leukocyte-rich zone. Beyond that a necrotic zone exists, and finally there is a zone in which spirochetes are seen infiltrating the surrounding tissues. This suggests active invasion of the tissues by the fusospirochetal flora under the conditions of acute infection.

Fusospirochetal forms, as well as other anaerobes from dental plaque, can also be found in abscessed or draining infections of the oral facial tissues. Infections may show only local signs or may be accompanied by systemic responses of fever, lymphadenopathy, and elevated blood leukocyte count. Infections can extend along facial plains to submandibular tissues, where inflammation and edema (Ludwig's angina) may close the pharynx, causing suffocation.

COMPLICATIONS. Organisms can also be carried by circulating blood from oral facial tissue infections to the brain, where abscesses or cavernous sinus thrombophlebitis can cause death. This is a potential of all severe infections of the head and neck.

Painful ulcerative fusospirochetal abscesses can develop from human bites.

Pulmonary infections are seen especially in alcoholics, apparently from aspiration of fusospirochetal flora. Pulmonary disease is similar during the first one to two weeks to that associated with pyogenic cocci. After several weeks clinical signs of pulmonary gangrene, a pulmonary abscess, or bronchiectasis appears.

While oral infections often respond rapidly to penicillin or erythromycin, the flora in oral facial abscesses and in pulmonary infections may contain other antibiotic-resistant anaerobic species. Antibiotic therapy should be verified by culture studies of samples taken when therapy is initiated.

While fusospirochetal disease that comes to the attention of physicians is accompanied by acute signs of disease, the flora found in clinical fusospirochetal infections is often indistinguishable from the flora observable in plaque masses that are associated with milder insidious forms of marginal gingivitis and/or periodontitis seen in most adults. The first sign of marginal gingivitis is recognized as gingiva that bleed easily upon brushing. Uncontrolled gingivitis results in long-term irritation of the gingiva, with gradual ulceration and recession of the gingival attachment to the teeth, forming pockets around the teeth that cannot be cleaned and frequently abscess. This entraps a flora that can easily be pumped into surrounding tissues, which abscess and can invade the circulating blood, risking injury to susceptible heart valves and other organs. Continued gingival inflammation results in an underlying breakdown of the periodontal ligament and bone that supports the teeth. Gingivitis and periodontitis result from prolonged stagnation of dental plaque and can be simply avoided by adequate training in preventive oral hygiene and preventive dental care.

Signs of gingival and periodontal disease are not dramatic for many years, and symptomatic mouth odors can be temporarily masked by use of commercial mouth washes. Despite the ease with which these diseases can be controlled by effective daily plaque removal, periodontal disease remains the most prevalent disease of mankind and the greatest cause of tooth loss with age among adults.

Transmission The source of the fusospirochetal organisms and accompanying mixed anaerobic species is indigenous in dental plaque, especially in the presence of gingivitis. However, outbreaks of Vincent's infection are seen at times in some school groups or dormitories housing young adults. This may be related to common tendencies of a group to neglect oral hygiene, good nutrition, and rest. Isolated instances have been observed in which the disease accompanies herpes gingivitis, which may account for apparent cross-infections.

Treatment For ANUG, warm water lavage with careful debriding and scaling of the teeth brings about dramatic relief and rapid healing. This is followed by frequent water rinses and improvement of home care, nutrition, and rest. When fever, lymphadenopathy, and other signs of systemic response to infections of the mucosa are present, antibiotics are considered a useful adjunct to therapy. Erythromycin is used for patients allergic to penicillin. Without control of other factors, however, antibiotics have little long-term value.

Diffusion of antibiotics into abscesses is very slow. These usually require surgical drainage plus intensive chemotherapy. Many anaerobic species that may resist penicillin, erythromycin, and even tetracyclines may be present in oral facial and pulmonary fusospirochetal abscesses. Drainage exudates should be cultured anaerobically and for bacteria commonly found in mixed anaerobic infections, such as *Bacteroides* and *Peptostreptococcus* species. These should be tested for susceptibility to these antibiotics plus cephalosporins and clindamycin.

While culture and antibiotic susceptibility testing is usually not necessary for diagnosis and treatment of mucosal surface lesions, cultural studies to demonstrate the absence of other pathogens, such as S. *pyogenes*, are indicated.

FURTHER READING

Books and Reviews

Buchanan RE, Gibbons NE: Bergey's Manual of Determinative Bacteriology, 8th ed. Baltimore, Williams & Wilkins, 1974

Department of Health, Education and Welfare. *Streptococcus mutans* and Dental Caries. Bethesda, Md, National Institutes of Dental Research, National Caries Program, 1973

Eastman Dental Center. Role of human foodstuffs in caries: proceedings of a workshop conference, supplement. J Dent Res 49:1201, 1283, 1970

Harris RS: Art and Sciences of Dental Caries Research. New York, Academic Press, 1968, pp 55-124

Harvard Conference. Current research concepts fundamental to the improvement of periodontal care: usefulness and limitations of model systems in studying periodontal disease; inflammation and repair, supplement. J Dent Res 50:236, 1971

University of Pennsylvania. Conference on the implication of immune reactions in the pathogenesis of periodontal disease. J Periodontol 41:196, 1970

Virginia Polytechnic Institute Anaerobe Laboratory. Outline of Clinical Methods in Anaerobic Bacteriology. Blacksburg, Virginia Polytechnic Institute and State University of Virginia, 1971

Selected Papers

Bahn AN: Microbial potential in the etiology of periodontal disease. J Periodontol 41:603, 1970

Crawford J, Sconyers J, Moriarty J, King R, West J: Bacteremia after tooth extractions studied with the aid of prereduced anaerobically sterilized culture media. Appl Microbiol 27:927, 1974

Felner JM, Dowell VR Jr: Anaerobic bacterial endocarditis. N Engl J Med 283:1188, 1970

Grainger RM, Jarrett TM, Honey SL: Swab test for dental caries activity: an epidemiologic study. J Can Dent Assoc 31:515, 1965

Hampp E, Mergenhagen S: Experimental intracutaneous

fusobacterial and fusospirochetal infections. J Infect Dis 112:84, 1963

Hampp, E: Experimental infections with oral spirochetes. J Infect Dis 109:43, 1961

Kennedy AE, Shklair IL, Hayashi JA, Bahn AN: Antibodies to streptococci in humans. Arch Oral Biol 13:1275, 1968

Keyes PH: Research in dental caries. J Am Dent Assoc 76: 1357, 1968

Keyes PH, Shern RJ: Chemical adjuvants for control and prevention of dental plaque. J Am Soc Prev Dent 1:18, 1971

Klinkhamer J: Human oral leukocytes. Periodontics 1: 109, 1963

Krasse B, Carlsson J: Various types of streptococci and experimental caries in hamsters. Arch Oral Biol 15:25, 1970

Listgarten M: Electron microscopic observations on the bacterial flora of acute necrotizing gingivitis. J Periodontol 36:326, 1965

McMinn MT, Crawford JJ: Recovery of anaerobic microorganisms from clinical specimens in prereduced media vs. recovery by routine clinical laboratory methods. Appl Microbiol 19:207, 1970

Myall RWT, Gregory HS: Current trends in the prevention of bacterial endocarditis in susceptible patients receiving dental care. Oral Surg 28:813, 1969

National Institutes of Health. Conference on specific questions related to periodontal diseases, supplement. J Dent Res 49:198, 256, 1970

O'Leary TJ, Nabers CL: Instructions to supplement teaching oral hygiene. J Periodontol 40:27, 1969

Sims W: The interpretation and use of Snyder tests and lactobacillus counts. J Am Dent Assoc 80:1315, 1970

Socransky S: Relationship of bacteria to the etiology of periodontal disease. J Dent Res (suppl to No 2) 49:203, 1970

Wilton J, Ivanyi C, Lehner T: Cell-mediated immunity and humoral antibodies in acute ulcerative gingivitis. J Periodont Res 6:9, 1971

57
Rickettsiae

Rickettsial infections have been significant factors in the history of western civilization. Epidemic typhus, which has been recognized as a distinct clinical entity since the sixteenth century, has always been intimately associated with wars, famine, and human suffering. It has played a decisive role in the outcomes of several major European wars. Charles I abandoned his plan to march on London in 1643 because of an epidemic of typhus fever. In 1741 Prague fell to the French army after 30,000 defenders had died of typhus. During the 1816-1819 epidemic in Ireland there were 600,000 cases of typhus among the population of 6,000,000. In both World Wars, typhus killed hundreds of thousands and caused suffering in many more thousands.

In spite of these and many other devastating epidemics, the first microbiologic description of rickettsia did not occur until the first decade of the twentieth century, when Dr. Howard Ricketts described the etiologic agent of Rocky Mountain spotted fever, cultivated the organism in laboratory animals, and deduced its natural ecology and epidemiology. Using similar experimental approaches, other investigators rapidly obtained a basic microbiologic understanding of other related rickettsial diseases. The family name Rickettsiaceae honors Ricketts for his brilliant experiments, which were performed with modest funds and simple laboratory equipment. Ricketts and a number of early rickettsiologists were eventually killed by the disease agents they were studying.

Once the importance of arthropod vectors was appreciated, outbreaks of the typhus fevers could be controlled using sanitary and vector control measures. The introduction of tetracycline and chloramphenicol has further brought the rickettsioses under man's control. In spite of these accomplishments, however, Hans Zinsser's comment in his book, *Rats, Lice and History,*[*] is as appropriate today as it was 40 years ago:

Typhus is not dead. It will continue to break into the open whenever human stupidity and brutality give it a chance, as most likely they occasionally will. But its freedom of action is being restricted, and more and more it will be confined, like other savage creatures, in the zoologic gardens of controlled diseases.

The rickettsiae are small pleomorphic coccobacilli, most of which are obligate intracellular parasites. They have a wide natural host range including various arthropods, birds, and mammals. Within the family Rickettsiaceae three genera contain organisms that have successfully adapted to a parasitic existence in man: *Rickettsia*, *Rochalimaea*, and *Coxiella*. Their ecology involves a complex interaction of arthropod vectors, animals, and/or man. Infection of animals and man is typically mediated by an arthropod vector, although *Coxiella burnetii* may also be transmitted by aerosols or by ingestion of contaminated dairy products. Natural reservoirs of infection may be maintained by transovarial passage in arthropod vectors (eg, *Rickettsia tsutsugamushi* in mites and *Rickettsia rickettsii* in ticks) or by infection in rodents (*Rickettsia typhi*) or man *Rickettsia prowazekii* and *Rochalimaea quintana*).

Pathogenic rickettsiae cause a number of diverse human diseases, including Rocky Mountain spotted fever, Q Fever, epidemic and endemic typhus, and scrub typhus.

MORPHOLOGY AND ULTRASTRUCTURE

Rickettsiae are pleomorphic rod-shaped to coccoid organisms that range in size from 0.3 to 0.6 μm in width to 0.8 to 2.0 μm in length. They stain poorly with gram stain but can be

[*]*Zinsser, H:* Rats, Lice and History. *Little, Brown and Company, 1935.*

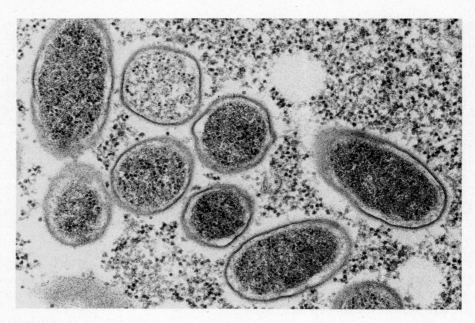

FIG. 57-1. *Rickettsia rickettsii,* the causative agent of Rocky Mountain spotted fever, in ovarian tissue of *Dermacentor andersoni.* ×66,000. (Courtesy of Dr. Lyle Brinton, Rocky Mountain Laboratory, USPHS, Hamilton, Montana)

visualized using both the Giemsa and Macchiavello methods. With the Gimenez modification of the Macchiavello method the organisms stain pink or red with carbolfuchsin and are visualized by counterstaining with malachite green.

The ultrastructure and chemical composition of rickettsiae resemble that of gram-negative bacteria. A characteristic three-layered cell wall, a trilaminar plasma membrane, and nuclear material have been observed by electron microscopy (Fig. 57-1). Ribosomelike particles and intracytoplasmic organelles have been observed in the granular cytoplasm, and in *R. prowazekii* an amorphous capsule surrounding the organism has been detected.

PHYSIOLOGY

Biochemistry Rickettsiae possess both RNA and DNA, have respiratory and synthetic capabilities independent of the cell, and divide by binary fission. The optimum temperature for growth is 32 to 35C. Pyruvate is the major energy source for *Coxiella,* whereas members of the genus *Rickettsia* utilize glutamate as their major carbon and energy source. Rickettsiae possess enzymatic mechanisms for the breakdown of carbohydrates, the formation of high-energy phosphate bonds, and the synthesis of lipids and proteins. Studies of DNA base composition have indicated wide differences in the G + C content of *Coxiella* and the typhus, spotted fever, and scrub typhus groups, although marked similarities exist among species of the same group.

Cultural Characteristics Except for *R. quintana* all rickettsiae require living cells for growth. They can be propagated in embryonated eggs, tissue culture, laboratory animals (guinea pigs, mice, meadow voles), and in certain arthropods. Because of the dangers of infection of laboratory personnel, cultural procedures should only be undertaken in specially equipped facilities.

Species differ in the location of intracellular multiplication both in vitro and in vivo. For example (with the exception of *Rickettsia canada*) both typhus group rickettsiae and *C. burnetii* characteristically grow only in the cytoplasm of infected cells, whereas spotted fever group organisms grow both in the cytoplasm and in nuclei. *R. quintana,* the agent of trench fever, is unique among the *Rickettsieae* in that it grows extracellularly in its arthropod vector (lice) and can be grown in vitro on cell-free media.

Resistance Members of the genus *Rickettsia* are unstable extracellularly under ordinary environmental conditions, and careful technique is required in the successful isolation of the organisms from body fluids and tissue. In contrast, *C. burnetii* is very resistant to heat and drying, a characteristic that is important to an understanding of its ecology and epidemiology. Rickettsiae remain viable for long periods when stored at −70C or lyophilized from appropriate media.

ANTIGENIC STRUCTURE

Differences in the antigenic composition of the rickettsiae have made possible their classification into genera, groups, and species. There is no common antigen for all members of the family Rickettsiaceae or for the tribe that contains the three genera of medical interest: *Rickettsia, Rochalimaea,* and *Coxiella.* Antigenically they are completely unrelated.

Two major kinds of antigens have been detected in rickettsiae: (1) the group-specific antigens that are soluble in ether and that represent stripped-off capsular material and (2) the type-specific antigens that are associated with the cell wall and that delineate species and the strains within a species. On the basis of antigenic analysis and the biologic properties discussed above, a single species comprises the genera *Rochalimaea* and *Coxiella: Rochalimaea quintana* (agent of trench fever) and *C. burnetii* (the agent of Q fever). Strains comprising the genus *Rickettsia* fall into three distinct groups or biotypes: typhus, spotted fever, and scrub typhus. Antigenic differences have permitted further speciation within the first two groups. Additional methods of separating various biotypes include cross-protection and toxin neutralization tests in laboratory animals and, more recently, DNA base ratio analyses.

Phase variation analogous to S → R variation in other bacteria has been observed in *C. burnetii* but in none of the other rickettsiae. Organisms isolated from natural infections of man and animals are in phase I, but repeated passage in the yolk sac elicits the emergence of phase II and changes in its antigenic makeup. Phase I can usually be re-established by passage in a laboratory animal. Phase I activity is attributable to a surface polysaccharide which is much more potent than phase II as an immunogen.

Serologic Diagnosis

Specific antibodies develop in response to rickettsial infection, and demonstration of an immune response during convalescence is the most widely used method of laboratory diagnosis. Complement-fixation antibodies are useful in identifying infection due to rickettsiae in different genera and groups. Cross-reactions of antibody with antigens of the same group occur. For example, complement-fixing cross-reactions occur between different members of the spotted fever group. However, this problem can be largely circumvented by using highly purified reagents and epidemiologic and clinical information. Microagglutination and fluorescent antibody tests have been developed, but they have not yet achieved widespread use in this country.

Weil-Felix Reaction Antibodies cross-reacting with certain strains of *Proteus vulgaris* (OX19 and OX2) or *Proteus mirabilis* (OXK) develop after certain rickettsial infections. This test, the Weil-Felix reaction, is based on cross-reactions between antirickettsial antibodies and *Proteus* polysaccharide O antigens. The test is inexpensive, widely available, and may provide an earlier clue to certain rickettsial infections than more specific complement-fixation tests. However, since a rise in Weil-Felix antibody titer may occur following *Proteus* infections (eg, urinary tract infections, bacteremia) and since some rickettsial diseases, such as rickettsialpox and Q fever, are not associated with Weil-Felix antibody rises and others, such as Rocky Mountain spotted fever, inconsistently elicit Weil-Felix agglutinins, caution should be exercised in interpreting either positive or negative tests.

DETERMINANTS OF PATHOGENICITY

In rickettsial diseases the microscopic pathology is characteristic. Multiplication of the organisms in the endothelial cells lining the small blood vessels causes endothelial proliferation and perivascular infiltration, resulting in leakage and thrombosis. Chick embryos, tissue cultures, and small laboratory animals have been successfully used as experimental models and have provided useful information on the penetration and multiplication of rickettsiae in host cells. Little is known, however, on how the organisms damage the host cell.

Only viable rickettsiae are capable of penetrating host cells. Organisms inactivated by heat, formalin, or UV irradiation lose their infectivity for mice. Unlike pathogenic bacteria, penetration by rickettsiae is an active process, requiring the expenditure of energy by the organism. Once inside the host cell the rickettsiae cause little detectable damage to the parasitized cell until the cell ruptures. However, when large numbers of viable rickettsiae are injected into a mouse the animal dies of acute toxemia within eight hours. This effect can be blocked by the administration of type-specific antibody but not by the antirickettsial drugs tetracycline or chloramphenicol. In order to be effective the immune serum must be administered before infection, suggesting that the attachment of the toxin to its primary binding site of action occurs very rapidly. The isolation and chemical characterization of a toxin from rickettsiae has not been accomplished, but there is evidence that at least one component possesses endotoxic activity. In addition, the typhus fever rickettsiae are capable of hemolyzing erythrocytes of several animal species. This hemolytic activity is correlated with infectivity of the rickettsiae and with their metabolic activity. The role, however, of toxic and hemolytic activities in human rickettsial disease remains conjectural.

Different isolates of the same rickettsial species may be shown to vary in virulence using a variety of in vitro systems. Over 40 years ago, Spencer and Parker showed that if ticks infected with a virulent strain of R. rickettsii are refrigerated for several months, they lose their virulence for guinea pigs, although they immunize the animal against challenge with a virulent strain. This phenomenon is not due to a difference in the number of rickettsiae in the tick or to a spontaneous mutation. Despite refrigeration, R. rickettsii retains its virulence for chick embryos, and a single egg passage re-establishes virulence for the guinea pig. Results of studies of Rocky Mountain spotted fever in monkeys suggest that the duration of the incubation period and severity of the disease may be related to the size of the inoculum of R. rickettsii.

There is not a satisfactory animal model that correlates consistently with virulence for humans. The mechanism of variations in virulence in naturally occurring human infections has been incompletely studied.

HOST DEFENSES

The relative importance of various host defense mechanisms in human beings with rickettsial infection is uncertain. Delayed hypersensitivity to typhus group antigens develops after human R. prowazekii infection, and lymphocyte-mediated hypersensitivity also can be demonstrated after vaccination or infection with C. burnetii. Lymphocytes collected from humans previously infected with R. rickettsii undergo blast transformation after in vitro exposure to spotted fever group antigens. Recent studies by Gambrel and Wesseman have shown that an interaction between humoral antibody (opsonins) and macrophages is required for effective killing of R. typhi in tissue culture systems.

CLINICAL INFECTION

Among the diverse clinical illnesses produced by rickettsiae are primary pneumonia (Q fever), fulminant vasculitis (Rocky Mountain spotted fever), a febrile illness associated with a vesicular rash (rickettsialpox), asymptomatic infection (trench fever), a recrudescent infection appearing many years after primary infection (Brill-Zinsser's disease), and endocarditis (Q fever).

Endothelial damage secondary to angiitis is a common finding in rickettsial infections, particularly in those due to spotted fever and typhus group organisms.

The Spotted Fever Group

The basic pathologic findings in severe spotted fever infections are proliferative and thrombotic lesions in small vessels, leading to microhemorrhages and in some cases areas of necrosis. A number of different organs and organ systems may be damaged by this general-

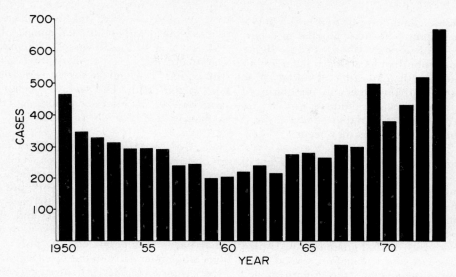

FIG. 57-2. Rocky mountain spotted fever. Reported cases by year, United States, 1950-1973. (From Morbidity and Mortality. CDC Weekly Report 23[53]:51, 1975)

ized infectious vasculitis, including the brain and myocardium.

Rocky Mountain Spotted Fever (American Spotted Fever, Tickborne Typhus) EPIDEMIOLOGY. *Prevalence.* Rocky Mountain spotted fever has been recognized as a distinct clinical entity for more than 70 years. Over 750 cases of RMSF in the United States were reported to the Center for Disease Control during 1974, and many other cases undoubtedly were either not reported or not diagnosed (Fig. 57-2). RMSF accounts for over 90 percent of the reported rickettsial disease in man in the United States. Cases have been reported from all except a few states, although over three-fourths of the reported cases in the past 10 years have been from the southeastern region of the country (Fig. 57-3).

Most cases of Rocky Mountain spotted fever in the eastern and southern United States occur in children and adolescents, whereas adult

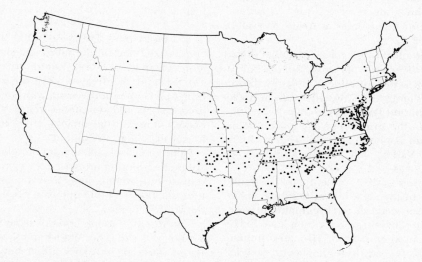

FIG. 57-3. Rocky mountain spotted fever. Reported cases by county, United States, 1973. (From Morbidity and Mortality. CDC Weekly Report 23[53]:51, 1975)

men are more commonly affected in the Rocky Mountain region. The peak months of occurrence are April through August. People living in rural and suburban locations are at a higher risk of infection than are urban dwellers. With increasing suburbanization and popularity of outdoor recreational activities, further increases in the incidence of spotted fever as well as other tickborne diseases may occur.

Ecology. R. *rickettsii*, the etiologic agent of RMSF, is cycled in nature through ticks, small rodents, and larger wild and domestic animals. Man is only accidentally infected. The ecology and epidemiology of spotted fever is directly related to the life cycle of four species of Ixodid (hard) ticks which are indigenous to the United States: the Rocky Mountain wood tick (*Dermacentor andersoni*), the American dog tick (*Dermacentor variabilis*), the Lone Star tick (*Amblyomma americanum*), and the rabbit tick (*Haemaphysalis leporispalustris*). *D. andersoni* is the major vector in the Rocky Mountain region, whereas the American dog tick is the major vector in the eastern and southeastern United States. The rabbit tick is found throughout the continental United States and rarely attaches to man but is thought to be important in maintaining a reservoir of infection in nature.

Ixodid ticks pass through four stages in their life cycle and can become infested by feeding on a rickettsemic animal; these ticks may in turn pass their infection to their progeny transovarially. Thus, infected ticks function both as a reservoir and as a vector of Rocky Mountain spotted fever.

A number of authors have speculated that strains of R. *rickettsii* vary in virulence. For instance, prior to the introduction of specific antimicrobial therapy, the mortality rate of Rocky Mountain spotted fever was known to be 70 to 80 percent in the Bitterroot Valley of Montana, but less than 5 percent in the nearby Idaho Snake River Valley.

Transmission. Most patients with spotted fever give a history of a recent tick bite. Infection may also occur through contamination of fingers while removing ticks which have fed on animals or another person. Human-to-human transmission of disease does not occur. Acquisition of infection by laboratory workers handling R. *rickettsii* is a well-known phenomenon.

PATHOGENESIS. R. *rickettsii* infection produces widespread endothelial damage, leading to occlusion of small vessels, microthrombi, microhemorrhages, secondary fluid and electrolyte changes, and in severe cases necrosis, shock, and death. The precise mechanism by which rickettsial infection produces endothelial damage is still largely unknown.

CLINICAL MANIFESTATIONS. The incubation period ranges from 3 to 12 days. The disease typically begins abruptly with headache, fever, and malaise. Chills may occur, and diffuse myalgias are common. Usually the rash appears two to four days after the onset and, in many cases, first appears on the ankles and wrists and then becomes generalized. The rash is usually maculopapular early in the disease but may later become petechial or hemorrhagic. Involvement of the palms and soles is common.

Gastrointestinal complaints, arthralgias, conjunctivitis, stiff neck, and periorbital edema are present in some cases. Splenomegaly is detected in approximately 25 percent of cases. Hyponatremia and thrombocytopenia are common, and overt disseminated intravascular coagulation syndrome may also occur.

Reported fatality rates have declined from approximately 20 percent in the 1940s to 5 to 10 percent in the past few years. Factors that increase the chance of a fatal outcome are increasing age, increasing length of time from onset to institution of effective chemotherapy, and, perhaps, virulence of the infecting organisms.

LABORATORY DIAGNOSIS. It should be emphasized that the initial diagnosis and treatment of spotted fever should be on clinical grounds and not delayed until laboratory confirmation is obtained. An appropriate constellation of signs and symptoms in a patient with a history of recent tick attachment is enough justification to begin treatment.

Isolation of rickettsiae from blood is possible, although isolation attempts are expensive and require trained personnel and specialized facilities that are available in only a few locations in the United States.

Confirmation of infection is usually based on serologic tests. The Weil-Felix test depends upon antigenic cross-reactions between antirickettsial antibodies and polysaccharide antigens from various strains of P. *vulgaris*. *Proteus* OX2 and/or OX19 agglutinins usually appear five to eight days after infection with *R. rickettsii*. A fourfold antibody rise is suggestive of recent infection. Type-specific complement-fixation tests (available through most state health departments) may not become positive until two to three weeks after onset. Paired sera should be tested in order to demonstrate a significant (fourfold) antibody rise. Either one or both serologic tests may remain negative in a small percentage of clinically diagnosed cases. It has been suggested that antibiotic treatment may blunt the complement-fixation or Weil-Felix antibody response.

Microagglutination, indirect hemagglutination, and fluorescent antibody tests have been developed but are not yet widely used in this country. Rickettsial mouse toxin neutralization tests and tests to detect erythrocyte-sensitizing substance have been described but require specialized laboratories and remain experimental tools.

Lymphocyte blast transformation occurs when lymphocytes from patients with Rocky Mountain spotted fever are exposed to killed *R. rickettsii* in vitro. The relative importance of different mechanisms of immunity (cell-mediated and humoral) in recovery from *R. rickettsii* infection is unknown.

TREATMENT. Tetracycline and chloramphenicol are both effective in the treatment of Rocky Mountain spotted fever. Tetracycline is safer and probably more widely used as treatment than chloramphenicol. However, the latter drug may be especially useful in treating severe cases in which differentiation from meningococcal infection may be difficult.

PREVENTION. Rocky Mountain spotted fever is much easier to treat than to prevent. Traditional measures of vector control are generally not practical. Protective clothing such as boots, leggings, and tightly buttoned shirts may be helpful in preventing tick attachment in persons exposed to heavily infested environments.

Individuals who are exposed to ticks and tick-infested environments should inspect their bodies regularly and remove attached ticks carefully. Experimental studies have shown that a poorly understood period of reactivation is required from the time an infected tick attaches and begins feeding until it transmits infection. Therefore, ticks removed within several hours of attachment may not transmit rickettsiae. When removing ticks, forceps and gentle traction are recommended. Alternately, the tick can be removed using paper or cloth to protect the fingers. Care should be used during removal to prevent crushing the tick and thereby contaminating the fingers, since both infected tick tissues and tick feces have been demonstrated experimentally to be capable of transmitting infection.

A vaccine is commercially available. Studies in human volunteers, however, have shown that killed vaccines are not completely effective in preventing spotted fever in man. There is little or no correlation between the presence of antibodies in serum and protection in volunteers given Rocky Mountain spotted fever vaccine. However, the incubation period is prolonged in subjects given vaccine and then exposed to virulent rickettsiae. The United States Public Health Service recommends that vaccine only be given to laboratory personnel working in the field of rickettsiology or to selected individuals who have unusual occupational exposure to ticks.

In geographic areas where the disease occurs frequently, both the public and physicians should be educated and periodically reminded of the signs, symptoms, and epidemiologic features of the disease.

Rickettsialpox Rickettsialpox is characterized by a local eschar, a papulovesicular rash, and a benign clinical course. It is caused by *Rickettsia akari*, a member of the spotted fever group that cross-reacts serologically with *R. rickettsii*.

EPIDEMIOLOGY. Rickettsialpox was first recognized in New York City in 1946. Since then, cases have been recognized in Boston, Cleveland, and Philadelphia. However, it is possible that the true distribution of rickettsialpox in the United States is wider, since the vector of the disease (*Allodermanyssus sanguineus*) is found throughout a large part of the country. Since the disease is typically mild and not usually reported to health departments, exact morbidity figures are not available.

An organism identical to *R. akari* has been isolated in urban areas in the Russian Ukraine, where the epidemiology and clinical features of the disease appear to be similar to rickettsialpox in the United States. *R. akari* has also been isolated from a wild Korean rodent (*Microtus fortis pelliccus*), which implies that there may also be a rural cycle of rickettsialpox in Korea.

Ecology. R. *akari* infects the mouse mite (*A. sanguineus*), which in turn is an ectoparasite of the common house mouse. The mite infects its progeny transovarially. As in several other rickettsial diseases, man only enters this cycle of infection accidentally. This is more apt to occur when the rodent population is initially reduced by vermin control programs. When murine hosts are scarce, *A. sanguineus* may feed on man and thus transmit disease. Most reported cases of rickettsialpox have been from urban areas where density of the murine mites and men is probably higher than in rural areas.

PATHOGENESIS.   Very little is known concerning the pathogenesis of R. *akari* infection. However, microscopically the maculopapular rash in rickettsialpox shows a mononuclear perivascular infiltrate and necrosis of epithelial cells resulting in intraepidermal vesicles.

CLINICAL MANIFESTATIONS.   The clinical hallmarks of rickettsialpox are a vesicular rash and a local eschar which is often associated with regional lymphadenopathy. The incubation period is not precisely known, since patients typically are unaware of receiving a mite bite. The first sign of disease is a local erythematous papule that evolves first into a vesicle and then into an eschar. Approximately three to seven days after the appearance of the eschar, chills and fever begin abruptly and may be associated with headache, malaise, and myalgia. Within 72 hours of the appearance of fever, a generalized maculopapular rash becomes apparent and soon evolves into a vesicular eruption. Differentiation of the rash of rickettsialpox from chickenpox is important and is based upon the fact that the rash of rickettsialpox occurs more often in adults and is associated with a primary eschar, and the cutaneous vesicles are surrounded by a papular ring. In contrast, the rash of chickenpox occurs most often in children, is entirely vesicular, and there is no primary lesion. Smallpox also does not have a primary eschar, is associated with an eruption that evolves into pustular lesions, and usually is a much more severe illness.

No fatalities due to rickettsialpox have been reported. Although a small scar may occur at the site of the primary lesion, the vesiculopapular eruption heals without scarring.

LABORATORY DIAGNOSIS.   Weil-Felix antibodies do not appear after infection with R. *akari*. However, complement-fixing antibodies can be measured one to two months after the onset of illness.

R. *akari* can be isolated from both the blood and the fluid from vesicular lesions of infected persons. Such isolations require the technical facilities of specially equipped laboratories and are accomplished by the inoculation of infected specimens into laboratory animals or embryonated hens' eggs.

TREATMENT AND PREVENTION.   Both tetracycline and chloramphenicol produce rapid defervescence and clinical improvement.

Measures aimed at controlling both rodent populations and their mite ectoparasites will prevent transmission of R. *akari* to man.

Other Tickborne Diseases   Other species of *Rickettsia* cause eastern hemisphere tickborne diseases that in many respects resemble Rocky Mountain spotted fever. *Rickettsia sibirica*, the agent of North Asian rickettsiosis, *Rickettsia australis*, the agent of Queensland tick typhus, and *Rickettsia conorii*, the agent of boutonneuse fever, are very similar to one another but, by the use of cross-immunity and mouse-toxin neutralization tests, can be shown to be separate organisms. North Asian tickborne rickettsiosis occurs in central Asia, Mongolia, and the Siberian region of the USSR; Queensland tick typhus occurs in Australia; and boutonneuse fever occurs in the Mediterranean region, Africa, and India. Boutonneuse fever has also been called "South African tick bite fever," "Kenya tick typhus," and "Indian tick typhus."

All three rickettsiae are maintained in nature in both Ixodid ticks and wild animals. Man only accidentally enters this natural cycle of infection and is not important in the maintenance of the rickettsiae in nature.

Diseases caused by these rickettsiae are characterized by local eschars or skin lesions at the site of tick attachment. All three produce diseases that are typically milder than Rocky Mountain spotted fever, although they have some of the same symptoms, namely, fever, headache, myalgia, malaise, and maculopapular eruptions that may become petechial.

Infection with any of the three rickettsiae is followed by the production of group-specific complement-fixing antibodies and inconstantly by *Proteus* OX19 or OX2 agglutinating antibodies. Type-specific complement-fixing antibodies can be measured after infection, although some serologic cross-reactivity with other members of the spotted fever group occurs. All three rickettsiae are sensitive to both chloramphenicol and tetracycline.

Rickettsia not Associated with Human Disease *Rickettsia parkeri* and *Rickettsia montana* are species serologically related to the spotted fever group but whose disease potentiality in humans is currently unknown. In 1939 Parker and his co-workers reported the isolation of a rickettsia form Gulf Coast ticks (*Amblyomma maculatum*) removed from cattle in eastern Texas. Isolations of this rickettsia were also made from the same tick species in Mississippi and Georgia. The name maculatum disease was given to the syndrome produced by experimental inoculation of guinea pigs, and the causal rickettsia was called the maculatum agent. In 1965, following extensive laboratory characterization of the organism, the name *R. parkeri* was proposed in honor of R.R. Parker, one of the founders of the Rocky Mountain Laboratory.

The name *R. montana* has been proposed for a rickettsia isolated by Bell and co-workers from ticks in eastern Montana. This organism is nonpathogenic in guinea pigs, and it can be distinguished from other members of the spotted fever group using serologic techniques.

The Typhus Group

These rickettsiae cause epidemic typhus (and its recrudescent infection, Brill-Zinsser disease) and murine typhus. Typhus group organisms are characterized by intracytoplasmic growth and a common, soluble, group-specific, complement-fixing antigen.

Epidemic Typhus (European Louseborne Typhus) Epidemic typhus, a louseborne disease caused by *R. prowazekii* (named after a Polish investigator, von Prowazek, who died of typhus contracted in the course of his studies), has had a great impact upon the history of man. According to Zinsser, Napoleon's retreat from Moscow "was started by a louse." In World War I, typhus was responsible for the death of over 150,000 Serbians and over 3,000,000 Russians and caused nonfatal illness in many additional millions.

EPIDEMIOLOGY. Epidemic typhus is worldwide in occurrence, but epidemics have disappeared in areas with high standards of living. In the United States, *R. prowazekii* infection occasionally occurs in its recrudescent form (Brill-Zinsser disease).

Ecology and Transmission. *R. prowazekii*, the etiologic agent of epidemic typhus, can infect both the human body louse (*Pediculus humanus corporis*) and the head louse (*Pediculus humanus capitis*), the former being the more significant vector. The body louse naturally feeds only on man, and all three stages of its life cycle (egg, nymph, and adult) can occur on the same host. Lice become infected after taking a blood meal from a rickettsemic human being. Several days later the ingested rickettsiae have multiplied sufficiently in the louse, and infective rickettsiae appear in the arthropod's feces. If the louse encounters a susceptible human being at this point, transmission of *R. prowazekii* may occur.

During each blood meal the louse defecates. The feeding process is irritating, and scratching by the host produces minor excoriations that function as portals of entry for the rickettsiae in the louse feces. Lice do not transmit *R. prowazekii* to their progeny but succumb to their infection within one to three weeks.

Since louse-man-louse transmission thrives under conditions in which individuals wear the same clothes repeatedly in crowded environments, it is not surprising that major epidemics have occurred in association with wars, poverty, and famines.

Persons in cold climates are more likely to acquire typhus infections, since they may be forced by poverty or unusually hard circumstances to wear the same clothes for long periods of time. Lice actively seek out locations where the temperature is approximately 20C, a temperature often found in the folds of clothing. Lice will abandon a host with a body temperature of 40C or greater as well as the body of a dead person.

CLINICAL MANIFESTATIONS. The incubation period typically ranges from 10 to 14 days. Prodromal symptoms of headache, malaise, and minimal temperature elevations sometimes occur, but usually the onset is abrupt, with generalized myalgias, chills, or chilliness, fever, and headache. Headache is characteristically frontal, severe, and unremitting. Other less specific symptoms are often present, including gastrointestinal complaints, weakness, and cough. Splenomegaly may be present, as may meningismus. The spinal fluid is typically normal.

A skin rash usually occurs from four to seven days after the onset of illness. It may first appear as a patchy cutaneous erythema and progress to maculopapular, petechial, or hemorrhagic forms. In contrast to Rocky Moutain spotted fever, the rash in typhus usually spares the palms, soles, and face and characteristically appears first on the trunk and later spreads to the extremities.

A wide variety of complications may occur in severe cases, including mental changes (stupor and delirium), hypotension, oliguria and azotemia, and even gangrene of the skin, genitalia, and digits.

Untreated, the disease may last up to three weeks. Mortality has varied from 10 to 40 percent in different outbreaks. Case fatality ratios have been shown to increase with increasing age. Survivors of epidemic typhus are generally immune for years following their primary infection, although mild recurrences of illness (Brill-Zinsser Disease) may occur years later.

LABORATORY DIAGNOSIS.   Once a clinical diagnosis is made, treatment should be instituted prior to laboratory confirmation. Substantiation of a clinical diagnosis can be obtained either by isolation of *R. prowazekii* or by serologic means. The former is difficult, potentially dangerous, expensive, and involves specialized personnel and equipment.

As in Rocky Mountain spotted fever, patients convalescent from typhus produce antibodies that agglutinate *Proteus vulgaris* OX polysaccharide antigens. These agglutinins usually appear in the second week after onset. Generally, agglutination is maximal with OX19 strains, although strongly positive reactions with OX2 antigens sometimes occur. Serial serum specimens should be tested rather than a single convalescent sample. A fourfold rise in agglutinating titer is suggestive of recent infection.

Antibodies against group-specific complement-fixing antigens (prepared from yolk sac-grown rickettsiae) typically appear in the third week after onset. Microagglutination and fluorescent antibody tests are also available through specialized laboratories.

TREATMENT.   Both chloramphenicol and tetracycline produce prompt defervescence and clinical improvement when given early in the course of the illness. Patients who develop circulatory and renal complications before receiving either tetracycline or chloramphenicol may die despite therapy.

PREVENTION AND CONTROL.   It is possible to rapidly and effectively interrupt epidemic louse-man-louse transmission of *R. prowazekii* by mass application of insecticides to human beings and their clothing. Once free of lice, patients with typhus are not infectious. Typhus vaccine prepared from infected yolk sacs is also an infective control measure. Vaccine lessens the severity and shortens the course of clinical disease.

Brill-Zinsser Disease Individuals who have previously had epidemic typhus may develop recrudescent infection many years later. This illness was named after Nathan Brill, who first recognized and described the clinical features, and Hans Zinsser, who first suggested in 1934 that the disease was a relapse of a prior epidemic typhus infection. A large amount of epidemiologic, clinical, and experimental evidence has since been published that confirms Zinsser's hypothesis.

EPIDEMIOLOGY.   In this country, recrudescent typhus occurs primarily in immigrants from previously endemic areas, such as eastern Europe. The disease may occur in an individual living in a lice-free environment, and many years may have passed since the patient's initial infection with *R. prowazekii*. However, lice that feed on a patient with recrudescent typhus can become infected, and if local conditions are right for louse-man-louse transmission, an outbreak of epidemic typhus may occur. Thus, latent human infection represents an interepidemic reservoir for epidemic typhus.

CLINICAL   MANIFESTATIONS.   Brill-Zinsser disease usually is a milder illness than classic epidemic typhus; a skin rash is often absent and the duration of disease is shorter (less than two weeks). Fever may be erratic instead of sustained. As in epidemic typhus and other rickettsial diseases, headache, malaise, and myalgias are common symptoms. Complications and fatalities are rare.

LABORATORY DIAGNOSIS. In this country, the clinical diagnosis of Brill-Zinsser Disease should be suspected when fever of obscure origin occurs in a foreign-born person who has previously resided in an area where epidemic typhus occurred and who complains of an intense headache and develops a maculopapular skin rash on the fourth to sixth day of his illness.

Weil-Felix agglutinins often do not develop in patients with Brill-Zinsser disease. As a general rule, the sooner recrudescent infection occurs after primary infection, the *less* likely are Weil-Felix antibodies to be present.

Complement-fixing antibodies are found in the second week after onset, which is earlier than in patients with epidemic typhus. Since some typhus patients may have detectable complement-fixing antibodies many years after primary infection, an isolated convalescent serum sample may yield confusing results. Therefore, a fourfold complement-fixing antibody rise should be sought in patients suspected of having recrudescent typhus.

Consistent with Zinsser's hypothesis, it has been found that patients with epidemic typhus initially have an IgM followed by an IgG antibody response, whereas patients with Brill-Zinsser disease initially have an anamnestic IgG antibody response.

The clinical history, epidemiologic setting, and dynamics of the antibody response are helpful in distinguishing among epidemic typhus, recrudescent typhus, and murine typhus.

TREATMENT AND PREVENTION. As in epidemic typhus, tetracycline and chloramphenicol are both effective in treatment. The ultimate prevention of Brill-Zinsser disease necessarily is dependent upon the prevention of epidemic typhus. If recrudescent typhus occurs in an environment where lice rarely infest man (as in the United States), no special precautionary public health measures are required. In areas where the potential for louse-man-louse transmission is high, delousing of both the patient and his contacts may be necessary to prevent an outbreak.

Murine Typhus (Endemic Typhus, Fleaborne Typhus, Rat Typhus) Murine typhus is a fleaborne illness caused by *R. typhi*, a member of the typhus group that is very similar to *R. prowazekii*. Typically, murine typhus is a mild illness characterized by fever, headache, and often by a generalized skin rash.

EPIDEMIOLOGY. *Prevalence.* Murine typhus is endemic in many countries, including the United States, where it occurs primarily in the Southeast and Gulf Coast region. During an investigation of murine typhus in Alabama and Florida over 40 years ago, Maxcy found that most cases occurred in individuals who worked in rat-infested shipyards and harbors. Cases have also more recently been reported from inland rural locations, presumably because infected rats and mice may occur in large numbers in areas where grains and feeds are stored. In the past decade, over half of all reported cases in the United States have occurred in Texas.

Although murine typhus is a reportable disease in the United States, considerable numbers of cases may be neither diagnosed nor reported. Despite this problem, it appears that the incidence of murine typhus has gradually decreased in the past two decades (Fig. 57-4).

Ecology. *R. typhi* is cycled in nature by the rat and two of its ectoparasites, the rat flea (*Xenopsylla cheopis*), and the rat louse (*Polyplax spinulosus*). The former is the more important vector. As in Rocky Mountain spotted fever, man only enters this arthropod-vertebrate-arthropod cycle accidently. *X. cheopis* acquires infection with *R. typhi* by feeding upon a rickettsemic mouse or rat. Once infected, the flea may infect other susceptible rodents, and thus a natural cycle or flea-rodent-flea infection may become established. Rodents infected with *R. typhi* do not succumb to their infection, despite the fact that viable rickettsia can be demonstrated in their brains for periods up to several months. Fleas do not transmit *R. typhi* transovarially.

Transmission. Transmission of *R. typhi* to man occasionally occurs. When infected fleas taking a blood meal defecate on the host, the host rubs the infected feces into small excoriations during scratching. Flea feces are also

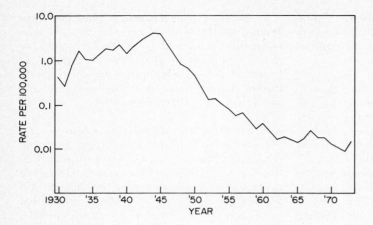

FIG. 57-4. Fleaborne (endemic, murine) typhus fever. Reported cases in the United States per 100,000 population. (From Morbidity and Mortality. CDC Weekly Report 23[53]:59, 1975)

infective if accidently transmitted to mucosal surfaces, such as the conjunctiva.

CLINICAL MANIFESTATIONS. Murine typhus is usually a mild illness with a mortality rate of less than 2 percent. The incubation period ranges from one to two weeks. The hallmarks of the disease are abrupt onset of fever, headache, malaise, and myalgias, and in most cases, a macular to maculopapular, nonpruritic skin rash that begins on the third to fifth day on the trunk and spreads to the extremities. As in epidemic typhus, involvement of the palms, soles, and face is rare. The rash may be fleeting or absent in some cases and may be inapparent in Blacks without careful inspection. Chills or chilliness, cough, nausea, vomiting, arthralgias, weakness, and extreme prostration may be associated symptoms. Untreated, the illness may last up to two weeks. Defervescence may occur by either abrupt crises or gradual lysis.

Fatalities are more likely to occur in the old and infirm. Such fatal cases may be heralded by peripheral vascular collapse and evidence of central nervous system involvement, such as stupor and coma.

Confusion between murine typhus and Rocky Mountain spotted fever may occur in this country, since both diseases are associated with rising titers against *Proteus* OX19 (and sometimes OX2) antigens. Spotted fever is usually a more severe illness and is often associated with an antecedent tick bite. The rash of murine typhus begins first on the trunk and spreads to the extremities, while the opposite evolution occurs in Rocky Mountain spotted fever. Since precise information on the evolution of the rash is often unavailable, this differ-

ential point is often not of use. Complement-fixation tests may be necessary to separate the two illnesses. In older, immigrant patients confusion between murine typhus and Brill-Zinsser disease may also occur (p. 732).

LABORATORY DIAGNOSIS. Agglutinins to *Proteus* OX19, and less commonly to OX2, appear in the second week of infection. Complement-fixing antibodies against *R. typhi* appear slightly later. With the complement-fixation test, serologic cross-reactions among members of the typhus group are common, but in patients with murine typhus much higher antibody titers are obtained with *R. typhi* than with *R. prowazekii*. The use of specific antigens in the complement-fixation test also permits differentiation of *R. typhi* and *R. prowazekii*. An indirect fluorescent antibody test using IgM and IgG fluorescent-labeled conjugates has been developed but has not been used extensively in this country.

Intraperitoneal inoculation of the patient's blood into a male guinea pig produces severe testicular lesions and scrotal swelling, in contrast to the very mild disease produced by the inoculation of blood from epidemic typhus patients.

TREATMENT AND PREVENTION. Both tetracycline and chloramphenicol are effective rickettsiostatic agents. Patients with laboratory-acquired murine typhus treated with chloramphenicol two to four days after onset have been shown by Wisseman et al to experience clinical relapses despite the presence of antirickettsial antibodies. These relapses responded to reinstitution of the same antimicrobials. Insecticides and rodenticides are both effective in reducing rat-flea-man transmission in endemic areas.

Rickettsia canada Infections *R. canada* was first isolated from rabbit ticks collected in Ontario, Canada, in 1967. Antigenically, *R. canada* belongs to the typhus group biotype. However, it grows in both the cytoplasm and the nuclei of infected cells, a characteristic of the spotted fever group.

The clinical spectrum of human infection with *R. canada* is still largely unknown. The organism has not yet been isolated from human sources. Bozeman and co-workers, however, have reported four patients with serologic evidence of *R. canada* infection who had symptoms typical of Rocky Mountain spotted fever. Bisno reported a similar case in which a patient with a clinical history consistent with spotted fever had a negative complement-fixation test using spotted fever group antigens but an antibody titer of 1:256 against *R. canada* antigen.

In complement-fixation tests, there are strong-cross reactions among *R. canada*, *R. prowazekii*, and *R. typhi* antigens. In experimental infections, *R. canada* produces fever but no scrotal reaction in guinea pigs.

Scrub Typhus (Chiggerborne Typhus) Tsutsugamushi Disease (Miteborne Typhus) Japanese River Fever, Rural Fever, Tropical Typhus

R. tsutsugamushi (also called *Rickettsia orientalis*) is actually a group of rickettsiae that produce one clinical illness in human beings despite the fact that different strains possess markedly different surface antigens. The name *tsutsugamushi* is derived from two Japanese words: *tsutsuga* (something small and dangerous) and *mushi* (creature). The appellation "scrub typhus" is derived from the fact that infection commonly occurs after exposure to terrain with secondary (scrub) vegetation in endemic areas. In the past several decades, it has been found that *R. tsutsugamushi* infection also occurs in a variety of habitats that cannot be described as scrub (including sandy beaches, mountain deserts, and equatorial rain forests). Therefore, Traub and Wisseman have suggested that scrub typhus is a misnomer and

that the term "chiggerborne typhus" is more descriptive.

Three major antigenic types of *R. tsutsugamushi* (Karp, Gilliam, and Kato) have been recognized.

EPIDEMIOLOGY. *Prevalence.* Chiggerborne typhus is endemic in a triangular geographic area of over 5,000,000 square miles, including Australia, Japan, Korea, India, and Vietnam. In World War II, it caused appreciable morbidity and mortality in both Japanese and American soldiers. In peacetime it occurs predominantly as a sporadic endemic illness. However, epidemics may occur when groups of people are brought into endemic mite-infested areas. Chiggerborne typhus occurred in sporadic form in United States troops in Vietnam.

Ecology. The vectors of chiggerborne typhus are several species of trombiculid mites. These mites have four-stage life cycles (egg, larva, nymph, and adult). The larva (chigger) is the only stage which feeds on vertebrates. After engorgement on a vertebrate host, chiggers detach and metamorphose into eight-legged nymphs, which in turn later develop into adults. The latter two stages are free living in the soil. Both transstadial (ie, from larva to nymph to adult) and transovarial (from adult to egg) transmission of *R. tsutsugamushi* occurs. Thus, similar to the role of several ixodid ticks in the ecology of Rocky Mountain spotted fever, trombiculid mites function as both vector and reservoir of chiggerborne rickettsiosis.

A natural cycle of *R. tsutsugamushi* transmission occurs between chiggers and small mammals (eg, field mice and rats) in endemic areas. Ground-feeding birds may also be important in the ecology of chiggerborne rickettsioses, especially as transporters of the disease agent over long distances. In chiggerborne typhus, as in rickettsialpox, Rocky Mountain spotted fever, and murine typhus, man only accidentally enters a natural cycle of rickettsial infection. Areas such as savannahs, forest clearings, riverbanks, grassy fields, and gardens may provide the proper conditions that allow infected mites to thrive and thus produce small focal geographic areas of high risk to human beings. Such mite-infested areas, which may be as small as a few meters in diameter, have been called "scrub typhus islands." Traub and Wisseman have suggested the term "zoonotic tetrad" to describe the coexistence and intimate relationship among *R. tsutsugamushi*, chiggers, rats, and secondary or transitional forms of vegetation. These four factors are essential components for the establishment of a microfocus of infection.

The seasonal incidence of the disease varies with the climate in different countries, occurring more frequently during the rainy season in the summer or fall.

Man-to-man transmission of infection does not occur.

CLINICAL MANIFESTATIONS.   Approximately one to three weeks after being bitten by an infected chigger, human beings develop, in an abrupt onset, chills, fever, and headache. Any or all of the following additional symptoms may also occur: cough, nausea, vomiting, myalgia, abdominal pain, and sore throat. The skin rash of scrub typhus is classically heralded by a local cutaneous lesion, which evolves from a small indurated or vesicular lesion into an ulcerated lesion present at the time of onset of symptoms when it is covered by a black scab (eschar). Lymphadenopathy may be prominent in the area proximal to the eschar. Five to eight days after the onset of fever, a macular or maculopapular eruption may appear on the trunk and later become generalized.

Although it is said that eschars are commonly found in Caucasians and less commonly in Asians, Berman et al found that only 46 percent of American servicemen in Vietnam with scrub typhus had an identifiable eschar and only 34 percent had a skin rash. Other signs sometimes found with scrub typhus include splenomegaly, conjunctivitis, and pharyngitis. During the first week of illness the pulse may be slow in relation to the amount of fever. In severe cases, deterioration in mental status (stupor, delirium), pneumonia, and/or circulatory failure may occur. Some patients may experience a second attack of scrub typhus, since infection with one strain of *R. tsutsugamushi* may not confer protection against another strain.

Fatality ratios in epidemics have varied from 0 to 50 percent. With prompt recognition and appropriate treatment, fatality rates are almost nil.

LABORATORY DIAGNOSIS.   Complement-fixation tests are of less value in the diagnosis of scrub typhus than in the diagnosis of infections due to rickettsiae of the spotted fever and typhus groups, since different strains have different surface antigens that do not cross-react with each other. Thus, if a complement-fixation test is to be used, a minimum of three different antigens (representing the Karp, Gilliam, and Kato strains) must be employed. Agglutinins to *Proteus* OXK antigens (but not OX2 and OX19) appear in the convalescent sera of many, but not all, patients with scrub typhus. These cross-reacting antibodies usually appear in the second week of illness, peak in the third to fourth weeks, and then disappear by about the fifth week after onset. As in other rickettsial serologic tests, paired sera should be collected in order to demonstrate a significant (fourfold) titer rise. A fluorescent antibody test employing pooled conjugates made from the three major strains of *R. tsutsugamushi* has also been a useful technique in some investigators' hands.

R. tsutsugamushi can be isolated by inoculating blood from patients into white mice.

TREATMENT.   As in other rickettsial diseases, both tetracycline and chloramphenicol are effective rickettsiostatic agents that usually produce prompt defervescence and clinical improvement. Relapses may occur when antibiotics are discontinued too quickly in patients treated within the first few days after onset. In patients first treated in their second week of illness, tetracycline or chloramphenicol can be discontinued one to two days after defervescence occurs. Fluorescent antibody levels are lower in those patients given early antibiotic treatment.

PREVENTION.   Because of strain variations, an effective scrub typhus vaccine has not been prepared. In endemic or hyperendemic areas, measures to prevent chigger bites (protective clothing, insect repellents) and to control mite populations (insecticides, clearing of vegetation, and chemical treatment of the soil) may be used to prevent chigger-man-chigger transmission.

Trench Fever (Shin Bone Fever, Five-day Fever, Quintana Fever)

Trench fever is caused by *Rochalimaea quintana* and is transmitted by the body louse (*Pediculus humanus corporis*) in a man-louse-man cycle of infection. *R. quintana* is the only rickettsia that can be grown on cell-free media.

Trench fever was first recognized in World War I as a five to six day febrile illness associated with pains in the shins and causing large epidemics in both German and Allied Armies. By the end of the war a wider spectrum of clinical illness and the louseborne transmission of infection had been recognized. The disease disappeared during the next two decades but reappeared in epidemic form in the armies on the Eastern Front during World War II. It has been rarely reported since 1945.

EPIDEMIOLOGY. Trench fever has been reported from England, France, Yugoslavia, Italy, Russia, Germany, and several other countries in eastern Europe. *R. quintana* has been isolated from lice in Mexico, an area where clinical trench fever has not yet been recognized.

Ecology. The body louse acquires infection by feeding on a rickettsemic human being. Once infected, the louse excretes *R. quintana* in its feces for the remainder of its life, which is not shortened by the rickettsial infection. Unlike all other members of the tribe Rickettsieae, *R. quintana* proliferates in an extracellular environment in the arthropod host, in the lumen of the gut rather than within the intestinal epithelial cells. Transovarial transmission of *R. quintana* to the louse's offspring does not occur.

No animal reservoir other than man has been identified, and man appears to be the principal reservoir of infection. Thus, like epidemic typhus, a louse-man-louse cycle of infection occurs. Little is known about the prevalence and distribution of *R. quintana* in nonepidemic intervals. *R. quintana* has been isolated from apparently healthy patients years after their original attack.

CLINICAL MANIFESTATIONS. The incubation period of trench fever in volunteers given intradermal inoculations of *R. quintana* ranges from 8 to 18 days. The clinical manifestations of the disease are highly variable and range from a mild afebrile disease to a moderately severe febrile disease with multiple relapses. The onset may be gradual or abrupt. Symptoms of acute disease include headache, malaise, fever,

chilliness, myalgias, and bone pain (especially in the tibial region). Fever curves vary widely among different patients. A macular rash resembling the rose spots of typhoid fever may occur.

LABORATORY DIAGNOSIS. Laboratory animals, such as guinea pigs, rabbits, or mice, are not suitable for the isolation of *R. quintana*, although they are in most rickettsioses. Instead, either xenodiagnosis (the feeding of uninfected lice on an infected patient and the later demonstration of rickettsia in the louse tissue) or primary isolation on enriched blood agar media are used for diagnosis. Like other members of the tribe Rickettsieae, the organism can also be grown in yolk sacs of embryonated hens' eggs. Complement-fixation and indirect immunofluorescent antibody tests have been developed and appear to be promising clinical and epidemiologic tools.

TREATMENT. Data on the efficacy of tetracycline and chloramphenicol in the treatment of trench fever are not available. Based, however, on in vitro sensitivity testing and the universal susceptibility of other Rickettsieae to these agents, both drugs are likely to be effective.

PREVENTION AND CONTROL. Measures to control human lice infestation will control the transmission of both tranch fever and epidemic typhus.

Q Fever

The name Q fever (the Q is short for "query") was first used in 1937 to describe an unusual febrile illness in Australian packinghouse workers. The causal agent, isolated from several of the affected workers, was identified as a rickettsia several years later by Burnet and Freeman. At about the same time, Davis and Cox identified the same organism in wood ticks collected in Montana. Cox, an American, and Burnet, an Australian, were honored for their early contributions by the selection of the name *Coxiella burnetii* for the etiologic agent of Q fever. Along with trench fever and epidemic typhus, Q fever caused epidemics in the armies fighting in Europe in World War II. In the past three decades, *C. burnetii* has been shown to have a worldwide distribution and a complex ecology and epidemiology.

EPIDEMIOLOGY. *Prevalence.* Exact morbidity figures on the incidence of Q fever are not available, although surveys have shown that many people throughout the world have serologic evidence of past infection with *C. burnetii*. In such surveys, the incidence of positive serologic tests far exceeds the incidence of clinical Q fever. The disease has been recognized in over 50 countries on 5 continents. In the United States outbreaks of Q fever, all associated with livestock or livestock products, have been recognized in California, Texas, and Illinois.

Ecology.   Several cycles of infection with *C. burnetii* exist in nature. One involves arthropods (including ticks, lice, and mites) and a large variety of vertebrates. The significance of arthropod-vertebrate transmission is still conjectural. Although man is not directly infected by ticks, these arthropods may transmit infection to domestic animals, especially sheep and cattle. Domestic animals have inapparent infections but may shed large quantities of infectious organisms in their urine, milk, feces, and especially their placental products. Because *C. burnetii* is unique among other Rickettsieae in its resistance to desiccation and exposure to light or temperature extremes, infectious organisms in placental products of domestic animals may become aerosolized after parturition and cause widespread outbreaks in human beings and other animals over a distance of several miles from their original origin. Dust in sheep and cattle sheds may become heavily contaminated and function as a reservoir of infection for susceptible human beings and animals. Once established, animal-to-animal spread is maintained primarily through airborne transmission.

Outbreaks of Q fever in human beings have also been traced to consumption of infected milk, to handling contaminated wool or hides, to soil contaminated by infected animal feces, to infected straw, and even to dusty clothing. Q fever may be an occupational risk in abattoir workers, sheep shearers, dairy and other farm workers, workers in tanneries, wool, and felt plants, and in technicians handling the organism in the laboratory.

C. burnetii may enter the body through the skin (eg, a contaminated minor abrasion), through the lungs (eg, inhalation of infectious aerosols), through mucous membranes (eg, conjunctival contact with infectious materials), or through the gastrointestinal tract (eg, ingestion of contaminated raw milk). Human-to-human transmission of Q fever has been reported but is probably rare.

CLINICAL MANIFESTATIONS.   *C. burnetii* is capable of causing inapparent infection, an influenzalike illness, pneumonia, prolonged fever, endocarditis, and hepatitis. Many mild or subclinical cases probably occur but are not diagnosed. Like most other rickettsial disease, clinically recognized Q fever usually begins abruptly with fever, chills or chilliness, headache, malaise, and myalgia. However, unlike most other rickettsial diseases, skin rash is not a part of the clinical syndrome, although evanescent macular rashes have been reported in a few cases. Patients may also complain of nonspecific gastrointestinal symptoms, sore throat, chest pain, nonproductive cough, and painful eyes.

Physical findings include hepatosplenomegaly, auscultatory evidence of pneumonic infiltration or consolidation, and a relative bradycardia. Chest x-rays may show unilateral or bilateral lower lobe infiltrates similar to infiltrates seen in viral and mycoplasma pneumonia and in psitticosis. Liver function tests are often minimally abnormal, but granulomatous hepatic lesions have been documented, with only mild liver function test abnormalities.

Q fever endocarditis may occur months or years after the acute attack and should be suspected when routine blood cultures are negative and unresponsiveness to antimicrobial therapy occurs in a clinical setting strongly suggestive of subacute bacterial endocarditis. Q fever endocarditis usually occurs on a previously damaged heart valve, often the aortic valve, and until recently was almost invariably fatal.

LABORATORY DIAGNOSIS.   The most definitive diagnostic procedure, isolation of *C. burnetii* from clinical specimens, can be accomplished by intraperitoneal inoculation of guinea pigs or mice or embryonated hens' eggs. However, unless there are available experienced personnel working in specialized facilities with stringent safeguards to prevent infection of laboratory personnel and other people in the vicinity of the laboratory, such primary isolations should not be attempted.

Complement-fixation tests utilizing highly purified antigens are available through most state health departments. Since *C. burnetii* exists in two phases, complement-fixing reagents prepared using phase I and phase II antigens can be useful in distinguishing acute from chronic (eg, endocarditis) or past infection. A microagglutination test has also been developed and appears to be a useful epidemiologic and clinical tool. Both the complement-fixation and microagglutination tests are sensitive and specific (ie, cross-reactions with other Rickettsieae do not occur). Weil-Felix antibodies do not appear in response to infection with *C. burnetii.*

TREATMENT. Many patients with mild or subclinical illnesses recover without antimicrobial therapy. However, all clinically diagnosed cases should be treated. Although tetracycline and chloramphenicol are both active against *C. burnetii*, patients with Q fever treated with these drugs do not respond as uniformly and as quickly as do patients with other rickettsial diseases. Tetracycline, which is less toxic and as effective as chloramphenicol, is the preferred drug for treatment. Therapy should be continued for five to seven days after defervescence.

Successful treatment of Q fever endocarditis has been reported after prolonged (10 months) therapy with tetracycline and with combined treatment using tetracycline and trimethoprim-sulfamethoxizole. Surgical replacement of the infected valve may be necessary.

PREVENTION AND CONTROL. Both live and killed Q fever vaccines elicit the production of complement-fixing antibodies and have been shown effective in guinea pigs. Their use in human beings has been hampered by the high rate of reactions (fever and pain and swelling at the site of injection). Recent work in both the United States and Russia using the M-44 strain of *C. burnetii* for the production of more effective vaccine has been encouraging, but a completely satisfactory vaccine has not yet been developed.

Measures to identify and decontaminate infected areas and to vaccinate domestic animal populations are difficult, expensive, and not generally done. Milkborne transmission, however, can be prevented by pasteurization.

FURTHER READING

Books and Reviews

Brezina, R, Murray ES, Tarizzo ML, Bozel K: Rickettsiae and rickettsial diseases. Bull WHO 49:433, 1974

Hahon NH: Selected Papers on the Pathogenic Rickettsiae, Cambridge, Mass, Harvard Univ Press, 1968

Ormsbee RA: Rickettsiae (as organisms). Annu Rev Microbiol 23:275, 1969

Swift HF: Trench fever. The Harvey Lectures, 1919-1920, Series IV. Philadelphia, Lippincott, 1921

Zinsser H: Rats, Lice and History. Boston, Little, Brown, 1935

Selected Papers

Berman SJ, Kundin WD: Scrub typhus in South Vietnam. A study of 87 cases. Ann Intern Med 79:26, 1973

Bozeman FM, Elisberg BL, Humphries JW, et al: Serologic evidence of *Rickettsia canada* infection of man. J Infect Dis 121:367, 1970

Brown GL: Clinical aspects of Q fever. Postgrad Med J 49:539, 1973

Burgdorfer W: Ecology of tick vectors of American spotted fever. Bull WHO 40:375, 1969

Dupont HL, Hornick RB, Dawkins AT, et al: Rocky Mountain spotted fever: A comparative study of the active immunity induced by inactivated and viable pathogenic *Rickettsia rickettsii,* J Infect Dis 128:340, 1973

Harell GT: Rocky Mountain spotted fever. Medicine 28:333, 1949

Hart RJ: The epidemiology of Q fever. Postgrad Med J 49:535, 1973

Hattwick MAW, Peters AH, Gregg MB, Hanson B: Surveillance of Rocky Mountain spotted fever. JAMA 225:1338, 1973

Maxcy KF: Clinical observations on endemic typhus (Brills' disease) in the United States. Public Health Rep 41:1213, 1926

Murray ES, Baehr G, Shwartzman G, et al: Brills' disease. I. Clinical and laboratory diagnosis. JAMA 142:1059. 1950

Murray ES, Gaon JA, O'Connor JM, et al: Serologic studies of primary endemic typhus and recrudescent typhus. J Immunol 94:723, 1965

Parker RR: Rocky Mountain spotted fever. JAMA 110:1185, 1273, 1938

Rose HM: The clinical manifestations and laboratory diagnosis of rickettsialpox. Ann Intern Med 31:871, 1949

Stuart BM, Pullen RM: Endemic murine typhus fever: Clinical observations. Ann Intern Med 23:520, 1945

Traub R, Wisseman CL Jr: The ecology of chigger-borne rickettsiosis (scrub typhus). J Med Entomol 11:237, 1974

Tyeryar FJ, Weiss E, Millar DB, et al: DNA base composition of rickettsiae. Science 180:415, 1973

Woodward TE: A historical account of rickettsial diseases with a discussion of unsolved problems. J Infect Dis 127:583, 1973

58
Bartonella

If there is truth in the notion that fact is stranger than fiction, it is to be found in bartonellosis or Carrion's disease. This exclusively human disease and its causative agent *Bartonella bacilliformis* are unique from nearly every point of view. The organism is an arthropodborne bacterium that causes two extraordinary and entirely different human syndromes: Oroya fever, a rapidly progressive, febrile, highly fatal, hemolytic anemia, and verruga peruana, a skin disease characterized by the eruption of bright red, angiomatous, wartlike lesions. Transmission is sharply confined geographically to certain areas on the western aspects of the Andes in Peru, Ecuador, and Colombia.

Verruga peruana quite probably was present in pre-Colombian Peru in essentially the same areas in which it may be found today. Oroya fever, however, was not clearly described until the mid-1800s. The verrucous form of the disease developed in some of the survivors of the hemolytic disease, and this gave rise to the suspicion that the two conditions might be etiologically related. It was soon after this, on August 27, 1885, that Daniel Carrion, a Peruvian medical student, inoculated himself with verrucous material in a quest for a better clinical definition of the earliest signs and symptoms of the skin disease. Just before his death from Oroya fever, 39 days later, he clearly stated his conviction," . . . that Oroya fever and the verruga have the same origin. . . ." While he soon became a national hero, his conclusion on the unity of causation of the two diseases was debated for many years. In 1905, Alberto Barton described the organism in erythrocytes in cases of Oroya fever. An expedition from Harvard in 1913, led by Richard Pearson Strong, confirmed and extended Barton's observations but failed to find the organism in histopathologic sections of verrugas. Strong concluded that the two diseases were unrelated and honored Barton by naming the organism *Bartonella bacilliformis*. In 1926, Hideyo Noguchi, working in New York, isolated the organisms from specimens sent from Peru. Of the major works for which this flamboyant microbiologist received worldwide adulation in the first decades of this century, only his work on bartonellosis, proving Carrion to be correct, has stood the test of time. He isolated identical organisms from blood specimens from Oroya fever patients and from verrugas excised from patients with the eruptive form of the disease. He was able consistently to produce verrugas in monkeys with organisms cultured from either source and to reisolate the organism in pure culture from the monkey lesions. His work has been confirmed repeatedly. In 1912, convincing epidemiologic evidence began to accumulate indicating that the organism is transmitted by certain species of flies of the genus *Phlebotomus*. In the 1940s, the findings that the organism is susceptible to penicillin and that DDT is highly effective against *Phlebotomus* flies provided the curative and preventive tools that are as effective today as when they were first used.

Morphology and Physiology

B. bacilliformis is the single species of the genus *Bartonella* and the only organism of the family Bartonellaceae of medical significance. Like other members of the family, however, it parasitizes red blood cells, possesses a cell wall, and has been cultured in vitro.

Bartonella are small, exceedingly polymorphic, motile, gram-negative bacteria. They range in shape from small coccoid and ring-shaped structures to long angular forms in chains and clusters. In erythrocytes they usually appear as short rods ranging from 1 to 3 μm in length by 0.25 to 0.5 μm in width (Fig. 58-1). The organisms stain weakly with aniline dyes but appear bright red to purple with Wright's or Giemsa's stain. They are not acid-alcohol-fast. The cultured organisms possess up to 10 terminal flagella (Fig. 58-2), but flagella have not been seen in fresh preparations of clinical specimens from man.

Under natural conditions *B. bacilliformis* is found in or on erythrocytes and in the cytoplasm of reticuloendothelial and vascular endothelial cells. In phlebotomus flies they are found in the lumen of the digestive tract.

Growth and maintenance in serial passage in the laboratory may be achieved in cell-free medium containing agar and fresh serum and hemoglobin from a number of species, including rabbit, horse, and man. Other culture systems include yolk and chorioallantoic fluids in the embryonated hen's egg and a variety of tissue cultures. In the latter, the organisms grow in the cytoplasm and extracellularly. In semisolid agar, colonies are 1 to 5 mm puffs of white that appear one to two weeks after inoculation. Temperatures around 30C favor growth and longevity. Cultures remain viable for long peri-

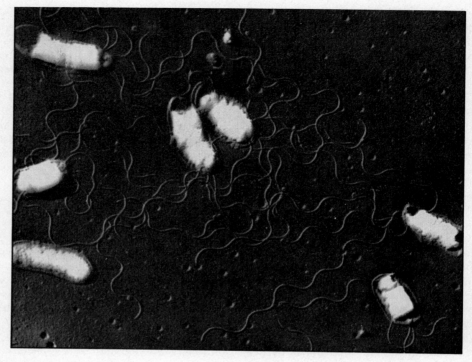

FIG. 58-1. Electron micrograph of culture of *B. bacilliformis* from seven-day culture. Note cell wall and terminal flagella apparently originating from protoplasts. ×15,000. (From Peters and Wigand: Z Tropenmed Parasitol 3:313, 1952)

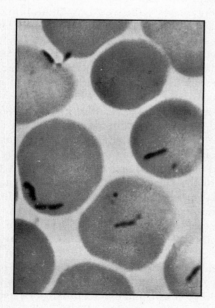

FIG. 58-2. *B. bacilliformis*. Human blood stained with Giemsa stain. ×3,000. (From Wigand, Peters, and Urtega: Z Tropenmed Parasitol 4:539, 1953)

ods when stored at −70C. Nutritional requirements for growth are satisfied in semisolid nutrient agar containing 10 percent rabbit serum and 0.5 percent rabbit hemoglobin. A number of specific nutrients, such as glutathione and ascorbic acid, have been identified.

No hemolysin has been demonstrated in vitro, and neither acid nor gas is produced in media containing a wide variety of sugars. The organisms are obligate aerobes. L forms have been shown to develop in hyperosmolar medium containing penicillin.

All strains appear to be similar in respect to morphology, growth characteristics, and antigenic reactivity. Organisms are agglutinated and complement is fixed by immune serum derived either from naturally infected man or from inoculated laboratory animals.

Clinical Infection

Epidemiology   Outbreaks of Oroya fever have been associated with the intrusion of non-immune persons into sharply demarcated areas on the western slopes of the Andes, where insect transmission occurs. In 1871, such an episode provided the first reported cases of the hemolytic disease, when expatriate laborers were building a railroad from Lima up into the mountains to the city of Oroya. Hundreds of cases occurred, and the case fatality reached 40 percent. The eruptive form of the disease subsequently appeared in some of the survivors and also in individuals who were not observed to have had the fever. Subsequent epidemics have been similar. Foci of endemic activity are notable for their stability over many years.

Transmission of bartonellosis is restricted by the habits and ecology of the *Phlebotomus* fly vector. The endemic area extends from 2 degrees north of the equator to 13 degrees south latitude, a distance of approximately 1,000 miles. It is further confined to a rather narrow band between 2,500 and 8,000 feet above sea level generally less than 100 miles in width, on the western slopes of the Andes in Peru, Colombia, and Ecuador. Major ecologic limitations include climatic conditions of temperature and humidity that are inimical to the fly. Transmission is at night when female flies take their blood meal. Even before insect transmission was seriously considered, disease was prevented in susceptible railroad workers by removing them from known endemic areas before nightfall.

The only known vertebrate reservoir is man, in spite of intensive search in many species of animals and plants. In some endemic areas, bacteremia may be detected in about 5 percent of apparently well individuals, and the duration of the bacteremia has been shown to be as long as a year, thus providing strong evidence for the suitability of man himself as the major reservoir.

There are many unsolved problems in the epidemiology of bartonellosis. Experimentally, transmission probably has been achieved by the transportation of flies caught in endemic areas to nonendemic areas and their feeding on laboratory monkeys. However, because of the difficulty of colonizing *Phlebotomus* in the laboratory and the incomplete expression of bartonella infection in laboratory animals, conclusive and complete transmission experiments have not been successful.

Pathogenesis In patients with Oroya fever organisms are found in large numbers of erythrocytes. The infected red blood cells are destroyed by an unknown mechanism. The organisms are also found in large clusters distending the cytoplasm of the endothelium of blood and lymph capillaries. In patients with verruga, the organisms are less easily found but are demonstrable in properly fixed sections of verruga stained with Giemsa's stain. The proliferative response of the vascular endothelium in these lesions is so intense and disorganized as to suggest sarcoma. The properties of insect transmission and invasion of and growth within erythrocytes and capillary endothelial cells are more often associated with protozoa and viruses than with bacteria.

Clinical Manifestations Oroya fever is a highly fatal illness characterized clinically by fever, diffuse and severe bone and muscle pains, and anemia. Most of the signs and symptoms of the disease are directly attributable to the rapidly progressive hemolysis and the resultant profound anemia. An incubation period of two to five weeks, hepatosplenomegaly, and terminal secondary infection with salmonella further typify the disease.

Verruga peruana is a chronic nonfatal illness that develops either in those who have recovered from Oroya fever or in persons with no prior clinical evidence of bartonellosis. Verruga peruana is best characterized by the presence of either localized or generalized angiomatous warts that vary in their size and degree of superficiality. Because of their histology, the more superficial ones may appear bright red. They reach the size of an egg. Systemic signs of fever, generalized pains, and malaise occur, although less frequently than in Oroya fever. The eruption lasts from a month to two years, averaging four to six months.

Infection results in an immunologic response that includes the production of complement-fixing antibodies and varying degrees of resistance to subsequent disease and infection. Oroya fever is believed to occur in the fully susceptible individual, while verruga peruana probably signifies a state of partial immunity.

Laboratory Diagnosis A laboratory diagnosis can be made by demonstration of the organism in erythrocytes in giemsa-stained films of peripheral blood or by blood culture. Serologic tests demonstrate the development of complement-fixing and agglutinating antibodies but are not major diagnostic tools.

Treatment   Penicillin, streptomycin, tetracyclines, and chloramphenicol have each been reported to reverse dramatically the downhill course in patients with Oroya fever. The bacteremia, however, may not be eradicated. Appropriate transfusion therapy often is useful. Antibiotics are reported to be less beneficial in verruga.

Control   Phlebotomus flies are exquisitely sensitive to DDT and can be controlled by its use. Antivector measures employing this chemical, the susceptibility of *B. bacilliformis* to a variety of antibiotics, plus unknown epidemiologic factors have all conspired to limit a more extensive distribution of what has at times been a local major public health problem. Vaccine development ceased in the 1940s when it became evident that antibiotics were curative and that the vector could be locally controlled by DDT.

FURTHER READING

Colichon HF, DeBedon C: Enfermedad de Carrion II. Nutrientes utilizables para el crecimiento de la *Bartonella bacilliformis*. Rev Lat Am Microbiol 15:75, 1973

Mandragon M: Verruga peruana. Evaluation of *Bartonella bacilliformis* in gel. Rev Lat Am Microbiol 16:1, 1974 (English abstract)

Schultz MG: A history of bartonellosis (Carrion's disease) Am J Trop Med Hyg 17:503, 1968

Sharp JT: Isolation of L-forms of *Bartonella bacilliformis*. Proc Soc Exp Biol Med 128:1072, 1968

Weinman D: Bartonellosis. In Weinman D, Ristic M (eds): Infectious Blood Diseases of Man and Animals. New York, Academic Press, 1968, Chap 15

59
Chlamydia

TABLE 59-1   CHARACTERISTICS DISTINGUISHING
CHLAMYDIA SPECIES

C. trachomatis	C. psittaci
Sensitive to sulfadiazine	Not sensitive to sulfadiazine
Sensitive to D-cycloserine	Not sensitive to D-cycloserine
Form compact microcolonies within cytoplasmic vesicles	Organisms tend to be dispersed throughout host cell cytoplasm
Iodine-staining carbohydrate and lipid produced by microcolony	Iodine-staining carbohydrate and lipid not produced
Low rate of heterologous DNA reassociation	

The Chlamydiaceae is a family of obligate intracellular bacterial parasites, characterized by a unique developmental cycle that is common to all members of the family.

Chlamydia infect a wide spectrum of vertebrate hosts; they are found in three major ecologic niches: birds, mammals, and man. Human diseases commonly caused by these organisms include trachoma, inclusion conjunctivitis, lymphogranuloma venereum, and psittacosis. Man occasionally is also infected with Chlamydia that are normally associated with disease of other animals, such as feline pneumonitis.

Only two distinct species of Chlamydia are recognized: (1) Chlamydia trachomatis, which is inhibited by sulfonamides and produces iodine-staining cytoplasmic inclusions, and (2) Chlamydia psittaci which is not inhibited by sulfonamides and does not produce iodine-staining inclusions in cytoplasmic vesicles (Table 59-1).

CHLAMYDIA

Morphology and Developmental Cycle

The unusual developmental cycle of chlamydiae is similar for both members of the genus. It consists of three major stages: (1) attachment and penetration of the elementary body into the host cell cytoplasm, (2) development of an inclusion body, and (3) synthesis of elementary body progeny. The elementary body, the minimal infecting unit of chlamydia, is a small dense spherical body 0.2 to 0.4 μm in diameter, which is phagocytosed by the host cell and surrounded by the invaginated host cell membrane to form the inclusion body. The elementary body then enlarges to 0.7 to 1 μm in diameter, to become an initial body, a granular and reticulated form that may be seen by light microscopy. The infectivity of the initial body is very low. Following a lag period of 12 hours after infection, initial bodies divide by binary fission, forming numerous, small, densely centered particles that do not themselves divide but that are highly infectious, the elementary bodies. Multiplication continues for several hours, accompanied by the formation of large numbers of elementary bodies. Intracellular inclusion bodies contain both large noninfectious initial bodies and elementary bodies that are capable of initiating infection. These inclusion bodies are intracellular bacterial microcolonies. The host cell with the inclusion body then ruptures, and the elementary bodies are released to begin a new infectious cycle (Fig. 59-1).

The initial body is the particle within the chlamydial inclusion that precedes the step of binary fission. These bodies are the precursors of elementary bodies and they lack a distinct nucleoid. Preceding the development of elementary bodies, initial body vesicles demonstrate a high rate of RNA and protein synthesis but a low rate of DNA synthesis.

In C. trachomatis the maturation of initial bodies into elementary bodies is accompanied by a rapid increase in the synthesis of DNA. The molecular weight of C. trachomatis DNA is approximately 660×10^6 daltons, which is greater than that of Mycoplasma hominis and approximately one-fourth that of Escherichia coli. Elementary bodies contain ribosomal subunits, transfer RNA, and messenger RNA. Host cell mitochondria are necessary for trachoma RNA synthesis. In addition, phospholipids that resemble those of the host cell may be found.

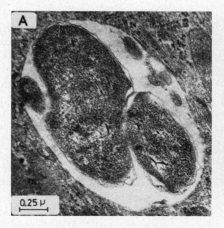
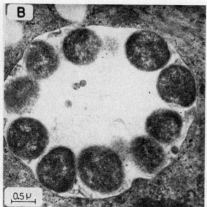
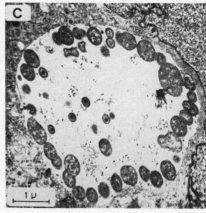

FIG. 59-1. The developmental cycle of *C. trachomatis* (TE55 strain) in FL cells. (A) An initial step in the formation of the inclusion body. (B) An inclusion body with initial bodies. (C) A developed inclusion body with initial bodies, dividing bodies, and elementary bodies. (From Becker: The agent of trachoma. Monogr Virol 7:31, 1974)

The elementary body is limited by a discrete cell wall and cell membrane. Enzymatic activity of trachoma elementary bodies includes DNA-dependent RNA polymerase, which is inhibited by rifampicin, polynucleotide phosphorylase, enzymatic pathways for glucose metabolism, and transaminase activity. The *Chlamydia* are unable, however, to synthesize their own high-energy phosphates, including ATP, and for this reason they are sometimes referred to as "energy parasites." The elementary body demonstrates an electron-dense nucleoid and a cell wall that firmly adheres to the cytoplasmic membrane. The cell wall stains gram-negative and contains traces of muramic acid and peptidoglycans.

Laboratory Identification

Isolation of *Chlamydia* may be accomplished by inoculation of infected material into embryonated eggs, into selected tissue culture cell lines, or into experimental animals.

The most common isolation procedure is inoculation of material into six- to eight-day-old chick embryo yolk sacs. All known strains of *Chlamydia* will infect the chick embryo, and characteristic inclusions and group-specific antigen are found in yolk sac material from infected embryos. Disadvantages in the use of the egg embryo yolk sac for diagnostic isolation include a long delay in confirmation of a result, inconvenience in culturing large numbers of specimens, and susceptibility of the embryo to superinfection with other bacteria.

Tissue cell culture methods for isolating *Chlamydia* have been improved by the use of centrifugation to enhance adsorption of *Chlamydia* to cells, by the use of new cell lines, and by the pretreatment of cells with DEAE-dextran to increase detection of inclusions. Cell lines commonly used to isolate *Chlamydia* include irradiated McCoy and HeLa cells. Isolation of *Chlamydia* from clinical sources is more frequently achieved in tissue cell cultures than from egg yolk sac inoculations.

Some strains of *Chlamydia* will infect mice; and the route of inoculation by which the infection may be established partially characterizes a strain. Lymphogranuloma venereum (LGV) strains will usually infect mice when inoculated intracerebrally, while *Chlamydia* causing trachoma and inclusion conjunctivitis will not infect mice by any route of injection. They will, however, cause a rapid toxic death in mice if injected intravenously. Mice may be protected against toxic death by prior immunization with the same strain. This phenomenon has been elaborated into a typing system called the "mouse toxicity prevention test."

Antigenic Structure

All *Chlamydia* possess a common heat-stable, group-specific antigen. This antigen is associated with the cell wall and is a carbohydrate-lipoprotein complex. The immunodominant group is a 2-keto-3-deoxyoctanoic acid. Since it is group specific, its presence cannot be used for identification of chlamydial strains or species. This group antigen may be detected by complement-fixation tests.

Species-specific and strain-specific antigens have been demonstrated. Wang has typed chlamydial isolates from ocular and genital sources by the indirect immunofluorescent test using homologous mouse antisera (Table 59-2). At least 11 types have been identified, which corresponds closely with the results of the mouse toxicity protection test. This test is itself a function of the development of strain-specific antibody. Another method of species identification is by infectivity neutralization using hyperimmune sera.

Frei Test   This is an intradermal skin test that has been used since 1925 primarily for the diagnosis of lymphogranuloma venereum (LGV). The test initially used boiled lymph node material excised from a patient with LGV; but at present it employs Lygranum antigen, prepared from infected chick embryo yolk sac material. The site of the skin test injection is examined at 48 and at 72 hours for the formation of a subcutaneous nodule. The test is not specific for LGV infection because group-specific antigen is involved in the reaction, and patients with other chlamydial infections may exhibit a positive Frei test. Similarly, intradermal tests using psittacosis antigen may be positive in patients with LGV. A modification of several of the antigens by acid extraction has resulted in a test of greater specificity, but because of difficulties in production it has not come into general use.

The Frei test is less sensitive than is complement fixation. Schachter found that four of six patients, all of whom were known to have LGV by recovery of *Chlamydia* from node biopsy, had a negative Frei test, but all developed complement-fixing antibody. The Frei test is a helpful confirmatory test for infection with chlamydia but is not as sensitive as a rise in complement-fixing antibody and not specific for LGV.

Antigenic subdivision of *C. trachomatis* types may be based upon immunofluorescent techniques (Table 59-2). Recent studies of strains isolated from eyes and the genital tract have revealed, using the mouse toxicity prevention test as well as the immunofluorescent test, that there are 11 or more distinguishable types. Types A, B, and C have been isolated primarily from eyes of persons with trachoma in trachoma endemic areas. Isolation of these types from genital sites is rare. Types D, E, F, G, H, I, J, and K have been isolated from the

TABLE 59-2   IMMUNOFLUORESCENT TYPES OF CHLAMYDIA TRACHOMATIS IN CLINICAL DISEASE

Immunofluorescent Type	Usual Disease	Geographic Distribution
A, B, C	Classical ocular trachoma	Primarily endemic in Asia and Africa
D, E, F, G, H, I, J, K	Inclusion conjunctivitis Genital trachoma	Worldwide, sporadic
LGV I, II, and III	Lymphogranuloma venereum Genital trachoma	Worldwide, sporadic

eyes of persons in areas where trachoma is nonendemic and most frequently from the genital tracks of adults. Included among strains D through K are isolates from infants who were born to mothers with cervical infection and developed inclusions conjunctivitis.

CHLAMYDIA TRACHOMATIS

Human infections caused by *C. trachomatis* include trachoma, inclusion conjunctivitis, and lymphogranuloma venereum. A characteristic of the species is the development of compact, clearly defined, glycogen-containing, intracellular microcolonies or inclusions known as "Halberstadter-Prowazek bodies." These are found in infected yolk sac preparations, infected animal tissue, inoculated tissue culture cells, and in conjunctival scrapings of persons with active trachoma or inclusion conjunctivitis. They are basophilic, stain mahogany with iodine stain, are gram-negative, and may be stained by fluorescent antibody or Giemsa stain. *C. trachomatis* is inhibited by sulfadiazine and usually by D-cycloserine.

Clinical Infection

Ocular Trachoma The name "trachoma," derived from the Greek word which means "rough," refers to the pebbled appearance of the infected conjunctiva. Naturally occurring trachoma is limited to man and continues to be a leading cause of blindness in underdeveloped areas.

EPIDEMIOLOGY Trachoma is a disease of poverty. In the United States, American Indians are the group most frequently infected. Trachoma is a disease optionally reported to the Center for Disease Control. Between 1969 and 1974 there were approximately 1500 cases reported annually, most of which were in the western United States.

PATHOGENESIS AND CLINICAL MANIFESTATIONS. The MacCallan classification is internationally accepted for describing trachoma. It provides four major stages of disease. Stage I is incipient trachoma. It may be relatively asympto-

matic, with little if any conjunctival exudate. Minimal keratitis is usually present. Stage II is established trachoma with follicular and papillary hypertrophy. Trachomatous pannus accompanies corneal infiltration. Stage III includes cicatricial complications with scarring of the conjunctiva; trichiasis, entropion, and further pannus develop. Stage IV represents healed trachoma without evidence of active inflammation. If no complications of trachoma develop during active infection, this stage may be asymptomatic.

Long periods of latent infection occur, and superinfection with other bacteria contributes to more advanced forms of the disease. Trachomatous persons living in conditions of good hygiene experience a mild course or clinical resolution of infection. Repeated exposure to ocular trachoma infection is associated with an increased incidence of marginal infiltration and neovascularization. This may have a late onset, after inclusions are no longer detectable in conjunctival scrapings, and represents host response to chlamydial antigen, which then contributes to the severe ocular damage.

The ocular exudate contains primarily polymorphonuclear leukocytes during the acute stage, although the subepithelial infiltrate is mainly mononuclear. Limbal follicles, neovascularization with pannus, interstitial keratitis, cicatrization of the tarsal conjunctiva, and corneal ulcers lead to impairment of vision. Recurrences often occur after apparent healing; the clinical course is variable.

IMMUNITY. Protective immunity conferred by a prior attack of trachoma is of a low order. Persons with ocular trachoma often develop neither complement-fixing antibody to the group antigen nor delayed sensitivity to the Frei antigen. However, detection of specific antibody in eye secretions and/or serum may be achieved with fluorescent antibody techniques.

LABORATORY DIAGNOSIS. *Serologic Tests.* The microimmunofluorescent technique has been modified to determine the type-specific antibody response to *C. trachomatis.* In the majority of patients for whom the identity of the infecting strain is known, there is a type-specific antibody response with a titer of 1:8 or greater. Exceptions include patients with LGV, in whom the antibody is frequently reactive with more than one type. Early antibody formation is of the IgM class and persists for approximately one month before being replaced by IgG. In the few instances in which serial antibody determinations have been made, type-specific antibody has been observed to decrease fairly rapidly after primary infection, often within one or two months.

Identification of Chlamydia trachomatis. Demonstration of the causative agent may be made by everting the tarsal plate, removing the exudate, and gently scraping epithelial cells from the surface. The inclusions in scrapings may stain with fluorescent antibody or Giemsa stain or may be cultured by inoculation into yolk sac or tissue cell culture preparations.

TREATMENT. Antibiotics may be used topically and systemically. In hyperendemic areas, their primary effect is to limit coexisting bacterial conjunctivitis, but in the United States this is probably not a significant factor. Studies of American Indians at a boarding school showed that although systemically administered tetracyclines and sulfonamides caused a regression of clinical trachomatous activity, the agent persisted in conjunctival scrapings, and subclinical disease among the children continued to spread. Nevertheless, treatment may limit complications and should be administered.

PREVENTION. Systemically administered vaccines may exacerbate the disease. Since the protection afforded by most vaccines is of a relatively low order and duration, they are usually not used in programs to control trachoma. Current research may provide a more satisfactory vaccine. Good standards of hygiene are essential in the control of trachoma.

Inclusion Conjunctivitis and Genital Trachoma IN THE INFANT. Inclusion conjunctivitis is often a disease of the newborn eye that is derived from infection of the adult genital tract. It is caused by an agent almost indistinguishable from that causing trachoma; the term "TRIC agent" historically encompasses both (Table 59-2).

The incidence of TRIC infection of the eyes of infants varies from one population to another, depending upon the prevalence of cervical infection in the mothers. In an English survey, 0.5 percent of infants had symptomatic disease of the eyes caused by these strains, while in South Africa 26 percent were infected.

The disease in the newborn is acquired during passage through an infected birth canal and usually becomes clinically apparent between 5 and 12 days after birth. It is characterized by a sticky exudate and conjunctivitis and may be unilateral. Vulvovaginitis, ear infection, and mucopurulent rhinitis may accompany ocular disease. Many children ascertained to have neonatal inclusion conjunctivitis are premature, but whether this represents increased susceptibility or longer observation of the infant due to hospitalization is unknown.

Inclusion conjunctivitis of the newborn eye had been considered benign and self-limited until recent studies showed a high incidence of micropannus, conjunctival scars, and late recurrence, which were prevented by local application of tetracycline before the twelfth day of life.

IN THE ADULT. Inclusion conjunctivitis in the adult is usually sporadic but may be epidemic following contamination of unchlorinated swimming pools. Inclusion conjunctivitis must be differentiated from epidemic keratoconjunctivitis, which is a viral disease.

The concept that these infections are harbored and transmitted sexually has received attention since the 1960s, although the association between neonatal inclusion conjunctivitis and maternal cervical disease was recognized much earlier. Jones demonstrated that adult ocular disease was associated with concomitant urethritis, cervicitis, and multiple sexual partners. Dunlop reported studies of patients whose infants had inclusion conjunctivitis. Salpingitis, cervicitis with cervical follicles, cervical discharge, prostatitis, proctitis, and nongonococcal urethritis afflicted their parents.

NONGONOCOCCAL URETHRITIS. Recovery of these agents and serologic evidence of infection with chlamydia occurs in 5 to 20 percent of males with nongonococcal urethritis and in a very high proportion of their contacts. The incidence of nongonococcal urethritis increased in England from 10,700 in 1951 to 32,300 in 1967. It occurs in men with a history of promiscuity and other venereal diseases and frequently in the consorts of women with cervical chlamydial infection. Infection with chlamydiae probably accounts for a large proportion of nongonococ-cal urethritis, but its exact position as the etio-logic agent has not been completely elucidated.

Lymphogranuloma venereum (LGV) Lym-phogranuloma inguinale, climatic bubo, tropi-cal bubo, and esthiomene are synonyms of a venereal disease which appeared from time to time throughout the eighteenth century. The distribution of this disease is now world-wide. It occurs more commonly in blacks than in whites and is recognized more frequently in males than in females. Man is the sole natural host. LGV should not be confused with gran-uloma inguinale, which is caused by *Calym-matobacterium granulomatis.*

ETIOLOGY. Organisms isolated from pa-tients with LGV differ from TRIC agents in that they fail to cause typical follicular conjunctivi-tis in the monkey eye, they cause death in mice which are infected intracerebrally, and they sometime cause rapid death of egg embryos. LGV isolates are divided by microimmuno-fluorescence into three antigenic types, LGV I, II, and III, which show cross-reactions with genital *Chlamydia* types E and D.

CLINICAL INFECTION. *Epidemiology.* LGV is grouped with the minor venereal diseases. Although the incidence of syphilis and gonor-rhea has been increasing during the past five years, the incidence of LGV has remained stable at about 500 reported cases per year. This may not remain the case, however, since recent reports suggest that importation of dis-ease from Southeast Asia has occurred. In this country, male homosexuals are particularly likely to experience LGV infection and consti-tute another major reservoir of disease. Patients with LGV commonly have other concomitant venereal diseases, especially syphilis. All pa-tients with LGV should be thoroughly exam-ined for evidence of other venereal disease.

Little is known about the infectivity of LGV or the duration of infection when untreat-ed. The observation that a man may infect his new wife many years after his initial infection and the frequency of relapse indicate that it may be a very long, indolent, and chronically active disease.

Clinical Manifestations. The usual incuba-tion period of LGV is one to four weeks. Early

constitutional symptoms such as fever, head-ache, and myalgia are common. The primary lesion is painless, small, inconspicuous, and vesicular and often escapes notice. Characteris-tically the presenting complaint concerns the enlarged matted inguinal and femoral lymph nodes. They are moderately painful, firm, and may become fluctuant. Aspiration of fluctuant nodes may be therapeutic and provide diagnos-tic material.

Women commonly experience proctitis, pre-sumably because the lymphatic drainage from the vagina is perirectal. Infection may cause diarrhea, purulent rectal drainage, tenesmus, anemia, abdominal pain, and the formation of infected sinuses. Rectal stricture and rectal per-foration are recognized late sequelae to LGV proctitis.

The course of the disease is variable. It may cause progressive destruction of the vulva and urethra. Lymphatic obstruction in women can lead to elephantiasis of the vulva, called "es-thiomene." Vulvar carcinoma is reported to be more common in women who have had LGV.

An unknown percentage of persons have asymptomatic infections or heal without com-plications. Serologic evidence of experience with *Chlamydia* at some time has been report-ed to be very common, especially among per-sons attending venereal disease clinics. These data do not indicate which strain of *Chlamydia* was present or when. Until more appropriate precise tests for routine use become available the extent of subclinical LGV will remain un-known.

Pathology. Autopsy of patients with chronic LGV infection has revealed lesions of the lymph nodes composed of aggregations of large mononuclear cells forming abscesses surround-ed by epithelioid cells. A few giant cells of the Langhans type may be found. Numerous plas-ma cells may invade the granuloma formation. Occasionally, necrotic lesions with few or no granulocytes but also surrounded by giant cells are present, usually in disease of long duration. Varying degrees of fibrosis occur, with bands of granulation and connective tissue and a thick-ened capsule.

Splenic changes resembling those of lymph nodes are reported, and fibrotic infiltration of the liver, especially in the portal areas, may lead to cirrhosis.

Hyperglobulinemia is common early after

infection, and a positive reaction for rheumatoid factor and cryoglobulins is frequent. A specific increase in IgA has been reported. Although a high incidence of biologic false positive reactions for syphilis has been claimed for patients with LGV, studies of patients who received careful examination revealed that most had early syphilis and that the rate of biologic false positive reactions was 3 percent or less, similar to that of many other acute infectious diseases.

Laboratory Diagnosis. Diagnosis depends upon (1) a compatible clinical presentation, (2) recovery of the organism from the site of infection and its identification as a *C. trachomatis* organism, (3) demonstration of rising LGV complement-fixation test (LGV-CFT) titer, microimmunofluorescent antibody titer rise, or (4) a reactive intradermal Frei test. In the interpretation of these parameters it must be recognized that the LGV-CFT is not specific for LGV and that the Frei test is both nonspecific and relatively insensitive. Recovery of the organism is the most satisfactory diagnostic aid, although the culture may fail to yield growth in situations that are in every other way typical of LGV, probably because of lack of sensitivity of the culture methods.

Treatment. Treatment may include sulfadiazine or tetracycline; penicillin has been effective when other drugs have failed. Meticulous follow-up for relapse or the development of complications is essential. A decrease in the LGV-CFT and reversion of the intradermal Frei test from positive to negative may follow treatment.

CHLAMYDIA PSITTACI

A severe febrile disease obviously contracted from parrots was recognized in Switzerland, France, and Germany in the last two decades of the nineteenth century. Worldwide interest in this infection dates from 1929-1930, when over 700 cases were found in 12 different countries, including the United States. Psittacosis caused endemic disease in parrots and parakeets and in a wide range of other birds, including ducks, chickens, and turkeys. Infection of flocks of turkeys in the United States

caused considerable human disease in the 1950s. Cattle and other animals may also experience endemic and epidemic psittacosis. Human disease transmitted from psittacine birds is called psittacosis and that transmitted from nonpsittacine birds is orthithosis. The diseases, however, are clinically indistinguishable.

Etiology

Four characteristics distinguish *C. psittacosis* from *C. trachomatis:* (1) The intracellular microcolonies contain little glycogen and do not stain recognizably with iodine. (2) The inclusions are not compact but are more diffuse and irregular in shape. They are called LCL (Levinthal-Cole-Lillie) bodies, and stain with Giemsa or Macchiavello methods. Fluorescent microscopy has not been adapted to the clinical diagnosis of psittacosis in human beings (3) The development of inclusions is not inhibited by sulfadiazine or cycloserine. (4) The DNA base composition differs from that of strains of *C. trachomatis*, and the degree of homology is low. However, few strains have been studied (Table 59-1).

Clinical Infection

Epidemiology The general prevalence of this disease is unknown, but a study in Wisconsin of sera referred for diagnostic studies on patients with respiratory disease found 2.8 percent positive for psittacosis. Relatively more cases occur in the autumn than in other seasons. Although only about 50 cases are currently reported annually, this reflects only the more severe disease and disease in bird handlers.

Between 1945 and 1951 an average of 28 cases of psittacosis per year were reported, after which there was a rapid increase to a peak of 568 in 1956. Some of the increase may be attributed to the relaxation of quarantine regulations for psittacine birds and some to the increased incidence of infections from turkeys. Since 1956 there has been a steady decline in the number of cases of psittacosis in the United States, and in 1973 there were 35 cases.

The respiratory tract is the main portal of entry, and inhalation of organisms from infected birds and their droppings is the usual source. Many, but not all, patients give a clear history of exposure to psittacine birds. Since pigeons, turkeys, chickens, and wild birds may harbor the disease, a patient may not recognize a possible exposure. In addition, person-to-person transmission occurs. Exposure to patients who will die of psittacosis in the next one or two days is especially likely to propagate a very severe or fatal secondary infection.

SPONTANEOUS DISEASE IN ANIMALS.   In parrots the naturally acquired disease is characterized by apathy, shivering, weakness, diarrhea, and respiratory symptoms. At necropsy, multiple areas of necrosis are found in the liver and spleen and occasionally in the lungs. Inapparent or subclinical infections occur in birds of the psittacine group and even more frequently in nonpsittacine birds. Small birds are often healthy carriers of the organism. Sheep in Colorado have a type of polyarthritis from which chlamydia have been isolated. Many other mammals experience arthritis, abortion, encephalitis, and conjunctivitis when infected with these agents.

Clinical Manifestations   The clinical disease was originally believed to be very severe, with 20 percent mortality rate. It is now recognized that the signs, symptoms, and severity vary greatly. For example, 10 percent of persons believed to have influenza in a British chest clinic were found probably to have psittacosis. Most cases are heralded by constitutional signs of fever, myalgia, and often a severe frontal headache. This precedes the pulmonary signs of the disease, which include nonproductive cough, rales, and consolidation. Hemoptysis and pleuritic chest pain are variable findings. The physical signs of pulmonary involvement are less prominent than is suggested by the patients' symptoms. Radiologic examination of the chest may suggest bronchopneumonia or primary atypical pneumonia, and inadequately treated patients may suffer repeated episodes of pneumonia.

The second most frequently involved organ system is the central nervous system. Symptoms are usually no more pronounced than a severe headache but encephalitis, coma, convulsions, and death may occur. The etiology is usually thought to be a toxic encephalitis rather than direct invasion of the central nervous system by *Chlamydia,* although LCL bodies have been identified in the meninges of involved cases.

Patients with psittacosis may also develop carditis, subacte bacterial endocarditis, hepatitis with or without formation of hepatic granulomata, erythema nodosum, and follicular keratoconjunctivitis. During the early phase of the illness, an acute biologic false positive test for syphilis may develop in a third of patients, and sera may be anticomplementary.

PATHOLOGY.   The pathology of psittacosis includes focal areas of necrosis in the liver and spleen, with a predominance of mononuclear cells. In the lungs, consolidation is characterized by thickening of alveolar walls, infiltration of mononuclear cells, and a gelatinous alveolar exudate also containing mononuclear cells.

Laboratory Diagnosis   *C. psittaci* may be isolated from infected material by methods similar to those used for other *Chlamydia,* including egg inoculation, tissue culture, and mouse inoculation intranasally, intraperitoneally, intracerebrally, and subcutaneously.

Treatment   Results of treatment of psittacosis are imperfect. Tetracyclines may be used with some success, and a good response has been achieved by the use of erythromycin. In one-half of the patients radiologic evidence of pulmonary infiltration persists for over six weeks. Fall of the peak complement-fixing titer may not occur for over a year. Asymptomatic persistence of infection in psittacosis has not been well studied, but one patient is known to have shed the organism in his sputum for 12 years, both before and after penicillin treatment. However, no secondary cases were attributed to him.

Prevention   Prophylactic treatment of psittacine birds with antibiotic-supplemented feed reduces the risk of disease in bird handlers. The recognition, however, that *C. psittaci* may infect many avian and mammalian species, sometimes causing subclinical communicable disease with occasional outbreaks involving human beings, widens the need for careful epidemiologic investigation of each case. Workers in poultry-processing plants should have excellent environmental protection, as they are in particular risk of heavy exposure to this infection.

Miscellaneous Diseases

Cat-scratch fever is a human disease of unknown etiology. It is characterized by contact with a kitten, development of a primary papule at the site of a scratch or injury, and subsequent lymphadenopathy central to the papule. Approximately 25 percent of persons with this disease exhibit an antibody response to chlamydial group antigens. However, *Chlamydia* sp. have not been recovered from excised tissue of infected persons, hence the suggestion that the disease is caused by a *Chlamydia* sp. is unproven.

REITER'S SYNDROME.   Patients with Reiter's syndrome characteristically exhibit a triad of recurring signs, including conjunctivitis or iridocyclitis, polyarthritis, and nonbacterial urethritis. The disease usually occurs in young white males and is frequently preceded by dysentery or gonococcal urethritis. Many organisms have been etiologically associated with Reiter's syndrome. Studies implicating *Chlamydia* strains have included isolation of *C. psittaci* from synovial fluid from a patient, and the demonstration that a higher proportion of Reiter's syndrome patients have antibody to *Chlamydia* group antigen than do comparable patients with gonorrhea or nongonococcal urethritis. The question of whether Reiter's syndrome patients react more vigorously to chlamydia antigen or whether the disease is caused directly by chlamydia infection has not been answered.

FURTHER READING

Books and Reviews

Becker Y: The agent of trachoma. Mongr Virol 7:31, 1974

Jawetz E: Chemotherapy of chlamydia infection. Adv Pharmacol Chemother 7:253, 1969

Sigel MM (ed): Lymphogranuloma Venereum. Miami, Fl, Univ of Miami Press, 1962

Storz J: Chlamydia and Chlamydia-Induced Diseases. Springfield, Ill, Charles C Thomas, 1971

Thygeson P: Trachoma Manual and Atlas. Washington, DC, Public Health Service Publication No 541, 1958

Trachoma. In Nichols PL (ed): Proceedings of the International Trachoma Conferences, Boston, 1970. Amsterdam, Excerpta Medica International Congress Series No. 223, 1971

Selected Papers

Chlamydia and genital infection. Lancet 2:264, 1974

Grayston JT, Wang SP: New knowledge of chlamydiae and the diseases they cause. J Infect Dis 132:87, 1975

Hilton AL, Richmond SJ, Milne JD, Hindley F, Clarke SKR: Chlamydia in the female genital tract. Br J Vener Dis 50:1, 1974

Jansson E: Ornithosis in Helsinki and some other localities in Finland. Ann Med Exp Biol Fenn 38[Suppl 4]:1, 1960

Schaffner W, Drutz DJ, Duncan GW, Koenig MG: The clinical spectrum of endemic psittacosis. Arch Intern Med 119:433, 1967

Wang SP, Grayston JT: Immunological relationship between genital TRIC, lymphogranuloma venereum, and related organisms in a new microtiter indirect immunofluorescent test. Am J Ophthalmol 70:67, 1970

Wang SP, Grayston JT: Human serology in *Chlamydia trachomatis* infection with microimmunofluorescence. J Infect Dis 130:388, 1974

60
Mycoplasma

Mycoplasmas are widespread in nature and are part of the indigenous microbial flora of the oropharynx and genitourinary tract of birds and mammals, including man. The type species of the genus *Mycoplasma, Mycoplasma mycoides.* was isolated in 1898 by Nocard and Roux from cattle that had pleuropneumonia. Similar microorganisms subsequently isolated from other animal species were referred to as pleuropneumonialike organisms (PPLO) until their taxonomic position was clarified. Individual *Mycoplasma* species tend to be species-specific in their host range.

The mycoplasmas are a heterogeneous group of unicellular, procaryotic organisms that lack a cell wall. They are bounded only by a single triple-layered membrane that is responsible for the cell's extreme plasticity and polymorphic appearance (Fig. 60-1). Mycoplasmas are intermediate in size between bacteria and viruses; their smallest reproductive units are within the range of the 100 nm theoretical minimal diameter of a free-living cell. Although mycoplasmas resemble in many ways the bacterial L forms, they lack any known or detectable derivation form a specific bacterium.

Two major groups of mycoplasmas are recognized, the Mycoplasmataceae that require sterol for growth, and the Acholeplasmataceae that do not require sterol.

The major human pathogen among the mycoplasmas is *Mycoplasma pneumoniae,* formerly known as the Eaton agent. This organism is the cause of primary atypical pneumonia, a syndrome of nonbacterial pneumonia first recognized as a clinical entity during World War II. Cold agglutinins, antibodies that agglutinate human red blood cells in the cold, appear in the serum of a portion of patients with atypical pneumonia. Cold agglutinin positive atypical pneumonia was the syndrome first linked epidemiologically with infection by a human mycoplasma. Also of medical importance are the T strains of mycoplasma that may cause nongonococcal urethritis.

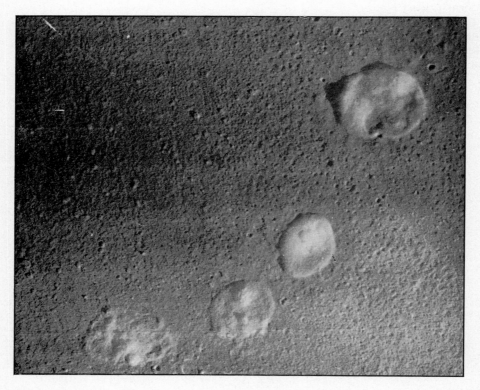

FIG. 60-1. Electron micrograph of mycoplasma. Note the obvious plasticity of the organism and the lack of a definite cell wall. ×20,000. (From Morton et al: J Bacteriol 68:697, 1954)

Morphology

Individual mycoplasma cells range in diameter from 125 to 330 nm for the spherical forms, to 150 μm in length for filaments. Although their shape can be greatly altered and deformed by various physical and chemical agents used in their preparation, five distinct morphologic types based on electron microscopy have been recognized: (1) coccoid cells, some forming streptococcuslike chains, (2) coccoid cells with membrane tubules, (3) filamentous cells, sometimes showing branching, (4) filamentous cells with terminal structures, and (5) pear-shaped cells with terminal structures. Most mycoplasmas replicate by binary fission, but filamentous species may fragment into several viable filamentous daughter cells.

Except for the absence of a cell wall, mycoplasma cells have an ultrastructure similar to that of other bacterial forms.

Physiology

Cultural Characteristics On solid media mycoplasmas produce very small colonies, 10 to 600 μm in diameter. They have an opaque, granular central area that grows down into the medium and a translucent peripheral zone. This biphasic growth gives the colony a fried-egg appearance. Colonies of *M. pneumoniae* are shown in Figure 60-2. On blood agar most organisms produce an α or β type of hemolysis.

Mycoplasma cultures follow typical bacterial growth curves. Most cells have a doubling time of one to six hours. Complex media containing peptones, yeast extract, and serum are required for growth. Species of the genus *Mycoplasma* also require sterol for growth and incorporate it into the cell membrane. The requirement of sterols for growth is of special interest, since sterols are not present in bacteria that possess cell walls or in their L form variants.

Metabolism Most species are facultative anaerobes, although growth is better in an aerobic environment. The classic mycoplasmas can be divided into two broad physiologic groups, the nonfermentative and the fermentative. The nonfermentative species obtain energy by the breakdown of arginine, 1 mole of arginine yielding 1 mole of ATP. Most fermentative

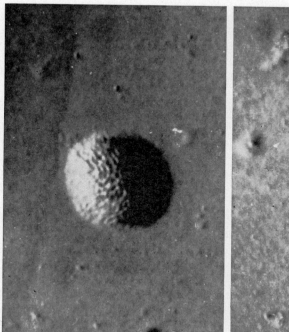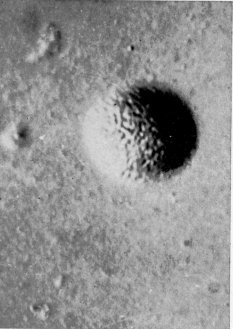

FIG. 60-2. Colonies of *M. pneumoniae*. Note the granular appearance. The organisms grow down into the agar beneath the surface colony. *M. pneumoniae*, on initial isolation, frequently does not have surrounding surface growth. (From Chanock, Hayflick, and Barile: Proc Nat Acad Sci USA 48:41, 1962)

species lack this pathway and obtain energy from sugars via the glycolytic pathway.

When grown in tissue culture, mycoplasmas cause significant biochemical changes in the host cell metabolism. Arginine is depleted in the tissue cell culture, and production of mycoplasma RNA species results in alterations in host nucleic acid metabolism.

Mycoplasmas produce a marked effect on the morphology of tissue cells. The nature of the effect, together with its extent, is determined by the species of mycoplasma and the cell type but may range from a zero effect to frank cytopathology. Characteristic morphologic changes in the nuclei are often observed; the most common of these are achromatic gaps and chromatid breaks. The T strain mycoplasmas also produce a progressive cytopathic effect in infected cells.

In their association with the host cell, mycoplasmas are present in the extracellular environment in close proximity to the cell membrane. Long cytoplasmic processes and microvilli often are observed to envelop the organism without actually phagocytosing it. Specific receptor sites are apparently responsible for the marked avidity of mycoplasmas for the cell membrane; sialic acid and glycoproteins are important binding sites. The intimate association of mycoplasma with host cells is assumed to be necessary in order to provide the essential nucleic acid precursors required for the organism's growth.

Mycoplasmas produce a number of extracellular products that contribute to their disease-inciting ability, among which are neurotoxins, hemolysins, and exoenzymes. Except for the two known neurotoxins produced by *Mycoplasma neurolyticum* and *Mycoplasma gallisepticum*, there is little information on toxins produced by the other species of *Mycoplasma*. A soluble hemolysin produced by some species (eg, *M. pneumoniae*) appears to be hydrogen peroxide. Among the exoenzymes are nucleases and enzymes that alter erythrocyte antigenic determinants.

MYCOPLASMA PNEUMONIAE

M. pneumoniae organisms are short filaments, 2 to 5 μm in length. The organism grows more slowly than most other mycoplasmas, with colonies appearing 5 to 10 days after inoculation. The organisms agglutinate guinea pig erythrocytes and adsorb red blood cells and tracheal epithelial cells from a number of animal species. Adsorption occurs most rapidly at 37C and less rapidly at 22C and is specifically inhibited by antiserum. Neuraminic acid is assumed to be the specific receptor site on the membrane for mycoplasma, since prior treatment with neuraminidase destroys the binding site. The pronounced affinity of *M. pneumoniae* for respiratory epithelium is important in the pathogenicity of the organism and may counteract rapid destruction of the mycoplasma peroxide by peroxidase present in extracellular fluids.

The major antigenic determinants of *M. pneumoniae* are present in lipid extracts of membranes, but their composition has not been defined. The organism is antigenically distinct from other species of human origin as determined by agglutination, complement fixation, and other immunologic procedures.

Clinical Infection

Epidemiology   *M. pneumoniae* is widely distributed in all parts of the world. Infection occurs throughout the year, with a tendency toward increased incidence during the late summer and fall. Illness due to *M. pneumoniae* is most prevalent in persons from 5 to 30 years of age. Atypical pneumonia in persons of this age is usually caused by *M. pneumoniae* except in specific outbreaks, such as an influenza epidemic or an outbreak of adenoinfection in a military camp. *M. pneumoniae* spreads slowly but efficiently through groups of persons having close contact, such as in the school, family, or barracks. Although the organism may be cultured from the throat for weeks after the illness, transmission is greatest during the acute phase of the disease.

Clinical Manifestations   The course of *M. pneumoniae* atypical pneumonia is illustrated in Figure 60-3. The incubation period after exposure is usually two to three weeks. Illness develops gradually over a few days and is characterized by fever, headache, malaise, fatigue,

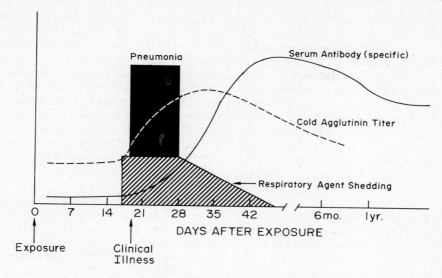

FIG. 60-3. The course of *M. pneumoniae* infection.

coryza and/or pharyngitis, and cough which is often paroxysmal with aching substernal discomfort. Sputum is usually small in amount, occasionally slightly purulent, and rarely blood streaked. Rales are heard on chest examination, but there may be less evidence of consolidation than chest roentgenograms suggest. A patchy interstitial infiltrate involving one or both lower lobes is the usual roentgenographic finding. Slight neutrophilia or a normal white blood cell count and differential may be found. Smear and culture of sputum for bacteria yield no predominant pathogen, and secondary bacterial infection is rare. The acute illness lasts one to two weeks in the untreated patient, but convalescence may be prolonged for several weeks.

Estimates of the proportion of persons who develop pneumonia during *M. pneumoniae* infection range from 1 in 30 to over 2 out of 3 depending on the population and methods of study. Illnesses which occur in the remainder include upper respiratory illness, pharyngitis, and bronchitis.

Other organ systems in addition to the respiratory tract may be affected during *M. pneumoniae* infection. Otitis media and bullous meningitis have been observed. Positive nongamma direct Coombs' tests and a slight increase in reticulocytes are frequently present, and an occasional patient may develop frank hemolytic anemia in association with very high cold agglutinin titers. A variety of skin rashes have been observed in a minority of patients, and a rare patient may develop erythema multiforme major. Several case reports describe neurologic diseases (meningoencephalitis, polyradiculitis). Additional organ involvements have been reported more rarely.

Laboratory Diagnosis SEROLOGIC TESTS. Differentiation between atypical pneumonia caused by *M. pneumoniae* and that caused by other agents, such as influenza virus, adenovirus, psittacosis, and Q fever, is ultimately dependent on laboratory diagnosis. Several serologic responses to infection with *M. pneumoniae* occur. Of historic interest is the nonspecific increase in titer of *Streptococcus* MG agglutinins that occurs in about 25 percent of patients. A more frequently used nonspecific serologic test is that for cold agglutinins. About two-thirds of patients with *M. pneumoniae* pneumonia will develop cold agglutinins for human red cells in a titer of 1:32 or greater, but about one-fifth of patients with adenovirus pneumonia may do similarly. Higher cold agglutinin responses are more likely to be associated with *M. pneumoniae* infection, but the proportion of patients having higher titers is decreased. An advantage of the cold agglutinin test is that titers may increase before a specific antibody response can be detected.

Tests most frequently used to assay for specific antibody to mycoplasmas are the metabolic inhibition (eg, tetrazolium reduction inhibition, glucose fermentation inhibition) and complement-fixation tests. Each will detect increases in antibody titer in appropriately collected sera from 80 percent or more of persons infected with *M. pneumoniae*. Other tests that can be used include indirect hemagglutination, latex fixation, indirect immunofluorescence, and the very sensitive complement-mediated mycoplasmacidal and radioimmunoprecipitation tests.

CULTURAL TECHNIQUES. *M. pneumoniae* can be cultured from sputum and throat swabs using special, enriched media. Growth can be achieved aerobically on a soft agar surface or in broth. Initial recovery may be enhanced by the use of diphasic medium (broth over agar). Inhibitors of bacterial growth (thallium acetate, penicillin) are routinely added to the media. Indicators for detection of growth (eg, 1 percent glucose and phenol red to detect fermentation) and inhibitors for the growth of mycoplasmas other than *M. pneumoniae* (eg, 0.001 percent methylene blue) may be added. Growth is slow, and media are usually observed for three to four weeks before being called negative. Colonies are small, and agar plates must be scanned microscopically with oblique lighting for detection of growth. *M. pneumoniae* can cause both hemagglutination (clumping of red blood cells by individual organisms) and hemadsorption (adsorption of red blood cells to colonies), apparently dependent on the presence of neuraminic acid-containing receptors on red blood cells. Another property frequently used for identifying *M. pneumoniae* colonies biologically on agar is rapid beta hemolysis of added guinea pig or sheep red blood cells due to production of a peroxide. Identity of the organism is established by testing for growth inhibition by specific antibody. This is conveniently done by placing antibody-impregnated paper disks on an agar plate that has been seeded with the organism and observing for zones of inhibition.

Treatment The laboratory diagnosis of *M. pneumoniae* infection usually cannot be achieved early enough to be of aid in guiding therapy, since methods for rapid diagnosis (eg, staining of specimens with fluorescein-labeled antibody) are not routinely available. Treatment must be instituted on the basis of the clinical diagnosis and epidemiologic data. Atypical pneumonia in adults is customarily treated with antibiotics directed against *M. pneumoniae*. In children, particularly those under age 5, the disease is usually treated only symptomatically because of the more frequent viral etiology and the desire to avoid the unnecessary use of antibiotics with their attendant dangers of toxicity and secondary infection with resistant bacteria.

Members of both the tetracycline and erythromycin groups of antibiotics reduce significantly the duration of fever and chest x-ray abnormalities in patients with mycoplasma pneumonia. Penicillins and cephalosporins are without effect. Improvement during therapy is not dramatic, and *M. pneumoniae* frequently persists in the throat after therapy. Antibiotic-resistant forms can be selected in the laboratory, but organisms recovered after treatment have remained sensitive to the antibiotic used.

Prevention There is no commonly accepted method available for preventing *M. pneumoniae* infection other than avoiding close contact with acutely ill patients. One approach to prophylaxis is the use of antibiotics in persons at high risk of infection. Use of prophylactic tetracycline in members of families with an index case of infection was reported to cause a significant reduction in clinical illness, although the incidence of infection was only minimally reduced.

Another approach has been through the development of vaccines. Trials with inactivated *M. pneumoniae* vaccines have shown them to be effective against both natural and artificially induced infection. However, in one study, illness appeared to be more severe in persons who failed to develop detectable antibody following vaccination than in controls. Strains of *M. pneumoniae* passed repeatedly on artificial media become attenuated and are effective vaccines, but they continue to produce illness in a portion of the vaccinees. Temperature-sensitive mutants restricted to growth in the upper respiratory tract have been developed recently and appear effective in preliminary animal studies.

OTHER MYCOPLASMAS

Diseases of human beings caused by mycoplasmas other than *M. pneumoniae* are infrequent and/or less well proven. *Mycoplasma fermentans* is a normal inhabitant of the genital tract, and *Mycoplasma orale* strains are normal inhabitants of the oropharynx. *Mycoplasma hominis* type 1 is a normal inhabitant of both the oropharynx and the genital tract, but a possible role in causing exudative pharyngitis and urethritis has been suggested. *M. hominis* type 1 has also been recovered from ovarian abscesses and from blood of patients with puerperal sepsis and febrile illness following gynecologic surgery. T strain mycoplasmas are normal inhabitants of the oropharynx and the genital trait, but they have been associated with venereally transmitted urethritis. Mycoplasmas have been detected in various specimens from patients with systemic lupus erythematosus, rheumatoid arthritis, and Reiter's syndrome. Whether mycoplasmas participate in causing such diseases, invade secondarily, or represent laboratory contaminants is uncertain. Similar uncertainty applies to mycoplasmas recovered from patients with leukemia and tumors. The organisms are common contaminants of tissue culture and may be falsely implicated in disease when isolation attempts involve tissue culture techniques.

FURTHER READING

Books and Reviews

Chanock RM, Musson MA, Johnson KM: Comparative biology and ecology of human virus and mycoplasma respiratory pathogens. Prog Med Virol 7:208, 1965

Couch RB: Mycoplasma pneumoniae. In Knight V (ed): Viral and Mycoplasmal Infections of the Respiratory Tract. Philadelphia, Lea & Febiger, 1973, p 217

Feizi T, MacLean H, Sommerville RG, et al: The role of mycoplasma in human disease: a symposium. Proc R Soc Med 59:1109, 1966

Grayston JT, Foy HM, Kenny GE: Mycoplasma (PPLO) in human disease. Disease-a-Month, Chicago, Year Book, Dec 1967

Hayflick O (ed): Biology of the mycoplasma. Ann NY Acad Sci 143:1, 1967

Hayflick L: Tissue cultures and mycoplasmas. Tex Rep Biol Med 23:285, 1965

Hayflick L, Chanock RM: Mycoplasma species of man. Bacteriol Rev 29:185, 1965

Hayflick L (ed): The Mycoplasmatales and the L-Phase of Bacteria. New York, Appleton, 1969

Kenny GE, Lemcke RM, Clyde WA (eds): Workshop on the Mycoplasmatales as Agents of Disease. J Infect Dis 127 (March Suppl), 1973, S1–S92

Stanbridge E: Mycoplasmas and cell cultures. Bacteriol Rev 35:206, 1971

Taylor-Robinson D: The biology of mycoplasmas. J Clin Pathol 21 [Suppl]:2, 1968

Selected Papers

Bak AL, Black FT, Christiansen C, Freundt EA: Genome size of mycoplasmal DNA. Nature 224:1209, 1969

Boatman ES, Kenny GE: Three-dimensional morphology, ultrastructure, and replication of Mycoplasma felis. J Bacteriol 101:262, 1970

Denny FW, Clyde WA Jr, Glezen WP: Mycoplasma pneumoniae in the community. Am J Epidemiol 93:55, 1971

Maniloff J: Electron microscopy of small cells: Mycoplasma hominis. J Bacteriol 100:1402, 1969

Murray HW, Masur H, Senterfit LB, Roberts RB: The protein manifestations of Mycoplasma pneumoniae infection in adults. Am J Med 58:229 1975

Shames JM, George RB, Holliday WB, Rasch JR, Mogabgab WJ: Comparison of antibiotics in the treatment of mycoplasmal pneumonia. Arch Intern Med 125:680 1970

SECTION 4
BASIC VIROLOGY

61
The Nature, Isolation, and Measurement of Animal Viruses

Many important infectious diseases afflicting mankind are caused by viruses. Some are important because they are frequently fatal; among these are rabies, smallpox, poliomyelitis, hepatitis, yellow fever, and various encephalitic diseases. Others are important because they are extremely contagious and create widespread discomfort; among these are influenza, the common cold, measles, mumps, and chickenpox, as well as respiratory–gastrointestinal disorders. Still other viruses, such as rubella, are teratogenic, and finally there are viruses that can cause tumors and cancer in animals and perhaps also in man.

There is little that can be done to interfere with the growth of viruses, since they multiply within cells, using the cells' synthetic apparatus. Only a limited number of highly specialized reactions are under their own control. Hopefully their selective inhibition will form the basis of a rational system of antiviral chemotherapy, thereby permitting virus diseases to be brought under effective control, just as antibiotics have brought most bacterial diseases under control.

In addition to their medical importance viruses provide the simplest model systems for many basic problems in biology. The reason is that viruses are essentially small segments of genetic material encased in protective shells. Since the information encoded in viral genomes differs from that in host cell genomes, viruses afford unrivaled opportunities for the study of the mechanisms that control the replication, transcription, and translation of genetic information. Knowledge of these mechanisms is fundamental to an understanding of the development and operation of differentiated functions in higher organisms and is therefore directly applicable to the practice of medicine and the improvement of human welfare.

HISTORICAL BACKGROUND

There are three major classes of viruses: animal viruses, plant viruses, and bacterial viruses. Since knowledge concerning each of these classes has accumulated along distinctive lines, extensive specialization has developed. Bacterial viruses are, therefore, only dealt with briefly in this book, and plant viruses are not considered at all. Yet, advances in our understanding of each of these virus classes have been profoundly dependent upon discoveries concerning the others.

The existence of viruses became evident during the closing years of the nineteenth century when, as the result of newly acquired expertise in the handling of bacteria, the infectious agents of numerous diseases were being isolated. For some infectious diseases this proved to be an elusive task until it was realized that the agents causing them were smaller than bacteria. Iwanowski in 1892 was probably the first to record the transmission of an infection (tobacco mosaic disease) by a suspension filtered through a bacteria-proof filter. This was followed in 1898 by a similar report by Loeffler and Frosch concerning foot-and-mouth disease of cattle. Beijerinck (1898) considered the infectious agents in bacteria-free filtrates to be living but fluid, that is, nonparticulate, and introduced the term "virus" (Latin, poison) to describe them. However, it quickly became clear that viruses were particulate, and the term "virus" became the operational definition of infectious agents smaller than bacteria and unable to multiply outside living cells. In 1911 Rous discovered a virus that produced malignant tumors in chickens, and during World War I Twort and d'Herelle independently discovered the viruses growing in bacteria, the bacteriophages.

During the next 25 years the experimental approaches in the three areas of virology diverged. Plant viruses proved easy to obtain in large amounts, thus permitting extensive chemical and physical studies. This work first led to the demonstration that plant viruses consisted only of nucleic acid and protein and culminated in the crystallization of tobacco mosaic virus by Stanley in 1935. This feat evoked great astonishment, since it cut across preconceived ideas concerning the attributes of living organisms and demonstrated that agents able to reproduce in living cells behaved under certain conditions as typical macromolecules.

Work with bacteriophages concentrated on their clinical application. It was hoped that bacteria could be destroyed inside the body by injecting appropriate bacteriophages. However, their activity in vivo never matched their activity in vitro, most probably because they are eliminated efficiently from the bloodstream.

Work with animal viruses concentrated on

the pathogenesis of viral infections and on epidemiology. Throughout this period fundamental studies on animal cell–virus interactions were severely hampered by the absence of rapid and efficient methods of quantitating viruses. The only method then available was the expensive and time-consuming serial end point dilution method using animals (p. 772).

Around the year 1940 came several breakthroughs. First, the advent of electron microscopy permitted visualization of viruses for the first time. As will become evident, not only is morphology an important criterion of virus classification, but also the study of the morphology of viruses has had a profound impact on our understanding of their behavior and function. Second, techniques for purifying certain animal viruses were being perfected, and a group of workers at the Rockefeller Institute headed by Rivers carried out some excellent chemical studies on vaccinia virus. Third, Hirst discovered that influenza virus agglutinated chicken red cells. This phemomenon, hemagglutination, was rapidly developed into an accurate method for quantitating myxoviruses, as a result of which this group of viruses became in the 1940s the most intensively investigated group of animal viruses. Finally, this period marked the beginning of the modern era of bacterial virology. Until then the interaction of bacteriophages with bacteria had been analyzed principally in terms of populations rather than at the level of a single virus partical interacting with a single cell. This conceptual block was removed by Ellis and Delbrück's study of the one-step growth cycle, as a result of which the bacteriophage–bacterium system became extraordinarily amenable to experimentation. Indeed, during the last three decades, most of the major advances in molecular biology have resulted from work in the bacteriophage field. Among these are the demonstration that initiation of viral infection involves the separation of viral nucleic acid and protein, the demonstration that the viral genome can become integrated into the genome of the host cell, the discovery of messenger RNA, and the elucidation of the factors that control initiation and termination of both the transcription and translation of genetic information.

Advances in animal virology during the last three decades have been due in large part to the development of techniques for growing animal cells in vitro. Strains of many types of mammalian cells can now be grown in media of defined composition. As a result, animal cell–virus interactions can now be analyzed with the same techniques that have proved so powerful in the case of bacteriophages.

THE NATURE OF VIRUSES

Viruses are a heterogeneous class of agents. They vary in size and morphology; they vary in chemical composition; they vary in host range and in effect on their hosts. However there are certain characteristics that identify viruses unequivocally.

(1) Viruses consist of a genome, either RNA or DNA, that is surrounded by a protective protein shell. Frequently this shell is itself enclosed in an envelope that contains both protein and lipid.
(2) Viruses multiply only inside cells. They are absolutely dependent on the host cells' synthetic and energy-yielding apparatus. They are parasites at the genetic level.
(3) The multiplication of all viruses involves as an initial step the separation of the genome from its protective shell.°

Viruses are therefore essentially elements of nucleic acid that can enter cells, where they replicate and code for proteins capable of forming protective shells around them.

Given this definition of viruses, are they to be regarded as living organisms or as lifeless arrangements of molecules? The answer to this question depends on whether one is concerned with viruses as extracellular suspensions of particles or as infectious agents. Isolated virus particles are arrangements of nucleic acid and protein molecules with no metabolism of their own and are no more active than isolated chromosomes. Within cells, however, virus particles are capable of reproducing their kind manyfold by virtue of precisely regulated sequences of reactions. Considered in this light viruses may indeed be said to possess at least some of the attri-

°*Recent work indicates that this rule is broken by reovirus (Chap. 65).*

butes of life. However such terms as "organism" and "living" are not really applicable to viruses, and it is preferable to refer to viruses as being functionally active or inactive, rather than living or dead.

THE ORIGIN OF VIRUSES

The question of the origin of viruses poses a fascinating problem. The two likeliest hypotheses are (1) viruses are the products of regressive evolution of free-living cells. An evolutionary pathway of this type has been suggested for mitochondria, which still retain vestiges of cellular organization, as well as a mechanism for replicating, transcribing, and translating genetic information. The largest animal viruses, the poxviruses, are so complex that one could imagine them also to be derived from a cellular ancestor. (2) Viruses are derived from cellular genetic material that has acquired the capacity to exist and function independently. It is impossible to decide between these two hypotheses, but the balance of evidence favors the latter.

THE CHARACTERISTICS OF CULTURED ANIMAL CELLS

The medical practitioner should understand not only how viruses affect the patient as a whole but also how viruses interact with cells. This understanding can be acquired far more readily by studying isolated infected cells than by examining infected cells in the intact organism. Animal virology provided the main impetus for the development of tissue culture, that is, the technique of growing cells in vitro, which is now used extensively for fundamental studies in areas ranging from growth, differentiation, and aging on the one hand to molecular biology and genetics on the other. Since knowledge concerning the normal cell is crucial to an understanding of the virus–cell interaction, we will first examine briefly the characteristics of animal cells cultured in vitro.

The Establishment of Animal Cell Strains

Cells of many organs can be grown in vitro. As a rule, small pieces of the tissue in question are dissociated into single cells by treatment with a dilute solution of trypsin, and a dilute suspension of the cells is then placed in a flask, bottle, or petri dish. There they attach to the flat surface, and provided they are supplied with a growth medium, they multiply. The essential constituents of the growth medium are physiologic amounts of 13 essential amino acids and 9 vitamins, salts, glucose, and a buffering system, generally consisting of bicarbonate in equilibrium with an atmosphere containing about 5 percent carbon dioxide. This medium is supplemented to the extent of about 5 percent with serum, the source of which is not predicated by the species from which the cells were derived: calf and fetal calf serum are the two most commonly employed. Antibiotics, such as penicillin and streptomycin, are also usually added in order to minimize the growth of bacterial contaminants, and a dye, such as phenol red, is generally included as a pH indicator. This medium, or slightly more complex versions of it, will permit most cell types to multiply with a division time of 24 to 48 hours.

When cells are brought into contact with a surface, they generally attach firmly and flatten so as to occupy the maximum surface area. The only time when they are not maximally extended is during mitosis, when they become round and are therefore easily dislodged from the substratum. Cells multiply until they occupy the whole available surface area, that is, until they are confluent, but no further. The reason for this is that cells cease dividing when they make contact with neighboring cells, a phenomenon known as "contact inhibition" (Chap. 69).

Animal cells can be cloned just like bacterial cells, although the efficiency of cloning is frequently less than 100 percent, and numerous genetically pure cell strains are now available. These fall into two morphologic categories, epithelial cells with a polygonal outline, and fibroblasts with a narrow spindlelike shape (Fig. 61-1).

The first cultures after tissue dispersion are known as "primary cultures." When such cul-

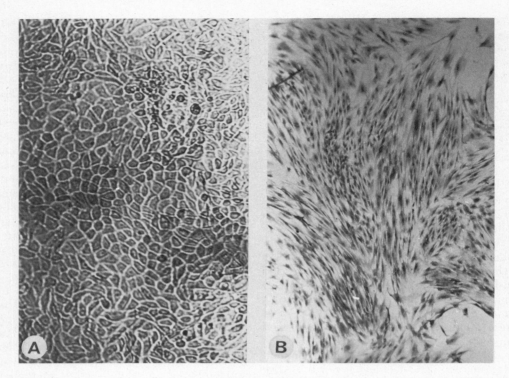

FIG. 61-1. Cultured mammalian cells. A. Unstained monkey kidney cells, which exhibit a typical epithelioid morphology. B. Chick embryo fibroblasts (Giemsa stain). Note characteristic spindle shape and orderly alignment. (A, from Eagle and Foley: Cancer Res 18:1017, 1958. B, courtesy of Dr. R. E. Smith).

tures are confluent, they are passaged by dislodgment from the surface by means of trypsin or the chelating agent ethylene diamine tetra-acetate (EDTA) and reseeded into several new containers, in which they form secondary cultures. Passaging can then be continued in this manner, provided that an adequate supply of growth medium is supplied at regular intervals.

The overall properties of cell strains are generally stable on continuous culturing. However, mutations occur constantly, so that one particular mutant, or variant, usually emerges as the dominant population component under any given set of conditions. As a result, the same cell strain cultured in two different laboratories may exhibit detectable phenotypic differences.

The Multiplication Cycle

The multiplication of each individual cell conforms to a regular pattern, which can be thought of as a cycle (Fig. 61-2). According to this scheme, the interval between successive mitoses is divided into three periods, namely, the G1 period preceding DNA replication, the S period during which DNA replicates, and the G2 period during which the cell prepares for the next mitosis. RNA and protein are not synthesized while mitosis proceeds, that is, during metaphase, but are otherwise synthesized throughout the multiplication cycle. Nongrowing cells are usually arrested in the G1 period; the resting state is often referred to as G 0 (G zero) . The relative durations of the various periods are quite variable, but metaphase rarely occupies more than one hour.

Under conditions of normal growth, the individual cells of a growing culture pass through this multiplication cycle in an unsynchronized fashion, so that cells at all stages of the cycle are always present. It is, however, possible to synchronize cells so that they multiply in step. Synchronized cultures are often very useful. For example, they permit the isolation of chromosomes in good yield, identification of the

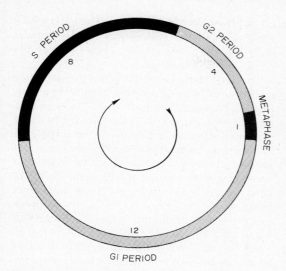

FIG. 61-2. The multiplication cycle of mammalian cells. The duration of the cycle illustrated here is 25 hours; the average lengths (in hours) of the individual periods is indicated by the numbers inside the cycle.

stage of the cell cycle when viral infection is most efficient, and so on.

The Aging of Cell Strains

Cells derived from normal tissue cannot be passaged indefinitely. Instead, after about 50 passages, which generally occupy about one year, their growth rate inevitably begins to slow. The amount of time that they spend in G 0 following each mitosis gradually increases, fewer and fewer cells enter the S period, and the cells' karyotype, that is, their chromosomal constitution, changes from the normal euploid (diploid) pattern characteristic of normal cells to an aneuploid one, characterized by the appearance of supernumerary chromosomes and chromosome fragments and by chromosomal aberrations, that is, changes in the structure of individual chromosomes. Finally, the cell strain dies out. Loss of cell strains in this manner is generally guarded against by growing large numbers of cells during the early passages and storing them at −196C, the boiling point of liquid nitrogen.

Continuous Cell Lines

While cells derived from normal tissues have the properties described thus far, malig-

nant tissues give rise to aneuploid cell lines that have an infinite life span and are referred to as "established cell lines." Very occasionally such cell lines seem to arise from euploid cell strains, but the possibility that malignant or premalignant cells were not present originally is difficult to rule out. In addition to being aneuploid and immortal, such cell lines usually have two other significant properties: they form tumors when transplanted into animals, and they can grow in suspension culture like bacteria. Cells growing in suspension are used extensively for studies of virus multiplication, since they are easier to handle experimentally than are cells growing as monolayers.

Pattern of Macromolecular Biosynthesis

Since virus multiplication consists essentially of nucleic acid and protein synthesis, a brief description of the pattern of macromolecular synthesis in animal cells is relevant. The essential feature of the animal cell is its compartmentalization. The DNA of the animal cell is restricted to the nucleus at all stages of the cell cycle except during metaphase, when no nucleus exists. All RNA is synthesized in the nucleus. The majority remains there, but messenger RNA and transfer RNA migrate to the cytoplasm. Ribosomal RNA is synthesized in the nucleolus; the two ribosomal subunits are assembled partly in the nucleolus and partly in the nucleus, and then they also migrate to the cytoplasm. All protein synthesis proceeds in the cytoplasm. The only exception to this brief summary concerns the mitochondria, which contain DNA-, RNA-, and protein-synthesizing systems of their own and which are located only in the cytoplasm.

THE DETECTION OF ANIMAL VIRUSES

The presence of viruses is recognized by the manifestation of some abnormality in host organisms or host cells. In the organism, symptoms of viral infection vary widely, from inapparent infections detectable only by the formation of antibody, the development of local lesions, or mild disease characterized by light febrile response, to progressively more severe disease culminating in death. Frequently the nature of the symptoms is profoundly influenced by the route of infection. For example, influenza virus causes pneumonia if instilled into the nose of a mouse, but if injected into the brain it causes toxic symptoms due to abortive multiplication, and poliovirus, administered orally, localizes preferentially in cells lining the intestinal tract and only rarely invades the central nervous system but, if injected intracerebrally, produces encephalitis. Such examples could be multiplied many times.

In cells, the symptoms of viral infection vary from changes in morphology and growth patterns to cytopathic effects, such as rounding, breakdown of cell organelles, the development of inclusion bodies, and general necrotic reactions, finally resulting in complete disintegration.

THE ISOLATION OF ANIMAL VIRUSES

Many techniques have been developed for isolating viruses. The source of virus may be excreted or secreted material, the bloodstream, or some tissue. Samples are collected and, unless processed immediately, sheltered from heat, preferably by storage at −70C, the temperature of dry ice. If necessary, a suspension is then prepared by grinding or sonicating in the presence of cold buffer solution, and this is then centrifuged in order to remove large debris and contaminating microorganisms.

This suspension is then tested for the presence of virus in several ways. First, it is injected back into the original host species in order to determine whether the first noted abnormality is produced. Second, the suspension is injected into other animals in order to establish whether more susceptible hosts exist in which the disease develops more rapidly, more severely, or in a more easily recognizable manner. Newborn or suckling animals, often mice or hamsters, or developing chick embryos, are hosts which permit many viruses to multiply more extensively than do adult animals and are accordingly widely used for virus isolation. Third, a search is conducted for a cultured animal cell strain or line in which the virus will multiply and in which it may actually be isolat-

ed and hopefully also assayed. The cells which will eventually be chosen will usually be ones in which the virus rapidly elicits readily observable cytopathic effects.

The final stage of the isolation procedures is a passage at limiting dilution in order to ensure that only a single unique virus is being isolated. This may be accomplished either by limiting serial dilution, when the virus suspension is diluted to such an extent that only one out of several aliquots inoculated gives a positive response, or by plaque isolation (p. 771). The latter is preferable wherever possible, since plaques originate from single virus particles, just as bacterial colonies originate from single bacterial cells.

While virus isolation from severely diseased hosts may present no difficulty, it may be a formidable task if the original source is merely suspected of containing a small amount of virus. As a result, no symptoms may result when the initial virus suspension is inoculated into the various test systems. In such cases one generally resorts to so-called blind passaging in the hope that gradual enrichment of virus will occur. In this procedure, cells are disrupted several days after inoculation even if they appear healthy and unaltered, and an extract of them is inoculated into fresh cells. This is repeated several times until symptoms appear. It is important that this procedure be adequately controlled by passaging extracts of uninfected cells under the same conditions, since animal cells are known to harbor latent viruses which may be induced to multiply and which may then be mistaken for the etiologic agent of whatever condition is under study.

Adaptation and Virulence   During the isolation of viruses, variants capable of multiplying more efficiently in the host cells used for this purpose than the original wild-type virus may emerge, a phenomenon known as "adaptation." Frequently, the new variants grow less readily in the original host and damage it less severely, that is, they are less virulent than the wild-type virus. Viruses are often purposely adapted in order to alter growth and virulence characteristics. A good example is provided by the attenuated vaccine virus strains, which are obtained by repeated passaging of virus virulent for one host in some different host until virus strains with decreased virulence for the original host are selected.

THE MEASUREMENT OF ANIMAL VIRUSES

Viruses are measured by several methods that can be divided into two categories. First, viruses may be measured as infectious units, that is, in terms of their ability to infect, multiply, and produce progeny. Second, viruses may be measured in terms of the total number of virus particles irrespective of their function as infectious agents.

Measurement of Viruses as Infectious Units

Measurement of the amount of virus in terms of the number of infectious units per unit volume is known as "titration." There are several ways of determining the titer of a virus suspension, all of them involving infection of host or target cells in such a way that each particle that causes productive infection elicits a recognizable reaction.

Plaque Formation In this method a series of monolayers of susceptible cells are inoculated with small aliquots of serial dilutions of the virus suspension to be titrated. Wherever virus particles infect cells, progeny virus is produced and released and then immediately infects adjoining cells. This process is repeated until, after a period ranging from 2 to 12 days or more, areas of infected cells develop which can be seen with the naked eye. These are called "plaques." In order to ensure that progeny virus particles liberated into the medium do not diffuse away and initiate separate (or secondary) plaques, agar is frequently incorporated into the medium.

The fundamental prerequisite for this method of enumerating infectious units is that the infected cells must differ in some way from noninfected cells: for example, they must either be completely destroyed, become detached from the surface on which they grow, or possess staining properties different from those of normal cells. In practice, the most common method of visualizing plaques is to apply the vital stain neutral red to infected cell monolayers after a certain number of days and to count the number of areas that do not stain (Fig. 61-3). Titers are expressed in terms of numbers of plaque-forming units (PFU) per ml.

There is a linear relationship between the amount of virus and the number of plaques produced, that is, the dose-response curve is linear. This indicates that each plaque is formed by a single virus particle. The viral progeny in each plaque therefore represents a clone, and virus stocks derived from single

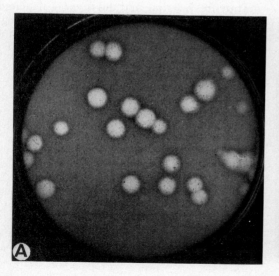
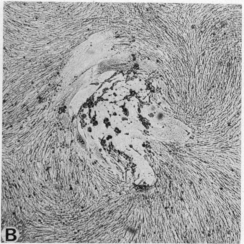

FIG. 61-3. Virus plaques. A. Plaques of influenza virus on monolayers of chick embryo cells, four days after inoculation. The monolayers were stained with neutral red on day 3. B. Photograph showing the microanatomy of a herpesvirus plaque on BHK 21 cells. (A, courtesy of Dr. G. Appleyard. B, courtesy of Dr. S. Moira Brown)

plaques are said to be plaque purified. Plaque purification is an important technique for the isolation of genetically pure virus strains.

Plaque formation is often the most desirable method off titrating viruses. It is economical of cells and viruses as well as technically simple. However, not all viruses can be measured in this way, owing to lack of cells that develop desired cytopathic effects. For these viruses alternate titration methods must be used.

Pock Formation   Many viruses cause macroscopically recognizable foci of infection or lesions on the chorioallantoic membrane of the developing chick embryo, which may be used in a manner similar to the cell monolayers employed for plaque assay. Its main advantage is its ready availability, wide virus susceptibility, and ease of handling. Its main disadvantage is variation in virus susceptibility among different eggs of even the same hatch, so that much larger numbers of eggs than cell tissue culture monolayers are necessary in order to attain the same level of statistical significance. The lesions caused by viruses are known as "pocks" and are generally recognizable as opaque white or red areas caused by cell disintegration, migration, and proliferation, as well as edema and hemorrhage (in the case of red pocks) (Fig. 61-4). The actual titration is carried out as described for plaques, with enumeration of pocks taking the place of plaque counting.

Focus Formation   Certain tumor viruses do not destroy the cells in which they multiply and therefore produce no plaques. However, they cause cells to change morphology and to multiply at a faster rate than uninfected cells. As a result, foci of transformed cells develop that gradually become large enough to be visible to the naked eye (Fig. 61-5). Assay by focus formation (counting the number of focus-forming units or FFU) is analogous to assay by plaque and pock formation.

Plaque and focus formation assays are generally performed on monolayers of cells growing in vitro but may be carried out in intact animals under special circumstances. For example, fowlpox virus may be assayed by inoculating the scalp of chickens and enumerating the number of local lesions produced, and certain mouse leukemia viruses may be assayed by injection into mice and counting the number of foci of transformed cells produced on the spleen.

The Serial Dilution End Point Method   Although many viruses destroy cells, they do not produce the type of cytopathic effects necessary for visible plaque formation. Such viruses may be titered by means of the serial dilution end point method. In this method serial dilutions of virus suspensions are inoculated into cell monolayers, which are then incubated until the cell sheet shows clear signs of cell destruction (Fig. 61-6). The end point is that dilution which gives a positive (cell-destroying) reaction, and the titer is calculated assuming that the last positive dilution originally contained at least one infectious unit.

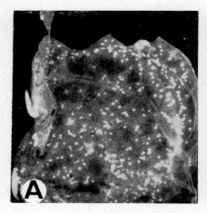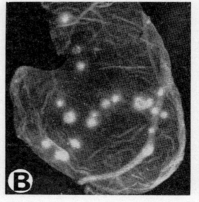

FIG. 61-4. Pocks on the chorioallantoic membrane of the developing chick embryo. The membrane is cut out two or three days after inoculation, washed and spread on a flat surface. A. Variola. B. Vaccinia. (From Kempe: Fed Proc 14: 468, 1955)

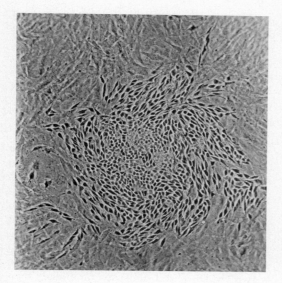

FIG. 61-5. Focus of NRK (normal rat kidney) cells transformed by Kirsten murine sarcoma virus. ×200. (Courtesy of Dr. S. A. Aaronson)

Considerable accuracy can be attained by the use of statistical methods of treating results.

The dilution end point method is also commonly employed when virus is titrated in laboratory animals. Examples are the titration of arboviruses in the brains of suckling mice, with death as the end point, and the titration of cer-

tain poxviruses on the backs of rabbits, the end point being the production of local lesions.

Enumeration of the Total Number of Virus Particles

It is universally true for all animal viruses that even though one virus particle is capable of causing infection, not all particles in a population actually do so. The total number of virus particles in a given preparation can be determined by either direct or indirect methods.

Counting by Means of Electron Microscopy
Direct counting of virus particles by means of electron microscopic examination is carried out according to either of two methods. The first involves mixing virus preparations with suspensions of latex spheres of similar size and known concentration and spraying the mixture onto coated electron microscope grids. The number of virus particles and spheres in individual spray droplets is then counted: knowing the concentration of the spheres, the number of virus particles can be calculated (Fig. 61-7). The second method involves centrifuging virus preparations onto electron microscope grids and counting the virus particles: Knowing what volume of the virus suspension was centrifuged, the virus concentration can again be calculated.

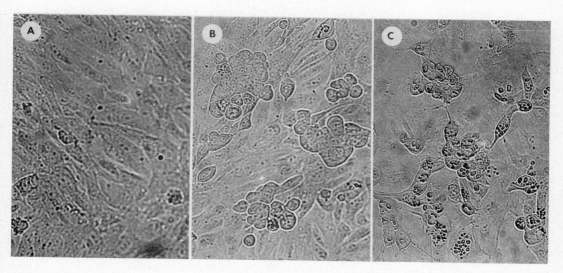

FIG. 61-6. The cytopathic effects caused by adenovirus type 7 in human embryonic kidney cells. A. Normal cell sheet. B. Partial cell destruction (five days after infection). C. Almost total cell destruction (seven days after infection). ×160. (Courtesy of Dr. C. M. Wilfert)

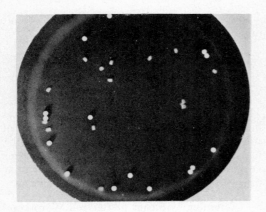

FIG. 61-7. An entire spray droplet containing 15 latex particles (spheres) and 14 vaccinia virus particles (slightly smaller brick-shaped particles). ×6,500. (From Dumbell, Downie, and Valentine. Virology 4:467, 1957)

Measurement of Optical Density The concentration of very highly purified virus preparations can be routinely determined by very simple methods once they have been standardized by electron microscopy. One of these methods is measurement of the optical density. For example, 1 ml of a suspension of reovirus particles which absorbs 90 percent of incident light at a wavelength of 260 nm (that is, 1 Optical Density unit or 1 OD_{260Nm} contains 2.1×10^{12} virus particles, and 1 OD_{260Nm} of vaccinia virus corresponds to 1.2×10^{10} particles.

The Hemagglutination Assay The most common indirect method of measuring the number of virus particles is the hemagglutination assay. Many animal viruses adsorb to the red blood cells of various animal species. Each virus particle is multivalent in this regard, that is, it can adsorb to more than one cell at a time. In practice, the maximum number of cells with which any particular virus particle can combine is two, because red cells are far bigger than viruses. In a virus–cell mixture in which the number of cells exceeds the number of virus particles, the small number of cell dimers that may be formed is generally not detectable, but if the number of virus particles exceeds the

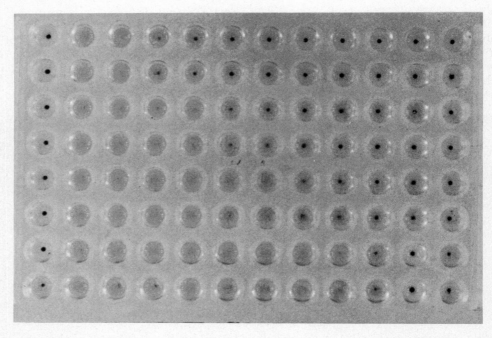

FIG. 61-8. Hemagglutination titration of influenza virus. In the bottom two rows a sample of influenza virus was diluted in serial twofold steps from left to right (except in the first tube, which served as a control). In the next two rows the amount of virus in the first virus tube was the same as in the third virus tube in the bottom rows, and so on up. The same number of red blood cells was then added to all tubes, and after mixing, the tray was placed at 4C for two hours. Unagglutinated cells form a dark button; where the virus has agglutinated cells, the resulting lattice has prevented button formation. The pattern developed in this tray attests to the reproducibility of the technique. (Courtesy of Dr. T. R. Cate)

number of cells, a lattice of cells is formed which settles out in a highly characteristic manner readily distinguishable from the pattern exhibited by unagglutinated cells.

The hemagglutination assay is performed by determining the virus dilution that will just hemagglutinate a given number of red cells (Fig. 61-8). Since the number of virus particles necessary for this is readily calculated, hemagglutination serves as a highly accurate and rapid method of quantitating virus particles. It was and still is particularly useful in studies with myxoviruses, particularly influenza virus, and many others.

The Significance of the Infectious Unit: Virus Particle Ratio   For all animal viruses the number of virus particles in any given preparation exceeds the number of demonstrably infectious units: usually the ratio of infectious units to particles is in the range of 1:10 to 1:1,000 or even less. There are two possible explanations for this situation. The first is that virus preparations contain a majority of noninfectious particles. Although this may be so sometimes, it is unlikely to be the general rule. It is more likely that although all virus particles in a given preparation are capable of causing productive infection, only a small proportion of them are actually successful in doing so. Two lines of evidence support this view. The first is that the titer of a given virus preparation varies markedly depending on the nature of the assay system. For example, the titer often differs with the route of inoculation, if the virus is assayed in whole animals, and with the type of cell, if it is assayed in tissue culture. Second, before a virus particle can manifest itself as a plaque, pock, focus, and so on, it must initiate a productive infection cycle that requires numerous reactions, many of which have a low probability of occurring (Chap. 65). Therefore, the number of infectious units cannot equal the total number of virus particles, and the ratio of the two may generally be regarded as a measure of the probability with which virus particles accomplish productive infection.

FURTHER READING

Books and Reviews

VIRUSES

Andrewes CH, Pereira HG: Viruses of vertebrates. Baltimore, Williams & Wilkins, 1972

Cooper PD: The plaque assay of animal viruses. In Maramorosch K, Koprowski H (eds): Methods in Virology, New York and London, Academic Press, 1967, p 243

Fenner F, McAuslan BR, Mims CA, Sambrook J, White DO: Animal Viruses, 2nd ed. New York, Academic Press, 1974

Higashi N: Electron microscopy of viruses in thin sections of cells grown in culture. Prog Med Virol 15:331, 1973

Joklik WK: Evolution in Viruses. Symp Soc Gen Microbiol 24:293, 1974

Kalter SS, Heberling RL: Comparative virology of primates. Bacteriol Rev 35:310, 1971

Luria SE, Darnell JE Jr: General Virology. New York, London, and Sydney, Wiley, 1967

Rosen L: Hemagglutination with animal viruses. In Habel K, Salzman NP (eds): Fundamental Techniques in Virology. New York and London, Academic Press, 1969, p 276

CELLS

Ambrose EJ, Easty B: Cell Biology. London, Nelson, 1970

Bautz EKF, Karlson P, Kersten H: Regulation of Transcription and Translation in Eukaryotes. New York, Heidelberg, and Berlin, Springer Verlag, 1974

Clarkson B, Baserga R (eds): Control of Proliferation in Animal Cells. New York, Cold Spring Harbor Laboratory, 1974

Giese AC: Cell Physiology, 4th ed. Philadelphia, Saunders, 1973

Ham RG: Unique requirements for clonal growth. J Natl Cancer Inst 53:1459, 1974

Harris H: Nucleus and Cytoplasm. Oxford, Clarendon Press, 1974

Hayflick L: Cell culture and the aging phenomenon. In Krohn PL (ed): Topics in the Biology of Aging. New York, Interscience, 1966, p. 83

Holper JC: Monolayer and suspension cell cultures. In Habel K, Salzman NP (eds): Fundamental Techniques in Virology. New York and London, Academic Press, 1969, p 3

Kaighn ME: "Birth of a Culture"—Source of postpartum anomalies. J Natl Cancer Inst 53:1437, 1974

Mueller GC, Kajiwara K: Synchronization of cells for DNA synthesis. In Habel K, Salzman NP (eds): Fundamental Techniques in Virology. New York and London, Academic Press, 1969, p 21

Pollack R (ed): Readings in Mammalian Cell Culture. New York, Cold Spring Harbor Laboratory, 1973

Taylor WG: "Feeding the Baby"—Serum and other supplements to chemically defined medium. J Natl Cancer Inst 53:1449, 1974

Selected Papers

Amsterdam A, Jamieson JT: Techniques for dissociating pancreatic exocrine cells. J Cell Biol 63:1037, 1974

Crissman HA, Tobey RA: Cell-cycle analysis in 20 minutes. Science 184:1297, 1974

Gilbert SF, Migeon BR: D-Valine as a selective agent for normal human and rodent epithelial cells in culture. Cell 5:11, 1975

Goldman RD, Lazarides E, Pollack R, Weber K: The distribution of actin in non-muscle cells. Exp Cell Res 90:333, 1975

Gospodarowicz D, Moran J: Effect of a fibroblast growth

factor, insulin, dexamethasone, and serum on the morphology of BALB/c 3T3 cells. Proc Natl Acad Sci USA 71:4648, 1974

Igarashi A, Mantani M: Rapid titration of dengue virus type 4 infectivity by counting fluorescent foci. Biken J 17:87, 1974

Kornberg RD: Chromatin structure: A repeating unit of histones and DNA. Science 184:868, 1974.

Kornberg RD, Thomas JO: Chromatin structure: Oligomers of histones. Science 184:865, 1974

Kuroki T: Colony formation of mammalian cells on agar plates and its application to Lederberg's replica plating. Exp Cell Res 80:55, 1973

Oudet P, Cross-Bellard M, Chambon P: Electron microscopic and biochemical evidence that chromatin structure is a repeating unit. Cell 4:281, 1975

Rheinwald JG, Green H: Growth of cultured mammalian cells on secondary glucose sources. Cell 2:287, 1974

Smith JR, Hayflick L: Variation in the life-span of clones derived from human diploid strains. J Cell Biol 62:48, 1974

Wheatley DN: Hypertonicity and the arrest of mammalian cells in metaphase: A synchrony technique for HeLa cells. J. Cell Sci 15:221, 1974

62

The Structure, Components, and Classification of Viruses

THE MORPHOLOGY OF ANIMAL VIRUSES

Although animal viruses differ widely in shape and size, they are nevertheless constructed according to certain common principles. Basically, viruses consist of nucleic acid and protein. The nucleic acid is the genome which contains the information necessary for virus multiplication; the protein is arranged around the genome in the form of a layer or shell that is termed the "capsid." The structure consisting of shell plus nucleic acid is the nucleocapsid. Many animal virus particles consist of a naked nucleocapsid, while others possess an additional envelope that is usually acquired as the nucleocapsid buds from the host cell. The complete virus particle is known as the "virion," a term that denotes both intactness of structure and the property of infectiousness.

Capsids

The essential feature of capsids is that they are composed of repeating subunits arranged in precisely defined patterns. The simplest form of such subunits is single protein molecules. More complex forms are morphologic subunits termed "capsomers" that can be seen by electron microscopy and that consist of several either identical or different protein molecules. The use of repeating subunits for capsid construction has two noteworthy consequences: (1) it minimizes the amount of genetic information necessary to specify capsids, and (2) it assures that they will be assembled efficiently. Capsid proteins exhibit a strong tendency to aggregate with each other, and much of the information necessary for the morphogenesis of nucleocapsids is inherent in their amino acid sequence.

Capsids (and envelopes) have a dual function. The first is to protect viral genomes from potentially destructive agents in the extracellular environment, such as enzymes, and the second is to introduce viral genomes into host cells. The need for this latter function stems from the fact that viral nucleic acids are often longer than cell diameters and cannot penetrate into cells by themselves. Capsids (and envelopes), on the other hand, adsorb readily to cell surfaces and can enter cells by several mechanisms (Chap. 65).

Envelopes

Only five groups of animal viruses exist as naked nucleocapsids. In all the remainder the nucleocapsids are enclosed by envelopes that consist of typical lipid bilayer membranes and that are acquired as the nucleocapsids bud through special patches of cell membrane on their way to the exterior of the cell. The source of the viral envelope membrane is most commonly either the outer cell plasma membrane or the vacuolar membrane. The membrane patches through which nucleocapsids bud are virus-modified: Usually the cell-specified proteins in them are completely replaced by virus-specified proteins, and virus-specified glycoprotein spikes are attached to their outer surface. However, there are exceptions: The envelopes of herpesviruses and RNA tumor viruses very probably still contain some host-coded proteins, and although herpesvirus envelopes contain glycoproteins, they do not form obvious spikes.

Viral envelopes generally lack rigidity. As a consequence they usually appear heterogeneous in shape and size when fixed for electron microscopy, and enveloped viruses are therefore often said to be "pleomorphic." There is little doubt, however, that in their native state most enveloped viruses are spherical, enclosing either icosahedral nucleocapsids or spherically coiled helical nucleocapsids. However, two types of enveloped viruses are not spherical. These are the rhabdoviruses, which possess a highly characteristic bulletlike shape, rounded at one end and flat at the other (Fig. 62-5), and certain strains of influenza virus, the helical nucleocapsids of which become enveloped not in a coiled but in an extended configuration, which causes the enveloped virus particles also to be long and filamentous (see Fig. 62-4).

Nucleocapsids

Viral nucleocapsids are constructed according to a small number of basic patterns.

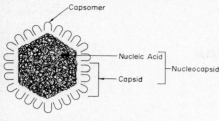

NAKED ICOSAHEDRAL NUCLEOCAPSID

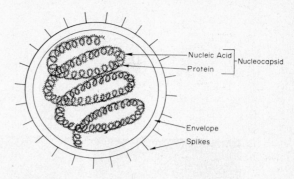

ENVELOPED HELICAL NUCLEOCAPSID

FIG. 62-1. The two basic patterns of animal virus structure. Left: the condensed genome is enclosed by a shell of capsomers arranged so as to display 5:3:2 rotational symmetry. Right: the extended genome is enclosed by protein molecules spaced so as to display helical symmetry. The resultant structure, the nucleocapsid, is enclosed in an envelope which is generally studded with spikes on its outer surface.

Two of these have been studied in great detail at both the structural and the molecular level: In one the nucleic acid is extended, in the other it is condensed (Fig. 62-1). Superimposed on these two patterns are variations dictated by both the size of the genome and the nature of the capsid polypeptides.

Nucleocapsids with Helical Symmetry   The prototype of nucleocapsids in which the nucleic acid occurs as an extended filament is a plant virus, tobacco mosaic virus (TMV), the structure of which has been studied extensively by x-ray diffraction. In this virus, the extended nucleic acid molecule is surrounded by protein molecules arranged helically so as to yield a structure with a single rotational axis (Fig. 62-2). The myxoviruses and rhabdoviruses possess nucleocapsids constructed in this manner, each with its own characteristic length, width, periodictiy, flexibility, and stability (Fig. 62-3). It should be noted that these nucleocapsids are not the complete virions: The virions of these virus families consist of the nucleocapsids coiled more or less tightly inside envelopes (Figs. 62-4 and 62-5).

Nucleocapsids with Icosahedral Symmetry In the second pattern of virus structure, the nucleic acid is condensed and forms the central portion of a quasispherical nucleocapsid. Here the capsid consists of a shell of protein molecules that are clustered into small groups called

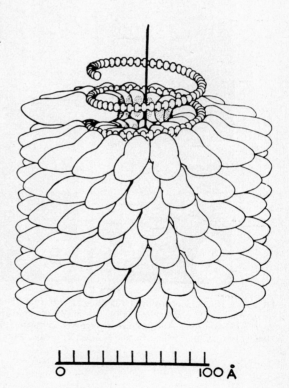

FIG. 62-2. Schematic representation of tobacco mosaic virus. As can be seen in the cutaway section, the ribonucleic acid helix is associated with protein molecules in the ratio of three nucleotides per protein molecule. (From Klug and Caspar: Adv Virus Res 7:225, 1960)

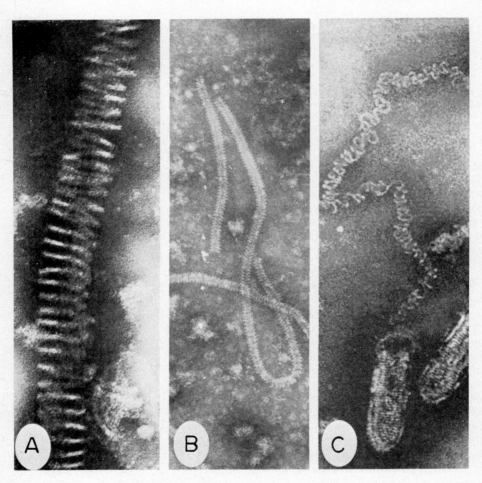

FIG. 62-3. The nucleocapsids of (A) influenza virus strain PR8 (×225,000), (B) measles virus (×150,000), and (C) vesicular stomatitis virus (VSV) (×160,000). The latter is emerging from a damaged virion. (From (A) Almeida and Waterson: In Barry and Mahy (eds): The Biology of Large RNA Viruses, 1970. Courtesy of Academic Press; (B) Finch and Gibbs: J Gen Virol 6:144, 1970; (C) Simpson and Hauser: Virology 29:660, 1966)

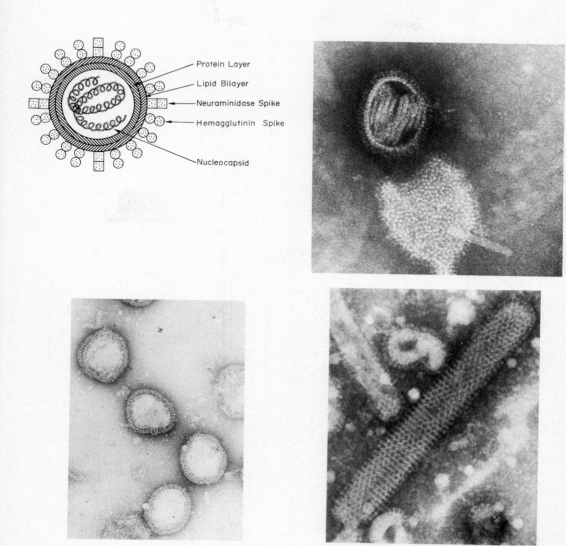

Protein Layer

Lipid Bilayer

Neuraminidase Spike

Hemagglutinin Spike

Nucleocapsid

FIG. 62-4. The structure of influenza virus. Top left. Model of influenza viral particle. The nucleocapsid is loosely coiled inside an envelope that consists of both protein and lipid and to which two different types of spikes, each consisting of two species of proteins, are attached. Hemagglutinin spikes are about five times as numerous as neuraminidase spikes. Top right. Influenza virus A$_2$, stained with phosphotungstate. One particle is penetrated by the stain, thereby revealing the arrangement of the internal nucleocapsid. ×155,000 (Courtesy of Dr. M.V. Nermut) Bottom left. Influenza virus A$_0$/WSN, stained with phosphotungstate, revealing the characteristic arrangement of spikes on the particle surface. ×135,000 (Courtesy of Dr. I.T. Schulze) Bottom right. A filamentous particle of an influenza C strain. Note reticular surface pattern of hexons and pentons and absence of spikes, which is reflected in the virtual inability of these strains to hemagglutinate. ×115,000. (From Apostolov and Flewett: J Gen Virol 4:366, 1969)

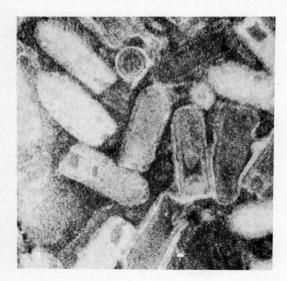

FIG. 62-5. Vesicular stomatitis virus (VSV) particles, some penetrated by stain, revealing the tightly coiled nucleocapsid. Note highly characteristic bullet shape. ×130,000. (From Hackett: Virology 24:55, 1964)

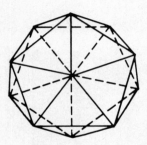 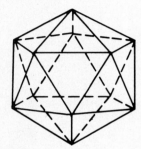 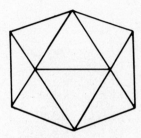

FIG. 62-6. The icosahedron viewed normal to 5-, 3-, and 2-fold rotational axes. Edges of the upper and lower surfaces are drawn in solid and broken lines respectively. The 5-fold rotational axes pass through the vertices (left); the 3-fold rotational axes pass through the centers of the triangular faces (center); and the 2-fold rotational axes pass through the edges (right). In this view, the edges on the upper and lower surfaces coincide. Note that the icosahedron possesses 12 vertices, 20 triangular faces, and 30 edges.

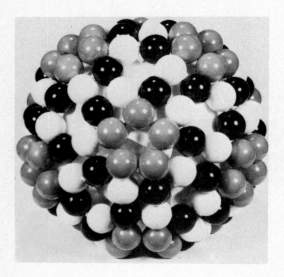

FIG. 62-7. Model of the picornavirus capsid. There are 60 capsomers, each consisting of three protein molecules, represented here by white, gray, and black balls. (From Johnston and Martin: J Gen Virol 11:77, 1971)

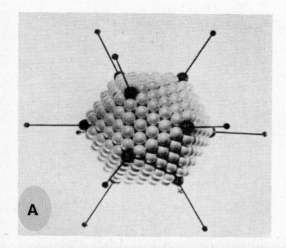

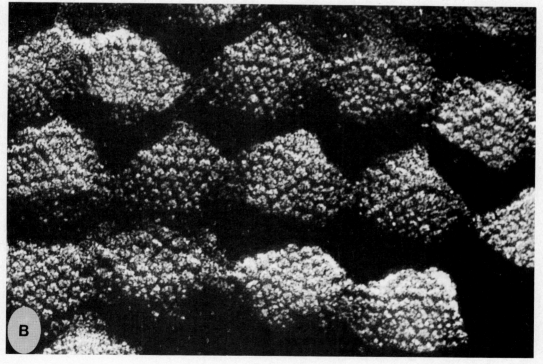

FIG. 62-8. A. Model of adenovirus constructed by R.C. Valentine. B. Adenovirus freeze-dried and shadowed with platinum. ×400,000 (Courtesy of Dr. M.V. Nermut)

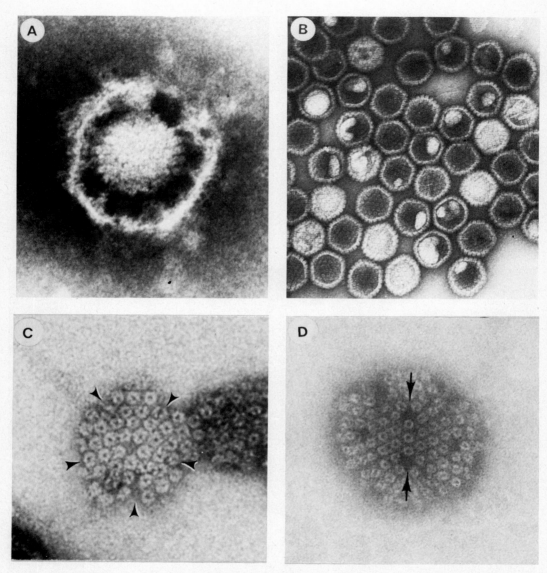

FIG. 62-9. The morphology of herpesviruses. A. Enveloped equine abortion virus (EAV) particle. ×125,000. B. EAV particles from which the envelope has been removed by treatment with detergent. ×75,000. C and D. Ultrastructure of partially disrupted herpesvirus nucleocapsids exhibiting 5-fold and 2-fold symmetry axes respectively. ×320,000. (A and B from Abodeely, Lawson, and Randall: J Virol 5: 513, 1970, C and D, courtesy of Dr. Erskine Palmer, Center for Disease Control, Atlanta, Georgia)

"capsomers," with the bonds between molecules within capsomers being stronger than those between capsomers. Capsomers are morphologic units which can often be seen with the electron microscope. They vary in size and shape from virus to virus: there are round as well as prismatic and solid as well as hollow capsomers.

X-ray diffraction analysis indicates that in this type of nucleocapsid the capsomers are arranged extremely precisely according to icosahedral patterns chracterized by 5:3:2-fold rotational symmetry (Fig. 62-6). Seven such patterns are found among animal viruses. The simplest is that exhibited by picornaviruses. Here 60 identical capsomers are situated equidistantly from a common center, which results in a spherical capsid (Fig. 62-7). The adenovirus capsid is constructed in the shape of an icosahedron with 6 capsomers along each edge and 252 capsomers altogether (Fig. 62-8). Of these, 240 are spherical and are situated along the edges and on the faces of the icosahedron; each has 6 nearest neighbors and is known as a "hexon" or "hexamer." The remaining 12 are situated at the 12 vertices of the icosahedron and have 5 nearest neighbors; these are known as "pentons" or "pentamers." They have a highly characteristic shape, consisting of a spherical base and a long fiber which may serve as the cell attachment organ.

The capsids of four other virus groups are constructed similarly. Iridovirus capsids possess 10 capsomers along each edge, and there are 1,112 capsomers altogether, 1,100 hexamers and 12 pentamers; herpesvirus capsids possess 5 capsomers along each edge and 162 capsomers altogether, 150 prism-shaped hexamers and 12 pentamers (Fig. 62-9); papovavirus capsids consist of 72 capsomers, 60 hexamers, and 12 pentamers (Fig. 62-10); and parvovirus capsids are probably made up of 32 capsomers, 20 hexamers, and 12 pentamers (Fig. 62-10).

Finally, the reoviruses fall into a special category, since they possess not one but two capsid shells. Both possess icosahedral symmetry, but it has so far proved impossible to discern either the total number of capsomers or the precise manner in which they are arranged (Fig. 62-11).

In the case of the picornaviruses, adenoviruses, papovaviruses, parvoviruses and reoviruses, the virions are the naked nucleocapsids. In the case of the herpesviruses and the sole iridovirus that is a mammalian virus, however, the naked nucleocapsids themselves are relatively noninfectious; here the virions consist of enveloped icosahedral nucleocapsids.

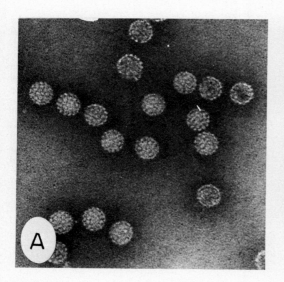 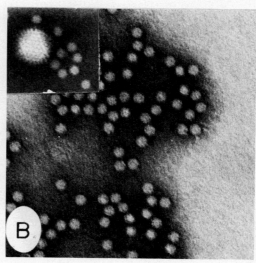

FIG. 62-10. A. The papovavirus SV40 (×160,000) and, B, the parvovirus adeno-associated virus (AAV) type 4 (×150,000). Insert. A virion of the simian adenovirus SV15, which enabled the AAV to multiply (Chap. 73). (A and B, Courtesy of Dr. Heather D. Mayor)

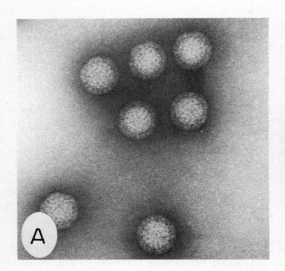

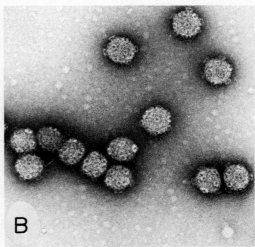

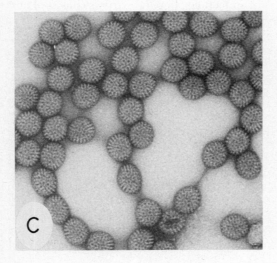

FIG. 62-11. Morphology of reovirus and infantile gastro-enteritis virus (Table 62-4 and Chap. 84). A. Reovirus. Note double capsid shell. The arrangement of capsomers is clearly discernible only at the periphery. ×120,000. B. Reovirus cores. Cores are derived from reovirions by digesting the outer capsid shell with chymotrypsin. Note the large spikes; there are 12, located as if situated on the 12 vertices of an icosahedron. C. Infantile gastroenteritis virus. There are 32 clearly defined capsomers. This structure is similar to, but not identical with, that of orbiviruses. ×136,000. (A and B, Courtesy of Drs. R. B. Luftig and W. K. Joklik, C, courtesy of Dr. Erskine Palmer, Center for Disease Control, Atlanta, Georgia).

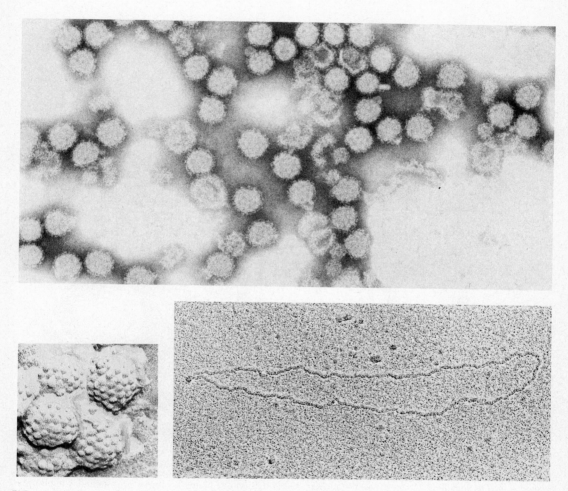

FIG. 62-12. The structure of togaviruses. Top. Sindbis virus, stained with phosphotungstate ×110,000. Bottom left. Sindbis virus, freeze-fractured and shadowed with platinum, to show the surface structure ×140,000. Bottom right. The circular nucleocapsid of the bunyavirus Uukuniemi virus, shadowed with platinum. The nucleocapsid was released from the virion with the nonionic detergent Triton X-100 ×60,000. (All micrographs courtesy of Dr. C.H. von Bonsdorff)

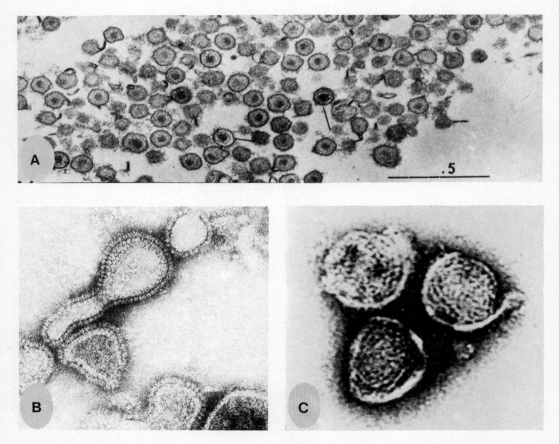

FIG. 62-13. The structure of RNA tumor viruses. A. Thin section of Rous sarcoma virus particles. Outer and inner membranes as well as nucleoids are clearly visible (arrows). ×52,000. B. Mouse mammary tumor virus stained with phosphotungstate, revealing the arrangement of surface glycoprotein spikes. ×160,000. C. Disrupted cores of Rauscher leukemia virus, revealing the circular arrangement of the internal component. ×200,000. (A, from Courington and Vogt: J Virol 1:400, 1967; B, courtesy of Dr. J.B. Sheffield; C, courtesy of Dr. R.B. Luftig)

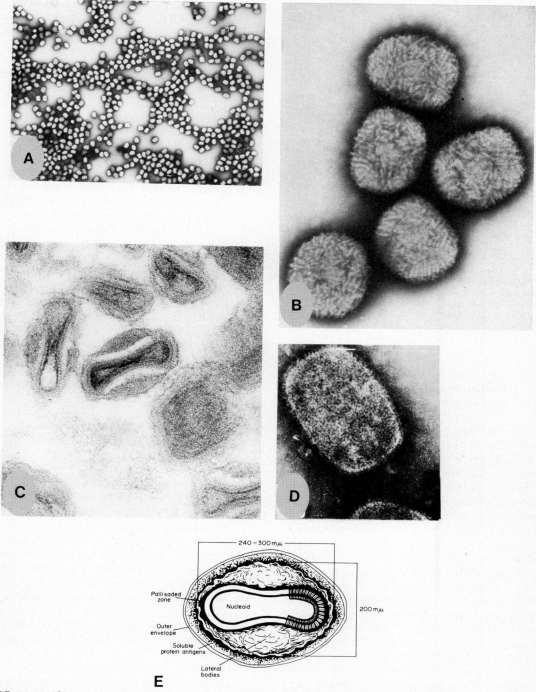

FIG. 62-14. The structure of vaccinia virus. A. A purified virus preparation. Note characteristic brickshape. ×6,000. B. Vaccinia virus particles stained with phosphotungstate to reveal surface structure. Note characteristic arrangement of rodlets or tubules. ×60,000. C. Cross-section of vaccinia virus particle. ×70,000. D. An isolated core, showing regular surface elements ×90,000. E. A. model of the vaccinia virus particle. (A, B and C, courtesy of Dr. Samuel Dales; D, from Easterbrook: J Ultrastruc Res 14:484, 1966; E, adapted from Westwood et al: J Gen Microbiol 34:67, 1964)

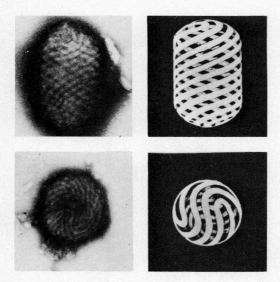

FIG. 62-15. Parapoxvirus particles. These are particles of contagious pustular dermatitis virus (ORF), negatively stained so as to reveal the crisscross arrangement of surface strands or tubules. ×90,000. (From Büttner, Giese, and Peters. Arch Ges Virusforsch 14:657, 1964)

The Structure of Togaviruses, Bunyaviruses, RNA Tumor Viruses, and Poxviruses

The structure of these viruses, particularly that of their nucleocapsids, is less well defined. There are two morphologic patterns within the Togavirus family. Alphaviruses (from the old Group A) consist of a condensed RNA molecule intimately associated with protein to form a nucleocapsid that possesses distinct icosahedral symmetry elements and that is surrounded by an envelope which, like most other viral envelopes, bears glycoprotein projections (Fig. 62-12). Flaviviruses (from the prototype strain *yellow* fever virus) possess a similar structure but are slightly smaller, and their nucleocapsids do not display obvious symmetry elements. The Bunyaviruses are much larger and possess circular helical nucleocapsids enclosed in similar envelopes.

RNA tumor viruses have a more complex structure. Their nucleocapsid seems to consist of a spirally or concentrically coiled filament in the central or core portion of the virion. This core is enclosed within a membrane which is closely associated with a capsid that possesses

icosahedral symmetry and that is itself bounded by a membrane that bears more or less prominent glycoprotein spikes (Fig. 62-13) (Chap. 69).

Poxviruses are the largest and most complex of all animal viruses. Morphologically, there are two classes of poxviruses. Most poxvirus particles are prolate ellipsoids that are often brick-shaped when fixed for electron microscopy. They are covered on their outer surface with tubules or filaments arranged in a characteristic whorled or mulberry pattern (Fig. 62-14). Within this outer layer there is a protein coat, which contains two lateral bodies of unknown composition and function, and a DNA-containing nucleoid or core bounded by a protein coat composed of well-defined subunits.

Parapoxviruses are somewhat smaller, ovoid rather than brick-shaped, and covered on their outer surface by tubules or filaments similar to those covering the poxvirus particles described above, except that they are arranged in a highly regular, crisscross pattern, which is in all probability caused by one continuous filament wound round each particle in 12 to 15 left-handed turns (Fig. 62-15). The internal components of parapoxvirus particles are similar to those of the poxvirus particles described above.

The Structure of Arenaviruses, Coronaviruses, and Some Miscellaneous Viruses

The morphology of these viruses is not well defined in structural terms and certainly not in molecular terms. Arenaviruses (Fig. 62-16) are enveloped virus particles that contain highly characteristic granules (Latin *arenosus*, sandy), which are thought to be ribosomes. Coronavirus particles (Fig. 62-17) are also enveloped, with characteristic large club-shaped or pear-shaped projections or spikes (which surround the virus particle like a halo, hence the name). The nucleocapsid structure of neither arenaviruses nor coronaviruses is known with certainty.

Finally, there are several viruses which have not yet been assigned to any virus family. Among these are hepatitis A and B viruses (infectious and serum hepatitis virus, respectively), which appear to be particles 27 nm and 42 nm (Dane particles) in diameter, respective-

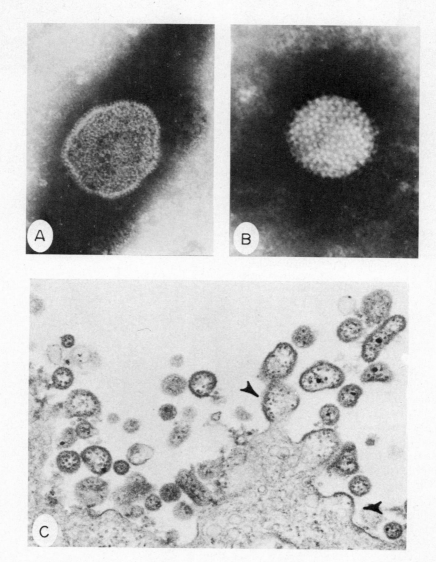

FIG. 62-16. Tacaribe virus, an arenavirus. A and B. Two virus particles, one of which has been partially penetrated by negative contrast medium, showing the close projections that cover the surface. ×135,000 and ×235,000, respectively. C. Thin section of Parana virus particles budding from the plasma membrane of Vero African Green Monkey kidney cells. Note the characteristic dense granules. ×45,000. (See Arenaviruses, Table 62-4.) (From Murphy et al: J Virol 6: 507, 1970)

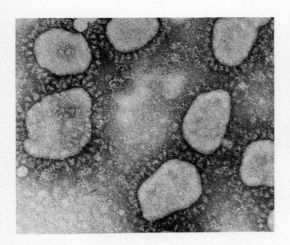

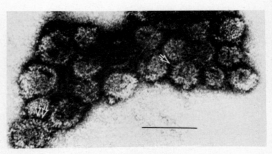

FIG. 62-18. Rubella virus. Note characteristic spicule surface subunits indicated by arrows. ×145,000. (From Smith and Hobbins: J Immunol 102:1016, 1969)

FIG. 62-17. Coronavirus particles. Note pleomorphic envelopes studded with characteristic widely-spaced club or pear-shaped surface projections. ×144,000. (From Kapikian, In Lennette EH, Schmidt NJ (eds): Diagnostic Procedures for Viral and Rickettsial Infections. American Public Health Association, Inc. 4th ed. 1969)

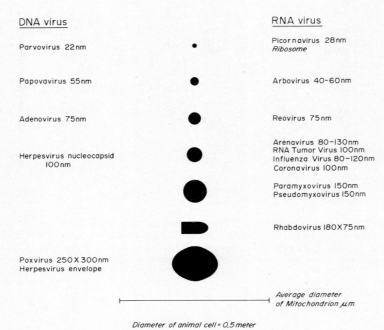

DNA virus

Parvovirus 22 nm

Papovavirus 55 nm

Adenovirus 75 nm

Herpesvirus nucleocapsid 100 nm

Poxvirus 250 X 300 nm
Herpesvirus envelope

RNA virus

Picornavirus 28 nm
Ribosome

Arbovirus 40-60 nm

Reovirus 75 nm

Arenavirus 80-130 nm
RNA Tumor Virus 100 nm
Influenza Virus 80-120 nm
Coronavirus 100 nm

Paramyxovirus 150 nm
Pseudomyxovirus 150 nm

Rhabdovirus 180X75 nm

*Average diameter
of Mitochondrion μm*

Diameter of animal cell = 0.5 meter

Length of DNA in poxvirus particle 5 meters

FIG. 62-19. The relative sizes of the principal families of animal viruses. Unless otherwise indicated, the scale is the same for all.

**TABLE 62-1   THE MORPHOLOGY
OF ANIMAL VIRUSES**

Virus	Morphology
DNA Viruses	
Poxvirus	Complex
Iridovirus	Enveloped icosahedral nucleocapsid
Herpesvirus	Enveloped icosahedral nucleocapsid
Adenovirus	Naked icosahedral nucleocapsid
Papovavirus	Naked icosahedral nucleocapsid
Parvovirus	Naked icosahedral nucleocapsid
RNA Viruses	
Picornavirus	Naked icosahedral nucleocapsid
Togavirus	Enveloped icosahedral or helical nucleocapsid
Bunyavirus	Enveloped helical circular nucleocaspid
Reovirus	Naked double-shelled icosahedral nucleocapsid
Orthomyxovirus	Enveloped helical nucleocapsid
Paramyxovirus	Enveloped helical nucleocapsid
Rhabdovirus	Enveloped helical nucleocapsid
RNA tumor virus	Enveloped nucleocapsid
Arenavirus	Enveloped nucleocapsid
Coronavirus	Enveloped nucleocapsid

ly (Chap. 80) and the chronic infectious neuropathic agents (see Table 62-4).

The relative sizes of some important animal viruses are illustrated in Figure 62-19. Their morphology is summarized in Table 62-1.

THE NATURE OF
THE COMPONENTS
OF ANIMAL VIRUSES

The Purification of Viruses

Little serious work on the properties, composition, and molecular biology of viruses is possible unless pure virus is available. The starting material for virus purification may be any material containing a sufficiently large amount of virus. This may be cellular material, such as infected organs or cultured cells, or it may be extracellular material, such as plasma, allantoic fluid, or cell culture medium. If the virus concentration in such material is not high enough, an initial concentration step employ-

ing either precipitation or centrifugation may be necessary. The next step is then generally designed to achieve a preliminary purification by removing the bulk of nonviral material. This may be achieved by treatment with detergents or emulsification with organic solvents followed by centrifugation or by adsorption to and elution from red blood cells (in the case of myxoviruses) or by passage through columns containing material capable of separating viral and cellular components. For the final purification step fractionation by means of density gradient centrifugation is almost always used. There are two modes of employing this technique (Fig. 62-20). In velocity density gradient or zonal centrifugation, the virus suspension is layered onto a density gradient composed of solutions of gradually increasing density containing either sucrose or glycerol or some salt, the maximum density being such that virus particles would migrate to the bottom of the tube if centrifuged long enough. If centrifuged for shorter periods, particles with the same sedimentation coefficient, which depends on size, density, and shape, sediment as homogeneous bands which may be collected. This step eliminates all impurities except those with the same sedimentation coefficient as virus par-

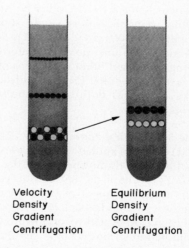

Velocity
Density
Gradient
Centrifugation

Equilibrium
Density
Gradient
Centrifugation

FIG. 62-20. Application of the technique of density gradient centrifugation to virus purification. A partially purified virus preparation is layered onto the density gradient on the left, which is then centrifuged so that particles with the same sedimentation coefficient form distinct bands. Three such bands are shown, one of which contains virus (open spheres). This band is then centrifuged to equilibrium in the gradient on the right, in which particles are separated according to their buoyant density.

ticles. In order to eliminate these impurities, the particles in the virus-containing band recovered from the first step are then centrifuged to equilibrium in a second density gradient composed of solutions of higher density. Here particles form bands where the density of the medium is identical to their own buoyant density. Since contaminants with both the same sedimentation coefficient and the same density as virus particles are rare, virus purified by two such density gradient centrifugation steps is generally considered to be pure.

The purification of icosahedral viruses generally presents no difficulties. Some enveloped viruses, however, are not easily purified because the amount of envelope per virus particle may be variable, causing them to be heterogeneous with respect to both size and density.

It is almost impossible to establish absolute criteria of purity for viruses, principally because small amounts of cellular constituents tend to adsorb to them. Absence of particulate impurities is best assessed by electron microscopic examination.

Viral Nucleic Acids

Animal virus nucleic acids are astonishingly diverse. Some are DNA, other RNA; some are double stranded, others single stranded; some are linear, others circular; some have plus polarity, others minus polarity. Information concerning these and other properties of viral nucleic acids is essential for an understanding of the key reactions during virus multiplication cycles.

The Size of Viral Nucleic Acids The nucleic acid content of animal viruses varies within wide limits. At the lower end of the scale, only 1 to 2 percent of the myxovirion is RNA, and only about 5 percent of the poxvirion is DNA; at the upper end, about 25 percent of the picornavirion is RNA. However, the proportion of nucleic acid in virions is not as significant as its absolute amount, which is the factor that determines the amount of genetic information that they contain. The smallest animal virus genomes are those of the picornaviruses, togaviruses, parvoviruses, and papovaviruses, the molecular weights of all of which are in the range from 1 to 3×10^6. Since the coding ratio, that is, the ratio of the molecular weight of sin-

gle stranded nucleic acid to the molecular weight of the protein for which it can code is about 9, these viral genomes can code for protein with a total molecular weight of from 100,000 to 350,000, which is equivalent to 3 to 10 average size proteins. The largest animal virus genomes, those of the poxviruses, are about 100 times larger; the estimates of their molecular weights range from 120 to 200×10^6. The molecular weights of viral genomes are listed in Table 62-2.

The Structure of Viral Nucleic Acids
STRANDEDNESS. Both double-stranded and single-stranded DNA as well as RNA can act as the genome of animal viruses (Table 62-2).

TERMINAL REDUNDANCY. Herpesvirus DNA is terminally redundant or repetitious, that is, its base composition may be represented as A, B, C . . . X, Y, Z, A, where A, B, C, and so on are nucleotide sequences. This is most readily demonstrated by digesting herpesvirus DNA with bacteriophage λ exonuclease, which attacks double-stranded DNA possessing 5'-terminal phosphates. In this way one end of one strand and the other end of the other strand are digested. On melting and reannealing, herpesvirus DNA digested in this manner circularizes, indicating that the two single-stranded regions at the two ends are complementary, hence the sequences are repetitious. The length of the repeated sequence is about 800 nucleotide base pairs, which is about 0.5 percent of the total length of the herpesvirus DNA molecule.

Adenovirus DNA is also terminally repetitious, but here the repeated sequence is inverted or reversed. This is indicated by the fact that here single-stranded DNA circles form upon melting and reannealing, without the need to first digest the ends with nuclease.

The significance of terminal redundancy is most probably related to the mode of DNA replication. This is discussed more fully in Chapter 70 in relation to bacteriophage DNAs.

CIRCULARITY. Most viral nucleic acids are linear (Fig. 62-21), but papovavirus DNA exists in the form of double-stranded supercoiled circles (Fig. 62-22). The reason for the supercoiling is a deficiency of 15 to 20 turns in their double helix, but the reason for the deficiency is not clear. Supercoiling is relieved either by the introduction of a single break or nick into

TABLE 62-2 CHARACTERISTICS OF VIRAL NUCLEIC ACIDS

Virus	Nature of Nucleic Acid	MW × 10^6	Strandedness	Structure	Number of Segments	Polarity	Infectivity of Naked Nucleic Acid
Poxvirus	DNA	120–200	Double	Linear	1		+
Herpesvirus	DNA	100	Double	Linear	1		+
Adenovirus	DNA	23	Double	Linear	1		+
Papovavirus	DNA	3.5*	Double	Supercoiled circular	1		+
Parvovirus	DNA	2	Single	Linear	1	+ and –	+
Picornavirus	RNA	2–3	Single	Linear	1	+	+
Togavirus	RNA	3–4	Single	Linear	1	+	+
Bunyavirus	RNA	?	Single	?†	?		?
Reovirus	RNA	15	Double	Linear	10		–
Orthomyxovirus	RNA	6	Single	Linear	8	–	–
Paramyxovirus	RNA	6	Single	Linear	1	–	–
Rhabdovirus	RNA	3–4	Single	Linear	1	–	–
RNA tumor virus	RNA	7	Single	Linear	2	+	?
Arenavirus	RNA	?	Single	?	?	?	?
Coronavirus	RNA	?	Single	?	?	?	?

* 5 × 10^6 for papilloma virus; 3.5 × 10^6 for all others

† The nucleocapsids of bunyaviruses are circular. It is not yet known whether their RNA is linear or circular.

FIG. 62-21. An electron micrograph of an intact herpesvirus DNA molecule, approximately 44 μm long. The small circular molecules are intact DNA molecules of the bacteriophage ΦX174 (Chap. 70), which were added to provide a size marker. (Courtesy of Dr. Edward K. Wagner)

one of the two strands, thus permitting unwinding to closed nicked circles, or by intercalation of substances, such as the acridine ethidium bromide (Fig. 62-23). The significance of circularity is not known. It is not essential for infectivity, since DNA in poxviruses, herpesviruses, and adenoviruses is linear. Conceivably, circularity is a prerequisite for integration into the host genome (Chap. 69), and adenovirus and herpesvirus DNAs circularize prior to being integrated.

CIRCULAR PERMUTATION. As will be discussed in Chapter 70 bacteriophage DNAs are frequently circularly permuted. Neither poxvirus nor herpesvirus nor adenovirus DNA appear to be circularly permuted.

SEGMENTATION. Until recently it was assumed that all viral genomes consisted of unbroken strands of nucleic acid. However, this is not always so. The genome of reoviruses consists of 10 segments of double-stranded RNA (Fig. 62-24), the genome of influenza viruses consists of 8 segments of single-stranded RNA, and the genome of RNA tumor viruses consists of 2 single-stranded RNA molecules. One of the consequences of segmentation is highly effi-

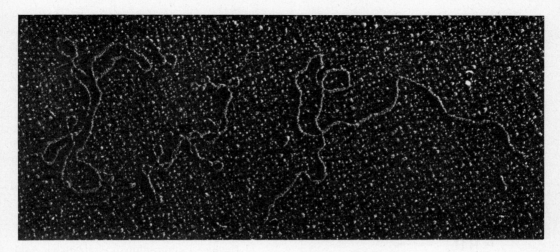

FIG. 62-22. The three forms of bovine papilloma virus DNA. Center, a supercoiled twisted circular molecule, which is the form in which the DNA exists within the virus. Left, a "relaxed" circular molecule, in which one strand has been "nicked" or broken by treatment with deoxyribonuclease, thereby relieving the supercoiling by permitting free rotation of the remaining intact strand. Right, a linear molecule, generated by the introduction of nicks close to one another in both strands. ×66,000. (Courtesy of Dr. H. J. Bujard)

cient formation of genetic recombinants caused by random assortment of segments in multiply infected cells (Chap. 67).

The Polarity of Viral Nucleic Acids   The single-stranded RNA molecules present in picornavirus and togavirus particles can combine with cell ribosomes and serve as messenger RNA, and all the genetic information necessary for the formation of progeny virus is translated directly from them. This is not the case for the RNA molecules present in myxovirus and rhabdovirus particles. These RNAs must first be transcribed into RNA strands of opposite polarity, and it is these transcripts that are then translated by the cell ribosomes. Since the

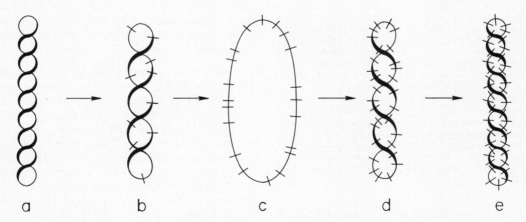

FIG. 62-23. Diagrammatic representation of the removal and reversal of supercoiling turns. The Watson-Crick helix is here represented as a single continuous line. The number of supercoiling turns in the original molecule (a) decreases as ethidium bromide molecules (represented by bars perpendicular to the helix axis) bind to the DNA (b) (Chap. 8). The drug molecules are inserted at random. At equivalence, the accumulated untwisting due to the number of drug molecules bound just balances the initial number of supercoiling turns (c). The untwisting caused by the binding of further drug molecules (d) leads to the introduction of supercoiling turns now in the opposite, left-handed, sense (e). (From Crawford and Waring: J Gen Virol 1:387, 1967)

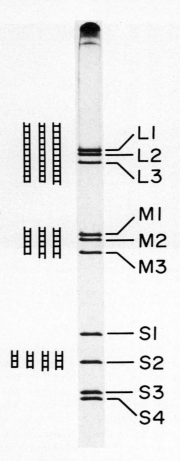

FIG. 62-24. The structure of the reovirus genome. RNA extracted from reovirions by treatment with the detergent sodium dodecyl sulfate (SDS) was subjected to electrophoresis in a polyacrylamide gel such as shown. In such gels molecules of various sizes migrate as discrete bands, the smallest ones moving fastest. The direction of migration in the gel shown here was from left to right. Bands of RNA were visualized by autoradiography.

The reovirus genome is seen to consist of ten molecular species that fall into three size classes, designated L, M, and S. Since the rate of migraton is inversely proportional to the square of the molecular weight, estimates of relative molecular weights can be made by measuring the distances traveled by the various bands. The relative sizes of the ten reovirus RNA segments are indicated underneath the gel.

polarity of messenger RNA is generally designated as plus, the polarity of picornavirus and togavirus RNA is plus, and that of the RNA in myxovirus and rhabdovirus particles is minus.

The adeno-associated satellite viruses, which belong to the Parvovirus family and contain single-stranded DNA, provide a unique situation. There are two kinds of these virus par-

ticles: One contains plus strands, the other minus strands. These two kinds of particles are always produced in equal amounts. When the DNA is extracted from them it tends to hybridize rapidly, thus giving the impression that it is double stranded. It is only when the DNA is extracted under conditions where the plus and the minus strands are prevented from hybridizing with each other that the true situation is revealed. All other parvoviruses contain single-stranded DNA of one polarity only, most probably plus.

The polarity of the RNA in RNA tumor virus particles is probably plus; that of the RNA in arenavirus and coronavirus particles is not known (Table 62-2).

The Base Composition of Viral Nucleic Acids
The molar base composition of viral genomes varies within wide limits. It is frequently of taxonomic significance: Thus all poxvirus DNAs so far examined contain about 36 percent guanidine + cytosine (G + C); all papovavirus DNAs contain about 48 percent G + C; there are three classes of adenoviruses, highly oncogenic, weakly oncogenic, and nononcogenic, the DNA of which contains about 48, 52, and 58 percent G + C; and among the herpesviruses, some oncogenic ones contain 42 percent G + C, while some that are not oncogenic contain as much as 68 percent G + C. In general, the G + C content of the DNA of oncogenic viruses is closer to that of the DNA of mammalian cells (about 45 percent G + C) than that of nononcogenic viruses, but there are notable exceptions where this is not the case.

The Genetic Relatedness of Viral Nucleic Acids   The genetic relatedness of animal virus nucleic acids is of interest for its taxonomic and evolutionary significance. For example, there are many viruses that are poxviruses, according to a variety of criteria (p. 790). The question naturally arises as to how closely related they are.

The best measure of genetic relatedness is determination of similarity of nucleic acid-base sequence. This is accomplished readily for double-stranded nucleic acids by measuring how extensively they can hybridize with each other. The two nucleic acids whose relatedness is to be determined are denatured to the single-stranded state, then mixed and allowed to reanneal. Single strands derived from the two genomes are thus presented with the opportunity of pairing with each other, and conditions are readily arranged so that such pairing can be quantitated. If the two genomes are very closely related, pairing will occur extensively; if there is no relatedness, no pairing will occur. For example, the genomes of the highly oncogenic adenoviruses referred to above hybridize with each other to the extent of 80 percent or more; in other words, they share over 80 percent of their base sequences. However, they share only 25 percent of base sequences with the genomes of the nononcogenic adenoviruses, which, however, share over 80 percent of base sequences among themselves.

It is much more difficult to measure similarity of base sequence content among viral genomes that consist of single-stranded nucleic acid, since at least one of them must be present as its double-stranded, or replicative, form (Chap. 65), which is usually very difficult to prepare in sufficient quantity.

Another measure of genetic relatedness employs comparison of proteins rather than of nucleic acids. Similarity of nucleic acid-base sequences signifies similarity of the amino acid sequences of the proteins coded by them. This in turn implies antigenic similarity, that is, ability of proteins to react with each others' antibodies. Ability of nucleic acids to hybridize and of the proteins coded by them to cross-react immunologically are thus measures of the same parameter.

The Infectivity of Animal Virus Nucleic Acids Viral nucleic acids contain all the information necessary for the formation of virus particles. This was first shown by Hershey and Chase in 1952, when they found that infection by bacteriophage is initiated by injection of viral DNA (along with a small amount of protein which has no genetic function) into the host cell. Later, in 1956, Gierer and Schramm showed that the same was true for plant viruses, when they found that RNA extracted from tobacco mosaic virions was infectious.

The nucleic acids of several groups of animal viruses, such as picornaviruses, togaviruses, papovaviruses, adenoviruses, and herpesviruses, are also infectious (Table 62-2). These are all nucleic acids that either can act as messenger RNA themselves or are transcribed into messenger RNA by host-coded RNA polymerases. Viral nucleic acids that are transcribed into messenger RNA by virus-coded polymerases, such as the minus-stranded RNAs of

myxoviruses and rhabdoviruses or the double-stranded RNA of reovirus, would not be expected to be infectious, as they could not possibly express themselves within the cell.

In all cases the naked nucleic acids are less infectious by factors varying from 10^3 to 10^6 than are the virions from which they were extracted. There are two principal reasons for this. First, naked viral nucleic acids are quickly degraded by nucleases that are generally present in extracellular fluids, as well as on outer cell membranes, and second, naked nucleic acids are taken up very poorly by cells. Uptake can be increased significantly by treating cells briefly with concentrated salt solutions, which promotes pinocytosis, thereby facilitating nucleic acid entry, or by complexing the naked nucleic acids with such polycations as protamine or DEAE-dextran, or by adsorbing them to precipitated calcium phosphate, which is taken up well by cells. The inefficiency with which naked viral nucleic acids penetrate into cells emphasizes the role of the viral capsid in this vital function.

The host range of naked viral nucleic acids is very much broader than that of the respective virions. This stems from the fact that the latter's host range is restricted by the specificity of the interaction between the capsid and cell surface receptors (Chap. 65). This is not the case for naked viral nucleic acids, which can apparently multiply in any cell into which they can penetrate without being degraded. For example, whereas poliovirions can only infect and therefore multiply in cells of human or primate origin, poliovirus RNA can also multiply in chicken cells and mouse cells.

Infectious viral nucleic acid can be extracted not only from infectious virus particles but also from all virus particles that contain undamaged nucleic acid. Among these are virus particles inactivated by heat, proteolytic enzymes, and detergents (Chap. 63).

The Presence of Host Nucleic Acids in Virions As a general rule, virus capsids enclose viral nucleic acids. However, sometimes segments of host nucleic acid become encapsidated instead. For example, particles exist that contain, within a papovavirus capsid, a linear piece of host DNA roughly the same size as the papovavirus genome. As far as is known, each particle, known as a "pseudovirion," contains a different piece of host DNA. Generally, pseudovirions make up only a small fraction of the yield, but in one cell line the majority of the particles formed as a result of infection with polyoma virus are pseudovirions. Another example is provided by virus particles that are formed when papovaviruses are passed repeatedly at high multiplicity, that is, in cells infected with many virus particles. These virus particles contain DNA molecules that consist partly of viral and partly of host cell sequences. They are formed when the viral genomes, which become integrated into host cell DNA prior to replication (Chaps. 67 and 69), are excised (or cut out of the host genome) imperfectly.

Virus particles that contain host DNA sequences have attracted attention because of their potential ability to transduce host genes from one cell to another, which could conceivably be exploited in correcting inborn errors of metabolism.

Viral Proteins

The principal constituent of all animal viruses is protein. Proteins are the sole component of capsids, they are the major component of envelopes, and they are also intimately associated, as internal or core proteins, with the nucleic acids of certain icosahedral viruses. All these proteins are referred to as "structural proteins," since their primary function is to serve as virion building blocks. They are almost always coded by the viral genome.

Viral proteins vary widely in size, from less than 10,000 daltons to more than 150,000 daltons. They also vary in number, some virions containing only 3 species, others more than 30. Viral proteins are characterized most conveniently by dissociating highly purified virus preparations and subjecting the resulting polypeptide mixtures to electrophoresis in polyacrylamide gels. The most commonly used dissociating agent is the detergent sodium dodecyl sulfate (SDS), which not only destroys the secondary structure of proteins but also forms complexes with them. These complexes carry numerous strong negative charges, so that upon electrophoresis in polyacrylamide gels they migrate strictly according to size. As a result SDS-polyacrylamide gel electrophoresis provides a very convenient method for determining not only the number of different polypeptide species that make up virus particles but

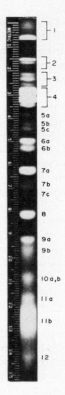

FIG. 62-25. Polyacrylamide gel of vaccinia virus structural polypeptides. Vaccinia virus labeled with ^{14}C-amino acids was dissolved in a buffer containing SDS, and the resulting solution electrophoresed in a 10 percent polyacrylamide gel. An autoradiogram was then prepared from it by exposing x-ray film to it. The direction of electrophoresis was from top to bottom. Some polypeptides are present in amounts too small to be seen after reproduction; over 30 polypeptides were discernible on the original photograph. (Courtesy Drs. I Sarov and W. K. Joklik)

also their sizes. The polyacrylamide gel electrophoresis profile of vaccinia virus polypeptides is shown in Figure 62-25.

All members of each of the major virus families (p. 804) display the same or almost the same highly characteristic electrophoretic polypeptide patterns. The patterns exhibited by reovirus, rhinovirus, ME-virus, and Sendai virus (a paramyxovirus) are illustrated in Figure 62-26.

Glycoproteins Viral envelopes often contain glycoproteins in the form of spikes or projections. Their carbohydrate moieties consist of oligosaccharides comprising 10 to 20 monosaccharide units, which are linked to the polypeptide backbone through N— and O—glycosidic bonds involving asparagine and

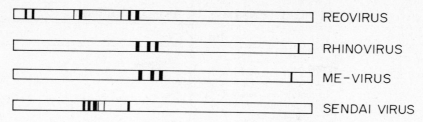

FIG. 62-26. Drawings of polyacrylamide gel patterns of the proteins of reovirus, rhinovirus, ME-virus, and Sendai virus. Highly purified preparations of these viruses were dissolved in a solution containing sodium dodecyl sulfate; the illustration shows gels in which the SDS complexes of the proteins of these four viruses had been electrophoresed from left to right. The location of each band is a measure of its molecular weight; thus the largest protein shown is the far left protein of reovirus (MW 150,000), the smallest the far right protein of rhinovirus (MW about 8,000). The relative amount of each protein is indicated by the thickness of the band representing it. It is clear from the gel patterns shown that the protein complements of rhinovirus and ME-virus, both picornaviruses, are very similar, and that they are quite different from those of reovirus and Sendai virus.

serine or threonine respectively. Their principal components are generally galactose and galactosamine, glucose and glucosamine, fucose, mannose, and neuraminic acid, which always occupies a terminal position.

The nature and sequence of the monosaccharides comprising the oligosaccharides of viral glycoproteins are characteristic of the host cell in which the virus multiplies. As a consequence, the oligosaccharides of the same virus grown in two different cell types are different. The infectivity of viruses, however, is not affected by differences in the carbohydrate portion of their glycoproteins.

Viral Proteins with Specialized Functions Some viral proteins have specialized biologic properties or functions. Among them are the following.

HEMAGGLUTININS. Many animal viruses, both naked and enveloped, hemagglutinate, that is, they agglutinate erythrocytes of certain animal species. Among them are picornaviruses, togaviruses, reoviruses, myxoviruses, adenoviruses, and papovaviruses. In the case of enveloped viruses, hemagglutination is the function of glycoprotein spikes located on the virion surface (Fig. 62-4).

ENZYMES. Virions often contain enzymes (Table 62-3). Among them are the following.

(1) Virions of the orthomyxovirus and paramyxovirus families contain an enzyme, neuraminidase, that hydrolyzes the galactose-N-acetylneuraminic acid bond at the termini of glycoprotein oligosaccharides, thereby liberating N-acetylneuraminic acid. Like the myxo-virus hemagglutinin, this enzyme is located on glycoprotein spikes: orthomyxoviruses possess two types of spikes, one with hemagglutinin and the other with neuraminidase activity (Fig. 62-4), while paramyxoviruses also possess two types of spikes on one of which both activities are located. When such myxovirus particles adsorb to cells, neuraminidase acts on the glycoproteins of the cell surface that serve as myxovirus receptors (Chap. 65) until the nucleocapsid has penetrated into the cell. If penetration is impossible, as in the case when the virus adsorbs to erythrocytes, the enzyme acts until N-acetylneuraminic acid has been removed from all receptor molecules, and the virus then elutes. The precise function of neuraminidase in virus multiplication is not clear. What evidence there is available suggests that it plays a role during virus release, rather than during adsorption and penetration.

(2) Many virions contain RNA polymerases. The necessity for such enzymes stems from the fact that the nucleic acid present in virions must be able to express itself once it has gained access to the interior of host cells. If this nucleic acid itself can act as messenger RNA, like picornavirus or togavirus RNA, then there is no problem. If it cannot, either because it is double stranded or because it is RNA with minus polarity, RNA with plus polarity must first be synthesized. There are two possible sources for the enzymes necessary for this purpose. The first is enzymes existing in the host cell. Herpesvirus, adenovirus, and papovavirus DNAs are probably transcribed into messenger RNA by host cell DNA-dependent RNA polymerases. The alternative is that the virus particle itself contains the enzyme. Examples of

TABLE 62-3   ENZYMES IN ANIMAL VIRUSES

Virus	Enzyme	Coded by
DNA Viruses		
Poxvirus	DNA-dependent RNA polymerase	Virus
	Nucleotide phosphohydrolase	?
	Poly A polymerase	Probably virus
	Capping enzymes	Probably virus
	Protein kinase	Probably virus
	Nucleases	Probably virus
Herpesvirus	ATPase*	Cell
Parvovirus	DNA polymerase	?
Hepatitis virus	DNA polymerase	?
RNA Viruses		
Picornavirus	None	
Togavirus	None	
Reovirus	RNA-dependent RNA polymerase	Virus
	Nucleotide phosphohydrolase	Virus
	Capping enzymes	Probably cell
Myxovirus	Neuraminidase	Virus
	RNA polymerase	Virus
Rhabdovirus	RNA polymerase	Virus
	Poly A polymerase	?
	Protein kinase	Probably cell
	Capping enzymes	Probably cell
RNA tumor virus	RNA-dependent DNA polymerase (reverse transcriptase)	Virus
	Ribonuclease H	Virus
	Other nuclease(s)	Probably cell
	Polynucleotide ligase	Probably cell
	ATPase*	Cell

This enzyme is present only if it is a component of the plasma membrane of the cells in which these viruses multiplied.

this type are the poxviruses which possess a DNA-dependent RNA polymerase in their cores, reoviruses which possess an RNA-dependent RNA polymerase in their cores, and myxoviruses and rhabdoviruses which contain RNA polymerases that synthesize plus RNA strands from the minus RNA strands present within them. These enzymes are not active in intact virus particles but are activated when the envelope or capsid is partially degraded, which generally occurs very soon after infection.

(3) RNA tumor viruses possess a DNA polymerase, the so-called reverse transcriptase, that transcribes their single-stranded RNA into double-stranded DNA (which is then in all probability integrated into the genome of the host cell—Chap. 69).

All these enzymes are virus-specified. The evidence for this conclusion is provided by the existence of virus strains that contain variant enzymes (as is the case for neuraminidase) and the fact that the enzyme in question often simply does not exist in the uninfected cell (as is the case for many of the polymerases).

Viruses also often contain other enzymes, and for many it is not quite clear whether they are virus-coded or host-coded. Among them are nucleases, nucleotide phosphohydrolases, protein kinases, and enzymes that modify both ends of the messenger RNA molecules synthesized by their polymerases (capping enzymes, that is, enzymes that add GMP to the 5′-termini and that methylate certain ribose and guanine residues near the 5′-termini, and poly A polymerases that add sequences of poly A ranging in length from 50 to 200 residues to the 3′-termini). While some of these enzymes are probably virus-coded, others appear to be cellular enzymes that become associated with virus particles by mechanisms that may possess a considerable degree of specificity.

Viral Lipids

Viral envelopes contain complex mixtures of neutral lipids, phospholipids, and glycolipids. As a general rule, the composition of these mixtures resembles that of the membranes of the host cells in which the virus multiplied. Since the lipid composition of membranes varies markedly from cell strain to cell strain, and even for the same cell strain depending on the composition of the medium, this means that the same virus grown in different cell strains may have widely differing neutral lipid, phospholipid, and glycolipid complements, even though its biologic properties, including its infectivity, are identical.

The nature and extent of the differences in composition that are encountered are best illustrated by the example of the paramyxovirus SV5. On the average, this virus contains about 20 percent total lipid, of which roughly 25 percent and 5 percent, respectively, are cholesterol and triglyceride, 55 percent is phospholipid, and 15 percent is glycolipid. If grown in cells the membranes of which have molar ratio of cholesterol to phospholipid of 0.81, the ratio for the viral envelope is 0.89. If the cellular ratio is 0.51, that for the viral envelope is 0.60. The same holds for the relative amounts of several phospholipids. If the ratio of phosphatidylcholine to phosphatidylethanolamine in host cell membranes is 3.55, the ratio in the viral envelope is 2.55. If the ratio in host cell membranes is 0.8, the ratio in the viral envelope is 0.6. However, for one cell the ratio is 1.6, while that in the viral envelope derived from it is 0.6, which suggests that within limits some selectivity of membrane lipids that are incorporated into viral envelopes is possible.

THE CLASSIFICATION OF ANIMAL VIRUSES

Attempts to devise a system of classification for animal viruses began almost as soon as their importance as pathogens became apparent. However, the criteria on which to base such a system have changed with advances in our knowledge of their nature and properties. For example, host range cannot be such a criterion: Not only is each animal species subject to infection by a wide variety of viral agents, but also virus strains exist which, although related genetically, infect different animal species. Similarly, the pattern of pathogenesis of the disease that is caused is an unreliable foundation on which to base a system of classification.

It has become more and more apparent that a system of classification must be based on the physical and chemical properties of the virus particles themselves.

Criteria for Classification

Morphology The primary criterion for classification is morphology. It is easy to apply because it does not require purified virus. Virus particles can be examined either within cells, that is, in thin sections of infected tissue, or in their extracellular state. Morphologic detail is usually brought out by shadowing with thin films of some heavy metal, such as uranium or tungsten, by staining with osmic acid or uranyl acetate, or by negative staining with phosphotungstic acid.

Most animal viruses conform to some 12 to 15 morphologic patterns; only very few viruses do not fit into any of these.

Physical and Chemical Nature of Virion Components Morphologic similarity correlates closely with similarity of virion components. For examples, all viruses with the morphology of adenoviruses contain double-stranded DNA genomes with a molecular weight of about 23 million, all papovaviruses contain circular supercoiled DNA genomes with a molecular weight of 3 to 5 million, and all reoviruses contain segmented double-stranded RNA genomes. In fact, a system of viral classification based on the structure and size of viral genomes yields the same grouping as one based on morphology. Similary, viruses with similar morphology are composed of similar collections of proteins, and a classification system based on polyacrylamide gel patterns, such as illustrated in Figure 62-26, again yields the same grouping.

Genetic Relatedness Although the members of each of the major virus families presumably derived from a common ancestor, genetic relationships among them are often no longer discernible today. For example, several groups of mammalian poxviruses exist (Table 62-4), the members of which are unrelated genetically as judged either by nucleic acid hybridization or by immunologic crossreactivity. The same applies to many members of the herpesvirus family, the human, simian, canine, and avian

TABLE 62-4 THE MAJOR FAMILIES OF ANIMAL VIRUSES

DNA-containing Viruses

I. POXVIRIDAE

All genera except *Parapoxvirus:* Brick-shaped complex particles, whorled surface filament pattern
Dimensions: 225 × 300 nm
Parapoxvirus: Ovoid complex particles, regular surface filament pattern
Dimensions: 150 × 200 nm

Strains pathogenic for many animal species exist. There are six genera, the members of each of which are closely related antigenically but which share only one antigen with members of the others. Poxviruses multiply in the cytoplasm.

	Host	Symptoms in man
A. Genus *Orthopoxvirus*		
Variola major	Man	Smallpox
Variola minor	Man	Alastrim
Vaccinia	Cattle	—
Cowpox	Cattle	—
Rabbitpox	Rabbit	—
Ectromelia (mousepox)	Mouse	—
Monkeypox	Monkey	—
B. Genus *Leporipoxvirus*		
Myxoma	Rabbit	—
Fibroma	Rabbit	—
C. Genus *Avipoxvirus*		
Fowlpox	Chicken	—
D. Genus *Capripoxvirus*		
Sheeppox	Sheep	—
Goatpox	Goat	—
E. Genus *Parapoxvirus*		
Orf (contagious postular dermatitis [CPD])	Sheep, goats, man	Nodules on hands
Pseudocowpox (milker's nodule virus)	Cattle, man	Nodules on hands
Bovine papular stomatitis	Cattle	—
F. Genus *Entomopoxvirus*		
Various strains	Arthropods	—
G. Ungrouped		
Molluscum contagiosum	Man	Benign epidermal tumors
Yaba monkey tumor virus	Monkey, man	Benign subcutaneous tumors

II. IRIDOVIRIDAE

Naked or enveloped icosahedral nucleocapsids
Diameter of naked nucleocapsids: 130 nm

Most iridoviruses are arthropod viruses and nonenveloped. The sole mammalian iridovirus is enveloped.

	Host	Symptoms in man
1. African swine fever virus	Swine	—
2. Frog virus 2	Amphibia	—
Frog virus 3		
3. Lymphocystis virus of fish	Fish	—
4. Tipula iridescent virus	Arthropods	—
Sericesthis iridescent virus		

III. HERPESVIRIDAE

Enveloped icosahedral nucleocapsids
Diameter of enveloped virions: 180 to 250 nm
Diameter of naked nucleocapsids: 100 nm

Herpesviruses are often classified into two groups depending on whether mature progeny is readily released from cells (Group A) or not (Group B). However recent studies have shown that this depends on the host cell rather than

TABLE 62-4 CONTINUED

on the virus. Some herpesviruses cause only mild symptoms in their natural hosts but severe disease in other species; for example, B virus produces transient herpetic facial lesions in monkeys but, almost invariably, fatal encephalitis in man. Few herpesviruses are closely related to each other as judged by DNA-DNA hybridization, but most show some relatedness (2-10 percent cross-hybridization). Almost all herpesviruses possess some common antigenic determinants. Herpesviruses cause type A nuclear inclusions (single large acidophilic inclusion bodies separated by a nonstaining halo from basophilic marginated chromatin).

	Host	Symptoms in man
A. Group A *Herpesvirus*		
1. *Herpes simplex virus* Type 1	Man	Stomatitis, upper respiratory infections, generalized systemic disease, severe and generally fatal encephalitis
2. *Herpes simplex virus* Type 2	Man	Genital infections
3. B virus	Monkey, man	Fatal encephalitis in man
4. Pseudorabies virus	Swine	—
5. Infectious bovine rhinotracheitis (IBR)	Cattle	—
6. Infectious bovine keratoconjunctivitis (IBKC)	Cattle	—
7. Equine herpesvirus Type 1 (equine abortion virus [EAV])	Horse	—
8. Equine herepsvirus Type 2 (LK Virus)	Horse	—
9. Feline rhinotracheitis	Cat	—
10. Infectious laryngotracheitis (ILT)	Chicken	—
B. Group B *herpesvirus*		
1. Varicella-zoster	Man	Chickenpox, herpes zoster
2. Cytomegalovirus: numerous strains	Man	Jaundice, hepatosplenomegaly, brain damage, death
	Monkey	
	Rodents	
	Swine	
C. Several herpesviruses either cause, or are strongly suspected of causing, tumors		
1. Lucké tumor virus	Frog	—
2. Marek's disease virus	Chicken	—
3. *Herpesvirus saimiri*	Squirrel monkey	—
4. *Herpesvirus ateles*	Spider monkey	—
5. *Herpesvirus sylvilagus*	Rabbit	—
6. Burkitt lymphoma agent (EB virus)	Man	Burkitt lymphoma (?) Nasopharyngeal carcinoma (?) Infectious mononucleosis (?)

IV. ADENOVIRIDAE
Naked icosahedral nucleocapsids
Diameter: 75 nm

Strains pathogenic for many animal species exist. All adenoviruses except avian ones share common group-specific complement-fixing antigenic determinants (on hexons) and in addition possess type-specific determinants (on pentons and fibers). They can be grouped into subgroups on the basis of antigenic cross-reactivity, DNA hybridization characteristics, ability to transform cells of various animal species, and ability to agglutinate rhesus monkey and rat erythrocytes. Some human and simian strains are very tumorigenic in certain rodents; all can transform cultured mammalian cells more or less efficiently (Chap. 69). Adenoviruses produce intranuclear Type B inclusions (basophilic masses sometimes connected to the nuclear periphery by strands of chromatin).

	Host	Symptoms in man
A. Human adenoviruses 31 serotypes	Man	Primarily respiratory (serotypes 4, 7, 14, and 21) and conjunctival (serotype 8) infections. Serotypes 1, 2, 5, and 6 cause acute febrile pharyngitis in infants and young children

TABLE 62-4   CONTINUED

	Host	Symptoms in man
B. Simian adenoviruses 23 serotypes	Monkey	—
C. Canine adenoviruses (infectious canine hepatitis [ICH])	Dog	—
D. Avian adenoviruses (GAL, gallus-adenolike; CELO, chicken-embryo-lethal- orphan)	Chicken Quail	— —

V. PAPOVAVIRIDAE

Naked icosahedral nucleocapsids
Diameter: 55 nm (papilloma viruses)
45 nm (all other papovaviruses)

*Papovaviruses (**pap**illoma-**po**lyoma-simian **vac**uolating agent) fall into two distinct groups on the basis of size; the viruses of genus A (the papilloma viruses) possess both larger capsids and larger genomes than the viruses of genus B. All except K virus have oncogenic potential; all produce latent and chronic infections in their natural hosts. None of the members of this family are antigenically related except SV40 and the viruses associated with PML in man. Polyoma and K virus agglutinate erythrocytes of certain animal species.*

	Host	Symptoms in man
A. Genus *Papovavirus A*		
1. Human papilloma (wart)	Man	Benign tumors (warts)
2. Shope rabbit papilloma	Rabbit	—
3. Various viruses pathogenic for other animal species	Cattle Dog	— —
B. Genus *Papovavirus B*	Hamster	—
1. Polyoma virus	Mouse	—
2. Simian vacuolating agent (SV40)	Monkey kidney cell cultures	—
3. Rabbit vacuolating agent	Rabbit	—
4. K virus	Mouse	—
5. BK virus	Man	Isolated from urine of patients following renal transplantation. Its DNA is 20–30% homologous with SV40 DNA. Transforms cultured cells
DAR virus	Man	Isolated from brain of patients with progressive multifocal leukoencephalo-pathy (PML). Its DNA is over 90% homologous with SV40 DNA
Unnamed virus	Man	Isolated from brain reticulum cell sarcoma and urine of patients with Wiskott-Aldrich syndrome. Related to BK virus and SV40
JC virus	Man	Isolated from brain of patients with PML. Only slightly related to SV40—causes brain tumors in hamsters

VI. PARVOVIRIDAE

Naked icosahedral nucleocapsids
Diameter: 22 nm

These viruses are grouped together on the basis of morphology and nucleic acid structure (single-stranded DNA). All multiply in the nucleus. Most are antigenically unrelated. AAV only multiply in cells simultaneously infected with adenoviruses (Chap. 67); RV only multiplies in cells that are themselves actively multiplying. Aleutian mink disease virus causes a slow disease characterized by hypergammaglobulinemia, systemic proliferation of plasma cells, glomeru-lonephritis, and hepatitis and is invariably fatal. The role of the immune response in causing the disease condition has been proved by the prevention of lesions by immunosuppression and by the enhancement of lesions following the administration of inactivated virus or passive antibody. Although it causes a slow disease, Aleutian mink disease virus replicates as rapidly as viruses that cause acute disease.

Table 62-4   Continued

	Host	Symptoms in man
A. Adeno-associated virus (AAV) 4 serotypes	Man	No known symptoms
B. Minute virus of mice (MVM)	Mouse	—
C. Hamster osteolytic viruses (H-1, H-3, rat virus [RV], X-14)		Latent viruses isolated from various hosts including human tumors; none are oncogenic or capable of transforming cultured cells. They produce a mongoloid osteolytic deformity in newborn hamsters
D. Aleutian mink disease virus	Mink	—
E. Densonucleosis virus	Arthropods	—

RNA-containing Viruses

I. PICORNAVIRIDAE   Naked icosahedral nucleocapsids
Diameter: 25–30 nm

Picornaviruses comprise a large number of virus strains pathogenic for many animal species. They are subdivided into three genera: Enterovirus, *members of which are acid-stable, and* Rhinovirus *and* Calicivirus, *members of which are acid-labile. The morphology of* Caliciviruses *differs slightly from that of the other members of this family, and they are slightly larger.*

	Host	Symptoms in man
A. Genus *Enterovirus*		
1. Human enteroviruses (a) Poliovirus 3 serotypes	Man, monkey	Poliomyelitis
(b) Coxsackie virus A 24 serotypes	Man, mouse	Differentiated from Group B Coxsackie viruses primarily on the basis of selective tissue damage: Group A, primarily general striated muscle damage; Group B, primarily fatty tissue and central nervous tissue damage. Group A viruses are associated with herpangina; aseptic meningitis, paralysis, and the common cold syndrome
(c) Coxsackie virus B 6 serotypes	Man, mouse	Pleurodynia (Bornholm disease), aseptic meningitis, paralysis, severe systemic illness of newborns
(d) ECHO viruses (*Enteric Cytopathogenic Human Orphan*) 33 serotypes	Man	Paralysis, diarrhea, aseptic meningitis
2. Simian enteroviruses Multiple serotypes	Monkey	—
3. Encephalomyocarditis viruses (a) Columbia SK (b) EMC (c) Mengo	Various species, including man	Mild febrile illness
4. Murine encephalomyelitis viruses Poliovirus muris (Theiler's virus) GDVII strain and others	Mouse	—
5. Bovine enteroviruses	Cattle	—

TABLE 62-4   CONTINUED

	Host	Symptoms in man

6. Porcine enteroviruses
   Teschen virus 1
   Teschen virus 2
	Swine	—

7. Nodamura virus	Mosquito, swine(?)	—

B. Genus *Rhinovirus*

	Host	Symptoms in man
1. Human rhinoviruses Multiple serotypes	Man	Common cold, bronchitis, croup, bronchopneumonia
2. Other Rhinoviruses Multiple serotypes	Strains pathogenic for horses, cattle, etc	—

3. Foot-and-mouth disease
   virus (FMDV)
   7 serotypes
	Cattle, swine,
	sheep, goats
		—

C. Genus *Calicivirus*

	Host	Symptoms in man
1. Vesicular exanthema of swine virus (VE)	Swine	—
2. San Miguel sea lion virus (SMSV)	Seals	—
3. Feline picornaviruses	Cat	—

II. TOGAVIRIDAE

Enveloped nucleocapsids
Diameter: 50-70 nm (alphaviruses)
         40-50 nm (flaviviruses)

Togaviruses include many of the viruses previously known as arboviruses (arthropodborne). They multiply in bloodsucking insects as well as in vertebrates; in their natural environment they alternate between an insect vector (usually a mosquito or tick) and a vertebrate reservoir, rarely producing disease in either. Many cause subclinical infections in man, particularly in the tropics, but several are among the most virulent and lethal of all viruses. They are commonly named for the geographic site where they were isolated. They are divided into two groups, primarily on the basis of antigenic relationships (neutralization, complement fixation, and hemagglutination inhibition). The alphaviruses and flaviviruses are the old arbovirus Groups A and B.

A. Genus *Alphavirus*
   (mosquitoborne)

	Reservoir	Symptoms in man
Eastern equine encephalitis (EEE)	Birds	Encephalitis: frequently fatal
Semliki forest virus	Monkey	Undifferentiated febrile illness
Sindbis	Monkey	None
Chikungunya	Monkey	Myositis-arthritis
O'Nyong-Nyong	?	Fever, arthralgia, rash
Ross river virus	Mammals	Fever, rash, arthralgia
Venezuelan equine encephalitis (VEE)	Rodents	Encephalitis
Western equine encephalitis (WEE)	Birds	Encephalitis

B. Genus *Flavivirus*

1. Mosquitoborne

	Reservoir	Symptoms in man
Yellow fever	Monkey	Hemorrhagic fever, hepatitis, nephritis, often fatal
Dengue (4 serotypes)	Man	Fever, arthralgia, rash
Japanese encephalitis	Birds	Encephalitis: frequently fatal
St. Louis encephalitis	Birds	Encephalitis
Murray Valley encephalitis	Birds	Encephalitis
West Nile	Birds	Fever, arthralgia, rash
Kunjin	Birds	

2. Tickborne

	Reservoir	Symptoms in man

Central European tickborne
   encephalitis (biphasic
   meningoencephalitis
	Rodents,
	hedgehog
		Encephalitis

Far Eastern tickborne
   encephalitis [Russian spring-
   summer encephalitis (RSSE)]
	Rodents	Encephalitis

TABLE 62-4   CONTINUED

	Reservoir	Symptoms in man
Louping III	Sheep	Encephalitis
Powassan	Rodents	Encephalitis
Omsk hemorrhagic fever	Mammals	Hemorrhagic fever
Kyasanur forest	Rodents	Hemorrhagic fever

C. Other togaviruses

Also included among the togaviruses are several viruses that are not transmitted by arthropod vectors. The first two resemble alphaviruses, the last three flaviviruses.

	Reservoir	Symptoms in man
1. Rubella virus	Man	Severe deformities of fetuses in first trimester of pregnancy. Like most togaviruses it multiplies in the brains of newborn mice
2. Riley's lactic dehydrogenase elevating virus (LDHV)	Mouse	[Produces lifelong chronic viremia in mice; elevates LDH levels by decreasing the rate of enzyme clearance]
3. Bovine diarrhea virus	Cattle	—
4. Hog cholera virus	Pig	—
5. Equine arteritis virus	Horse	—

III. BUNYAVIRIDAE

Enveloped nucleocapsids
Diameter: about 100 nm

Bunyaviruses include all former arbovirus Group C viruses as well as several previously ungrouped arboviruses. They comprise a family separate from the togaviruses since they are larger and possess a fundamentally different structure: Their nucleocapsids possess helical rather than icosahedral symmetry and are circular.

Bunyamwera	Mammals	—
Former Group C arboviruses	Mammals	
California encephalitis	Mammals	Encephalitis
Other likely members		
Uukuniemi	Birds	
Rift Valley fever	Sheep, cattle	Fever, arthralgia, retinitis
Congo-Crimean hemorrhagic fever viruses	Mammals	Hemorrhagic fever
Phlebotomus fever virus—various strains	Sandfly	Facial erythema

IV. REOVIRIDAE

Naked nucleocapsids possessing two capsid shells (except genus *Cytoplasmic Polyhedrosis Virus*), each with icosahedral symmetry
Diameter: 75 nm

The primary criterion for inclusion in this family is possession of a genome consisting of 10 or 12 segments of double-stranded RNA. There are five genera with widely differing host ranges and somewhat differing morphologies. The (vertebrate) reoviruses possess two clearly defined capsid shells; the orbiviruses (which are transmitted by arthropods and are functionally arboviruses) possess a structurally featureless outer shell and an inner shell composed of 32 large ring-shaped capsomers (hence the name, Latin orbis, ring). The cytoplasmic polyhydrosis viruses possess only one capsid shell with clearly defined icosahedral symmetry, and members of one of the two plant reovirus genera (A) closely resemble the vertebrate reoviruses, while those of the other (B) possess a structure more reminiscent of cytoplasmic polyhydrosis viruses. The members of the five genera are not related antigenically.

A. Genus *Orthoreovirus* (respiratory-enteric-orphan)	Host	Symptoms in man
Mammalian reoviruses 3 serotypes	Man, other animals	Pathogenicity not established
Avian reoviruses 5 serotypes	Chicken, duck	—
B. Genus *Orbivirus*		
Bluetongue virus	Culicoides, sheep	—
Eubenangee virus	Mosquitoes	—

TABLE 62-4 CONTINUED

	Host	Symptoms in man
Komarovo	Ticks	—
African horse sickness virus	Culicoides, horses	—
Colorado tick fever	Ticks, man	Encephalitis

C. Genus *Cytoplasmic Polydrosis Virus*

Numerous strains	*Bombyx mori* (silkworm) and other Lepidoptera, Diptera, and Hymenoptera	—

D. Genus *Plant Reovirus (A)*

Wound tumor virus	Plants, leaf	—
Rice dwarf virus	hoppers	

E. Genus *Plant Reovirus (B)*

Maize rough dwarf virus	Plants, leaf hoppers	—
Fiji disease virus		

F. *Also included in this family are a newly discovered, immunologically related group of viruses that cause gastrointestinal disorders in the young of a variety of animal species, including man, which may form a sixth genus within this family when more details concerning their RNA and protein complements are known.*

Human infantile enteritis virus	Man	Diarrhea in infants
Neonatal (Nebraska) calf diarrhea virus	Calf	—
Epizootic diarrhea of infant mice	Mouse	—
Similar agents	Monkey	—
	Piglet	—
	Sheep	—

V. ORTHOMYXOVIRIDAE

Enveloped helical nucleocapsids
Diameter: 80–120 nm

The term myxovirus was coined originally to denote the unique affinity of influenza viruses for glycoproteins, which they partially degrade by means of the enzyme neuraminidase. Nowadays members of this family are characterized by possession of nucleocapsids with helical symmetry that reside within lipid-containing envelopes, to the outer surface of which glycoprotein spikes of two types are attached: One is the hemagglutinin, the other the neuraminidase. Members of the genus influenzavirus C differ from those of the other two genera in that their buoyant density is lower, the receptors for their hemagglutinins do not appear to contain sialic acid, and in the specificity of their receptor-destroying enzyme (that is, their enzyme seems to cleave some bond other than the -gal-neuraminic acid bond).

A. Genus Influenzavirus A	Host	Symptoms in man
Influenza virus		
(a) Type A		
i. Human subtypes	Man	Acute respiratory disease
A_0 1933–1947*		ʺ
A_1 1947–1957		ʺ
A_2 1957–1964 (Asian)		ʺ
A_2 1968– (Hong Kong)		ʺ
ii. Swine influenza virus	Swine	ʺ
iii. Avian subtypes		

*In 1971 a WHO Study Group adopted a new nomenclature for influenza type A viruses. In this system virus strains are described in terms of both the hemagglutinin (HA) and neuraminidase (NA) antigens. A_0 strains are now designated as HON1; A_1 strains as H1N1; the Asian type A_2 of 1957 as H2N2; and the Hong Kong type A_2 of 1968 as H3N2.

TABLE 62-4 CONTINUED

	Host	Symptoms in man
Fowl plague virus and numerous other strains	Chicken, duck, turkey, and others	—
iv. Equine subtypes	Horse	—
B. Genus Influenzavirus B		
Human subtypes		
B$_0$ 1940–1945	Man	Acute respiratory disease
B$_1$ 1945–1955		—
B$_2$ 1962–1964		—
B$_3$ 1962 (Taiwan)		—
C. Genus Influenzavirus C	Man	Acute respiratory disease

VI. PARAMYXOVIRIDAE

Enveloped helical nucleocapsids
Diameter: about 150 nm

Members of this family were until recently grouped with the orthomyxoviruses in the family Myxoviridae. They have been placed in a separate family because they differ from orthomyxoviruses in the following characteristics: Their genomes are not segmented; and the hemagglutinin and neuraminidase are located on the same glycoprotein spike, the other type of spike being responsible for the cell-fusing and hemolyzing activities. Members of the genus Pseudomyxovirus do not possess neuraminidase activity and some do not hemagglutinate.

A. Genus *Paramyxovirus*	Host	Symptoms in man
(a) Parainfluenza virus—1		
i. Sendai virus (hemagglutinating virus of Japan [HVJ])	Man, pig, mouse	Croup, common cold syndrome
ii. HA-2 (hemadsorption virus)	Man	Mild respiratory disease
(b) Parainfluenza viruses—2 to 5		
Numerous strains including HA-1, SV5	Man and other animals	Respiratory tract infections
(c) Newcastle disease virus (NDV)	Chicken	—
(d) Mumps	Man	Parotitis, orchitis, meningoencephalitis
B. Genus *Pseudomyxovirus*		
1. Measles	Man	Measles, subacute sclerosing panencephalitis (SSPE)
Distemper	Dog	—
Rinderpest	Cattle	—
2. Pneumonia virus of mice (PVM)	Mouse	—
3. Respiratory syncytial virus (RSV) Numerous strains	Man	Pneumonia and bronchiolitis in infants and children, common cold syndrome

VII. RHABDOVIRIDAE

Bullet-shaped, enveloped helical nucleocapsids
Dimensions: 180 × 75 nm

This group comprises all viruses with the unique bullet-shaped morphology. It includes VSV, rabies, and some viruses isolated from insects that do not appear to cause disease in vertebrates, but antibodies to them are found in birds and mammals, including man.

	Host	Symptoms in man
A. Vesicular stomatitis virus (VSV)	Cattle, horse, swine	—
B. Rabies virus	All warm-blooded animals	Encephalitis, invariably fatal
C. Marburg virus	Monkey, man	Hemorrhagic fever, frequently fatal

TABLE 62-4 CONTINUED

	Host	Symptoms in man
D. Hart Park and Flanders viruses	Mosquitoes, birds	—
E. Kern Canyon and several other viruses	Bats	—
F. Cocal virus	Mites	— —
G. Sigma virus	Drosophila	
H. Several plant viruses		

VIII. RETRAVIRIDAE (RNA tumor viruses) Enveloped nucleocapsids (perhaps with helical symmetry)
Diameter: about 150 nm

The RNA tumor virus family comprises a large group of viruses characterized by possession of a segmented RNA genome, a common morphology and a reverse transcriptase. There are four genera. The first (genus Oncornavirus C) comprises the C-type viruses. Many C-type viruses, the so-called sarcoma and leukosis/leukemia viruses, cause a variety of neoplasms when injected into animals and may also transform cultured cells in vitro; there are also many endogenous viruses which, although constantly produced by cells, cause no discernible effect when introduced either into the host from which they were isolated or into any other animal species. Most mammalian species, and perhaps most vertebrate species, have C-type viruses associated with them. The second genus (genus Oncornavirus B) comprises the B-type viruses, or mammary tumor viruses, which differ slightly from C-type viruses in morphology and are not related to them antigenically. Several B-type virus strains of mice are known. Viruses with characteristics intermediate between those of C- and B-type viruses have recently been isolated from primates and guinea pigs; they should perhaps be placed in a separate genus. The third genus (genus Lentivirus) comprises the Visna group of viruses. They resemble C- and B-type viruses with respect to morphology, nature of the genome, and possession of a DNA polymerase, and can transform cultured cells in vitro, but they have not yet been shown to possess oncogenic potential. The fourth genus (genus Spumavirus) consists of the foamy viruses, which are found in spontaneously degenerating monkey and chimpanzee (and other) kidney cell cultures, causing the formation of multinucleated vacuolated giant cells that have a highly characteristic appearance. Foamy viruses resemble RNA tumor viruses in morphology and in certain key characteristics of their mode of replication.

	Host	Symptoms in man
A. Genus *Oncornavirus C*		
(I) Subgenus *Oncornavirus C avian*		
1. Avian sarcoma viruses (ASV)	Chicken	—
(a) Rous sarcoma virus (RSV) Several strains		
(b) B77 virus		
(c) Fujinami sarcoma virus		
2. Avian leukosis viruses (ALV)	Chicken	—
(a) Rous-associated viruses Several strains, such as RAV-1, RAV-2		
(b) Avian myeloblastosis virus (AMV)	Chicken	
(c) Avian erythroblastosis virus (AEV)	Chicken	
(d) Avian myelocytomatosis virus (MC29)	Chicken	
(e) Avian lymphomatosis virus—RPL-12 and other strains	Chicken	
3. Reticuloendotheliosis virus (Duck infectious anemia virus)	Duck	—
(II) Subgenus *Oncornavirus C mammalian*		—
1. Murine sarcoma viruses (MSV) Harvey sarcoma virus Moloney sarcoma virus Kirsten sarcoma virus	Mouse	

TABLE 62-4 CONTINUED

	Host	Symptoms in man
2. Murine leukemia viruses (MLV) Numerous strains, such as Gross, Friend, Graffi, Kirsten, Moloney, Rauscher, etc	Mouse	—
3. Feline sarcoma and leukemia viruses	Cat	—
4. Feline endogenous viruses (RD 114 and CCC)	Cat	—
5. Primate sarcoma viruses (gibbon ape, woolly monkey)	Primates	?
6. Primate endogenous viruses (baboon)	Primates	—
7. Viruses of hamsters, rats, cattle, guinea pigs, pigs, and other species	Mammals	—
(III) Subgenus *Oncornavirus C reptilian* Viruses of reptiles	Reptiles	—
B. Genus *Oncornavirus B*		
1. Mouse mammary tumor virus (Bittner virus [milk factor])	Mouse	—
2. Viruses of guinea pigs, baboons, and possibly other mammals	Mammals	—
3. Possible separate subgenus:		
(a) Mason-Pfizer monkey virus (MPMV)	Rhesus monkey	—
(b) Viruses from primates, including human cells	—	?
(c) Guinea pig virus	Guinea pig	—
C. Genus *Lentivirus*		
1. Visna	Sheep	
2. Maedi	Sheep	
3. Progressive pneumonia virus	Mice	
D. Genus *Spumavirus*		
1. Simian foamy viruses 7 serotypes	Monkey kidney cells	—
2. Canine foamy virus	Dog kidney cells	
3. Bovine foamy virus	Bovine kidney cells	

VII. ARENAVIRIDAE   Enveloped nucleocapsids
                               Diameter: 80–130 nm

This group comprises viruses characterized by well-defined envelopes bearing closely spaced projections, enclosing an unstructured interior containing a variable number of characteristic electron-dense granules about 25 nm in diameter. They share a group-specific antigen, but antisera do not cross-neutralize.

	Host	Symptoms in man
A. Lymphocytic choriomeningitis (LCM)		Latent infection in mice, may produce fatal meningitis in many other species, including man
B. Tacaribe complex of viruses: several viruses including Argentinian (Junin) and Bolivian (Machupo) hemorrhagic fever	Isolated from insects and rodents	Hemorrhagic fever, Machupo frequently fatal

TABLE 62-4   CONTINUED

	Host	Symptoms in man
C. Lassa virus	?	Hemorrhagic fever, frequently fatal

X. CORONAVIRIDAE — Enveloped helical nucleocapsids
Diameter: about 100 nm
Nucleocapsids probably helical, loosely coiled, characteristic club-shaped surface projections. There is some antigenic relationship between certain human and murine strains.

	Host	Symptoms in man
i. Infectious bronchitis virus (IBV)		
(a) Avian strains	Chicken	—
(b) Human strains	Man	Isolated from patients with acute upper respiratory disease
ii. Mouse hepatitis virus	Mouse	

XI. MISCELLANEOUS VIRUSES
Several viruses do not fit into any of the families listed so far. The most important are:
A. Hepatitis virus. *Clinically, two types of viral hepatitis are distinguished, one characterized by a short incubation (infectious hepatitis, or epidemic jaundice), the other by a long incubation and usually requiring parenteral transmission (serum hepatitis). The etiologic agent of the former, hepatitis virus A, appears to be a particle about 27 nm in diameter; that of the latter (hepatitis virus B) is probably a particle about 40 nm in diameter that contains DNA and a DNA polymerase (Dane particles).*
B. Chronic infectious neuropathic agents (CHINA viruses). *These agents have a preclinical period lasting months to several years, succeeded by a slowly progressing, usually fatal disease. Most of them affect the central nervous system. Degenerative diseases of other organs and tissues may be caused by similar agents. They include the agents that cause* kuru *and* Creutzfeldt Jakob disease *in man,* scrapie *in sheep, and* transmissible mink encephalopathy *in mink. All are slow degenerative disorders of the central nervous system marked by ataxia and wasting, ending in death. The etiologic agents have been transmitted, but not yet isolated or even visualized.*

adenoviruses, and so on. However, within each major virus family there are viruses that *are* related to varying degrees, and it is this relatedness that forms the basis of ordering viruses within the major families into subgroups.

The Major Families of Animal Viruses

Table 62-4 presents a summary of the distinguishing characteristics of the major families of animal viruses, together with a list of the most important animal and human pathogens in each. It is based in large part upon a series of recommendations that have recently been made by the International Committee on Taxonomy of Viruses.

FURTHER READING

Books and Reviews

Brakke MK: Density-gradient centrifugation. In Maramorosch K, Koprowski H (eds): Methods in Virology, New York and London, Academic Press, 1967, pp 93-108

Caspar DLD, Klug A: Physical principles in the construction of regular viruses. Cold Spring Harbor Symp Quant Biol 27:1, 1962

Choppin PW, Compans RW: Reproduction of paramyxoviruses. In Fraenkel-Conrat H, Wagner RR (eds): Comprehensive Virology. New York and London, Plenum Press, 1975, vol 4, p 95

Compans RW, Choppin PW: Reproduction of myxoviruses. In Fraenkel-Conrat H, Wagner RR (eds): Comprehensive Virology. New York and London, Plenum Press, 1975, vol 4, p 179

Dalton AJ, Hagenau F (eds): Ultrastructure of Animal Viruses and Bacteriophages: An Atlas. New York, Academic Press, 1973

Diener TO: Viroids. Adv Virus Res 17:295, 1972

Horne RW, Wildy P: Virus structure revealed by negative staining. Adv Virus Res 10:102, 1963

Horzinek MC: The structure of togaviruses. Prog Med Virol 16:109, 1973

Joklik WK: Reproduction of reoviridae. In Fraenkel-Conrat H, Wagner RR (eds): Comprehensive Virology. Vol. 2, New York and London, Plenum Press, 1974, vol 2, p 231

Kaplan AS (ed): The Herpesviruses. New York and London, Academic Press, 1973

Knight CA: Chemistry of Viruses, 2nd ed. New York and Vienna, Springer Verlag, 1975

Lehmann-Grube F (ed): Lymphocytic Choriomeningitis Virus and other Arenaviruses. Berlin, Heidelberg and London, Springer Verlag, 1973

Levintow L: Reproduction of picornaviruses. In Fraenkel-Conrat H, Wagner RR (eds): Comprehensive Virology.

New York and London, Plenum Press, 1974, vol 2, p 109

Maizel JV Jr: Acrylamide gel electrophoresis of proteins and nucleic acids. In Habel K, Salzman NP (eds): Fundamental Techniques in Virology. New York and London, Academic Press, 1969, p 334

Maramorosch K, Kurstak E (eds): Comparative Virology. New York, Academic Press, 1971

Moss B: Reproduction of poxviruses. In Fraenkel-Conrat H, Wagner RR (eds): Comprehensive Virology, New York and London, Plenum Press, 1974, vol 3, p 405

Pfefferkorn ER, Shapiro D: Reproduction of togaviruses. In Fraenkel-Conrat H, Wagner RR (eds): Comprehensive Virology. New York and London, Plenum Press, 1974, vol 2, p 171

Philipson L, Lindberg U: Reproduction of adenoviruses. In Fraenkel-Conrat H, Wagner RR (eds): Comprehensive Virology. New York and London, Plenum Press, 1974, vol 3, p 143

Roizman B, Furlong D: The replication of herpesviruses. In Fraenkel-Conrat H, Wagner RR (eds). Comprehensive Virology. New York and London, Plenum Press, 1974, vol 3, p 229

Rose JA: Parvovirus reproduction. In Fraenkel-Conrat H, Wagner RR (eds): Comprehensive Virology. New York and London, Plenum Press, 1974, vol 3, p 1

Schulze IT: Structure of the influenza virion. Adv Virus Res 18:1, 1973

Stott EJ, Killington RA: Rhinoviruses. Annu Rev Microbiol 26:503, 1972

Theiler M, Downs WG: The Arthropod-borne Viruses of Vertebrates. New Haven and London, Yale Univ Press, 1973

Tinsley TW, Longworth JF: Parvoviruses. J Gen Virol 20[Suppl]:7, 1973

Wagner RR: Reproduction of rhabdoviruses. In Fraenkel-Conrat H, Wagner RR (eds): Comprehensive Virology. New York and London, Plenum Press, 1975, vol 4, p 1

White DO: Influenza viral proteins: Identification and synthesis. Curr Top Microbiol Immunol 63:2, 1974

Wilner BI: A Classification of the Major Groups of Human and Other Animal Viruses, 4th ed. Minneapolis, Burgess, 1969

Selected Papers

POXVIRUSES

Geshelin P, Berns KI: Characterization and localization of the naturally occurring cross-links in vaccinia virus DNA. J Mol Biol 88:785, 1974

Kates JR, McAuslan BR: Messenger RNA synthesis by a "coated" viral genome. Proc Natl Acad Sci USA 57:314, 1967

Moss B, Rosenblum E, Garon CF: Glycoprotein synthesis in cells infected with vaccinia virus. III. Purification and biosynthesis of the virion glycoprotein. Virology 55:143, 1973

Paoletti E, Rosemond-Hornbeak H, Moss B: Two nucleic acid nucleoside triphosphate phosphohydrolases from vaccinia virus. J Biol Chem 249:3273, 3281, 1974

Rosemond-Hornbeak H, Paoletti E, Moss B: Single-stranded deoxyribonucleic acid-specific nuclease from vaccinia virus. J Biol Chem 249:3287, 3292, 1974

Sarov I, Joklik WK: Studies on the nature and location of

the capsid polypeptides of vaccinia virions. Virology 50:579, 1972

HERPESVIRUSES

Graham FL, Veldhuisen G, Wilkie NM: Infectious herpesvirus DNA. Nature [New Biol] 245:265, 1973

Heine JW, Honess RW, Cassai E, Roizman B: Proteins specified by herpes simplex virus. XII. The virion polypeptides of Type 1 strains. J Virol 14:640, 1974

Huang E, Pagano JS: Human cytomegalovirus. II. Lack of relatedness to DNA of herpes simplex I and II, Epstein-Barr virus and nonhuman strains of cytomegalovirus. J Virol 13:642, 1974

Palmer EL, Martin ML, Gary GW: The ultrastructure of disrupted herpesvirus nucleocapsids. Virology 65:260, 1975

Wadsworth S, Jacob RJ, Roizman B: Anatomy of herpes simplex virus DNA. II. Size, composition, and arrangement of inverted terminal repetitions. J Virol 15:1487, 1975

ADENOVIRUSES

Garon CF, Berry KW, Hierholzer JC, Rose JA: Mapping of base sequence heterogeneities between genomes from different adenovirus serotypes. Virology 54:414, 1973

Lacy S, Green M: The mechanism of viral carcinogenesis by DNA mammalian viruses: DNA-DNA homology relationships among the "weakly" oncogenic human adenoviruses. J Gen Virol 1:413, 1967

Nermut MV: Fine structure of adenovirus type 5. I. Virus capsid. Virology 65:480, 1975

Roberts RJ, Arrand JR, Keller W: The length of the terminal repetition in adenovirus-2 DNA. Proc Nat Acad Sci USA 71:3829, 1974

PAPOVAVIRUSES

Finch JT: The surface structure of polyoma virus. J Gen Virol 24:359, 1974

Finch JT, Klug A: The structure of viruses of the papilloma-polyoma type. J Mol Biol 13:1, 1968

Gibson W: Polyoma virus proteins: A description of the structural proteins of the virion based on polyacrylamide gel electrophoresis and peptide analysis. Virology 62:319, 1974

Grady L, Axelrod D, Trilling D: The SV40 pseudovirus: its potential for general transduction in animal cells. Proc Nat Acad Sci USA 67:1886, 1970

Sen A, Levine AJ: SV40 nucleoprotein complex activity unwinds superhelical turns in SV40 DNA. Nature 249:343, 1974

PARVOVIRUSES

Berns KI, Kelley TJ: Visualization of the inverted terminal repetition of adeno-associated DNA. J Mol Biol 82:267, 1974

Chesebro B, Bloom M, Hadlow W, Race R: Purification and ultrastructure of Aleutian disease virus of mink. Nature 254:456, 1975

Mayor HD, Torikai K, Melnick JL: Plus and minus single-stranded DNA separately encapsidated in adeno-associated satellite virions. Science 166:1280, 1969

Rose JA, Maizel JV, Inman JK, Shatkin AJ: Structural proteins of adenovirus-associated viruses. J Virol 8:766, 1971

PICORNAVIRUSES

Burroughs JN, Brown F: Physico-chemical evidence for the re-classification of the caliciviruses. J Gen Virol 22: 281, 1974

Medappa KC, McLean C, Rueckert RR: On the structure of rhinovirus 1A. Virology 44:259, 1971

Young NA: Size of the gene sequences shared by polioviruses Types 1, 2, and 3. Virology 56:400, 1973

Young, NA: Polioviruses, coxsackieviruses, and echoviruses: Comparison of the genomes by RNA hybridization. J Virol 11:832, 1973

TOGAVIRUSES

von Bonsdorff CH, Harrison SC: Sindbis virus glycoproteins form a regular icosohedral surface lattice. J Virol 16:141, 1975

Hirschberg CB, Robbins PW: The glycolipids and phospholipids of Sindbis virus and their relation to the lipids of the host cell plasma membrane. Virology 61:602, 1974

Horzinek MC, van Wielink PS, Ellens DJ: Purification and electron microscopy of lactic dehydrogenase virus of mice. J Gen Virol 26:217, 1975

de Madrid AT, Porterfield JS: The flaviviruses (group B arboviruses): A cross-neutralization study. J Gen Virol 23:91, 1974

Murphy FA, Harrison AK, Whitefield SG: Bunyaviridae: Morphologic and morphogenetic similarities of Bunyamwera serologic supergroup viruses and several other arthropod-borne viruses. Intervirology 1:297, 1973

Pedersen CE, Eddy GA: Separation, isolation, and immunological studies of the structural proteins of Venezuelan equine encephalomyelitis virus. J Virol 14:740, 1974

Petterson RF, von Bonsdorff CH: Ribonucleoproteins of Uukuniemi virus are circular J Virol 15:386, 1975

REOVIRUSES

Furuichi Y, Morgan M, Muthukrishnan S, Shatkin AJ: Reovirus mRNA contains a methylated, blocked 5'-terminal structure: m^7G (5')ppp(5')G^mpCp$^-$. Proc Nat Acad Sci USA 72:262, 1975

Furuichi Y, Muthukrishnan S, Shatkin AJ: 5'-terminal m^7G(5')ppp(5')G^mp in vivo: Identification in reovirus genome RNA. Proc Nat Acad Sci USA 72:742, 1975

Gillies S, Bullivant S, Bellamy AR: Viral RNA polymerases: Electron microscopy of reovirus reaction cores. Science 174:694, 1971

Luftig RB, Kilham SS, Hay AJ, Zweerink HJ, Joklik WK: An ultrastructural study of virions and cores of reovirus type 3. Virology 48:170, 1972

Martin SA, Zweerink HJ: Isolation and characterization of two types of bluetongue virus particles. Virology 50: 495, 1972

Shatkin AJ, Sipe JD, Loh P: Separation of ten reovirus genome segments by polyacrylamide gel electrophoresis. J Virol 2:986, 1968

Smith RE, Zweerink HJ, Joklik WK: Polypeptide components of virions, top component and cores of reovirus type 3. Virology 39:791, 1969

MYXOVIRUSES

Bishop DHL, Roy P, Bean WJ Jr, Simpson RW: Transcription of the influenza ribonucleic acid genome by a virion polymerase. III. Completeness of the transcription process. J Virol 10:689, 1972

Etkind PR, Krug RM: Influenza virus messenger RNA. Virology 62:38, 1974

Kolakofsky D, Boy de la Tour E, Bruschi A: Self-annealing of Sendai RNA. J Virol 14:33, 1974

Scheid A, Choppin PW: Identification of biological activities of paramyxovirus glycoproteins. Activation of cell fusion, hemolysis, and infectivity by proteolytic cleavage of an inactive precursor protein of Sendai virus. Virology 57:475, 1974.

Shimizu K, Shimizu YK, Kohama T, Ishida N: Isolation and characterization of two distinct types of HVJ (Sendai virus) spikes. Virology 62:90, 1974

Stanley P, Crook NE, Streader LG, Davidson BE: The polypeptides of influenza virus. VIII. Large-scale purification of the hemagglutinin. Virology 56:640, 1973

Wrigley NG, Skehel JJ, Charlwood PA, Brand CM: The size and shape of influenza neuraminidase. Virology 51:525, 1973

RHABDOVIRUSES

Bishop DHL, Repik P, Obijeski JF, Moore NF, Wagner RR: Reconstitution of infectivity to spikeless vesicular stomatitis virus by solubilized viral components. J Virol 16: 75, 1975

Emerson SU, Wagner RR: L protein requirement for in vitro RNA synthesis by vesicular stomatitis virus. J Virol 12:1325, 1973

Etchison JR, Holland JJ: Carbohydrate composition of the membrane glycoprotein of vesicular stomatitis virus grown in four mammalian cell lines. Proc Nat Acad Sci USA 71:4011, 1974

Imblum RL, Wagner RR: Protein kinase and phosphoproteins of vesicular stomatitis virus. J Virol 13:113, 1974

Wagner RR, Prevec L, Brown F, et al: Classification of rhabdovirus proteins: A proposal. J Virol 10:1228, 1972

HEPATITIS VIRUSES

Barker LF, Almeida JD, Hoofnagle JG, et al: Hepatitis B core antigen: Immunology and electron microscopy. J Virol 14:1552, 1974

Krugman S, et al: Nomenclature of antigens associated with viral hepatitis B. Intervirology 2:134, 1974

Provost PJ, Wolanski BS, Miller WF, et al: Physical, chemical and morphologic dimensions of human hepatitis A virus strain CR326. Proc Soc Exp Biol Med 148:532, 1975

Robinson WS, Greenman RL: DNA polymerase in the core of human hepatitis B virus. J Virol 13:1231, 1974

63
The Inactivation of Viruses

Knowledge of the nature of the interaction of viruses with the chemical and physical components of the extracellular environment is of significance for three reasons: it is important to know (1) how to inactivate viruses when the object is to eliminate them and (2) how to preserve them when the object is to avoid loss of infectivity. (3) Analysis of the mode of action of specific reagents on virions often throws light on the nature of viral capsids and of their association with nucleic acids.

ENZYMES

All viral genomes are protected from nucleases by virtue of the capsids that enclose them. Animal viruses are generally resistant to attack by the proteases of higher animal, such as pepsin, trypsin, and chymotrypsin. Some, such as the enteroviruses, are completely resistant, while others, such as the poxviruses and reoviruses, possess susceptible outer shells but resistant cores. Glycoprotein spikes of enveloped viruses can generally be removed by treatment with proteolytic enzymes, and the resulting bald particles lack infectivity. Phospholipases usually inactivate enveloped viruses by hydrolyzing their phospholipids.

CHEMICAL REAGENTS

Many types of chemical compounds inactivate viruses. Among them are oxidizing agents, salts of heavy metals, and most reagents that interact with proteins chemically. Many of these reagents are of little importance for the selective destruction of viral infectivity, and the study of their interaction with viruses has not contributed significantly to our knowledge of virion structure. However, there are several chemical reagents whose action on viruses is of great interest.

Detergents (1) Nonionic detergents (such as Nonidet P-40, Triton X-100, and the like), which are usually polyoxyethylene ethers or sorbitans, solubilize lipid components of viral envelopes, thereby releasing undenatured internal components and glycoprotein spikes, which can then be examined further with respect to morphology, antigenic constitution, and enzymatic activity.

(2) Anionic detergents, the most important of which is sodium dodecyl sulfate, not only solubilize viral envelopes but also dissociate capsids into their constituent polypeptides. The use of sodium dodecyl sulfate for the characterization of these polypeptides by means of polyacrylamide gel electrophoresis has already been discussed (Chap. 62).

(3) Cationic detergents have so far found little use in virology.

Protein Solvents Guanidine, urea, and phenol are powerful protein solvents that are used extensively to dissociate viral capsids into their constituent polypeptide chains. In contrast to sodium dodecyl sulfate, they do not form complexes with polypeptides but act by minimizing the formation of hydrogen bonds on which protein structure is largely dependent. Phenol is the most commonly used reagent for liberating viral nucleic acids.

Formaldehyde Formaldehyde destroys infectivity without significantly affecting antigenicity and has therefore been used extensively for preparing inactivated virus vaccines. It destroys infectivity primarily by reacting with those amino groups of adenine, guanine, and cytosine that are not involved in hydrogen bond formation. Viruses containing single-stranded nucleic acid are therefore inactivated readily, while those that contain double-stranded nucleic acid are resistant to formaldehyde It also reacts with amino groups of proteins, forming addition compounds of the Schiff's base type and cross-linking polypeptide chains without, however, significantly disturbing protein conformation. Reaction with protein is most probably responsible for the occasional generation of a formaldehyde-resistant infectious virus fraction, which appears to be caused by such extensive cross-linking of capsid proteins that formaldehyde cannot reach and inactivate the viral nucleic acid. Careful control of reaction conditions and rigorous checks for residual infectious virus are mandatory for the preparation of formaldehyde-inactivated virus vaccines.

pH Viruses differ greatly in their resistance to acidity. For example, enteroviruses are very resistant to acid conditions, while rhinoviruses are very susceptible. All viruses are disrupted under alkaline conditions.

PHYSICAL AGENTS

Heat Viruses differ enormously in heat stability. In general, icosahedral viruses, such as enteroviruses, reoviruses, papovaviruses, and adenoviruses, as well as poxviruses, are reasonably heat stable: their infectivity decreases by no more than twofold to fourfold during six hours at 37 C. By contrast many enveloped viruses, especially myxoviruses and RNA tumor viruses, are very heat labile: Their half-life at 37 C is sometimes no more than one hour. The infectivity titer of the former group of viruses remains stable for months at 4C. Viruses of the latter group must be stored at −70C, the temperature of dry ice, or in liquid nitrogen (−196C).

The initial rate of heat inactivation is exponential, that is, a constant fraction of virus is inactivated in each unit of time. This is most readily explained in terms of an energy distribution, with those molecules that possess more than a certain minimal energy of activation having a significant probability of undergoing an inactivating change. As the temperature increases, so does the proportion of molecules with this minimal amount of energy.

Heat stability is strongly influenced by environmental conditions. Proteins stabilize all viruses to greater or lesser extent, as do metal ions, especially diavalent cations such as Mg^{++} and Ca^{++}. Measurement of heat inactivation therefore requires careful standardization of suspension media.

Radiation All viruses are inactivated by electromagnetic radiation, especially x-radiation or gamma-radiation and ultraviolet (UV) radiation. X-rays inactivate viruses primarily by causing scissions (breaks) in nucleic acid strands. If the viral genome consists of single-stranded nucleic acid, every scission is lethal; if the genome consists of double-stranded nucleic acid, scissions in both strands located near to each other are required for inactivation. X-rays, therefore, inactivate viruses containing single-stranded nucleic acid much more efficiently (about ten-fold) than they do those containing double-stranded nucleic acid.

Ultraviolet radiation also damages nucleic acids (Chap. 8). In particular, it causes the formation of covalent bonds between adjacent pyrimidine molecules, thereby giving rise to cyclobutane derivatives. In DNA, the most commonly formed pyrimidine dimers are those between adjacent thymine rings; in RNA, dimers are formed between any adjacent uracil and cytosine rings. Dimer formation inactivates viral genomes by preventing replication and probably also transcription and translation.

Dimers are removed from DNA by several mechanisms. These have been studied mainly in bacteria, but there is evidence that they operate in animal cells as well. One involves an enzyme system that utilizes radiation of longer wavelengths, particularly those of visible light, for dissociating dimers: This is the so-called photoreactivating repair systems. Another mechanism (the dark or excision repair mechanism) involves nucleases that recognize dimers and excise them, the gaps then being repaired by a DNA polymerase acting in conjunction with polynucleotide ligase: This is the host cell reactivating system.

Ultraviolet radiation also induces cross-linking of the two strands of double stranded DNA by a mechanism that is not clear. No doubt this also contributes to virus inactivation.

Ultraviolet radiation also causes the addition of water molecules across the C5-C6 double bond of pyrimidines in both DNA and RNA, which results in the formation of photohydrates (6-hydroxy-5,6-dihydro derivatives). These photohydrates represent a major portion of the lethal damage caused by ultraviolet light in many RNA-containing viruses.

The most radiation-sensitive property of a virion is its infectivity. The reason is that infectivity requires expression of the genome's entire information content and thus presents the largest target. Sometimes virus particles that have lost the ability to reproduce can still express some special function or group of functions that originate from cistrons that have not sustained radiation damage. Examples of such functions are the ability to synthesize early enzymes (Chap. 65) and the ability to transform cells (Chap. 69). At very high radiation doses damage to capsid proteins becomes important. This causes loss of the ability to interfere with the multiplication of related viruses, loss of ability to hemagglutinate, and loss of antigenicity.

Photodynamic Inactivation Virions interact with certain organic dyes in such a manner that illumination with visible light inactivates them. One such dye is methylene blue. When methylene blue is added to vaccinia virus and the mixture is kept dark, infectivity is not affected. However, if it is illuminated with white light in the presence of oxygen, the virus is inactivated. The mechanism of this inactivation is not well understood. Presumably the dye must penetrate into the virus and become associated with the nucleic acid.

The acridine dye, neutral red, acts in a similar manner. Acridines characteristically intercalate between the stacked hydrogen-bonded base pairs of double-stranded nucleic acids, and they also intercalate, although more weakly, between base pairs of double-helical regions of single-stranded nucleic acids (Chap. 8). If a virus, such as poliovirus, is allowed to multiply in the presence of neutral red, the viral RNA together with intercalated dye becomes enclosed in capsids, forming virions that are fully infectious unless they are illuminated with white light. This phenomenon is of practical importance for two reasons. First, neutral red is a vital dye that is commonly used for the enumeration of plaques (Chap. 61). Plates on which plaque titrations are performed must be protected from bright white light once neutral red is added to them, since otherwise progeny virus is inactivated, and visible plaques do not form. Second, the fact that neutral red-containing virus is photosensitive provides a very useful method for inactivating infectious virus, which finds application in several types of studies.

FURTHER READING

Books and Reviews

Bachrach HL: Reactivity of viruses in vitro. Prog Med Virol 8:214, 1966

Luria SE, Darnell JE: General Virology. New York, London, and Sydney, Wiley, 1967, pp 149-172.

Selected Papers

Cooper PD: Studies on the structure and formation of the polioviruses: Effect of concentrated urea solutions. Virology 16:485, 1962

Gard S: Theoretical considerations in the inactivation of viruses by chemical means. Ann NY Acad Sci 83:638, 1960

Ito Y: A tumor-producing factor extracted by phenol from papillomatous tissue (Shope) of cottontail rabbits. Virology 12:596, 1960

Oster G, McLaren AD: The ultraviolet light and photosensitized inactivation of tobacco mosaic virus. J Gen Physiol 33:215, 1950

Papaevangelou GJ, Youngner JS: Thermal stability of ribonucleic acid from poliovirus mutants. Virology 15:509, 1961

Salk JE: Considerations in the preparation and use of poliomyelitis virus vaccine. JAMA 158:1239, 1955

Shapiro AL, Viñuela E, Maizel JV: Molecular weight estimation of polypeptide chains by electrophoresis in SDS-polyacrylamide gels. Biochem Biophys Res Commun 28:815, 1967

64
Viruses and Viral Proteins as Antigens

Many proteins coded by viruses are good antigens. This is of vital significance both medically and scientifically. Although great strides have been made during the last decade in defining the biochemistry and molecular biology of the multiplication cycles of animal viruses, the chemotherapeutic control of virus diseases is not yet a practical proposition. In fact, with very few exceptions, there is no way in which virus infections can be controlled; in almost all cases one relies on the natural ability of the host to form antibody to the invading virus. When the spread of viral infection to essential organs is too rapid, or when for some reason antibody formation does not take place early enough, the patient may succumb. Gamma globulin from hyperimmune sera is sometimes administered as a last resort: Even then one must rely on antibodies, not on drugs. By the same token, the only presently practical form of antiviral prophylaxis is provided by antibodies produced in response to vaccines (Chap. 68).

Structural viral proteins stimulate the formation of antibodies not only as components of virions but also as components of virion subunits, such as capsomers or nucleocapsids, and also in the free state. The principal antigenic determinants are often the same in all three forms, but extra antigenic sites are sometimes generated as individual proteins become part of more complex structures; for example, adenovirus hexons exhibit antigenic determinants not expressed by free hexon proteins.

The range of antiviral antibodies formed under conditions when viruses can and cannot multiply differs greatly. If a virus cannot multiply, either because it has been inactivated or because the host is not susceptible, only antibodies to surface components of the virus particle are usually formed. However, if the virus can multiply, not only is far more antibody formed because progeny virus will also act as antigen, but also the range of antibodies produced is much wider, since antibodies are then also formed to the unassembled and partially assembled virion components that are synthesized as a result of virus multiplication, as well as to nonstructural virus-coded proteins. For example, antisera to inactivated vaccinia virus contain only a few species of antibody directed against its surface components; but antisera from animals in which vaccinia virus has multiplied contain antibodies against at least 25 different viral proteins in readily detectable amounts.

The most specific, or individual, components of a virion's antigenic complement are its surface antigens, which usually vary from strain to strain and are known as the "type-specific antigens." Internal proteins of virus strains belonging to the same subgroup (or species) often possess common antigenic determinants, which are therefore known as "group-specific (gs) antigens." In the case of mammalian RNA tumor viruses (Chap. 69), some of the proteins that possess group-specific determinants also possess antigenic specificities common to several groups; these are said to be "interspecies-specific" antigenic determinants."

Possession of group- and type-specific antigenic determinants is of great taxonomic significance and provides an important tool for epidemiology. On the one hand, newly isolated virus strains usually receive their preliminary characterization as a result of tests against a variety of antisera of known specificity. On the other hand, it is possible to determine whether a given human or animal population has been exposed to a particular virus strain by testing serum samples for antiviral antibody.

The interaction of viruses and viral proteins with antibodies can be recognized and measured in several ways. The three most important follow.

THE INTERACTION OF VIRUS WITH NEUTRALIZING ANTIBODY

Antibodies to virus surface components neutralize infectivity; these are the neutralizing antibodies that protect against disease. They usually persist in the body for many years, and even when their level drops, a secondary or anamnestic response to virus generally boosts their titers to very high levels, so that no second cycle of infection ensues. This explains the fact that animals generally contract any particular virus disease only once. Exceptions, such as the common cold and influenza, are due to special circumstances; the reason for the frequent recurrence of the common cold syndrome is that it is elicited by a very large group of viruses, among which are rhinoviruses, enteroviruses, adenoviruses, and myxoviruses, and the reason for recurrent epidemics caused by the influenza virus is its genetic and therefore, immunologic variability (Chap. 67).

The reaction between neutralizing antibody and virus follows first order kinetics, which indicates that one antibody molecule can inactivate one virus particle. It does so by interfering with one of the initial events of the virus multiplication cycle, most probably uncoating. As we shall see, under conditions of normal infection, viral genomes are liberated into the interior of the cell, ready to start multiplication; but virus–antibody complexes are apparently engulfed and inactivated in phagocytic vacuoles, so that no intact viral genomes are able to reach the interior of the cell (Chap. 65).

In practice, a small fraction of virus, varying from 0.1 to 10 percent, generally remains infectious even in the presence of a large excess of antibody. The reason for this is that the virus–antibody union is reversible. Simple dilution causes dissociation, and so does contact with cells. Different cell types differ in their ability to reactivate virus-antibody complexes, so that the titers of virus–antibody mixtures tend to vary with the type of cell used for assay. A contributing factor to the formation of a persistent non-neutralizable virus fraction is the fact that antisera generally contain antibody molecules with diverse avidities which compete with each other for virus, so that some virions are usually combined with low avidity antibody. The lower the avidity, the less perfect is the fit between the antigenic site on the virus and the antibody-combining site, and the more readily reversible is the antigen-antibody union.

COMPLEMENT-FIXING ANTIGEN AND ANTIBODY

The virus–antibody interaction can also be measured by taking advantage of the fact that the complex of viral protein and antibody often fixes complement. Since sensitive methods for titrating complement are available, this provides a very convenient and accurate method of measuring either the amount of viral antigen (complement-fixing antigen or CFA) or of antibody to such antigens. The chief advantage of this method of detecting viral antigens is that any virus-coded protein may be a complement-fixing antigen. Both structural and nonstructural virus-coded proteins, such as the T antigens formed in cells infected with adenovi-

ruses and papovaviruses (Chap. 69), as well as viral subunits and virions themselves, may form complexes with antibody that fix complement. This method of quantitating viral proteins is particularly useful for detecting abortive virus infections when only part of the genetic information present in the viral genome is expressed and no virions are produced (Chap. 66). It is also of great importance in epidemiology, since it is often far easier to classify newly isolated virus strains by determining whether extracts of cells infected with them fix complement with antisera of known specificity than by measuring the ability of such antisera to neutralize infectivity.

VIRUS-CODED CELL SURFACE ANTIGENS

As will be described in Chapters 65 and 69, new antigenic determinants frequently appear on the surfaces (outer plasma membranes) of infected cells. In some cases these new determinants are probably on host membrane polypeptides that are normally masked or covered, and that become unmasked because outer cell membrane components are lost or because the membrane undergoes configurational changes. Much more commonly, however, these new determinants are on virus-coded polypeptides. In the case of enveloped viruses these polypeptides become, in due course, part of the viral envelope; in the case of nonenveloped viruses they are nonstructural polypeptides that are synthesized early during the infection cycle. In either case virus-coded cell surface polypeptides provide a clear signal to the immune mechanism that a cell is infected, and antibodies are formed against them.

GEL IMMUNODIFFUSION AND IMMUNO-ELECTROPHORESIS

Under appropriate conditions of antigen–antibody equivalence, antigen-antibody complexes are insoluble. This property is used in gel immunodiffusion and gel immunoelectrophoresis, techniques that are widely used for resolving mixtures of viral antigens such as occur in extracts of infected cells.

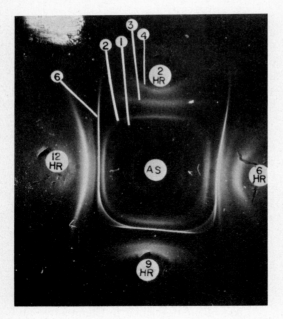

FIG. 64-1. The use of gel diffusion analysis to detect virus-specified proteins in extracts of infected cells. Antiserum to vaccinia virus was placed into the center well (AS) of a petri dish containing a layer of agar. Extracts of HeLa cells infected for 2, 6, 9, and 12 hours with vaccinia virus were placed into the other four wells, and the antibodies and antigens were allowed to diffuse toward each other. Precipitin lines, formed as described in the text, were then stained with Poinceau S. The pattern becomes increasingly complex with increasing time after infection, as more virus-specified proteins are revealed without the necessity for purification. (From Salzman and Sebring: J Virol 1:16, 1967)

The most widely used modification of gel immunodiffusion is the Ouchterlony method, which employs petri plates containing agar into which a number of wells are cut, one being situated centrally and the others equidistantly

from it and from each other. Antiserum or antibody is placed in the center well, antigen is placed in the outer ones, and diffusion is then allowed to proceed. Where the concentration of antigen–antibody complexes exceeds their solubility product, precipitin lines form, the location of which depends on the relative diffusion rates, and therefore on the relative sizes, of antigen and antibody. Identity of antigens is revealed by the familiar fusion of precipitin lines (Chap. 15) (Fig. 64-1).

In the gel immunoelectrophoresis technique, antigens are not separated by free diffusion but by electrophoresis in agar slabs, after which antiserum is applied in a trough cut parallel to the direction of electrophoresis. After diffusion, precipitin lines form as above (Fig. 64-2). The concentrations of antibody and antigen used in both these techniques are generally adjusted so that the precipitin lines are very thin, thus permitting great resolution.

THE VISUALIZATION OF VIRAL ANTIGENS USING TAGGED ANTIBODY

There are many occasions when direct visual localization of viral antigens is desired. This can be achieved by using antibody that is tagged, conjugated, or labeled with some material that can be visualized with either the light microscope or the electron microscope.

Antibody labeled with the dye fluorescein fluoresces brightly when viewed with a microscope equipped with a source of ultraviolet light (Fig. 64-3). Such antibody is a sensitive

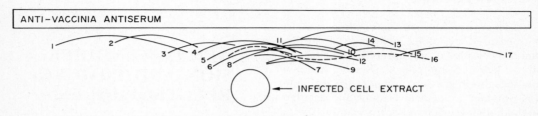

FIG. 64-2. Diagrammatic representation of an immunoelectrophoretic pattern of the virus-specified proteins present in an extract of chicken cells infected with vaccinia virus. In this technique the cell extract is placed in a circular well cut into an agar slab, and an electric field is applied, causing antigens to migrate at rates governed by their charge and size. After electrophoresis, antiserum to vaccinia virus is placed in a trough cut parallel to the direction of electrophoresis and allowed to diffuse toward the separated cell extract components. Virus-specified proteins able to react with antibodies in the antiserum form precipitin lines. Seventeen such proteins can be detected in the extract shown here. (From Rodriguez-Burgos et al: Virology 30:569, 1966)

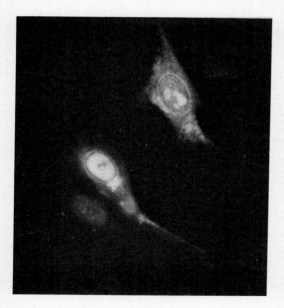

FIG. 64-3. Visualization of viral antigens by means of immunofluorescence. Cells infected with herpes simplex virus were washed, fixed in acetone, and allowed to react either with herpesvirus antibody conjugated with fluorescein isothiocyanate (direct immunofluorescence) or with herpesvirus antibody prepared in rabbits, followed by antirabbit globulin conjugated with fluorescein isothiocyanate (indirect immunofluorescence). Cells were then examined under ultraviolet light. The cells shown here were stained by the indirect method. The top cell shows fluorescent nuclear patches as well as fluorescence at the nuclear membrane and some diffuse cytoplasmic fluorescence. The other cell shows bright fluorescence of practically the whole nucleus, as well as cytoplasmic fluorescence. ×550. (From Ross, Watson, and Wildy: J Gen Virol 2: 115, 1968)

research tool in viral pathogenesis, that is, in studies on the route of infection and the spread of virus within the organism, since it can reveal a small number of infected cells in large populations of uninfected ones. It is also useful for measuring the proportion of infected cells in a variety of experimental situations, and it can serve as a rapid diagnostic tool, since minute amounts of infected biopsy material can be treated with fluorescein-labeled antibodies to several suspected viruses, one of which will cause the infected cells to fluoresce. Finally, since fluorescein-labeled antibody can also reveal the pattern of viral antigen distribution within infected cells, and since this pattern is often highly characteristic (nuclear or cytoplasmic, diffuse or highly localized), it can also serve in this way as a useful adjunct to virus identification.

Antibody molecules can also be tagged with large molecules or particles that can be seen with the electron microscope. Among these are ferritin, a large iron-containing protein, bacteriophage or virus particles with characteristic shapes, and latex spheres. Use of such antibody permits observation of the distribution of viral antigen in infected cells in exquisite detail. It is, therefore, invaluable in studies aimed at establishing the exact location of the sites of synthesis, accumulation, and assembly of viral protein components (Fig. 64-4).

THE IMMUNE RESPONSE TO VIRAL INFECTION

During viral infection antibodies are formed against all classes of virus-coded antigens. Those that are most important for eliminating virus from the body are those that are directed against virion components and virus-coded cell surface antigens. The former include the neutralizing and complement-fixing antibodies that prevent virus particles from infecting cells (p. 822). As for the latter, their combination with virus-coded antigens on cell surfaces renders the cell subject to destruction by at least two mechanisms: combination with complement followed by lysis, and attack by activated macrophages, again followed by lysis. In either case the infected cell is eliminated as a source of progeny virus.

Usually these mechanisms for destroying infectious virus and infected cells are beneficial to the host. However, it is now recognized that sometimes they may be very harmful. Let us consider first the destruction of infected cells. As a rule the number of cells that are destroyed is not large enough to cause serious problems for the host organism, but there are exceptions. A good example is provided by lymphocytic choriomeningitis virus (LCM), which causes encephalitis in mice and also in man. LCM, an enveloped virus, is not a very "lytic" virus; cells infected with it are not severely damaged and may survive for long periods of time. In mice, LCM produces no overt disease if the immune mechanism is not operative (in immunosuppressed or tolerant animals). However, in immunologically competent mice, LCM causes a fatal meningitis within a week,

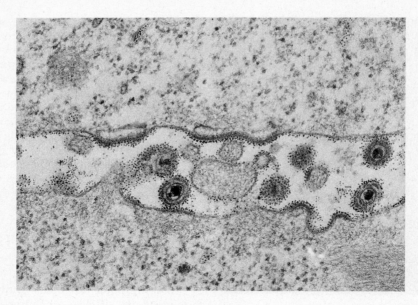

FIG. 64-4. Visualization of viral antigens by means of ferritin-conjugated antibody. This electron micrograph reveals the localization of virus-specified proteins on the surface of cells infected with herpes simplex virus. Infected cells were allowed to react with herpesvirus antibody conjugated with ferritin and then washed, fixed, embedded, and sectioned. The surfaces of two adjacent cells are seen, both with intensely labeled patches. Budding virus particles and detached cytoplasmic fragments are also labeled. ×48,000. (From Nii et al: J Virol 2:1172, 1968)

that is, as soon as antibody begins to be formed, death being due to the destruction of infected cells by activated macrophages. The disease is thus not caused by the destruction of the host's cells by the virus but by the destruction of infected cells by the host's immune mechanism. A similar interaction between immune lymphocytes and virus-coded cell surface antigens may account for the symptoms associated with some viral diseases of man, for example, hepatitis.

There is a second mechanism for destroying infected cells: Combination with antibody and complement will destroy infected cells long before cells break down as a direct result of viral infection. This mechanism also, though no doubt generally very valuable as a defense against infection, may sometimes cause severe damage to the host, for it appears that the sometimes fatal hemorrhagic shock syndrome associated with dengue fever is caused by sudden increases in vascular permeability that may be triggered by the interaction of immune complexes with the complement and clotting systems.

Although virus–antibody complexes are usually eliminated from the body without difficulty either before or after combination with complement, they may cause diseases quite unrelated to those caused by viruses alone. This realization has come from studies of several viral infections in animals, particularly LCM and lactic dehydrogenase virus (LDHV). Infection with both of these viruses results in the presence in the bloodstream of large amounts of virus–antibody complexes; it is also characterized by the development of glomerulonephritis and the presence in kidney capillaries of large amounts of virus-antibody-complement complexes. Similar observations have been made with respect to Aleutian mink disease and equine infectious anemia, in which the inflammatory changes are not confined to the kidneys but also involve the blood vessels (with the development of arteritis) and other parts of the body. Clearly, human glomerulonephritis may also be caused by virus–antibody complexes. Further, it is known that some virus–antibody complexes, such as complexes between adenovirus and antibody to hexon (but not to penton or fiber), are cytotoxic even in the absence of complement, and although this has so far been demonstrated only in vitro, the possibility exists that such complexes also cause tissue damage in the body.

Finally, it is now suspected that autoimmune diseases, such as rheumatoid arthritis and lupus erythematosus, are also caused by the interaction of viruses and the immune mechanism.

FURTHER READING

Books and Reviews

Almeida JD, Waterson AP: The morphology of virus-antibody interactions. Adv Virus Res 15:307, 1969

Casals J: Immunological techniques for animal viruses. In Maramorosch K, Koprowski H (eds): Methods in Virology. New York and London, Academic Press, 1967, vol 3 pp 113-198

Dent PB: Immunodepression by oncogenic viruses. Prog Med Virol 14:1, 1972

Howe C, Morgan C, Hsu KC: Recent virologic application of ferritin conjugates. Prog Med Virol 11:307, 1969

Notkins A (ed): Viral Immunology and Immunopathology. New York and London, Academic Press, 1976

Oldstone MBA: Virus neutralization and virus-induced immune complex disease. Prog Med Virol 19:85, 1975

Porter DD: Destruction of virus-infected cells by immunological mechanisms Annu Rev Microbiol 25:283, 1971

Sommerville RG: Rapid diagnosis of viral infections by immunofluorescent staining of viral antigens in leukocytes and macrophages. Prog Med Virol 10:398, 1968

Svehag S: Formation and dissociation of virus-antibody complexes with special reference to the neutralization process. Prog Med Virol 10:1, 1968

Selected Papers

Brown F, Smale CJ: Demonstration of three specific sites on the surface of FMDV by antibody complexing. J Gen Virol 7:115, 1970

Dales S, Kajioka R: The cycle of multiplication of vaccinia virus in Earle's strain L cells. I. Uptake and penetration. Virology 24:278, 1969

Fazekas de St Groth S, Webster RG: Disquisitions on original antigenic sin. J Exp Med 124:331, 347, 1966

Norrby E: The relationship between the soluble antigen and the virion of adenovirus type 3. 4. Immunological complexity of soluble components. Virology 37:565, 1969

Oldstone MBA: Immune complexes in cancer: Demonstration of complexes in mice bearing neuroblastomas. J Natl Cancer Inst 54:223, 1975

Pettersson U: Structural proteins of adenoviruses. 6. On the antigenic determinants of the hexon. Virology 43:123, 1971

Radwan AI, Burger D: The complement-requiring neutralization of equine arteritis virus by late antisera. Virology 51:71, 1973

Stollar V: Immune lysis of Sindbis virus. Virology 66:620, 1975

Wallis C, Melnick JL: A persistent fraction of herpesvirus caused by insufficient antibody. Virology 42:128, 1970

Woodroofe GM, Fenner F: Serological relationships within the poxvirus group: an antigen common to all members of the group. Virology 16:334, 1962

Yoshiki T, Mellors RC, Strand M, August JT: The viral envelope glycoproteins of murine leukemia virus and the pathogenesis of immune complex glomerulonephritis of New Zealand mice. J Exp Med 140:1011, 1974

65
The Viral Multiplication Cycle

Virions represent the static or inert form of viruses. Their very existence generally is only recognizable in terms of their interaction with cells, which is the central theme of virology.

The interaction of virus and cell generates a novel entity, the virus–cell complex, the fate of which varies widely, since it depends both on the nature of the cell and on the nature of the virus. The two most commonly observed virus–cell interactions are (1) the lytic interaction, which results in viral multiplication and lysis of the host cell, and (2) the transforming interaction, which results in the integration of the viral genome into the host genome and the permanent transformation or alteration of the host cell with respect to morphology, growth habit, and the manner in which it interacts with cells with which it comes in contact.

In studying the virus–host interaction, one can focus primarily either on the fate and functioning of the invading virus particle and on the production of virus progeny or on the reaction of the host cell to viral infection. Both approaches are of fundamental importance to the medical practitioner. The former is particularly relevant to the development of a rational approach to antiviral chemotherapy, the latter to an understanding of chronic viral infection and cancer. In this chapter we will focus on the invading virus particle, in the next on the response of the cell.

THE LYTIC VIRUS–CELL INTERACTION

The lytic virus-cell interaction is best thought of in terms of a cycle, the infection or multiplication cycle, during which the virus enters cells, multiplies, and is released. This cycle is repeated many times when a virion infects an organism, until either further multiplication is arrested for one reason or another or the host dies.

One of the principal goals of virology is the definition in molecular terms of all the various reactions that proceed during the virus multiplication cycle. As an example, when a poliovirion infects a cell, one RNA molecule and about 200 protein molecules are introduced into it. How does this RNA molecule replicate? What are the proteins for which it codes, and

what are their functions? How are mature virus particles assembled? What is the fate of the 200 parental protein molecules? What effect do they have on the host cell? What are the reactions that cause the host cell to die?

It is impossible to answer these and many other questions by studies in the intact organism. Instead, simple experimental systems are required that can be manipulated at will. Such systems are provided by cloned strains of cultured animal cells that grow in vitro and can be infected under any desired set of conditions with pure (plaque purified) strains of virus. Among their many advantages is the fact that they permit focusing on one multiplication cycle rather than on many repeated cycles, which is achieved by infecting all cells at the same time. In fact, one of the major conceptual breakthroughs in virology occurred when Ellis and Delbrück demonstrated, about 35 years ago, how very much simpler the analysis of the one-step growth cycle is than that of numerous successive unsynchronized cycles. In populations of cultured cells infected at high multiplicity—that is, with many virus particles per cell—so as to ensure that infection commences at the same time in all cells, the various reactions that together comprise virus multiplication proceed synchronously according to a regulated progressive pattern that is amenable to study by the techniques of biochemistry, biophysics, and cellular and molecular biology.

THE ONE-STEP GROWTH CYCLE: GENERAL ASPECTS

The virus multiplication cycle can be divided into several phases, using events of critical importance as markers (Fig. 65-1). As we shall see, infectivity is destroyed or eclipsed when virus adsorbs; the initial phase of the cycle is therefore often referred to as the "eclipse period." This phase ends with the formation of the first mature progeny virus particle, which marks the beginning of the rise period. Alternatively, the synthesis of the first progeny genome is often taken to divide the multiplication cycle into the early and late periods. The eclipse and early and the rise and late periods overlap substantially, with the interval between the beginning of the late and rise peri-

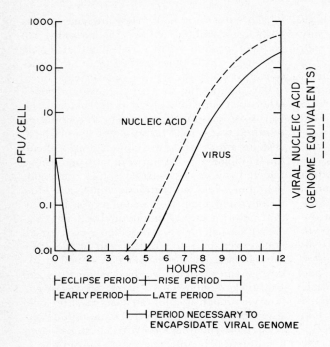

FIG. 65-1. The one-step growth cycle. Its essential features are as follows. After adsorption, viral infectivity is abolished or eclipsed, which is caused by uncoating of the infecting virus particles. Then follows the eclipse or early period, which can last from a few minutes to many hours, during which the stage is set for viral nucleic acid replication. The appearance of the first progeny genome marks the beginning of the late period, and the appearance of the first mature progeny virus particle the beginning of the rise period. It should be noted that the interval between the beginning of the late and rise periods represents the average time necessary for virus maturation, that is, the incorporation of a free nucleic acid molecule into a mature virus particle. The lengths of all periods, as well as the extent of virus multiplication, vary greatly for different viruses and cells.

ods representing the time necessary for the incorporation of a viral genome into a mature virion.

The Eclipse Period

Adsorption The first step of the virus–cell interaction is adsorption, which can itself be separated into several stages. The first of these is ionic attraction. Both cells and virus particles are negatively charged at pH 7, and positive ions are therefore required as counterions. As a rule this requirement is met most efficiently by magnesium ions. The second stage involves an accurate aligning of virus particles with the cell surface by virtue of interaction with specific receptor molecules, the existence of which is particularly apparent in the case of enteroviruses. There are two lines of evidence. First, poliovirus adsorbs only to cells of human or primate origin. In fact, in the body, poliovirus adsorbs only to cells of the central nervous system and to cells lining the intestinal tract. Other human and primate cells develop the ability to adsorb poliovirus only after being cultured in vitro, which causes unmasking of receptors. Second, the receptors for different enteroviruses, particularly for certain strains of

ECHO virus and Coxsackie virus, can be either removed or inactivated differentially. Furthermore, virus particles that do not combine with the same species of receptor molecule can nevertheless, by steric hindrance, inhibit each other's ability to adsorb.

A further example of virus receptors is provided by the oligosaccharide groups of the glycoproteins of the outer cell membranes of mammalian cells. These groups frequently terminate in the disaccharide galactose-N-acetyl-neuraminic (sialic) acid, which is hydrolyzed by the enzyme neuraminidase (sialidase), a component of orthomyxoviruses and paramyxoviruses (Chap. 62). The affinity between neuraminidase and its substrate appears to be one of the factors operating in the adsorption of these myxoviruses, since they elute from cells when all substrate has been hydrolyzed.

The time course of virus adsorption follows first order kinetics. The rate of adsorption is independent of temperature if suitable corrections for changes in the viscosity of the medium are made, but it is directly proportional to the amount of surface to which virus can adsorb, that is, to the cell concentration. The kinetics of adsorption are described by the relation

$$\frac{V_t}{V_0} = e^{-Ktc}$$

where V_0 and V_t are the concentrations of free virus at time 0 and after t minutes, respectively, c is the cell concentration, t is the time in minutes, and K is the adsorption rate constant.

The number of virus particles or infectious units adsorbed per cell is referred to as the "multiplicity of infection" (moi). Animal cells are generally capable of adsorbing very large amounts of virus; its has been shown, for example, that cells contain about 100,000 receptor sites for Sindbis virus (Fig. 65-2).

Penetration and Uncoating The second stage of the virus multiplication cycle involves penetration and uncoating, which are considered together because although they are separated both temporally and spatially for some viruses, they occur simultaneously for others. Penetration refers to the entry into the cytoplasm of either the whole virus particle or that part of it that contains the genome. Uncoating signifies the physical separation of viral nucleic

acid from viral protein. Viral genomes are invariably uncoated, a fact that is of taxonomic significance, since viruses are the only intracellular infectious agents or parasites for which this is an obligatory step of the multiplication cycle. (However, this is not true for reoviruses, which form an exception.)

Penetration itself, sometimes referred to as viropexis, is best observed directly by means of the electron microscope. Alternatively it may be followed by measuring the loss of the ability of antiviral antiserum to arrest initiation of virus multiplication. The reason for this is that as long as the virion remains outside the cell, combination with antibody significantly decreases its ability to cause productive infection, but once virus is within the cell, it is no longer accessible to antibody. Uncoating, on the other hand, is best assessed by measuring physical and chemical changes in the adsorbed virus particles. Among these are progressive labilization of the capsid structure as judged by loss of its ability to shield the viral genome

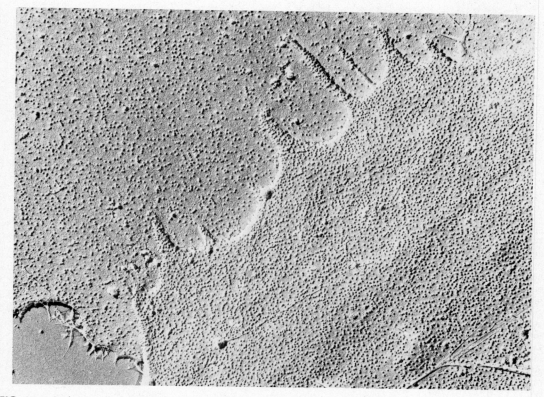

FIG. 65-2. Surface replica of Sindbis virus adsorbed to the surface of two chicken cells. ×9300. (From Birdwell and Strauss: J Virol 14:672, 1974)

from hydrolysis by nucleases, loss of some antigenic determinants, and progressive loss of capsid protein.

The actual pathways of penetration and uncoating of the several different types of viral particles differ markedly, which is not surprising in view of the great diversity of virus structure.

PENETRATION AND UNCOATING OF VIRIONS WITH NAKED ICOSAHEDRAL NUCLEOCAPSIDS.   There is morphologic evidence for two quite distinct pathways of penetration. On the one hand, virus particles aligned with the outer surface of the cell seem to be engulfed by the cell membrane, which in essence flows over them. They are thus drawn into the cell within phagocytic vacuoles, which subsequently break down, liberating more or less intact virus particles into the cytoplasm. On the other hand virus particles

may be able to pass directly across the cell membrane without becoming engulfed in phagocytic vacuoles (Fig. 65-3).

Physical changes in the structure of the capsid become evident very soon after adsorption. First, structural rearrangements of capsomers cause the capsid to become susceptible to reagent, such as urea and sodium dodecyl sulfate, to which intact virions are resistant. Virus particles then lose their ability to react with antibody, indicating further changes in capsid conformation, and finally the genome is liberated. There is no evidence for the involvement of enzymes in any of these changes; rather it seems that combination of the virion with receptor molecules causes conformational changes in the capsid that finally result in the liberation of the genome. The total time from adsorption to final uncoating ranges from several minutes to about two hours.

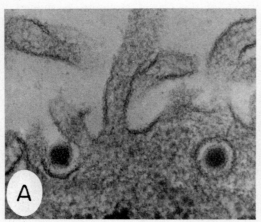

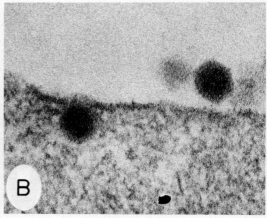

FIG. 65-3. The penetration and uncoating of adenovirus. Two alternative pathways are illustrated. A. The virus particle is engulfed by the cell membrane and enters the cytoplasm inside a phagocytic vacuole or vesicle which will break down and release the intact particle without its fibers. B. The virus particle passes directly across the cell membrane by a mechanism not yet understood. C. Diagrammatic representation of the uptake and uncoating of adenovirions. Once inside the cell, they migrate toward the nucleus where they are gradually degraded. Free viral DNA only appears in the nucleus. (A, from Chardonnet and Dales: Virology 40:462, 1970; B, from Morgan, Rosenkranz, and Mednis: J Virol 4:777, 1969)

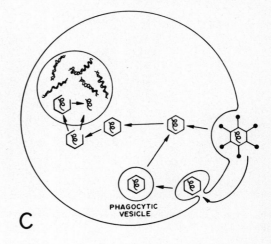

PENETRATION AND UNCOATING OF POXVIRIONS. Poxvirus particles have a highly specialized mechanism for penetration and uncoating. They enter cells by engulfment in phagocytic vacuoles and are broken down within them to cores that are liberated into the cytoplasm. The degradation of these cores, which results in the uncoating of the viral DNA, requires the synthesis of a special uncoating protein (Fig. 65-4).

PENETRATION AND UNCOATING OF ENVELOPED VIRIONS. Just as in the case of the naked icosahedral viruses, there seem to be two mechanisms by which enveloped viruses gain access to the interior of cells. The first involves fusion of the viral envelope with the outer cell membrane, thereby liberating the naked nucleocap-

sid into the cytoplasm, where the RNA is then either fully uncoated or transcribed (p. 844). There are several lines of evidence for this pathway, including direct morphologic evidence, the fact that the viral envelope was once part of the host cell membrane and is known to be capable of fusing with membranes, and the observation that enveloped viruses frequently possess the ability to fuse cells and hemolyze erythrocytes. The second mechanism, for which there is also good morphologic evidence, is identical with that described above, namely, engulfment of the entire virus particle into phagocytic vacuoles and liberation of the nucleocapsid within the cytoplasm rather than at the outer cell membrane. It is conceivable that both these penetration and uncoating

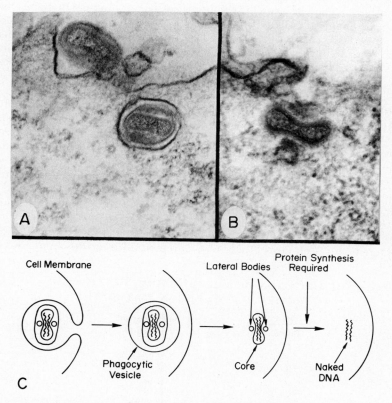

FIG. 65-4. The penetration and uncoating of vaccinia virus. Three stages are shown. A. One of the two virus particles is aligning itself with the cell membrane, which is preparing to flow around it. The other particle is already inside the cytoplasm, enclosed within a phagocytic vacuole. B. The phagocytic vacuole has broken down, as has the virion's outer protein coat. The core is now free, and the two lateral bodies have moved some distance away. The final stage of uncoating is the breakdown of the core, which results in the liberation of the DNA. This step is not achieved if protein synthesis is inhibited. It is therefore assumed that the synthesis of a special uncoating protein is required. Poxviruses are the only viruses that require the synthesis of a special protein for uncoating. This whole process is shown diagrammatically in C. A and B, ×80,000. (A and B, from Dales: J Cell Biol 18:63, 1963; C, modified from Joklik: J Mol Biol 8:277, 1964)

mechanisms are operative, and that the factors that determine which is used are primarily the nature of the virus and the nature of the cell.

Eclipse Adsorption, penetration, and uncoating result in loss of infectivity, which is referred to as "eclipse." The only residual infectivity is that due to the viral nucleic acid itself, which, however, is never more than a small fraction of that of the virus particles themselves.

The first three stages of infection are usually inefficient processes. Virus particles often adsorb to portions of the cell surface at which penetration will not proceed, viral genomes are damaged by ribonuclease which is frequently associated with outer (or plasma) cell membranes, and virus particles may fail to be released from the phagocytic vacuoles in which they have become engulfed. All these inefficiencies account in large part for the fact that the ratio of infectious to total animal virus particles is almost always far less than 1 (Chap 61).

The Synthetic Phase of the Viral Multiplication Cycle

Once the viral genome is uncoated, the synthetic phase of the viral growth cycle commences. In essence, this encompasses the replication of the viral genome and the synthesis of capsid proteins, followed by the formation of mature progeny virus particles.

The location where the viral genome replicates is characteristic for each virus (Table 65-

1). There is no correlation between this location and any other property, such as chemical nature or size of genome. Viral protein is always synthesized in the cytoplasm on polyribosomes composed of viral messenger RNA, host cell ribosomes, and host cell transfer RNA.

The Early Period The early period of the synthetic phase is devoted primarily to the activation of reactions that are prerequisite for the initiation of viral genome replication. This activation proceeds as the result of the virus's exercising certain eary functions. In spite of much intensive work, little is yet known concerning their nature. However, it is either known or likely, that the following are early functions: (1) the inhibition of host DNA, RNA, and protein synthesis, which may involve the synthesis of virus-coded proteins that alter the specificities of the DNA-replicating, RNA-transcribing, and polypeptide-synthesizing systems, so that viral rather than host cell genetic information is processed, (2) the synthesis of proteins that form the matrix of inclusions, either within the nucleus or within the cytoplasm, within which viral nucleic acids replicate and viral morphogenesis proceeds, (3) the synthesis of certain enzymes, primarily DNA and RNA polymerases, which is true for all RNA-containing viruses except RNA tumor viruses, as well as for the large DNA-containing viruses, and (4) the synthesis of some capsid proteins, which is the exception rather than the rule, since capsid proteins are generally late proteins.

The extent to which early functions are expressed varies greatly from virus to virus. Some

TABLE 65–1 THE LOCATION OF VIRAL GENOME REPLICATION, NUCLEOCAPSID FORMATION, AND VIRION MATURATION

Virus	Genome Replication	Nucleocapsid Formation	Virion Maturation
Poxvirus	Cytoplasm	Cytoplasm	Cytoplasm
Herpesvirus	Nucleus	Nucleus	At nuclear and cytoplasmic membranes
Adenovirus	Nucleus	Nucleus	Nucleus
Papovavirus	Nucleus	Nucleus	Nucleus
Poliovirus	Cytoplasm	Cytoplasm	Cytoplasm
Togavirus	Cytoplasm	Cytoplasm	At membranes
Reovirus	Cytoplasm	Cytoplasm	Cytoplasm
Ortho myxovirus	Nucleus	Nucleus (?)	At membranes
Paramyxoviruses	Cytoplasm	Cytoplasm	At membranes
Rhabdovirus	Cytoplasm	Cytoplasm	At membranes
RNA tumor virus	Nucleus	Cytoplasm	At membranes

viruses possess so little genetic information that only very few early functions are expressed. Others, for example, poxviruses, possess so much that they may express from 30 to 50 early functions. Early functions are expressed through (early) virus-coded proteins that are transcribed from early viral messenger RNA species. Those viral genomes that are plus-stranded RNA themselves serve as messenger RNA. For all other viruses, plus-stranded messenger RNA must first be transcribed from infecting parental genomes by means of the polymerases present within them.

The Late Period During the late period, the late viral functions are expressed. The late viral proteins are primarily the components of progeny virus particles and the enzymes and other nonstructural proteins that function during viral morphogenesis. Late viral proteins are coded by late viral messenger RNA molecules. Since there are always more late viral messenger RNA molecules than early ones (because there are more progeny genomes than parental ones), the amount of late proteins that are synthesized always greatly exceeds that of the early ones. For most RNA viruses the nature of the various early and late protein species is the same, although their relative amounts may differ, but for the double-stranded DNA-containing viruses the early and late protein species are different and are coded from different portions of the viral genome. Activation of the portion of the viral genome that codes for late functions may or may not be accompanied by deactivation of the portion that codes for early functions. In either case, a mechanism exists that specifies that one set of genes (the early set) is transcribed from parental genomes, while a different set (the late set) is transcribed only from progeny genomes. The basis of this mechanism probably lies in the specificity of the enzyme(s) that transcribes DNA. Indeed, work with certain bacteriophages has indicated that the host-specified, DNA-dependent RNA polymerase is modified early during infection to a form that can transcribe those sites on the phage genome that code for early functions, and that at the beginning of the late period, its specificity is altered again so as to enable it to respond to those signals that specify late functions (Chap. 70). Similar mechanisms may also operate in the case of animal viruses.

During the late period, the newly formed viral genomes and capsid polypeptides are assembled into progeny virus particles, a process that is known as "morphogenesis." This is a spontaneously occurring process, and most of the information for virus assembly resides in the amino acid sequence of the capsid polypeptides, a fact demonstrated by the occurrence among the yield of most icosahedral viruses of empty virus particles—that is, virus particles that contain no nucleic acid—that are morphologically indistinguishable from mature virions.

The duration of the late period is generally limited by the ability of the host cell to supply energy for macromolecular synthesis. This is a critical factor, since infecton with lytic viruses invariably interferes with the functioning of the host cell by multiple mechanisms that will be discussed in Chapter 66. As a result, synthesis of viral genome and viral capsid proteins slows down progressively, limiting the amount of viral progeny.

The Release of Progeny Virus

The final step of the infection cycle is the release of progeny. There is no special mechanism for the release of unenveloped viruses and poxviruses: Infected cells simply disintegrate more or less rapidly, liberating the viral progeny that has accumulated within them. The amount of cell-associated virus therefore exceeds the amount of released virus until the very last phase of the multiplication cycle (Fig. 65-6). A special mechanism does, however, exist for the enveloped viruses, for which release is the final stage of morphogenesis. Here virus-coded envelope proteins are incorporated into certain areas of host cell membranes while nucleocapsids are being synthesized. They then bud through these modified membranes and become enveloped by them (p. 778). Budding occurs both at the outer plasma cell membrane and at the membranes lining intracytoplasmic vacuoles, which then transport the virus to the exterior of the cell. These viruses do not exist in the mature infectious form within cells, and the amount of extracellular virus, therefore, greatly exceeds the amount of cell-associated virus at all stages of the multiplication cycle (Fig. 65-5).

The duration of the phases of the viral multi-

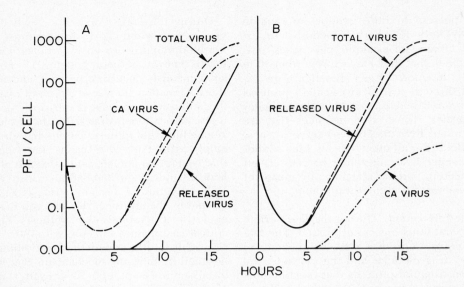

FIG. 65-5. The relationship between virus multiplication and release. A. This graph refers to viruses with icosahedral nucleocapsids. Such viruses are not released readily from cells. Viral progeny accumulates within the cell so that for much of the rise period the amount of cell-associated (CA) virus greatly exceeds the amount of released virus. Release of virus only occurs when cells break down at the end of the rise period. B. This graph refers to all enveloped viruses. Such viruses only mature in the process of being released, since it is only then that they acquire their envelope. The amount of liberated virus, therefore, always greatly exceeds the amount of cell-associated virus. The only cell-associated virus particles are those in the process of budding from the plasma membrane and those that bud into intracytoplasmic vacuoles.

plication cycle varies greatly, depending on the nature of the virus and the nature of the host cell. Table 65-2 gives the minimum length of the eclipse period and of the complete multiplicaton cycle of some well-studied viruses.

TABLE 65–2   APPROXIMATE DURATION OF THE ECLIPSE PERIOD AND OF THE ENTIRE MULTIPLICATION CYCLE

Virus	Eclipse Period (Hr)	Total Multiplication Cycle (Hr)
Poxvirus: vaccinia virus	4	24
Herpesvirus: herpes	3–5	12–30
simplex virus	8–10	48
Adenovirus		
Papovavirus: polyoma	12–14	48
virus	1–2	6–8
Poliovirus	2	10
Togavirus: Sindbis virus	4	15
Reovirus	3–5	18–36
Myxovirus: influenza virus		
Rhabdovirus: vesicular	2	8–10
stomatitis virus		

THE MULTIPLICATION CYCLE OF DOUBLE-STRANDED NUCLEIC ACID-CONTAINING VIRUSES

We will now consider in more detail the growth cycles of those animal viruses that contain double-stranded nucleic acid, those that contain single-stranded RNA and possess no envelopes, and those that contain single-stranded RNA and are enveloped. The growth cycles of each of these three types of viruses possess some fundamentally distinguishing features.

Although the multiplication cycles of poxviruses, herpesviruses, adenoviruses, and papovaviruses differ in many details, the same overall principles are involved in all. We will consider vaccinia virus as their prototype and indicate where the others exhibit divergent behavior. Papovaviruses will be considered in greater detail in Chapter 69.

The Early Period

As soon as it is uncoated, 40 to 50 percent of the vaccinia virus genome and a similar fraction of the herpesvirus, adenovirus, and papovavirus genomes is transcribed into early messenger RNA. Only very few of the corresponding proteins, which may number more than 50 in the case of vaccinia virus, are known. Some are the so-called early enzymes, such as thymidine kinase, DNA polymerase, and several nucleases, all of which are probably required for viral DNA replication. A few vaccinia virus (and herpesvirus) structural proteins are also early proteins. However, many more vaccinia virus and herpesvirus and all adenovirus and papovavirus structural proteins are late proteins. Interestingly enough, the few early structural vaccinia virus proteins are assembled into virus precursor particles that are spherical, bounded by a membrane, and possess little internal structure (Fig. 65-6).

Other early vaccinia virus proteins perhaps include a protein that causes rapid cessation of host DNA replication and a protein that prevents host cell messenger RNA from combining with ribosomes (Chap. 66). In fact, a striking feature of infection with vaccinia virus is the rapidity with which the synthesis of host protein is inhibited; under suitable conditions well over half of the protein synthesized as early as one hour after infection is viral. This changeover from host-specified to virus-specified protein synthesis is much more rapid than the rate of decay of cellular messenger RNA and implies the existence of an active mechanism for

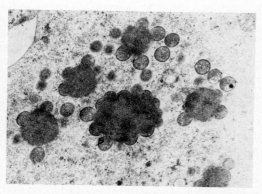

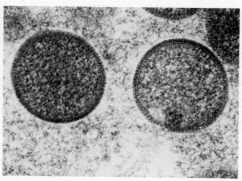

FIG. 65-6. Immature vaccinia virus particles in the cytoplasm of infected cells. Top. Particles developing from intracytoplasmic inclusions after reversal of vaccinia virus morphogenesis arrest by rifampicin (Chap. 68). ×15,000. Characteristic structure of immature vaccinia virus particles, ×80,000. Bottom. For photos of mature vaccinia virions, see Chapter 62. (Photos courtesy of Dr. T. H. Pennington)

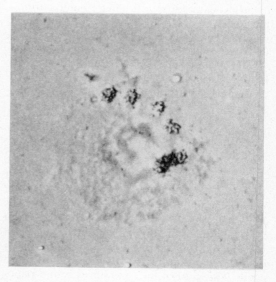

FIG. 65-7. Vaccinia virus factories in the cytoplasm of a HeLa cell. Cells growing on a coverslip were infected at a multiplicity of 6 PFU per cell. At six hours after infection, tritiated thymidine was added, and at seven hours the cells were fixed. Autoradiographic stripping film was then applied, and the slide was stored for two weeks. On developing, the picture shown here was obtained. There are no grains (indicative of thymidine incorporation and therefore DNA replication) over the nucleus, but there are five areas or factories in the cytoplasm (one is actually composed of two coalesced areas) that are labeled. This cell had been stained with vaccinia antibody coupled to fluorescein before autoradiography, and it was thereby demonstrated that the only areas in the cell that contained appreciable amounts of vaccinia antigens were the factories. Both viral DNA replication and virus morphogenesis, therefore, proceed within the factories. (From Cairns: Virology 11:603, 1960)

preventing the translation of cellular messenger RNA.

Finally, the proteins that form the matrix of the inclusions within which vaccinia DNA replicates and is subsequently incorporated into progeny virions may also be early proteins. These inclusions are easily visible with the light microscope, and they are composed of fibrillar material and may be located anywhere within the cytoplasm. Their number per cell is proportional to the multiplicity of infection, which suggests that each infecting virion initiates its own factory (Fig. 65-7).

Herpesviruses and adenoviruses form inclusions in the nucleus. Herpesviruses form Type A inclusions, which are characteristically single homogeneous eosinophilic bodies that occupy the central area of the nucleus and are clearly separated from the marginated chromatin. Adenoviruses form Type B inclusions, which are formed by condensation of basophilic material, including nuclear chromatin, into a single central mass or into multiple discrete bodies. Papovaviruses also multiply in the nucleus, but they form no clearly defined inclusions.

The Replication of Viral DNA

Vaccinia DNA replication starts at about 1.5 hours after infection and is complete about 3 hours later. This is in contrast to herpesvirus DNA replication, which generally starts about 2 to 6 hours after infection, rapidly reaches a maximal rate, and then continues at a gradually decreasing rate until the end of the replication cycle. The pattern for adenoviruses and papovaviruses is similar, except that replication does not commence until about 8 to 12 hours after infection (Fig. 65-8). In all cases, viral DNA is synthesized in large excess. For example, about 20,000 molecules of vaccinia virus DNA may be synthesized per cell, but only a fraction of it, sometimes as small as one-quarter, is usually encapsidated into progeny virions.

The Switch-off Phenomenon

When the late period of the vaccinia virus multiplication cycle commences, the expression of some, but not of all, early functions is inhibited. For example, synthesis of the early enzymes ceases, but synthesis of at least some of the early structural proteins continues. Cessation of the synthesis of early enzymes is due to the so-called switch-off phenomenon (Fig. 65-9), which is of great interest, since it provides one of the few well-documented examples of regulation of gene expression at the translational level. In essence, cessation of the synthesis of early enzymes is not due to inhibition of the transcription of the cognate genes, to instability of the corresponding messenger RNA species, or to instability of the enzymes themselves. Rather it is due to a suddenly developing inability of the messenger RNA species that code for early enzymes to be translated. If viral DNA replication and protein synthesis are inhibited, this inability does not develop. It is thought, therefore, that one of the first late proteins to be synthesized specifically prevents the translation of the messenger RNA molecules that code for early enzymes. This mechanism of controlling protein synthesis is obviously highly selective, since many other viral messenger RNA molecules, for example, those that code for structural proteins, continue to be translated (p. 839). It is of great potential significance for antiviral chemotherapy, since it implies the existence of a chemical difference between those messenger RNA molecules that continue to be

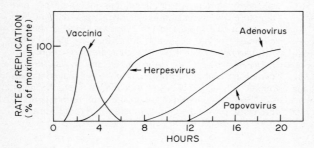

FIG. 65-8. The replication of vaccinia virus, herpesvirus, adenovirus, and papovavirus DNA. Vaccinia DNA is atypical in replicating during a brief period of time very early during the multiplication cycle, well in advance of virus maturation. However, irrespective of the length of the interval by which viral DNA replication precedes virus maturation, progeny DNA molecules always form a pool from which individual molecules are selected at random for incorporation into progeny virus particles.

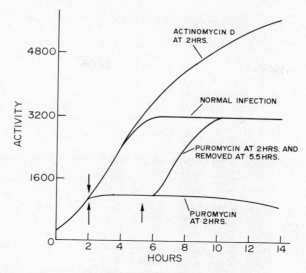

FIG. 65-9. The switch-off phenomenon. This graph depicts the synthesis of "early" enzymes, such as thymidine kinase and DNA polymerase, during vaccinia infection. Under normal conditions these enzymes begin to be formed soon after infection and their synthesis is "switched-off" at four to five hours. If actinomycin D, which inhibits messenger RNA formation, is added at two hours, "switch-off" does not occur. This demonstrates, first, that the messenger RNAs from which these enzymes are translated are very stable, and, second, that switch-off itself requires the synthesis of some other messenger RNA. If protein synthesis is inhibited with puromycin at two hours, enzyme synthesis immediately ceases; if puromycin is removed at five and one-half hours, enzyme synthesis resumes and is again switched off after a time interval equivalent to that between addition of puromycin and the onset of normal switch-off. This indicates that switch-off is due to the accumulation of a certain amount of some specific protein. (Modified from McAuslan: Virology 21:383, 1963)

translated and those that are switched off. It may prove possible to exploit this difference (Chap. 68).

Another class of vaccinia proteins whose synthesis is switched off comprises certain late proteins that are formed only for a period of several hours starting at about the time when viral DNA synthesis reaches its maximum. Together with the early and late proteins, the synthesis of which is never switched off, there are thus at least four different vaccinia virus (and herpesvirus) protein translation patterns, and there may be many more. Indeed, there is good evidence for more such classes among bacteriophage-specified proteins (Chap. 70). The implication of all this evidence is clear: the viral genome expresses itself according to a strictly regulated temporal pattern.

The Late Period

Somewhat more than one-half of poxvirus, herpesvirus, adenovirus, and papovavirus DNA codes for late proteins. By far the quantitatively most important of these are the capsid proteins, most of which, like DNA, are usually formed in large excess. The remainder are synthesized in small amounts only, and little is known concerning their nature. Presumably they function during morphogenesis.

The number and size of virus-specified proteins that are synthesized in infected cells can often be determined by autoradiography of polyacrylamide gels in which extracts of infected radioactively labeled cells were electrophoresced. The patterns that are obtained are particularly clear if the virus shuts down host cell protein synthesis completely. One of the viruses that does this is herpes simplex virus type 2 in HEp-2 cells. Figure 65-10 shows the viral proteins that are synthesized at various stages of the viral multiplication cycle; clearly different proteins are synthesized at different stages of the cycle. Proteins can be grouped into several major synthesis patterns, summarized in Figure 65-11 for the case of vaccinia virus.

Progeny genomes of all DNA viruses replicate faster than they are incorporated into virus

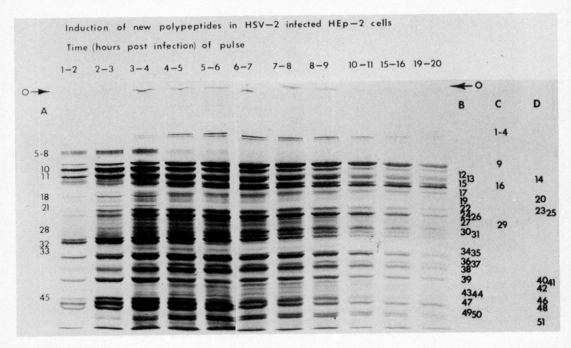

FIG. 65-10. Autoradiogram of the polyacrylamide gel in which the proteins synthesized at various stages of the herpesvirus infection cycle (1 to 2 hours, 2 to 3 hours, 3 to 4 hours, and so on) had been electrophoresced. The direction of electrophoresis was from O (origin) downward. A, B, C, and D refer to kinetic groups to which individual polypeptides can be assigned. (Courtesy of Dr. Richard J. Courtney)

particles. They, therefore, accumulate to form pools from which individual genomes are withdrawn at random in order to be encapsidated. Whereas some may be withdrawn very soon after they are formed, others may remain naked for long periods of time. This is so particularly in the case of the vaccinia virus multiplication cycle, where DNA replication ceases at about 5 hours after infection, while virion morphogenesis continues until about 25 hours. The time

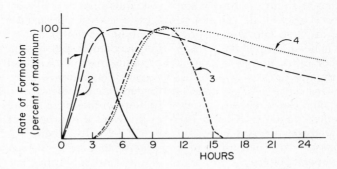

FIG. 65-11. The synthesis of four classes of vaccinia-specified proteins. First, there are some early proteins, the synthesis of which is switched off when DNA replication commences. Early enzymes and two structural vaccinia proteins belong to this class. Second, there are those early proteins, the synthesis of which continues throughout the multiplication cycle. One of the principal components of immature virus particles belongs to this class. Third, there are late proteins that are synthesized for some time following DNA replication and are then switched off, and, finally, there are those late proteins that are synthesized throughout the entire late period of the multiplication cycle. Most structural components of vaccinia virus particles belong to this class. (Modified from Holowczak and Joklik: Virology 33:726, 1967)

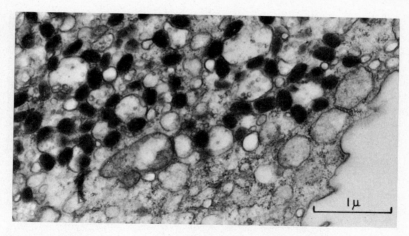

FIG. 65-12. Mature vaccinia virus progeny accumulating in the cytoplasm of infected cells. ×20,000. (From Dales and Siminovitch: J Biochem Biophys Cytol 10:475, 1961)

necessary for a complete virus particle to be assembled around a vaccinia DNA molecule is about one hour.

The morphogenesis of vaccinia virus proceeds in the cytoplasm, where mature virions accumulate until they are liberated as cells disintegrate (Fig. 65-12). The other three DNA-containing viruses are all assembled in the nucleus, where they often form paracrystalline arrays consisting of both complete virions and empty virus particles (Fig. 65-13). Excess protein also tends to form paracrystalline masses, particularly in the case of adenovirus (Fig. 65-14), and long tubular particles that have the same diameter as virions are often found in cells infected with papovaviruses.

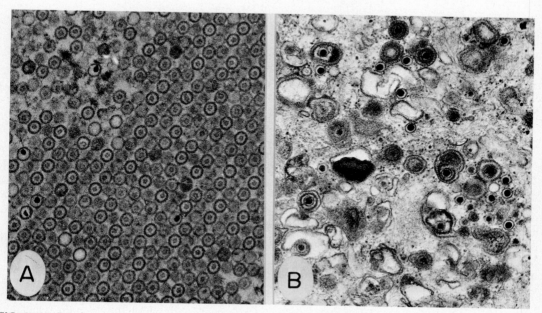

FIG. 65-13. Development and accumulation of herpes simplex virus. A. Typical intranuclear crystal composed of capsids and cores. ×35,000. B. Virus in the cytoplasm at various stages of acquiring its envelope. Note naked nucleocapsids and virus particle budding into vacuole. ×28,000. (From Nii, Morgan, and Rose: J Virol 2:517, 1968)

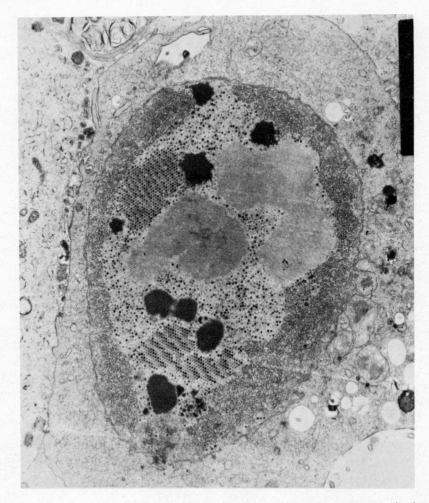

FIG. 65-14. The nucleus of a Vero African Green Monkey kidney cell 70 hours after infection with adenovirus type 2. Paracrystalline arrays of virions, crystals of vertex or core proteins, and intranuclear inclusions (the densely strained masses) are all visible. ×10,000. (From Henry et al: Virology 44:215, 1971)

Double-stranded RNA-containing Viruses

The multiplication cycle of reoviruses has two unique features. First, reoviruses are the only viruses whose genomes are not uncoated. Once reovirus has gained access to the interior of the cell, probably via phagocytic vacuoles, its outer capsid shell is partially degraded so that a subviral particle is formed, with the viral RNA still inside. An RNA polymerase in this particle then transcribes all 10

genome segments, each of which corresponds to a gene, into messenger RNA molecules, which are translated into proteins. The parental double-stranded RNA never escapes from the subviral particles.

The second unique feature relates to the mode of formation of progeny double-stranded RNA: After several hours the single-stranded messenger RNA molecules begin to serve as the templates for the synthesis of complementary strands with which they remain associated, thereby giving rise to progeny double-stranded

RNA molecules. In other words, the stages of the infection cycle when the plus and minus strands of reovirus double-stranded RNA are synthesized are separated by an interval of several hours. Double-stranded RNA is thus synthesized by a mechanism that is quite different from that by which double-stranded DNA is formed, for the two progeny DNA strands are synthesized either simultaneously or virtually simultaneously.

THE MULTIPLICATION CYCLE OF PICORNAVIRUSES

The principles involved in the multiplication of the small, single-stranded RNA-containing picornaviruses, such as poliovirus, differ in several respects from those described for the double-stranded, nucleic acid-containing viruses.

After uncoating, the parental poliovirus genome itself functions as messenger RNA and is translated into one single very large protein with a molecular weight of between 200,000 and 300,000. This protein, the polyprotein, is then cleaved into several smaller proteins, among which are the enzyme or enzymes necessary to replicate poliovirus RNA, and the capsid proteins. Poliovirus RNA is thus a monocistronic messenger RNA, with only one site at which translation is initiated. It resembles in this regard all animal cell messenger RNAs that have been examined. It is of interest in this regard that post-translational cleavage of viral proteins occurs frequently, for there are numerous examples of vaccinia virus, reovirus, myxovirus, togavirus, and other viral proteins being synthesized in the form of precursors larger than themselves. The reason for this may be that precursors are the form in which capsid proteins must exist prior to assembly so as to present the configuration necessary for interacting correctly with other proteins. Alternatively, the cleavage of precursors to capsid proteins may provide the driving force for morphogenesis.

The early phase of the poliovirus multiplication cycle is very short, for replication of viral RNA seems to start as soon as the necessary polymerase(s) has been synthesized. It pro-ceeds by a mechanism similar to, but not identical with, that responsible for the replication of the RNA of bacteriophages such as Qβ, MS2, R17, and f2 (Chap. 70) (Fig. 65-15).

Progeny poliovirus RNA molecules fulfil a dual function: they serve both as messenger RNA for the synthesis of capsid proteins and as genomes for progeny virus particles (Fig. 65-15). It is not clear what determines whether any given molecule will serve as template or become encapsidated. The choice may well be determined by the environment, that is, it may depend on whether the particular RNA molecule happens to combine first with capsid protein or with ribosomes (Chap. 62). For the population of progeny RNA molecules as a whole, the average time between formation and encapsidation is about 30 minutes.

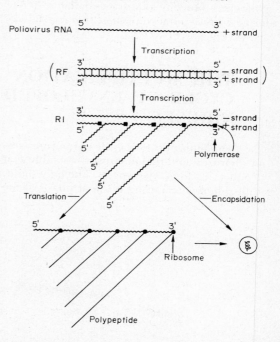

FIG. 65-15. Replication and functioning of poliovirus RNA. Parental viral RNA strands first code for polymerase (not shown) and are then transcribed into a strand of opposite polarity to yield a double-stranded replicative form (RF) (which may exist only very briefly). Progeny strands are then transcribed repeatedly from the minus-strand template by a peeling-off type mechanism. The structure consisting of minus-strand template and several plus-strand transcripts in various strages of completion is known as the replicative intermediate (RI). Early during the infection cycle the number of RFs and therefore of RIs increases, so that the rate of formation of progeny RNA molecules first increases and then becomes constant.

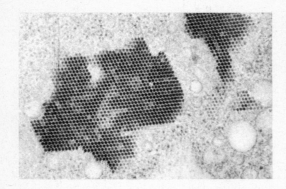

FIG. 65-16. A large crystal of poliovirus in the cytoplasm of a HeLa cell infected seven hours. ×50,000. (From Dales et al: Virology 26:379, 1965)

As is the case for other icosahedral viruses, poliovirus progeny often accumulates in the form of large, intracytoplasmic, paracrystalline arrays (Fig. 65-16).

THE MULTIPLICATION CYCLE OF ENVELOPED VIRUSES

The multiplication cycles of togaviruses, myxoviruses, and rhabdoviruses resemble that of poliovirus in many respects. The only significant differences during the first phase of the cycle are that the genomes of myxoviruses and rhabdoviruses possess minus polarity and must first be transcribed into plus strands before they can express themselves, and that an early stage of the influenza virus multiplication cycle is inhibited by actinomycin D, the only known function of which is prevention of the transcription of DNA into RNA. It is likely, therefore, that some host cell function is essential for successful influenza virus multiplication.

The unique feature of the multiplication cycles of enveloped viruses is the manner of their morphogenesis. These viruses code for two classes of structural proteins, nucleocapsid proteins and envelope proteins. The latter are incorporated into cell membranes, primarily the outer plasma membranes and the membranes lining cytoplasmic vacuoles, where they completely replace host-specified proteins in progressively enlarging discrete areas (Fig. 65-17). The nucleocapsids, which can often be seen free in the cytoplasm, migrate to these modified membrane areas, which they seem to recognize with great specificity, and align themselves with them. Next the glycoprotein spikes characteristic of viral envelopes are added to the outer surface of the membrane, and the nucleocapsids then bud through these modified membrane patches, becoming coated with them in the process (Fig. 65-18). Since the nucleocapsids of enveloped viruses are noninfectious, the rise period of their multiplication

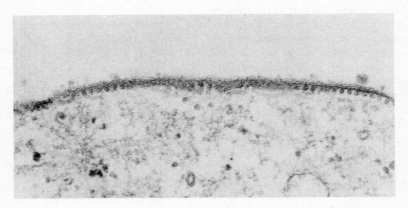

FIG. 65-17. Modification of the plasma membrane of a monkey kidney cell infected with SV5. A layer of dense material resembling the spikes present on viral envelopes is present on the outer surface of the membrane. Nucleocapsid strands, many seen in cross section, are aligned immediately beneath large segments of the cell membrane. In due course they will bud through these modified membrane patches, and will become coated by them in the process. ×67,000. (From Compans et al Virology 30:411, 1966)

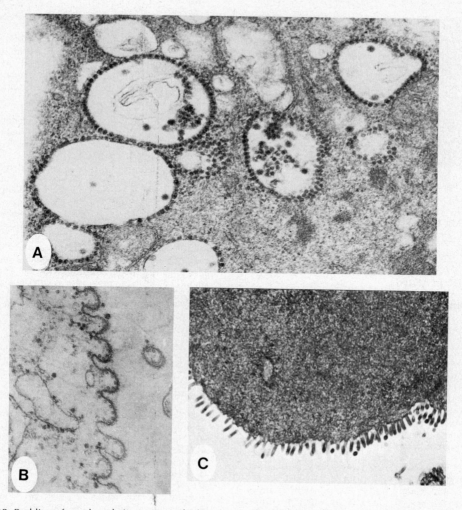

FIG. 65-18. Budding of enveloped viruses. A. A chick embryo cell infected with the togavirus Semliki forest virus (SFV). Numerous nucleocapsids lining cytoplasmic vacuoles prior to budding into them can be seen. ×22, 000. B. A row of SV5 particles budding from the plasma membrane of a monkey kidney cell, showing many cross sections of nucleocapsids. ×50,000. C. VSV budding from the plasma membrane of a mouse L cell. In L cells the majority of VSV particles bud from the plasma membrane; in other cells, such as chick embryo fibroblasts and pig kidney cells, almost all VSV buds into cytoplasmic vacuoles. ×21, 500. (A, from Grimley, Berezesky, and Friedman: J Virol 2:1326, 1968; B, from Compans et al: Virology 30:411, 1966; C, from Zee, Hackett, and Talens: J Gen Virol 7:95, 1970)

cycles starts not when the first nucleocapsid is formed but when the first one buds.

While budding is very efficient in some strains of cells, it is very inefficient in others. This sometimes leads to the intracytoplasmic accumulation of very large numbers of nucleocapsids (Fig. 65-19).

The budding process itself does not harm the host cell significantly. In numerous cases of persistent infections, for example by mumps or measles virus, cells remain normal in appearance and continue to multiply for many generations while viruses bud from their surfaces. However, some enveloped viruses, such as VSV, are highly cytopathic and quickly kill the cells which they infect; and others, such as Sendai virus, strongly promote cell fusion so that giant syncytia are formed (Chap. 66).

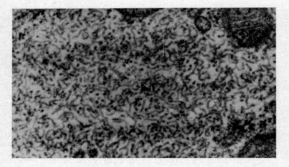

FIG. 65-19. Accumulation of SV5 nucleocapsids in the cytoplasmic matrix of BHK-21 cells. Such accumulation does not occur in monkey kidney cells from which nucleocapsids bud as rapidly as they are synthesized. ×34,000. (From Compans et al: Virology 30:411, 1966)

FURTHER READING

Books and Reviews

Baltimore D: The replication of picornaviruses. In Levy HB (ed): The Biochemistry of Viruses. New York and London, Marcel Dekker, 1969, p 101

Bishop JM, Levintow L: Replicative forms of viral RNA. Structure and function. Prog Med Virol 13:1, 1971

Choppin PW, Compans RW: Reproduction of paramyxoviruses. In Fraenkel-Conrat H, Wagner RR (eds): Comprehensive Virology. New York and London, Plenum Press, 1975, vol 4, p 95

Ciba Foundation Symposium. Strategy of the Viral Genome. Edinburgh and London, Churchill Livingstone, 1971

Cohen SS: Virus-induced Enzymes. New York and London, Columbia Univ Press, 1968

Compans RW, Choppin PW: Reproduction of myxoviruses. In Fraenkel-Conrat H, Wagner RR (eds): Comprehensive Virology. New York and London, Plenum Press, 1975, vol 4, p 179

Dales S: Early events in cell-animal virus interactions. Bacteriol Rev 37:103, 1973

Hershko A, Fry M: Post-translational cleavage of polypeptide chains: Role in Assembly. Annu Rev Biochem 44:775, 1975

Joklik WK: Reproduction of reoviridae. In Fraenkel-Conrat H, Wagner RR (eds): Comprehensive Virology. New York and London, Plenum Press, 1974, vol 2, p 231

Joklik WK, Zweerink HJ: The morphogenesis of animal viruses. Annu Rev Genet 5:297, 1973

Kaplan AS (ed): The Herpesviruses. New York and London, Academic Press, 1973

Kingsbury DW: Replication and function of myxovirus ribonucleic acid. Prog Med Virol 12:49, 1970

Kohn A, Fuchs P: Initial effects of viral infection in bacterial and animal host cells. Adv Virus Res 18:159, 1973

Levintow L: Reproduction of picornaviruses. In Fraenkel-Conrat H, Wagner RR (eds): Comprehensive Virology. New York and London, Plenum Press, 1975, vol 2, p 179

McAuslan BR: The biochemistry of poxvirus replication.

In Levy HB (ed): The Biochemistry of Viruses. New York and London, Marcel Dekker, 1969, p 361

Moss B: Reproduction of poxviruses. In Fraenkel-Conrat H, Wagner RR (eds): Comprehensive Virology. New York and London, Plenum Press, 1974, vol 3, p 405

Pfefferkorn ER, Shapiro D: Reproduction of togaviruses. In Fraenkel-Conrat H, Wagner RR (eds): Comprehensive Virology. New York and London, Plenum Press, 1974, vol 2, p 171

Philipson L, Lindberg U: Reproduction of adenoviruses. In Fraenkel-Conrat H, Wagner RR (eds): Comprehensive Virology. New York and London, Plenum Press, 1974, vol 3, p 143

Roizman B, Furlong D: The replication of herpesviruses. In Fraenkel-Conrat H, Wagner RR (eds): Comprehensive Virology. New York and London, Plenum Press, 1974, vol 3, p 229

Rose JA: Parvovirus reproduction. In Fraenkel-Conrat H, Wagner RR (eds): Comprehensive Virology. New York and London, Plenum Press, 1974, vol 3, p 1

Schlesinger RW: Adenoviruses: the nature of the virion and of controlling factors in productive or abortive infection and tumorigenesis. Adv Virus Res 14:2, 1969

Singh KRP: Growth of arboviruses in arthropod tissue culture. Adv Virus Res 17:187, 1972

Wagner RR: Reproduction of rhabdoviruses. In Fraenkel-Conrat H, Wagner RR (eds): Comprehensive Virology. New York and London, Plenum Press, 1975, vol 4, p 1

Selected Papers

POXVIRUSES

Esteban M, Metz DH: Early virus protein synthesis in vaccinia-infected cells. J Gen Virol 19:201, 1973

Fil W, Holowczak JA, Flores L, Thomas V: Biochemical and electron microscopic observations of vaccinia virus morphogenesis in HeLa cells after hydroxyurea reversal. Virology 61:376, 1974

Katz E, Moss B: Vaccinia virus structural polypeptide derived from a high molecular weight precursor: formation and integration into virus particles. J Virol 6:717, 1970

McAuslan BR: The induction and repression of thymidine kinase in the poxvirus-infected Hela cell. Virology 21:383, 1963

Oda K, Joklik WK: Hybridization and sedimentation studies on "early" and "late" vaccinia messenger RNA. J Mol Biol 27:395, 1967

Pennington TH: Vaccinia virus polypeptide synthesis: Sequential appearance and stability of pre- and post-replicative polypeptides. J Gen Virol 25:433, 1974

Pogo BGT, Dales S: Biogenesis of vaccinia: Separation of early stages from maturation by means of hydroxyurea. Virology 43:144, 1971

HERPESVIRUSES

Ben-Porat T, Kervina M, Kaplan AS: Early functions of the genome of herpesvirus: V. Serological analysis of "immediate-early" proteins. Virology 65:335, 1975

Frenkel N, Silverstein S, Cassai E, Roizman B: RNA synthesis in cells infected with herpes simplex virus. VII. Control of transcription and of transcript abundancies of unique and common sequences of herpes simplex virus 1 and 2. J Virol 11:886, 1973

Honess RW, Roizman B: Regulation of herpesvirus macromolecular synthesis: 1. Cascade regulation of the synthesis of three groups of viral proteins. J Virol 14:8, 1974

Honess RW, Roizman B: Regulation of herpesvirus macromolecular synthesis: Sequential transition of polypeptide synthesis requires functional viral polypeptides. Proc Natl Acad Sci USA 72:1276, 1975

Kit S, Dubbs DR, Anken M: Altered properties of thymidine kinase after infection of mouse fibroblast cells with herpes simplex virus. J Virol 1:238, 1967

Kozak M, Roizman B: Regulation of herpesvirus macromolecular synthesis: Nuclear retention of nontranslated viral RNA sequences. Proc Natl Acad Sci USA 71: 4322, 1974

Nii S, Morgan C, Rose HM, Hsu KC: Electron microscopy of herpes simplex virus. IV. Studies with ferritin-conjugated antibodies. J Virol 2:1172, 1968

ADENOVIRUSES

Brown DT, Burlingham BT: Penetration of host cell membranes by adenovirus 2. Virology 12:386, 1973

Burger H, Doerfler W: Intracellular forms of adenovirus DNA. III. Integration of the DNA of adenovirus 2 into host DNA in productively infected cells. J Virol 13:975, 1974

Chardonnet Y, Dales S: Early events in the interaction of adenoviruses with HeLa cells. Virology 40:462, 478, 1970

Ishibashi M, Maizel JV: The polypeptides of adenovirus. VI. Early and late glycopolypeptides. Virology 58:345, 1974

Philipson I, Lonberg-Holm K, Pettersson N: Virus-receptor interactions in an adenovirus system. J Virol 2:1064, 1968

Tal J, Craig EA, Raskas HJ: Sequence relationships between adenovirus 2 early RNA and viral RNA size classes synthesized at 18 hours after infection. J Virol 15: 137, 1975

van der Vliet PC, Levine AJ: DNA-binding proteins specific for cells infected by adenovirus. Nature [New Biol] 246:170, 1973

Wall R, Weber J, Gage Z, Darnell JE: Production of viral mRNA in adenovirus-transformed cells by the posttranscriptional processing of heterogeneous nuclear RNA containing viral and cell sequences. J Virol 11: 953, 1973

PICORNAVIRUSES

Butterworth BE, Rueckert RR: Kinetics of synthesis and cleavage of encephalomyocarditis virus-specific proteins. Virology 50:535, 1972

Cooper PD, Steiner-Pryor A, Wright PJ: A proposed regulator for poliovirus: The equestron. Intervirology 1:1, 1973

Fernandez-Thomas CB, Baltimore D: Morphogenesis of poliovirus. II. Demonstration of a new intermediate, the provirion. J Virol 12:1122, 1973

Lawrence C, Thach RE: Identification of a viral protein involved in posttranslational maturation of the encephalomyocarditis capsid precursor. J Virol 15:918, 1975

Medrano L, Green H: Picornavirus receptors and picornavirus multiplication in human-mouse hybrid cell lines. Virology 54:515, 1973

Rekosh D: Gene order in poliovirus capsid proteins. J Virol 9:479, 1972

Summers DF, Maizel JV, Darnell JE: Evidence for virus-specific noncapsid proteins in poliovirus-infected HeLa cells. Proc Natl Acad Sci USA 56:505, 1965

TOGAVIRUSES

Birdwell CR, Strauss EG, Strauss JH: Replication of Sindbis virus. III. An electron microscopic study of virus maturation using the surface replica technique. Virology 56: 429, 1973

Birdwell CR, Strauss JH: Distribution of the receptor sites for Sindbis virus on the surface of chicken and BHK cells. J Virol 14:672, 1974

Schlesinger MJ, Schlesinger S: Large-molecular-weight precursors of Sindbis virus proteins. J Virol 11:1013, 1973

Strauss JH, Burge BW, Darnell JE: Sindbis virus infection of chick and hamster cells: synthesis of virus specific proteins. Virology 37:367, 1969

REOVIRUSES

Bellamy AR, Joklik WK: Studies on reovirus RNA. J Mol Biol 29:19, 27, 1967

Both GW, Lavi S, Shatkin AJ: Synthesis of all the gene products of the reovirus genome in vivo and in vitro. Cell 4:173, 1975

Chang C, Zweerink HJ: Fate of parental reovirus in infected cell. Virology 46:544, 1971

Schonberg M, Silverstein SC, Levin DH, Acs G: Asynchronous synthesis of the complementary strands of the reovirus genome. Proc Natl Acad Sci USA 68:505, 1971

Silverstein SC, Schonberg M, Levin DH, Acs G: The reovirus replicative cycle: conservation of parental RNA and protein. Proc Natl Acad Sci USA 67:275, 1970

Watanabe Y, Millward S, Graham AF: Regulation of transcription of the reovirus genome. J Mol Biol 36:107, 1968

Zweerink HJ: Multiple forms of SS → DS RNA polymerase activity in reovirus-infected cells. Nature 247: 313, 1974

Zweerink HJ, McDowelll MJ, Joklik WK: Essential and nonessential noncapsid reovirus proteins. Virology 45: 716, 1971

MYXOVIRUSES

Compans RW, Holmes KV, Dales S, Choppin PW: An electron microscopic study of moderate and virulent virus-cell interactions of the parainfluenza virus SV5. Virology 30:411, 1966

Dourmashkin RR, Tyrrell DAJ: Electron microscopic observations on the entry of influenza virus into susceptible cells. J Gen Virol 24:129, 1974

Follett EAC, Pringle CR, Wunner WH, Skehel JJ: Virus replication in enucleate cells: Vesicular stomatis virus and influenza virus. J Virol 13:394, 1974

Klenk H, Choppin PW: Plasma membrane lipids and parainfluenza virus assembly. Virology 40:939, 1970

Meier-Ewert H, Compans RW: Time course of synthesis

and assembly of influenza virus proteins. J Virol 14: 1083, 1974

Mountcastle WE, Compans RW, Lackland H, Choppin PW: Proteolytic cleavage of subunits of the nucleocapsid of the paramyxovirus Simian virus 5. J Virol 14: 1253, 1974

Palese P, Schulman JL, Bodo G, Meindl P: Inhibition of influenza and parainfluenza virus replication in tissue culture by 2-deoxy-2,3-dehydro-N-trifluoroacetylneuraminic acid (FANA). Virology 59:490, 1974

Schwarz RT, Klenk H: Inhibition of glycosylation of the influenza virus hemagglutinin. J Virol 14:1023, 1074

RHABDOVIRUSES

Birdwell CR, Strauss JH: Maturation of vesicular stomatitis virus: Electron microscopy of surface replicas of infected cells. Virology 59:587, 1974

Both GW, Moyer SA, Banerjee AK: Translation and identification of the mRNA species synthesized in vitro by the virion-associated RNA polymerase of vesicular stomatitis virus. Proc Natl Acad Sci USA 72:274, 1975

Schloemer RH, Wagner RR: Mosquito cells infected with vesicular stomatitis virus yield unsialylated virions of low infectivity. J Virol 15:1029, 1975

Scholtissek C, Rott R, Ham G, Kaluza G: Inhibition of the multiplication of vesicular stomatitis and Newcastle disease virus by 2-deoxy-glucose. J Virol 13:1186, 1974

Zee YC, Hackett AJ, Talens L: Vesicular stomatitis virus maturation sites in six different host cells. J. Gen Virol 7: 95, 1970

66

The Effect of Virus Infection on the Host Cell

The effect of virus infection on host cells is far more difficult to study in molecular terms than is the process of virus multiplication. Study of the latter requires merely the ability to recognize and measure virus-specified macromolecules; study of the former requires a detailed knowledge of the functioning of the normal host cell. In fact, studies that have focused attention on the effect of virus infection on host cells have widened our knowledge of the functioning of uninfected cells, and the acquisition of such knowledge has been one of the important spin-offs of the study of cell–virus interactions.

Whatever the reason that lytic viruses destroy their host cells, several causes can be ruled out. One is that virus synthesis creates an excessive demand for protein and nucleic acid precursors, so that competition causes a shortage of building blocks that prevents synthesis of host cell macromolecules. This is unlikely, since the amount of viral material synthesized rarely exceeds 15 percent of total host cell material. Considerations of this nature also rule out the necessity for breakdown of host cell material in order to provide precursors for synthesis of viral macromolecules.

Since both nucleic acid and protein synthesis are absolutely dependent on the supply of energy, the largest virus yields would be expected in cells that are damaged least for the longest periods of time. Many highly lytic viruses are, however, very successful. This is primarily because they take over the host cell's synthetic apparatus very rapidly and multiply extensively in the brief period of time for which it can function.

CYTOPATHIC EFFECTS

The most easily detected effects of infection with lytic viruses are the cytopathic effects, which can be observed both macroscopically and microscopically. Plaque formation is due to the cytopathic effect of viruses: Viruses kill the cells in which they multiply, and plaques are the areas of killed cells. The light microscope, as well as the electron microscope, often reveals changes in a variety of cell organelles soon after infection. Frequently the nucleus is affected first, with pyknosis, changes in nucleolar structure, and margination of the chromatin. This is often followed by changes in the cyto-

plasm, where granular or fibrillar masses may develop. Distinct foci then often appear either in the nucleus or in the cytoplasm, generally composed of masses of fibrillar material that gradually spread: these are the classic inclusion bodies that have long been described by cytologists and that represent the sites of virus-directed biosynthesis and morphogenesis.

Cell Fusion   Changes also develop in the cell membrane. Early changes frequently include cell rounding and diminished ability to adhere to supporting surfaces. Frequently, plasma cell membranes of infected cells develop a tendency to fuse with each other, which results in the formation of giant syncytia, masses of cytoplasm bounded by one membrane that may contain hundreds and even thousands of nuclei. This type of response is induced primarily by certain enveloped viruses, such as herpesviruses and paramyxoviruses (SV5 and Sendai virus) (Fig. 66-1). Fusion seems to be caused by changes induced in cell membranes by interaction with viral envelopes and can therefore be induced not only with active but also with inactivated virus, and it can be induced not only among identical but also among different cells. The products of fusion are either heterokaryons—cells containing several nuclei

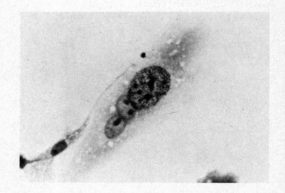

FIG. 66-1. Cell fusion induced by UV-inactivated Sendai virus. Three chick embryo fibroblasts have fused to yield the heterokaryon shown here, which contains three nuclei. The two small ones are normal chick nuclei, while the large one is from a chick cell transformed with Rous sarcoma virus. It has been labeled with ^{3}H-thymidine and the grains which it seems to contain are actually silver grains caused by the disintegration of ^{3}H atoms in a thin layer of photographic emulsion which overlies this cell. Detection of radioactive label by this technique is known as autoradiography. ×400. (From Svoboda and Dourmashkin: J Gen Virol 4:523, 1969)

of different types—or hybrid cells containing the fused nuclei of the parents. The hybrid cells are frequently viable and have, therefore, become widely used for studies in somatic cell genetics. They are usually produced by fusing mixtures of the two cell lines to be hybridized with UV-inactivated Sendai virus and are then cloned. They are particularly useful for determining the chromosomal location of specific genes: Hybrid cells often lose chromosomes, and one can readily correlate loss of a specific chromosome with loss of a particular gene function. Many human genes have been assigned to chromosomes in this manner in recent years, using human-mouse cell hybrid cells that lose human chromosomes. Further applications of hybrid cells in genetic research are: (1) Hybrids of mutant cells permit genetic complementation analysis, (2) hybridization of virus-transformed cells with normal cells permits the rescue of tumor virus genomes integrated into the host cell genome (Chap. 69), (3) hybrid cells can be used to determine whether events such as the induction of the synthesis of specific proteins are under positive or negative control, and (4) the genetic factors that control susceptibility to virus infection and the expression of tumorigenicity are being studied with the aid of somatic cell hybrids.

Cell Necrosis Later in the infection cycle necrotic and degradative changes become noticeable. This may be attributed to at least four causes. First, by this time interference with host cell macromolecular biosynthesis is generally complete. It is known that all host cell macromolecules turn over to a greater or lesser extent, that is, there is a continual breakdown and resynthesis of most types of macromolecules that is essentially independent of the growth rate. Inhibition of resynthesis in the presence of continuing breakdown could clearly lead to structural and functional failure. Second, as infection progresses, the inclusion bodies in which virus morphogenesis proceeds often become so large that their presence creates mechanical problems, since they displace host cell organelles, interfere with intracellular transport, and so on. Third, loss of plasma membrane function, possibly induced by interference with host cell biosynthesis and replacement of host proteins by viral ones, results in failure to maintain the proper intracellular ionic environment and in diminished transport of

essential nutrients into the cell and of waste products out of it. Finally, failure of the membranes of lysosomes may well cause the degradative hydrolytic enzymes that they contain to leak out into the cytoplasm, thereby exacerbating the effects caused by other mechanisms.

The net result of these necrotic changes is to facilitate the release of those viruses that do not bud from the cell membrane. In general, the smaller the virus, the more readily it is released. Large viruses, such as poxviruses, are often retained in the ghosts of infected cells for considerable periods of time. In the body, the situation may be different, for damaged cells may become phagocytosed, thereby providing an additional mechanism for the dissemination of viral progeny.

Induction of Chromosomal Aberrations Certain viruses induce chromosomal aberrations. This effect is not usually exhibited by lytic viruses in permissive cells, that is, in cells that permit extensive viral multiplication, since cytopathic effects then usually develop too rapidly. However, chromosome damage is frequently observed in cells that are not too permissive and that are infected at low multiplicities with measles, mumps, adenoviruses, varicella, cytomegaloviruses, and other viruses. Usually, there is no clear correlation between damage to a specific chromosome and infection with some particular virus strain. However, chromatid gaps and breaks in human chromosome 17 occur frequently in cells infected with adenovirus type 12 and type 31. It should be noted that the conditions favoring the development of chromosomal aberrations are those most likely to occur under conditions of natural infection, for there are many cells in the body that are not fully permissive for any given virus, and the multiplicity of natural infection is also likely to be low. The induction of chromosomal aberrations by slowly replicating viruses may therefore have far-reaching consequences for the health of the host.

INHIBITION OF HOST MACROMOLECULAR BIOSYNTHESIS

While cytopathic effects caused by viruses are easily observed and often spectacular, they provide little insight into the primary and specific mechanisms that inhibit essential host cell functions. Such insight can only be provided by biochemical investigations. The first effect of infection with most lytic viruses is generally inhibition of DNA replication. Host cell RNA synthesis is also quickly arrested by many lytic viruses; this seems to be caused less by a direct effect on the DNA-dependent RNA polymerases than by changes that are induced in the physical state of the DNA that apparently decrease its efficiency as a template. For example, it has already been pointed out above that among the earliest detectable cytopathic effects there are often margination of chromatin and changes in nucleolar structure. As a result, not only is progressively less and less host cell messenger RNA synthesized, but the supply of new ribosomes is also quickly interrupted, so that the only ribosomes available for protein synthesis during the viral multiplication cycle are those present in the cytoplasm at the time of infection.

Since less and less host cell messenger RNA reaches the cytoplasm, the rate of host protein synthesis also gradually declines. However, in many virus infections the rate of host protein synthesis decreases far more rapidly than would be expected on the basis of the decay rate of messenger RNA in uninfected cells. For example, infection with high multiplicities of vaccinia virus inhibits host protein synthesis by well over 90 percent within two hours (Fig. 66-2). This is not a general toxic effect on the host cell, since viral protein is already being synthesized vigorously at this time. Rather, inhibition of host messenger RNA translation is another early direct consequence of viral infection. The mechanism responsible for this effect is not yet understood. Some viruses may code for special proteins that have this function, but such proteins have not yet been found. Alternatively, viral structural proteins may be responsible. In support of this hypothesis, it is known that inactivated viruses that are unable to multiply and are unable to express any of the information encoded in their genomes can kill cells; for example, as few as 10 heat-inactivated vaccinia viral particles can kill a cell. There is also at least one example of a structural protein, the adenovirus fiber, that is strongly cytotoxic by itself. Further, the degree of inhibition of host macromolecular biosynthesis frequently increases greatly when viral capsid protein

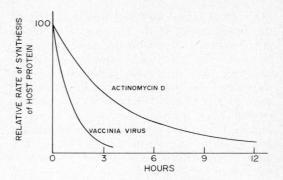

FIG. 66-2. Effect of infection with vaccinia virus, as well as of actinomycin D, on cellular protein synthesis in mouse L fibroblasts. Actinomycin D inhibits RNA transcription; the decrease in the rate of host protein synthesis in its presence therefore reflects the stability of messenger RNA, the average half-life of which is about three hours. Infection with vaccinia virus inhibits host protein synthesis much more rapidly: Presumably it either causes host messenger RNA to be inactivated or it actively prevents it from being translated.

synthesis reaches its peak. Although all this evidence implicates structural virus proteins themselves as being at least partially responsible for the cytopathogenicity of viral infection, there is also evidence to the contrary: Empty reovirus particles, even at high multiplicity, fail to inhibit cellular DNA, RNA, or protein synthesis.

CHANGES IN THE REGULATION OF GENE EXPRESSION

Viral infection may also affect the regulation of host genome expression. Thus the activity of certain enzymes on the pathway of nucleic acid biosynthesis often increases after infection. While these increases are sometimes caused by the formation of virus-coded enzymes, they are on other occasions caused by increases in the rate of synthesis of cellular enzymes. For example, infection with the papovaviruses polyoma and SV40 causes increases in the activity of at least six enzymes, for which the small viral DNA cannot possibly contain the genetic information. Further, infection with almost all viruses leads to the synthesis of a new protein, interferon, which will be discussed in Chapter 68. These lines of evidence suggest that infection may upset the mechanism that usually prevents the expression of a large portion of the cellular DNA and that there may be a period of time during the early part of the infection cycle when more of the cell's genome expresses itself in infected than in uninfected cells.

APPEARANCE OF NEW ANTIGENIC DETERMINANTS ON CELL SURFACE

Sooner or later following infection, the outer cell membrane is modified. Usually this manifests itself in two ways: The cells become more agglutinable by the lectin concanavalin A (Chap. 69), and/or new antigenic determinants appear on the cell surface. When the infecting virus is an enveloped virus, these new determinants are likely to be viral envelope proteins that have become incorporated into the cell membrane (Chap. 65), but new antigenic determinants also appear on the surfaces of cells that are infected with nonenveloped viruses, such as poxviruses and papovaviruses. These determinants may be either virus-coded proteins or cellular proteins that are normally present on the cell membrane in a form masked by other macromolecules or cellular proteins whose synthesis is induced by infection. When they are virus-coded, their presence serves to alert the immune mechanism that the cells are infected and should therefore be eliminated (Fig. 66-3). They will be discussed further in Chapter 69 in relation to tumor and transplantation antigens.

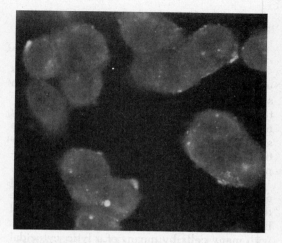

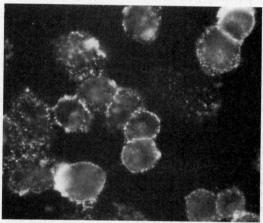

FIG. 66-3. Virus-specified surface antigen on HeLa cells infected with vaccinia virus. Top. Uninfected cells. Bottom. Cells infected for 8 hours. The cells were unfixed and were stained with rabbit antiserum to vaccinia virus-infected rabbit cells. (Courtesy of Dr. Yoshiaki Ueda)

ABORTIVE INFECTION

Most of the changes described so far relate to the lytic multiplication cycle under conditions of productive infection, that is, when virus multiplies to high titer in permissive cells. However, viruses can also infect cells that are not fully permissive and even cells that are nonpermissive. In such cells, viruses cannot multiply because some essential step of the multiplication cycle cannot proceed. Examples of this type are the abortive infection of HeLa cells by influenza virus, of dog kidney cells by herpes simplex virus, of pig kidney cells by certain mutants of rabbitpox virus, of monkey cells by human adenovirus, and many others. Furthermore, the infection of permissive cells in the presence of antiviral agents, such as IBT or interferon (Chap. 68), is also abortive. In all such cases the viral genome begins to express itself, but no mature progeny virus is produced. The significant feature of most such abortive infections is that the alterations in the host cell that were described above do occur and that the host cell generally dies (unless the multiplicity of infection is very low).

67
The Genetics of Animal Viruses

Viruses are encapsidated segments of genetic material; and like other genetic systems, viral genomes are not invariate but are subject to change by mutation. Spontaneous mutations occur constantly in the course of virus multiplication; and while many are lethal, others are not. Virus populations, therefore, always contain an assortment of viral genomes, only one of which will usually have all the attributes that enable it to predominate under a given set of conditions. Therefore, when virologists refer to "vaccinia virus" or "rhinovirus" it must be clearly kept in mind that there are many different strains of vaccinia virus or rhinovirus which, although closely related genetically, may differ markedly phenotypically.

TYPES OF VIRUS MUTANTS

Mutant virus strains can also be generated in the laboratory as a result of mutagenesis. Among the procedures for mutagenizing RNA-containing viruses are treatment of virus particles with nitrous acid, hydroxylamine, N-methyl-N′-nitro-N-nitrosoguanidine (NTG), or ethane methane sulfonic acid, and propagation in the presence of 5-fluorouracil, 5-azacytidine, or proflavine (for the double-stranded RNA-containing reovirus). For DNA-containing viruses, treatment of virus particles with nitrous acid, hydroxylamine, or ultraviolet irradiation, and growth in the presence of 5-bromodeoxyuridine, NTG, or proflavine have been used.

Conditional Lethal Mutants

Among the many different types of mutants that can be obtained, there is one that, although capable of multiplying under some conditions, nevertheless cannot multiply under other conditions when wild-type virus can do so. These are the so-called conditional lethal mutants, which are extremely useful for defining the nature of the numerous reactions involved in virus multiplication. There are two classes of these mutants. The first comprises mutants that are temperature-sensitive (ts) with respect to their ability to multiply. Wild-type animal viruses can generally multiply over a temperature range that extends from a lower

limit of about 20 to 24C to an upper one of about 39.5C for mammalian viruses and 1 to 2C higher for avian viruses. In ts mutants there is a nucleic acid base substitution that causes an amino acid replacement in some virus-coded protein, as a result of which it cannot assume or maintain the structural conformation necessary for activity at elevated or nonpermissive (restrictive) temperatures, though it can still do so at lower or permissive temperatures. The typical ts mutation thus causes the formation of an enzyme or a structural protein that cannot function in a temperature range (typically from about 36 to 41C) where the corresponding protein of the wild-type strain can function. The reason why ts mutants are so important in studies seeking to define the reactions essential for virus multiplication is that they permit study of the virus multiplication cycle with one, and only one, reaction unable to proceed. Use of such mutants, therefore, permits both the assessment of the role of any particular known reaction in the course of virus multiplication and also the detection of hitherto unknown functions.

Cold-sensitive mutants of animal viruses also exist. They have not been investigated intensively, but presumably the basis of their defect is similar (in the opposite sense) to that of ts mutants.

The second class of conditional lethal mutants are the host–dependent mutants. Such mutants have been studied extensively among the bacteriophages; they are the amber (and ochre and opal) mutants (Chap. 7 and 8). Among animal viruses, mutants of this type are far less well characterized. The best known are a series of rabbitpox virus mutants that are blocked at different stages of their multiplication cycles in pig kidney cells, although they are able to multiply normally in other cells. Elucidation of the nature of these mutations may provide important information concerning the regulation of gene expression in mammalian cells.

Many other types of virus mutants have been obtained. Among them are the following.

Plaque Size Mutants

Many virus strains give rise to spontaneous mutants that form smaller plaques than wild-type virus because their adsorption is

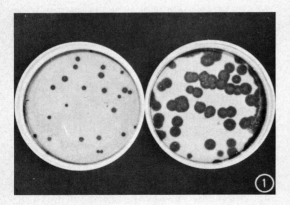

FIG. 67-1. Comparative sizes of two Mengovirus plaque size variants, S-Mengo (left) and L-Mengo (right). The plaques are 48 hours old. The L mutant is more virulent in animals and more cytopathic in cell cultures. (From Amako and Dales: Virology 32:184, 1967)

inhibited by sulfated polysaccharides present in agar (Fig. 67-1). Large plaque mutants are also known, and in this case the ability of wild-type virus to absorb is inhibited by the polysaccharides, whereas that of the mutant is not. In either case, the site of the mutation is in a capsid polypeptide that functions in adsorption.

Drug-resistant Mutants

Drugs capable of inhibiting the multiplication of certain viruses are known (Chap. 68), and mutants exist that are resistant to them. Examples are poliovirus mutants resistant to guanidine and vaccinia virus mutants resistant to rifampicin and IBT. Poliovirus mutants dependent on guanidine and vaccinia virus mutants dependent on IBT also exist.

Enzyme-deficient Mutants

Viruses code for several enzymes essential for virus multiplication, and mutations that result in the loss of this ability are obviously lethal. Some viruses also code for enzymes that are not essential, and mutants lacking the ability to code for them are viable. For example, poxviruses and herpesviruses code for enzymes that phosphorylate thymidine (thymidine kinases). Virus mutants that are deficient in the ability to induce the synthesis of these enzymes are known; they multiply well, demon-

strating that the survival advantage conferred by the ability to code for them is small.

Hot Mutants

These are mutants that can grow at temperatures higher than wild-type virus. For example, whereas 41C is near the upper limit of the temperature growth range of wild-type poliovirus, mutant strains exist that grow as well at 41C as at 37C, or even better. Not surprisingly, such strains are very virulent, since they can multiply rapidly in patients with higher fever, when the multiplication of wild-type virus is at least partially inhibited.

INTERACTIONS AMONG VIRUSES

Under conditions of multiple infection, cells may become infected with two or more virus particles with different genomes. If they are sufficiently closely related—that is, if they belong to the same virus family—they may be able to interact. There are several types of such interactions.

Recombination

The detection of recombination between two virus strains depends on the availability of techniques that permit the differentiation of the phenotypes of the two parents from those of the recombinants. If the two parents are single-step mutants of some wild-type strain, each differing from it in some recognizable manner, some of the recombinants will have the wild-type genotype and, therefore, its phenotype and will be easily detectable. The detection of other recombinants, such as the reciprocal recombinants or recombinants between viruses that differ in several loci, is usually more difficult and requires the use of selective conditions.

Viruses differ greatly in the ease with which they undergo recombination, the principal relevant factor being the nature of their genomes. With the exception of poliovirus and foot-and-mouth-disease virus, viruses that possess a single molecule of single-stranded RNA do not recombine. Viruses that contain a single mole-

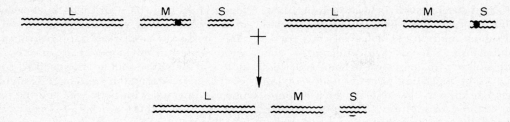

FIG. 67-2. Generation of wild-type genomes by reassortment of damaged genome segments. Two genomes, each consisting of three segments of double-stranded nucleic acid, are shown. One carries a mutation in an M segment, the other in an S segment. When they are introduced into same cell, sets of undamaged segments are generated by reassortment. This type of mechanism can account for the generation of new genotypes among reoviruses, influenza viruses, and RNA tumor viruses.

cule of double-stranded DNA recombine efficiently, most probably by a mechanism analogous to that by which the genomes of bacteria and higher organisms recombine. The most efficiently recombining animal viruses are those whose genomes consist of several nucleic acid segments. In such cases recombination proceeds not by classical recombination involving breakage and reformation of covalent bonds, but by simple reassortment of segments into new sets (Fig. 67-2). Both single-stranded and double-stranded RNA segments participate in this type of recombination, as shown by the fact that pairs of both reovirus and influenza virus mutants generate wild-type virus with high frequencey. Recombination of this type may account for the marked antigenic variability of influenza virus, which is illustrated by the fact that influenza A_0, A_1, and A_2 virus strains prevalent during the periods from 1933 to 1947, 1947 to 1957, and since 1957 possess quite different hemagglutinins and neuraminidases (H0N1, H1N1, and H2N2 as well as H3N2, respectively, Chap. 62). It is known that influenza virus strains pathogenic for man can recombine with strains pathogenic for other animal species, and it has been suggested that new human pathogens have arisen in this manner. In fact, the Hong Kong influenza virus strain of 1968 may have derived part of its genome from an equine or duck influenza virus.

Multiplicity Reactivation

Viruses containing double-stranded nucleic acid frequently exhibit multiplicity reactivation after being subjected to ultraviolet irradiation. This phenomenon is recognized by the fact that the frequency of survivors increases sharply with multiplicities of infection above 1. It is due to cooperation between viral genomes that have been damaged by the irradiation and that can therefore no longer multiply on their own. The nature of the cooperation is probably recombination, that is, the damaged genomes recombine until an intact genome arises, which can then replicate and form progeny.

Complementation

Viral genomes can also interact indirectly by means of complementation. A typical example of this type of interaction is provided by infection of cells at the restrictive temperature with two virus mutants that bear temperature-sensitive mutations in different cistrons and neither of which can multiply alone. If complementation occurs, progeny comprising both mutants is produced. The explanation of this phenomenon is that each mutant produces functional gene products of all cistrons except the one bearing the temperature-sensitive mutation, so that in cells infected with both mutants all gene products necessary for virus multiplication are formed, and both mutants can therefore multiply. Complementation plays a major role in permitting the survival of viruses with genomes that contain damaged or nonfunctional genes.

A special case of complementation is the phenomenon of poxvirus reactivation. As outlined in Chapter 65, the second stage of poxvirus uncoating, that is, the uncoating of the viral core, requires the synthesis of an uncoating protein. This protein is not formed if the infecting virus has been subjected to protein-denaturing conditions, such as heat: heat-inactivated poxvirus particles are therefore not uncoated and cannot multiply. If, however, cells are simultaneously infected with denatured and undenatured virus particles, both are uncoated because the uncoating protein elicited by the latter also uncoats the former, which is therefore enabled to multiply. This phenomenon was initially interpreted as reactivation of the denatured virus by the active virus, hence its name.

Phenotypic Mixing and Phenotypic Masking

Another special case of complementation is the dual phenomenon of phenotypic mixing and phenotypic masking. When two closely related viruses, for example, poliovirus type 1 and poliovirus type 3, infect the same cell, the two resulting sets of progeny genomes may become encapsidated not only by their own capsids but also by hybrid capsids, that is, capsids composed of polypeptide chains characteristic of both genomes (phenotypic mixing), or even by capsids entirely specified by the other genome (phenotypic masking or transcapsidation) (Fig. 67-3). This situation is most readily detected by antigenic analysis, for the former class of virions is neutralized by antiserum to either of the two parents, while virions of the latter class are neutralized by antiserum to one of the parents, and their progeny is neutralized by antiserum to the other.

A similar phenomenon occurs among enveloped viruses. In particular, the nucleocapsid of the rhabdovirus vesicular stomatitis virus (VSV) possesses a remarkable ability to become encapsidated in envelopes that are only partially, or sometimes not at all, specified by it. For example, among the yield of cells simultaneously infected with both VSV and the paramyxovirus SV5 there are bullet-shaped particles that contain VSV nucleocapsids encased in envelopes that bear not only VSV-specified glycoprotion spikes but also both types of SV5-specified spikes. Another example of great current interest is provided by VSV nucleocapsids completely encased in RNA tumor virus envelopes. Since such particles are easily and rapidly quantitated, they have great potential for studies on RNA tumor virus host range (which is specified by the envelope) and for the detection of the presence of RNA tumor virus-specified envelope proteins, particularly in connection with the search for human tumor viruses (Chap. 69). Finally, VSV nucleocapsids can even be encased in herpesvirus envelopes.

DEFECTIVE VIRUS PARTICLES

Several types of virus particles exist that cannot multiply on their own but can multiply in cells simultaneously infected with some infectious virus. They can be subdivided into two classes: those that interfere extensively with the multiplication of their helper virus, and those that do not.

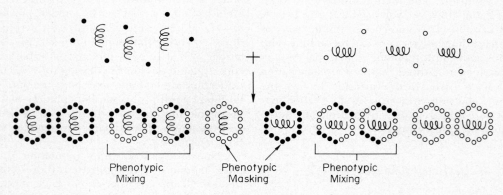

FIG. 67-3. Phenotypic masking and phenotypic mixing. Simultaneous infection with two related viruses is illustrated. Either genome can be encapsidated in capsids that are composed exclusively of homologous capsomers, or mixed capsomers (phenotypic mixing), or of exclusively heterologous capsomers (phenotypic masking). The method of detecting the latter two classes of particles is described in the text.

Defective Interfering (DI) Virus Particles

When viruses are passaged repeatedly at high multiplicity, the progeny frequently includes, in addition to mature virions, defective virus particles that are capable of interfering with the multiplication of homologous virus. Such virus particles have the following properties: (1) They contain the normal structural capsid proteins, (2) they contain only a part of the viral genome, (3) they can only reproduce in cells infected with homologous virions, which act as helpers, (4) although unable to reproduce on their own, they can nevertheless express a variety of functions in the absence of helper, such as inhibition of host biosynthesis, synthesis of viral proteins, and transformation of cells, and (5) they specifically interfere with the multiplication of homologous virus.

The following are some examples of defective interfering virus particles that have been characterized in some detail.

Defective Interfering Influenza Virus Particles Under conditions of repeated passaging at high multiplicity, the infectivity of successize influenza virus yields gradually decreases a millionfold or even more, though the total number of virus particles produced remains

roughly the same; in other words, noninfectious, defective virus particles gradually replace virions in the yields. This phenomenon was first described in 1952 by von Magnus and bears his name. Defective particles are not formed if influenza virus is passaged at low multiplicity, and they are readily eliminated from virus stocks by passaging at a multiplicity of less than 1, which shows that defective particles cannot multiply on their own. The ability of the defective particles to inhibit the multiplication of infectious virus is readily demonstrated by the fact that the addition of defective particles to influenza virus preparations free of them immediately reduces the yields of infectious virus in most types of cells.

The essential difference between infectious and defective influenza virus particles is that the latter lack one of the genome segments. Defective particles are thus deletion mutants whose ability to multiply is complemented by influenza virions, and which have a survival advantage over virions.

Defective particles that lack one (or even two) genome segments are also known among the reoviruses.

Defective Interfering Particles of Other Viruses Defective interfering particles are produced not only by viruses with segmented

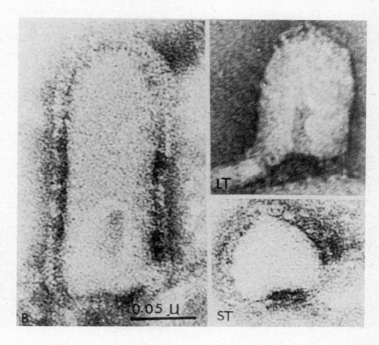

FIG. 67-4. Defective interfering particles of VSV. B, a bullet-shaped virion; LT, a *long truncated* particle; ST, a *short truncated* particle. LT particles are about one half, ST particles (which are round) about one-third the length of virions. They contain RNA molecules that are proportionately shorter than the RNA molecules in virions. (Courtesy of Dr. C. Y. Kang).

genomes but also by viruses with genomes that consist of a single nucleic acid molecule. The defective particles then contain nucleic acid molecules that are shorter than those of infectious virus particles. For example, when VSV is passaged at high multiplicity, virions among the progeny are gradually replaced by particles that are about one-third as long and contain RNA molecules about one-third as long as VSV genomes (Fig. 67-4). These particles, the so-called T (for "truncated") particles, can only multiply in the presence of virions but interfere extensively with their multiplication.

Defective interfering particles analogous to those of VSV occur also in high passage yields of poliovirus, pseudorabies virus, the papovaviruses polyoma and SV40, and probably most other viruses. In each case the morphology of the defective particles is indistinguishable from that of the corresponding virions, but their nucleic acid molecules are up to 20 percent shorter than intact genomes.

The reason that defective virus particles interfere with the multiplication of infectious virus is not known for certain. The best explanation is that their shortened nucleic acid molecules have a higher affinity for the enzymes that replicate viral nucleic acids than do intact genomes, so that they are synthesized preferentially and therefore gradually replace the latter.

Other Defective Virus Particles

Several kinds of defective virus particles exist that do not interfere significantly with their helpers. Their origin and relationship with their helper viruses is quite different from that of the particles just described.

Particles Aiding the Replication of Adenovirus (PARA)   Human adenoviruses cannot multiply in monkey cells but will do so in the presence of the simian papovavirus SV40, which performs some helper function. The progeny of such mixed infections sometimes includes particles that contain, within an adenovirus capsid, a hybrid DNA molecule that contains both adenovirus and SV40 DNA sequences but does not contain *all* the sequences of either. In one example of such particles, those of the E46+ strain of adenovirus type 7, about 10 percent of the adenovirus genome is replaced by about 75 percent of the SV40 gen-

ome (Fig. 67-5). These particles cannot, of course, multiply on their own, since they contain neither a complete adenovirus genome nor a complete SV40 genome, but they can perform that function which enables human adenoviruses to multiply in monkey cells. Further, they themselves can multiply in the presence of the human adenovirus, which presumably supplies the function(s) that is coded by that piece of adenovirus DNA which is missing in PARA DNA. Thus, here are two types of virus particles, human adenovirus and PARA, neither of which can multiply in monkey cells by itself but which can both multiply if they infect monkey cells simultaneously.

Several other types of adenovirus-SV40 hybrids are also known. One example is provided by hybrids between adenovirus type 2 and SV40 that contain not partial but complete SV40 genomes covalently linked to incomplete adenovirus genomes. Such hybrids enable adenovirus type 2 to multiply in monkey cells and are themselves complemented by adenovirus type 2. In addition they yield infectious SV40, since they contain the entire SV40 genome.

Even more interesting adenovirus-SV40 hybrids are the *infectious* adenovirus type 2-SV40 hybrids, five of which have been characterized in detail (Fig. 67-6). In these hybrids, a portion of the adenovirus genome is deleted from a region that is not essential for virus multiplication. This region comprises from 4.5 to 7.1 percent of the adenovirus genome and, in all hybrids, starts at a position that is 14 percent from one of its ends. In its place is inserted a portion of SV40 DNA that codes for early functions; this portion varies from 7 to 43 percent of the SV40 genome and also starts at the same position in all five hybrids. The largest piece

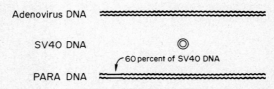

FIG. 67-5. PARA DNA, which is enclosed in an adenovirus capsid, consists of an adenovirus DNA molecule from which the segment that lies between 0.05 and 0.15 fractional genome lengths from one end has been deleted and substituted by about 60 percent of an SV40 genome. It may have been generated by two recombination events, one that led to the insertion of a complete SV40 genome, and a second, intramolecular event that deleted some adenovirus as well as some SV40 DNA.

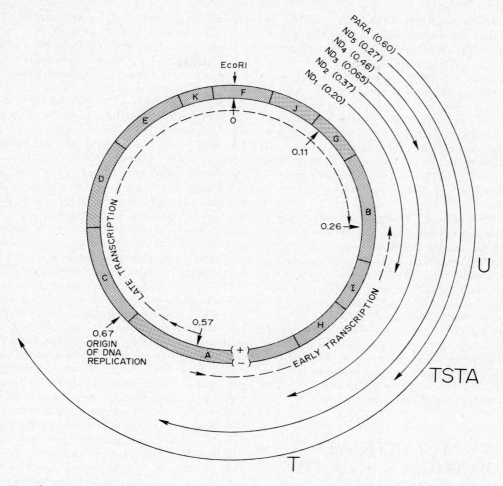

FIG. 67-6. The nature of the SV40 sequences in the DNA of certain nondefective SV40-adenovirus type 2 hybrids as well as of PARA particles. The SV40 genome is represented by the hatched circle. The segments A-K are the fragments that result when it is cleaved with the Hin restriction endonuclease from Hemophilus influenzae, ordered with respect to the single site that is susceptible to cleavage by the *E. coli* R1 restriction endonuclease (which is marked 0). The lengths, in fractional SV40 genome lengths, of the SV40 sequences present in the hybrids Ad²+ND$_{1-5}$, as well as in PARA particles of the E46 + strain of adenovirus type 7 (see text and Fig. 67-5), are indicated in brackets. Note that the SV40 sequence in all six hybrids starts at the same site on the SV40 genome, about 0.11 fractional genome lengths from 0. Note also that all the sequences then extend into that portion of the SV40 genome that is transcribed during the early period of the lytic multiplication cycle (between 0.26 and 0.57 units on the map). The three proteins that are coded by this region are the U, TSTA (tumor-specific transplantation antigen) and T antigens (see Chap. 69). It can be seen from the map that all hybrids except ND$_3$ code for the U antigen, and that only ND$_5$ and PARA code for the T antigen.

(43 percent) of SV40 DNA expresses *all* early SV40 functions, while the smallest piece (7 percent) can code for no more than 10,000 to 15,000 daltons of protein, yet this is sufficient to endow even this hybrid with the capacity to multiply in monkey cells.

Since these five hybrids provide a set of virus particles with different but precisely defined amounts of SV40 genetic material, they have been very useful in detailed studies of the arrangement of genetic information in the SV40 genome and of how it expresses itself. These studies will be described below in the section dealing with the application of restriction endonucleases to the structural and functional analysis of viral genomes (p. 865).

Adeno-associated Virus (AAV)   AAV is a virus that can multiply only in cells that are infected with adenovirus. The morphology of AAV, a parvovirus, is quite distinct from that of adenovirus, and AAV is not related genetically to it or to any other virus. By all criteria, AAV is a distinct virus with a uniquely narrow host range, namely, cells infected with adenovirus. The nature of the helper function that is performed by adenovirus is not known. It may well be that adenovirus does not provide a specific gene product but rather that it modifies the cell in some way essential for AAV multiplication.

RNA Tumor Viruses: Sarcoma Viruses   Other examples of viruses that require helpers are found among the RNA tumor viruses. In particular, many mammalian sarcomagenic viruses usually depend on leukemia viruses for the provision of their envelopes. These viruses will be discussed in detail in Chapter 69.

Viruses that can multiply only in cells also harboring other viruses may be of great importance in causing human diseases of as yet undefined etiology. They are very difficult to detect, but detailed studies of such systems as those described above may provide valuable clues in the search for additional ones.

TS MUTANTS, DI PARTICLES AND THE ETIOLOGY OF PERSISTENT VIRAL INFECTIONS

The mechanisms that underlie the persistence of viral infection in chronic disease, the basic characteristics of which were described in Chapter 66, have long been investigated intensively. Recently, two significant observations have added new dimensions to our understanding of them. First, many of the virus strains that have been isolated from persistently infected cells and animals have been found to be temperature-sensitive. For example, foot-and-mouth disease virus isolated from carrier cattle 2 to 12 months after exposure to virus was unable to multiply at 40 to 41C, a temperature at which the original wild-type FMDV multiplied normally; and recently a virus similar to Sendai virus, but with a much lower optimum growth temperature (33C as against 37C), was isolated from the brain of a patient with multiple sclerosis. These findings have been paralleled by the results of studies with persistently infected cultured cells. It has been known for some time that virus recovered from such cells differs from the virus with which they were originally infected in being less virulent and less cytopathic, and recently it was recognized that such virus also frequently possesses a lower optimum growth temperature. This has now been found for Coxsackie virus, Sindbis virus and WEE, influenza virus, Newcastle disease virus, Sendai virus, mumps and measles virus, VSV, and herpesvirus. Clearly, attempts to isolate viruses from the tissues of patients with suspected chronic and persistent viral infections should be made at incubation temperatures of 31 to 33C rather than 37C.

The second new factor is the realization of the potential importance of defective interfering virus particles in dampening the effects of viral infections. Indeed, it has been demonstrated that the highly lethal and cytocidal VSV can establish persistent infection in cultured cells if its T particles (p. 862) are inoculated at the same time; and that inoculation of T particles into animals, together with infectious VSV, converts otherwise rapidly fatal disease to a slowly progressive infection. The formation of defective interfering particles has now been implicated in chronic infections with Sendai virus, NDV and measles, lymphocytic choriomeningitis virus, Sindbis virus, and WEE.

In summary, the replacement of virulent by less virulent virus strains and the inhibition of the multiplication of virulent virus by defective interfering particles are both of major importance for the establishment and maintenance of persistent viral infection.

USE OF RESTRICTION ENDONUCLEASES FOR STRUCTURAL AND FUNCTIONAL ANALYSIS OF VIRAL GENOMES

The basic aims of virologists are to characterize the various functions involved in virus multiplication and to identify the portions of the viral genomes that code for them. Biochemical studies and, to an increasing degree, the availability of temperature-sensitive (ts) mutants have permitted rapid advances toward the first of these aims, but until recently no techniques were available for realizing the second. True, recombination analysis of ts mutants in different cistrons permits the construction of genetic maps that establish the order of gene functions on viral genomes, but not nearly enough ts mutants of any animal virus are yet available to construct any but the most rudimentary genetic maps. [However, this is not true for several bacteriophages, detailed genetic maps of which have been assembled (Chap. 70)]. In any case, these genetic maps relate only to the order of genes rather than to their location on physical portions of viral nucleic acids.

Recently this situation has changed with the discovery of the bacterial restriction endonucleases, which are components of the restriction–modification systems of bacteria (Chap. 8). These enzymes are extremely specific for palindromic sequences of double-stranded DNA, that is, sequences that are symmetrical around one or more axes. The palindromic sequences recognized by some restriction endonucleases are as simple as 5′ GG CC , but CC GG 5′ they may be more complex, such as, for example, 5′ (A/T) G AATT C(T/A) . Several of (T/A) C TTAA G(A/T) 5′ these restriction endonucleases cleave double-stranded viral DNAs in a relatively small number of locations. The most intensive analysis of this kind has been carried out with the smallest DNA-containing animal viruses, the papovaviruses, especially with SV40. The EcoRI restriction endonuclease [coded by the RTF 1 plasmid of *Escherichia coli* (Chap. 8)] cleaves SV40 DNA in one location; the *Haemophilus parainfluenzae* restriction endonuclease I cleaves it in 3 locations; and the mixture of *Haemophilus influenzae* restriction endonucleases II and III cleaves it in 11 locations. The resulting fragments can be isolated by polyacrylamide gel electrophoresis, their component strands can be separated, and they can be ordered within the viral genome. A restriction endonuclease fragment map of SV40 DNA is included in Figure 67-6. These fragments provide a series of extremely precise reagents of less than cistron size for the entirety of both viral DNA strands, and any mutant, variant, or related viral DNA molecule, as well as all mes-

senger RNA molecules transcribed both from them and from wild-type viral DNA, can be precisely identified by measuring their ability to hybridize with them. The following are examples of the types of analyses that have been performed with their aid.

(1) The origin of replication of SV40 DNA has been identified (Fig. 67-6).

(2) The region of SV40 DNA from which early and late mRNA molecules are transcribed during lytic infection, and the strands from which they are transcribed, have been identified.

(3) The regions of SV40 DNA that are transcribed in a variety of cells transformed by SV40 (Chap. 69) have been identified.

(4) The nature and size of the SV40 DNA sequences in the adenovirus-SV40 hybrids described previously, and in others like them, have been identified.

(5) Serial passage of SV40 at high multiplicity of infection leads to the accumulation of defective virus particles, the DNA of which contains deletions and duplications or reiterations of viral sequences, and their substitution by cellular DNA sequences. The sequences that are deleted and duplicated or reiteracted in such particles can be identified.

(6) Papovaviruses have recently been isolated from the brains of patients with progressive multifocal leukoencephalopathy (PML) and from the urine of renal transplant recipients (Chap. 62). The relation between these viruses and SV40 has been explored by the use of restriction endonuclease fragments (Fig. 67-7).

(7) The restriction endonuclease fragments can be used to map ts mutants. The procedure is to hybridize endonuclease fragments derived from wild-type virus to single-stranded circular DNA derived from the mutants. The resulting partial heteroduplexes are then tested for infectivity at nonpermissive temperatures. It is found that the ts defect of each mutant can be corrected by a specific DNA fragment, which indicates that the mutation is localized in it. To the extent that the damaged functions of the various mutants are known, this type of analysis also serves to assign functions to endonuclease cleavage fragments.

This list of important fundamental questions that are now being answered attests to the power of restriction endonuclease fragment analysis. This type of analysis, first applied to SV40 (and polyoma), is now also being used to

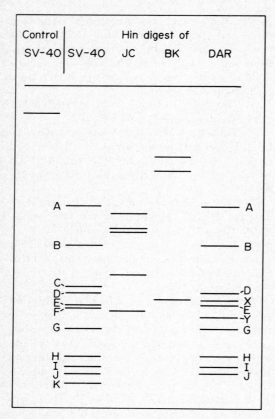

FIG. 67-7. An example of the usefulness of restriction endonuclease analysis. Polyacrylamide gel patterns of the fragments produced when the DNA of SV40, JC, BK, and DAR (Chap. 62) is digested with the Hin restriction endonuclease. The direction of electrophoresis was from top to bottom. Pattern 1 is the product obtained by cleaving SV40 DNA with restriction endonuclease EcoRI, which only cleaves at one site, that is, it yields the SV40 DNA in linear form. DAR and JC viruses were isolated from the brains of patients with progressive multifocal leukoencephalopathy (PML), BK virus from the urine of kidney transplant recipients. The restriction endonuclease fragment patterns yielded by SV40 and DAR are obviously very similar; this agrees with the finding that they are antigenically very closely related, and they may be regarded as variants of the same virus. The patterns yielded by JC and BK are quite different from SV40/DAR, as well as from each other. This agrees with the fact that they are much less closely related antigenically and that nucleic acid hybridization analysis indicates that their relatedness to SV40/DAR is no more than 10 and 20 to 30 percent, respectively. (Adapted from Osborn et al: J Virol 30:614, 1974; Sack et al: Virology 51:345, 1973)

characterize the genomes and transcription patterns of the larger adenoviruses and herpesviruses and may find application in answering specific questions concerning the organization of the human genome.

INTERFERENCE BETWEEN VIRUSES

It has been known for a long time that when two different viruses infect the same cell, they may not only increase each other's ability to multiply but they may also interfere with each other and diminish each other's yield. Generally, the first infecting virus is the one that interferes, but the precise nature of the interference is known only in very few instances. Sometimes the first virus inhibits the ability of the second virus, the challenging virus, to adsorb, by either blocking or destroying its receptors: this is the case for certain pairs of enteroviruses and myxoviruses, respectively. In other cases, it prevents the early messenger RNA of the challenging virus from being translated: this is the case when vaccinia virus infects cells infected with adenovirus. However, in most cases there is no explanation for the interference, as, for example, in the case of cells infected with rubella virus, which become completely resistant to NDV, although they remain susceptible to a variety of other viruses.

Although the results of studies that are directed specifically at determining why certain pairs of viruses interfere with each other's ability to multiply have been meager so far, it does seem that there is great potential for using one virus to interfere with some specific reaction essential for the multiplication of another. Such studies may become increasingly feasible as we learn more about the ability of viruses to interfere with the expression of genomes other than their own.

FURTHER READING

Books and Reviews

Cooper PD: The genetic analysis of polioviruses. In Levy HB (ed): The Biochemistry of Viruses. New York and London, Marcel Dekker, 1969, pp 177-218

Ghendon YZ: Conditional-lethal mutants of animal viruses. Prog Med Virol 14:68, 1972

Huang AS: Defective interfering viruses. Annu Rev Microbiol 27:101, 1973

Meselson M, Yuan R, Heywood J: Restriction and modification of DNA. Annu Rev Biochem 41:447, 1972

Nathans D, Smith HO: Restriction endonucleases in the analysis and restructuring of DNA molecules. Annu Rev Biochem 44:273, 1975

Takemoto KK: Plaque mutants of animal viruses. Prog Med Virol 8:314, 1966

Selected Papers

VIRUS MUTANTS

Dubbs DR, Kit S: Isolation and properties of vaccinia mutants deficient in thymidine kinase inducing activity. Virology 22:214, 1964

Sambrook JF, Padgett BL, Tomkins JKN: Conditional lethal mutants of rabbitpox virus. 1. Isolation of host cell-dependent and temperature-dependent mutants. Virology 28:592, 1966

INTERACTIONS AMONG VIRUSES

Choppin PW, Compans RW: Phenotypic mixing of envelope proteins of the parainfluenza virus SV5 and vesicular stomatitis virus. J Virol 5:609, 1970

Huang AS, Palma EL, Hewlett N, Roizman B: Pseudotype formation between enveloped RNA and DNA viruses. Nature 252:743, 1974

Joklik WK, Woodroofe GM, Holmes IH, Fenner F: The reactivation of poxviruses. I. The demonstration of the phenomenon and techniques of assay. Virology 11:168, 1960

Joklik WK, Abel P, Holmes IH: Reactivation of poxviruses by a nongenetic mechanism. Nature 186:992, 1960

Lake JR, Priston RAJ, Slade WR: A genetic recombination map of foot-and-mouth disease virus. J Gen Virol 27:355, 1975

Laver WG, Webster RG: Studies on the origin of pandemic influenza: Evidence implicating duck and equine influenza viruses as possible progenitors of the Hong Kong strain of human influenza. Virology 51:383, 1973

Trautman R, Sutmoller P: Detection and properties of a genomic masked viral particle consisting of foot-and-mouth disease virus nucleic acid in bovine enterovirus protein capsid. Virology 44:537, 1971

DEFECTIVE VIRUS PARTICLES

Ben-Porat T, Demarchi JM, Kaplan AS: Characterization of defective interfering viral particles present in a population of pseudorabies virions. Virology 61:29, 1974

Choppin PW, Pons MW: The RNAs of infective and incomplete influenza virions grown in MDBK and HeLa cells. Virology 42:603, 1970

Cole CN, Baltimore D: Defective interfering particles of poliovirus. II. Nature of the defect. III. Interference and enrichment. J Mol Biol 76:325, 345, 1973

Cole CN, Smoler D, Wimmer E, Baltimore D: Defective interfering particles of poliovirus. I. Isolation and physical properties. J Virol 7:478, 1971

Huang AS, Greenawalt JW, Wagner RR: Defective T particles of vesicular stomatitis virus. Virology 30:161, 173, 1966

Huang AS, Baltimore D: Defective viral particles and viral disease processes. Nature 226:325, 1970

Kingsbury DW, Portner A: On the genesis of incomplete Sendai virus. Virology 42:872, 1970

Uchida S, Watanabe S: Transformation of mouse 3T3 cells by T antigen-forming defective SV40 virions (T particles). Virology 39:721, 1969

Weiss BE, Goran D, Cancedda R, Schlesinger S: Defective interfering passages of Sindbis virus: Nature of the intracellular defective viral RNA. J Virol 14:1189, 1974

Yoshiike K: Studies on DNA from low-density particles of SV40. Virology 34:391, 402, 1968

ANALYSIS OF VIRAL GENOMES USING RESTRICTION ENDONUCLEASES (see also Chapters 8 and 69)

Khoury G, Fareed GC, Berry K, et al: Characterization of a rearrangement in viral DNA: Mapping of the circular Simian virus 40-like DNA containing a triplication of a specific one-third of the viral genome. J Mol Biol 87:289, 1974

Osborn JE, Robertson SM, Padgett BL, et al: Comparison of JC and BK human papovaviruses with Simian virus 40: Restriction endonuclease digestion and gel electrophoresis of resultant fragments. J Virol 13:614, 1974

INTERFERENCE BETWEEN VIRUSES

Aubertin A, Guir J, Kirn A: The inhibition of vaccinia virus DNA synthesis in KB cells infected with frog virus 3. J Gen Virol 8:105, 1970

Bablanian R, Russell WC: Adenovirus polypeptide synthesis in the presence of non-replicating poliovirus. J Gen Virol 24:261, 1974

Dales S, Silverberg H: Controlled double infection with unrelated animal viruses. Virology 34:531, 1968

Giorno R, Kates JR: Mechanism of inhibition of vaccinia virus replication in adenovirus-infected HeLa cells. J Virol 7:208, 1971

Marcus PI, Carver DH: Intrinsic interference: a new type of viral interference. J Virol 1:334, 1967

68

Antiviral Chemotherapy, Interferon, and Vaccines

THE RATIONAL APPROACH TO ANTIVIRAL CHEMOTHERAPY

Virus multiplication consists of the synthesis of viral nucleic acids and proteins and their assembly into virions. Any rational approach to antiviral chemotherapy should examine whether and where these processes can best be interrupted without detriment to the host. The following is a brief analysis along these lines.

THE REPLICATION OF VIRAL NUCLEIC ACIDS. The replication of the nucleic acids of many viruses is catalyzed by enzymes that do not exist in uninfected cells. This is true especially for all RNA-containing viruses, as well as for the poxviruses. It should be possible to isolate and characterize these enzymes and to find specific inhibitors for them.

THE SYNTHESIS OF VIRAL PROTEINS.   Several lines of evidence suggest that viral messenger RNAs differ in some fundamental way from host messenger RNAs. Viral messenger RNAs are as a rule translated in preference to host cell messenger RNAs. Furthermore, translation of host messenger RNAs often ceases entirely several hours after infection, when translation of viral messenger RNAs proceeds rapidly and extensively. This suggests that viral messenger RNAs differ in some recognizable, presumably chemical, manner from host messenger RNAs, and this difference should be exploitable. In fact, two of the most successful antiviral agents known, isatin-β-thiosemicarbazone and interferon (p. 872), act by preventing viral messenger RNAs from being translated but have no detectable effect on the translation of most host cell messenger RNAs. Analysis of the features that differentiate viral from host cell messenger RNAs is therefore a promising avenue of approach.

It is unlikely that inhibitors specific for viral protein synthesis itself will be found, since viral proteins are synthesized by the same ribosomes that synthesize host proteins and since they present no unusual features in their primary amino acid sequence.

VIRAL MORPHOGENESIS.   Viral morphogenesis proceeds at several levels. Many viral capsid polypeptides are now known to be synthesized in the form of precursors that are cleaved to furnish the actual polypeptides used for the formation of virions. The nature of the enzymes that cleave these precursors is not known. It may be fruitful to isolate and characterize them and to design inhibitors for them.

No way of specifically inhibiting the assembly of virions exists. It is conceivable that budding could be prevented when more is known about the properties of cell membranes, but it seems that the cell membrane is such an important cell organ that it may be unwise to attempt to prevent virion formation at this point. By the same token, inhibition of virion uptake and penetration at the beginning of the multiplication cycle has not been attempted seriously. As will be discussed below, the drug α-adamantanamine does inhibit the uptake of certain myxoviruses, but it does not do so by directly affecting the functioning of the cell membrane.

In summary, the two most promising avenues of approach for specifically inhibiting virus multiplication are inhibition of viral genome replicases and exploitation of the chemical differences between viral and host cell messenger RNAs.

THE MODE OF ACTION OF CERTAIN ANTIVIRAL CHEMOTHERAPEUTIC AGENTS

No antiviral chemotherapeutic agent capable of inhibiting virus multiplication efficiently in either man or animal is yet available. However several chemicals have been used more or less successfully in clinical trials, either as prophylactic agents or as inhibitors of virus multiplication under special conditions. Their mode of action is of considerable interest, since some of them act through one or another of the mechanisms discussed above. However, most of them were first used for empirical reasons.

Isatin-β-thiosemicarbazone (IBT)   IBT is a potent inhibitor of poxvirus multiplication (Fig.

68-1). It also inhibits adenovirus multiplication, and some of its derivatives inhibit the multiplication of certain enteroviruses. Only its antipoxvirus activity has been investigated in detail.

At a concentration of 3 mg per liter, IBT inhibits vaccinia virus multiplication in cultured cells by over 90 percent but has no detectable effect on the host cells themselves. In its presence, the early period of the poxvirus multiplication cycle, viral DNA replication and transcription of late messenger RNA all proceed normally. However, the translation of late messenger RNA is inhibited, and the synthesis of late proteins, which include most of the viral capsid proteins, is therefore prevented and no progeny virions are formed.

Mutants resistant to and dependent on the presence of IBT have been isolated. In cells infected with the latter in the absence of IBT, one of the core proteins that is normally formed by cleavage of a precursor is not produced.

It seems clear that the mechanism through which IBT exerts its effect is capable of exploiting the chemical differences between host cell and early viral messenger RNA on the one hand, and late viral messenger RNA on the other. Perhaps this mechanism is related in some way to the switch-off mechanism, which causes cessation of the translation of early viral messenger RNA at the beginning of the late period (Chap. 65). IBT may conceivably interfere with the ability of this mechanism to discriminate between early and late viral messenger RNAs and thereby cause the translation of both types of messenger RNA to be inhibited.

The effectiveness of IBT in inhibiting the multiplication of vaccinia virus, coupled with its low toxicity, has excited interest both in it and in derivatives that could be used to control smallpox. In field trials in India and Pakistan, N-methyl-IBT (Marboran), administered by mouth to known smallpox contacts, has reduced the incidence of infection.

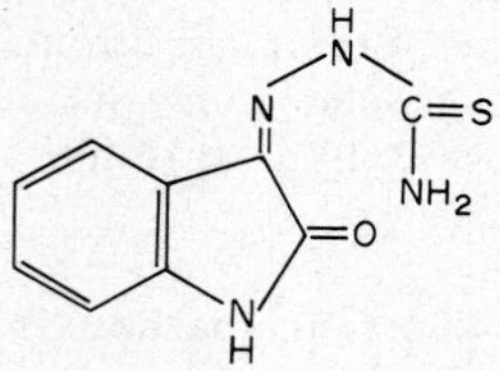

2-Hydroxybenzylbenzimidazole (HBB) and Guanidine These two reagents (Fig. 68-2) inhibit the multiplication of many picornaviruses, such as poliovirus, echoviruses, Coxsackie viruses, and foot-and-mouth disease virus. They are examples of reagents that interfere with the replication of viral RNA, either by preventing initiation of the synthesis of progeny plus strands or by preventing progeny plus strands from separating from the replicative form-replicase complex (Chap. 65). The precise manner in which this is accomplished is not known.

Neither HBB nor guanidine alone nor both together are useful antiviral agents in the intact host, since both resistant and dependent viral mutants emerge very rapidly.

Although these two compounds appear to inhibit picornavirus multiplication by similar mechanisms, these mechanisms are not identical. This is shown by the fact that (1) there is little cross-resistance among the mutants to either (although guanidine can replace HBB in promoting the growth of HBB-dependent mutants), (2) their antiviral spectra are not identical (for example, there are guanidine-sensitive but no HBB-sensitive rhinovirus strains), and (3) simple methyl donors, such as choline and methionine, rapidly and efficiently reverse the inhibitory effect of guanidine (by an entirely unknown mechanism) but have no effect on the inhibition caused by HBB.

Rifampicin Rifampicin (Fig. 10-16) and related rifamycin derivatives bind to bacterial RNA polymerases, thereby preventing the initiation of transcription. Rifampicin does not bind to animal RNA polymerases, but it does

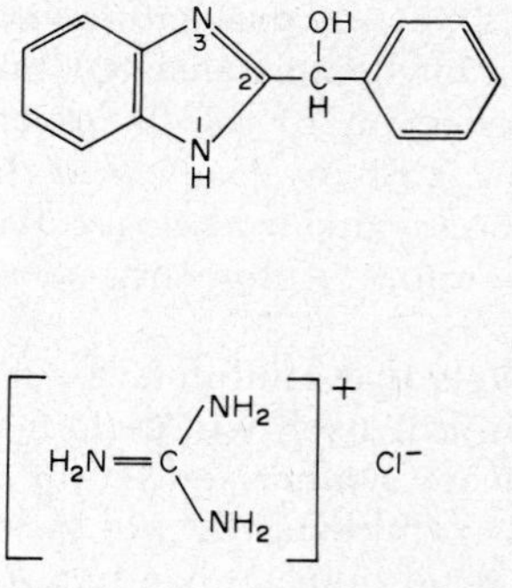

FIG. 68-1. Isatin-β-thiosemicarbazone (IBT).

FIG. 68-2. 2-Hydroxybenzylbenzimidazole (HBB) and guanidine hydrochloride.

inhibit the multiplication of poxviruses and adenoviruses. The mechanism by which it achieves this has been studied most intensively in vaccinia virus-infected cells. Inhibition of viral RNA polymerase is not involved, since both early and late messenger RNAs are transcribed normally. Rather, the mechanism involves some event in viral morphogenesis, for in the presence of the drug, immature virus particles of the type illustrated in Figure 65-12 accumulate. As a result of this block in morphogenesis, one of the viral capsid polypeptides that normally arises during maturation as a result of cleavage of a precursor (Chap. 65) is not formed. The specific nature of the step that is inhibited is not known. However, it is clear that it involves a diffusible product, most probably a protein, since wild-type virus sensitive to rifampicin matures normally in cells simultaneously infected with mutants resistant to it. Presumably the latter code for a protein that is unaffected by the drug and can therefore function when the normal wild-type protein cannot. As a result, resistant mutants rescue sensitive virus.

Although rifampicin does not inhibit the vaccinia DNA-dependent RNA polymerase, the RNA-dependent DNA polymerase of RNA tumor viruses (the reverse transcriptase, Chap. 69) is very sensitive to it and to certain of its derivatives.

α-Adamantanamine α-Adamantanamine (amantadine, Symmetrel) (Fig. 68-3), a substance with a remarkably rigid structure, inhibits the penetration, uptake, and perhaps also the release of certain myxoviruses and arenaviruses. It probably acts by combining with the outer plasma cell membrane and interfering with the penetration processes by which these viruses gain access to the interior of the cell. α-Adamantanamine has been specifically recommended for the prevention of disease caused by influenza virus type A on the basis

of large-scale trials that demonstrated that it had a statistically significant prophylactic effect. It has been used extensively in the Soviet Union and is presently the only drug for viral respiratory disease that is licensed in the United States. However, it is not used greatly in this country because it seems impractical to control, through chemoprophylaxis in an open population, a disease that is generally mild and that the individual patient has a good chance of avoiding anyway. As for the problem of protecting individuals at high risk and in whom the disease may be potentially dangerous, there is a choice between this drug and the influenza vaccine (p. 874). At least at this time, the vaccine would seem to be preferred.

5-Iododeoxyuridine (IDU) 5-Iododeoxyuridine (Fig. 68-4) has been used successfully in the treatment of keratoconjunctivitis caused by herpesvirus and adenovirus. It is worthwhile examining its mode of action in some detail, since it is not a specifically antiviral reagent in the sense outlined above.

In the cell IDU is phosphorylated to 5-iododeoxyuridine triphosphate, which is then incorporated into DNA, with 5-iodouracil replacing thymine. Since 5-iodouracil does not pair with adenine as faithfully as does thymine, mismatching occurs during both the replication and the transcription of substituted DNA. In addition, both IDU itself and its phosphorylated derivatives inhibit competitively the reactions involved in the synthesis of thymidine triphosphate, thereby reducing the overall rate of DNA synthesis. The net result is that IDU reduces the amount of DNA that is formed and interferes with the functioning of those DNA molecules into which it has been incorporated.

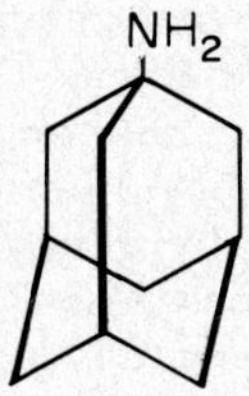

FIG. 68-3. α-Adamantanamine.

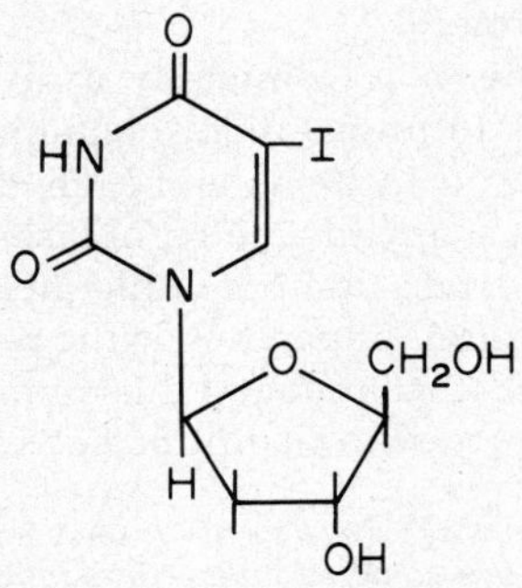

FIG. 68-4. 5-Iododeoxyuridine (IDU).

There is little evidence that IDU interferes with virus-specified reactions more than with those specified by the host genome, although its presence in certain DNAs (or genes) may well be more detrimental than in others. However, this is not a major effect, nor is it at all predictable. IDU acts as a successful antiviral chemotherapeutic agent in the eye because the cells in which herpesvirus and adenovirus replicate in the eye do not multiply, so that the only DNA with the synthesis and function of which IDU can interfere is viral DNA. In essence, the clinician here takes advantage of a rare situation and uses a nonspecific inhibitor in order to control virus multiplication.

INTERFERON

Properties and Mode of Action of Interferon

The antiviral agent on which interest is currently focused most intensely is one that is elaborated by living cells themselves. Animal cells infected with viruses very often produce a substance which, when added to uninfected cells, protects them against viral infection or, more precisely, greatly decreases the chance that subsequent viral infection will initiate a productive multiplication cycle. This substance is called "interferon." The key facts that are known concerning its nature, formation and mode of action are as follows.

(1) Interferon is species specific but not virus specific. For example, interferon secreted by human cells in response to infection with any virus inhibits the multiplication of any virus in human cells but not in other cells.* This is strong evidence that interferon is a host-specified protein.

(2) Interferon is commonly assayed by exposing cells to preparations containing it for a period of 12 to 24 hours and then challenging them with a standard amount of virus known to produce a certain number of plaques. The titer of the interferon preparation is the reciprocal of that dilution that reduces this number by 50 percent. The media of cultured cells stimulated

---

Recently, several examples of cross-species interferon activity have come to light—for example, human interferon has been found to be very active in protecting bovine and porcine cells against viral infection.

---

to produce it commonly contain in the order of 10^5 PRD_{50} (50 percent plaque reduction doses) of interferon per milliliter.

(3) Numerous attempts have been made to purify interferon, but until very recently none have been successful, primarily because interferon is extraordinarily active biologically. As a result, although very high titers of it can be produced, these titers correspond to no more than small amounts of interferon in physical terms. Interferon preparations have been obtained with about 10^9 PRD_{50}/ml protein, but such preparations still seem to contain impurities.

(4) The best evidence shows that human interferon is a glycoprotein with a molecular weight of about 25,000. Individual interferon molecules probably possess different numbers of sialic acid residues. Recent evidence indicates that the interferons produced by human fibroblasts and leukocytes differ significantly from each other, which suggests that the human genome contains at least two interferon genes, only one of which, however, expresses itself to any significant extent in any given cell.

(5) The principal distinguishing feature of interferon is its resistance to low pH. The commonly used operational definition of interferon is that is is that protein that protects cells against viral infection after it has been exposed to pH 2 for 48 hours at 4C.

(6) Normal cells do not as a rule contain interferon. Interferon released by infected cells is synthesized after virus infection. Its synthesis is induced as a result of virus infection, and it is generally produced most rapidly at about the time when replication of the viral genome proceeds most rapidly.

(7) Interferon itself is not the protein that inhibits virus multiplication. It only protects cells if RNA and protein synthesis are permitted to proceed. Interferon, therefore, appears to be an inducer that causes the cell to synthesize a protein that prevents virus multiplication. This protein has not yet been isolated. It confers onto the cells in which it is produced a virus-refractory state that generally lasts for several days. Further evidence that interferon and antiviral protein are different comes from genetic mapping studies. Interferon formation in man is controlled by genes on two chromosomes (chromosomes 2 and 5), while expression of the antiviral state is controlled by a gene on chromosome 21.

(8) The precise mode of action of interferon is not known, but it seems clear that the basic

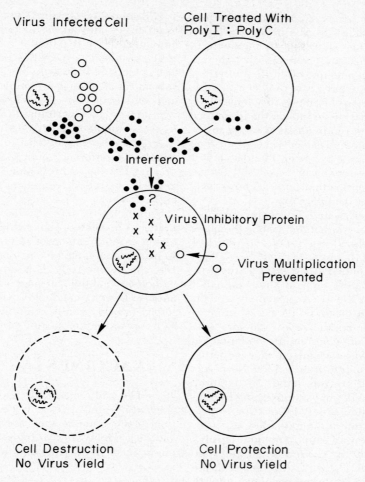

FIG. 68-5. Diagrammatic representation of the induction and mode of action of interferon. Interferon is formed either as a result of viral infection (left) or as a result of the action of an inducer like poly I: poly C, a copolymer of polyinosinic acid and polycytidylic acid (right). When interferon is added to cells, it induces the formation of a protein that prevents challenging virus from multiplying. As a result, the infection becomes abortive, which in some cells results in death, in others in survival.

mechanism involves interference with the ability of parental or early viral messenger RNA to be translated. As a result, no virus-specified proteins are synthesized, no progeny viral genomes are formed, and infection is abortive (Fig. 68-5).

(9) Finally, although in general host macromolecular synthesis is not detectably inhibited by interferon, some host cell functions do appear to be affected by it. Examples are the multiplication of certain tumor cells, the expression of certain cell surface antigens, the response to mitogenic stimuli, and modification of the immune response. It is conceivable that all these functions are mediated by messenger RNAs that share certain sequences, and that the

primary function of interferon is to regulate the expression of these *cellular* messenger RNAs rather than those of viral messenger RNAs (which may be inhibited because they are structurally similar). Thus interferon may have evolved as a cellular regulatory, rather than as an antiviral defense, mechanism.

The Induction of Interferon

The lack of toxicity of interferon, coupled with its extraordinarily high biologic activity, has placed it into the forefront of potentially useful antiviral agents, particularly for prophylaxis. There are two possible approaches to the induction of high levels of circulating interferon in man. The first is to administer interferon by injection. This approach is impractical, since interferon is cleared very rapidly from the bloodstream. The amounts of purified interferon that would be necessary to protect a population would therefore be impossibly large. The alternative approach is to induce the formation of interferon in the individuals who are to be protected. This method is receiving a great deal of attention, since it has been found that the formation of interferon can be caused by inducers other than infectious virus. Among such other inducers are the following.

(1) Viruses inactivated by agents such as heat or ultraviolet irradiation. Among them are inactivated influenza virus, NDV, reovirus, and bovine enterovirus.

(2) Double-stranded RNA, such as reovirus RNA, the replicative form of single-stranded viral RNAs, and the RNA present in certain fungal viruses. In fact, a crude extract of *Penicillium stoloniferum* known as "statolon" was known to be an inducer of interferon formation long before it was recognized that its active principle is the double-stranded RNA of a virus that is harbored by this mold. In addition, certain synthetic double-stranded polyribonucleotides, in particular poly I: poly C, are effective inducers of interferon formation, especially under conditions of superinduction. This is a phenomenon that is elicited when cells are treated with poly I: poly C together with the protein synthesis inhibitor, cycloheximide. If, after five hours, actinomycin D is added, followed one hour later by reversal of the inhibition of protein synthesis, about 50 times more interferon is produced than if cycloheximide had not been added initially. The basis of this phenomenon is thought to be inhibition of the synthesis of a regulatory protein that interferes with the translation of interferon messenger RNA. Further enhancement may result from the fact that interferon messenger RNA would not be translated in the presence of cycloheximide and would therefore accumulate. Single-stranded RNA and single-stranded or double-stranded DNA are inactive as interferon inducers, as are double-stranded RNA-DNA hybrid molecules. Free $2'-OH$ groups (on ribose) on both strands are essential for interferon-inducing activity.

(3) Certain synthetic polycarboxylic acids and pyran copolymers are inducers of interferon formation at relatively high concentrations,

as is bacterial endotoxin. The feature common to all these substances, including the polyribonucleotides, is that they are polyanions.

The mechanism by which interferon formation is induced is unclear. Nor is it known why substances as diverse as double-stranded RNA and endotoxin can both induce interferon, while a substance as similar to double-stranded RNA as double-stranded DNA cannot. However, it is clear that at least in the mouse, the extent of interferon production, and therefore presumably the expression of the interferon gene, is controlled by a single codominant locus.

Unfortunately, none of the three types of inducers discussed above fulfills both of the essential requirements of an interferon inducer in man, namely, effectiveness and low toxicity. Interest is currently focused both on nonpathogeic viral inducers and on synthetic polyanions. Development of a satisfactory interferon inducer would certainly mark a major step forward in the conquest of viral disease.

VACCINES

The only currently feasible means of preventing viral disease is through mobilization of the immune mechanism by means of vaccines. There are two types of antiviral vaccines: inactivated virus and attenuated active virus.

Inactivated Virus Vaccines

The primary requirements for an effective vaccine of this type are complete inactivation coupled with minimum loss of antigenicity. These requirements are not easily met simultaneously, since few reagents are available that inactivate viral genomes, the source of infectivity, without also affecting viral protein, the source of antigenicity. Ultraviolet irradiation could accomplish this best but is generally inapplicable because the virus preparations generally used for vaccine production contain large amounts of nonviral material that absorbs radiation, thereby shielding virus. In addition, genomes inactivated by ultraviolet irradiation may become reactivated by means of multiplicity reactivation (Chap. 67). Formaldehyde satisfactorily inactivates viruses containing single-stranded nucleic acid [although care must be exercised to avoid formation of a resistant viral fraction (Chap. 63)] but, it does not inactivate viruses containing double-stranded nucleic acid. Beta-propiolactone is a potentially useful inactivating agent but has been used only rarely because it is a potent carcinogen. Photodynamic inactivation (Chap. 63) inactivates viral nucleic acids efficiently and irreversibly without damaging viral proteins, which therefore retain full immunogenicity. However, it has recently been found that herpesvirus inactivated in this manner can still transform cultured cells in vitro and may therefore be tumorigenic. Further work is therefore necessary if this mode of inactivating virus is to provide a safe vaccine.

Inactivated virus vaccines are generally made from unpurified virus preparations that contain much host cell material. Since inactivated virus cannot multiply, relatively large amounts of this type of vaccine must be administered so as to provide sufficient antigen. As a result, a great deal of nonviral material that may cause undesirable side effects is also introduced into the body.

Although the inactivated vaccines that are currently used perform satisfactorily, they could, nevertheless, be improved by the application of new approaches. In the first place, vaccines should be prepared from highly purified virus rather than from the crude preparations currently in use. Not only would far less undesirable nonviral material be administered, but the likelihood of introducing into the body infectious passenger viruses would also be greatly diminished. Looking further ahead, it may very well be feasible to use as antigen not whole virus but that portion of the virus that elicits the formation of neutralizing antibody. The technology for achieving this is already available, since viral capsids can now be dissociated into their component proteins, which can be separated by several methods. Vaccines consisting of such material would certainly be more costly to produce than those currently in use, but their absolute safety and freedom from side effects would make their development well worthwhile.

Attenuated Active Virus Vaccines

The second method of immunizing against viral pathogens is by administering attenuated virus strains, antibody to which is capable of neutralizing the pathogen (Chap. 64). This is the principle on which Jenner's vaccination procedure against smallpox in 1798 was based. Since then many attenuated vaccine strains have been developed, among them Theiler's yellow fever vaccine strain, the attenuated Sabin poliovirus vaccine strains, and attenuated measles and rubella virus strains. The most commonly used method of producing such attenuated virus strains is by repeated passage of the human pathogen in other host species, which causes the selection of variants with drastically reduced virulence for man.

Attenuated virus vaccines are effective in very small amounts, since the attenuated virus can multiply. This provides a powerful amplification effect; it is viral progeny rather than the virus in the inoculum that acts as the antigen. Since only small quantities of this type of vaccine need be administered, the virus is usually not purified. However, just as in the case of the inactivated vaccines discussed above, the use of purified virus would yield important benefits. In particular, it would greatly reduce the likelihood of the presence of other, potentially dangerous, viruses in vaccines, which would in turn permit vaccine viruses to be produced more efficiently than is currently advisable. Attenuated vaccine virus strains are usually grown in cultured cells derived from a variety of animal species and organs. Great care is always taken that these cells display none of the characteristics of cells transformed by tumor viruses (Chap. 69). In particular, the cells must be euploid, display a high degree of contact inhibition, and contain no particles that may be virus particles. Generally cells that have not been passaged long in vitro are preferred, so as to reduce the likelihood of transformation in vitro and the selection of transformed cells. The disadvantage of such contact-inhibited, euploid cells is that they usually do not grow rapidly and do not achieve high population densities, and that therefore the amounts of virus that they yield are relatively low. By contrast, cells of established continuous cell strains display superior growth capabilities in vitro and permit the production of larger amounts of virus, but they are often derived from cells that are preneoplastic or neoplastic in character, are usually aneuploid, and often contain particles that may be virus particles. Such cells are therefore not used for the production of attenuated virus vaccine strains. However, the potential danger of the presence of tumor viruses and passenger viruses in general in attenuated virus vaccines could be virtually eliminated by routinely purifying all such vaccines by techniques such as density gradient centrifugation. If this were done, the easily cultured, high-yielding, established cell lines could be used safely for the growth of attenuated virus vaccines.

Several potential hazards associated with the use of active attenuated virus vaccines have not caused difficulties as yet but should be kept in mind. First, there is the danger that attenuated virus strains will, by mutation, revert to more virulent strains. This has not happened, probably because the attenuated virus strains are multistep rather than single-step variants. Second, administration of active attenuated vaccines involves infecting humans with virus. The only desired effect of this virus is to elicit the formation of antibodies, but this may not always be their only effect. For example, attenuated viruses, like their pathogenic parents, may in rare instances multiply in cells that are not their usual host cells. If these cells are those of an organ such as the brain, serious damage may result. This is in fact what happens in postvaccination encephalitis (Chap. 72). Third, the vaccine virus may activate latent viruses: models for such interactions are provided by AAV, which only multiplies in cells infected with adenovirus and by the PARA particles (Chap. 67). Finally, as discussed in Chapters 66 and 67, virus strains that are less virulent than wild-type virus have been implicated in the establishment and maintenance of persistent infections. This applies particularly to temperature-sensitive variants, some of which have directly been shown to cause chronic infections. Proposals to develop attenuated vaccine virus strains on the basis of selecting virus strains with lower optimum growth temperatures should therefore be evaluated very carefully, and any such strains should be tested exhaustively before being certified for general use.

This discussion of the potential hazards associated with the use of inactivated and attenuated active virus vaccines is in no way intended to discourage their development and use. Indeed, it has already been emphasized that such vaccines currently provide the only practical defense against infection. However, it should serve as a warning against the indiscriminate use of antiviral vaccines, and medical practitioners should be clearly aware of the potential dangers as well as of the undoubted benefits of vaccination. For example, although in absolute numbers the incidence of harmful sequelae following administration of a given vaccine may be very low, a serious public health issue may develop if 100 deaths were to result from vaccinating 100 million human beings. A decision as to whether to continue using such a vaccine would then have to be weighed in terms of the situation that would arise if the vaccine were not used. Furthermore, this discussion is intended to emphasize the fact that the application of modern techniques for virus purification could render antiviral vaccines appreciably safer and that these techniques should be applied irrespective of the economic factors involved.

FURTHER READING

Books and Reviews

Cockburn WC: The programme of the World Health Organization in medical virology. Prog Med Virol 15:159, 1973

Collins FM: Vaccines and cell-mediated immunity. Bacteriol Rev 38:371, 1974

Colby C, Morgan MJ: Interferon induction and actions. Annu Rev Microbiol 23:333, 1974

Foege WH, Eddins DL: Mass vaccination programs in developing countries. Prog Med Virol 15:205, 1973

Gresser I: Antitumor effects of interferon. Adv Cancer Res 16:97, 1972

Hilleman MR: Toward control of viral infections of man. Science 164:506, 1969

Horstman DM: Need for monitoring vaccinated populations for immunity levels. Prog Med Virol 16:216, 1973

MacKenzie JS, Houghton M: Influenza infections during pregnancy: Association with congenital malformations and with subsequent neoplasms in children, and potential hazards of live virus vaccines. Bacteriol Rev 38:356, 1974

Prusoff WH, Goz B: Potential mechanisms of action of antiviral agents. Fed Proc 32:1679, 1973

Selected Articles

CHEMOTHERAPEUTIC AGENTS

Bauer DJ, Sadler PW: The structure-activity relationships of the antiviral chemotherapeutic activity of isatin-β-thiosemicarbazone. Br J Pharmacol 15:101, 1960

Kato N, Eggers HJ: Inhibition of uncoating of fowl plague virus by 1-adamantanamine hydrochloride. Virology 37:623, 1969

Katz E, Margalith E, Winter B: The effect of isatin-β-thiosemicarbazone (IBT)-related compounds on IBT-resistant and on IBT-dependent mutants of vaccinia virus. J Gen Virol 25:239, 1974

Katz E, Moss B: Formation of a vaccinia virus structural polypeptide from a higher molecular weight precursor:

inhibition by rifampicin. Proc Natl Acad Sci USA 66: 677, 1970

Moss B, Rosenblum EN: Protein cleavage and poxvirus morphogenesis: Tryptic peptide analysis of core precursors accumulated by blocking assembly with rifampicin. J Mol Biol 81:267, 1973

Moss B, Rosenblum EN, Grimley PM: Assembly of virus particles during mixed infection with wild-type vaccinia and a rifampicin-resistant mutant. Virology 45:135, 1971

Woodson B, Joklik WK: The inhibition of vaccinia virus multiplication by isatin-β-thiosemicarbazone. Proc Natl Acad Sci USA 54:946, 1965

INTERFERON

Brodeur BR, Merigan TC: Suppressive effect of interferon on the humoral immune response to sheep red blood cells in mice. J Immunol 113:1319, 1974

Claes P, Billiau A, de Clercq, E, et al: Polyacetal carboxylic acids: a new group of antiviral polyanions. J Virol 5: 313, 321, 1970

Dianzani F, Pugliese A, Baron S: Induction of interferon by nonreplicating single-stranded RNA viruses. Proc Soc Exp Biol Med 145:428, 1974

Dorner F, Scriba M, Weil R: Interferon: Evidence for its glycoprotein nature. Proc Natl Acad Sci USA 70:1981, 1973

Friedman RM, Sonnabend JA: Inhibition of interferon action by p-fluorophenylalanine. Nature 203:366, 1964.

Gresser I, Brouty-Boye D, Thomas M, Macieira-Coelho A: Interferon and cell division. 1. Inhibition of the multiplication of mouse leukemia L 1210 cells in vitro by interferon preparations. Proc Natl Acad Sci USA 66:1052, 1970

Hallum JV, Thacore HR, Youngner JS: Factors affecting the sensitivity of different viruses to interferon. J Virol 6: 156, 1970

Havell EA, Berman B, Ogburn CA, et al: Two antigenically distinct species of human interferon. Proc Natl Acad Sci USA 72:2185, 1975

Joklik WK, Merigan TC: Concerning the mechanism of action of interferon. Proc Natl Acad Sci USA 56:558, 1966

Lampson GP, Tytell AA, Field AK, Nemes MM, Hilleman MR: Inducers of interferon and host resistance. I. Double-stranded RNA from extracts of *Penicillium funiculosum*. Proc Natl Acad Sci USA 58:782, 1967

de Mayer E, de Mayer-Guignard J: Gene with quantitative effect on circulating interferon induced by Newcastle disease virus. J Virol 3:506, 1969

Mozes LW, Vilcek J: Distinguishing characteristics of interferon induction with Poly(I)-Poly(C) and Newcastle disease virus in human cells. Virology 65:100, 1975

Repik P, Flamand A, Bishop DHL: Effect of interferon upon primary and secondary transcription of vesicular stomatitis and influenza viruses. J Virol 14:1169, 1974

Rousset S: Refractory state of cells to interferon induction. J Gen Virol 22:9, 1974

Samuel CE, Joklik WK: A protein synthesizing system from interferon-treated cells that discriminates between cellular and viral messenger RNAs. Virology 58:476, 1974

Stewart WE, Gosser LB, Lockhart RZ: Priming: a nonantiviral function of interferon. J Virol 7:792, 1971

Stewart WE, de Somer P, Edy VG, et al: Human interferons: Requirements for stabilization and reactivation of human leukocyte and fibroblast interferon. J Gen Virol 26:327, 1975

Tan YH: Chromosome 21-dosage effect on inducibility of anti-viral gene(s). Nature 253:280, 1975

Tan YH, Creagan RP, Ruddle FH: The somatic cell genetics of human interferon: Assignment of human interferon loci to chromosomes 2 and 5. Proc Natl Acad Sci USA 71:2251, 1974

Thacore HR, Youngner JS: Rescue of vesicular stomatitis virus from interferon-induced resistance by superinfection with vaccinia virus. I. Rescue in cell cultures from different species. II. Effect of UV-inactivated vaccinia and metabolic inhibitors. Virology 56:505, 512, 1973

69
Tumor Viruses

Tumor viruses are considered separately from lytic viruses in order to focus attention on the role of viruses in carcinogenesis. Both RNA-containing and DNA-containing viruses can cause various types of neoplasms in animals, and evidence is mounting that they may act similarly in man. Awareness of the principles of tumor virology will therefore be important for medical practitioners in the decades ahead.

THE ORIGIN OF TUMORS

Tumor etiology, the study of the causes of tumors, has brought to light a bewildering variety of tumorigenic agents that fall into three classes: chemical substances, physical stimuli, and biologic agents. The chemical substances include compounds of the most diverse constitution, ranging from polycyclic hydrocarbons such as methylcholanthrene, benzo(a)pyrene, and dimethylbenzanthracene on the one hand, to multifunctional compounds such as dimethylnitrosamine, nitrosomethylurea, and 4-nitroquinoline-1-oxide on the other. The physical agents include both x-rays and ultraviolet irradiation, and the most important biologic agents are viruses.

The concept that infectious agents might be involved etiologically in the cancer process was advanced as early as 1908 by Ellerman and Bang, who observed that the mode of transmission of leukemia in the fowl was similar to that of an infectious disease. Shortly thereafter, Rous demonstrated that the infectious agent in avian sarcomas could pass through a filter that would not permit passage of bacteria. This discovery remained an isolated finding for many years, until in 1932 Shope discovered a viral agent in wild cottontail rabbits that transmitted a wartlike growth not only to cottontails but also to domestic rabbits. While most warts in cottontails remained benign or regressed, those in domestic rabbits sometimes developed into highly malignant carcinomas. Then, in 1938, Bittner discovered a virus in mammary gland tumors of mice, the milk factor, which is passed from mother to offspring through suckling. The finding which, more than any other, elicited the upsurge of interest in viruses as carcinogenic agents was the discovery by Gross in 1951 of a

virus that induced leukemia in mice, a disease that is remarkably similar to leukemia in man. Efforts to develop animal models applicable to the human disease have resulted in the isolation of a large number of viruses that cause many kinds of cancers in every major group of animals.

THE CHARACTERISTICS OF VIRUS-TRANSFORMED CELLS

Viruses are unique among carcinogens in that their tumorigenic activity is expressed efficiently in vitro and can therefore be studied under controlled conditions. Discussion of the virus-cell interaction up to this point has been focused on the lytic interaction, which involves multiplication of the virus and destruction of the host cell. However, certain DNA viruses can interact with cells not only by means of the lytic interaction but also by means of an interaction in which virus multiplication is repressed and the host cell is not destroyed. The viral DNA then becomes closely associated with or integrated into the cellular genome, thereby giving rise to a new entity, the transformed or tumor cell, which can multiply indefinitely. In addition, a group of RNA-containing viruses, the RNA tumor viruses (oncornaviruses), can also transform cells and cause tumors. Until recently, the problem of how viral RNA could be integrated into the host genome presented a major conceptual hurdle. However, this has now been overcome by the discovery in RNA tumor viruses of a DNA polymerase that can transcribe RNA into DNA; this is the so-called reverse transcriptase. DNA transcribed from viral RNA by this enzyme is integrated into the cellular genome, conceivably by a mechanism analogous to that which integrates the genomes of the DNA-containing viruses.

In both cases the infected cells are altered in several fundamental characteristics and are said to be "transformed;" and since these changes are at the genetic level, they are passed on to their descendants. The principal properties in which virus-transformed cells differ from normal ones are as follows.

Possession of the Viral Genome   Transformed cells contain the genome of the virus that causes the transformation. More often than not, this genome is integrated into the cell DNA, but in some transformed cell nuclei it may exist as a free plasmidlike entity (Chap. 8). The extent to which the viral genome expresses itself in transformed cells varies widely, from full expression, with resultant formation of progeny virions, to complete silence, as judged by the absence of messenger RNA transcribed from it or polypeptides coded by it.

Morphology   Normal and transformed cells differ in morphology. There are two major changes. First, transformed cells are usually more rounded and refractile than are normal cells. Second, normal and transformed cells differ in the orientation of cells relative to each other. Normal cells usually arrange themselves in regular patterns, while transformed cells tend to orient themselves randomly (Fig. 69-1). These changes are often virus specific. There are mutants of Rous sarcoma virus and polyoma virus that give rise to transformed cells with morphologies that differ from those induced by the corresponding wild-type viruses.

Changes in Growth Patterns   Most types of untransformed cells grow in vitro to a certain cell density and then stop (or almost stop) dividing when a monolayer of uniformly spread cells has formed. Under the same conditions, the corresponding transformed cells continue to multiply until they reach very much higher cell densities.

This alteration of growth patterns is primarily due to two factors.

LOSS OF CONTACT INHIBITION.   When an untransformed cell comes into contact with another cell, the ceaseless rapid movement of the pseudopodia (ruffled edges) that are constantly extended and retracted ceases, and forward movement is arrested. At the same time the cell stops dividing. This dual phenomenon is known as "contact inhibition." It is the ability to respond to contact with other cells that ensures that any given cell only grows in its appropriate location within the complete organism and does not proliferate unless it receives a signal that more of its kind are needed for the organism's orderly growth or maintenance.

While cell strains differ appreciably in their susceptibility to contact inhibition, transformed cells are always much less susceptible than are their untransformed counterparts. This loss of contact inhibition represents release from one of the normal controls over multiplication, which may account in part for their unregulated growth in the organism. Some transformed cells, such as cells of benign tumors, have only lost the ability to respond to contact with each other but are still inhibited by contact with other cell types; while other cells, such as those of metastasizing tumors, respond to contact neither with each other nor with other types of cells.

REDUCTION OF THE REQUIREMENT FOR SERUM.   Contact inhibition is not the only factor that limits cell growth. The addition of serum to a nondividing contact-inhibited monolayer of untransformed cells results in further rounds of division, so that cells may actually pile up on top of one another. Virus transformation markedly reduces cellular serum dependence; transformed cells require much less serum to initiate division than do untransformed cells. For example, 3T3 cells, a line of mouse fibroblasts, will not grow optimally unless the serum concentration is greater than 5 percent. By contrast, 3T3 cells transformed with SV40 can divide to a small but significant extent in serum concentrations as low as 0.5 percent. The nature of the factors in serum and how they act is not known. Hopefully, the recognition of their

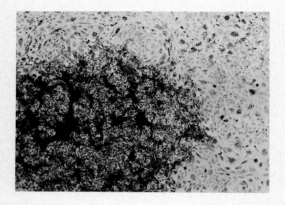

FIG. 69-1. Focus of hamster embryo cells transformed by murine sarcoma virus. The focus consists of small, densely packed, randomly oriented cells. (From Za'Vada and McPherson: In Barry and Mahy (eds): The Biology of Large RNA Viruses, 1970. Courtesy of Academic Press)

existence will hasten the deciphering of the signals that guide cells through their growth cycles.

Ability to Form Colonies in Agar Suspension

Untransformed cells of fibroblast origin must attach to a solid surface before they can divide; this requirement is known as "anchorage dependence of multiplication." By contrast, transformed cells will divide in suspension culture. In particular, ability to grow and form colonies when suspended in soft (0.5 percent) agar (Fig. 69-2) provides not only a very useful test for the stably transformed state but also the basis for a selective procedure that permits the isolation of transformed cells from populations of predominantly untransformed cells.

Tumorigenicity   Transformed cells generally give rise to tumors when injected into animals. Like naturally occurring tumors, different lines of virus-transformed cells exhibit wide variation in invasiveness. Some transformed cells, even when injected in large numbers, merely produce benign tumors at the site of inoculation, while even small numbers of others give rise to highly invasive cancers.

Secretion of Protease   Most transformed cells secrete a protease that converts plasmino-gen into plasmin, the enzyme that digests fibrin. This enzyme is not secreted to any extent by untransformed cells except those of lung or kidney origin. The significance of protease production is not clear. Although this property correlates well with ability to form tumors in immunosuppressed hosts, ability to grow in soft agar, and increased agglutinability by lectins (p. 882), the untransformed phenotype is not restored by inhibitors of protease activity. On the other hand, the protease may be responsible for the fact that transformed cells release more glycoproteins into the surrounding medium than do untransformed cells.

Cell Membrane Changes   Many of the altered properties of transformed cells have their origin in changes in the outer cell surface membrane.

CHANGES IN ANTIGENIC COMPOSITION.   The surfaces of virus-transformed cells possess antigenic determinants not present on untransformed cells. These new surface antigens can be detected by immunofluorescence or by tests for cytotoxic and cell-mediated immunologic response. Indeed, their presence causes transformed cells to be recognized as foreign and subject to immunologic surveillance (that is, destroyed by lymphocytes with the appropriate

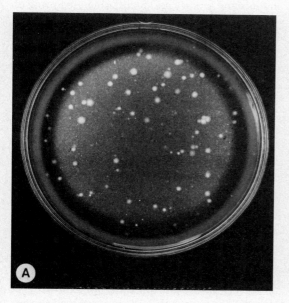
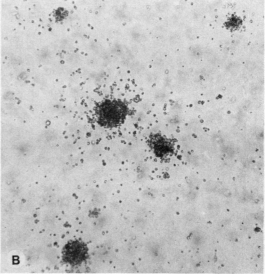

FIG. 69-2. Suspension colonies in soft agar of chick embryo fibroblasts transformed by Rous sarcoma virus. A. Appearance of a petri plate with numerous colonies (14 days after infection and plating). B. Enlargement of several colonies (8 days after infection and plating). (Courtesy of Dr. Thomas Graf)

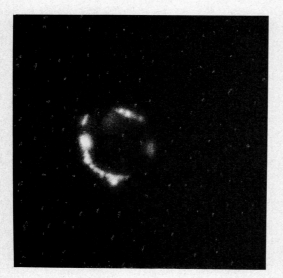

FIG. 69-3. Demonstration, by means of immunofluorescence, of the surface antigen [tumor-specific transplantation antigen (TSTA)] on a cell derived from a tumor induced in hamsters with adenovirus type 12. The cell was treated first with a hamster antiserum to such cells and then with rabbit antihamster globulin conjugated with fluorescein isothiocyanate. The antiserum was prepared by repeated injection of adenovirus type 12, followed by one injection of tumor cells. Note the annular pattern of specific fluorescence on the cell membrane. TSTA on cells transformed with papovaviruses can be demonstrated by analogous procedures. (From Vascencelos-Costa: J Gen Virol 8:69, 1970)

surface configuration). Some of these new antigenic determinants are virus-specified. This is true for antigens present on the surface of cells transformed by many RNA tumor viruses, and it may also be true for the tumor-specific transplantation antigens (TSTA) (Fig. 69-3) that elicit the formation of antibodies that protect animals against challenge by transformed cells. These antigens are present on the surface of cells transformed by papovaviruses and adenoviruses (and probably by other viruses also) and are not structural viral polypeptides. Others of these new antigenic determinants may be coded by the host genome. Among the several mechanisms that might cause new host-specified antigens to manifest themselves following transformation are derepression of segments of the host cell genome that do not ordinarily express themselves and unmasking or exposure of determinants that are not normally apparent.

INCREASED AGGLUTINABILITY BY LECTINS.
Many animal cells are agglutinated by certain glycoproteins (and proteins) that are present in plant seeds, snails, crabs, and some fish and that are collectively known as "lectins" (or agglutinins). Some of these lectins preferentially agglutinate spontaneous tumor cells and cells transformed by viruses (as well as by chemical carcinogens). The two lectins that best discriminate between normal and transformed cells are the jack bean agglutinin concanavalin A (Con A) and wheat germ agglutinin (WGA). At first it was thought that transformed cells are agglutinated more readily than are nontransformed ones because they bind more lectin molecules. However, it is now known that this is not so; rather, the reason seems to lie in the arrangement of the lectin-binding sites which are dispersed in untransformed cells and clustered in transformed ones. Further, it is now known that both Con A and WGA can agglutinate untransformed cells under certain conditions: They will agglutinate cells in metaphase and cells exposed briefly to proteases, such as trypsin. Interestingly, contact-inhibited protease-treated cells escape from growth control for brief periods of time, probably until the proteins that are removed by proteases are regenerated. The reason why treatment with proteases renders cells more agglutinable is not known, and one explanation is that proteases split off surface glycopeptides, thereby increasing membrane fluidity and facilitating clustering of lectin receptor sites.

CHANGES IN CHEMICAL COMPOSITION. Whereas the protein composition of membranes appears to be fairly constant, their lipid, glycolipid, and glycoprotein carbohydrate components are notoriously variable; they are exquisitely sensitive to changes in the medium, changes in the cell growth rate, and changes in growth conditions in general. It is difficult, therefore, to pick out changes attributable to transformation, but the following appear to be significant.

(1) When untranformed cells become density-(contact-) inhibited, their glycolipids become larger and more complex; fucose, galactose, N-acetylgalactosamine, and N-acetylneuraminic acid (NANA) are then added to them covalently. Apparently the transferases responsible for these extensions are not expressed in rapidly growing cells but are expressed in contact-inhibited cells. Transformed cells do not exhibit this cell density-dependent glycolipid

extension response. Fucose-, galactose-, and NANA-containing glycolipids are present in transformed cells in smaller amounts than in untransformed cells and are smaller in size.

(2) Strangely enough, changes of a similar but opposite nature occur in the oligosaccharides of glycoproteins: in transformed cells these groups are larger than in untransformed cells, and they contain more NANA (which always occupies a terminal position).

(3) As discussed previously, the antigenic compositions of cell surface membranes of untransformed and transformed cells are not identical. This is reflected in their polypeptide compositions as revealed by electrophoresis in polyacrylamide gels. Transformed cells generally contain fewer very large (over 150,000 daltons) glycoproteins than do untransformed cells—which are perhaps released by the protease that is produced by transformed cells (p. 881)—and contain several polypeptides in the 50,000 to 100,000 dalton range that are not present in untransformed cells.

MEMBRANE TRANSPORT PROPERTIES. Simple sugars and other nutrients are transported several times more rapidly across the outer membrane of transformed than of untransformed cells. This is generally the earliest observable change following transformation. It is conceivable that increased sugar transport into transformed cells is responsible, at least in part, for the increased rate of glycolysis that is generally observed in transformed cells.

Chromosomal Changes Transformation generally results in changes in chromosomes. Among the most common changes are deletion of portions of some chromosomes and duplication of portions of others. Less commonly, extra copies of entire chromosomes are incorporated in a stable manner into the cellular genome. The fact that independent transformants often exhibit the same deletions and duplications has prompted the formulation of a gene balance theory of virus-induced malignancy that postulates that some genes promote malignancy, while others tend to suppress it.

Members of five families of virus are now known to be tumorigenic and capable of transforming cells in culture. The manner in which transformation by these viruses is established, maintained, transmitted, and detected will now be described.

DNA TUMOR VIRUSES

Papovaviruses

Most members of the papovavirus family are oncogenic. First, there are the papilloma viruses. They include rabbit papilloma virus, which causes benign or malignant tumors depending on the host (Chap. 62), and the human wart virus, which almost always induces benign tumors that grow for some time, then often remain static for a period of years, and then disappear for reasons that are understood poorly. Little is known concerning the interaction of these viruses with cells because no in vitro system has been available in which they transformed and/or multiplied in cultured cells. However, it has now been reported that human papilloma virus will infect and multiply in human epithelioid cells and that the viral genome can persist for many months in infected, phenotypically normal (and non-virus-producing) cells. The ubiquitous human wart virus will, therefore, have to be given serious consideration as a possible agent of neoplastic disease in man.

Second, there is polyoma virus which was originally isolated from mouse cell extracts used for the transmission of leukemia. It is only rarely responsible for tumors in nature. When injected into newborn mice or hamsters, it produces a wide variety of histologically distinguishable tumors, hence its name.

Then there is simian virus 40 (SV40) which was first isolated from apparently normal cultures of monkey kidney cells. The only host in which it causes tumors is the baby hamster. Lymphocytic leukemia, lymphosarcoma, reticular cell sarcoma, and osteogenic sarcoma are all produced.

Finally, there are the papovaviruses that have recently been isolated from man, among them BK, JC, and DAR (Chap. 62), some of which can transform cultured cells, and one of which, DAR, causes tumors in hamsters.

By far the most intensively studied of all these viruses are SV40 and polyoma, and the following discussion will deal almost exclusively with them.

The importance of papovaviruses for studies of viral oncogenesis lies in the small size of their DNA, which can only code for about 1,500 amino acids. Since mutants of these viruses exist that are temperature-sensitive with respect to ability to initiate and maintain the transformed cell state, transformation is apparently a viral function, and since the genome of these viruses can code for no more than four to six proteins, it will hopefully soon be possible to identify the nature of the function that transforms normal cells into tumor cells.

Both polyoma and SV40 not only transform cells but also interact with cells by means of the lytic pathway. Cells are transformed if they are nonpermissive, that is, if polyoma and SV40 cannot multiply in them; or, if they are permissive, they can be transformed when infected with defective virus particles, such as the deletion mutants that arise upon repeated passage at high multiplicity (Chap. 67), or with inactivated virus particles [for example, by photodynamic inactivation (Chap. 63)]. In other words, if polyoma and SV40 *can* multiply in a given cell, that cell will generally not be transformed; if they *cannot* multiply, the cell will often be transformed.

The Lytic Cycle In order to understand how polyoma and SV40 transform cells, it is first necessary to examine the nature of their lytic interaction with cells. The lytic growth cycle of polyoma and SV40 can be divided into a well-defined early and late phase. During the early phase, which lasts a surprisingly long time, about 12 to 14 hours, the viral genome exercises at least two functions. First, it in-duces the appearance of several new antigens. Among them is the T (tumor) antigen, which accumulates in the nucleus in large amounts (Fig. 69-4). The function of this T antigen, which binds to polyoma and SV40 DNA at the site where replication originates, is not known. A second antigen, known as the U antigen, also appears at this time; it is located at the nuclear membrane rather than within the nucleus. Whereas the T antigen is known to be virus-coded (since a ts mutant of polyoma codes for a T antigen that is itself temperature-sensitive), the U antigen has not yet been proved to be a product of a viral gene. Finally, the new antigens also appear at the cell surface. These antigens may be identical with the tumor cell-specific transplantation antigens (TSTAs, p. 882) detectable on the surface of transformed or tumor cells. Although they are known to be virus specific, they have not yet been proved to be viral gene products.

Second, the polyoma and SV40 genome induces the synthesis of cellular DNA. Substantial amounts of DNA are formed, and, generally, the DNA replicates at least once. At the same time, the activity of several enzymes involved in DNA synthesis increases. These must be cellular enzymes, since polyoma and SV40 DNA are far too small to code for them.

Finally, viral DNA is integrated into cellular DNA during the early period. The significance of integration during the lytic cycle is not clear,

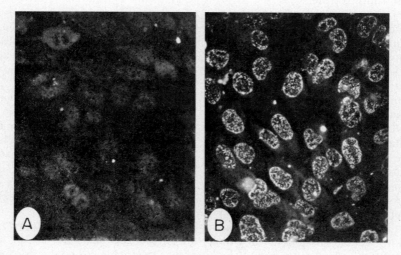

FIG. 69-4. Demonstration of the SV40 T antigen by means of immunofluorescence. Cells from a tumor induced by SV40 in a hamster were exposed to fluorescein-conjugated serum from a non-tumor-bearing hamster (A) and a tumor-bearing hamster (B). ×280. (From Rapp, Butel, and Melnick: Proc Soc Exptl Biol Med 116:1131, 1964)

since it has not yet been established, and is technically very difficult to establish, whether integration is a *necessary* event during the lytic cycle of these viruses. It is conceivable, for example, that viral genomes that become integrated never give rise to infectious progeny.

During the late phase, viral DNA and capsid proteins are synthesized, and progeny virus particles are assembled. Since the proteins synthesized during the early and late phases of the multiplication cycle are different, the corresponding messenger RNAs are also different. The papovavirus transcription program has been extensively characterized by hybridizing messenger RNA molecules to restriction endonuclease-generated viral genome fragments (Chap. 67). Its essential features are as follows

(Fig. 69-5): (1) About one-third of the papovavirus DNA is transcribed during the early period (E mRNA), and all of it is transcribed during the late period [late messenger RNA, therefore, comprises E mRNA together with some RNA that is only transcribed during the late period (L mRNA)], (2) the actual amount of early mRNA is no more than 2 to 10 percent of late messenger RNA, (3) as isolated from polyribosomes, E mRNA and L mRNA hybridize to opposite strands of papovavirus DNA. There is, however, evidence that substantial regions of the DNA are transcribed symmetrically, that is, that both strands are transcribed simultaneously. This would imply the existence of selective post-transcriptional degradation and/or transport from the nucleus to the cytoplasm.

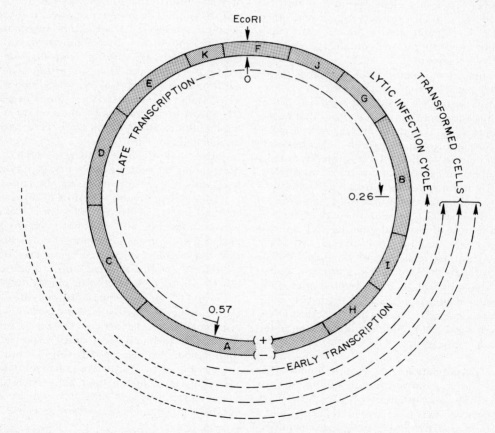

FIG. 69-5. The transcription program of SV40 in productively infected cells (lytic multiplication cycle) and in three clones of SV40-transformed BSC-1 African Green Monkey kidney cells. In the former the region between 0.26 and 0.57 fractional genome lengths (relative to the EcoR1 cleavage site) is transcribed during the early period from one DNA strand, while the remainder is transcribed only during the late period from the other strand. In the clones of transformed cells, all the early region is transcribed, together with varying amounts of the late region from the *wrong strand*. However, the amount of extra RNA transcribed in this manner is generally small compared with the amount of early type RNA. (Adapted from Khoury, et al: Virology 63:263, 1975)

The virus particles that are formed present several interesting features. First, the basic proteins that are intimately associated with the viral DNA within the particle core comprise three cellular histone species (F3, F2b, and F2a,). Second, some particles contain not viral but host DNA. Toward the end of the late period, host DNA begins to be extensively fragmented into molecules similar in size to papovavirus DNA, and some of these molecules are encapsidated to form particles known as "pseudovirions." The extent of pseudovirion formation depends on the nature of the host cell; in some cells more pseudovirions than virions are formed. Pseudovirions have attracted some attention because of their potential ability to transfer cellular genes from one cell to another. However, it is not clear whether it will be possible to put this ability to good use, since the DNA is fragmented randomly, and each pseudovirion, therefore, contains a different cell DNA fragment.

Pseudovirions are not the only progeny papovavirus particles that contain host DNA. Frequently, particles are formed with DNA that contains segments of cellular DNA that correspond to some 5 percent of the viral genome. The formation of such particles also depends on the nature of the cell and probably results from aberrant excision of integrated viral DNA. Finally, upon repeated passage at high multiplicity, defective virus particles begin to be formed (Chap. 67). Some of these particles still contain most of the viral genome and can still express some viral functions on their own, such as transforming cells, coding for the synthesis of T antigen (the so-called T particles), and so on. Others, especially those formed after many passages at high multiplicity, contain nucleic acid molecules that consist mostly of host DNA, the only viral DNA being the region around the origin of replication.

Transformation The establishment of the transforming papovavirus-cell interaction requires high multiplicities of infection (10^6 to 10^7 particles per cell) (since the cells must either be nonpermissive or at least semipermissive, or the particles defective). There is evidence that the frequency of transformation is enhanced, by some as yet unknown mechanism, by treating cells with chemical carcinogens, such as 4-nitroquinoline-1-oxide. The

initial stages of the transforming virus-cell interaction are the same as those during the early phase of the lytic cycle: certain enzymes are synthesized at an increased rate, certain new enzymes are synthesized,° and host DNA is induced to replicate. Its essential feature is that parental viral DNA is stably integrated into the DNA of the host cell, and that in distinction to events in the lytic multiplication cycle, it is not excised from it. As a result it cannot multiply, and no infectious progeny virus is produced. By no means are all infected cells transformed in this manner; the majority are transformed abortively, that is, they escape from growth control for a few cell generations but then revert to the normal uninfected state for reasons that are not understood. The fixation of stable transformation requires at least one cell division. The number of sites in the host genome where viral DNA can be integrated is strictly limited, as can be shown readily by exposing cells to varying concentrations of wild-type virus and then inquiring whether additional viral genomes can still be integrated. The number of integrated viral genomes generally varies from 1 to 3 (with some reports ranging as high as 10 to 20), and all are located in human cells on chromosome 7. The fact that it is entire viral genomes that are integrated, and not genome portions or segments, is proved by two types of experiments. First, the papovavirus genome, particularly that of SV40, can be rescued from transformed cells — cells that contain no infectious virus and not even any viral capsid polypeptides — by fusing them with uninfected permissive cells. Fusion may be effected by simple cocultivation or, much more efficiently, by treatment with inactivated Sendai virus (Chap. 66). Apparently only the *cytoplasm* of permissive cells is necessary, since enucleated cells have been shown to rescue SV40. The mechanism of virus rescue is not understood. Among the possibilities are that the cytoplasm of permissive cells facilitates or effects excision of the viral from the host genome, or replication of viral DNA, or the synthesis and translation of viral messenger RNA. Not

---

°*One example is provided by thymidine kinase. The thymidine kinase present in human adult tissue differs from that present in fetal tissue. When adult human cells are infected with SV40, it is the fetal form of thymidine kinase that is synthesized, that is, a gene that is silent is derepressed.*

all lines of cells transformed by SV40 yield virus when fused to permissive cells. The reason why virus can quite often not be rescued is not known and it does not appear to depend on the number of viral genome copies that the cell harbors nor on the extent to which it is transcribed (p. 885). Sometimes virus is rescued from transformed cell lines by fusing not with uninfected permissive cells but with other lines of transformed cells (that also fail to yield virus on fusion with normal cells). The explanation here is probably that these are cells that are transformed by defective viral genomes and that on fusion they complement each other and recombine to yield wild-type virus.

The second line of evidence that shows that transformed cells harbor the entire viral genome is that infectious viral DNA can be extracted from them. This is a simpler and more efficient way of assaying for the presence of the intact viral genome in transformed cells than rescue of infectious virus by fusion. In fact, infectious viral DNA can be extracted from several cell lines in which rescue of virus cannot be effected by fusion.

Although viral DNA in stably transformed cells does not multiply except as part of the host genome, it does express itself. In fact, substantial amounts of mRNA are generally transcribed from it by the α-amanitin-sensitive cellular RNA polymerase II. The nature of this RNA has been analyzed in numerous independently isolated clones of transformed cells, using the techniques outlined in Chapter 67. Although it differs slightly in various clones, the major portion of it in all transformed cells corresponds to the early mRNA sequences transcribed in productively infected cells (Fig. 69-5).

While all cells transformed by papovaviruses exhibit the characteristics just discussed, individual clones of transformed cells display wide variations in biologic properties that span the entire range from normal cells on the one hand to standard transformants on the other. The reasons for these variations have not even begun to be explored.

Transformation by one papovavirus does not preclude transformation by another papovavirus nor by unrelated viruses. Thus, double transformants by SV40 and polyoma, as well as SV40 and adenovirus and SV40 and various RNA tumor viruses, have been isolated and studied. Rat cells infected (but not transformed) by Rauscher leukemia virus are more sensitive to transformation by SV40 than are normal cells.

REVERTANTS OF TRANSFORMED CELLS. Numerous attempts have been made to isolate revertants of transformed cells. Among the techniques that have led to the selection of cell lines that exhibit growth control comparable to that of normal cells are selection for serum dependence, passage at high dilution, resistance to nucleic acid-base analogs at high cell density (ie, inability to multiply at high cell density and resistance to con A. All these methods yield cells that display contact inhibition of growth and resemble normal cells morphologically. However, almost always they still synthesize the T antigen, display unaltered virus-specific transcription patterns, and contain the entire viral genome. Reversion is, therefore, due to a change in the cellular, rather than in the viral, genome. Revertants cannot be retransformed with the virus whose genome they already harbor but can be retransformed by other tumor viruses. Finally, revertant cell lines often contain more chromosomes than their transformed antecedents, which has suggested a hypothesis that the cell phenotype is modified as a result of changes in the relative amounts of chromosomes with genes that promote and genes that oppose transformation.

TEMPERATURE-SENSITIVE PAPOVAVIRUS MUTANTS. Several classes of ts mutants of SV40 and polyoma that are useful for studying their interaction with cells have been isolated. The most interesting is a class that is temperature-sensitive with respect to ability to maintain the transformed cell phenotype. Cells transformed with such mutants display the transformed phenotype at the permissive temperature (typically about 33C) and the normal phenotype at the restrictive temperature (typically about 39C), and they can be switched from one temperature to the other at will, with appropriate changes in phenotype. Expression of the transformed state is thus clearly dependent on the correct functioning of a viral gene product. Identification of this protein and definition of its mode of action are two of the primary aims of cancer research.

Adenoviruses

Adenoviruses also can transform animal cells in vitro, and some but not all cause tumors in animals. Many of the phenomena described for papovaviruses also hold for adenoviruses. For example, cells transformed by adenoviruses contain adenovirus DNA that is integrated into the host genome and that expresses itself partially as judged by the presence of viral messenger RNA and the synthesis of adenovirus-specific T antigen. Like papilloma virus they are noninducible. The adenovirus genome has not been rescued from transformed cells by any technique tested so far, including cell fusion.

Human adenoviruses comprise 31 serotypes that can be divided into three groups on the basis of their oncogenicity. Serotypes 12, 18, and 31 are highly oncogenic; when injected into newborn hamsters, they cause tumors rapidly and with high frequency. Serotypes 3, 7, 14, 16, and 21 are weakly oncogenic; they produce tumors in newborn hamsters with low frequency and after a long latent period. Most of the remaining serotypes, exemplified by serotypes 2 and 5, are nononcogenic, but even they can transform rodent cells in culture. All adenoviruses can also interact with cells by means of the lytic interaction, with growth cycles of rather long duration (peak titers at about 48 hours).

Human adenoviruses can also be divided into three subgroups according to the base composition of their DNA. The grouping so obtained coincides exactly with that obtained on the basis of their tumorigenic potential: The DNA of the highly oncogenic, weakly oncogenic, and nononcogenic groups of adenoviruses contains, on the average, 48, 52, and 58 percent G + C. The members within each group are very closely related, as judged by the ability of their genomes to hybridize with each other, but the three groups are only distantly related among themselves. In terms of numbers of genes, the adenovirus genome contains about 30 genes, the equivalent of at least 25 of which are shared by the members within each group, but only about 3 to 5 of which seem to be common to any two adenovirus subgroups.

Cells transformed by adenoviruses, or cells derived from tumors caused by adenoviruses, generally contain a small number, probably no more than one to three, adenovirus genomes. This corresponds to about 0.001 percent of the DNA in the cell. These integrated genomes are transcribed with very high frequency, for about 1 percent of the messenger RNA transcribed in such cells is adenovirus messenger RNA. The nature of this messenger RNA is currently being characterized with respect to the location on the adenovirus genome of the sequences from which it is transcribed. Under conditions of lytic infection, 10 to 20 percent of adenovirus DNA is transcribed during the early phase of the infection cycle. These segments are widely dispersed throughout the genome, and some are located on one DNA strand, others on the other. In transformed cells, between one-half and almost all of these early sequences, depending on the cell type, are transcribed, and no late mRNA sequences are ever transcribed in transformed cells. Interestingly enough, the sequences that are transcribed in cells transformed by highly, weakly, and nononcogenic adenoviruses are quite unrelated. The corresponding portions of the adenovirus genomes have evidently diverged very extensively during the course of evolution.

The demonstrated oncogenicity of human adenoviruses in rodents raises the possibility that they may cause neoplasia in man. This has been investigated using the exquisitely sensitive hybridization techniques that provided the quantitative data just discussed. This technique can be refined to such an extent that 1 part of viral DNA can be detected in the presence of 10^6 parts of host DNA, which corresponds to less than 1 adenovirus genome per cell. So far no human neoplasms have been found that contain adenovirus DNA.

Herpesviruses

Numerous herpesviruses are either oncogenic in animals, are associated with tumors, or can transform cells in vitro. At present, there is more evidence for a herpesvirus causing malignant disease in man than for any other virus.

Six herpesviruses are oncogenic in animals (Table 69-1). As for the situation in man, evidence is mounting that some forms of malignant disease may be caused by the following herpesviruses.

Epstein-Barr Virus   Burkitt lymphoma is a rather common disease in children of East Afri-

TABLE 69-1 ONCOGENIC ANIMAL HERPESVIRUSES

Virus	Host	Malignancy
Marek's disease virus (MDV)	Chicken	Neurolymphomatosis
Frog herpesvirus	Frog	Lucké adenocarcinoma
herpesvirus saimiri	Squirrel monkey	Lymphoma in marmoset
herpesvirus ateles	Spider monkey	Lymphoma in marmoset and owl monkey
herpesvirus sylvilagus	Cottontail rabbit	Lymphoma
Guinea pig virus	Guinea pig	Lymphocytic leukemia

ca, and it also occurs with low frequency in other parts of the world. In the body, the tumor cells contain no virus, but cell lines established from tumor cells almost always contain some 5 to 20 percent of cells that produce virus particles with the morphology, capsid protein constitution, and genome characteristics of a herpesvirus that is antigenically distinct from all known herpesviruses. This virus is known as Epstein-Barr virus (EB virus) after its discoverers.

EB virus causes lymphoma in marmosets and transforms human leukocytes. Normal human peripheral blood leukocytes do not multiply in vitro, but when exposed to EB virus, they are transformed into lymphoblastlike cells capable of indefinite growth. Such cells do not usually produce EB virus, but they can be stimulated to do so by arginine deprivation. Such treatment will also cause the proportion of producer cells in established lines of Burkitt lymphoma cells to increase and will also induce the virus to multiply in some Burkitt lymphoma cell lines that do not produce it spontaneously. EB viral DNA is present in Burkitt lymphoma cells in the body, as well as in the leukocytes transformed by it in vitro. This is readily demonstrated by DNA–DNA hybridization analysis. Usually, from 1 to 10 viral genome equivalents of DNA are present per cell. Interestingly, this DNA may not be integrated into the host cell genome as is papovavirus or adenovirus DNA but may exist free in a plasmidlike form.

EB virus DNA is present not only in Burkitt lymphoma cells but also in the cells of nasopharyngeal (postnasal) carcinoma, which occurs with rather high frequency in the Orient. It has not been found in numerous other human tumors.

EB VIRUS AND INFECTIOUS MONONUCLEOSIS. Sera from patients with Burkitt lymphoma and nasopharyngeal carcinoma contain antibodies to EB virus particles. Very surprisingly, about one-third of the normal adult population of the United States are also positive for EB virus antibodies. Conversion from the negative to the positive state occurs during the acute phase of infectious mononucleosis. Apparently, therefore, EB virus is the etiologic agent of infectious mononucleosis. Presumably, most infections with it are so mild as to go unnoticed, some others cause clinical mononucleosis of varying severity, and, very rarely, Burkitt lymphoma or nasopharyngeal carcinoma ensue. The reason why these tumors occur much more frequently in some parts or some populations of the world than in others is not known.

Herpes simplex virus Two types of Herpes simplex virus infect man: type 1, which causes primarily oral lesions, and type 2, which is associated with genital infections. Several lines of epidemiologic and serologic evidence suggest that carcinoma of the cervix may be caused by Herpes simplex virus type 2. Women with genital herpetic infections have a higher than average incidence of cervical carcinoma, women with cervical carcinoma have a higher than average incidence of antibodies to Herpes simplex virus type 2, and cervical carcinoma cells often contain antigens that react with antisera to Herpes simplex virus type 2. Further, there is one report of a cervical carcinoma containing about 40 percent of the Herpes simplex virus type 2 genome and RNA transcripts corresponding to about 5 percent of the viral DNA. It has also been found that Herpes simplex virus (as well as cytomegalovirus) can transform cultured cells when inactivated by UV irradiation (so as to preclude the productive, lytic virus-cellular interaction).

Although suggestive, all this evidence is not yet sufficient to establish a definitive causal relationship between herpes simplex virus and malignant disease in man. In fact, such a relationship will be very difficult to establish for two reasons: herpesviruses are ubiquitous, and herpesviruses tend to establish latent and persistent infections. Since experimentation with man is not feasible, the most direct evidence is likely to be provided by a vaccine that markedly reduces the incidence of some form of cancer.

Poxviruses

Two poxviruses are tumorigenic: fibroma virus (including the classical Shope fibroma virus, which is pathogenic for rabbits, as well as several closely related viruses pathogenic for deer, squirrels, and hares), and Yaba monkey tumor virus (pathogenic for several species of monkeys and man). Both produce benign tumors that soon regress (especially in the case of fibroma virus).

The interest in poxvirus tumorigenicity derives from the fact that poxviruses are DNA-containing viruses that have always been thought to multiply exclusively in the cytoplasm. Very recently acquired evidence suggests, however, that while vaccinia virus does not have an *obligatory* nuclear phase in its multiplication cycle (since it can multiply in enucleated cells), some viral DNA and RNA is often present in the nucleus early during the infectious cycle. Poxvirus DNA may therefore have the opportunity to become integrated into the host cell genome or to become otherwise stably associated with it, and when that happens, cell transformation may result. When fibroma virus transforms cells, host DNA replication is first arrested, and viral DNA replication is initiated. However, it quickly ceases, host DNA replication recommences, and the cells become transformed. They then multiply more rapidly than before, exhibit an altered morphology, are less sensitive to contact inhibition, and display new antigens on their surface. While the precise nature of the association of the fibroma and the host cell genome is not known, it is clear that it is not a very stable one, since the tumors often regress and contain fibroma virions when they do so.

RNA TUMOR VIRUSES

Interest in RNA tumor viruses has increased greatly in recent years because they cause leukemias and solid tumors in many animal species, including chickens, mice, hamsters, cats, and primates, that are often strikingly similar to certain human neoplasms. Indeed, evidence is coming to hand that antigenic determinants and nucleic acid sequences related to those of RNA tumor viruses of various animal species, as well as particles similar to typical RNA tumor virus particles, are present in a variety of human neoplasms.

RNA tumor viruses are enveloped particles that bud from the surface of the cells in which they multiply. They fall into two major classes on the basis of morphology. The first comprises the so-called C-type virus particles characteristic of most leukemia and sarcoma viruses. No free intracellular nucleocapsids are ever seen, and cores, presumably containing nucleocapsids and already bounded by a membrane, can only be detected immediately prior to budding. The released particles, the immature C-type particles, are characterized by three distinct layers or shells surrounding an electronlucent nucleoid. During the next several hours the morphology of these particles changes as they become converted to stable mature C-type particles that have an electron-dense nucleoid surrounded by two shells (Fig. 69-6). The first, or inner, shell consists of a membrane closely associated with a layer composed of regularly, seemingly icosahedrally, arranged capsomers. The second shell consists of a membrane, and spikes are attached to it.

The second class comprises the so-called B-type viral particles that are characteristic of the mammary tumor viruses (MTV). Here cores or nucleoids, the A particles, are often apparent in infected cells. B-type particles also mature extracellularly, as described above. The principal feature in which they differ from C-type particles is the eccentric rather than central location of their nucleoid in thin sections. Both B-type and C-type particles are covered with regularly spaced knobs, projections, or spikes. Those on the former are larger and more easily demonstrable.

The exact number of polypeptide species that make up RNA tumor viral particles is not known, and it is difficult to determine, since they contain much cell-derived membrane in which not all host proteins may be replaced by viral proteins. It is clear, however, that they contain at least seven species of virus-coded polypeptides (Table 69-2), two of which are glycoproteins that form the envelope glycopro-

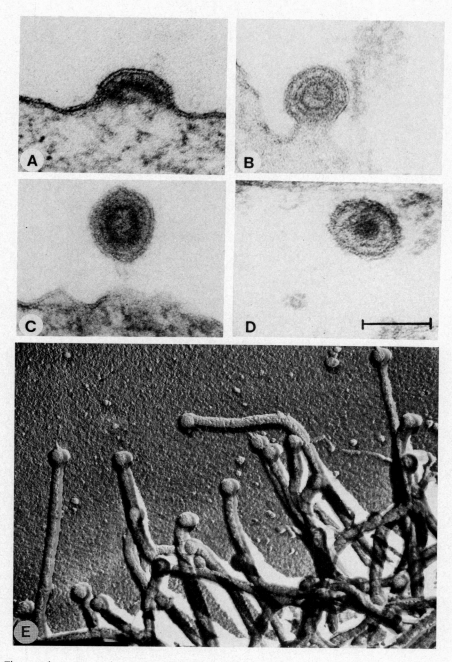

FIG. 69-6. The morphogenesis and structure of RNA tumor viruses. A–D. Four stages in the budding of a C-type (avian) RNA tumor virus. Note the electronlucent center or core in immature particles (B and C) and the electron-dense core in the mature particle (D). E. A micrograph of a surface replica of a GR cell that is producing murine mammary tumor virus (MMTV) particles (B-type RNA tumor virus). It shows the cell margin with microvilli, from the tips of which the virus buds. (Panels A–D, courtesy of Dr. Heinz Bauer; panel E, courtesy of Dr. J.B. Sheffield)

TABLE 69-2 C-Type RNA Tumor Viral Structural Proteins*

Protein†	Number per Virion‡	Location in Virion	Neutralizing Antibody	Antigenic Specificity§		
				Type	Group (Species)	Interspecies¶
Avian Viruses						
p10	1,250	Surface	−	?	?	?
p12	5,800	Core:RNA-associated	−	−	+	?
p15	3,200	Between core shell and surface	−	−	+	?
p19	3,600	Interior	−	+	+	?
p27	4,100	Core shell	*	−	+	?
gp37	350	Surface spike stalk		+	+	?
gp85	450	Surface spike knob	+	+	+	?
Mammalian Viruses						
p10		Core: RNA-associated	−	−	+	−
p12		Surface (?)	−	+	±	−
p15		Core	−	+	−	+
p15E		Surface	−	−	+	+
p30		Core shell	−	+	+	+
gp45		Surface (?)	?	?	?	?
gp71		Surface spike knob	+	+	+	+

*In principle, the structure of B-type RNA tumor viruses is similar to that of the C-type viruses. The major B-type viral structural proteins are p12, p18, p28, gp34, p42, gp55, and gp68. Gp55 is the major group-specific surface antigen; p28 is the major internal group-specific antigen. The number indicates the approximate size in daltons $\times 10^{-3}$. In addition to the seven proteins that are listed, each virion also contains about 70 molecules of the RNA-dependent DNA polymerase (reverse transcriptase)

†gp = glycoprotein; p = protein.

‡The numbers are approximate. The numbers of protein molecules with similar functions in mammalian and avian RNA tumor virus particles are comparable

§Type-specific: determinants that differentiate virus strains from each other

Group (species)-specific: determinants that are common to groups of viruses, such as those with the same host species

Interspecies-specific: determinants that are common to viruses with different host species

Note that the same protein may have one, two, or all three types of antigenic determinants

¶Not yet determined for avian RNA tumor viruses

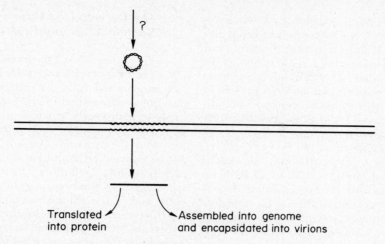

FIG. 69-7. Diagram depicting the molecular virology of RNA tumor viruses. The viral genome consists of two segments, each about 10,000 nucleotides long. These segments are transcribed into DNA on primers that are tRNA$_{trp}$ molecules, one of which is apparently hydrogen-bonded to each genome RNA segment, presumably at one end. The single-stranded DNA transcript covalently linked to tRNA$_{trp}$ is then converted, by unknown pathways, to circular double-stranded DNA molecules about 10,000 nucleotide base pairs long. The double-stranded circular DNA is then integrated into host DNA. The viral DNA genome expresses itself by being transcribed into RNA that can function as messenger RNA. When virus replicates, these RNA transcripts become encapsidated and reform the viral genome.

tein spikes. These polypeptides possess a variety of antigenic determinants, some of which are restricted to individual viral strains, others of which are common to groups of viruses with common hosts, while still others of which are present (in the case of mammalian C-type viruses) in all viruses (Table 69-2).° Antibody to the larger glycoprotein neutralizes the virus and can be used to immunize. Finally, RNA tumor viruses also contain a DNA polymerase capable of transcribing RNA, the so-called reverse transcriptase, which has been extensively purified and characterized.

The genome of all RNA tumor viruses is single-stranded RNA with a molecular weight of about 7×10^6, which, when subjected to denaturing conditions such as heating or exposure to dimethyl sulfoxide, dissociates into three to four subunits of about 3.5×10^6 daltons and several molecules of tryptophan-accepting transfer RNA. The two subunits are in all probability identical. In addition, RNA tumor viri-

°*However, there are no antigenic determinants common to mammalian C-type viruses, avian C-type viruses, and B-type viruses.*

ons generally contain about 100 other molecules of transfer RNA representing about 14 different amino acid-accepting species. The significance of their presence is not clear.

The Molecular Virology of RNA Tumor Viruses

There has long existed a conceptual difficulty concerning the role of RNA-containing viruses as oncogenic agents. Transformation represents a heritable alteration of cellular biosynthetic patterns that is most plausibly accounted for by a change in genetic capabilities. Mechanisms whereby a viral DNA genome might cause such changes after being integrated are conceivable, but how can a viral RNA genome achieve this? Furthermore, many cells transformed by RNA tumor viruses always produce virus for generation after generation — what type of mechanism could ensure that host and viral genome replication will proceed in step? In 1964 Temin advanced a revolutionary hypothesis: he proposed that on infection the viral RNA genome was transcribed into DNA by a reversal of the usual flow of information transfer, that this DNA was then integrated into the host cell genome, and that progeny viral genomes were transcribed from it just as all other RNA is normally transcribed. In essence, the hypothesis implied that the RNA present in RNA tumor viruses is not the genome but rather the messenger RNA of a genome that only exists intracellularly.

This scheme was supported by some experimental evidence. In particular, successful infection by and multiplication of all RNA tumor viruses was found to be absolutely dependent on DNA replication during the first five hours, and RNA tumor virus multiplication is always sensitive to agents that inhibit the transcription of DNA into RNA. The reason for these requirements became apparent when it was discovered that each RNA tumor virus particle contains about 70 molecules of a DNA polymerase, the so-called reverse transcriptase, that can transcribe RNA into DNA (Fig. 69-7). When RNA tumor viruses infect cells, this enzyme transcribes the viral RNA into double-stranded circular DNA molecules 6 to 7 $\times$ 10^6 daltons in size, the provirus, each apparently representing a transcript of an entire RNA subunit. These circles, which are synthesized in the cytoplasm, are then transported to the nucleus, where they are integrated into the host genome during the next several hours. Inhibitor studies have shown that circularization is a prerequisite for integration and that integration is a prerequisite for cell transformation and progeny virus formation. In general only one or two viral genome DNA equivalents are integrated into the host DNA, apparently adjacent to unique rather than repetitive sequences. Both free and integrated provirus DNA is infectious.

The RNA of progeny RNA tumor virus particles is most probably transcribed from the integrated proviral DNA and functions as messenger RNA. At least some of the polypeptides translated from it are synthesized in the form of larger precursors that are subsequently cleaved (Chap. 65).

RNA tumor viruses are generally not cytocidal but multiply in and bud from cells that are capable of continuous growth, both in the body and in vitro, either after causing morphologic transformation or without causing any detectable change.

The Detection of Virus-specific Nucleic Acids and Proteins in Cells

The extent to which integrated proviral DNA expresses itself varies widely. In infected and transformed cells that produce virus, the provirus is transcribed freely, but provirus also exists in many cells in which no virus is produced (p. 898), and in such cells either only a portion of the provirus is transcribed, or it may not be transcribed at all (that is, it may be completely silent). Definition of the amount and nature of RNA tumor viral genetic material in cells, and of the extent to which it expresses itself, is currently in the forefront of research aimed at identifying human tumor viruses. The techniques that are being used for this purpose are highly sensitive and sophisticated. For the detection of virus-specific nucleic acids, the ability of either highly labeled virion RNA or of highly labled DNA transcribed from it in vitro by the reverse transcriptase to hybridize with cellular DNA or with cellular messenger RNA is measured (Table 69-3). Conditions are readily arranged so that the amounts of nucleic acid

TABLE 69-3   MEASUREMENT OF VIRUS-SPECIFIC INTRACELLULAR NUCLEIC ACID

Nucleic Acids to be Measured	Technique
Virus-specific DNA integrated into the host genome	a. Measure the *rate* and *extent* of hybridization with highly labeled SS DNA transcribed from virion RNA (DNA probe). The rate is related to the amount of intracellular DNA and provides a measure of the *number* of viral genome equivalents present in each cell; the extent indicates whether the intracellular DNA corresponds to the entire, or to only part, of the viral genome
	b. Measure *rate* and *extent* of hybridization with highly labeled virion RNA by analogous techniques
Viral RNA transcripts	Measure *rate* and *extent* of hybridization with highly labeled DNA probe, as described above in a

that are detected can be expressed in terms of viral genome equivalents per cell. For the detection of virus-coded proteins, radioimmunoassays using pure viral polypeptides have been developed that can detect minute amounts of several structural capsid polypeptides and glycopolypeptides. As will be detailed on page 902, these techniques are now being applied intensively to the detection of the footprints of RNA tumor viruses in human cancers. They are also being used extensively in another very important area of viral oncology, namely, that of determining the genetic relationships among the many different RNA tumor viruses that have been, and that are still being, discovered.

The Pathology of RNA Tumor Viruses

The best studied RNA tumor viruses are the avian and mammalian ones. They cause primarily tumors of connective tissue (sarcomas) and of the hematopoietic and reticuloendothelial systems. The latter manifest themselves either as leukemias, when the blood contains large amounts of circulating tumor cells, or they may be aleukemic, the neoplasm being a solid mass of tumor cells in some organ. In chickens and cattle the leukemic and aleukemic hematopoietic neoplasms are often referred to as "leukoses." In many animals, such as fowl, rodents, cattle, cats, and so on, such neoplasms are the commonest malignancies, and sarcomas and leukemias are also the commonest neoplasms in young human beings. In human adults, carcinomas (malignant tumors of epithelial origin) are responsible for most cancer deaths, and the same is also true of other animals that often survive into old age (such as dogs and horses). RNA tumor viruses are implicated here also. It has long been known that the mouse mammary tumor virus, a B-type RNA tumor virus, causes mammary carcinoma, and renal adenocarcinomas occur in chickens infected with certain C-type RNA tumor viruses.

Biologic Properties of RNA Tumor Viruses

As pointed out in the preceding discussion, during an obligatory phase of the multipli-

cation cycle of RNA tumor viruses, their genome is proviral DNA integrated into the genome of the host. Numerous, and perhaps all, animal species harbor both C-type and B-type RNA tumor proviruses, which are transmitted vertically as dominant genetic traits, as are cellular genes. Frequently these viral genes express themselves during embryonic life, even to the extent of virion formation, without causing disease. They are then repressed, and virus is virtually undetectable in most young adults. Later on in life, however, they often begin to express themselves again. Virus particles then begin to be formed, and malignant disease results, probably because the newly produced virus particles transform the appropriate target cells into tumor cells. This process of spontaneous induction has been most intensively studied for both C-type and B-type RNA tumor viruses in the mouse, using for this purpose the large number of highly inbred mouse strains that are available, many of which were in fact bred specifically for the purpose of studying leukemia and mammary carcinoma. For C-type viruses, the ease with which virus can be induced is determined by at least two loci in the mouse genome, as well as by the nature of the virus. Mice of some strains, such as the C58 and Ak strains, develop leukemia between 6 and 18 months of age, and C3H mice develop mammary tumors early in life; these are so-called high-incidence mouse strains. Mice of other strains, such as the BALB/c and DBA strains, develop malignant disease only late in life and with low frequency; these are low-incidence mouse strains. Finally, mice of some strains, such as the NIH Swiss and NZB strains, do not develop leukemia at all.

Numerous both C-type and B-type RNA tumor virus strains have been isolated from spontaneously induced leukemias and mammary carcinomas, respectively. They are identified by the names of their discoverers (Table 62-4) and constitute the *exogenous* RNA tumor viruses. Numerous other proviruses of RNA tumor viruses do *not* express themselves spontaneously but can be induced to do so by a variety of inducing agents (p. 898), these are the *endogenous* RNA tumor viruses. Each of these two classes of C-type RNA tumor viruses will now be examined briefly in turn; for the B-type RNA tumor viruses, both will be considered together.

Exogenous C-type RNA Tumor Viruses

Leukemia/Leukosis Viruses　These are viruses that cannot transform cultured fibroblasts in vitro. Some leukemia/leukosis viruses can transform other types of cultured cells, but most cannot, and for most the primary target cell that is transformed in vivo is not known. The most studied leukemia/leukosis viruses are the avian and murine ones and, to a lesser extent, the feline ones. Avian leukemia/leukosis viruses are very widely spread, and many chickens are congenitally infected with them. They multiply in various cells of the body, causing a moderate viremia but no detectable ill effects. Eventually certain cells become transformed, giving rise to a variety of neoplasms. Among them are visceral lymphomas, leukemias (myeloblastosis and erythroblastosis), myelocytomas, nephroblastosis, and osteopetrosis.

The various strains of murine leukemia virus cause several types of leukemia, depending on a variety of factors, such as the age, sex, genetic constitution, and physiologic state of the animals when inoculated. Among them are erythroblastic leukemia of the spleen, myeloid leukemia of the spleen, lymphoblastic or lymphocytic leukemia of the thymus, and reticulum cell sarcoma of intestinal lymph nodes.

As for the feline leukemia viruses, they have created much interest because of their ability to cross species barriers. Leukemia, which generally takes the form of generalized lymphosarcoma, is one of the most frequent cancers in cats. Feline leukemia viruses also cause leukemia in dogs, and feline sarcoma viruses (p. 897) cause solid tumors in young rabbits, marmosets, and monkeys. This virus also readily grows in human cells.

The genetic relationships among the various leukemia/leukosis viruses are only now beginning to be explored. As judged by nucleic acid hybridization there are four distinct subgroups of murine leukemia viruses, whose prototypes are the Friend, Gross, Moloney, and Kirsten strains. Simian leukemia virus is related to these viruses, as is feline leukemia virus, to a lesser extent. The avian viruses are completely unrelated (Table 69-4).

Another method of grouping the avian, murine, and feline leukemia/leukosis viruses is according to host range, ability to interfere with each other's growth, and antigenic properties. This is illustrated particularly well in the case of chicken RNA tumor viruses, which, according to these criteria, fall into five subgroups. A, B, C, D, E.

Host Range.　The susceptibility of chick cells to infection depends upon the presence of receptor sites specific for each subgroup, which is determined in simple Mendelian manner by dominant alleles of autosomal loci. If receptors are lacking, the virus can adsorb but not penetrate, and the cells are therefore resistant. The phenotype of a cell is designated according to

TABLE 69-4　Genetic Relationships among Certain RNA Tumor Viruses*

Source of RNA†	Woolly Monkey Sarcoma Virus	KiSV	Source of DNA Probe Gross MLV	Rauscher MLV	FeLV	MMTV	AMV
	%	%	%	%	%	%	%
Woolly monkey sarcoma virus	100	82	10	8	2–5	0	0
KiSV	85	100	100	10	10	0	0
Gross MLV	6–10	47	100	10	14	0	0
Rauscher MLV	8	14	8	100	10	0	0
FeLV	1–3	4	6	6	100	0	0
MMTV	0	0	0	0	0	100	0
AMV	0	0	0	0	0	0	100

*KiSV is a sarcoma-leukemia virus with both rat and mouse history; MLV = murine leukemia virus; FeLV = feline leukemia virus; MMTV = mouse mammary tumor virus; AMV = avian myeloblastosis virus
†In each case the ability of virus-specific RNA to hybridize with single-stranded DNA probe complementary to the RNA of other viruses was measured. The numbers given are percentages, and the value for each homologous pair was taken to be 100 percent
Adapted from Gillespie and Gallo: Science 188:802, 1972

the virus subgroups that are excluded; thus C/O cells are susceptible to viruses of all five subgroups, C/A cells are susceptible to all except those of subgroup A, and so on.

ABILITY TO INTERFERE. The same grouping is obtained if the criterion is interference with the ability to multiply: Prior infection with a virus of the same subgroup prevents RNA tumor virus multiplications, apparently by preventing the superinfecting virus from penetrating effectively. Historically, this interference was discovered when a factor was detected in chickens that interfered with the ability of Rous sarcoma virus to form foci of transformed cells. This factor was first called RIF (Rous inhibitory factor) and was subsequently identified as one of several avian leukosis virus strains that were present in chickens as the result of congenital infection. RIF is now always avoided by screening cells for its absence.

ANTIGENIC PROPERTIES. The grouping of chick RNA tumor viruses into the five subgroups defined above is upheld by their immunologic properties, as judged by cross-reactions among their neutralizing antibodies. This suggests that all three criteria are expressions of the presence and functioning of the same macromolecules. Indeed, the antigen that gives rise to neutralizing antibody is the large glycoprotein gp85, and it is in all probability also the virus component that reacts with the host cell receptor system. It should be noted that while the three criteria just described separate viruses into subgroups, the members of each subgroup can be subdivided further, since their gp85s are not identical; they possess not only *subgroup* specificity but also individual *type* specificity, which can be detected and measured by immunofluorescence and radioimmunoassay procedures.

Among the feline leukemia viruses the situation is quite analogous. There are three subgroups, A, B, and C, as determined by host range and interference patterns. Among the murine RNA tumor viruses, however, the situation is different. Murine leukemia viruses fall into two serologic subgroups, the Gross-AKR subgroup and the Friend-Moloney-Rauscher (FMR) subgroup. Both belong to a single interference group, since virus infection with any mouse leukemia virus interferes with the mul-

tiplication of any subsequently infecting challenge virus. However, they belong to three host range subgroups on the basis of their ability to grow in NIH Swiss mice (N-tropic), in BALB/c mice (B-tropic), or in both (NB-tropic). These host ranges are *not* determined by the presence of specific virus envelope antigens, as in the avian virus system. Furthermore, in the mouse system, resistance, rather than susceptibility, is dominant.

Defective Leukemia Viruses Some leukemia viruses cannot multiply on their own, apparently because they cannot synthesize envelope antigens. They therefore require helper viruses to supply this missing function, and, as a consequence, they acquire the envelope of their helper as they bud through the plasma membrane. Examples of such viruses exist both among the avian and among the murine leukemia viruses. Thus, the murine Friend leukemia virus consists of two viruses, namely, the defective spleen focus-forming virus (SFFV), which causes erythroid cell transformation, and its helper, the nondefective lymphoid leukosis virus (LLV), which causes lymphoid leukemia.

Sarcoma Viruses Whereas cell transformation in vitro by leukemia/leukosis viruses is seldom if ever observed, sarcoma viruses readily transform cultured cells, especially fibroblasts. The efficiency with which they do so approaches 100 percent in 48 to 72 hours, which is far higher than the efficiency with which DNA tumor viruses transform cells.

Most avian sarcoma viruses are complete, that is, infectious on their own. However, there is one notable exception, the Bryan strain of Rous sarcoma virus (RSV). Consideration of the nature of its defect is of considerable interest and may well be relevant to the search for human cancer viruses.

The Bryan strain of RSV (BH-RSV) is a double-deletion mutant. It is defective in ability to code for reverse transcriptase, and it is defective in ability to code for its envelope antigens, especially gp85. When it infects chick cells in which the endogenous viral genome that all chick cells contain (Rous-associated virus-O[RAV-O]) does *not* express itself, particles, designated α, are produced in small numbers that lack reverse transcriptase and envelope glycoproteins and that are, therefore, not infectious. When it infects chick cells in which RAV-O does express itself at least to the extent of coding for its reverse transcriptase and its envelope glycoproteins (chick-helper factor-positive or chf⁺ cells) (p. 899), infectious viral particles, designated β, are produced—again in small numbers—that consist of the BH-RSV genome and the internal proteins, the gs antigens, for which it codes, and the reverse transcriptase and the envelope glycoproteins coded by RAV-O; such particles are described by the notation BH-RSV (RAV-O). Finally, when BH-RSV infects either chf⁻ or chf⁺ cells that are also infected with some avian leukosis virus (many of which have been isolated and which are designated RAV-1, RAV-2, RAV-3, and so on), large yields of a mixture of two types of virus particles are produced: the leukosis virus in question and BH-RSV particles that contain the reverse transcriptase and envelope glycoproteins of the leukosis virus, and that are therefore designated as BH-RSV (RAV-1, -2, -3, and so on).

It is important to note that, as in the case of defective DNA tumor viruses, BH-RSV transforms cells no matter whether the helper is present or not.

All mammalian sarcoma viruses are also defective; they transform fibroblasts in vitro, giving rise to cells that do not produce progeny virus (nonproducer cells). If such cells are superinfected with a leukemia virus, the sarcoma virus genome is rescued with the formation of particles that contain the sarcoma virus genome and gs antigens, and the leukemia virus envelope [MSV (MLV) and FeSV(FeLV) in the case of murine and feline viruses, respectively]. Rescue can be effected not only by leukemia viruses of the same species but also by those of different species [eg, MSV can be rescued by FeLV, giving rise to MSV (FeLV) particles that have the host range, interference patterns, and antigenic properties characteristic of FeLV but interact with cells genetically as MSV]. All mammalian sarcoma viruses are therefore pseudotypes, that is, viruses that possess their own genome and internal components but envelopes characteristic of a helper, and all mammalian sarcoma virus strains consist of two types of particles, the sarcoma virus pseudotype and the helper.

TRANSFORMATION-DEFECTIVE MUTANTS OF SARCOMA VIRUSES.   The ability of avian sarcoma viruses to transform chick embryo fibroblasts in vitro is correlated with possession of RNA subunits that are larger than those of leukemia-leukosis viruses. As described above, the RNA of RNA tumor viruses consists of two subunits that are probably identical. However, the subunits of sarcoma viruses, the *a* subunits, are some 5 to 10 percent larger than those of leukemia/leukosis viruses, the *b* subunits. The latter viruses only contain *b* subunits; the former frequently contain only *a* subunits, particularly when recently cloned, but also often contain *b* subunits. Two possibilities concerning the origin of these *b* subunits in sarcoma viruses are either that they represent subunits of an endogenous leukosis virus or that they arise from *a* subunits by deletion. It is known in this respect that transformation-defective variants of sarcoma viruses exist that possess only *b* subunits. Much interest is currently focused on the nature of genetic information that is present in *a* but absent in *b* subunits and the function of which appears to be the transformation of cultured fibroblasts.

Endogenous C-type RNA Tumor Viruses

Endogenous viral genomes can be induced by a variety of agents, including infection with some other RNA tumor virus, x-rays and ionizing radiation, inhibitors of protein synthesis, bromo- and 5-iododeoxyuridine (which must be incorporated into DNA before they will induce), chemical mutagens, and carcinogens. Often the efficiency of induction is enhanced by adrenal corticosteroid hormones. Endogenous viral genomes are also activated during skin graft rejection reactions, during the mixed lymphocyte culture reaction, when cells are transplanted into foreign species, and after prolonged culture in vitro. Strenuous efforts are currently being made along these lines to induce putative RNA tumor viruses in human neoplasms, so far without success.

There are two classes of endogenous RNA tumor viruses. The first consists of viruses that readily infect the cells from which they were induced; these are the ecotropic viruses. The second comprises viruses that cannot infect the cells from which they were induced but only cells of other species; these are the xenotropic viruses. Examples of both kinds are known among chicken, mouse, rat, hamster, pig, guinea pig, cat, and primate viruses. They are best studied in the mouse, where the availability of highly inbred, genetically pure, or almost pure, strains permits their detailed genetic analysis. Different mouse strains differ in the number of these viruses that they contain. There are some mouse strains with very few endogenous viruses, and indeed some, like the NIH Swiss strain, appear to contain no ecotropic viruses (although they do contain xenotropic ones), while other mouse strains harbor six or more ecotropic and xenotropic viruses. These viruses are usually under independent cellular genetic control, since they are often induced to different degrees in different cells, as well as by

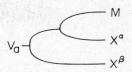

FIG. 69-8. Scheme depicting the relationships among the various groups of endogenous murine C-type RNA tumor viruses. V_a = the viral ancestor; M = ecotropic viruses; X^α = xenotropic viruses from BALB/c, AKR, and so on, mouse strains; X^β = xenotropic viruses from NIH Swiss and NZB/BINJ mouse strains. (After Callahan R, et al: J Virol 15:1378, 1975)

different inducing agents. Thus, inhibitors of protein synthesis and bromodeoxyuridine induce different endogenous viruses in some mouse cells. Endogenous RNA tumor viruses are of the leukemia/leukosis type; there are several that cause lymphoblastic leukemia, others that cause myelogenous leukemia, and so on. One endogenous virus transforms the cells in which it can be induced and produces carcinomas when injected into syngeneic mice. Interestingly, endogenous RNA tumor viruses induce high levels of neutralizing antibodies after induction.

Recently it has been found that mouse strains with different incidences of spontaneous leukemia possess different numbers of endogenous RNA tumor virus genomes (Table 69-5). High-incidence mice contain several leukemia virus genomes as well as 7 to 8 partially related ones, low-incidence mice contain only one to two leukemia virus genomes and seven to eight partially related ones, while mice from which no ecotropic virus can be induced, such as NIH Swiss mice, contain only the latter type of genomes. Presumably, these genomes, which share only some sequences with leukemia viruses, are the genomes of xenotropic viruses.

All these viruses are now beginning to be examined by nucleic acid hybridization and serologic techniques in order to establish their genetic relationships. It appears that although all endogenous murine viruses are quite closely related, they do fall into three even more closely related groups, one comprising all the ecotropic viruses, and the other two the xenotropic ones (Fig. 69-8). Other xenotropic RNA tumor viruses are quite unrelated to the exogenous and ecotropic viruses to which the cells in which they exist are susceptible; for example, the cat endogenous viruses RD114

TABLE 69-5 NUMBER OF RNA TUMOR VIRAL GENOMES PRESENT IN THE GENOMES OF VARIOUS MOUSE STRAINS

Mouse Strain*	Type M†	Type L‡
High-virus Strains		
AKR-J	7 – 8	3 – 4
C3H/FgLw	7 – 8	3 – 4
Low-virus Strains		
BALB/cN	7 – 8	1 – 2
DBA/2N	7 – 8	1 – 2
C3H/HcN	7 – 8	1 – 2
C57BL/6J	7 – 8	1 – 2
Nonvirus Strains		
NIH Swiss	7	0
129/J	10	0
NZB/N	7 – 8	0

*High-virus and low-virus strains are those in which spontaneous leukemia occurs with high and low frequency (high and low incidence), respectively; nonvirus strains are those in which leukemia neither occurs nor can be induced

†SS DNA complementary to AKR virus RNA was used as the probe (Table 69–3). Type M (for more abundant) genomes, which most probably comprise several different species, are partially related to AKR virus; not only are there some sequences that are not shared at all, but many of the sequences that are shared do not match exactly

‡SS DNA complementary to AKR RNA was used as the probe here also. Type L (for less abundant) genomes are identical to AKR RNA as far as one can tell

All mice thus contain RNA tumor virus genomes that are related to AKR virus. All mice contain 7–8 copies of genomes that are only partially related; presumably these are the xenotropic ones. In addition high- and low-virus mice also contain viral genomes of the AKR type, the former containing 2–3 times as many as the latter.

Adapted from Lowy et al. Proc Natl Acad Sci USA 71:355, 1974

TABLE 69-6   NATURE OF THE ENDOGENOUS TUMOR VIRUS GENOMES PRESENT IN THE DNA OF VARIOUS BIRDS

Species	Extent of Hybridization*	Copies per Haploid Genome
	%	
Chicken	100	1–2
Japanese quail	8	3
Pigeon	12	0.5
Peking duck	10	6
Ring-necked pheasant	50	10

Adapted from Tereba et al: Virology 65:524, 1975
*The DNA probe (Table 69-3) that was used here was that of RAV-0, the principal, if not the only, endogenous (ecotropic) RNA tumor virus of chickens. The extent of hybridization measures the fractions (in percent) of RAV-0 sequences that are present in the various cellular genomes

and CCC are unrelated to feline leukemia/sarcoma viruses but very closely related to a baboon endogenous virus (which is itself unrelated to the ecotropic woolly monkey/gibbon ape viruses), as well as to an endogenous virus isolated from a fetal mouse. The presence of such very closely related viral genomes in the DNA of such dissimilar animal species poses fascinating problems in evolutionary history.

The Existence of Provirus Fragments in Cellular Genomes

Cellular genomes contain not only intact proviruses, but also provirus fragments. This has been well studied in several avian species. Table 69-6 shows that pheasants, Japanese quail, ducks, and pigeons all contain small numbers (0.5 to 10 per cell) of provirus fragments of the endogenous chicken virus RAV-O. The significance of the presence of such provirus fragments is not clear at this time.

Mouse Mammary Tumor Virus (MMTV)

Several strains of MMTV exist that differ slightly genetically but differ markedly in the extent to which they express themselves. The most familiar is the milk factor of Bittner (1936), a strain that is resident in C3H and A mice (high-incidence strains), expresses itself in all cells of its hosts, and is present in particularly large amounts in lactating mammary tissue and, therefore, in milk. As a result, it is passed on

readily to progeny animals, in which it produces mammary adenocarcinomas with high frequency early in life (generally at between 6 and 12 months). It is also passed on to animals of low-incidence strains when they are reared by foster mothers of the C3H and A strains and produces tumors with high frequency in them also.

The other MMTV strains express themselves far less readily; they are not present in large amounts in milk and are transmitted vertically through the gametes. They are also much less oncogenic; they cause tumors with low frequency late in life. They are resident in both low- and high-incidence mouse strains; their presence in the latter is demonstrated by the fact that they develop adenocarcinomas late in life even when they are freed of the milk factor by being nursed by foster mothers of low-incidence strains.

Until very recently, no cultured cell line was known in which MMTV could be grown. As a result, it had to be assayed by injecting virus into newborn mice and waiting for the 6 to 12 months before tumors developed. Recently it has been found that MMTV will multiply in a feline kidney cell line, and it should now be possible to develop a much more efficient and rapid assay in them.

Mice of high- and low-incidence strains contain similar numbers of MMTV proviruses in their genomes (2 to 10). However they are transcribed to very different degrees. In virus-producing tumors and lactating mammary tissue of high-incidence mouse strains there are from 100 to 1,000 genome equivalents of MMTV RNA per cell, in tumors of low-incidence mouse strains only 1 to 2, and in livers and spleens from either high- or low-incidence mouse strains, that is, in cells that never become transformed and never produce MMTV, there are 0.1 to 1 genome equivalents of viral RNA per cell. These levels of transcription correlate with the extent of virus production and indicate that the primary control of MMTV gene expression occurs at the level of transcription. The factors that actually regulate the transcription of MMTV provirus are both host genetic and hormonal. A mendelian gene with a dominant allele for MMTV expression is known. Estrogens enhance the development of mammary cancer (which normally occurs only in female mice but can be induced by estrogens in male mice of high-incidence strains), and glucocorticoids increase greatly the degree of MMTV provirus transcription and the level of

MMTV formation in lactating mammary tissue cells, and mammary tumor cells but are unable to effect significant increases in other mouse cells.

A-type Particles

Certain mouse cells contain particles with toroidal (ring-shaped) nucleoids enclosed by a membrane (Fig. 69-9). These particles occur in two locations. In cells that produce B-type RNA tumor virus particles, they are found in the cytoplasm; these intracytoplasmic particles have long been thought to be the precursors of B-type particles, but strong evidence in favor of this hypothesis is lacking. In fact, there are recent reports that their RNA, although 70 S, does not hybridize with the RNA of the B-

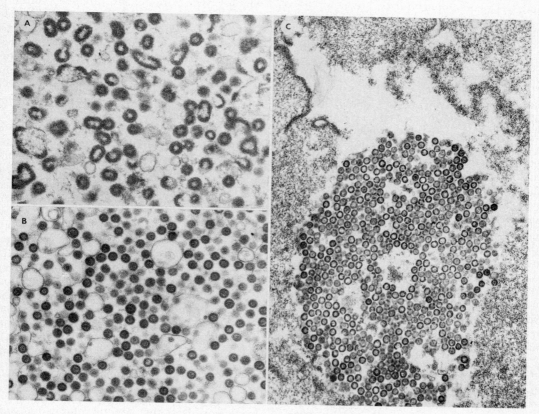

FIG. 69-9. A-type particles. A. Intracisternal A particles, extracted from mouse plasma cell tumor MOPC 104E and partially purified by sucrose density gradient centrifugation. × 70,000. B. Intracytoplasmic A particles from a mouse mammary tumor and partially purified by sucrose density gradient centrifugation. ×53,000. C. Intracytoplasmic A particle inclusion in the nuclear pellet fraction of a homogenate of a mouse mammary tumor. ×35,000 (Courtesy of Dr. N. A. Wivell)

type particles produced by the cells in which they occur.

The second common location in which A-type particles occur is in myeloma cells, in which they are located intracisternally. These intracisternal A-type particles contain a DNA polymerase as well as 70 S RNA which has been reported to be partially homologous to the RNA of murine sarcoma virus/leukemia viruses. Their biologic significance is not known.

Neither class of A-type particles has yet been found to be infectious.

THE ROLE OF VIRUSES IN ONCOGENESIS

A large number of both RNA-containing and DNA-containing viruses are now known that can cause cancer in animals. Nevertheless, viruses can rarely be demonstrated in the majority of naturally occurring cancers. Even in those cases where a virus can be shown to cause tumors reproducibly and with high efficiency and where it can then be recovered from the tumor, we are totally ignorant of how the virus actually transforms cells. The most hopeful approach to defining the specific role of the viral genome in the transformation process is probably provided by studies of virus mutants that are temperature-sensitive with respect to their ability to maintain the transformed phenotype. Since these are in all probability single-step mutants, their lesions presumably reside in a single polypeptide coded by them, and it should be possible to characterize it. Unfortunately, no assay for this protein has yet been devised, and nothing is known concerning the regulation of its expression and the conditions necessary for it to function. Nor is it known what its target is. A much fuller understanding of the animal cell will be required before any of these questions can be answered.

A further level of complexity is introduced by the discovery that genetic material harboring information for triggering oncogenic transformation in the form of proviruses is part of the genomes of many, if not all, animal species. The potential for developing malignant disease is thus quite clearly passed on vertically from generation to generation. This mode of trans-

mitting the potential for cancer is far more important in nature than is horizontal spread of malignant disease in all except very few cases (such as mammary tumors in mice induced by the milk factor, feline leukemia, and Marek's disease and Rous sarcomas in chickens).

The significance of the induction of proviruses in tumorigenesis is only imperfectly understood. The induction of tumors by chemical carcinogens is often accompanied by the induction of proviruses and the appearance of mature RNA tumor virus particles. It has therefore been proposed that the carcinogens merely induce the virus and that the tumor is caused by the virus. However, chemical carcinogens can sometimes induce malignancy without inducing a provirus. It should also be noted in this connection that induction of proviruses is not invariably followed by tumorigenesis. Thus, as noted before (p. 895), many cells are known in which C-type particles are produced continuously, yet they are not transformed, and lactating mouse mammary tissue produces large amounts of B-type particles, yet it is not tranformed. Clearly the induction of cancer requires target cells in which the viral protein that induces and maintains the tumor cell phenotype is not only formed but can also function.

Two theories have been advanced that seek to account for the origin of RNA tumor viruses and their role in oncogenicity. The oncogene theory of Huebner and Todaro proposes that all cells contain in their DNA information necessary for the synthesis of RNA tumor viruses. This is the virogene, parts of which may be expressed normally, for example, in development. Part of the virogene is the oncogene, which is responsible for most tumors. This information is normally repressed, presumably by cellular factors, but when this regulation breaks down, the oncogene function is expressed, and the cell is transformed. Oncogene and virogene are postulated to be independently regulated, which would account for the existence of tumor cells that do not contain or produce virus and normal cells that release RNA tumor virus particles.

The protovirus theory of Temin, on the other hand, postulates that genetic information constantly flows from RNA to DNA as well as from DNA to RNA, thereby providing the opportunity for gene duplication and gene modification.

The protovirus would arise if genetic information at some state acquired an independently stable form, and mutation and recombination might then lead to the appearance of genes capable of transforming cells. The protovirus theory thus postulates that oncogenes are generated continuously.

There is some evidence in favor of each of these two theories, but it is not sufficient to permit a clear-cut decision to be made as to which, if either, is correct.

Do Viruses Cause Cancer in Man?

What assessment can be made at this time of the role of viruses in carcinogenesis in man? No causal relationship has been demonstrated, and it may well be that the most direct evidence concerning the etiologic role of some virus will be the demonstration that vaccination against it lowers the incidence of some form of cancer.

In the meantime, attention is focused on attempts to detect the presence of viral genetic material or of its expression in human tumor cells. As pointed out previously (p. 888), the evidence is best concerning the herpesvirus EB virus, the genome of which is certainly present in Burkitt lymphoma and nasopharyngeal carcinoma cells, but the greatest effort is being directed at the possible involvement of RNA tumor viruses. The evidence currently is as follows.

(1) C-type RNA tumor viruses have been isolated from monkeys and apes, both from spontaneous neoplasms and from normal tissue. None have yet been shown to be tumorigenic, and some are clearly xenotropic. They fall into two groups of closely related viruses, those from old world monkeys (baboon virus (M7) /RD114 group) and those from new world monkeys (the woolly monkey/gibbon ape group). Further, viruses with characteristics intermediate between those of B-type and C-type particles have been isolated from mammary carcinomas in Rhesus monkeys (MP virus).

(2) Particles that contain 70 S RNA and a reverse transcriptase appear to occur in many human neoplasms. In some cases, these have been reported to possess the morphology of typical C-type particles, and there is one report of a *normal* human tissue (placenta) containing such particles.

(3) Human leukemic cells have been reported to possess DNA sequences at least partially homologous to murine leukemia viral RNA. It has also been shown that the DNA of leukemic twins contains sequences not present in nonleukemic twins, a result that implies that the malignancy was the result of an infection, rather than activation of an oncogene. Further, the RNA of both groups of monkey/primate C-type viruses, that is, the baboon (M7)/RD114, as well as the woolly monkey/gibbon ape groups, hybridizes weakly but unmistakably with human DNA.

(4) Normal human tissue contains antigens that cross-react with gs proteins of viruses of both these groups. Malignant human tissue contains similar amounts of the same antigens, which suggests that the virus that codes for them is not the etiologic agent of the malignant disease. However, tissues of patients with systemic lupus erythematosus contain markedly elevated levels of these antigens. A possible role for RNA tumor viruses in the etiology of this disease in mice has been suggested on the basis of a close correlation between the occurrence and expression of endogenous RNA tumor viruses and the severity of the lupus syndrome.

(5) A C-type RNA tumor virus closely related to woolly monkey/gibbon ape virus was recently isolated from cutured human acute myelogenous leukemia (AML) cells. In fact, this virus has now been isolated twice from human AML cells and only once from a woolly monkey. It may therefore be a human, rather than a monkey, virus.

(6) Particles containing 70 S RNA and the reverse transcriptase have been found in human milk. DNA synthesized by such particles has been reported to possess homology to murine mammary tumor virus (MMTV) RNA. Further, RNA from malignant human breast tumors possesses sequence homology with the RNA of the MP viruses of rhesus monkeys.

In summary, while no RNA tumor virus with oncogenic potential has yet been isolated from human tissue, evidence is mounting that man does harbor endogenous RNA tumor viruses, just like all other mammalian and avian species that have been examined. Continued intensive attempts to isolate these viruses and to assess their tumorigenic potential will constitute one of the most important segments of our attempt to conquer cancer.

FURTHER READING

Books and Reviews

GENERAL

Cairns HJF: Mutation, selection and the natural history of cancer. Nature 255:197, 1975

Eckhart W: Genetics of DNA tumor viruses. Annu Rev Genetics 8:301, 1974

Gillespie D, Gallo RC: RNA processing and RNA tumor virus origin and evolution. Science 188:802, 1975

Gross L: Facts and theories on viruses causing cancer and leukemia. Proc Natl Acad Sci USA 71:2013, 1974

Lindenmann J: Viruses as immunological adjuvants in cancer. Biochim Biophys Acta 355:49, 1974

McAllister RM: Viruses in human carcinogenesis. Prog Med Virol 16:48, 1973

Tooze J (ed): The Molecular Biology of Tumor Viruses. Cold Spring Harbor Laboratory, 1973

Tooze J, Sambrook J (eds): Selected Papers in Tumor Virology. Cold Spring Harbor Laboratory, 1974

CELL TRANSFORMATION

Dulbecco R: Cell transformation by viruses. Science 166:962, 1969

Hakomori SI: Glycolipids of tumor cell membranes. Adv Cancer Res 18:265, 1973

Rafferty KA Fr: Epithelial cells: Growth in culture of normal and neoplastic forms. Adv Cancer Res 21:249, 1975

Rapin AC, Burger MM: Tumor cell surfaces: General alterations detected by agglutinins. Adv Cancer Res 20:1, 1974

PAPOVAVIRUSES

Levine AJ: The replication of papovavirus DNA. Prog Med Virol 71:1, 1974

Salzman NP, Khoury G: Reproduction of papovaviruses. In Fraenkel-Conrat H, Wagner RR (eds): Comprehensive Virology. New York and London, Plenum Press, 1974, vol 3, p 63

ADENOVIRUSES

Merkow LP, Slifkin M (eds): Oncogenic Adenoviruses. Basel, S. Karger, 1972

Philipson L, Lindberg U: Reproduction of papovaviruses. In Fraenkel-Conrat H, Wagner RR (eds): Comprehensive Virology. New York and London, Plenum Press, 1974, vol 3, p 143

HERPESVIRUSES

Epstein MA, Achong BG: The EB Virus. Annu Rev Microbiol 27:413, 1973

Kaplan AS (ed): The Herpesviruses. New York and London, Academic Press, 1973

Rapp F: Herpesviruses and cancer. Adv Cancer Res 19:265, 1974

Roizman B, Furlong D: Reproduction of herpesviruses. In Fraenkel-Conrat H, Wagner RR (eds): Comprehensive Virology. New York and London, Plenum Press, 1974, vol 3, p 229

RNA TUMOR VIRUSES

Bader JP: Reproduction of RNA tumor viruses. In Fraenkel-Conrat H, Wagner RR (eds): Comprehensive Virology. New York and London, Plenum Press, 1975, vol 4, p 253

Bauer H: Virion and tumor cell antigens of C-type RNA tumor viruses. Adv Cancer Res 20:275, 1974

Bolognesi DP: Structural components of RNA tumor viruses. Adv Virus Res 19:315, 1974

Hirsch MS, Black PH: Activation of mammalian leukemia viruses. Adv Virus Res 19:265, 1974

Lilly F, Pincus T: Genetic control of murine viral leukemogenesis. Adv Cancer Res 17:231, 1973.

Moore DH: Evidence in favor of the existence of human breast cancer virus. Cancer Res 34:2322, 1974

Schafer W, Demsey A, Frank H, et al: Morphological, chemical and antigenic organization of mammalian C-type viruses. In Ito Y, Dutcher RM (eds): Comparative Leukemia Research 1973, Leukemogenesis. Tokyo, Univ of Tokyo Press, and Basel, Karger, 1975, p 497

Temin HM: On the origin of RNA tumor viruses. Annu Rev Genetics 8:155, 1974

Selected Papers

CELL TRANSFORMATION

Christman JK, Acs G: Purification and characterization of a fibrinolytic factor associated with oncogenic transformation: The plasminogen activator from SV40-transformed hamster cells. Biochim Biophys Acta 340:339, 1974

Dulbecco R, Elkington J: Conditions limiting multiplication of fibroblastic and epithelial cells in dense cultures. Nature 246:197, 1973

Greenberger JS, Aaronson SA: Morphologic revertants of murine sarcoma virus transformed nonproducer BALB/3T3: Selective techniques for isolation and biologic properties in vitro and in vivo. Virology 57:339, 1974

Holly RW, Kiernan JA: Control of the initiation of DNA synthesis in 3T3 cells: Serum factors. Proc Natl Acad Sci USA 71:2908, 1974

Nomura S, Dunn KI, Mattern CFT, Hartley JW, Fischinger PJ: Revertants of mouse cells transformed by murine sarcoma virus: Flat variants without a rescuable sarcoma virus from a clone of BALB/3T3 transformed by Kirsten MSV. J Gen Virol 25:207, 1974

Otten J, Johnson GS, Pastan I: Regulation of cell growth by cyclic adenosine 3',5'-monophosphate. J Biol Chem 247:7082, 1972

Stone KR, Smith RE, Joklik WK: Changes in membrane polypeptides that occur when chick embryo fibroblasts and NRK cells are transformed with avian sarcoma viruses. Virology 58:86, 1974

Yogeeswaran G, Hakomori S: Cell contact-dependent ganglioside changes in 3T3 fibroblasts and a suppressed sialidase activity on cell contact. Biochemistry 14:2151, 1975

PAPOVAVIRUSES

Brockman WW, Gutai MW, Nathans D: Evolutionary variants of simian virus 40: Characterization of cloned, complementing variants. Virology 66:36, 1975

Eisinger M, Kucarova O, Sarkar NH, Good RA: Propagation of human wart virus in tissue culture. Nature 256: 432, 1975

Frenkel N, Lavi S, Winocour E: The host DNA sequences in different populations of serially passaged SV40. Virology 60:9, 1974

Khoury G, Martin MA, Lee TNH, Nathans D: A transcriptional map of the SV40 genome in transformed cell lines. Virology 63:263, 1975

Koprowski H, Jensen FC, Steplewski Z: Activation of production of infectious tumor virus SV40 in heterokaryon cultures. Proc Natl Acad Sci USA 58:127, 1967

Lai C, Nathans D: Mapping temperature-sensitive mutants of simian virus 40: Rescue of mutants by fragments of viral DNA. Virology 60:366, 1974

Lancaster WD, Meinke W: Persistence of viral DNA in human cell cultures infected with human papilloma virus. Nature 256:434, 1975

Lebowitz P, Kelly TJ, Nathans D, Lee THN, Lewis AM: A colinear map relating the simian virus 40 (SV40) DNA segments of six adenovirus-SV40 hybrids to the DNA fragments produced by restriction endonuclease cleavage of SV40 DNA. Proc Natl Acad Sci USA 71: 441, 1974

Pett DM, Estes MK, Pagano JS: Structural proteins of simian virus 40. 1. Histone characteristics of low-molecular-weight polypeptides. J Virol 15:379, 1975

Risser R, Pollack R: A nonselective analysis of SV40 transformation of mouse 3T3 cells. Virology 59:477, 1974

Sambrook J, Sugden B, Keller W, Sharp PA: Transcription of simian virus 40. III. Mapping of "early" and "late" species of RNA. Proc Natl Acad Sci USA 70:3711, 1974

Sambrook J, Westphal H, Srinivasan PR, Dulbecco R: The integrated state of viral DNA in SV40-transformed cells. Proc Natl Acad Sci USA 60:1288, 1968

Shani N, Huberman E, Aloni Y, Sachs L: Activation of simian virus 40 by transfer of isolated chromosomes from transformed cells. Virology 61:303, 1974

ADENOVIRUSES

Doerfler W: Integration of the deoxyribonucleic acid of adenovirus type 12 into the deoxyribonucleic acid of baby hamster kidney cells. J Virol 6:652, 1970

Gallimore PH, Sharp PA, Sambrook J: Viral DNA in transformed cells. II. A study of the sequences of adenovirus 2 DNA in nine lines of transformed rat cells using specific fragments of the viral genome. J Mol Biol 89:49, 1974

Graham FL, van der Eb AJ, Heijneker HJ: Size and location of the transforming region in human adenovirus type 5 DNA. Nature 251:687, 1974

Lewis JB, Atkins JF, Anderson CW, Baum PR, Gesteland RF: Mapping of late adenovirus genes by cell-free translation of RNA selected by hybridization to specific DNA fragments. Proc Natl Acad Sci USA 72:1344, 1975

Mulder C, Sharp PA, Delius H, Pettersson U: Specific fragmentation of DNA of adenovirus serotypes 3, 5, 7, and 12, and adeno-simian virus 40 hybrid virus Ad2+ND1 by restriction endonuclease R *Eco* RI. J Virol 14:68, 1974

HERPESVIRUSES

Adams A, Lindahl T: Epstein-Barr virus genomes with properties of circular DNA molecules in carrier cells. Proc Natl Acad Sci USA 72:1477, 1975

Anzai T, Dressman GR, Courtney RJ, et al: Antibody to herpes simplex virus type 2-induced nonstructural proteins in women with cervical cancer and in control groups. J Natl Cancer Inst 54:1051, 1975

Duff R, Rapp F: Oncogenic transformation of hamster embryo cells after exposure to inactivated herpes simplex virus type 1. J Virol 12:209, 1973

zur Hausen H, Schulte-Holthausen H, Klein G, et al: EBV DNA in biopsies of Burkitt tumor and anaplastic carcinomas of the nasopharynx. Nature 228:1056, 1970

zur Hausen H, Schulte-Holthausen H, Wolf H, Dörries K, Egger H: Attempts to detect virus-specific DNA in human tumors. II. Nucleic acid hybridization with complementary RNA of human herpes group viruses. Int J Cancer 13:657, 1974

Henle G, Henle W, Diehl V: Relation of Burkitt's tumor-associated herpes-type virus to infectious mononucleosis. Proc Natl Acad Sci USA 59:94, 1968

Klein G, Giovanella BC, Lindahl T, et al: Direct evidence for the presence of Epstein-Barr virus DNA and nuclear antigen in malignant epithelial cells from patients with poorly differentiated carcinoma of the nasopharynx. Proc Natl Acad Sci USA 71:4737, 1974.

RNA TUMOR VIRUSES

Aaronson SA, Hartley JW, Todaro GJ: Mouse leukemia virus: "spontaneous" release by mouse embryo cells after long-term in vitro cultivation. Proc Natl Acad Sci USA 64:87, 1969

Benveniste RE, Todaro GJ: Evolution of type C viral genes: I. Nucleic acid from baboon type C virus as a measure of divergence among primate species. Proc Natl Acad Sci USA 71:4513, 1974

Callahan R, Lieber MM, Todaro GJ: Nucleic acid homology of murine xenotropic type C viruses. J Virol 15: 1378, 1975

Chattopadhyay SK, Lowy DR, Teich MM, Levine AS, Rowe WP: Evidence that the AKR murine-leukemia-virus genome is complete in DNA of the high-virus AKR mouse and incomplete in the DNA of the "virus-negative" NIH mouse. Proc Natl Acad Sci USA 71:167, 1974

Chattopadhyay SK, Rowe WP, Teich NM, Lowy DR: Definitive evidence that the murine C-type virus inducing locus *Akv-1* is viral genetic material. Proc Natl Acad Sci USA 72:906, 1975

Colcher D, Spiegelman S, Schlom J: Sequence homology between the RNA of Mason-Pfizer monkey virus and the RNA of human malignant breast tumors. Proc Natl Acad Sci USA 71:4775, 1974

Cooper GM, Temin HM: Infectious Rous sarcoma virus and reticuloendotheliosis virus DNAs. J Virol 14:1132, 1974

Duesberg PH, Vogt PK: RNA species obtained from clonal lines of avian sarcoma and from avian leukosis virus. Virology 54:207, 1973.

East JL, Knesek JE, Chan JC, Dmochowski L: Quantitative nucleotide sequence relationships of mammalian RNA tumor viruses. Virol 15:1396, 1975

Fischinger PJ, Nomura S: Efficient release of murine xenotropic oncornavirus after murine leukemic virus infection of mouse cells. Virol 65:304, 1975

Gallagher RE, Gallo RC: Type C RNA tumor virus isolated from cultured human acute myelogenous leukemia cells. Science 187:350, 1975

Gerard GF, Loewenstein PM, Green M, Rottman F: Detection of reverse transcriptase in human breast tumours with Poly (Cm) · Oligo (dG). Nature 256:140, 1975

Greenberger JS, Stephenson JR, Moloney WC, Aaronson SA: Different hematological diseases induced by type C viruses chemically activated from embryo cells of different mouse strains. Cancer Res 35:245, 1975

Hayward WS, Hanafusa H: Recombination between endogenous and exogenous RNA tumor virus genes as analyzed by nucleic acid hybridization. J Virol 15:1367, 1975

Huebner RJ, Todaro GJ: Oncogenes of RNA tumor viruses as determinants of cancer. Proc Nat Acad Sci USA 64:1087, 1969

Huebner RJ, Kelloff GJ, Sarma PS, et al: Group-specific antigen expression during embryogenesis of the genome of the C-type RNA tumor virus: Implications for ontogenesis and oncogenesis. Proc Natl Acad Sci USA 67:366, 1970

Igel HJ, Huebner RJ, Turner RC, Kotin P, Falk HL: Mouse leukemia virus activation by chemical carcinogens. Science 166:1624, 1969

Kalter SS, Helmke RJ, Heberling RL, et al: C-type particles in normal human placentas. J Natl Cancer Inst 50:1081, 1973

Lieber MM, Sherr CJ, Todaro GJ, et al: Isolation from the Asian mouse *Mus caroli* of an endogenous type C virus related to infectious primate type C viruses. Proc Natl Acad Sci USA 72:2315, 1975

Parks WP, Ransom JC, Young HA, Scolnick EM: Mammary tumor virus induction by glucocorticoids. Characterization of specific transcriptional regulation. J Biol Chem 250:3330, 1975

Proffitt MR, Hirsch MS, Black PH: Murine leukemia: A virus-induced autoimmune disease? Science 182:821, 1973

Rapp UR, Nowinski RC, Reznikoff CA, Heidelberger C: Endogenous oncornaviruses in chemically induced transformation. 1. Transformation independent of virus production. Virology 65:392, 1975

Schincariol AL, Joklik WK: Early synthesis of virus-specific RNA and DNA in cells rapidly transformed with Rous sarcoma virus. Virology 56:532, 1973

Sherr CJ, Todaro GJ: Primate type C virus p30 antigen in cells from humans with acute leukemia. Science 187:855, 1975

Sherr CJ, Fedele LA, Benveniste RE, Todaro GJ: Interspecies antigenic determinants of the reverse transcriptase and p30 proteins of mammalian type C viruses. J Virol 15:1440, 1975.

Shoyab M, Markham PD, Baluda MA: Host induced alteration of avian sarcoma virus B-77 genome. Proc Natl Acad Sci USA 72:1031, 1975

Strand M, August JT: Structural proteins of mammalian oncogenic RNA viruses: Multiple antigenic determinants of the major internal protein and envelope glycoprotein. J Virol 13:171, 1974

Strand M, August JT: Type-C RNA virus gene expression in human tissue. J Virol 14:1584, 1975.

Strand M, August JT: Structural proteins of mammalian RNA tumor viruses: Relatedness of the interspecies antigenic determinants of the major internal protein. J Virol 15:1332, 1975

Tereba A, Skoog L, Vogt PK: RNA tumor virus-specific sequences in nuclear DNA of several avian species. Virology 65:524, 1975

Vaidya AB, Black MM, Dion AS, Moore DH: Homology between human breast tumor RNA and mouse mammary tumor virus genome. Nature 249:565, 1974

Vogt PK: A virus released by "nonproducing" Rous sarcoma cells. Proc Natl Acad Sci USA 58:801, 1967

Weiss RA, Friis PR, Vogt PK: Induction of avian tumor viruses in normal cells by physical and chemical carcinogens. Virology 46:920, 1971

70

The Bacteriophages

TABLE 70-1 CHARACTERISTICS OF SOME WELL-STUDIED BACTERIOPHAGES

Phage	Host	Particle Dimensions (nm) Head	Particle Dimensions (nm) Tail	Structure	Type	Strandedness	Nucleic Acid MW $\times 10^6$	Structure
T1	E. coli	50	10×150	Hexagonal head, simple tail	DNA	DS	27	Linear
T2, T4, T6	E. coli	80×110	25×110	Prolate icosahedral head, complex tail with fibers	DNA	DS	105	Linear, circularly permuted and terminally redundant, contains glucosylated 5-hydroxymethylcytosine
T3, T7	E. coli	60	10×15	Hexagonal head, short tail	DNA	DS	25	Linear
T5	E. coli	65	10×170	Hexagonal head, simple tail	DNA	DS	66	Linear, one strand segmented
λ	E. coli	54	10×140	Hexagonal head, simple tail	DNA	DS	31	Linear, cohesive ends
SP01	B. subtilis	90	30×210	Hexagonal head, complex tail	DNA	DS	105	Linear, contains 5-hydroxymethyluracil
PM2	Pseudomonas BAL-31	60	None	Hexagonal head, envelope contains lipid	DNA	DS	6	Circular
φX174, S13, M12	E. coli	27	None	Icosahedral	DNA	SS	1.7	Circular
f1, fd, M13	E. coli	$5–10 \times 800$	None	Filamentous	DNA	SS	1.3	Circular
φ6	Pseudomonas phaseolica	65	None	Polyhedral head, envelope contains lipid	RNA	DS	9.5	3 linear segments (2.2, $2.8 \times 4.5 \times 10^6$)
MS2, f2, fr, Qβ	E. coli	24	None	Icosahedral	RNA	SS	1.2	Linear

In 1915 Twort published a note describing the infectious destruction of micrococcal colonies and offered three possible explanations for this phenomenon: First, the destroyed colonies represented a stage in the bacterial life cycle that induced normal colonies to undergo a glassy transformation; second, the lytic agent was an enzyme that caused both cell destruction and the production of more enzyme; and third, the causative agent was a virus that grew in and destroyed bacteria. All of these explanations could be reconciled with the original finding that the agent would not grow on any medium, passed through bacteria-proof filters, and was inactivated by heating to 60C for one hour. d'Hérelle, who discovered this phenomenon independently, soon demonstrated the particulate nature of what he called "bacteriophages." The elegant pioneering work of Burnet and of Schlesinger in the 1930s confirmed the viral nature of the Twort-d'Hérelle agents.

Early hopes of using the action of phage on susceptible bacteria as a means of preventing and treating infectious diseases was not fulfilled (Chap. 61). However, in the early 1940s, Delbrück and a group of investigators around him realized that the availability of viruses multiplying in cloned populations of rapidly growing host cells provided an ideal tool for gaining an insight into the mechanisms of biologic self-replication. Their expectation was amply borne out. The bacteriophage–bacterium system proved to be highly amenable to experimentation, and intensive investigation of it over the last three decades has provided many of the fundamental concepts concerning molecular genetics, nucleic acid replication, and the transcription and translation of genetic information. These concepts are applicable not only to bacterial viruses but also to animal viruses and to cells in general. Thus, although bacteriophages were a failure as therapeutic agents, they have proved invaluable for the elucidation of the reactions most basic to life.

The purpose of this chapter is to review the mechanisms involved in the multiplication of several classes of bacteriophages, emphasizing in particular those that already have been or may in the future be shown to operate also during animal virus multiplication.

THE STRUCTURE OF BACTERIOPHAGES

Bacteriophages for every bacterial species exist. Only very few have been investigated in detail, but intense concentration on a small number of them has permitted rapid progress. Almost all well-studied phages are active either on *Escherichia coli, Bacillus subtilis,* or *Pseudomonas* (Table 70-1).

The Structure of Phage Capsids

The structure of bacteriophages is governed by the same principles as were described in Chapter 62. Some of the smaller phages, such as ϕX174 and MS2, have icosahedral capsids (Fig. 70-1); others, such as phage f1, are filamentous and possess helical symmetry (Fig. 70-6). Larger phages generally consist of a head, that comprises the phage genome enclosed within a single capsid shell that is generally hexagonal in outline and may or may not be elongated, and a tail, that serves both as the cell attachment organ and as a tube through which phage DNA passes into the host cell. The complexity of this tail varies greatly from phage to phage, but in most phages it conforms to one of three morphologic patterns. In the first, exemplified by coliphages T3 and T7, the tail is very short (Fig. 70-2). In the second, exemplified by coliphages T1 and λ, the tail is

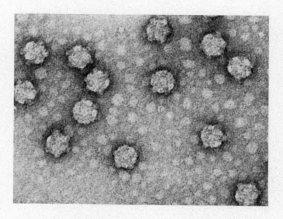

FIG. 70-1. Bacteriophage ϕX 174. ×225,000. (Electron micrograph by Dr. R. B. Luftig)

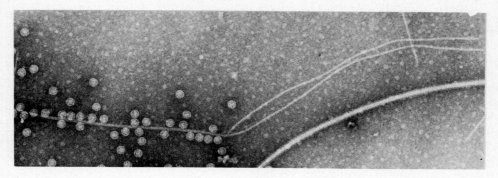

FIG. 70-2. An F-pilus with two types of male-specific phage attached: icosahedral RNA-containing MS2, and filamentous DNA-containing fl. The former are attached along the entire length of the F-pilus; the latter are adsorbed by their ends to the tip of the pilus. (From Caro and Schnos: Proc Natl Acad Sci USA 56:128, 1968)

long but rather simple in construction: It consists essentially of a noncontractile flexible tube that may or may not possess either a knob or one or several spikes or fibers at its distal end (Fig. 70-3). The third morphologic tail pattern, exhibited by the coliphages T2, T4, and T6, the so-called T-even phages, is almost staggeringly intricate (Figs. 70-4, 70-5). These tails consist of a hollow core, which is attached at one end to the head and bears at its distal end a hexagonal base plate to which six pins and six long tail fibers bent in the middle are attached. This core has a thin collar situated close to the head and is surrounded for most of its length by a

sheath composed of 24 rings of helically arranged capsomers. These tails, which consist of about 20 different protein species, serve as syringes by means of which phage DNA is injected into the cell (p. 913).

Very few phages are enveloped. Among the enveloped phages is the *Pseudomonas* phage PM2, which is being studied as a model for enveloped animal viruses (Fig. 70-6). The hope is that, given the ease with which almost any desired mutant of both host cell and virus can be obtained in the bacterial system, study of the morphogenesis of PM2 will yield new insight into both the formation and the structure

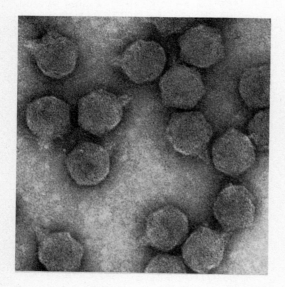

FIG. 70-3. Bacteriophage T7. Magnification: ×225,000. (Electron micrograph by Dr. R. B. Luftig)

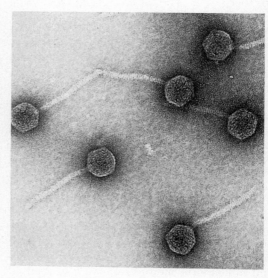

FIG. 70-4. Bacteriophage λ. ×135,000. (Electron micrograph by Dr. R. B. Luftig.)

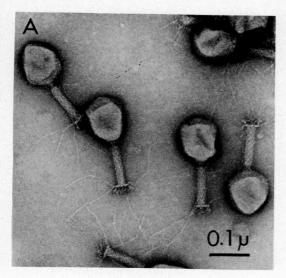

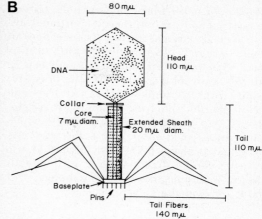

FIG. 70-5. A. Bacteriophage T4. ×100,000. B. Model of phage T4. (Electron micrograph by Dr. R. B. Luftig.)

of viral envelopes and of membranes in general.

The Structure of Phage Nucleic Acids

Bacteriophage genomes take several forms (Table 70-1). Most of them consist of single, linear, double-stranded DNA molecules that vary in molecular weight from about 1 million to more than 100 million. Some of them, in particular those of the T-even phages, exist in a form which is both circularly permuted and terminally redundant. In them the nucleotide sequence of some molecules is A, B, C, D, . . .

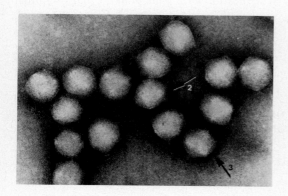

FIG. 70-6. The enveloped phage PM2 fixed with glutaraldehyde and negatively stained with phosphotungstate. The numbered arrows indicate axes of 2-fold and 3-fold symmetry. ×120,000. (From Silbert, Salditt, and Franklin: Virology 39:666, 1969)

W, X, Y, Z, A, B; of others B, C, D, . . . W, X, Y, Z, A, B, C; of others still C, D, . . . W, X, Y, Z, A, B, C, D; and so on. In other words, all molecules contain the same nucleotides, but the terminal nucleotide sequences differ in individual genomes and a few nucleotides are reiterated at the ends of the molecules. This situation is due to the fact that their replication seems to proceed via a structure which may be represented as A, B, C, D, . . . W, X, Y, Z, A, B, C, D, . . . W, X, Y, Z, A, B, C, D, . . . which is then cut at random so as to yield molecules of identical size (p. 918). It is of interest in this connection that adenovirus and herpesvirus DNAs are not circularly permuted.

Other phage genomes, such as that of PM2, consist of circular double-stranded DNA molecules, others, such as those of phages ϕX174 and fd, consist of single-stranded circular DNA molecules possessing plus polarity, while still others are linear single-stranded nonpermuted RNA molecules with plus polarity, analogous to poliovirus RNA. Recently a phage of *Pseudomonas phaseolica*, ϕ6, has been discovered that contains double-stranded RNA. Like the double-stranded RNA-containing genomes of animal viruses, ϕ6 RNA is segmented: it consists of three unique segments, the molecular weights of which are 2.2, 2.8, and 4.5 million.

Phage nucleic acids are infectious, just as are the nucleic acids of animal viruses. The bacterial cell wall, however, presents a more formidable barrier to the entry of nucleic acids than does the plasma membrane of animal cells, and infection by naked phage nucleic acids, termed "transfection," can only be demonstrated under special circumstances. Transfection of whole bacterial cells is rare: cells of *B. subtilis* that are competent for transformation (Chap. 8) can be transfected, and so can cells of *E. coli* treated with Ca^{++} (only with λ DNA). The more readily transfectible bacterial forms are spheroplasts (Chap. 3) and frozen-thawed cells, which can be transfected not only with the small single-stranded phage RNAs and DNAs but also with the double-stranded DNAs of numerous phages, including those of the coliphages T1 and λ, and even the T-even phages.

Unusual Nucleic Acid Bases   Whereas the genomes of animal viruses contain only the normal nucleic acid bases adenine, guanine, cytosine, and uracil or thymine, phage genomes sometimes contain unusual or substituted ones. For example, the DNA of the T-even bacteriophages contains not cytosine but 5-hydroxymethylcytosine; the DNA of certain *B. subtilis* phages contains not thymine but uracil, 5-hydroxymethyluracil, or 5-(4′,5′-dihydroxypentyl) uracil, and in the DNA of a *Pseudomonas acidovorus* phage, thymine is partially replaced by 5-(4-aminobutylaminomethyl) uracil (also known as α-putrescinylthymine).

Glucosylation and Methylation   The bases of bacteriophage DNA are often glucosylated and/or methylated in highly characteristic patterns. Both 5-hydroxymethyluracil and particularly 5-hydroxymethylcytosine are frequently linked by phage-coded enzymes to either one or two glucose residues via α or β bonds. The situation concerning the T-even phages is summarized in Table 70-2. In addition, a small proportion of the bases in phage DNAs is generally methylated by host-specified enzymes. Both

types of substitution confer resistance to degradation by nucleases. As discussed in Chapter 8, bacteria guard themselves against foreign DNAs by degrading them, and in order to prevent their own DNA from being destroyed, they cause methyl groups to be attached to it in specific locations, thereby rendering it resistant to their own restricting nucleases. Since phage nucleic acids also become methylated, highly specific restriction patterns, known as "host-induced modifications," exist among bacteriophages. For example, the DNA of a phage grown in host A will be methylated by that host's enzymes in such a manner that it will be resistant to that host's restricting nucleases, but most of the DNA of this phage will be degraded by the restricting nucleases of many other bacteria. However, any DNA molecules that escape degradation in such hosts can replicate, and their progeny is then modified by the methylating enzymes of the new hosts, acquiring new specificities in the process.

THE PHYSIOLOGY OF LYTIC PHAGE INFECTION

Like animal viruses, some bacteriophages lyse their hosts, while others integrate their genomes into the host genome. The former are known as virulent phages, the latter as temperate or lysogenic phages. We will consider first the lytic phage one-step multiplication cycle which is formally analogous to that of animal viruses (Chap. 65) but proceeds very much more rapidly. For example, whereas the length of the latent period (the interval between infection and release of progeny virus) is at least 4 hours for poliovirus and 12 hours for vaccinia

TABLE 70-2   EXTENT OF GLUCOSYLATION OF 5-HYDROXYMETHYLCYTOSINE IN T-EVEN PHAGES[*]

Phage	Not Glucosylated	α-Glucosyl	β-Glucosyl	β-1:6-Glucosyl-α-Glucosyl
T2	25	70	0	5
T4	0	70	30	0
T6	25	3	0	72

From Lehman and Pratt: J Biol Chem 235:3254, 1960
[*]*Figures represent percentages*

virus, it is 13 minutes for phages T1, T3, T7, and φX174, and 21 to 25 minutes for the T-even phages and MS2.

Adsorption

The initial step of the phage multiplication cycle illustrates particularly clearly the existence of virus-specific receptors on host cells. Phages are usually highly specific for a limited number of bacterial host strains. This specificity resides in the complementarity of molecular configurations on phage attachment organs and receptor molecules on the bacterial surface. The nature of the phage attachment organ varies from phage to phage: small icosahedral phages, such as φX174 and MS2, have multiple attachment sites, filamentous phages, such as f1, absorb with their ends (Fig. 70-2), and tailed phages adsorb with the knobs, spikes, or fibers that are located at the tips of their tails. Phage receptors on the bacterial surface are sometimes on lipopolysaccharide, at other times on lipoprotein, and sometimes on F pili (Chap. 3), which causes the phages that adsorb to them, typically single-stranded DNA-containing and RNA-containing phages, to be male-specific (Fig. 70-2).

Mutations in bacteria that destroy the complementarity of the phage-receptor interaction result in resistance. Phage populations usually contain mutants that are themselves altered in such a way as to restore the necessary complementarity. These are known as "host-range mutants" and can grow in the mutated bacteria.

Since phage receptors are surface components, bacteria capable of adsorbing the same phage are often antigenically related. This observation has found diagnostic application in the practice of phage typing. In this method the sensitivity/resistance patterns of bacterial strains to a series of bacteriophages are determined. Since these patterns are both readily determined and highly characteristic, they are useful tests for identification. For example, some phages of *Salmonella typhi* are specific for strains possessing the Vi antigen, which is characteristic of virulent strains (Chap. 38), and these phages are used for the identification of virulent strains of typhoid vacilli. Several other phage-typing systems exist, the best known being that of staphylococci.

Injection and Uncoating

The events immediately following phage adsorption are involved with the injection of phage nucleic acid into the cell and provide an excellent illustration of the general principle that uncoating of viral genomes involves the physical separation of genome and capsid. This was first shown in 1952 by Hershey and Chase in an experiment that represents one of the milestones of virology. They infected bacteria with phage T2 labeled in the protein with the radioisotope ^{35}S. Following an incubation period of several minutes, the mixture of phage and bacteria was sheared by blending in a Waring Blendor: after blending, only a small amount of radioactive label was associated with the bacteria. When this experiment was repeated with phage in which the DNA had been labeled with the radioisotope ^{32}P, the converse was true, that is, the radioactive label was now associated with the cells. This experiment was correctly interpreted as signifying that the DNA passed into the interior of the cell, while the protein coat remained attched to the outer cell surface, from which it could be dislodged by shearing forces. Since the bacteria from which phage coats were removed by shearing yielded normal phage progeny, this experiment also clearly showed that viral DNA itself contained all the information necessary for phage multiplication.

The actual infection process has been best studied for the T-even phages. Following adsorption by means of the tail fiber-receptor interaction, the six tail pins make contact with the host surface and firmly anchor the phage tail plate to it. The conformation of the tail plate, which is an extremely complex structure consisting of at least 12 different polypeptide species, then changes, caused, apparently, by the interaction of one of its components, the enzyme dihydrofolate reductase, with pyridine nucleotides (such as NADPH) that temporarily leak from cells in response to infection (Fig. 70-7). The tail plate conformation change in turn triggers a change in the manner in which the protein subunits of the tail sheath are arranged, as a result of which the sheath contracts, thereby driving the tail core about 12 nm into the bacterial cell wall (Fig. 70-7). The phage DNA then passes through the tail core into the bacterial cell. The role of the host cell in DNA injection is obscure; on the one hand, it is known

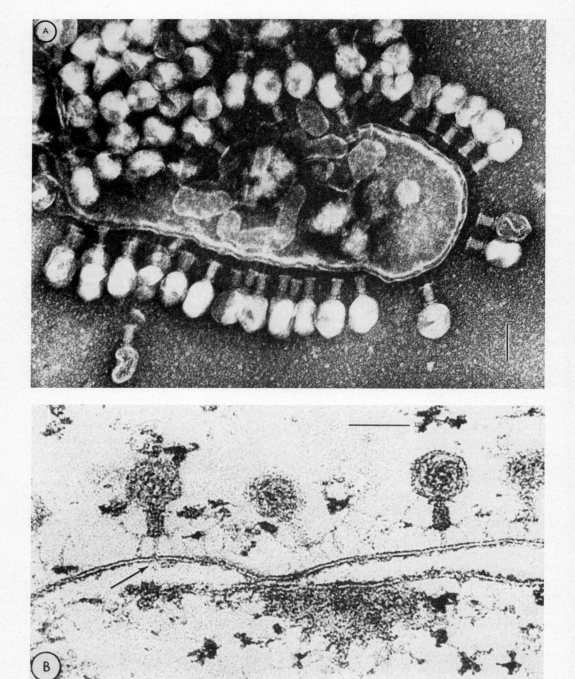

FIG. 70-7. Bacteriophage T4 adsorbed to *Escherichia coli*. A. The phages' sheaths are contracted, and their base plates are 30 to 40 nm from the cell wall. B. The phages visible in this section are seen to be attached to the cell wall by the tail fibers; the cell wall appears as two continuous electron-opaque lines separated by an electron-transparent space. The arrow indicates where the needle (tail core) of an adsorbed phage may have penetrated the cell wall. (From Simon and Anderson: Virology 32:279, 1967)

that if T2 phages are mixed with cell wall fragments, the DNA is ejected into the medium, suggesting a passive role for the host, but, on the other hand, there is evidence that host protein synthesis is necessary for the transfer of the entire genome from the phage head into the cell. Most probably, cooperation between virus and host is required. The holes created in the cell (Fig. 70-8). Most probably, cooperation between virus and host is required. The holes created in the cell surface by the phage tail cores are normally quickly sealed by cell wall material newly synthesized under the control of a phage gene called "spackle." Clearly, it would not be to the advantage of the phage to permit these holes to remain, since cell contents would leak out through them. In fact, if the multiplicity of infection is too high, excessive leakage does occur, resulting in a phenomenon known as "lysis from without," and the multiplication cycle is aborted.

As pointed out previously, most phages do not possess tails with contractile sheaths, and still others possess no tails at all. Nevertheless, here also the phage protein coat remains on the outside, and only the nucleic acid is introduced into the cell.

The Multiplication Cycle of Phages Containing Double-stranded DNA

The Nature of the Information Encoded in the Phage Genome   During the phage multiplication cycle the genetic information encoded in the viral genome expresses itself. The nature of this information is much more completely defined for several phage systems than for most animal viruses. The principal reason for this is the ease with which phage mutants deficient or recognizably altered in a variety of genes can be selected, characterized, and mapped. The most useful class of mutants for this purpose are the conditional lethal mutants, that is, mutants that can function under one set of conditions but not under others. The nature of one class of such mutants, the temperature-sensitive mutants, has already been described (Chap. 67). Another class of conditional lethal mutants are the so-called amber mutants, in which codons normally coding for certain amino acids are mutated to UAG, which signifies termination of translation (Chap. 67). Only protein fragments, which are rarely functional, can be specified by genes containing such codons. However,

bacterial mutants exist in which transfer RNA molecules are mutated in such a way that they recognize UAG not as chain-terminating but as amino acid-specifying codons. In such host cells the mutated phage genes can be translated into complete protein molecules, and as a result the amber mutants can multiply. Since they suppress the consequences of amber mutations, such mutant bacterial strains are known as "suppressor strains" (Chap. 8). A third type of mutant that has found application in the analysis of the phage multiplication cycle are deletion mutants, which simply lack portions of phage DNA.

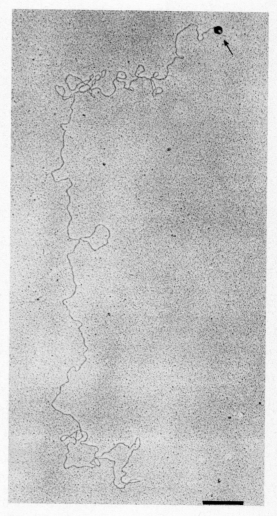

FIG. 70-8. A T7 phage particle ejecting its DNA. Almost the entire DNA molecule (12 nm long) has been ejected. The DNA was caused to eject by treatment with formamide. The bar is 0.3 nm long. (Courtesy of Dr. Kaoru Saigo)

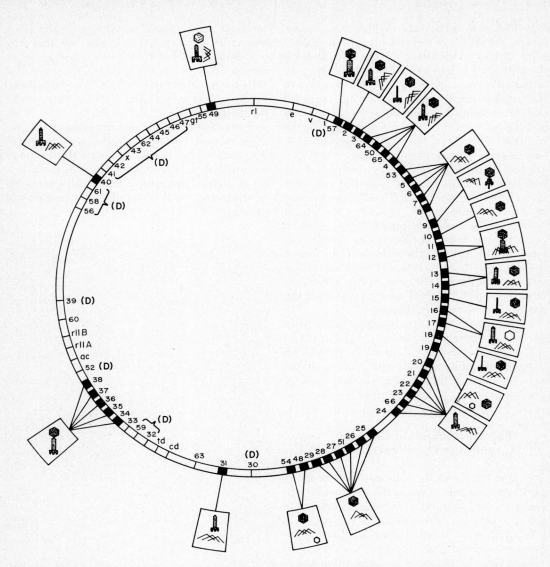

FIG. 70-9. The genetic map of T4. The solid segments indicate late genes with morphogenetic functions, while the short bars represent early genes with enzymatic or regulatory functions. Genes with functions in DNA replication are identified by "D." The boxes indicate viral components, such as heads, tails, and tail fibers that are present in extracts of cells infected with conditional lethal mutants under restrictive conditions. (Adapted from Edgar and Wood: Proc Natl Acad Sci USA 55:498, 1966)

Thousands of phage mutants have by now been obtained and characterized with respect to the function in which they are defective. For example, there are mutants that fail to synthesize some early proteins, mutants that fail to replicate phage DNA, mutants that fail to form mature phage particles, and so on. Over 100 such functions, each corresponding to a specific gene, have so far been discovered for bacteriophage T4, which is probably about one-half of the total number of T4 genes, and for smaller, less complicated phages, this proportion is considerably higher. Most of the known T4 genes have been mapped: all lie on a circular linkage group, which agrees with the finding that although T4 DNA is linear, it is circularly permuted (Fig. 70-9). Similar maps have been prepared for several other phages, notably T7, λ, and the small phages that contain single stranded nucleic acid (p. 909).

The proteins specified by the genes of the large complex phages, such as the T-even phage, have a wide variety of functions. Most of them can be grouped into eight classes.

(1) Membrane proteins
(2) Enzymes that degrade host DNA
(3) Enzymes that synthesize nucleic acid precursors
(4) Proteins that function in phage DNA replication
(5) Proteins that program transcription of the phage genome
(6) Proteins that are structural phage components
(7) Proteins that function catalytically in phage morphogenesis
(8) Proteins that repair the bacterial cell wall and cell membrane early in infection and degrade them during the late stages of the multiplication cycle.

In addition, the T-even phages code for eight species of transfer RNA, the genes for which are clustered in a small region of the phage genome where they may form a single transcription unit or operon. Mutants lacking these genes can multiply, but their burst size, or yield, is smaller than that of wild-type phage. This suggests that the phage-coded transfer RNAs supplement the reading capacity of those codons that are used more commonly by the virus than by the host, thereby ensuring optimum rates of protein synthesis in the maximum number of hosts.

We will now consider each of the eight categories of proteins in turn and examine their role in phage multiplication.

The Functions of Various Categories of Phage Gene Products

MEMBRANE PROTEINS. Infection causes the bacterial cell membrane to become permeable to cellular contents, which begin to leak out. Within several minutes sealing occurs and preinfection permeability is restored. The precise mechanism by which this is achieved is not clear, but it is known that at least five phage-coded proteins are synthesized early during the infection cycle and incorporated into the cell membrane.

ENZYMES THAT DEGRADE HOST DNA. Among the earliest effects of phage T4 infection is the breakdown of host DNA (Fig. 70-10), which has several consequences. First, it provides a source of nucleic acid precursors, which may be limiting under certain conditions. More important, transcription of host-specified messenger RNA ceases abruptly, and since most bacterial messenger RNAs are very short lived, this not only leads to the sudden cessation of host-specified protein synthesis but also quickly provides ribosomes for the translation of phage-specified messenger RNA. The following is a graphic example of the consequences of the cessation of host protein synthesis. If a culture of *E. coli* grown in glucose-containing medium and infected with T4 is transferred to medium containing lactose, phage infection is aborted. The reason is that lactose utilization requires the induction of the synthesis of certain proteins, among them a permease

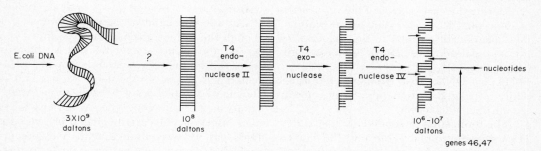

FIG. 70-10. A tentative scheme to account for the degradation of *E. coli* DNA after infection with phage T4. An enzyme which has not yet been isolated first degrades *E. coli* DNA to fragments about one-tenth its size, which are then nicked by endonuclease II. The nicks are then thought to be widened by an exonuclease and the single-stranded stretches so produced are then cleaved by endonuclease IV. The products are duplex DNA molecules which are more than 100 times smaller than the original *E. coli* genome. Since fragments of this size accumulate in cells infected with phage mutants carrying lesions in genes 46 and 47 but not in cells infected with wild type phage, these genes presumably code for enzymes that function in their further degradation. (Adapted from Warner et al: J Virol 5:700, 1970)

and the enzyme β-galactosidase. T4 infection halts host protein synthesis. Therefore, lactose cannot be metabolized, energy production is prevented, and no phage progeny can be formed.

ENZYMES THAT SYNTHESIZE NUCLEIC ACID PRECURSORS.   Numerous enzymes function in the synthesis of nucleic acid precursors, particularly when the phage DNA contains both unusual bases and substituted bases. For example, in the case of T4, which contains glycosylated 5-hydroxymethylcytosine instead of cytosine, the following enzymes are required: (1) enzymes to destroy deoxycytidine triphosphate (so that cytosine is not incorporated into phage DNA), (2) an enzyme that hydroxymethylates deoxycytidylic acid, and (3) enzymes that glucosylate 5-hydroxymethylcytosine residues in polymerized DNA. In addition, numerous enzymes, among them enzymes that function in the synthesis of the other three deoxyribonucleoside triphosphates, are specified by the T-even genome. They are not absolutely essential but increase the yield of progeny phage.

PROTEINS THAT FUNCTION IN PHAGE DNA REPLICATION.   The mechanism by which double-stranded phage DNA replicates is exceedingly complex, and although an enormous amount of effort has been devoted to its elucidation, no clear picture has yet emerged (Chap. 7). The following facts are pertinent.

(1) Phage DNA replicates by a semiconservative mechanism.
(2) During the early stages of the replication of some phage DNAs, extensive recombination occurs. This results in the dispersal of the parental genome among numerous progeny genomes.
(3) Phage DNA most probably replicates while associated with membrane in some as yet unspecified manner.
(4) The replication of some double-stranded DNA genomes, notably those of the T-even phages, proceeds via the formation of intermediates that are considerably larger than the genome itself and that contain repeats of the mature phage DNA sequence. The possible significance of this intermediate in the formation of circularly permuted and terminally redundant genomes has already been discussed.

(5) Progeny phage genomes form a pool from which individual molecules are withdrawn at random for encapsidation into virions (Chap. 65).

Items (1) and (5) are also true for animal viral DNAs. The other three may apply as well.

Among the enzymes known to function in the replication of T4 DNA are a DNA polymerase (coded by gene 43), a polynucleotide ligase, and, most probably, several nicking enzymes (nucleases). A protein that facilitates unwinding of DNA may well participate also.

PROTEINS THAT FUNCTION IN TRANSCRIPTION PROGRAMMING.   Phage genomes, like all other genomes, express themselves via messenger RNA. In fact, it is worth noting that messenger RNA was discovered in phage-infected cells. In 1956 Volkin and Astrachan noted that the base composition of newly synthesized RNA in T2-infected E. coli resembled that of T2 DNA rather than that of host DNA, and in 1959 Brenner, Jacob, and Meselson firmly established the concept of messenger RNA by showing that this RNA combines with ribosomes and is responsible for the synthesis of phage proteins.

Phage-specified proteins, like those specified by animal virus genomes (Chap. 65), are synthesized in a strictly ordered sequence. The necessity for this is obvious: for example, enzymes breaking down host DNA should be synthesized first, and viral structural proteins should by synthesized last. There are two ways of achieving programmed protein synthesis: either the entire viral genome is transcribed continuously and translation is programmed, or transcription is programmed, and messenger RNAs are translated as they are formed. Although the former mechanism may apply to a few species of messenger RNA, it is primarily transcription that is programmed in phage-infected and animal virus-infected cells. This is shown most readily by hybridization experiments of the following type. At various times after infection, cells are incubated for brief periods, say for two minutes, with RNA precursors labeled with some radioisotope. On extraction such cells yield labeled messenger RNA populations synthesized from 0 to 2, 2 to 4, 4 to 6, and so on, minutes after infection. These messenger RNA populations are then allowed to hybridize with denatured phage DNA in the presence of excess unlabeled messenger RNA extracted from cells at various stages of infection. If the labeled and unlabeled RNA populations are identical, the large excess of unlabeled RNA will, by simple competition, almost completely prevent the labeled RNA from hybridizing. If the two populations are completely different, the presence of unlabeled RNA will have no effect on the ability of labeled RNA to hybridize to DNA.

Early studies on transcriptional control of T4 gene expression revealed the existence of two main classes of phage-coded messenger RNAs: those that are transcribed immediately after infection (early) and those that are only transcribed late in the infection cycle. To a first approximation, the former are mainly transcribed from the *l* strand of DNA, the latter from the *r* strand.

Subsequent work has shown that the situation is often more complex. The messenger RNAs of the smaller, simpler phages, like T7, indeed fall into merely two transcription classes, but those of the larger phages, like the T-even coliphages, or the *B. subtilis* phage SP01, are far more complex. Here the early and late messenger RNA classes can be further subdivided into subclasses, each with its own transcriptional pattern. Eight distinct classes of T4 messenger RNA molecules have been characterized with respect to when during the phage multiplication cycle they are transcribed, and six such subclasses have been identified in bacteria infected with SP01. Conceivably the actual transcription programs are still more complex.

How are such complex transcription programs managed? Elucidation of this problem is currently one of the most exciting areas in biology, since it could help to answer fundamental questions concerning embryogenesis and differentiation in higher organisms. The complete answer is not yet evident, but it seems that one of the factors of critical importance is the specificity of the transcribing enzymes.

Since phages do not contain RNA polymerases, the first phage genes are always transcribed by the host RNA polymerase. As discussed in Chapter 7, the *E. coli* RNA polymerase is a complex enzyme that consists of four subunits—2 α subunits, 1 β subunit, and 1 β' subunit—and has associated with it one protein molecule, the σ factor, which controls its specificity. The fraction of the phage genome that is transcribed by this enzyme is usually not large, and it is governed by the presence of initiation and termination signals that it can recognize.

The messenger RNAs transcribed by it are known as early or immediate early (in the case of very complex programs).

The remainder of the transcription program is managed by phage-coded proteins (specified by early messenger RNAs). There are two principal means by which this is accomplished. The first, employed by the simpler phages, such as T7, involves the synthesis of a new RNA polymerase: this new enzyme consists of only a single polypeptide chain, and its specificity is such that it transcribes its homologous DNA more efficiently than any other. The second, employed by the more complex phages, such as T4 and SP01, involves the synthesis of a series of polypeptides that modify the host RNA polymerase in a series of successive steps. Among these modifications are adenylation of the α subunits and, perhaps, proteolytic cleavage of small portions from the β and β' subunits, as well as the replacement of the σ factor by several phage-coded polypeptides. If the ability to recognize and react with promoters and transcription termination signals of each of these modified RNA polymerase species is different, they could readily effect transcription programs such as those described above.

STRUCTURAL PHAGE COMPONENTS. The messenger RNAs that code for the proteins described so far are generally transcribed only from parental DNA. Those that code for the proteins to be described now are usually transcribed only from progeny DNA. These proteins are known as the "late proteins," and the quantitatively most important class of late proteins is the structural components of progeny phage particles (compare Chap. 65). Tailed phage particles are complex structures composed of a relatively large number of polypeptide species, for example, T4 contains at least 30 protein species; and even simple phages like T7 and λ contain 10 to 15 different species.

PROTEINS THAT FUNCTION CATALYTICALLY IN MORPHOGENESIS. Phage genomes usually code for several proteins that function in a catalytic capacity during morphogenesis (p. 920). For example, in addition to the 30-odd structural protein species, T4 DNA codes for at least 17 additional proteins that are also essential for the formation of mature phage particles. Their nature and the precise manner in which they function is largely unknown (but see p. 920 for the scaffolding protein). The genes for tail proteins are clustered in the T4 genome (Fig. 70-9) into three sets: one for proteins that are needed in very few copies, one for proteins needed in intermediate numbers of copies, and one for proteins needed in very many copies per cell. The situation seems to be similar for several ther phages. The genetic apparatus for the formation of phage tails is thus very highly refined.

Enzymes Necessary for Progeny Phage Liberation: Cell Lysis Most virulent phages are liberated from their hosts by a mechanism that differs fundamentally from any employed by animal viruses (Chap. 65). The bacterial cell lyses suddenly, over a period of about one minute, thereby liberating the entire progeny. This is known as cell lysis and, in the case of the T-even phages, is the result of the function of two late phage-coded proteins. One is an enzyme, probably a lipase, coded by the t gene, which attacks the cell membrane, thereby halting metabolic processes; the other is the enzyme lysozyme, coded by the *e* gene, which then hydrolyzes the cell wall.

Phage Morphogenesis Phage morphogenesis has been studied most intensively for the T-even coliphages, in particular T4, and for the lysogenic coliphage λ. The most successful approach has been to study the products of infection of a large number of conditional lethal mutants, both temperature-sensitive and amber (p. 915), under restrictive conditions. Cells infected with numerous mutants in genes, whose location on the phage chromosome is precisely known as a result of recombination analysis, accumulate not mature phage particles but phage components, such as partially complete or complete heads, such tail components as fibers, cores, sheaths, and so on, partially complete tails, and so on. As a result, it has been possible to link defects in both structural and catalytic proteins to particular genes.

As for the study of the morphogenetic pathway itself, one of the most useful approaches has been to examine the ability of extracts of cells infected with such mutants to complement each other. In other words, pairs of such extracts are mixed, and one determines whether infectious phage particles are formed from the components present in each. By such means,

the scheme for T4 tail assembly shown in Figure 70-11 has been worked out.

As for the assembly of phage heads and the insertion of DNA into them, current evidence indicates that these processes are achieved with the aid of a catalytic head assembly or scaffolding protein. Heads of the phage P22 (a *Salmonella typhimurium* phage that resembles phage λ in many respects) do not self-assemble. Instead, 200 to 300 molecules of a scaffolding protein catalyze the accurate polymerization of the coat protein into a head precursor shell that contains both proteins. The scaffolding protein then exits and is replaced by the DNA. Possibly the exit of the protein exposes charge sites that serve to collapse the DNA. The actual amount of DNA that is inserted into the phage head is determined by the so-called headful cutting mechanism, that is, the DNA, in the form of large replicative intermediates (p. 918), is inserted until the head is full, and the DNA is then cut.

Clearly, much remains to be discovered in clarifying how proteins interact with each other to form large structures, but the basic principles are beginning to emerge. Here, as in many other fields, phages are proving to be most valuable model systems for answering fundamental questions. It is now becoming clear that the assembly of proteins into stable large structures involves their processing. Two kinds of processing have been observed: protein fusion (during λ head assembly) and, more commonly, proteolytic cleavage (during T4 and P2 head assembly, as well as during T5 and λ tail assembly), which results in the removal of (generally) a small portion of polypeptide. Perhaps cleavage provides the energy necessary to drive protein rearrangements, resulting in the formation of protein complexes irreversibly locked into stable configurations.

The Multiplication Cycle of Phages Containing Single-stranded DNA

Several *E. coli* phages contain not double-stranded but single-stranded DNA (Table 70-1). Since they may serve as a model for parvoviruses, it is worth examining their mode of replication in some detail.

The principal problems posed by their discovery were (1) how do single DNA strands

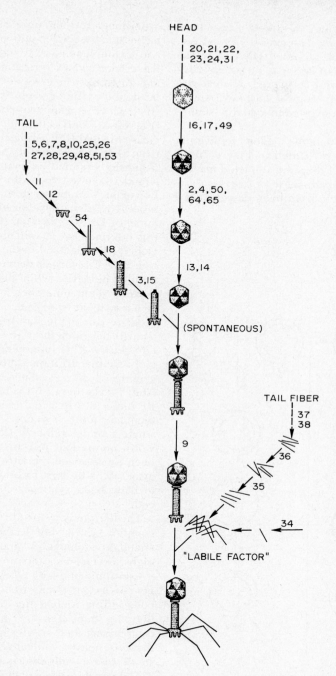

HEAD

20,21,22,
23,24,31

16,17,49

TAIL

5,6,7,8,10,25,26
27,28,29,48,51,53

11
12
54

18

2,4,50,
64,65

3,15

13,14

(SPONTANEOUS)

9

TAIL FIBER

37
38

36

35

34

"LABILE FACTOR"

FIG. 70-11. The morphogenetic pathway of T4. There are three principal branches leading independently to the formation of heads, tails, and tail fibers, which then combine to form complete virus particles. The numbers refer to the gene product(s) involved in each step. (Adapted from Wood and Edgar: Sci Am 217:74, 1967 Courtesy of Freeman and Co.)

replicate and still obey the rules of base pairing, and (2) since all messenger RNAs are transcribed from double-stranded DNA, how can single-stranded DNA serve as their template? These questions were answered when it was found that upon entering the host cell, single-stranded DNA is converted to a double-stranded replicative form.

A scheme describing the mode of replication of φX174 DNA is presented in Figure 70-12. Although several of the steps depicted may be greatly oversimplified, most of the key elements of the scheme have been demonstrated

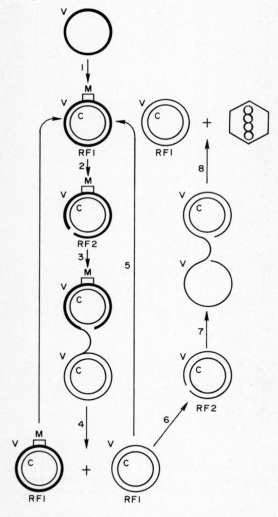

FIG. 70-12. A scheme to account for the replication of φX 174 DNA. V represents the DNA strand present in phage; C represents the complementary strand. The heavy V strand is that in the parental particle.

experimentally. The parental DNA (V) first attaches to a host cell membrane component (M), and a complementary strand is synthesized by bacterial enzymes (presumably a polymerase and a ligase) so as to yield a supercoiled circular double-stranded replicative form known as RF1, which is analogous to papovavirus DNA (Fig. 62-22). This is then nicked by an endonuclease to yield RF2, a related circular molecule (step 2). In step 3 the V strand is then elongated using the C strand as template, and a new C strand is synthesized with the elongated portion of the V strand serving as its template. This process is a modification of the rolling circle mode of DNA replication (Chap. 7). In step 4 this intermediate is split into a membrane-attached RF1 identical to the original one and a free RF1. The former than repeats steps 2 to 4, forming new RFs, while the latter has two options. If membrane sites are available, it can attach to them (step 5) and then also generate progeny RFs, or it may be converted to RF2 (step 6), on which the V strand is again elongated (step 7). This intermediate is then split to yield another RF2 (possibly via RF1) and a V strand, which is immediately encapsidated (step 8). The net result is that double-stranded RF molecules first replicate and then serve as templates for the synthesis of large numbers of single-stranded progeny DNA molecules. It is worth noting that infectious φX174 DNA has been synthesized in vitro with purified enzymes. It is the first functioning DNA genome to have been synthesized outside the living cell.

The enzymology of all these steps is very complex. Even step 1, the synthesis of a C strand on a template V strand, requires at least eight host enzymes and protein factors.

Concomitantly with DNA synthesis, messenger RNAs are transcribed from membrane-bound RFs. Among the proteins into which they are translated are the structural phage components, one species of which attaches to the loose ends of progeny V strands arising in step 7, thereby initiating encapsidation.

The infection cycle of the filamentous phages fl, fd, and M13 differs somewhat from that of φX174. Whereas nascent φX174 DNA is immediately encapsidated, forming progeny that accumulates within the cell and is eventually liberated when the cells lyse, large amounts of free viral DNA accumulate intracellularly in the case of the filamentous phages. These mole-

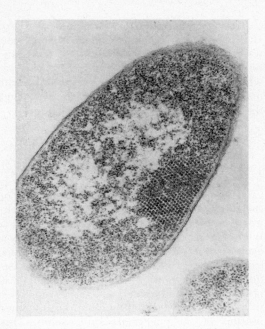

FIG. 70-13. An *E. coli* cell 50 minutes after infection with MS2. Note the paracrystalline viral particle array. The virus is slightly larger than the ribosomes that are present throughout the cell. This cell is about to lyse. ×000. (Courtesy of Dr. M. Van Montagu)

cules are then encapsidated at the cell membrane, and virus particles are released without cell lysis in a process that is in part analogous to that by which enveloped animal viruses are released from their host cells (Fig. 70-13).

The Multiplication Cycle of Phages Containing Single-stranded RNA

Single-stranded RNA-containing phages are small icosahedral viruses that closely resemble picornaviruses Like them, their capsids consist of 180 protein molecules, but whereas there are 60 molecules each of three different protein species present in picornaviruses, all 180 protein molecules are identical in the case of the RNA phages. In addition, each phage particle contains one molecule of an additional protein, the maturation or A protein, which is necessary both for proper assembly and for ability to adsorb. The RNA of these phages has a molecular weight of just over 1 million, which is less than one-half the size of the picornavirus genome.

Most of the known RNA phages are coli-phages. They fall into three or four serologic groups. Most of the well-studied RNA phages (f2, fr, MS2, R17, and so on) belong to one group, while one, Qβ, belongs to another. All RNA phages are male-specific because their receptor sites are on F pili.

The study of the multiplication cycle of these phages has provided important clues for investigations of animal viruses that contain RNA. In addition, their extraordinary simplicity—they are the simplest viruses known—has made them fascinating objects for the elucidation of fundamental biologic processes.

The genomes of RNA phages comprise only three genes. These are, from the 5'-terminus of the RNA, the genes for the A protein, the coat protein, and the RNA polymerase. The latter is actually only one of four polypeptides that together make up the functional RNA polymerase, the others being three bacterial polypeptides that are normally located on ribosomes, namely, factor i, elongation factor Tu, and elongation factor Ts. The precise function of these host-coded polypeptides as components of the viral RNA polymerase is not known, but it has been suggested that they somehow control specificity and affinity for initiation sites and that they are essential for maintaining the enzyme complex in its active conformation.

The genome of RNA phages possesses plus polarity and starts functioning as a messenger very soon after it enters the cell. After coding for the RNA polymerase, it replicates by a mechanism similar to that described for poliovirus (Fig. 65-15). This involves, first, the formation of complementary minus strands and then their successive transcription into progeny plus strands. Coat protein then begins to be synthesized in large amounts together with some A protein, and as soon as their concentrations are sufficiently high, encapsidation of RNA commences and mature progeny phage accumulates. These events are quite analogous to those that occur during the picornavirus multiplication cycle (Chap. 65).

The Programming of the RNA Phage Multiplication Cycle The multiplication cycle of RNA phages, like that of other viruses, is programmed, with the various reactions necessary for morphopoiesis taking place in a regularly progressing sequence. Yet, the genome of RNA phage is too small to code for proteins with a purely regulatory function. How then does it happen that coat protein, which is present in virions in 180-fold excess over A protein, is in fact synthesized in vastly greater amounts than A protein? How is it arranged that the RNA polymerase polypeptide is synthesized early during the infection cycle, when it is required, and not throughout the cycle? And since parental RNA genomes must be both translated and transcribed, what mechanism prevents collisions between ribosomes, which traverse messenger RNA from the 5′- to the 3′-terminus, and RNA polymerase molecules, which traverse templates in the opposite direction?

The genomes of RNA phages are polycistronic messenger RNAs; there are three ribosome attachment sites, one at the start of each cistron. Like other RNAs, they possess a pronounced secondary structure that is determined by base pairing between homologous nucleotide sequences, probably rather like that exhibited by tRNA molecules, and, as a result, the accessibility of individual sequences to approaching molecules or particles differs markedly. The most accessible ribosome binding site in the naked phage RNA is that at the beginning of the cistron that codes for the coat protein, which would therefore be formed in the greatest amount. However, attachment of ribosomes there renders the site at the beginning of the polymerase cistron also accessible to ribosomes, so that during the initial stages of infection, both coat protein and polymerase are formed freely. Coat protein itself, however, can bind to the ribosome binding sites at the beginning of the A protein and polymerase cistrons, thereby preventing ribosome attachments, so that as it accumulates, it gradually inhibits translation of these two cistrons more and more strongly. The net result is that the A protein cistron is translated only infrequently throughout most of the infection cycle and the polymerase cistron is translated frequently during the early stages of the infection cycle but only very infrequently during the later stages.

The collision problem is solved in the following manner. When a polymerase molecule attaches to the 3′-terminus of the RNA strand, it also binds to the coat protein cistron ribosome attachment site, thereby preventing further ribosome attachment. When ribosomes have cleared from the region between these two points, the polymerase molecule can then progress along the RNA strand unimpeded.

It is clear therefore that, although it is very simple and small, the RNA phage genome can nevertheless regulate a sophisticated transcription and translation program. The means by which this is achieved is by several of the four macromolecules that it controls (the RNA and the three proteins) serving dual functions.

LYSOGENY

Not all phage infections result in lysis of the host cell. There are some phages which, upon entering a sensitive cell, elicit either a lytic response, that is a typical multiplication cycle such as already described, or repress the expression of almost all their genetic information and integrate their genome into that of the host cell. The integrated phage genome, the prophage, behaves from then on like any other portion of the bacterial chromosome. This phenomenon is known as lysogeny: Bacteria harboring prophages in their chromosomes are known as lysogens, and phages capable of integrating their genomes into those of their host cells are known as lysogenic, or temperate, phages.

When it was discovered that some animal viruses could enter into a similar relationship with their hosts (Chap. 69), the analogy between them and temperate phages was quickly recognized, and although there are differences in the manner in which tumor viruses and temperate phages interact with their host cells, the concepts which have evolved from studies with the latter have profoundly influenced our thinking concerning the former.

The Prophage

The frequency of lysogenization varies both with the phage-host system and with the multiplicity of infection. It is greater the higher the multiplicity, which suggests that each phage genome has a finite probability of lysogenization. The number of any particular species of prophage per lysogen is generally the same as the number of bacterial genomes, suggesting that the prophage attachment site is restricted to a particular locus on the bacterial chromosome. That a unique location generally exists can be demonstrated by genetic studies, such as the interrupted mating technique (Chap. 8). However, occasionally there is more than one attachment site for the same prophage, and all may be occupied simultaneously. Superinfection may result in the integration of two prophages at the same site, inserted either into each other or tandemly (adjacent to each other). Further, bacterial chromosomes generally contain prophage attachment sites for several different unrelated prophages, and all of these may be occupied at the same time. Finally, a temperate phage, phage μ, exists that has no specific integration site but that can insert its genome anywhere in the bacterial chromosome.

The Concept of Immunity

Under normal conditions prophage is stable. Termination of the lysogenic state does, however, occur spontaneously with low frequency (of the order of 10^{-5}), the phage genome is excised from the host chromosome (p. 926), and a normal lytic multiplication cycle then ensues. As a result, cultures of lysogenic bacteria generally contain low titers of infectious virus. A variety of agents that inhibit host DNA replication, notably irradiation with ultraviolet light and chemical compounds capable of alkylating DNA, increase the frequency of termination of the lysogenic state, or induction, to almost 1. That is, almost 100 percent of lysogenic bacteria in a culture can be induced at the same time under appropriate conditions.

Although cultures of lysogenic bacteria always contain infectious phage, they are not lysed by it. They are immune. This is not because the phage cannot adsorb and inject its DNA, but it is due to the inability of the injected DNA to express itself and replicate. The reason for this is that one of the prophage genes codes for a repressor that prevents transcription of all other phage genes, both those on prophage and those on superinfecting phage genomes. Immunity is highly specific and bacteria lysogenic for one phage are not immune to other temperate phages unless they are closely related.

The Nature of Phage λ

By far the most intensively studied of the many temperate bacteriophages that are known to exist is the coliphage λ, which is probably the most intensively studied of all viruses. The exquisite and intricate mechanism that controls its interaction with the host and its multiplication represents the system par excellence with which to study biologic control. We will therefore discuss the mechanisms operating in lysogeny in terms of the λ system.

Phage λ possesses a simple noncontractile tail with one terminal tail fiber and is composed of about 10 polypeptide species. Its DNA, which contains no unusual bases, is linear and has a molecular weight of 31×10^6, representing about 50 genes. Figure 70-14 shows a simplified genetic map of λ. About 20 genes code for its structural proteins and for proteins that function in its morphogenesis. These genes, which include genes A to J, are in the left arm of the DNA, which contains 55 percent guanine plus cytosine. Some 30 other genes have been identified as regulating in one way or another the interaction of the λ genome with that of the host cell and its transcription and translation. These genes are located in the right arm of the DNA, which contains 45 percent guanine plus cytosine. Not all genes are transcribed from the same DNA strand. As shown in Figure 70-14, some genes are transcribed from one strand, while others are transcribed in the opposite direction from the other strand.

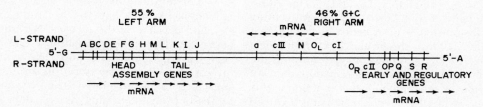

FIG. 70-14. A simplified genetic map of phage λ. (Adapted from Taylor, Hradecna, and Szybalski: Proc Natl Acad Sci USA 57:1618, 1967)

The ends of the two strands of λ DNA are not equal in length. Each 5′-terminus has an unpaired single-stranded region 12 nucleotides long. The base sequence at the left arm 5′-terminus is GGGCGGCGACCT, and that at the right arm terminus is complementary to this. Phage λ DNA cyclizes readily because these two sequences, known as "cohesive" or "sticky" ends, tend to hybridize. The origin of the sticky ends is as follows: Just like the DNA of T4 and φX174, λ DNA replicates via an intermediate that is longer than it is itself. Whereas the T4 intermediate is split into random headful portions of DNA, causing T4 DNA to be circularly permuted, λ DNA is split at specific locations, and the scissions in the two strands do not coincide but are 12 nucleotides apart.

Events Leading to Lysogeny: Integration

When λ DNA enters the cell, it cyclizes, and the two nicks are sealed by polynucleotide ligase, thus forming covalently closed circles. The decision whether a lytic multiplication cycle is to be initiated or whether the phage genome is to become integrated is then made within a brief critical period. It appears to be influenced principally by the relative rates with which several viral gene products reach critical concentrations and by their ability to function. Two of these gene products are the proteins specified by genes N and cI. The N gene product, which apparently modifies the host RNA polymerase, is essential for the switching on of all early λ genes. If it is not synthesized, or if it is defective, phage λ cannot multiply, and the lytic response to λ infection is precluded. The protein specified by gene cI is the λ repressor, a protein with a molecular weight of about 30,000, which in dimeric and perhaps also in monomeric and tetrameric form binds to two operators, O_R and O_L, on either side of gene cI (Fig. 70-14), thereby preventing the transcription of all λ genes, including that of gene N. While the cI and N gene products are of critical importance in determining the outcome of the phage-host interaction, they are by no means the only ones that function in this manner. In fact, the mechanism that is involved is extraordinarily complex. The reason for this is that phage-coded proteins are required for integration, and the phage must therefore not impose repression before these proteins are synthesized but must shut off viral development before an irreversible commitment to lytic growth is made. Among several other proteins that are also important is determining the outcome of infection and those specified by gene Q, which provides for the rapid synthesis of head, tail, and lysis proteins and therefore promotes lytic development, and those specified by genes cII and $cIII$, which provide for rapid synthesis of the repressor.

If sufficient N and Q gene products are formed, the λ genome can express itself, and a lytic infection cycle ensues. This also happens in the case of mutants with mutations in gene cI that render the repressor defective and which are therefore obligatorily virulent. If, however, the repressor accumulates, the λ genome cannot express itself. In that case the λ genome has two options. (1) It is integrated into the host genome by a mechanism that is illustrated schematically in Figure 70-15. The region aa′ between genes J and $cIII$ aligns itself with the region bb′, the prophage attachment site on the bacterial chromosome, which is situated between the galactose and biotin genes. Enzymes coded by the phage int system then make scissions in all four nucleotide strands, the phage DNA is inserted by means of double crossing over, and covalent bonds are then reformed. The λ genome is now integrated. It should be noted that the gene order on prophage is the reverse of that on vegatative λ DNA. (2) If the aa′ and bb′ regions do not match, most commonly because of a deletion, the phage genome cannot become integrated. It then multiplies in the host cell as an episome (Chap. 8). In either event, the only λ gene that is transcribed is gene cI.

Release from Repression: Induction

The termination of the lysogenic state, or induction, requires both release from repression and excision of the phage DNA from the host DNA. The cellular signal for release from repression is inhibition of host DNA synthesis (p. 924), which apparently causes an inducing substance to be generated that prevents the repressor from functioning. As a result enzymes specified by the int and xis phage genes can be synthesized which excise the phage DNA from the host DNA. Excision proceeds essen-

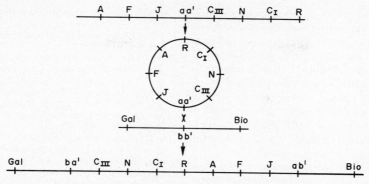

FIG. 70-15. The Campbell model for prophage integration. After circularization of λ DNA by joining of cohesive ends, reciprocal recombination between phage aa' and bacterial bb' recognition sites provides for linear insertion of the viral DNA into that of the host. (Adapted from Echols and Joyner: In Fraenkel-Conrat (ed): Molecular Basis of Virology, 1968. Courtesy of Reinhold Book Corp.)

tially via reversal of the integration process and yields a circular DNA molecule, which then replicates in the normal manner characteristic of virulent λ infection.

The juxtaposition of bacterial and phage genes in the chromosome of the lysogen sometimes leads to excision occurring in such a manner that some bacterial DNA is excised together with phage DNA. This provides an opportunity for the transfer of genetic material from one bacterium to another via phage DNA, which is known as "transduction." Transduction discussed in Chapter 8.

The Significance of Lysogeny

Every bacterium may well carry one or more prophages. Numerous defective or cryptic prophages are known, that is, prophages that lack the complete set of information necessary for phage multiplication, so that even when induced and therefore excised, no infectious phage particles are formed. Bacteria harboring such prophages are analogous in some respects to cells transformed by defective SV40 virus (Chap. 69). Even if they possess complete genomes, lysogenic phage cannot be detected unless nonimmune bacterial indicator strains are available that lack prophage attachment sites and that can be infected by the lytic pathway.

Lysogenic Phage Conversion Although in most cases the phenotype of bacteria that carry prophage is indistinguishable from that of bacteria that do not, there are several interesting examples where there is a clear difference. These bacteria exhibit the phenomenon known as "lysogenic conversion."

One case of lysogenic conversion involves the phage-mediated conversion of the somatic O antigen of *Salmonella*. This antigen forms part of the lipopolysaccharide structure of the cell wall and is composed of highly esterified lipid (lipid A) linked to a polysaccharide core to which side-chains consisting of repeating sequences of a variety of sugars are attached (Chap. 6). The antigenic specificity resides in the sugars and can be modified by altering their nature.

A wide variety of temperate phages of *Salmonella* can modify the antigenic properties of the somatic O antigen. For example, the O antigen of *Salmonella anatum* normally has the antigenic formula 3,10 (based on its response pattern to various antisera) and carries terminal O-acetyl-D-galactosyl groups linked by means of α-1:6 linkages to D-mannosyl residues. When lysogenized by the temperature phage ϵ^{15}, antigenic specificity 10 is lost, and specificity 15 is acquired. This is due to loss of the O-acetyl group and replacement of the α-1:6 bond by a β-1:6 bond. Cells lysogenized by phage ϵ^{15} can themselves be lysogenized by phage ϵ^{34}, which causes a further change in antigenic specificity, this time due to the addition of D-glucosyl residues by means of α-1:4 linkages. There are numerous other examples.

There is no doubt that the chemical alterations in *Salmonella* polysaccharides are phage-induced since ϵ^{15} causes repression or inhibition of the α-1:6-galactosyl transferase and acetylase and codes for a β-1:6-galactosyl trans-ferase. These converting functions are, how-ever, not essential to the phage, since mutants defective in them grow well. On the other hand, it is significant that ϵ^{15} cannot adsorb to cells with antigenic specificity 3,15, that is, cells carrying ϵ^{15} cannot be infected by it. The significance of this type of lysogenic conver-sion, therefore, lies most probably in the speci-fication of host range patterns, possibly in order to augment phage immunity systems.

A second example of lysogenic conversion concerns *Corynebacterium diphtheriae.* Toxi-genic strains carry the prophage β, and nontoxi-genic strains can be made toxigenic by lysogeni-zation. It is clear that the structural gene for toxin is located on the phage genome, since phage mutants coding for defective toxin have been isolated. However, it is not clear what ad-vantage the phage gains by coding for a poly-peptide with the remarkable biologic and enzymatic properties of the toxin (Chap. 33). Most probably the advantage relates not to the phage but to the bacterial lysogen. In other words, corynebacteria that can synthesize toxin most probably have a survival advantage over those that can not do so.

A third example involves *Clostridium botu-linum* types C and D, which only produce toxin when demonstrably infected with (and yield-ing) phages CE β and DE β respectively. How-ever, in their case, the relation between host cell and phage may not be true lysogeny, since infected *C. botulinum* becomes nontoxigenic (and nonvirogenic) when treated with antiser-um to phage.

FURTHER READING

Barksdale L, Arden SB: Persisting bacteriophage infec-tions, lysogeny, and phage conversions. Annu Rev Microbiol 28:265, 1974

Borek E, Ryan A: Lysogenic induction. Prog Nucleic Acid Res Mol Biol 13:239, 1973

Bradley DE: Ultrastructure of bacteriophages and bacter-iocins. Bacteriol Rev 31:230, 1967

Cairns J, Stent GS, Watson JD: Phage and the Origins of Molecular Biology. New York, Cold Spring Harbor Laboratory of Quantitative Biology, 1966.

Casjens S, King J: Virus assembly. Annu Rev Biochem 44: 555, 1975

Cohen SS: Virus-induced Enzymes. New York, Columbia University Press, 1968

Echols H: Developmental pathways for the temperate phage: lysis vs. lysogeny. Annu Rev Genetics 6:157, 1972

Eiserling FA, Dickson RC: Assembly of viruses. Annu Rev Biochem 41:467, 1972

Eklund MW, Poysky FT, Reed SM, Smith CA: Bacterio-phage and the toxinogenicity of Clostridium botulinum type C. Science 172:482, 1971

Eoyang L, August JT: Reproduction of RNA bacterio-phages. In Fraenkel-Conrat H, Wagner RR (eds): Com-prehensive Virology, New York and London, Plenum Press, 1974, vol 2, p 1

Fox TD, Pero J: New phage-SP01-induced polypeptides associated with Bacillus subtilis RNA polymerase. Proc Natl Acad Sci USA 71:2761, 1974

Gottesman ME: The integration and excision of bacterio-phage λ. Cell 1:69, 1974

Hausmann R: The genetics of T-odd phages. Annu Rev Microbiol 27:51, 1973

Hershey AD (ed): The Bacteriophage Lambda. Cold Spring Harbor Laboratory, 1971

Herskowitz I: Control of gene expression in bacteriophage lambda. Annu Rev Genetics 7:289, 1973

Jazwinski SM, Lindberg AA, Kornberg A: The gene H spike protein of bacteriophages φX 174 and S13. 1. Functions in phage-receptor recognition and in transfection. Virol-ogy 66:283, 1975

Jazwinski SM, Marco R, Kornberg A: The gene H spike protein of bacteriophages φX 174 and S13. II. Relation to synthesis of the parental replicative form. Virology 66:294, 1975

King J, Casjens S: Catalytic head assembling protein in virus morphogenesis. Nature 251:112, 1974

King J, Laemmli UK: Bacteriophage T4 tail assembly: Structural proteins and their genetic identification. J Mol Biol 75:315, 1973

Kozak M, Nathans D: Translation of the genome of a ri-bonucleic acid bacteriophage. Bacteriol Rev 36:109, 1972

Lemke PA, Nash CH: Fungal viruses. Bacteriol Rev 38:29, 1974

Lindberg AA: Bacteriophage receptors. Annu Rev Micro-biol 27:205, 1973

Male CJ, Kozloff LM: Function of T4D structural dihydro-folate reductase in bacteriophage infection. J Virol 11: 840, 1973

Mathews CK: Bacteriophage Biochemistry. New York, Cincinnati, Toronto, London, and Melbourne, van Nostrand-Reinhold, 1971

Siegel PJ, Schaechter M: The role of the host cell mem-brane in the replication and morphogenesis of bacterio-phages. Annu Rev Microbiol 27:261, 1973

Sternberg N, Weisberg R: Packaging of prophage and host DNA by coliphage λ. Nature 256:97, 1975

Studier FW: Bacteriophage T7. Science 176:367, 1972.

Summers WC: Regulation of RNA metabolism of T7 and related phages. Annu Rev Genetics 6:191, 1972

Vanderslice RW, Yegian CD: The identification of late bacteriophage T4 proteins on sodium dodecyl sulfate polyacrylamide gels. Virology 60:265, 1974

Weissman C, Billeter MA, Goodman HM, Hindley J, Weber H: Structure and function of phage RNA. Annu Rev Biochem 42:303, 1973

SECTION 5
CLINICAL VIROLOGY

71
Diagnostic Virology

TREATMENT OF SPECIMENS
IDENTIFICATION OF VIRUS
TISSUE PATHOLOGY
ELECTRON MICROSCOPIC EXAMINATION

Specific diagnosis of viral infection is essential if antiviral therapy is to be practical, and it should also enhance the development of more rapid diagnostic methods. Viral diagnostic facilities vary greatly, and the clinician must determine what specific resources are available in his hospital or community. The facilities of the municipal or state health departments are accessible and without direct patient costs, and through these laboratories referral of clinical materials can be made to the Center for Disease Control in Atlanta, Georgia. In addition, laboratories within community hospitals and associated with medical schools are accessible in some areas.

There are viral diseases where the diagnosis will be of extreme importance to the patient, his family, or his community. For example, the possibility of a traveler importing smallpox has increased with the expansion of world air travel. However, the World Health Organization's global program for eradication of smallpox has resulted in a dramatic reduction in the number of countries reporting this disease and in the number of cases in these countries. This increases the difficulty of the accurate clinical diagnosis of smallpox by physicians who have had no personal experience with the disease. It also increases the importance of understanding how the laboratory can efficiently assist the clinician. Similarly, the correct diagnosis of an initial case of paralytic poliomyelitis can allow effective immunization to be instituted, thereby preventing a sizable outbreak of disease. This requires isolation, identification, and typing of the virus in the laboratory.

In particular instances an appropriate viral diagnosis will allow cessation of unnecessary therapy and may shorten hospitalization. For example, a cerebrospinal fluid pleocytosis may commit a patient with viral meningitis to hospitalization and at least 10 days of antimicrobial therapy for possible bacterial infection. Many of the enteroviruses can be isolated and recognized in the laboratory within several days after obtaining the spinal fluid specimen, thus permitting an early reevaluation of the need for therapy and hospitalization.

When rubella infection is suspected in the first trimester of pregnancy, the currently available accurate serologic means of identification are mandatory to confirm the diagnosis prior to any consideration of pregnancy interruption.

The serologic assessment of rubella immunity should become an integral part of the female premarital examination, since attenuated rubella vaccine offers a means of establishing immunity in susceptible women prior to pregnancy.

Finally, diagnostic virology provides an excellent means for training young physicians to become familiar with viral illnesses, institute appropriate control measures when necessary, and provide appropriate prophylaxis for others when this is available. Laboratory documentation of viral illness that confirms the clinical impression on the one hand, or provides an unsuspected diagnosis on the other, will improve the judgment of these physicians who will be providing patient care for many years to come.

TREATMENT OF SPECIMENS

A basic understanding of laboratory procedures is necessary to utilize optimally the available virus laboratory facilities. Whenever a specimen is submitted, adequate information must accompany the request. This information is essential, as specimens are often processed in the laboratory according to their source and the physician's provisional diagnosis. Commonly needed information includes patient identification and age, the clinical diagnosis, the referring physician, the source of the specimens, and the date when they were obtained. In addition, it is often helpful to know whether the patient has recently received viral vaccines. The laboratory that is responsible for processing these materials should be consulted whenever questions arise, since they will be able to specify the optimal handling of the materials.

Patient materials are cultured for the presence of viruses to detect a specific etiologic agent (Table 71-1). Such specimens are inoculated into tissue cultures, embryonated eggs, or animals. Tissue culture systems are usually more readily available, less cumbersome, and less expensive than are embryonated eggs or animals. The type of cells that are utilized is dictated in part by the facilities available in the particular laboratory and by the suspected type of infection. It is usually advisable to collect specimens as early as possible in the course of a

TABLE 71–1 SUGGESTED SPECIMENS TO BE SUBMITTED FOR VIRAL DIAGNOSIS

Diagnosis	Specimen Source for Culture							Serology	
	N-P	Stool	Urine	CSF	Skin°	Pleural Fluid	Pericardial Fluid	Acute Serum	Convalescent† Serum
Respiratory disease‡	X	X				X (if present)		X	X
Enteric illness	X	X						X	X
Exanthema	X	X	+		X			X	X
Aseptic meningitis	X	X	+	X				X	X
Myocarditis–pericarditis	X	X					X (if present)	X	X
Vesicular eruption	X§	+§	+§		X			X	X
Newborn baby with suspected intrauterine infection	X	X	X	X	+‖			X#	
Orchitis–parotitis**	X		X					X	X
Hepatitis–infectious mononucleosis group of illnesses	X		X					X††	X††

X, denotes usual sites of culture
+, denotes sites that may also be useful
°Vesicle fluid, pustules, or skin scrapings
†Convalescent serum 2–4 weeks after onset of illness
‡Agents include respiratory syncytial virus, adenoviruses, enteroviruses, influenza, parainfluenza viruses, and coronaviruses
§In cases of generalized eruption
‖Mother's cervix can be examined by Papanicolaou stain
#Blood in newborn period and 6–9 months after birth. Mother's serum may also be evaluated
**Usually mumps; occasionally Coxsackie virus or lymphocytic choriomeningitis virus
††Peripheral leukocytes from heparinized blood may yield EB virus or CMV. HB$_s$Ag determinations should be performed on sera

clinical illness. Since viral agents are not affected by antimicrobial agents, cultures may be obtained even if therapy for potential bacterial pathogens has previously been initiated. Such materials are obtained from the same site(s) as specimens for bacterial cultures. Throat secretions, stool, urine, cerebrospinal fluid, pleural fluid, pericardial fluid, blood, bone marrow, vesicle fluid, and skin scrapings may be utilized in attempted viral isolations. Tissue specimens from biopsies or postmortem examinations are suitable for attempted viral isolation if fresh or frozen but not in formalin.

The principles adhered to in the collection of bacterial specimens are applicable to specimens submitted for viral culture. Containers must be clean and sterile and handled accordingly. The more stable viral agents include vaccinia, variola, the enteroviruses, and the adenoviruses. As it is rarely possible to know the particular etiologic agent until the virus is isolated, all specimens should be treated as though the agent were potentially labile. Most viruses are unstable at an acid pH or at temperatures greater than 4C. Attempts to culture such agents as respiratory syncytial virus may fail if the material has previously been frozen or allowed to stand at refrigerator temperatures for more than a few hours. All patient specimens should be transported as rapidly as possible to the laboratory. If a delay of hours occurs, the material should be refrigerated at 4C; longer delays prior to inoculation usually necessitate freezing of the specimens, preferably at −70C.

In addition to their heat and acid lability, many viruses do not withstand drying. Thus, specimens other than body fluids (blood, cerebrospinal fluid, urine) should be placed in a transport medium that provides both a protein source and a buffered salt solution for preserving infectious virus. Several such media are easily made and readily available from any microbiology laboratory. A 1 percent solution of skimmed milk in distilled water or Hanks' balanced salt solution with 10 percent fetal calf serum or bovine albumin have been used successfully. Each of these media has antibiotics (penicillin 50 units/ml, amphotericin 1 μl/ml, streptomycin 5 μg/ml) included to prevent overgrowth by resident host bacterial flora and to decrease exogenous specimen contamination.

IDENTIFICATION OF VIRUS

Isolation of an agent from a patient does not always prove an etiologic relationship to his illness. For this reason, patients being evaluated for viral disease should have both acute and convalescent sera drawn for antibody determinations. The commonly accepted serologic confirmation of acute infection is a fourfold or greater rise in antibody titer. The acute specimen of blood is obtained from the patient as early as possible in his illness, and the convalescent specimen is drawn two to three weeks later. The serum is separated and kept at refrigerator or freezer temperature. Whole blood should not be frozen, as the erythrocytes lyse and the subsequent assay of hemolyzed serum is difficult and inaccurate. Serologic demonstration of antibody response may provide evidence of infection in the absence of recovery of virus from culture. Serology may also be used to assay the immune status of an individual following previous infection or vaccination.

The most frequently used techniques for assaying virus antibodies include complement fixation (CF), hemagglutination inhibition (HI), and neutralization of the viral cytopathic effect. Complement fixation offers a relatively rapid, efficient way of screening sera for a number of viral antibodies. It is particularly useful for determining whether recent infection has occurred. As a general rule the antibodies thus detected are group-specific and not type-specific (Chap. 64). For example, adenovirus antibody can be distinguished from poliovirus antibody, but antibody to type 1 adenovirus cannot be distinguished from antibody to types 7, 8, 12, or any other adenovirus CF antibody. CF antibodies usually decline more rapidly than specific neutralizing antibodies, so that their absence does not necessarily denote susceptibility.

Hemagglutination-inhibition (HI) studies are limited by the fact that not all viruses possess a hemagglutinin. Agents with recognized hemagglutinins are influenza, mumps, measles, the parainfluenzae, rubella, vaccinia, variola, the arboviruses, and some of the adenoviruses and ECHO viruses. The limitations of the test itself are primarily technical, as it is often difficult to eliminate nonspecific inhibitors of hemagglu tination from the serum being tested. The HI antibodies are type-specific, and the test is quite sensitive, correlating well with the antibodies observed in the neutralization test.

Neutralizing antibodies are highly specific for the virus type, appear early in the course of the illness, and persist for a long time thereafter. The determination of neutralizing antibody requires the growth of an agent in a cell culture or an animal system. The serum in question is incubated with the suspected etiologic agent and is then placed into the appropriate culture system. The results are commonly unavailable for at least a week, as the appearance of the cytopathic effects in the cell culture or illness in the animal determines the length of time necessary for the performance of the test.

In recent years adaptation of several immunologic techniques has been of great assistance in the viral diagnostic laboratory. In the case of serum hepatitis, immunoprecipitation has been employed to detect viral antigen in the secretions or sera of individuals. Countercurrent immunoelectrophoresis has increased the speed with which such determinations can be performed and has made the test available on a large scale. This technique and the radioimmunoassay (RIA) are examples of rapid, accurate diagnostic procedures that are already of practical value.

Immunofluorescent staining is available for specific situations. The basic techniques are simple, but interpretation of results requires persons skilled and familiar with the materials and methods. Technical problems have hindered the utilization of the techniques by many general microbiology laboratories.

TISSUE PATHOLOGY

Any hospital where tissue pathology is done can examine tissues microscopically, and this may facilitate a viral diagnosis. Histologic examination of pertinent clinical specimens with hematoxylin and eosin or Giemsa stains may disclose pathognomonic features of viral infection, such as inclusion bodies or multinucleate giant cells.

Measles infection, either that of natural disease or of attenuated virus, may produce multinucleate giant cells in the urine as well as intranuclear and intracytoplasmic inclusions. Such findings have also been described in the sputum or throat scrapings of patients with giant cell pneumonia or in malnourished patients with measles. Rubella, mumps, Coxsackie viruses, and variola have been reported to produce eosinophilic cytoplasmic inclusions in the cells of the urine sediment. Agents, such as cytomegalovirus and herpes simplex virus, have been observed to produce intranuclear inclusions in cells in the urine. Such positive findings in the urine, sputum, or tissues will point toward the probability of viral infection but, without laboratory culture of the virus, cannot identify the specific agent involved. The absence of such findings does not exclude viral disease, and it is very important to recognize that many agents (for example, the enteroviruses) may not cause specific hallmarks of viral infection.

Cutaneous lesions, such as vesicles, macules, or pustules, can also be examined for the presence of multinucleate giant cells and inclusion-bearing cells. Materials obtained from such lesions can be examined easily and quickly. The vesicle is sponged with alcohol (if no viral cultures are being taken from the lesion), and the roof of the vesicle is reflected. The fluid is blotted, the base of the lesion is scraped, avoiding gross bleeding where possible, and the cellular material is spread on a glass slide and air dried. It can be fixed with methyl alcohol and stained with Wright's or Giemsa stain. Giant cells are readily apparent, and with carefully made preparations inclusions may be seen. The presence of such giant cells will exclude vaccinia and variola from the differential diagnosis but will not distinguish between herpes simplex and varicella-zoster. Similarly, the diagnosis of herpes simplex infection of the female genital tract can be approached by obtaining a swab of the cervix and examining by Papanicolaou stain for giant cells and/or intranuclear inclusions.

ELECTRON MICROSCOPIC EXAMINATION

The electron microscope has been utilized recently to assist in viral diagnosis. Examination of materials from vesicular lesions by experienced personnel can readily distinguish a viral agent of the Herpesviridae family from one of the Poxviridae family. Another example of the use of the electron microscope has been the detection of previously unrecognized viral particles in stool specimens. These observations have led to identification of several agents of the Reoviridae family now considered causative in acute gastrointestinal disease. Other refinements of methodology have broadened the diagnostic applications of the electron microscope. For example, the use of specific antiserum causes adherence of virions to the antibody and results in clumps of virus particles. This clumping may permit detection of virus particles previously too few to be recognized in specimens. Such immune electron microscopy may evolve into a practical, rapid mode of serologic identification of tissue culture isolates.

The information provided in this brief discussion can be applied in the diagnosis of all the virus infections discussed in the chapters that follow.

FURTHER READING

Bradstreet CMP, Pereira MS, Pollock TM: The organization of a National Virological Diagnostic Service. Prog Med Virol 16:242, 1973

Herrmann EC Jr: New concepts and developments in applied diagnostic virology. Prog Med Virol 17:222, 1974

Hsiung GD: Diagnostic Virology. New Haven and London, Yale Univ Press, 1973

Lennette EH, Spaulding EJ, Truant JP: Manual of Clinical Microbiology, 2nd ed. Washington, DC, The American Society for Microbiology, 1974

Schmidt NJ, Lennette EH: Advances in the serodiagnosis of viral infections. Prog Med Virol 15:244, 1973

72
Poxviruses

Poxviruses cause disease associated with skin lesions in many species of animals: examples are cowpox, vaccinia, mousepox (ectromelia), rabbitpox, sheeppox, swinepox, fowlpox, myxoma, fibroma, and contagious pustular dermatitis (Table 62-4). In addition, several poxviruses are human pathogens. Two of these, smallpox (variola) and molluscum contagiosum, are specifically human infections, while the others, vaccinia, orf, milker's nodules (pseudocowpox), cowpox, and Yaba monkey tumor virus are primarily animal pathogens that may be transmitted to man. By far the most important of these is smallpox, which has been one of the principal scourges of mankind throughout history until the last 50 years.

SMALLPOX

History Smallpox was recognized as a specific entity in Africa and Asia as early as 1000 BC. It probably spread to Europe during the Arab expeditions of the sixth century: the term "variola" was applied to the disease by Marius of Avenches in 570 AD, and the clinical illness was described by Bishop Gregory of Tours in 582 AD. Dissemination of the disease into all parts of Europe was a product of the accelerated commerce with Africa and Asia beginning with the voyages of the Vikings into the Mediterranean in the eighth through tenth centuries and continuing with the Crusades. Steady urbanization of the population in Europe created a sufficient density of susceptible people to permit disastrous epidemics in the seventeenth and eighteenth centuries. In the 1760s in London one-tenth of all deaths and one-third of all deaths in children were due to smallpox. Eighty percent of the population living in England during the eighteenth century probably contracted the disease at some time during their lives.

Epidemiology Until recently, smallpox was a major problem throughout the entire world. As recently as 1920 over 200,000 cases of smallpox occurred annually in the United States alone. The widespread use of vaccination in developed countries and the enforcement of rigid laws requiring recent vaccination of international travelers gradually eradicated smallpox from most parts of the world until by the mid-1950s the disease occurred primarily in the Indian subcontinent, Indonesia, and parts of Africa. The World Health Organization then initiated an intensive campaign, based upon mass vaccination, to eradicate smallpox from these areas also. This campaign has been so successful that in 1974 only 15 cases of smallpox (all in Bangladesh) were reported in the entire world, and no cases at all were reported in 1975.

Transmission of the disease occurs by contact with an infected patient during the eruptive phase of the illness (p. 938). Most infections are acquired by inhalation, although inoculation through breaks in the integument may occur occasionally. The virus is resistant to desiccation and persists in an infectious state for long periods of time in scabs or on bedding and clothing.

Diagnosis In countries from which smallpox has been eradicated, its rapid diagnosis is essential, since immediate and far-reaching public health procedures must be initiated if it is introduced. Several diseases, especially chickenpox and vaccinia (p. 939), resemble smallpox in their early stages. Differentiation between chickenpox and smallpox can now be achieved very rapidly in the laboratory by any one of several methods. First, material derived from epithelial lesions or smears of vesicle fluid can be examined by means of the electron microscope for the presence of the highly characteristic poxvirus particles which are easily distinguishable from the enveloped icosahedrons of chickenpox virus, a herpesvirus. Second, samples of such material may be treated with fluorescein-labeled antibody directed against vaccinia virus or chickenpox virus: Staining with the former but not with the latter is indicative of smallpox. Third, complement-fixation or gel diffusion tests using vesicle fluid as antigen against a hyperimmune vaccinia antiserum also permit rapid diagnosis (Chap. 64). All these methods are capable of providing a diagnosis within a matter of hours.

Differentiating variola from vaccinia virus takes longer. It is best accomplished by observing the nature of the pocks produced on the chorioallantoic membrane of the developing chick embryo (Fig. 61-4) or by inoculating onto monolayers of chick embryo fibroblasts, on which vaccinia virus produces plaques, while variola virus does not.

Clinical Features   Variola exists in two clinically and epidemiologically distinct forms, caused by two different viruses which can be differentiated by their growth characteristics on the chorioallantoic membrane of the developing chick embryo at 38C and in the mouse brain. Variola major (smallpox) is a severe disease with a mortality that can exceed 50 percent, whereas variola minor (alastrim) is a much milder disease with a mortality of no more than 1 percent. Both cause specifically human generalized infections.

The course of smallpox infection is shown in Figure 72-1.

During the incubation period the virus replicates in unknown loci, probably in the respiratory epithelia and regional lymph nodes. After 8 to 14 days of local replication, during which patients are not infectious, virus particles enter the bloodstream. Viremia, which coincides with the onset of fever and prostration, results in secondary inoculation of target cells in the skin, mucous membranes, and internal organs. Two to four days later the characteristic eruptions appear. Lesions may occur over the entire body, including the palms and soles. Characteristically they progress from a maculopapular eruption to vesiculation and finally to rupture, with crusting of the residual lesions. The lesions usually erupt simultaneously over the entire body, in distinction to chickenpox, which shows multiple crops of lesions. Fever usually subsides with the appearance of the skin lesions, though it may return with secondary bacterial infection of the lesions.

The mortality rate is highly variable and depends on the nature of the virus strain, the previous health of the patient, the presence of secondary infection, and the availability of medical care. In most epidemics, the death rate is approximately 25 percent, but confluent or hemorrhagic smallpox bears a much graver prognosis.

Treatment and Prevention   Until recently no effective therapy existed to abort the illness during the incubation period or to abbreviate the clinical illness. Vaccination has no effect if it is performed during the incubation period. Hyperimmune vaccinia antiserum or gamma globulin possesses a limited effect in aborting the disease but accomplishes nothing once the disease is manifest. N-methyl isatin-β-thiosemicarbazone (methisazone) (Chap. 68) suppresses the disease in contacts, suggesting that it may be of some value after the lesions of smallpox have appeared.

Public Health Measures   Smallpox is a quarantinable disease. Suggestive symptoms coupled with a history of sojourn in or passage through endemic areas within the preceding two weeks should lead to a suspicion of smallpox. Doubtful cases should be referred promptly to the Public Health authorities for laboratory diagnosis. If the diagnosis is positive, the patient must be removed immediately to an appropriate quarantine facility, and all objects with which he has come into contact must be disinfected. All human contacts should either receive hyperimmune vaccinia gamma globulin or be vaccinated or revaccinated, given methisazone, and kept under surveillance for 16 days.

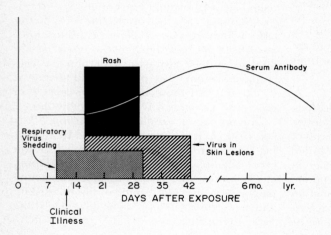

FIG. 72-1. The course of infection with smallpox virus.

Patients with smallpox should be isolated with utmost care. All medical personnel engaged in treatment of patients should have been vaccinated within the preceding six months. After the patient has been removed from quarantine, the quarters should be cleaned meticulously and exposed to germicidal lamps or to formaldehyde gas before being used again.

Vaccination   The use of variolation was introduced into Europe from Asia in the seventeenth century. This first recorded use of immunization in man was accomplished by removing infectious material from the lesions of a patient with smallpox and inoculating the material into the skin of another individual. This practice generally produced only limited disease, though classic smallpox was produced occasionally, and the mortality from this procedure was about 1 percent. Benjamin Franklin was interested in it and wrote a pamphlet describing the results of this practice in London in 1759.

Protective vaccination with cowpox was described by Edward Jenner in 1798 in a paper entitled "An Inquiry into the Causes and Effects of the Variola Vaccinae." Though initial opposition to this revolutionary practice existed, Jenner's findings were soon recognized as being valid, and by 1805 Napoleon ordered that all his troops should be vaccinated.

Today the virus used for vaccination is always vaccinia virus. Its origin is uncertain; it may have been derived from Jenner's original strain of cowpox virus, or it may have evolved from recombination of cowpox and smallpox. Its importance lies in the fact that intradermal inoculation of it into man produces a localized infection in the skin followed by the development of neutralizing antibodies for related poxviruses, including smallpox. Vaccination every 6 to 12 months produces a high level of protection against smallpox infection.

Vaccinia virus for use in man is prepared by inoculating one of a number of strains into the scarified skin of calves and allowing the lesions to reach maturity in five to seven days. At a suitable stage the animal is sacrificed and the crusts are harvested by scraping. Glycerol and brilliant green are added and the tissue is disrupted by grinding. Preparations suitable for vaccination must contain 10^6 to 10^8 pockforming units per 0.05 ml as assayed on the chorioallantoic membrane. In the form of suspensions in liquid, the vaccine must be kept frozen. In lyophilized form, vaccinia virus prepared in this manner remains active for at least a month at room temperature. This form of the vaccine is essential for use in underdeveloped areas. Recently, vaccinia virus for vaccination purposes has been prepared to an increasing extent in the chorioallantoic membrane of the developing chick embryo. For suggestions for the further improvement of vaccines, including smallpox vaccine, see Chapter 68.

METHODS OF VACCINATING.   Vaccination against smallpox is achieved as a result of intradermal inoculation. A drop of the vaccine is applied to a small sterilized area of the skin, and the epidermis beneath it is then rapidly punctured about 30 times by means of a sharp sterile needle. The point should not be driven into the skin, but at each pressure the elasticity of the skin should pull a fraction of an inch of the epidermis over the point of the needle, so that the vaccine is carried into the deeper layers of the epidermis. There should be no bleeding, and all evidence of trauma should fade out in less than six hours. Immediately after the pressures have been made, the remaining vaccine is gently wiped off with sterile gauze.

In mass vaccination campaigns, jet guns are often used.

Response to Vaccination   The extent of multiplication and spread of virus from the inoculated site depend on the state of immunity and hypersensitivity of the host. Normally three types of response are noted.

VACCINIA OR PRIMARY REACTION.   When there is no antibody, a papule appears on the third to the fifth day and rapidly becomes a vesicle, which reaches its greatest development on the eighth to tenth day and develops a secondary erythema. Often there may be some axillary lymphadenitis and mild febrile reactions. After the tenth day the pustule dries up, and a scab forms, which then separates. Immunity develops on about the tenth day.

VACCINOID OR ACCELERATED REACTION.   This reaction is seen in those retaining partial immunity from a previous attack of smallpox or a previous vaccination. The whole reaction is less pronounced and more rapid than the primary reaction, with the papule appearing on the third day or fourth day and vesicle formation by the fifth. Pustulation is frequent. The height of the reaction occurs on the sixth or seventh day, after which it subsides rapidly.

IMMEDIATE OR ALLERGIC REACTION. This reaction is usually seen in solidly immune individuals. A red area is obvious at the site of inoculation by 24 hours, increases in size until the third day, and then begins to subside without a vesicle forming. This type of reaction, formerly interpreted as indicating immunity, is more likely to be a delayed type of allergic reaction and can be induced with equal or greater frequency with heat-inactivated virus. It is in effect a hypersensitivity response. Such a reaction does not always indicate immunity, nor does it necessarily lead to immunity, since individuals giving such reactions may be allergic and nonimmune or allergic and immune. Individuals giving this response who are likely to be exposed to smallpox should be revaccinated with fresh virus.

Adverse Reactions to Primary Vaccination Ordinarily no untoward results follow vaccination, particularly revaccination. However, primary vaccination does occasionally entail serious complications. Fortunately these are rare (1 to 3 per 10,000), and the mortality rate is less than 1 per 100,000 vaccinations. However, even this low number is too high when millions are being vaccinated. In most Western countries routine compulsory vaccination has now been abandoned.

The complications which may follow primary vaccination are as follows.

POSTVACCINATION ENCEPHALITIS. This is characterized by the development of headaches, fever, and confusion 10 to 13 days after vaccination. The spinal fluid may contain 100 to 200 mononuclear cells per cu mm at this time. The pathogenesis of the disease is unknown. It is uncertain whether vaccinia virus invaded the neural tissue directly or whether this complication is a form of allergic encephalopathy. Recovery from the illness may be incomplete, with residual mental deficiency, and the mortality rate is generally between 25 and 50 percent.

ECZEMA VACCINATUM. This condition may occur when patients with generalized dermatitis are vaccinated or exposed to a family member who has recently been vaccinated. The illness is characterized by generalized vesiculation, fever, and prostration beginning 5 to 10 days after exposure (Fig. 72-2). The mortality rate is 30 to 40 percent. This complication is readily avoidable in most instances by avoiding vaccination of individuals with dermatitis. If they must be vaccinated, they should be given antivaccinial immunoglobulin and/or methisazone at the time of vaccination.

PROGRESSIVE VACCINIA OR VACCINIA GANGRENOSUM. This is a very rare condition which occurs most frequently in individuals who have some immunologic defect, such as those seen in leukemia, Hodgkin's disease, giant follicular lymphoma, and occasionally in patients with agammaglobulinemia. This complication is characterized by a marked and inexorable increase in the size of the vaccination lesion, with

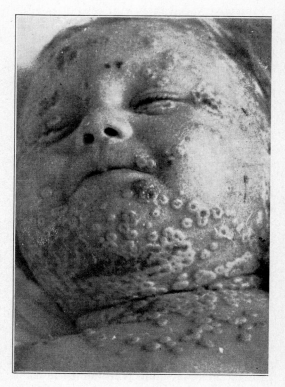

FIG. 72-2. Eczema vaccinatum. (From Perry and Maritneau: JAMA 141:657, 1949)

excavation and gangrene extending into the deep tissue. Fresh vesicles may appear, and there may be viral ulceration of the nasopharynx. The mortality rate exceeds 50 percent.

GENERALIZED VACCINIA.   This condition occurs when viremia is established, and typical secondary vesicles appear over body surfaces remote from the inoculation site in a healthy individual. The cornea may be involved, and permanent scarring may result. Most cases of generalized vaccinia are usually mild, though death occurs in 10 to 20 percent of cases.

Abortion may occur in pregnant women due to intrauterine infection of the fetus. Vaccination during pregnancy should therefore be avoided.

OTHER POXVIRUSES

Several other poxviruses occasionally produce disease symptoms in man.

Molluscum Contagiosum

This is a specifically human disease spread by direct contact and inoculation of the virus into minute abrasions in the skin. Two to eight weeks after inoculation a small papillomatous lesion appears at the site of inoculation (Fig. 72-3). These lesions are easily distinguished from other papillomata by their umbilicated appearance produced by central

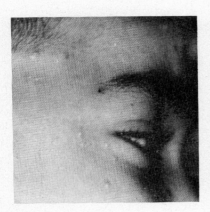

FIG. 72-3. Molluscum contagiosum lesions on the face. (From Neva: Arch Intern Med 110:720, 1962)

degeneration and by the formation of satellite nodules at the periphery of the parent lesion. On pathologic examination the epidermis shows ballooning degeneration, acanthosis, hyperplasia, and the presence of large acidophilic inclusions (molluscum bodies) in superficial epithelial cells. Ordinarily the lesions, which are white in color and painless, disappear after a few months and require no therapy. The incubation period varies widely from 14 to 50 days. The disease is worldwide but much more common in some localities than in others. Swimming pools may be a source of infection.

Orf

This old Saxon term refers to the infection of man with the virus of contagious pustular dermatitis (scabby mouth) of sheep, which is not a true poxvirus, but a parapoxvirus. In lambs the disease is characterized by the development of watery papillomatous lesions on the cornea, lips, and mouth, which usually resolve in four to six weeks without consequence. In man vesicles usually develop at the site of abrasions on the hand or face, which may evolve into hyperplastic nodular masses accompanied by regional lymphadenopathy. Ordinarily the lesions require no treatment. Since parapoxviruses and orthopoxviruses are only very distantly related immunologically, vaccination provides no protection. Orf is an occupational disease associated with handling of sheep, particularly in shearers.

Milker's Nodules (Pseudocowpox)

This conditions is also caused by a parapoxvirus. It is a cutaneous disease of cattle that may be transmitted to man by contact. Lesions appear one to two weeks after contact and are similar to those produced by contagious pustular dermatitis. Recovery is complete in four to eight weeks. Reinfection may occur, indicating that immunity does not last long.

Cowpox

Cowpox produces a vesicular eruption on the udders of cattle from which it may be transmitted to man. Usually the illness in man is a limited vesicular eruption of the skin, though rarely the disease develops into a widespread eruption with systemic symptoms. The disease occurs occasionally in Europe but appears to be virtually unknown in the United States.

Yaba

Yaba monkey tumor virus causes a disease accompanied by the formation of numerous masses of densely packed histiocytes in the skin measuring 25 to 50 mm in diameter. After a period of 6 to 12 weeks the nodules usually regress spontaneously. Accidental or experimental but no spontaneous infection in man has been reported.

FURTHER READING

Baxby D: Identification and interrelationships of the variola/vaccinia subgroup of poxviruses. Prog Med Virol 19:216, 1975

Bedson HS, Dumbell KR: Smallpox and vaccinia. Br Med Bull 23:119, 1967

Cho CT, Wenner HA: Monkeypox virus. Bacterial Rev 37:1, 1973.

Dick G: Smallpox: a reconsideration of public health policies. Prog Med Virol 8:1, 1966

Dixon CW: Smallpox. London, Churchill, 1962

Downie AW: Poxvirus group. In Horsfall FL, Tamm I (eds): Viral and Rickettsial Infections of Man, 4th ed. Philadelphia, Lippincott, 1965, p 932

Downie AW, Kempe CH: Poxviruses. In Lennette EH, Schmidt NJ (eds): Diagnostic Procedures for Viral and Rickettsial Infections, 4th ed. New York, American Public Health Association, 1969, p 281

Kaplan C: Immunization against smallpox. Br Med Bull 25:131, 1969

Kemp CH, St. Vincent L: Variola and vaccinia viruses. In Lennette EH, Schmidt NJ (eds): Diagnostic Procedures for Viral and Rickettsial Disease, 3rd ed. New York, American Public Health Association, 1964, p 665

Lane JM, Ruben FL, Neff JM, Millar JD: Complications of smallpox vaccination, 1968. N Engl J Med 281:1201, 1969

Marsden JP: Variola minor: a personal analysis of 13,686 cases. Bull Hyg 23:735, 1948

McCarthy K, Downie AW, Bradley WH: Antibody response in man following infection with viruses of the pox group: antibody response following vaccination. J Hyg (Camb) 56:466, 1958

73
Herpesviruses

The herpesviruses of man include Herpes simplex virus, the varicella-zoster virus, cytomegalovirus (CMV), and the Epstein-Barr virus (EBV). While not closely related, they nevertheless cross-react serologically to a significant extent. Herpesviruses in general (though not EBV) have a tendency to infect derivatives of the ectoderm, and it is not surprising, therefore, to find that their infections manifest skin/or nervous system involvement. Herpesviruses also possess oncogenic potential; at least two of the human herpesviruses are strongly suspected of causing cancer in man. The other fascinating characteristic of herpesviruses is that they may establish latent infections, with reactivation possible after variable periods of quiescence.

HERPES SIMPLEX VIRUS

Infections induced by Herpes simplex virus were recognized and described by early physicians. The word "herpes" derives from the Greek, *herpos,* to creep. Hippocrates probably knew and described herpetic infections, Galen may have used the name herpes to describe zoster, and Richard Morton, who gave us the name "chickenpox," also wrote a good account of herpes simplex infections.

Herpes simplex virus infections commonly involve the skin, mucous membranes, eyes, and central nervous system. The initial or primary infection is generally acquired through the mouth, mucous membranes, or broken skin. Infection may also be acquired by venereal contact. Most primary infections are unrecognized or subclinical. In many (and perhaps all) cases the virus becomes latent, and the patient develops antibody. Subsequently, in response to a variety of stimuli, the latent virus may be reactivated. Reactivation is not usually accompanied by a significant antibody change and may occur with or without recognizable accompanying lesions. The spread of recrudescent herpes simplex virus very likely occurs cell-to-cell, since otherwise it is difficult to imagine how the virus would avoid the neutralizing effects of circulating antibody.

Recurrent herpes infections may be stimulated by fever, menstruation, exposure to sunlight (ultraviolet irradiation), emotional upsets, or intercurrent infections. Not all febrile diseases are equally efficient in stimulating reactivation of these recurrences. Herpetic lesions are very

common in malaria and in pneumococcal pneumonia, less frequent in brucellosis, and rare in typhoid fever.

Primary Herpes simplex virus Infections

Gingivostomatitis This condition affects children between the ages of 1 and 6 years. It occurs without any seasonal distribution and is accompanied by fever and a sore mouth. The gums become painful and swollen and then vesiculated. Ultimately the vesicles ulcerate, and the gingival surface bleeds readily. Vesicles also appear on the buccal mucosa, tongue, and lips. The lesions may less commonly involve the tonsillar pillars and pharynx. The child remains febrile and ill for about one week, though the ulcers may require a longer time to heal completely.

It is apparent that the most heavily involved tissues are those of ectodermal derivation. In contrast, herpangina, a reflection of enterovirus (Coxsackie A) infection, is accompanied by painful vesicular lesions, involving primarily the posterior oropharynx (tissues of endodermal origin). This distinction is not absolute, however, and herpangina and herpetic gingivostomatitis are commonly confused. It is noteworthy that Coxsackie infections have a seasonal incidence, with marked prevalence in the summer and early fall months.

The major problems encountered by children with herpetic gingivostomatitis relate to the extreme discomfort, as well as the difficulty in maintaining fluid balance and adequate nutrition during the acute phase of disease. Topical anesthetics may be applied to permit some oral ingestion of fluids, but care must be taken not to anesthetize the posterior pharynx and epiglottis, since this may interfere with swallowing.

Vulvovaginitis In this case the primary lesions involve the mucous membranes and skin of the labia and lower vagina. The ulcers are accompanied by fever and regional lymphadenopathy. Primary vulvovaginitis is recognized more frequently than is its counterpart in males, herpes progenitalis.

Meningoencephalitis Many   cases   of hepetic meningoencephalitis follow a primary infection of the central nervous system. However, in some instances this illness follows viral recurrence in individuals with preexisting antibodies. These illnesses are severe and quite damaging. They are accompanied by significant swelling, necrosis, and destruction of the involved brain. The mortality may be as high as 70 to 80 percent, and survivors frequently manifest residual brain damage.

Keratoconjunctivitis The eye represents an important site of serious herpetic infection. Corneal ulcerations induced by herpesvirus may be quite deep and can result in blindness. Primary herpetic involvement of the eye can be severe and should be treated promptly.

Eczema Herpeticum (Formerly called Kaposi's varicelliform eruption. This confusing eponym, which was also applied to eczema vaccinatum, should not be used.) This condition is a complication of eczema or severe atopic dermatitis. The abraded weeping and denuded skin is inoculated with virus, which spreads widely in the absence of the protective cornified epithelium. The onset of disease is heralded by fever and nonspecific symptoms, followed by the appearance of vesicles which evolve and crust in a fashion similar to those of varicella. A Tzanck preparation (pp. 946 and 947) may distinguish herpetic infections from vaccinial involvement. Lesions may appear for more than one week. The course is variable, ranging from a mild illness to a severe fulminant and fatal disease.

Involvement of Abraded and Injured Skin Herpetic infections may occur in the skin of burned patients, in wrestlers (herpes gladiatorum), and at the site of injured cuticles on the fingertip (herpetic whitlow). The latter condition is an occupational hazard if personnel do not wear gloves when providing mouth care to debilitated patients.

Disseminated, Visceral, and Congenital Herpes Simplex Virus Infections When a primary herpesvirus infection occurs in a pregnant woman, the fetus is at risk just as in the case of maternal rubella or CMV infection. Unprotected by maternal antibodies, the fetus may become infected in utero and develop stigmata of severe disseminated congenital viral infection.

In the case of herpes simplex virus, the major involvement is of the liver and the central nervous system.

If the maternal infections involve the cervix or the labia, the infant may be infected during passage through the birth canal. In this case, the manifestations of infection may be delayed several days postnatally. It has been suggested that if a significant maternal genital infection is recognized prepartum, it is an indication for caesarean section, although in some instances even operative removal of the fetus has failed to prevent evolution of the disease, suggesting that transmission occurred earlier by an ascending route or due to a maternal viremia.

Disseminated herpes simplex virus infections in the newborn carry a grave prognosis. Although most of these babies succumb, a few survive, making difficult the evaluation of the few (uncontrolled) trials of systemic therapy.

Individuals other than the fetus and neonate subject to disseminated herpes simplex virus infections include these patients severely debilitated and or malnourished, individuals receiving immunosuppressive therapy or having a severe underlying immunologic deficit, and occasional patients undergoing certain intercurrent infections (such as measles) which abrogate normal cellular immune mechanisms.

Recurrent Herpes simplex virus Infections

Individuals who experience recurrent herpes simplex virus infections always have preexisting serum antibody to the virus. The manifestation of recurrence is most frequently a skin eruption—grouped vesicles surrounded by a halo of erythema. Prior to the appearance of the vesicles the patient may experience a burning or itching sensation at the site. Most often these eruptions occur on the face at mucocutaneous junctions, such as the nostrils or, more frequently, the lips (herpes labialis). The vesicles evolve, crust, and fade in approximately one week.

Recurrent herpetic eruptions may also occur at the site of traumatic virus inoculation of the skin. In addition, the vesicles may appear in other areas of mucocutaneous junction, including the penis (herpes progenitalis), the urethral orifice, and the vulva.

Although eruptions recur in the same site

with little variation, latent virus does not reside in the skin. Areas of affected skin have been excised between recurrences, and fresh unaffected skin has been transplanted. After this procedure, the recurrent disease may return at the original site. It is likely that virus may be latent in the ganglia of sensory nerves innervating the affected area of skin. In support of this concept, recurrent herpetic lesions of the skin occasionally follow the distribution of sensory nerves, imitating zoster in appearance (zosteriform herpes). In this regard, herpes simplex virus has been recovered from explanted neural ganglia in man and experimental animal hosts. It has been proposed that the virus remains latent in sensory nerve ganglion cells and, under certain circumstances, travels down the associated neural axons to involve the skin and associated organs of the innervated dermatome.

Since occasionally herpetic recurrence may involve the central nervous system, not all recurrent herpes infections are benign. Herpetic encephalitis is accompanied by a high mortality. Encephalitis frequently involves the temporal lobe and may present as a mass lesion of the brain. Indeed, radiologic studies may suggest the presence of a brain tumor.

Corneal herpes may also recur, with resultant repetitive attacks of keratoconjunctivitis. These repeated episodes of herpetic activation may result in progressive corneal injury and, finally, blindness.

The pathogenesis of recurrent herpes infections has been extensively studied. Rabbits are subject to recurrent herpes infection and have been used as experimental models. A proportion of inoculated animals will develop a herpetic encephalitis. Surviving rabbits appear entirely well, and yet induction of anaphylactic shock or treatment with epinephrine can reactivate the latent virus and produce fatal encephalitis.

EPIDEMIOLOGY.   Herpes simplex virus infections are virtually universal, and there are no appreciable seasonal patterns. Most people are infected by the age of 6 or 7 years. Only about 1 percent of those infected experience a recognizable associated illness. A much larger percentage of the general population possessing antibodies will develop recurrent herpetic eruptions at some time. Herpetic infection is more common in lower socioeconomic groups.

Spread appears to be primarily by direct contact.

Two subtypes of herpes simplex virus have been distinguished: herpes simplex virus Type 1, which usually infects the mouth, throat, respiratory tract, eyes, and central nervous system; and herpes simplex virus Type 2, which involves primarily the genitalia. These types are commonly termed "oral" and "genital" strains. Although either strain may involve the oral or genital mucosa, there is a striking tendency for oral strains to produce infections above the waist, while herpetic infection below the waist is usually caused by genital strains. These subtypes may be distinguished on the basis of serologic and biologic studies. These variants can also be clearly distinguished biochemically.

For a discussion of the role of herpes simplex virus in the etiology of cancer, see Chapter 69.

DIAGNOSIS.   Diagnosis   of   herpesvirus infections may usually be made on clinical grounds. However, where uncertainty or therapeutic considerations arise, virologic and serologic techniques are available. Because of the rapid replication of *H. simplex* in vitro, a more prompt diagnostic study may be performed in this instance than in the case of most viruses.

A Tzanck smear (scrapings of the vesicle base stained with Giemsas stain) will reveal multinucleated giant cells and intranuclear inclusions in the case of herpesvirus infections. One cannot by this means, however, distinguish between varicella-zoster virus and herpes simplex virus infections.

A skin test of the delayed hypersensitivity type has been developed for herpes simplex virus but its clinical usefulness is limited.

TREATMENT.   Recurrent herpes infections had been treated for years with a vast variety of preparations. In this case, as in most instances, a diversity of therapeutic approaches indicates that none were actually very effective. In 1962 Kaufman demonstrated that herpetic keratitis could be ameliorated with the topical use of 5-iodo-2′-deoxyuridine (IDU). This halogenated pyrimidine competes with thymidine for incorporation into DNA, thus yielding a biologically inactive nucleic acid (Chap. 68). These studies gave vast impetus to the field of antiviral chemotherapy. However, although treatment with IDU did have a significant effect on the superficial keratitis, it did not actually cure the disease or heal deep lesions. Recurrences were not prevented, and after prolonged therapy resistant mutants appeared.

Topical treatment of recurrent herpetic skin vesicles has also been attempted. Results were generally disappointing, although herpes progenitalis was said to be ameliorated, and application of IDU to skin by a spraygun applicator appeared to have some effect upon recurrent lesions.

In several severe life-threatening hypersvirus infections, systemic IDU treatment has been attempted, and some amelioration may have been accomplished. Treatment has been applied to neonatal and adult herpes virus simplex encephalitis. In a controlled double-blind study, six patients were treated with a full course of systemic IDU. Four survived without residual damage. Of seven untreated patients, only one survived without serious residual.

Whereas steroids are helpful in certain viral infections or postviral immunologic diseases, these substances are contraindicated during most herpes virus simplex infections. Whether applied topically or administered systemically, they appear to enhance virus spread and should ve avoided. Steroids may be administered to patients with herpetic encephalitis, in which case their role may be to reduce brain swelling and edema.

VARICELLA (CHICKENPOX)

CLINICAL COURSE. In nosocomial outbreaks the incubation period is between 15 and 18 days. The existence and severity of the prodrome is variable, ranging from nothing recognizable in the pre-eruptive phase to a moderate period of fever, headache, anorexia, and malaise. In most children systemic symptoms and the exanthem appear simultaneously. The course of the disease is illustrated in Figure 73-1.

The characteristic rash of varicella may be preceded by a brief scarlatiniform eruption. Thereafter the exanthem appears abruptly, usually first on the trunk, then spreading to involve the extremities. Macules evolve quickly

into papules and then into superficial clear watery vesicles surrounded by an erythematous area. These water dropletlike vesicles are in contrast to the lesions of variola and vaccinia, which are more firm and deeply seated. Lesions frequently appear on the scalp as well as on the palms and soles. Where creases of the skin are involved the vesicles may become oval and elongated. The vesicles are usually not umbilicated and do not feel hard except occasionally over areas of heavy cornification, such as the palms and soles. The vesicular fluid becomes cloudy (bacteria and inflammatory cells) for two to three days and subsequently dries as the vesicles crust (after approximately one week). The lesions evolve rapidly and continue to spread, with new vesicles making their appearance for up to one week. For this reason, the varicella patient characteristically appears with crops of lesions in a variety of stages.

The concentration of lesions is generally heavier on the trunk and the central portion of the extremities. In contrast to variola and vaccinia, the vesicles and pustules of chickenpox tend to involve the axillae and in general favor covered, protected areas of the trunk. Varicella lesions concentrate in body hollows rather than on prominences. The palate and tonsillar areas may also be involved.

Pathologically, varicella skin lesions consist of ballooned injured and degenerating cells in the deeper layers of epidermis, accompanied by a massive outpouring of extracellular fluid. In the base of the lesion giant cells may be found, some multinucleated, with intranuclear inclusions. In contrast, scrapings from the vesicles of vaccinia or variola yield cells with cytoplasmic inclusions only. These observations form the basis of the Tzanck test, in which scrapings from the base of fresh vesicles are prepared with Giemsa stain and examined microscopically.

When varicella occurs in the adult, systemic symptoms may be severe, the rash very profuse, and the entire disease much more intense than in childhood. The rash may become hemorrhagic, and occasionally bullous lesions appear. Varicella pneumonitis is rare in children, and though also uncommon in adults, this complication is much more frequent in older individuals. In (rare) fatal cases of varicella pneumonia an associated hepatitis may be found at autopsy. Varicella pneumonia may be followed

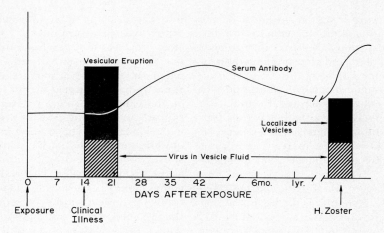

FIG. 73-1. The course of varicella virus infection.

by the appearance of scattered calcified nodules visible on chest x-ray.

Significant secondary bacterial infection of varicella lesions may occur. These are usually staphylococcal or streptococcal infections. In the latter instance, complications of the streptococcal invasion may occur, including septicemia and acute glomerulonephritis. Acute rheumatic fever does not occur following streptococcal invasion of varicella skin lesions.

Reye has described the syndrome of acute hepatic failure, encephalopathy, and hypoglycemia which may appear following several infectious entities. The syndrome, which has now been recognized by many additional clinicians, has in a significant number of cases followed varicella, in some instances accompanied by a history of the administration of large doses of salicylates.

Rarely varicella is accompanied by encephalitis, which may appear before, coincident with, or following the eruption. Although most individuals with varicella encephalitis survive and recover without sequelae, there is an incidence of mortality (about 5 percent) and brain damage (7 of 59 in the series of Applebaum reported in 1953).

In recent years, several new problems have been posed for certain special patients exposed to the varicella virus. These individuals include those being treated with high doses of corticosteroids, cytotoxic, or immunosuppressive drugs and patients with disseminated malignancies, who, with the benefit of chemotherapy, are maintained alive although with severely compromised immunologic functions. Patients receiving immunosuppressive therapy may develop herpes zoster, which can in some cases spread to become generalized. Generalized zoster is, essentially, the same condition as varicella. Very elderly and/or debilitated patients may develop varicella even in the presence of a definite past history of childhood varicella.

EPIDEMIOLOGY. Varicella is primarily a disease of children. There is a peak incidence between the ages of 2 and 8 years. Cases do occur in adults who have escaped infection during childhood and occasionally in individuals with compromised cellular immunity on the basis of disseminated malignancies, extreme age and disability, or immunosuppressive drug therapy. If a primary infection occurs during pregnancy, the virus is capable of crossing the placenta and infecting the fetus. Congenital infections may be associated with the appearance at birth or shortly thereafter of varicella. Neonatal varicella may be severe, and it carries a significant mortality. There is some suggestive evidence, however, that if the eruption is present at birth or shortly thereafter, the illness is more often mild, possibly reflecting the transmission of some maternal antibody. It has been recognized recently that primary maternal varicella occurring early in gestation may result in congenital infection manifested at birth by cicatrizing lesions of the extremities as well as neuromuscular disorders.

The disease is worldwide in distribution and

occurs throughout all seasons, with a somewhat higher incidence in winter and spring in temperate climates. Large fluctuations in case occurrence and significant epidemics do not occur. The illness occurs sporadically and endemically in most urban centers in the United States. Microepidemics occur especially within families and schools, reflecting the lability of this agent and the need for relatively close direct contact to effect transmission. With direct contact varicella is a highly transmissible infectious disease. Although there exists some evidence for transmission of varicella by the respiratory route, the virus has been very difficult to recover from the nasopharynx, possibly because the presence of virus in the mouth and pharynx occurs very early during the incubation period.

DIAGNOSIS. The diagnosis of chickenpox is usually made on clinical grounds. The features of the rash already described will usually serve to distinguish this exanthem. The differentiation of varicella and variola remains important, especially in an era when jet travel permits importations of smallpox rather early during incubation. It has been recognized that electron microscopic survey of phosphotungstic acid-stained vesicle contents provides a rapid diagnosis, since the virions of herpesviruses are readily distinguished from those of poxviruses.

The viruses of varicella and zoster are almost certainly one and the same, and the agent is frequently called V-Z virus. The identity of these viruses is based upon their behavior in tissue cultures, the interchangeable results of cross-immunologic studies, and inoculation studies. In the latter, susceptible children inoculated in the skin with vesicle fluid from zoster and varicella patients develop typical chickenpox. In the presence of a past history of chickenpox or zoster, inoculation with either fluid is without effect.

TREATMENT AND PREVENTION. Treatment of varicella is usually symptomatic and revolves in most cases around control of fever and itching. Other than this, the therapy of varicella is directed at the complications of this infection. Steroids have been advised in the treatment of varicella encephalitis as well as in hemorrhagic chickenpox. The latter seems paradoxical,

since hemorrhagic varicella has occurred as a complication of long-term steroid therapy. There exists no good evidence for the efficacy of steroids in treating these complications, although steroid therapy does not appear hazardous. The key factors here are apparently the dose and duration of steroid therapy. Intercurrent varicella in a patient on long-term steroid medication is frequently severe. Short-term therapy instituted after the onset of disease is apparently, in contrast, without significant danger.

Exposed individuals are usually not protected by administration of pooled gamma globulin. Brunell and associates prepared zoster immune globulin (ZIG) from the plasma of patients recovering from herpes zoster and found that a 2 ml dose of ZIG given within 72 hours after the initial exposure prevented varicella. Infection was apparently prevented rather than modified (failure of antibody rise). It has been shown that ZIG is protective when administered to varicella-exposed susceptible adults as well as to patients with cancers, those under therapy with corticosteroids or antimetabolites, and exposed newborns whose mother contracted chickenpox at or near term.

Prolonged isolation of infected children is generally not indicated, although in order to protect the highly susceptible patients who populate modern hospitals, individuals with varicella should only be admitted to a general medical ward when absolutely necessary and then under strict isolation precautions.

After the prodromal symptoms develop or the eruption of varicella appears, preventive measures have no effect. In the face of life-threatening varicella infections the use of experimental drugs is justified. Drugs that inhibit DNA synthesis, developed in the course of cancer chemotherapeutic studies, have been applied, and encouraging preliminary reports have been obtained in disseminated severe varicella infections occurring in patients with malignancies and immunologic deficiencies.

HERPES ZOSTER (SHINGLES)

CLINICAL COURSE AND EPIDEMIOLOGY. It is thought that herpes zoster in most cases probably represents a reactivation of latent virus (acquired during an earlier bout of varicella). The length of the incubation period is thus uncertain. It is thought that in some patients, after chickenpox, the V-Z virus remains latent in host nerve root cells, in most cases cells of the posterior root ganglia or cranial nerve roots. The factors that reactivate the virus are ill defined. Cold and trauma have been cited. Since zoster may appear following exposure to varicella, some authors propose that the condition may also follow invasion of a partially immune host by virus newly acquired. That altered immunity plays a role in any case seems likely, since zoster frequently appears in patients with diminished immunologic competence. Zoster may appear in a newborn or young child after maternal chickenpox. The latter infection probably was transmitted to the fetus and resulted in a partial or inadequate degree of immunity.

Once activated, the virus apparently moves down the sensory nerves to the innervated skin. The most common site of sensory nerve involvement is the skin innervated by the thoracic ganglia. The most frequently affected cranial nerve is the fifth (trigeminal).

The outstanding prodromal symptom of zoster is pain. The eruption appears following three or four days of pain. The skin lesions resemble those of varicella, but their distribution is strictly along the course of the affected sensory or cranial nerve(s). The evolution of vesicles is identical to that described for varicella. Regional nodes may be enlarged and painful.

The distribution of lesions is usually unilateral. When the ophthalmic branch of the trigeminal nerve is involved, the uvea may become inflamed. Involvement of the mandibular branch may lead to the appearance of vesicles on the mouth and tongue, while maxillary branch zoster may yield vesicles on the uvula and tonsil. When the geniculate ganglion is involved, the Ramsay-Hunt syndrome appears (ear pain, facial paralysis, and vesicles in the external auditory canal). It is of interest that an identical syndrome may be produced by infection with herpes virus simplex.

Pathologically, the involved skin is indistinguishable from that seen in the case of varicella. Infected sensory nerves may show axonal degeneration and demyelination.

DIAGNOSIS.   In most cases the diagnosis is readily made on the basis of the clinical findings. It should be noted that herpes virus simplex may cause identical (zosteriform) eruptions. Giemsa stain of vesicular scrapings cannot distinguish V-Z infection from that of herpes virus simplex, but V-Z virus may be grown in tissue culture and can be serologically differentiated from herpes virus simplex. Serologic studies may be helpful, since zoster patients develop high levels of antibody very rapidly after the appearance of lesions (immunologic recall).

TREATMENT.   During the acute stages of zoster, treatment is directed primarily at control of pain. Occasionally, this pain may persist, leading to a severe painful neuralgia. Extreme measures have been attempted to control this postinfectious neuralgia. These include injection of the involved ganglion with alcohol, leukotomy, or application of cold to the affected area. The number and variety of therapeutic maneuvers employed is a reflection of the lack of consistent success resulting from the use of any one.

CYTOMEGALOVIRUS

HISTORY.   At the turn of the century several pathologists reported the presence of large swollen cells in the liver, kidney, and lungs of infants dying with presumed congenital syphilis. These cells were so odd in appearance that they were thought to represent invasive amebae rather than altered host cells. By 1910 the ameba had actually been classified and named *Entamoeba mortinatalium*.

It remained for Goodpasture and Talbot in 1921 and Lipschütz in the same year to recognize that these cells resembled the swollen, injured inclusion-bearing cells seen in some virus infections. Goodpasture and Talbot were so impressed by the massive swelling of the infected cells that they coined the term "cytomegaly."

Farber and Wolbach recognized salivary gland cytomegaly in an astonishing 12 percent of infants dying of all causes. Infants with overwhelming CVM infection were said to have cytomegalic inclusion disease (CID). At the same time, the concentration of observations on the salivary glands led to the designation of the virus as "salivary gland virus." To prevent confusion with other salivary gland-associated viruses and in recognition of its potential spread to many organs, the virus was finally re-named "cytomegalovirus (CMV)." At least three serotypes which share complement-fixing antigens can be distinguished by neuralization tests.

CLINICAL COURSE. A broad spectrum of clinical illnesses has been associated with CMV infections. The picture emerging from epidemiologic surveys is that of a ubiquitous virus which may be shed persistently by infected hosts. In the face of persistence and widespread occurrence, it has been difficult to assign to CMV etiologic responsibility even when the virus is recovered in simultaneous association with a clinical entity. Certain conditions have, however, been definitely or tentatively associated with CMV infections.

Congenital Infections When a primary CMV infection occurs during gestation, the virus may invade the placenta. The infection then spreads to involve the fetal villi, followed by a viremia in the developing fetus. The results of fetal CMV infection, reminiscent of congenital rubella invasion, may be dependent upon the timing and extent of the virus invasion.

Many babies survive to term though infected and damaged. The length of gestation may not be altered, although the infants are small and were in the past termed "premature." They may bear clinical resemblance to infants born after congenital infections with rubella, toxoplasmosis, herpes simplex virus and syphilis.

Typically the baby manifesting congenital CMV infection is small-for-dates and has hepatosplenomegaly and associated abnormalities of liver function. Petechial rash is common (Fig. 73-2), associated with a moderate thrombocytopenia and hemolytic anemia. The most common and devastating injuries and abnormalities are those of the central nervous system. Infected infants may be microcephalic or (less commonly) hydrocephalic. There may be additional intense involvement of the central nervous system, such as chorioretinitis, infantile seizures, intracerebral calcifications, and, occasionally, massive necrosis of the brain. Deafness has been reported as have microphthalmia, cataracts, and glaucoma. Although these latter abnormalities occur less frequently than they do in association with congenital rubella, their occurrence emphasizes the difficulties which

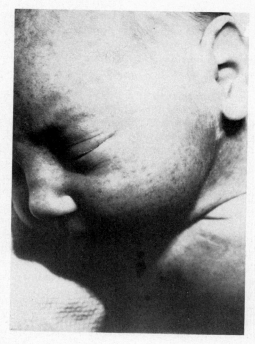

FIG. 73-2. Fine macular and petechial rash in a neonate with congenital cytomegalovirus infection.

may be encountered in distinguishing these conditions.

In addition to arrested and/or abnormal development, some organs of affected infants manifest evidence of active or burned-out inflammation and injury. Thus one may find bile stasis associated with periportal inflammatory infiltrates, giant-cell hepatitis, focal pancreatic fibrosis, and pulmonic and renal infiltrates.

In general, recognizable congenital CMV infection occurs only following a primary maternal infection. However, several investigators have reported the birth of two successive CMV infected babies to one mother. Reactivated CMV may, therefore, in some instances be transmitted congenitally.

Recognition of congenital CMV infections was originally based upon pathologic studies of fatal cases, which created the impression that CMV infection was rare and usually fatal. More recent studies, using virologic as well as exfoliative techniques, have shown that cytomegaloviruria can be detected in 1 to 2 percent of neonates. Between 15 and 20 percent of these infants eventually exhibit evidence of central nervous system damage.

Hepatitis   Acquired CMV infections are frequently associated with hepatitis. The manifestations of CMV hepatic disease are usually milder than those associated with hepatitis A or B.

Mononucleosis   In 1965 Klemola and associates reported the association with CMV of a heterophil-negative, mononucleosislike syndrome. Affected patients may exhibit high spiking fevers and chills associated with a mild hepatitis, enlarging spleen, and large numbers of atypical lymphocytes. A similar syndrome occurring in approximately 3 to 5 percent of patients following cardiopulmonary bypass perfusion during open-heart surgery was also found to be associated with CMV infection. Blood transfusions seem to be incriminated, with the implication that CMV may be carried in the blood of asymptomatic blood donors. As many as 50 to 60 percent of seronegative patients undergoing perfusion or receiving multiple transfusions of blood develop virologic and/or serologic evidence of CMV infection. In one study, CMV was recovered from the blood of 2 of 35 asymptomatic blood donors.

Opportunistic Infections   Patients with disseminated malignancies, those with immunologic deficiencies, especially of the cellular variety, and individuals receiving steroids and/or immunosuppressive therapy experience clinically significant CMV infections very frequently. As many as 90 percent of recipients of organ transplants exhibit evidence of CMV infection during life or at autopsy. Although some of these infections are apparently recently acquired and primary, there is evidence that many represent reactivation of latent virus. Some patients develop interstitial pneumonia terminally, and at autopsy evidence may be found of extensive CMV involvement of the liver, kidneys, and central nervous system.

Epidemiology.   Anywhere from 20 to 80 percent of a population possess CF antibody by adulthood. Cytomegalovirus spreads slowly and apparently requires close contact for transmission. It is presumed that CMV is transmitted in salivary secretions, and it has been suggested that venereal infections also occur. Virus may be recovered from the saliva, the urine, and from the uterine cervix. Lang and Kummer have demonstrated the prolonged presence of CMV in semen in the absence of urologic symptoms or significant alterations in the composition of semen. Virus was recovered from semen when simultaneous urine specimens were negative for CMV. In addition, virus may be present in blood, and it has also been recovered from human milk.

The persistence of viruria following an initial infection has made assessment of the role of CMV in associated illnesses difficult. Viruria has been demonstrated in as many as 40 percent of children living in institutions. Surveys of children from 2 to 8 years of age living at home have revealed as many as 5 to 10 percent excreting CMV in the urine. Beyond the age of 10, however, recovery of virus from urine becomes infrequent.

Studies of pregnant women have shown an increasing incidence of viruria during gestation until, by term, as many as 3 percent of women surveyed may exhibit a viruria. Cultures of the cervix also demonstrate an increase in the number of positive cultures during the final trimester of gestation. Younger women tend to have a higher incidence of viruria, of virus recovered from the uterine cervix, and of symptomatic infected babies.

Congenitally infected infants may excrete CMV in the urine indefinitely, and viruria of four and five years duration has been documented. During early infancy these babies may have very high titers of virus in the urine and can be an efficient source of contagion to contacts.

Diagnosis.   Identification of CMV is usually made on the basis of its characteristic cytopathology, inability to replicate in cells derived from other species, and serologic studies, most of which employ the complement-fixation test, which is usually performed with a crude CMV antigen. Indirect fluorescent antibody (FA) techniques have also proved useful in the study of CMV. Based upon the observation that the fetus and neonate produce IgM antibodies which do not ordinarily cross the placenta, a CMV-specific IgM FA test has been developed which permits the identification of congenital CMV infection with the analysis of a single serum. The presence of specific CMV IgM antibody in initially asymptomatic CMV-infected infants correlates closely with the recognition later of significant central nervous system dam-

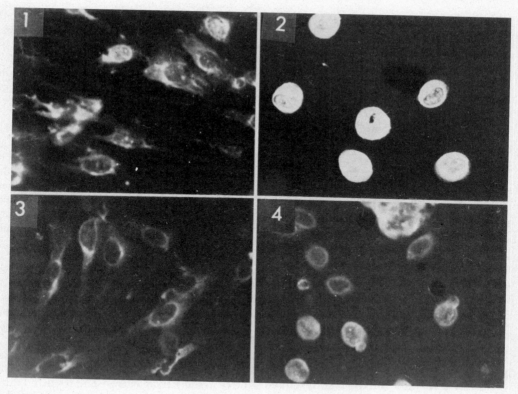

FIG. 73-3. Indirect fluorescent antibody demonstration of CMV-specific IgM antibody. IgM positive serum on (1) uninfected and (2) infected cells. IgM negative serum on (3) uninfected and (4) infected cells. (Courtesy of Drs. S. Harwood and D. Lang)

age. A positive CMV IgM FA test is depicted in Figure 73-3.

When available, laboratory isolation of CMV is the most sensitive method to identify the presence of an active infection. Urine should be collected for this purpose in a sterile fashion, maintained cold, and transported promptly to the viral laboratory. If nasopharyngeal secretions are obtained on a cotton or nylon swab, this should be immersed in transport medium. Blood specimens for isolation should be heparinized to facilitate removal and inoculation of the leukocyte-rich plasma.

When no virus laboratory is available, urine specimens may be examined in the cytology laboratory for the presence of characteristic inclusion-bearing cells (Fig. 73-4). Absence of such cells does not rule out CMV infection.

PREVENTION AND TREATMENT. The development of antitumor drugs that inhibit DNA synthesis has been exploited by virologists and clinicians to treat certain DNA virus infections, including CMV infections. Systemic administration of drugs, such as the halogenated pyrimidine derivatives and cytosine arabinoside, has been tried cautiously. Phosphonoacetic acid, a compound that seems to interfere with the function of herpesvirus DNA polymerase, has yielded encouraging results in the treatment of murine CMV infections.

Experimental CMV vaccines are presently under study in the United Kingdom and continental Europe, although some workers feel that this approach is premature.

ONCOGENIC POTENTIAL. Ultraviolet-inactivated CMV can induce malignant transformation of hamster cells, and human cells infected with active CMV transiently acquire some characteristics of transformed cells. CMV may therefore possess oncogenic potential. This possibility is being investigated actively in several laboratories.

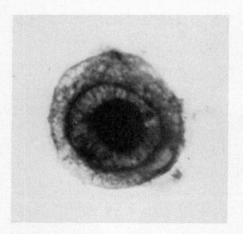

FIG. 73-4. Typical inclusion-bearing cell found in the urine of CMV-infected individual (Papanicolaou stain). ×400.

EPSTEIN-BARR VIRUS (EBV)

HISTORY.   In 1958 Burkitt first described a malignant lymphomatous disease which affected children and occurred with a peculiarly high frequency in Central and West Africa. These tumors were found to constitute about 50 percent of all malignancies seen in African children. The neoplasm, which frequently involved the jaw and abdomen, had a characteristic cytopathology termed by pathologists a "starry sky" appearance, reflecting descriptively the presence of diffuse, primitive, poorly differentiated, large, immature cells of lymphoblastic type. Epidemiologic features suggested that a transmissible agent might be involved. For example, the age distribution of the tumor resembled that seen in common virus diseases of childhood, the tumor was often multifocal, suggesting the rapid dissemination of an invading agent, clusters of cases occasionally occurred in villages and even within families, and cases occurred frequently in adult immigrants from tumor-free areas.

In 1964 Epstein, Achong, and Barr noted that a proportion of cultured cells derived from a Burkitt lymphoma contained a herpeslike virus visible on electron microscopy (Chap. 69). This virus was named the Epstein-Barr Virus (EBV).

A lymphoma similar to Burkitt's occurs in the United States, although infrequently. An American patient with a Burkitt-type lymphoma was found to possess EBV antibody. However, EBV antibody was also found widely distributed among normal healthy individuals; it appeared early in life, but without recognizable association with a specific illness.

In August 1967, a 21-year-old technician working in the laboratory of Gertrude and Werner Henle became ill. Her leukocytes, placed in culture, proliferated and established a cell line. This was in contrast to most normal peripheral white cell cultures, which usually fail to establish permanent cell lines. Fortunately, her serum was on file in the laboratory from an earlier date. This earlier serum was EBV antibody-negative, while the serum obtained during her illness manifested antibody to this virus. Meanwhile the patient was sent home with a fever, sore throat, and extreme fatigue. Her private physician subsequently made a diagnosis of infectious mononucleosis (IM).

Extensive serologic studies since have confirmed that seroconversion from the EBV-negative to the EBV-positive state occurred during IM. The significance of EBV as the etiologic agent of Burkitt's lymphoma, nasopharyngeal carcinoma and IM is discussed in Chapter 69. Although EBV has not absolutely been proven to be the etiologic agent of IM, the association is very strong, and the illness is considered here on that basis.

Infectious Mononucleosis

HISTORY.   In 1889 Pfeiffer described a glandular fever, "Drüsenfieber," which probably encompassed a melange of febrile disorders associated with lymphoid proliferation, including IM. The disease is still occasionally called Pfeiffer's disease.

In the 1920s Sprunt and Evans coined the name "infectious mononucleosis," described the clinical features more exactly, and identified the presence of the associated atypical lymphocytes. In 1932 Paul and Bunnell described the presence in IM patients of agglutinins for sheep red blood cells, heterophil antibodies. Precedence for the recognition of the sheep agglutinins in IM is claimed by a Roumanian named Haganutziu in 1924 and also independently by a German investigator Deicher in 1926. Subsequently, it was noted that similar agglutinins may be present in the sera of normal persons. The specificity of the heterophil test was markedly improved by Howard and Davidsohn, who noted that the heterophil antibodies of IM were absorbed by beef cells but not by an extract of guinea pig kidney. Heterophil antibodies in normal sera were found to be absorbed by guinea pig kidney but not by bovine erythrocytes, while an additional antibody occasionally encountered in serum sickness was absorbed by both the kidney preparation and the beef cells.

CLINICAL COURSE. Since the exact mode of transmission is uncertain, the time of infection is usually unknown, and so the incubation period is indeterminate. Guesses range from 4 to 50 days.

The initial symptoms are usually headache, fatigue, fever, chills, anorexia, and general malaise, followed by lymphoid proliferation and sore throat. Various of these features may predominate, leading some authors to subclassify IM into glandular, febrile, and aginose (sore throat) types.

The fever may be as high as 104 to 105F (40C) and accompanied by sweats and shaking chills. The patient does not appear markedly ill between bursts of fever but simply worn and exhausted. When fever prevails, the similarity of its course to that of typhoid has led some workers to designate this phase or variety of IM as "typhoidal."

The illness may be brief, or it may persist for weeks. The sore throat can be quite severe and is occasionally accompanied by a striking membranous exudate. Cases of IM are recorded in the literature which were initially diagnosed as diphtheria. Lymph nodes are frequently enlarged and tender, particularly in the cervical chain, and splenic enlargement is almost always present.

The most common additional clinical features include a mild hepatitis, transient skin eruptions, and, less frequently, pneumonitis, hematologic disorders (thrombocytopenia), and central nervous system involvement.

A high incidence of skin rash has been observed in IM patients who are treated with ampicillin, which is frequently prescribed by physicians in undiagnosed fevers. Thus, such patients might be labeled as "penicillin-sensitive" if this possible association is not kept in mind.

EPIDEMIOLOGY. Infectious mononucleosis is thought of as a disease of young adults of higher socioeconomic strata, thus college students. Cases do occur among children, although the course in younger patients is usually less severe. Infection early in life is probably frequently inapparent and may occur more often among lower socioeconomic groups.

The age-associated attack rates (per 100,000) for recognized IM in the United States are approximately as follows:

45 in the nation as a whole
66 betwen the ages of 10 and 14
343 between 15 and 19 years
123 for individuals between 20 and 24

No definite large epidemics have been noted. Hoagland suggested that close contact is required for transmission and, partially on the basis of the age distribution, hypothesized that the agent was acquired by kissing. This suggestion captured the imagination of the general public as well as physicians and the illness is sometimes called the "kissing disease," an as yet unproven, though romantic, notion.

DIAGNOSIS. The diagnosis may be suspected on clinical grounds alone. The occurrence of fever, malaise, sore throat, enlarged lymph nodes, and splenomegaly in an otherwise healthy adolescent or young adult should arouse the suspicion of IM. The finding of a lymphocytosis and the presence of significant numbers (10 to 50 percent) of atypical lymphocytes further support the diagnosis. Occasionally IM patients manifest a leukopenia with diminished granulocytes. Thrombocytopenia is sometimes present, although in IM the diminished platelet count is rarely associated with clinically significant bleeding. The presence of heterophil antibodies absorbed by bovine cells and not by guinea pig kidney completes the identification of heterophil-positive IM. The heterophil test has recently been modified by the substitution of horse erythrocytes (formalinized) which permits a sensitive, rapid spot test performed upon a very small sample of serum.

TREATMENT AND PREVENTION.   Although no definite treatment or prevention is available for IM, there has been a good deal of attention directed to the use of short-term steroid therapy for symptomatic relief and reduction of the length of required bedrest.

FURTHER READING

Herpes simplex virus

BOOKS AND REVIEWS

Docherty JJ, Chopan M: The latent herpes simplex virus. Bacteriol Rev 38:337, 1974
Kaplan AS (ed): The Herpesviruses. New York, Academic Press, 1973
Nahmias AJ, Roizman B: Infection with herpes-simplex viruses 1 and 2. N Engl J Med 289:667, 719, 781, 1973
Rapp F: Herpesviruses and cancer. Adv Cancer Res 19: 265, 1974

SELECTED PAPERS

Baringer JR: Recovery of herpes simplex virus from human sacral ganglions. N Engl J Med 291:838, 1974
Bastian FO, Rabson AS, Yee CL, Tralka TS: Herpes-virus hominis: isolation from human trigeminal ganglion. Science 178:306, 1972
Hanshaw JB: Herpesvirus hominis infections in the fetus and newborn. Am J Dis Child 126:546, 1973
Kaufman HE: Clinical cure of herpes simplex keratitis by 5-iodo-2'-deoxyuridine. Proc Soc Exp Biol Med 109: 251, 1962
Kaufman HE, Brown DC, Ellison EM: Recurrent herpes in the rabbit and man. Science 156:1628, 1967
Nahmias AJ, Naid ZN, Josey WE: Herpesvirus hominis Type II infection — associated with cervical cancer and perinatal disease. Perspect Virol 7:73, 1971
Stevens JG, Cook ML: Maintenance of latent herpetic infection: An apparent role for anti-viral IgG. J Immunol 113:1685, 1974

Varicella-Zoster

BOOKS AND REVIEWS

Brunell PA, Gershon AA: Passive immunization against varicella-zoster infections and other modes of therapy. J Infect Dis 127:415, 1973
Burgoon CF Jr, Burgoon JS, Baldridge GD: Natural history of herpes zoster. JAMA 164:265, 1975
Downie AW: Chicken pox and zoster. Br Med Bull 15: 197, 1959

SELECTED PAPERS

Brunell PA, Wolman SR, Steinberg S: Propagation of varicella-zoster virus in a diploid strain of embryonic thyroid cells from the rhesus monkey. J Infect Dis 125:545, 1972
Dodion-Fransen J, Dekegel D, Thiry L: Congenital varicel-

la-zoster infection related to maternal disease in early pregnancy. Scand J Infect Dis 5:149, 1973
Haggerty RJ, Eley RS: Varicella and cortisone. Pediatrics 18:160, 1956
Jordan GW, Merigan TC: Cell-mediated immunity to Varicella-zoster virus: In vitro lymphocyte responses. J Infect Dis 130:495, 1974
Judelsohn RG, Meyers JD, Ellis RJ, Thomas EK: Efficacy of zoster immune globulin. Pediatrics 53:476, 1974
Newman CGH: Perinatal varicella. Lancet 2:1159, 1965
Pinkel D: Chickenpox and leukemia. J Pediatr 58:729, 1961
Rifkind D: The activation of varicella-zoster virus infections by immunosuppressive therapy. J Lab Clin Med 68:463, 1966
Sargent EN, Carson MJ, Reilly ED: Varicella pneumonia: Report of 20 cases with postmortem examination in six. Calif Med 107:141, 1967
Weller TH, Wilton HM: Etiologic agents of varicella and herpes zoster: Serologic studies with viruses as propagated in vitro. J Exp Med 108:869, 1958

Cytomegalovirus

BOOKS AND REVIEWS

Krech U, Jung M, Jung F: Cytomegalovirus infections of man. Basel, Karger, 1971, pp 18-35
Plummer G: Cytomegaloviruses of man and animals. Prog Med Virol 15:92, 1973
Weller TH: The cytomegaloviruses. N Engl J Med 203, 267, 1971

SELECTED PAPERS

Abrect T, Rapp F: Malignant transformation of hamster embryo fibroblasts following exposure to ultra-violet-irradiated human cytomegalovirus. Virology 55:53, 1973
Elek SD, Stern H: Development of a vaccine against mental retardation caused by cytomegalovirus infection in utero. Lancet 1:1, 1974
Lang DJ: Cytomegalovirus infections in organ transplantation and posttransfusion: An hypothesis. Arch Gesamte Virusforsch 37:365, 1972
Lang DJ, Kummer JF: Cytomegalovirus in semen: observations in selected populations. J Infect Dis 132:472 October, 1975)
Numazaki Y, Yano N, Morizuka T, et al: Primary infection with human cytomegalovirus; virus isolation from healthy infants and pregnant women. Am J Epidemiol 91:410, 1970
Stagno S, Reynolds DW, Lakeman A, Charamella LJ, Alford CA: Congenital cytomegalovirus infection: Consecutive occurrence due to viruses with similar antigenic compositions. Pediatrics 52:788, 1973
Starr JG, Bart RD Jr, Gold E: Inapparent congenital cytomegalovirus infection. N Engl J Med 282:1075, 1970

EB Virus and Infectious Mononucleosis

BOOKS AND REVIEWS

Dalrymple W: The present status of infectious mononucleosis: A selective review. J Am Coll Health Assoc 18: 265, 1970

Editorial: EB virus, infectious mononucleosis and Burkitt lymphoma. Lancet, 2:887, 1969

Epstein MA: Aspects of the EB virus. Adv Cancer Res 13: 383, 1970

Joncas JH: Clinical significance of the EB herpesvirus infection in man. Prog Med Virol 14:200, 1972

Miller G: The oncogenicity of Epstein-Barr virus. J Infect Dis 130:187, 1974

SELECTED PAPERS

Burkitt D: Etiology of Burkitt's lymphoma—an alternative hypothesis to a vectored virus. J Natl Cancer Inst 42:19, 1969

Burkitt D, O'Coner GT: Malignant lymphoma in African children. I. A clinical syndrome. Cancer 14:258, 1961

Chang RS, Lewis JP, Abildgaard C: Prevalence of oropharyngeal excreters of leukocyte-transforming agents among a human population. N Engl J Med 289:1325, 1973

Henle G, Henle W, Diehl V: Relation of Burkitt's tumor-associated herpes-type virus to infectious mononucleosis. Proc Natl Acad Sci USA 59:94, 1968

Kieff E, Levine S: Homology between Burkitt herpes viral DNA and DNA in continuous lymphoblastoid cells from patients with infectious mononucleosis. Proc Natl Acad Sci USA 71:355, 1974

McCollum RW: Infectious mononucleosis and the Epstein-Barr virus. J Infect Dis 121:347, 1970

Nonoyama M, Huang CH, Pagano JS, Klein G, Singh S: DNA of Epstein-Barr virus selected in tissue of Burkitt's lymphoma and nasopharyngeal carcinoma. Proc Natl Acad Sci USA 70:3265, 1973

Sawyer RN, Evans AS, Niederman JC, McCollum RW: Prospective studies of a group of Yale University freshmen. I. Occurrence of infectious mononucleosis. J Infect Dis 123:263, 1971

74

Adenoviruses and Adenovirus-associated Viruses

ADENOVIRUSES

Adenoviruses were first recovered from human beings almost simultaneously in the early 1950s by two groups of investigators, one finding them in surgically removed tonsils and adenoids, the other in army recruits with acute respiratory disease. Viruses with similar physicochemical and morphologic properties have since been recovered from many animal species. All except the chicken adenovirus share a common group-specific antigen that can be detected in complement-fixation tests with appropriate antisera. Adenoviruses are relatively species-specific in their host range. Only human strains comprising 31 different serotypes will be considered here (Table 62-4).

Disease Adenoviruses assemble in the nucleus of infected cells, producing early eosinophilic inclusions that evolve into a large basophilic mass. Adenoviruses show a predilection for infecting conjunctival, respiratory, and intestinal epithelium, and regional lymphoid tissue. The incubation period for disease is one to two weeks where discernible. Latent tissue infections, healthy persons shedding virus, and prolonged virus shedding (particularly intestinal) following illness have all been described.

Adenovirus types 1, 2, 5, and 6 have been recovered from surgically removed tonsils and adenoids and have also been associated with sporadic mild respiratory illness of infants and children. Types 3 and 7 cause similar illness sporadically or sometimes in epidemics. Characteristically, the patient is febrile, with pharyngitis, cervical adenitis, and conjunctivitis. Coryza and cough are frequently present. Atypical pneumonia may occur, and adenoviruses have been recovered from the lungs of fatal cases. The whooping cough syndrome has also been associated with adenovirus infection. Gastrointestinal symptoms are occasionally prominent, and it is thought that adenovirus-induced lymphoid hyperplasia in the gastrointestinal tract can in some cases serve as a focus promoting intussusception.

Adenovirus types 3, 4, 7, 14, and 21 have been associated with epidemics of febrile respiratory illness in institutional populations, particularly among military recruits. Syndromes include an influenzalike illness, febrile pharyngitis, and atypical pneumonia. The conjunctival mucosa is frequently involved, and occasionally there are gastrointestinal symptoms.

Epidemic keratoconjunctivitis is most commonly caused by adenovirus type 8, although other types may sometimes be responsible. The disease is characterized by the acute onset of tearing, erythema, suffusion, lymphoid follicles beneath the conjunctiva, and preauricular adenopathy. As the conjunctivitis begins to subside after one to two weeks, discrete corneal infiltrates appear. The latter may persist for one or two years.

Several other syndromes have been associated with adenovirus infection. Among them are acute hemorrhagic cystis and generalized exanthems. Many of the higher adenovirus serotypes have been recovered from persons with inapparent infections, and their significance in disease is uncertain. Several human adenoviruses have been shown to induce tumors when injected into animals, such as hamsters, particularly types 12, 18, and 31, but evidence for a role in human cancer has thus far been negative.

Epidemiology Human adenoviruses spread from person to person with no other known reservoir. Serologic evidence of infection with one or more low-numbered serotypes is very common by age 5. Approximately 5 to 10 percent of civilian respiratory disease appears to be due to adenovirus infection. Occasional outbreaks of infection have been associated with swimming pools, but most have no such association. Adenovirus disease occurs throughout the year, with a tendency toward a higher incidence in winter and spring.

The method of acquisition of adenovirus appears to be important in determining disease. Attempts to induce conjunctivitis artificially in volunteers are unsuccessful unless the conjunctival surface is mildly irritated by swabbing. Dusty environments, swimming pools, and optical instruments, such as tonometers, can all provide the necessary conjunctival irritation and in some cases transmit the virus as well.

Nasopharyngeal inoculation of volunteers with adenovirus and ingestion of the virus usually result in asymptomatic infection or mild, afebrile illness. However, inhalation of adenovirus aerosols into the lower respiratory tract has resulted in the full range of clinical syndromes. It is thus suggested that the epidemic adenovirus disease seen in army recruits is the result of airborne spread facilitated by close contact of a large group of susceptible people.

Diagnosis The differential diagnosis of the clinical syndromes caused by adenoviruses includes infections with several bacteria, *Chlamydia* species, *Mycoplasma pneumoniae*, and several viruses. A frequent differential diagnosis that is important for therapeutic reasons is between streptococcal and adenoviral pharyngitis. Characteristics more common for adenoviral pharyngitis include exudate on the pharyngeal wall (as opposed to tonsils), a granular appearance to the mucosa, only moderate tenderness of the enlarged cervical nodes, and a normal or minimally elevated white blood cell count. However, culture for streptococci must be done to be certain.

The atypical pneumonia caused by adenoviruses cannot be clinically distinguished from that caused by mycoplasma. As many as one in five persons with adenoviral atypical pneumonia has modest elevations in cold agglutinins. One must depend on epidemiologic data to guide therapy and on cultural and serologic data for retrospective diagnosis.

Adenoviruses can be recovered from respiratory secretions, throat swabs, conjunctival swabs, and feces of infected persons. Virus in specimens is stable for days under ordinary environmental conditions. The specimen is inoculated into a continuous human cell line (HeLa, Hep2, KB) and/or human embryonic kidney tissue culture. Virus growth may be slow, necessitating passage into fresh tissue culture tubes so that three to four weeks of observation can be achieved. Typical adenovirus cytopathic effects consist of clusters of rounded, refractile cells. Identification of the agent as an adenovirus can be accomplished using hyperimmune antiserum to detect the group-specific antigen in a complement-fixation test. Adenoviruses can be subgrouped according to their hemagglutination reaction with rhesus and rat blood cells. Serotype identity is accomplished using specific antisera in hemagglutination-inhibition and/or neutralization tests.

Because adenoviruses can be recovered from healthy persons, increases in antibody titer between acute and convalescent sera should be sought to document recent acute infection. This may be done using the complement-fixation test and any adenovirus serotype. Neutralization or hemagglutination-inhibition tests may also be used if the adenovirus serotype causing infection is available. Sera to be used for the hemagglutination-inhibition test must be pretreated to remove nonspecific inhibitors.

Treatment Treatment of adenovirus infections is symptomatic and supportive. Secondary bacterial infection is not common.

Prevention Immunity following adenovirus infection is serotype-specific and appears to be long-lasting. Because adenovirus infections are a particular problem in military recruit camps, vaccines have been developed and tested in this setting. Experience with subcutaneous inoculation of an inactivated polyvalent vaccine containing types 3, 4, and 7 indicated that such vaccines could control infection. Use of this vaccine was discontinued because of problems of variation in potency, contamination with SV40, and oncogenicity of types 3 and 7 in hamsters.

More recently, infectious adenovirus type 4 and type 7 vaccines have been developed for oral administration. The virus is encased in an enteric-coated capsule and is released in the intestine where it causes an asymptomatic, nontransmissible infection. Good protection has been provided by these vaccines, particularly when both are used simultaneously, so that the vaccine-suppressed serotype is less likely to be replaced by a nonsuppressed serotype. Efforts are being directed toward the development of additional infectious vaccines, new ways of vaccine administration, and vaccines composed of purified viral antigens.

ADENOVIRUS-ASSOCIATED VIRUSES

Electron microscopy of several adenovirus preparations has revealed small, icosahedral virus particles 20 to 25 nm in diameter, much smaller than adenovirus particles, the diameter of which is about 70 nm. These small virus particles, which are unable to multiply except in cells simultaneously infected with adenoviruses, are referred to as adeno-associatd viruses (AAV) or adeno-satellite viruses (Chaps. 62 and 67). Their growth in tissue culture cannot be followed by cytopathic effect. Instead electron microscopy, complement fixation or immunofluorescence with specific antisera, and hemagglutination with type 4, the only hemagglutinating AAV, must be used. Cultural and serologic data indicate that types 1, 2, and 3 are of human origin and cause natural infection, while type 4 is of simian origin. The relationship of AAV infection to acute disease, if any, is obscured by the concomitant occurrence of adenovirus infection and also by inadvertent immunization with AAVs that contaminate various monkey kidney-grown vaccines.

FURTHER READING

ADENOVIRUS

Belshe RB, Mufson MA: Identification by immunofluorescence of adenoviral antigen in exfoliated bladder epithelial cells from patients with acute hemorrhagic cystitis. Proc Soc Exp Biol Med 146:754, 1974.

Brandt CD, Kim HW, Vargosko AJ, et al: Infections in 18,000 infants and children in a controlled study of respiratory tract disease. I. Adenovirus pathogenicity in relation to serologic type and illness syndrome. Am J Epidemiol 90:484, 1969

Clarke EJ, Phillips IA, Alexander ER: Adenovirus infection in intussusception in children in Taiwan. JAMA 208: 1671, 1969

Couch RB, Cate TR, Douglas RG Jr, Gerone PJ, Knight V: Effect of route of inoculation on experimental respiratory viral disease in volunteers and evidence for airborne transmission. Bacteriol Rev 30:517, 1966

Dudding BA, Top FH Jr, Winter PE, et al: Acute respiratory disease in military trainees. The adenovirus surveillance program, 1966–1971. Am J Epidemiol 97:187, 1973

Ginsberg HS, Dingle JH: The adenovirus group. In Horsfall FL, Tamm I (eds): Viral and Rickettsial Infections of Man, 4th ed. Philadelphia and Montreal, Lippincott, 1965, p 860

Jackson GG, Muldoon RL: Viruses causing common respiratory infection in man. IV. Reoviruses and adenoviruses. J Infect Dis 128:811, 1973

Knight V, Kasel JA: Adenoviruses. In Knight V (ed): Viral and Mycoplasmal Infections of the Respiratory Tract. Philadelphia, Lea & Febiger, 1973, p 65

McAllister RM, Gilden RV, Green M: Adenoviruses in human cancer. Lancet 1:831, 1972

Nelson KE, Gavitt F, Batt MD, et al: The role of adenoviruses in the pertussis syndrome. J Pediat 86:335, 1975

Numazaki Y, Kumasaka T, Yano N, et al: Further study on the hemorrhagic cystitis due to adenovirus type II. N Engl J Med 289:344, 1973

Sprague JB, Hierholzer JC, Currier RW, Hattwick MAW, Smith MD: Epidemic keratoconjunctivitis. A severe industrial outbreak due to adenovirus type 8. N Engl J Med 289:1341, 1973

ADENOVIRUS-ASSOCIATED VIRUS

Atchison RW, Casto BC, Hammon W McD: Adenovirus-associated defective virus particles. Science 149:754, 1965

Blacklow NR, Hoggan MD, Kapikian AZ, Austin JB, Rowe WP: Epidemiology of adenovirus-associated virus infection in a nursery population. Am J Epidemiol 88:368, 1968

Boucher DW, Melnick JL, Mayor HD: Nonencapsidated infectious DNA of adeno-satellite virus in cells coinfected with herpesvirus. Science 173:1243, 1971

Hoggan MD, Blacklow NR, Rowe WP: Studies of small DNA viruses found in various adenovirus preparations: physical, biological, and immunological characteristics. Proc Natl Acad Sci USA 55:1467, 1966

Mayor HD: Satellite viruses. In Busch H (ed): Methods in Cancer Research. New York, Academic Press, 1973, vol 8, p. 203

Mayor HD, Ito M: Distribution of antibodies to type 4 adeno-associated satellite virus in simian and human sera. Proc Soc Exp Biol Med 126:723, 1967

Mayor HD, Kurstak E: Viruses with separately encapsidated complementary DNA strands. In Kurstak E, Maramorosch K (eds): Viruses, Evolution and Cancer. New York, Academic Press, 1974, p 55

Parks WP, Boucher DW, Melnick JL, Taber LH, Yow MD: Seroepidemiological and ecological studies of the adenovirus-associated satellite viruses. Infect Immun 2: 716, 1970

Melnick JL, Rongey R, Mayor HD: Physical assay and growth cycle studies of a defective adenosatellite virus. J Virol 1:171, 1967

Rosenbaum MJ, Edwards EA, Pierce WE, et al: Serologic surveillance for adeno-associated satellite virus antibody in military recruits. J Immunol 106:711, 1971

Rowe WP, Baum SG: Evidence for a possible genetic hybrid between adenovirus type 7 and SV40 viruses. Proc Natl Acad Sci USA 52:1340, 1969

Smith KO, Gehle WD, Thiel JF: Properties of a small virus associated with adenovirus type 5. J Immunol 97:754, 1966

75

Picornaviruses

ENTEROVIRUSES

Those members of the picornavirus group that infect man are the rhinoviruses and the enteroviruses. The former are responsible mainly for acute upper respiratory tract infection and are recovered from the nose and throat. The enteroviruses are composed of three subgroups, the polioviruses, Coxsackie viruses, and ECHO viruses. These three were originally grouped together because their common portal of entry included the gastrointestinal tract, wherein they replicated and initiated many different forms of disease. There are 3 distinct poliovirus serotypes, 33 ECHO viruses, 23 Coxsackie A, and 6 Coxsackie B viruses.

History   Sporadic cases of paralytic disease are as old as recorded history. A famous Egyptian stele from the period 1580 to 1350 BC depicts a priest with a flail atrophic lower limb typical of paralytic polio. Sir Walter Scott underwent an illness in 1772, which was probably the earliest and most renowned case of polio described in the British Isles. Acute paralytic illness in children was first described by Underwood in his textbook in 1789, while the name "anterior poliomyelitis" is attributed to Kussmaul in the late nineteenth century. The term "poliomyelitis" was derived from the Greek for gray marrow of the spinal cord and the Latin *(itis)* for inflammation; the location of the involved cells in the anterior horns of the spinal cord contributed the designation "anterior." Outbreaks of illness were regularly identified in the nineteenth and twentieth centuries by the observation of paralysis among young children. The first isolations of poliovirus were achieved in 1908 by the inoculation of central nervous system tissue into susceptible monkeys by the intracerebral route. In 1949 Enders, Robbins, and Weller reported their classic experiments on the cultivation of poliovirus in tissue cultures of nonneural human cells. These techniques paved the way for rapid development of the fields of animal and human virology.

In contrast to the centuries old descriptions of poliovirus infections, the histories of the other enteroviruses are relatively short. In 1948 Dalldorf and Sickles isolated a filterable agent from the stool of a patient with paralytic illness from Coxsackie, New York. They utilized suckling mice to test for the presence of this virus.

Subsequently, a large group of antigenically related agents has been characterized and designated as the Coxsackie viruses. The division into subgroups A and B was based on differing pathology in the infected suckling mice. The members of the A group produced paralysis with extensive degeneration of skeletal muscle and the B viruses produced focal myositis and inflammatory lesions in many viscera plus fat necrosis. The ECHO viruses were also isolated initially from human fecal specimens, frequently from patients without overt disease and their name represented an acronym (*Enteric Cytopathogenic Human Orphan*). With increasing experience, they have been associated with a wide variety of clinical illness, so that they no longer are orphans. They replicated in monkey kidney cell cultures but were not pathogenic for mice or monkeys. As distinct antigenic serotypes were identified, they were assigned sequential numbers. With further refinement of the physical and biochemical features of viruses, these features have now been utilized for more accurate assignment of viruses to different groups. As a result, several of the agents originally listed as ECHO viruses have been reallocated to other groups.

Epidemiology   The epidemiology of all human enteroviruses is quite similar. The pattern is most clearly defined for the polioviruses because paralytic disease has been so readily identifiable. As early as 1916 the clinical epidemiologic features were defined on the basis of an outbreak which occurred in New York City. These principles were (1) that poliomyelitis is, in nature, exclusively a human infection, transmitted from person to person without the necessary intervention of a lower animal or insect host, (2) that the infection is far more prevalent than is apparent from the incidence of clinically recognized cases, since a large majority of persons infected become carriers without clinical manifestations. It is probable that during an epidemic, such as that in New York City, a very considerable proportion of the population became infected, adults as well as children, (3) that the most important agencies in disseminating infection are the unrecognized carriers and perhaps mild abortive cases ordinarily escaping recognition. It is fairly certain that frank paralytic cases are a relatively minor factor in the spread of infection, and (4) that an epidemic of 1 to 3 recognized cases per 1,000, or even less, immunizes the general population to such an extent that the epidemic declines spontaneously, due to the exhaustion or thinning out of infectable material. Apparently an epidemic incidence relatively small in comparison to that prevailing in an epidemic may produce a population immunity sufficient to definitely limit the incidence rate in a subsequent epidemic.

The utilization since the mid-1950s of poliovirus vaccines has dramatically reduced the occurrence of paralytic disease in this country and in other nations. Certain tropical countries, especially in Central and South America, Africa, and parts of Asia, have had problems with the utilization and distribution of vaccine, which has prevented such a dramatic decrease. The annual case rates for the Western Hemisphere are shown in Figure 75-1. The existence of only three distinct serotypes of poliovirus, in contrast to the large numbers of serotypes of the other enteroviruses, made poliovirus vaccine development possible.

In temperate climates the recognized, reported numbers of patients with enterovirus infections are greatest during the summer and early autumn. In tropical zones they may occur year round. Because the usual route of transmission appears to be a fecal-oral one, improvements in sanitation and hygiene alter the usual epidemiology. Epidemics of polio originally occurred almost exclusively in children less than 6 years of age. In the early twentieth century, outbreaks were reported which involved teenagers and adults. Improvement in sanitation and living conditions was felt to have been responsible for this, as childhood exposure with resultant infection and immunity was less likely

to occur. In the presence of crowding and less optimal hygiene, infants and young children were infected early in life with the enteroviruses. With improved sanitation, exposure to the agent was postponed, so that children, in the absence of the immunizing experience of early life infection, became susceptible adults. Paralytic disease more frequently resulted from poliovirus infection of an adult than of a child.

Many outbreaks with other enteroviruses have been studied over the past several decades. Coxsackie B epidemics tend to recur every two to five years. Young infants constitute the largest susceptible population and are the most commonly affected. Older children and adults are most likely to be immune to a given agent if it has circulated in the community within the past five years. The characteristic features of an outbreak of a specific agent will vary considerably. With virologic studies it is possible to show a range of clinical manifestations from occult infection to overt disease with varying clinical symptoms (Table 75-1). Transmission of virus occurs most readily under intimate contact situations. These include household settings, day care centers, nurseries, children's institutions, and other similar environments. Early in the infection, both pharyngeal secretions and stools will be positive for virus. The pharynx after a few days will be free of infectious material, but the virus will persist in stools for periods as long as six to eight weeks. Studies of families indicate nearly a 100 percent infection rate among children and only slightly lower rates among the adult members. Monitoring of community sewage has been

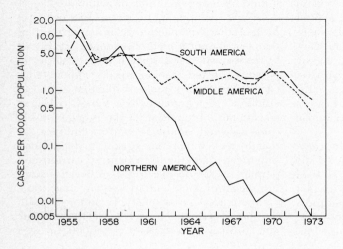

FIG. 75-1. Reported cases of polio (per 100,000 population) in the Western Hemisphere by regions, 1955-1973. (Adapted from the World Health Organization Bulletin)

TABLE 75–1 CLINICAL MANIFESTATIONS OF ENTEROVIRUS INFECTIONS

Clinical Syndrome	Polio	Coxsackie A	Coxsackie B	ECHO
Asymptomatic infection	X	X	X	X
Nonspecific febrile illness	X	X	X	X
Respiratory Disease		X	X	X
Exanthems		X	X	X
Enanthems		X		
Pleurodynia			X	
Orchitis			X	
Myocarditis			X	
Pericarditis			X	X
Aseptic meningitis and meningoencephalitis	X	X	X	X
Disseminated neonatal infection			X	
Transitory muscle paresis	X		X	X
Paralytic disease	X			

X = involvement of multiple serotypes

used as an epidemiologic tool to study community spread of the various enteroviruses.

Clinical Illness The broad spectrum of clinical disease produced by the enteroviruses overlaps among groups. A listing of various syndromes is included in Table 75-1. The more common manifestations associated with infection are discussed briefly.

FEBRILE ILLNESS. The great majority of infections with enteroviruses produce no specific etiologic hallmarks. In young children febrile illness, nonspecific malaise, and myalgias are frequently associated with enterovirus infection. There is nothing unique about this type of clinical presentation. Some infants and young children have had vomiting and diarrhea with ECHOvirus infections, but it is dubious whether these agents have an important etiologic role in gastroenteritis.

RESPIRATORY DISEASE. Mild upper respiratory tract illness has been associated with several of the Coxsackies and ECHO viruses. A very few cases of pneumonia have been attributed to Coxsackie infection.

EXANTHEMS AND ENANTHEMS. Various enteroviruses (particularly ECHO 9 and 16, Coxsackie A9 and A16, Coxsackie B5) have been associated with outbreaks of febrile rash disease. Younger children are more likely to develop exanthem, and they vary widely in their characteristics. Vesicular lesions have been described on the hands and feet in association with ulcers of the buccal mucosa (hand-foot-mouth disease), particularly with Coxsackie A16. Macular and maculopapular eruptions indistinguishable from rubella have been observed with a number of the Coxsackie and ECHO viruses. Petechiae have accompanied some rashes, especially with ECHO virus 9. The presence of virus has been demonstrated in the skin lesion themselves. Some of the syndromes include an associated enanthem. Herpangina, one of these, is most commonly associated with Coxsackie A infections. Ulcerative lesions of the mucosa are seen in the posterior pharynx and soft palate. The associated discomfort, fever, and sore throat are prominent. Because many different serotypes of the ECHO and Coxsackie groups can cause identical clinical pictures, viral isolation is necessary to identify the specific etiologic agents.

PLEURODYNIA (BORNHOLM DISEASE). This is a febrile illness with extreme myalgia, pleuritic chest pain, and headache. Most often it has been associated with Coxsackie B viruses, but other agents have occasionally been recovered from patients.

ORCHITIS. Although viral orchitis most often is due to mumps, it has accompanied infections with the Coxsackie B viruses.

MYOCARDITIS, PERICARDITIS. Newborn infants may have severe myocarditis as a part of generalized Coxsackie B viral infection. Isolated myocarditis and/or pericarditis in older children and adults has been shown to result from Coxsackie B or ECHO virus infections. The spectrum has ranged from benign, self-limited pericarditis to severe, fatal myocardial disease.

VIRAL MENINGITIS AND MENINGOENCEPHALITIS. Many of the enteroviruses have been isolated from the cerebrospinal fluid (CSF) of patients suffering from aseptic meningitis and/or encephalitis. These illnesses are characterized by fever, headache, malaise, and varying degrees of altered central nervous system function. The most severely affected patients may be obtunded or comatose. The least involved patients may complain only of mild headache and/or stiff neck. A CSF pleocytosis is detected, with usually less than 500 cells per cu mm. Early in the disease these are likely to be predominantly polymorphonuclear leukocytes, but after 24 to 48 hours of illness mononuclear cells are the majority. The CSF protein is moderately elevated, but the glucose is normal. The prognosis for such patients is far better than that for similar pyogenic infections of the central nervous system and meninges. Even the youngest infants appear to recover completely, but there are few longitudinal studies of such patients to determine their eventual intellectual, motor, and emotional function.

CONGENITAL AND NEONATAL INFECTIONS. Transplacental and neonatal transmission has been demonstrated with Coxsackie B viruses, resulting in a serious disseminated disease that may include hepatitis, myocarditis, meningoencephalitis, and adreno-cortical involvement. Myocarditis as an isolated phenomenon has also been observed with Coxsackie B virus infection of the newborn. Several clusters of such cases have been noted in nurseries, suggesting postnatal transmission. Many of these infections have been fatal. When poliovirus infections were common, examples of transmission from infected mother to fetus were apparent by the birth of a paralyzed infant. Several ECHO viruses have been associated with neonatal hepatic necrosis, usually fatal.

PARALYTIC DISEASE. Poliovirus infection, especially with types 1 and 3, was responsible for almost all the paralytic disease associated with the enteroviruses. Occasional cases of transient paralysis and muscle weakness have been noted with other members, particularly the *Coxsackie B* agents, but these are very few in number. With classic paralytic polio, there is a two to six day incubation period with an initial nonspecific febrile illness. This probably coincides with early replication of virus in the pharynx and gastrointestinal tract. With the subsequent hematogenous spread of virus, central nervous system involvement may result in meningitis and the anterior horn cell infection. Anywhere from 1 to 4 percent of susceptible patients infected with polioviruses will develop central nervous system involvement. The spectrum of paralytic disease is enormously variable and may involve only an isolated muscle group or extensive paralysis of all extremities. Characteristically the picture is one of asymmetrical distribution, the lower extremities involved more frequently than the upper. Large muscle groups are more often affected than are the small muscles of the hands and feet. Involvement of cervical and thoracic segments of the spinal cord may result in paralysis of the muscles of respiration. Infection of cells in the medulla and the cranial nerve nuclei results in bulbar polio, with compromise of the respiratory and vasomotor centers. With the return of the patient's temperature to normal, the progress of paralysis ceases, and the subsequent weeks and months may see a varying spectrum of recovery ranging from full return of function to significant residual paralysis. Recovery may be exceedingly slow, and its full extent cannot be judged for 6 to 18 months. Atrophy of involved muscles becomes apparent more rapidly, after four to eight weeks.

Pathology Because most Coxsackie and ECHO virus infections are nonfatal, little is known of their histology. The pathologic changes of poliovirus in the central nervous system are most prominent in the spinal cord, medulla, pons, and midbrain. After initial cytoplasmic alterations in the Nissl substance of the motor neurons, nuclear changes develop next, and pericellular infiltrates of polymorphonuclear and mononuclear cells accumulate. The final stage is destruction, with neuronophagocytosis and dropping out of the necrotic cells.

Immunity Enterovirus replication within the gastrointestinal tract results in the production of local secretory immunoglobulin A at the site of contact of virus with lymphoid cells. The polioviruses have been extensively investigated, and the localized nature of the antibody response has been carefully documented. Serum antibody specific to the virus is found shortly after onset of the clinical syndrome, as shown in Figure 75-2. Development of type-specific antibody provides lifelong protection against clinical illness caused by the same agent. Local reinfection of the gastrointestinal tract may recur, but this is accompanied by only a brief and abbreviated period of virus replication and without clinical illness. Serum antibodies to the enteroviruses can be demonstrated in three immunoglobulin classes, IgM, IgG, and IgA. Usually the earliest response is in the IgM fraction, overlapping with the development of IgG antibodies. Complement fixation, virus neutralization, immunoprecipitation, and, in a few instances, hemagglutination inhibition are the most widely used techniques for assaying enterovirus antibodies. Neutralizing antibodies are type-specific, whereas complement fixation demonstrates group-reactive antibodies. In the course of his lifetime, man sustains multiple infections, occult or overt, with a variety of enteroviruses. A specific infection elicits the production of antibody specific to that virus type but also may prompt an anamnestic response demonstrated by an increase in group-reactive antibody and by parallel rises in antibodies to serotypes of some of the other enteroviruses previously encountered. The concomitant serologic rises in antibody titer create some problems with serologic

surveys, rendering the complement-fixation test inadequate to define a specific infection. Virus-neutralizing antibody is a far more precise technique.

The aspects of cellular immunity for enterovirus infection are not well defined. Circulating peripheral white blood cells have been a source of virus isolation during acute illness. The infected cells are probably lymphocytes or macrophages, but this has not been determined with certainty. There are also several in vitro assays of white blood cell response to enterovirus infection, but no extensive evaluation of host cell-mediated immunity to these agents has been accomplished. The abnormal response of some children with immunodeficiency disease to infection with attenuated polioviruses may offer some further insight into the immune processes normally stimulated by enterovirus infection. These are discussed further on page 969.

Diagnosis The clinical illness in some instances may permit a presumptive diagnosis of enterovirus infection. As shown in Table 75-1, the spectrum of illness is wide. The time of year may also be helpful, with a predilection for summer and early autumn circulation of enteroviruses in communities in the temperate zones. Specimens for virus isolation should be obtained early in the course of illness from various sites. The cerebrospinal fluid of patients with aseptic meningitis and/or meningoencephalitis has been an abundant source of enteroviruses, except for the three polio types. Materials, such as pleural and pericardial fluid,

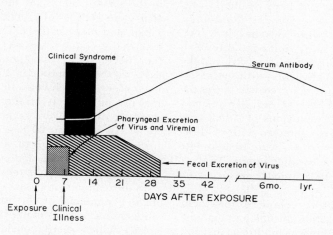

FIG. 75-2. The course of typical enterovirus infection.

should also be cultured when available and appropriate to the clinical illness. Various simian and human cell culture systems will support replication of most of the enteroviruses, with cytopathic effects revealing their presence. However, some of the Coxsackie A viruses are more fastidious and may require the inoculation of suckling mice. The specimens submitted most often for attempted virus isolations are nasopharyngeal swabs and stool specimens. As noted, an enterovirus may be excreted in fecal material for several weeks after a clinical illness. Recovery of an enterovirus from throat or stool of a patient does not in itself signify that this is the etiologic agent of the illness observed. The temporal association of illness, virus recovery, and an antibody rise specific to that agent provide firmer evidence of a significant infection.

Acute and convalescent serum samples obtained from 7 to 21 days apart will help to define quantitative changes in antibody titers. The isolation of a specific virus provides the opportunity for assessment of the patient's antibody against his own viral agent. In the absence of the recovery of a virus, one faces the problem of seeking specific antibody rises against the whole family of enteroviruses which might have been responsible for the clinical illness.

Prevention   Because there is no specific treatment for enterovirus infections, efforts have focused on means of prevention. The multiple antigenic types and the usually benign, self-limited course of most ECHO viral and Coxsackie viral infections have resulted in little stimulus for the development of vaccines. The story of the poliovirus vaccines, however, has been one of the most exciting and rewarding sagas in microbiologic history. Prior to the work of Enders and colleagues with successful tissue culture techniques for growth of the polioviruses, there had been several ill-fated vaccines prepared from emulsions of spinal cord removed from monkeys infected with wild poliovirus. These preparations were treated with formalin or other inactivating agents. Trials of these vaccines in 1935 proved unsuccessful and unacceptable.

Enders' tissue culture techniques lent themselves to the propagation of sufficient amounts of relatively pure poliovirus in vitro so that controlled formaldehyde inactivation could be used to produce noninfectious virus which retained its antigenicity. Salk and his colleagues pursued this line of research and, by 1954, were able to embark on a field trial which established the efficacy of an inactivated poliovirus vaccine in the prevention of paralytic disease. This was a trivalent preparation incorporating the three poliovirus types. After an initial series of two or three injections spaced several weeks to months apart, followed by a booster 6 to 12 months later, there was demonstrable serum antibody to all three polio serotypes. The vaccine was widely used in the United States during the five years from 1956 through 1960. The results were dramatic. Previous years had seen from ten to twenty thousand cases of paralytic disease reported annually. With the widespread use of Salk vaccine, this rapidly dropped to 2 or 3 thousand cases annually, as increasingly large numbers of susceptible individuals were immunized.

By the early 1960s, a second vaccine was available. Strains of poliovirus which Sabin had selected and studied in his laboratory were attenuated for monkey and man. Although their ingestion resulted in intestinal infection and virus excretion, humoral and gastrointestinal tract immunity developed without any illness. Because these could be administered more readily, by the oral route, and because their multiplication in the gastrointestinal tract more closely mimicked natural infection, they offered certain selected advantages which led to their replacing the injectable Salk vaccine. Over the first five years of the 1960s, more than 400 million doses of vaccine were distributed in the United States. At the same time, trials also were successfully conducted in Europe, Japan, and other nations. The use of oral vaccine in this country was accompanied by a further decrease in the annual reported polio cases, so that beginning in 1966 fewer than 100 have occurred each year. In 1975, with continued use of the oral vaccines, only six cases of paralytic disease were recorded in the United States. In less than 20 years, a disease which had claimed thousands of victims annually and which had been the source of indescribable community anxiety, was reduced to a rarity.

In the complex processes of vaccine development, commercial production, and widespread utilization a number of unexpected events transpired which merit consideration. After the highly successful field trials of 1954, commercial manufacture of the Salk type vaccine was licensed. Within a few weeks of its use, paralytic disease was observed in April-June 1955 among children in California and Idaho who had received some of the first lots of commercial vaccine manfuactured by the Cutter Laboratories. By the time this had been fully investigated and resolved, it was learned that there were 204 cases of vaccine-associated disease. Seventy-nine were among children who had received the vaccine, 105 were among their family contacts, and 20 were in community contacts. Nearly three-quarters of the cases were paralytic, and there were 11 deaths. The virus isolated from these patients was type 1. Laboratory tests on vaccine distributed by Cutter Laboratories revealed viable type 1 poliovirus in 7 of 17 lots tested. Revisions of the federal regulations governing the steps in vaccine manufacture were promptly promulgated and implemented to prevent recurrence of such a tragic episode.

Manufacturers faced further difficulties in maintaining the fine balance between complete elimination of infectious live virus from the production process and retention of effective antigenicity of the inactivated components. A number of lots of vaccine subsequently proved to be poorly antigenic for type 3 poliovirus. As a result, when community polio outbreaks occurred among well-immunized groups, there were breakthroughs with paralytic disease, especially due to type 3 virus, in previously immunized subjects. Such an outbreak was studied in 1959 in Massachusetts, where an analysis of polio cases revealed that 47 percent (62 of 137) of the patients had previously received three or more inoculations of inactivated vaccine.

With the availability of attenuated oral vaccine, enthusiasm for its use was enhanced by the aforementioned unfortunate episodes with inactivated vaccine. A final unanticipated discovery in 1960 was the detection of SV40 as a contaminant of the simian cell cultures utilized in preparation of both inactivated and oral attenuated vaccines. Once again, a revision of standards for preparing and testing the tissue cultures was necessary to exclude this previously unrecognized agent. In the United States, inactivated vaccine has been used sparingly over the past decade. Almost all immunization has been conducted with the oral attenuated material. A number of European countries, especially those in Scandinavia, have adhered to the use of inactivated vaccine. With successful production of fully potent antigens, their record of achievement in the control of polio has been parallel to that of this country.

With the marked decrease in paralytic disease due to wild polioviruses, there has emerged a small but significant number of cases of oral vaccine recipients who have developed paralytic illness in temporal association to the ingestion of vaccine. In addition to these few cases among recipients of vaccines, there have also been paralytic episodes reported among susceptible family or community contacts of the vaccine recipients. These have been few in number and are difficult to characterize with complete clarity at this time. A small portion of these patients have been found to be immunodeficient children, particularly those with congenital hypogammaglobulinemia. One concern has always been that the attenuated strains of virus might prove genetically unstable in human intestinal passage, so that increased neurovirulence might result from widespread dissemination. This has not been demonstrated. Monovalent oral polio vaccine (MOPV) was used extensively until 1964, when it was supplanted by trivalent vaccine (TOPV). With MOPV the risk of vaccine-associated illness in recipients was estimated to have been 0.19 per million doses distributed. With TOPV an over-all figure of risk to recipients and their contacts has been calculated at 0.28 per million or 1 case per 3.6 million doses.

The achievements with poliovirus vaccination have been impressive in the United States, Canada, most of Europe, Australia, and some Asian and African nations. Polio remains an endemic disease in many tropical lands. It is premature, therefore, to relax the use of poliovirus vaccination in those parts of the world where disease has been nearly eradicated. The possibility of the inadvertent introduction of virulent virus is omnipresent. A number of such episodes have occurred already on the Texas-Mexico border. Although polio immunization is now confined principally to infants and children, it is recommended that adult Americans traveling abroad to endemic areas receive polio vaccine prior to departure. Armed Forces recruits are routinely administered oral poliovirus vaccine. Its major use remains that for infants and children in the first 18 months of life.

RHINOVIRUSES

Rhinoviruses (nose viruses) are important in causing acute respiratory infections with predominant involvement of the upper airway passages. Over 100 different serotypes have been recognized, the first one being recovered in 1956 and initially classified as ECHO virus type 28.

Clinical Illness   The usual symptoms of a rhinovirus common cold are nasal obstruction and discharge, sneezing, scratchy throat, mild cough, and malaise. Severe tracheobronchitis and even atypical pneumonia may occur occasionally in adults, but fever and significant lower respiratory tract involvement are more likely with rhinovirus infection in children. Rhinovirus infection has been associated in a few studies with acute exacerbations of chronic obstructive pulmonary disease in adults.

Epidemiology   Rhinovirus infections have been documented in all populations studied. They occur throughout the year with a tendency toward increased incidence in the fall. Occasional epidemics with a single serotype have been described, but more often multiple serotypes appear to be circulating at the same time. The viruses spread among close associates by uncertain means. Aerosol spread has been shown to be possible. Children frequently serve to introduce rhinoviruses into the family unit, with subsequent illnesses occurring within two or three days to a week.

Diagnosis   Acute upper respiratory infections can be caused and/or simulated by multiple viruses, bacteria, allergies, and so on. To distinguish rhinovirus infection from other etiologic factors requires virus isolation and demonstration of a rise in antibody titer between acute and convalescent sera. Assays for antibody must be done with neutralization tests against the specific rhinovirus causing the infection. Specific serologic identification requires multiple cross-neutralization tests and is impractical for general use.

Rhinoviruses are generally recovered by inoculating specimens from the nose and/or throat into human embryonic fibroblast or human embryonic kidney tissue cell cultures. They are almost never recovered from stool or rectal swabs. An isolate can be identified as a rhinovirus by its physicochemical properties, especially acid lability, which serve to distinguish rhinoviruses from enteroviruses. Rhinoviruses can be further subdivided into H strains that grow well only in tissues of human origin, and M strains that will also grow in monkey kidney tissue.

Treatment   Treatment of rhinovirus infection is aimed at prevention of secondary bacterial infections and relief of symptoms. Hydration and preventing obstruction of airways, paranasal sinuses, and eustachian tubes are the mainstays of therapy.

Prevention   Resistance to reinfection with the same rhinovirus serotype can be shown following an initial infection. An important element of this resistance appears to be secretory antibody, which is not induced well by parenteral killed-virus vaccines. For this reason, as well as because of the existence of a multiplicity of rhinovirus serotypes, vaccination appears unlikely to be a successful method of prophylaxis against the rhinovirus common cold.

Nonspecific resistance to reinfection with virus lasting one to two months appears to follow acute respiratory virus infection. The mechanism responsible for this resistance is uncertain, but attempts to simulate it using interferon inducers or other chemotherapeutic agents are underway. High doses of vitamin C have been advocated as a prophylactic measure, but the efficacy is unproven.

Further Reading

ENTEROVIRUSES

Berkovich S, Pickering JE, Kibrick S: Paralytic poliomyelitis in Massachusetts, 1959. N Engl J Med 264:1323, 1961

Editorial: Simian virus 40 and polio vaccine. JAMA 185:723, 1963

Enders JF, Weller TH, Robbins FC: Cultivation of the Lansing strain of poliomyelitis virus in cultures of various human embryonic tissues. Science 109:85, 1949

Forman ML, Cherry, JD: Exanthems associated with uncommon viral syndromes. Pediatrics, 41:873, 1968

Fraumeni JF Jr, Stark CR, Gold E, Lepow ML: Simian virus 40 in polio-vaccine: follow-up of newborn recipients. Science 167:59, 1970

Gear JHS, Measroch V: Coxsackievirus infections of the newborn. Prog Med Virol 15:42, 1973

Horstmann DM: Viral exanthems and enanthems. Pediatrics 41:867, 1968

Kibrick S: Current status of Coxsackie and ECHO viruses in human disease. Prog Med Virol 6:27, 1964

Linneman CC Jr, Steichen J, Sherman WG, Schiff GM: Febrile illness in early infancy associated with ECHOvirus infection. J Pediatr 84:49, 1974

Montefiore DG: Problems of poliomyelitis immunization in countries with warm climates. Pan American Health Organization Scientific Publication No 226. Conference on the Application of Vaccines against Viral, Rickettsial, and Bacterial Diseases of Man, Washington, DC, 1971

Nathanson N, Langmuir AD: The Cutter incident, I, II, III. Am J Hyg 78:16, 1963

Ogra PL: Effect of tonsillectomy and adenoidecetomy on nasopharyngeal antibody response to poliovirus. N Engl J Med 284:59, 1971

Paul JR: A History of Poliomyelitis. New Haven, Yale Univ Press, 1971

Poliomyelitis Annual Summary. Atlanta, George, Center for Disease Control, Neurotropic Diseases Surveillance. US Dept HEW. 1975

Sabin AB: Pathogenesis of poliomyelitis. Science 123:1151, 1956

Salk JE: Antigenic potency of poliomyelitis vaccine. JAMA 162:1451, 1956

Sanders DY, Cramblett HC: Antibody titers to polioviruses in patients ten years after immunization with Sabin vaccine. J Pediatr 84:406, 1974

Sells CJ, Carpenter RL, Ray, CG: Sequelae of central-nervous system enterovirus infections. N Engl J Med 293:1, 1975

Sweet BH, Hilleman MR: The vacuolating virus, SV40. Proc Soc Exp Biol Med 105:420, 1960

Weinstein L: Poliomyelitis — a persistent problem. N Engl J Med 288:370, 1973

Wilfert CM, Lauer BA, Cohen M, Costenbader ML, Meyers E: An epidemic of ECHOvirus 18 meningitis. J Infect Dis 131:75, 1975

RHINOVIRUSES

Cate TR: Rhinoviruses. In Knight V (ed): Viral and Mycoplasmal Infections of the Respiratory Tract. Philadelphia, Lea and Febiger, 1973, p 141

George RB, Mogabgab WJ: Atypical pneumonia in young men with rhinovirus infections. Ann Intern Med 71:1073, 1969

Gwaltney JM JR: Rhinoviruses. Yale J Biol Med 48:17, 1975

Hamre D: Rhinoviruses. Monogr Virol 1:1, 1968

Higgins PG: The rhinoviruses. Practitioner 199:633, 1967

Hilleman MR: Present knowledge of the rhinovirus group of viruses. Curr Top Microbiol Immunol 41:1, 1967

Hilleman MR: Toward control of viral infections of man. Science 164:506, 1969

Jackson GG, Muldoon RL: Viruses causing common respiratory infections in man. J Infect Dis 127:328, 1973

Stenhouse AC: Rhinovirus infection in acute exacerbations of chronic bronchitis: a controlled prospective study. Br Med J 3:461, 1967

Tyrrell DAJ: Common Cold and Related Diseases. Baltimore, Williams & Wilkins, 1965

Tyrrel, DAJ: Rhinoviruses. Virol Monogr 2:67, 1968

Tyrell DAJ: Chanock RM: Rhinoviruses: a description. Science 141:152, 1963

76
Arboviruses and Certain Arenaviruses

Arboviruses (*arthropodborne*) are maintained in nature by cyclical transmission between susceptible vertebrates and blood-sucking arthropods, with the virus multiplying in both. In vertebrates, arboviruses produce, after an incubation period, a viremia of sufficient titer and duration to permit infection of arthropods. In arthropods, viral multiplication results in the capacity to transmit virus by bite to new vertebrates after a period of time known as the "extrinsic incubation period." This biologic transmission, which depends upon multiplication of virus in the arthropod, is in contrast to mechanical transmission, which occurs as the result of rapid carriage of virus by an arthropod from one host to another. The consequences of infection of the vertebrate range from total absence of disease to major illness and death; with rare exception, no effect on the arthropod has been detected.

Most arboviruses are members of the family Togaviridae, but some are Reoviridae, and at least one belongs to the Picornaviridae. Proof of biologic transmission has not been obtained for many arboviruses. Moreover, the discipline or arbovirology customarily deals with some viruses, such as certain arenaviruses, that are probably not arthropodborne and for which other modes of transmission have been demonstrated. This latter situation has resulted from an initial presumption of arthropod transmission based on clinical and epidemiologic similarities to known arbovirus disease.

The year 1900 marked the beginning of arbovirology, when Walter Reed demonstrated the biologic transmission of yellow fever by the mosquito *Aedes aegypti*. The facts, so convincingly elucidated by the commission of which Reed was chairman, proved the remarkable perception of Dr. Carlos Finlay and the essentials of the basic definition of arboviruses.

During ensuing decades other viruses, many of which are human pathogens, were recognized to possess life cycles that involve arthropod–vertebrate transmission. By the end of the 1930s there were approximatey 30 arboviruses. Since World War II hundreds more have been discovered, so that now there are in excess of 300 known arboviruses. Some 90 may infect man, and most produce disease.

Beginning in the 1920s with the yellow fever program of its International Health Division, the Rockefeller Foundation has provided the major physical and intellectual base of arbovirology. In 1964 the Rockefeller Foundation Virus Program became the Yale Arbovirus Research Unit. Besides developing the conceptual base, much of the basic technology, and most of the facts of arbovirology, the Foundation's conquest of yellow fever by the development of the first, tissue culture attenuated, live virus vaccine stands as a major achievement.

CLASSIFICATION AND NOMENCLATURE

Initially, arboviruses were named for the disease that they caused, for example, dengue and yellow fever. Later, combined names were devised that comprised both geography and disease, such as St. Louis encephalitis. Names currently derive from the place of collection of the specimen from which the first isolation was made, especially for those agents for which no disease is recognized. Most arboviruses fall into this group.

Arboviruses are classified according to serologic relationships based on tests employing complement fixation, hemagglutination inhibition, and infectivity neutralization. At first, serogroups were designated A, B, and C. More recently, groups are given the name of the first virus isolated. More than 40 serogroups have been identified, and more than 60 viruses are as yet ungrouped.

There are several other ways of grouping arboviruses that may be useful in certain circumstances. These include classification according to vector, geographic range, type of disease, or combinations, such as "tickborne hemorrhagic fevers." Because this text is intended primarily for medical students, it seems appropriate to use a clinically oriented classification (Tables 76-1, 76-2, and 76-3).

TECHNOLOGY

The epidemiologic and clinical study of arboviruses involves two basic technologies, virus isolation and measurement of antibodies. The major culture medium for isolation is the infant mouse, in which nearly all arboviruses are pathogenic when inoculated intracerebrally. Cell cultures are the next most useful medium, especially for the study of many established

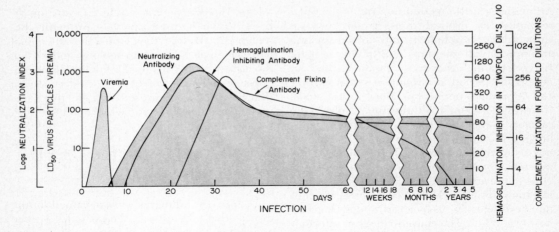

FIG. 76-1. Hypothetical diagnostic virologic and serologic features of arbovirus infections of man. (From Work: Hunter, Swartzwelder JC, and Clyde DF (eds): Tropical Medicine, 5th ed., 1976. Courtesy of W. B. Saunders Co)

isolates. In the usual search for arboviruses, serum or tissue specimens from man or other vertebrates, as well as aqueous suspensions of ground-up arthropods, are routinely inoculated intracerebrally into each infant mouse in a litter. The mice are observed for signs of illness over the next month. Brain tissue from mice that become sick during this time is used for further passage. Serial passages are made until mouse pathogenicity is constant, at which time a large pool of infected brain tissue is stored frozen for use in biologic, physical, chemical, and serologic characterization of the agent.

Serum antibody measurements are usually essential in diagnosis of individual patients (Fig. 76-1). Antibodies also provide a record of past infection that permits detection of the involvement of specific populations of man and other vertebrates in the transmission cycle. These seroepidemiologic investigations are of great value to the understanding of the geographic distribution of arboviruses. Geographic distribution also is delineated through the use of sentinel animals, such as caged mice or chickens placed in the forest; presence of virus in these animals is revealed by disease or by a rise in serum antibodies.

The techniques of viral isolation and antibody measurement may be applied to captured or colonized vertebrates and arthropods to determine their potential as natural hosts for a given virus. Experts in field and laboratory zoology and entomology are, therefore, essential.

As a result, the arbovirus laboratory is staffed by a broad-based medical zoology group.

ECOLOGY, EPIDEMIOLOGY, AND THE PUBLIC HEALTH

Arboviruses are distributed throughout the world. While most exist in the tropics and subtropics, some have also been isolated from arthropods and vertebrates in climatically less hospitable areas, such as Finland, Canada, Siberia, and Alaska. Their epidemic potential continues to surprise us. Outbreaks of major and often new clinical disease in the savannahs, forests, and swamps of the tropical world provide episodes of romance and high adventure as well as tragedy and misery.

The conceptual and technical base of arbovirus ecology grew from the work in the late 1920s and 1930s on yellow fever. Yellow fever initially was thought to be entirely a problem of man to man transmission by the relatively domestic mosquito A. aegypti. When the entirely nonhuman jungle cycle was discovered and the study broadened zoologically, several arthropod-transmitted viruses were discovered that were not yellow fever. After World War II an extraordinary global effort was made to study these agents. Arbovirus laboratories were established around the tropical world in such places as Jamaica, Trinidad, Egypt, India, Malaya, Taiwan, Brazil, Panama, Nigeria, and Uganda. The hundreds of arboviruses that we know today were discovered in this effort.

Arboviruses generally maintain themselves in nature by constant and fairly frequent transmission between an arthropod and a vertebrate host (Fig. 76-2). Many variables influence the likelihood and frequency of successful transmission. For example, the frequency of feeding of an arthropod on a vertebrate host depends upon numerous innate and behavioral factors of each animal that may be environmentally determined. These factors may differ from time to time and from place to place. Arthropod longevity, a major determinant, depends in turn upon climatic factors, such as humidity and temperature, availability of food, and the prevalence of predators, as well as on noxious physical chemical, and biologic agents. Many other complex factors similarly influence transmission. Clearly, a systems analysis approach is needed to assess the effect of any change in any variable. Such an approach in malariology has been nicely expressed both in words and mathematically by the late Professor George Macdonald. Because of the large number of agents, the numerous nonhuman hosts, and the great gaps in our knowledge, this approach has not yet come into its own.

Although viremia is usually of sufficient intensity for transmission only for a matter of days, there is evidence that long-lasting infections in some vertebrates, such as turtles infected with Eastern equine encephalitis virus, may permit a virus to remain in an area during a period of unsuitable climate, such as the New England winter, and to be transmitted again when arthropod feeding resumes. Transovarial transmission through generations of arthropods occurs with some viruses and provides the prospect of indefinite survival of virus without cyclical transmission. The important subject of how arboviruses survive periods when cyclical transmission cannot occur has been reviewed recently by Reeves. Arthropod to arthropod transmission probably does not occur other than transovarially. However, direct transmis-

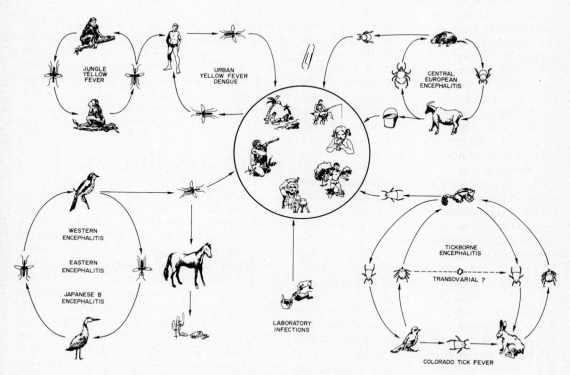

FIG. 76-2. Some basic arbovirus transmission cycles showing their relationship to man. (From Work: In Hunter, Swartzwelder JC, and Clyde DF (eds): Tropical Medicine, 5th ed., 1976. Courtesy of W. B. Saunders Co)

sion may occur between vertebrate hosts, as in the case of Eastern equine encephalitis virus, which is passed from pheasant to pheasant under crowded conditions of commercial pheasant farms.

Man is generally an incidental host and a dead end for virus transmission. A notable exception is the man–mosquito cycle of dengue and urban yellow fevers. As a rule, arboviruses are clinically silent as they cycle in nature. Disease occurs in unnatural hosts, such as man and equines in Eastern equine encephalitis virus, and these hosts are of no consequence to viral transmission.

There are two basic ecologic mechanisms that ensnare man and other animals: either man enters the geographic area of the transmission cycle, or the cycle changes and moves closer to man. Yellow fever ecology provides examples of both. The former occurs when a person enters a forest where yellow fever virus is cycling between monkeys and the tree-top mosquitoes. Without the intrusion these mosquitoes might never feed on man. When the infected person returns to town, he may introduce yellow fever virus into a cycle involving man and the peridomestic mosquito *A. aegypti,* and an urban epidemic may result. Some viruses may come to man by another mechanism, the amplification cycle. These viruses have a basic cycle away from man that involves arthropods that feed almost exclusively on animals. With seasonal buildup of populations of different arthropods and, let us say, birds, another cycle is started that carries the virus closer to man and arthropods that are more likely to bite man.

From time to time an arbovirus disease appears where it has been previously unknown. Bolivean hemorrhagic fever, Lassa fever in West Africa, hemorrhagic fever of southeast Asia, Kyasanur forest disease in India, and Chikungunya and O'nyong-nyong fevers in East Africa are all examples of new disease situations that have been recognized within the past two decades. Did O'nyong-nyong fever virus became more pathogenic for man as a result of passage in anopheline mosquitoes? This is a possibility, since all other group A arboviruses (Alphaviruses) are transmitted by culicenes. Was pick-up and transmission by a certain genus of tick responsible for human pathogenicity of Kyasanur forest disease virus? It is difficult to prove that pathogenicity for man may be enhanced by a change in the transmission cycle, but the question is of great importance as we persist in meddling with our environment. The possibility that the clinical consequences of infection may be affected by sensitization from prior infection by a related virus has been raised to explain the hemorrhagic fever syndromes in the Philippines and southeast Asia caused by dengue viruses. Dengue virus previously was known only in connection with classical dengue, a relatively benign disease characterized by fever and nonhemorrhagic rash. Thus, one disease may change as a result of a change in the ecology of another infection. Whatever the reasons prove to be, we are clearly in an unstable situation, with some surprises in the future.

Arboviruses cause disease and death in thousands of persons each year. From year to year and decade to decade the epidemic potential results in wide swings in incidence in a given geographic area. In the United States there are approximately 100 cases of arboviral encephalitis annually. In the 1960s, there was an epidemic of yellow fever in remote areas of Ethiopia that is believed to have killed 10,000 persons. Hemorrhagic fever in the Philippines and southeast Asia affects thousands each year, with substantial mortality. Laboratories must not be overlooked in a discussion of epidemiology. Man's curiosity about arboviruses has resulted in more than 400 reported laboratory infections, of which 18 caused the deaths of investigators.

HUMAN DISEASE

Arboviruses cause acute febrile illnesses that range from minimal severity to highly fatal diseases with devastating sequelae for the survivors. There are three general types of disease. One type is characterized by undifferentiated fever that may or may not be accompanied by rash and arthralgia (Table 76-1). In another type there is viral invasion of the central nervous system productive of an often severely damaging encephalitis (Table 76-2). The third category includes the viral hemorrhagic fevers (Table 76-3). There follow brief descriptions of representatives of each of these categories, somewhat arbitrarily selected because they occur within the United States or because of their significance to the public health.

TABLE 76-1 SUMMARY OF SELECTED HUMAN ARBOVIRUS DISEASES CHARACTERIZED BY FEVER WITH OR WITHOUT RASH

Virus Name*	Antiserogroup	Geography	Maintenance Hosts Vertebrate	Arthropod	Clinical (Other than Fever) and Epidemiologic Features
Dengue	B	Tropics and sub-tropics through-out world	Man	Mosquito	Headache, myalgia, rash, arthralgia; endemic and epidemic
Colorado tick	Ungrouped	Western North America	Small mammals	Tick	Headache, myalgia, rash, biphasic rash; spring and summer focal endemnicity
West Nile	B	Mediterranean, Middle East, Russia, and Asia	Birds	Mosquito, ticks	Headache, lymphadenopathy, rash; endemic and epidemic
Sandfly	Phlebotomus fever group	Mediterranean, Asia, tropical America	Man, monkeys, small mammals	Phlebotomus flies	Myalgia, rash, conjunctivitis; seasonally epidemic and sporadically endemic
Rift Valley	Ungrouped	Africa	Large mammals	Mosquito	Headache, myalgia, photophobia, retinal damage may occur; sporadic from mosquito or by contact with tissue from infected animals
O'nyong-nyong	A	Africa	Man	Mosquito	Like dengue; epidemic
Chikungunya	A	Africa	Man	Mosquito	Like dengue; epidemic
Mayaro	A	South and Central America	Monkeys and marsupials	Mosquito	Like dengue; forest-associated endemic
Ross River	A	Australia	Mouse	Mosquito	Like dengue, arthritis; endemic and seasonal epidemic

*Disease name is generally the viral name plus fever, eg, Colorado tick fever

TABLE 76-2 SUMMARY OF SELECTED HUMAN ARBOVIRAL DISEASES CHARACTERIZED BY ENCEPHALITIS

| Virus | | Geography | Maintenance Hosts | | Clinical (Other than Encephalitis) and Epidemiologic Features |
Name*	Antiserogroup		Vertebrate	Arthropod	Case Fatality (F) and Sequelae (S)
Western equine	A	North and South America	Birds	Mosquito	Summer epidemics North America; equine epizootics; F = high, S = severe
Eastern equine	A	Eastern and North America and Caribbean	Birds	Mosquito	Summer epidemics and equine and bird epizootics; F = high, S = severe
Venezuelan	A	South and Central America, USA, Caribbean	Rodents, birds, equines	Mosquito	Influenzalike. CNS involvement far less common. Encephalitis epizootics in equines; F = low, S = moderate
St. Louis	B	Western hemisphere especially USA	Birds	Mosquito	Summer epidemics in U.S.A.; F = high, S = severe
California (LaCrosse)	California	USA	Small mammals	Mosquito	Summer outbreaks and sporadic cases; F = low, S = ?
Japanese B	B	Asia, Japan, Pacific Islands	Birds, pigs	Mosquito	Summer and fall epidemics in temperate areas; F = high, S = severe
Murray Valley	B	Australia and New Guinea	Bird	Mosquito	Epidemic; F = high
Powassan	B	U.S.A. and Canada	Small mammals	Tick	Two cases of human disease recognized, one fatal
Russian spring-summer	B	Russia	Birds, mammals	Tick†	Diphasic pattern. Bulbospinal paralysis; F = high, S = severe
Central European	B	Europe	Birds, mammals	Tick†	Diphasic pattern
Kyasanur forest disease	B	India	Birds, mammals	Tick†	Hemorrhagic manifestations more common; F = low, S = 0
Louping ill	B	British Isles	Birds, mammals	Tick†	Diphasic pattern; F = 0, S = 0

*Disease and virus name is name listed plus, usually, encephalitis, eg, St. Louis encephalitis
†Transovarially transmitted

Arboviruses that Cause Fevers/Rash Arthralgia Undifferentiated arbovirus fevers with or without rash and arthralgia are generally of low mortality, and recovery is complete with rare exceptions. Classical dengue fever is the prototype, and many of the other members of the group often are described as denguelike. Members of the group that are transmitted in the United States include Colorado tick fever and vesicular stomatitis virus fever.

Dengue fever is a disease of rapid onset, with the temperature rising suddenly to high levels and persisting for several days. Accompanying the fever are headache and aching in the muscles and joints. There is an associated macular rash that blanches with pressure; later in the disease it may become papular and morbilliform, sparing only the palms and soles. After 5 to 10 days the acute symptoms disappear, but generalized weakness and lassitude may delay complete recovery for weeks. In the midst of the acute disease there may be one or several days when manifestations of illness disappear. This provides the biphasic course that characterizes many arboviral diseases. Leukopenia is the most striking and consistent laboratory abnormality. Etiologic diagnosis is confirmed by virus isolation from the blood or by the demonstration of a rise in serum antibody titer. Death is rare, and most patients recover completely. The disease occurs throughout the tropical world. Epidemics may be widespread, affecting a very high proportion of the population. Typically, the virus cycles between man and *Aedes* mosquitoes, especially *A. aegypti*. In some areas there may be a jungle cycle involving primates.

O'nyong-nyong, Chikungunya, Mayaro, and *Ross River* are four related, mosquitoborne viruses that cause denguelike disease in Africa, southern Asia, South and Central America, and Australia.

Colorado tick fever is characterized by fever, headache, and myalgia. Photophobia and a history of tickbite are common. A biphasic disease pattern occurs in approximately half of the cases and does not occur in any other infectious disease that is endemic in the United States. In approximately 10 percent of cases there is a maculopapular rash that is sometimes petechial. There is no particular distribution to the rash. The disease lasts almost a week and occurs in the far western states from April through August. The arthropod host is *Dermacentor andersoni,* in which transovarial passage occurs.

Arboviruses that Cause Encephalitis The arthropodborne viral encephalitides are a group of serious illnesses that occur sporadically or in epidemic form throughout the tropical and subtropical world. Infected persons are at varying risk of death or severe central nervous system damage depending on their age and on the type of virus. In the United States since 1955, there have been an average of 250 arboviral encephalitis cases reported to the Center for Disease Control annually, ranging from a low of 45 in 1959 to a high of 625 cases in 1956. In recent years, California and St. Louis encephalitis viruses account for most of these cases, followed by Western, Eastern, and Venezuelan equine encephalitis viruses, with Powassan virus making its appearance in human disease for the first time in single cases in 1971 and 1972.

In Britain, Louping ill is a tick-transmitted encephalitis of sheep and man. Central European and Russian spring-summer encephalitis are found in Europe and Russia, while Japanese B encephalitis occurs in Japan, Asia, and the Pacific. Kyasanur Forest disease in India entails signs of central nervous system involvement as well as abnormal bleeding and thus is classified both as an encephalitis and a hemorrhagic fever. Murray valley encephalitis is found in Australia.

Western equine encephalitis is an acute generalized illness characterized by fever, meningeal signs, somnolence, coma, convulsions, and paralysis. Fatality is high, and permanent brain damage is common, especially in children. The virus cycles in nature between a variety of small birds and the mosquito *Culex tarsalis.* Man and equines are dead-end hosts because viremia adequate for mosquito infection does not occur. Overwintering may occur as a result of chronic viremia in snakes, but annual return of the virus to temperate areas is probably more often by way of migratory birds. Diagnosis depends upon demonstration of rise in antibodies between acute and convalescent serum specimens. Virus isolation attempts from human tissue are rarely successful. The disease is confined to the western hemisphere and in North America occurs in epidemic form in spring and later summer.

Eastern equine encephalitis is an acute gen-

TABLE 76-3 VIRAL HEMORRHAGIC FEVERS: ETIOLOGIC AND EPIDEMIOLOGIC CONSIDERATIONS

Fever	Causative Agents	Vector(s)	Vertebrate Host(s)	Geographic Distribution	Epidemiologic Features of Involvement of Man	Control	Remarks
Yellow fever (urban)	YF virus, a group B arbovirus	Aedes aegypti in cities	Man	Human populations (usually urban in tropics of South and Central America	Person to person passage by Aedes	Aedes aegypti control: vaccination	Sylvan YF can spread to cities
Yellow fever (sylvan)	YF virus, a group B arbovirus	Haemagogus mosquitoes in New World, Aedes species in Africa	Monkeys of several genera and species	Forests and jungles of South and Central America and West, Central, and East Africa	Man infected by exposure in jungles (ie, wood-cutters, hunters, etc)	Vaccination	Human cases sporadic and unpredictable, disease often a silent endemic in forests
Dengue hemorrhagic fever	Dengue viruses of four types, group B arboviruses	Aedes aegypti	Man (involvement of other primates has been postulated)	Tropical and subtropical cities of Southeast Asia and Philippines	Small children usually involved in cities where Aedes aegypti densities are high	Aedes aegypti control: mosquito repellent, screens, etc	Disease may represent an immunologic overresponse to a sequential infection with a different dengue strain
Omsk hemorrhagic fever	Two distinguishable subtypes of HF virus	Ticks of genus Dermacentor	Small rodents and muskrats	Omsk region of USSR, northern Romania	People exposed in fields and wooded lands	Tick repellents and protective clothing	
Kyasanur Forest disease	KFD virus, a group B arbovirus	Ticks of several species in genus Haemaphysalis	Monkeys (rhesus and langur) and small rodents and birds	Mysore State, India	People exposed in fields and wooded lands	Tick control: tick repellents and protective clothing	Monkey mortality signals epidemic

Disease	Etiologic Agent	Arthropod Vector	Reservoir	Geographic Distribution	Persons at Risk	Control	Comments
Argentine hemorrhagic fever	Junin virus, an arenavirus, LCM-related	None proved, mites suspected	Small rodents: Akodon, *Calomys laucha, musculinus*	Argentina: NW of Buenos Aires extending west to Province of Cordoba	Field workers at harvest time are particularly at risk	Rodent control in fields	Infected rodents contaminate environment with urine
Bolivian hemorrhagic fever	Machupo virus, an arenavirus, LCM-related	None recognized	Small rodent: Calomys callosus	Beni Province of Bolivia	Residents of small rodent-infested villages and homes, 1971 nosocomial outbreak in Cochabamba, Bolivia	Rodent control in fields	High mortality in man
Lassa fever	Lassa virus, an arenavirus LCM-related,	None required	Small rodent: Mastomys natalensis	West Africa; Nigeria, Liberia, Sierra Leone	Residents of small rodent-infested villages, dramatic nosocomial outbreaks	None known, possibly rodent control	High mortality in man
Crimean hemorrhagic fever	CHF Congo virus, an ungrouped arbovirus	Ticks of several genera	Larger domestic animals implicated, also African hedgehog	Southern USSR, Bulgaria, East and West Africa	Cowhands and field workers in USSR, nosocomial outbreaks reported	Tick control relating to livestock, full isolation in patient care	Human disease important in USSR, importance to man in Africa not known
Korean hemorrhagic fever (hemonephroso-nephritis)	Not known; virus suspected	Not known	Possibly small mammals	Korea, northern Eurasia to and including Scandinavia	Rural or sylvan exposure (military, forest occupations, farmers)	None	A baffling epidemiologic and clinical entity

(From Johnson: In Beeson and McDermott (eds): Textbook of Medicine, 14th ed, 1975, p 239. Courtesy of W.B. Saunders Co.)

eralized illness characterized by fever and central nervous system signs and symptoms, including those of meningeal irritation, lethargy, coma, pareses, and convulsions. Death is frequent, and in survivors residual central nervous system damage is common and severe. A striking polymorphonuclear leukocytosis occurs in blood and in cerebrospinal fluid. Etiologic diagnosis depends upon virus isolation from brain tissue or the demonstration of an increase in serum antibody. Mosquitoborne epidemics and equine epizootics occur in late summer along the eastern strip of North America from Florida to Canada and the Caribbean.

California encephalitis is an acute febrile illness of 7 to 10 days duration, characterized by headache, vomiting, lethargy, disorientation, seizures, and focal neurologic signs. Although convalescence may be prolonged, fatality and morbidity are low. The cerebrospinal fluid contains abnormally high protein and increased numbers of white blood cells during acute phase. Etiologic diagnosis depends on either viral isolation or demonstration of rise of specific antibodies. It is a disease of children and occurs during summer months in wide areas of midwestern and southern United States. Mosquitoes of the genus *Aedes* transmit the virus to man. Vertebrate hosts include small animals.

St. Louis encephalitis is an acute febrile illness that occurs in a small percentage of those infected. It is usually characterized by fever and headache, and abnormalities of coordination and motor cranial nerve function may be common, especially in children. Signs of urinary tract inflammation may occur. Fatality may reach 25 percent, and mental and emotional sequelae are common. Cerebrospinal fluid changes are consistent with viral infections. Diagnosis depends on demonstration of serum antibody rise, and viral isolation is rarely achieved from human specimens. The virus cycles between birds and *Culex* mosquitoes. Large urban and suburban outbreaks occur in the United States.

Japanese B encephalitis is an acute illness that occurs in a small percentage of those infected with the virus. The usual consequence of infection is either inapparent or mild, undifferentiated disease. The encephalitis disease is similar to St. Louis encephalitis, with more severe neurologic involvement. Fatality is high, especially in older persons. Diagnosis is

confirmed serologically, and viral isolation from human specimens is unusual. The virus cycles annually between *Culex* mosquitoes and birds or pigs in temperate areas including Japan, Siberia, Korea, Taiwan, Pacific islands, and in tropical areas of southeast Asia.

The tick-borne group B viruses comprise a group of related agents that are found, each in a circumscribed domain, in North America, Britain, Europe, Russia, and Asia. The most common ones are Powassan, Russian spring-summer, central European and Louping ill encephalitides, and Omsk hemorrhagic fever and Kyasanur forest disease. The clinical spectrum includes hemorrhagic fever or encephalitis or a combination of the two. For this reason, they are listed in both Tables 76-2 and 76-3. The diseases vary greatly in fatality and in the severity of permanent neurologic damage. Diagnosis is by viral isolation from blood or brain tissue and by serologic tests.

Arboviruses and Arenaviruses that Cause Hemorrhagic Fevers The viral hemorrhagic fevers comprise 10 distinct diseases with widely differing epidemiologies and geographic loci. They are caused by viruses representing several taxonomic groups (Table 76-3). Some are mosquitoborne, others are tickborne, and the arthropod vectors of a third group are unknown or nonexistent. One disease is only presumed to have a viral etiology, and its mode of transmission is unknown. In addition to man himself, vertebrate hosts generally include primates or small mammals or rodents. The diseases are severe, with high fatality, but are self-limited, and survivors usually recover completely. None of these diseases is transmitted within the United States. The clinical picture comprises fever, bleeding often from the gastrointestinal tract, and a hypovolemic shock syndrome that is out of proportion to the blood loss and is probably due to leakage of noncellular components of blood from the vascular space. Depending on the virus, other organs and tissues may be involved, as for example, the liver in yellow fever. Dengue hemorrhagic fever illustrates a special point, in that apparently identical viruses can cause classical dengue throughout most of the tropical world, while in southeast Asia and the Philippines a hemorrhagic fever occurs. This may occur because the patient's immunologic status has been modified by prior infections with related arboviruses (Chaps. 18 and 64). Because of their historical significance, virulence, and public health importance, yellow fever and the arenavirus hemorrhagic fever are selected for further description as representative of the group.

YELLOW FEVER.   In spite of the presence of a safe, effective, attenuated vaccine that has been available since the 1930s, yellow fever remains today a real or potential public health problem for many peoples of the tropical world. Clinically, the disease is marked by the sudden onset of fever associated with severe headache, myalgia, back pain, conjunctivitis, and photophobia. As the disease progresses, prostration increases, and there are signs of involvement of the liver, kidneys, and heart with hepatomegaly, albuminuria, and a striking slowing of the heart rate. A hypovolemic shock phase associated with bleeding gums, hematemesis, oliguria and jaundice follows. Case fatality is high; recovery is complete. Diagnosis is confirmed by the isolation of the virus from the blood or from the liver, or by demonstration of a specific serologic response.

The characteristic histopathology of midzonal necrosis in the liver lobule has given rise in some areas to an epidemiologic method wherein mandatory postmortem corings of the liver are obtained from all deaths and sent in fixative to a central examining point, thus permitting an assessment of the proportion of deaths that are due to yellow fever.

Yellow fever has two distinct cycles in nature. One is an *A. aegypti*-man cycle that is operative in the large urban epidemics that are now, fortunately, history. The virus also cycles in the forest involving monkeys and different genera of mosquitoes. The virus is carried from the forest cycle to the urban cycle by infected people. Transmission can be effectively interrupted, in the case of the urban cycle, by *A. aegypti* control measures. Such measures, used prior to the recognition of the sylvan cycle, rid the urban centers of the Western hemisphere of dreadful epidemics that affected cities as far north as Philadelphia into the first decade of the present century. These same measures permitted completion of the Panama Canal. They are, however, relatively useless when one is dealing with zoophilic forest mosquitoes. As if in defiance of man's best effort, yellow fever epidemics occur today in areas where lack of logistic underpinnings of society prevent vector control or immunization programs.

ARENAVIRUS HEMORRHAGIC FEVERS.   The related viruses Machupo, Junin, and Lassa cause, respectively, the diseases Argentine hemorrhagic fever, Bolivian hemorrhagic fever, and Lassa fever, which occurs in Nigeria. Although many of the persons infected with these viruses suffer undifferentiated febrile illnesses, a fatal, hemorrhagic fever frequently occurs. Disease typically comprises headache, myalgia, and conjunctivitis. After several days, hemorrhagic manifestations appear and include petechiae as well as hemorrhages from the gastrointestinal and genitourinary tracts. As in other hemorrhagic fevers, a hypotensive crisis occurs which, if survived, is followed by complete recovery. Neurologic signs may occur in Argentine and Bolivian disease. Fatality is high; sequelae in survivors are not a problem. Diagnosis is confirmed by viral isolation as well as demonstration of an increase of specific antibodies. The agents are probably not arthropodborne. The reservoir is chronically infected rodents, as evidenced by viremia of long standing. It is suspected that man is infected as a result of contact with infected rodents or their virus-containing excreta. In the laboratory these agents are dangerous and should be studied only under conditions permitting maximum microbiologic security.

TREATMENT, CONTROL, AND PREVENTION

There are no therapeutic agents that are specific for arboviruses. The management of patients with disease comprises measures designed to restore and maintain nutrition and reasonably normal physiology. The latter might include, for example, restoration of intravascular volume during the hypovolemic shock phase of hemorrhagic fever or measures to reduce destructive degrees of cerebral edema in patients with encephalitis.

With the exception of the highly effective, safe, attenuated, tissue culture vaccine that has been in use since the 1930s for yellow fever, there are no arbovirus vaccines in general use.

Many experimental vaccines are under trial or laboratory development.

For arboviruses with limited host range and an accessible vector, there have been instances of effective prevention based on vector control. Urban yellow fever was eradicated in the early decades of this century by measures against *A. aegypti*. The task becomes infinitely more complex when one considers arboviruses that cycle silently in a variety of natural settings in birds, mammals, and arthropods. In these situations the possibilities may be restricted to lessening man's exposure to the ecosystem in question. Such a measure may fail because of anticipated and unacceptable consequences as, for example, might beset a woodcutter denied access to the forest.

FURTHER READING

Berge TO: International Catalogue of Arboviruses, 2nd ed. Dept of Health, Education, and Welfare, Washington DC, US Gov Printing Office, 1975

Blaskovic D, Nosek J: The ecological approach to the study of tick-borne encephalitis. Prog Med Virol 14: 275, 1972

Casals J: Arboviruses, arenaviruses and hepatitis. In Hellman A, Oxman MN, Pollack R (eds): Biohazards in Biological Research. Cold Spring Harbor Laboratory, 1973, p 223

Hammon W McD, Suther GE: Arboviruses. In Lennette EH, Schmidt NJ (eds): Diagnostic Procedures for Viral and Rickettsial Infection. American Public Health Association, 1969, p 227

Henderson PE, Coleman PH: The growing importance of California arboviruses in the etiology of human disease. Prog Med Virol 13:404, 1971

Johnson KM, Meiklejohn G, Downs WG: Arthropod-borne viral fevers, viral encephalidites and viral hemorrhagic fevers. In Beeson PB, McDermott W (eds): Textbook of Medicine, 14th ed. Philadelphia, Saunders, 1975, p 223

McDonald G: The Epidemiology and Control of Malaria. London, Oxford Univ Press, 1957

Monath TP, Newhouse VF, Kemp GE, Setzer HW, Cacciapuoti A: Lassa virus isolation from *Mastomys natalensis* rodents during an epidemic in Sierra Leone. Science 185:263, 1974

Reeves WC: Overwintering of arboviruses. Prog Med Virol 17:193, 1974

Strode GK: Yellow Fever. New York, McGraw-Hill, 1951

Theiler M, Downs WG: The Arthropod-Borne Viruses of Vertebrates. New Haven, Yale Univ Press, 1973 (See also review of this book, Work TH: Science 182:273, 1973)

US Public Health Service: Morbidity and Mortality Weekly Report. Atlanta Ga, Center for Disease Control

US Public Health Service: Neurotropic Viral Diseases Surveillance, Annual Summary. Atlanta Ga, Center for Disease Control

Work TH: The expanding role of arthropod-borne viruses in tropical medicine. In: Industry and Tropical Health IV. Boston, Harvard School of Public Health, 1961, p 225

Work TH: Exotic virus diseases. In Hunter GW, Swartzwelder JC, Clyde DF (eds). Tropical Medicine 5th ed. Philadelphia Saunders, 1976, p 1.

77
Orthomyxoviruses and Paramyxoviruses

INFLUENZA VIRUSES

Epidemics of the acute respiratory disease known as influenza have been described for centuries. Knowledge of the viruses causing this disease began with the isolation of influenza virus A in ferrets in 1933. By 1941 the development of the highly efficient technique for culturing influenza viruses in embryonated eggs and the discovery of hemagglutination by Hirst had provided the means for modern studies of influenza epidemiology.

Clinical Features Influenza viruses are respiratory pathogens, their primary target being ciliated respiratory epithelium. Infected cells release virus, undergo necrosis, and slough, leaving behind only a basal layer of cells. The virus spreads from the initial site of infection with progressive involvement of the respiratory tract via direct infection and/or toxic effects. The extent of damage to epithelium, submucosal inflammation, and extravascation of fluid determine the severity of influenza illness. When influenza pneumonia occurs, one may find intraalveolar hemorrhage and/or edema, sometimes with denuded alveolar walls, hyaline membranes, and capillary thrombosis. Macrophages containing virus antigen have been observed with immunofluorescent staining at all stages of the infection. Whether these cells combat infection, spread virus, or merely clear out virus-laden debris is uncertain. Bacterial superinfection occurs frequently, probably because of impaired mucociliary clearance, denuded surfaces, presence of rich extravascated fluid to serve as culture medium, and impairment of macrophage phagocytosis and bactericidal activity. Organs other than the respiratory tract may be involved in overwhelming influenza, particularly the heart. Central nervous system malfunction, neuropathies, and myopathy occur rarely. They follow the respiratory illness by a few days and may be asociated with few pathologic findings.

Characteristic clinical manifestations of influenza virus infection are the rather sudden onset of cough and coryza with a mild sore throat and prominent constitutional complaints, such as malaise, myalgias, headache, anorexia, and shivering. The patient is febrile, with a flushed face, conjunctival injection, nasal obstruction, nasal discharge, pharyngeal injection, and cough which may be paroxysmal. About a third of patients with uncomplicated influenza will produce some whitish sputum. Occasionally rales and rhonchi will be heard, and rarely a small pulmonary infiltrate may be seen on chest x-ray. The incubation period of this illness is one to two days (Fig. 77-1). Most acute symptoms in previously healthy individuals are over in three to four days, but cough and weakness may persist for a week or more.

Much more ominous is the acutely dyspneic, cyanotic patient who produces a thin, hemorrhagic sputum. Râles are heard diffusely, and though dullness to percussion may be only slight, chest x-ray reveals a patchy, fluffy infiltrate extending out from the hila. Although one must always look closely at the sputum smear, peripheral white blood cell count, and blood and sputum cultures for evidence of bacterial superinfection, the picture described can be produced by influenza infection alone. Influenza pneumonia is more likely to occur in patients with preexisting cardiac and/or pulmonary disease, especially rheumatic mitral disease. Pregnancy also carries a less well defined risk. The mortality rate with diffuse

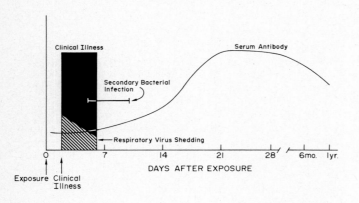

FIG. 77-1. The course of influenza virus infection.

influenza pneumonia is very high. Death is primarily due to respiratory insufficiency, although congestive heart failure secondary to myocarditis has been described.

Bacterial superinfection may occur early and be superimposed on the acute virus illness. More commonly the bacterial infection occurs later as a recrudescence of illness in the patient who seemed to be recovering. The bacteria involved are primarily pneumococci and staphylococci. Staphylococcal pneumonia is infrequent except following viral infections, such as influenza.

The disease described thus far is that which is characteristically recognized during influenza epidemics when such indicators as school and work absences and mortality due to influenza and pneumonia increase. Between epidemics when influenza virus is minimally active in a partially immune population, infection may be associated with much milder disease which passes as a common cold. Similar mild illness occurs in a portion of persons during epidemics, probably dependent on host defense mechanisms and degree of exposure.

Epidemiology Influenza viruses comprise three groups (A, B, and C), each with its own group-specific nucleoprotein (NP) antigen, also called the S (for soluble) antigen. Reaction of this antigen with specific antibody is usually studied by means of the complement-fixation test. Antibody to NP antigen does not neutralize infectivity or toxicity of influenza viruses.

In the viral envelope are two strain-specific viral (V) antigens: the hemagglutinin (H), whose reaction with antibody is commonly studied by means of hemagglutination-inhibition (HI) assays, and the neuraminidase (N), the activity of which can be inhibited by specific antibody. Antibody to H antigen neutralizes infectivity (as measured by a reduction in the number of plaques on susceptible tissue culture monolayers), while antibody to the N antigen interferes with infectivity by what is thought to be inhibition of the release of virus from infected cells (for example, similar number of plaques but reduced plaque size) (Chap. 62).

Major genetically determined changes in H antigens of group A influenza viruses over the past four decades have led successively to the establishment of influenza A types A_0, A_1, and A_2. However, genetically determined minor antigenic drift or major change can occur independently in both V antigens. Current nomenclature of the influenza viruses includes not only the NP antigen group, the animal source if other than man, the geographic origin, the strain number if assigned, and the year of isolation, but also the antigenic identity of both H and N subtypes. For example, the original Hong Kong influenza recovered in 1968 is designated A/Hong Kong/1/68(H3N2) and exhibited a major change in only the H antigen from the 1957 Asian influenza, A/Jap/305/57(H2N2), formerly called A_2 influenza. Antigenic differences exist among the various influenza B virus strains, but the differences have not been sufficiently major to necessitate the designation of subtypes. Similarly, only one type of influenza C virus is recognized.

Much of the periodicity of influenza over the world seems to be a function of antigenic changes in V antigens and the level of immunity in the population. Localized epidemics or outbreaks of influenza occur every two to three years, mostly with A strains and occasionally with B strains. Influenza virus C causes sporadic infection and is not important epidemiologically. The worldwide influenza pandemics are all associated with subtypes of influenza virus A which have abruptly undergone major shifts in V antigens.

Influenza viruses having group A NP antigen have been recovered from swine, horses, and birds. Swine influenza virus has been shown to persist in lungworms and earthworms, but the importance of this cycle in natural disease is uncertain.

Whether animal strains play a role in human influenza is also uncertain. It is of interest that antigenic shifts in influenza A strains may be cyclical. For example, serologic studies suggest that 1957 A_2 strains are related to those which caused the pandemic of 1889 to 1890, and 1968 Hong Kong influenza strains appear related to those that circulated at the turn of the century. Serologic studies also suggest that swine influenza is related to the 1918 pandemic strain. Moreover, Hong Kong influenza has been found to be antigenically related to an influenza strain from horses and identical with a strain from pigs. It has been hypothesized that major epidemic strains of influenza may arise from animals and that intermittent two-way transmission of influenza A strains between animals and man may lead to the periodic reappearance in man of strains which seemed to have disappeared.

Diagnosis   The clinical diagnosis of influenza virus infection is difficult in interepidemic periods. Other agents which might cause an illness mimicking moderately severe influenza include adenoviruses, *Mycoplasma pneumoniae*, psittacosis, and Q fever in adults, and a large variety of viruses in patients under 5 years of age.

Rapid virologic diagnosis can be accomplished using immunofluorescent staining of respiratory epithelial cells. Antibody against group-specific NP antigen can be used for this purpose, so that variation in V antigens does not interfere. However, the test is available in only a few laboratories.

Recovery of influenza virus is best accomplished by use of both embryonated eggs and primary monkey kidney tissue culture. Influenza virus usually does not produce a characteristic cytopathic effect in monkey kidney tissue culture, but its growth may be detected by hemadsorption (adsorption of red blood cells to tissue culture cells that are releasing virus). Virus may be detected in allantoic or tissue culture fluid by its ability to agglutinate red blood cells. Both hemadsorption and hemagglutination with influenza virus are carried out at 4C, since viral neuraminidase destroys red blood cell receptors on warming (Chap. 62). Identification of the virus can be accomplished using specific antisera in hemagglutination-inhibition or complement-fixation tests.

Increases in serum antibody titer between the times of collection of acute and convalescent sera can be detected using complement-fixation or hemagglutination-inhibition tests. For the complement-fixation test sera need only be heat-inactivated in order to destroy their own complement (56C for 30 minutes), and the influenza virus used need only be of the same group as that which caused infection, and not necessarily the same strain. For the hemagglutination-inhibition test, sera must be specifically treated to destroy nonspecific mucopolysaccharide inhibitors of influenza hemagglutination, and the virus strain used must have the same or a closely related H antigen. Virus infectivity neutralization tests for antibody can also be used, but they are much more expensive and cumbersome.

Once influenza activity has been documented during an epidemic, the major diagnostic problem in the individual patient is concerned with bacterial superinfection. The white blood cell count in influenza usually is normal or very nearly so, and it may not increase in the presence of bacterial superinfection. However, if the blood cell count rises above 15,000/mm³, bacterial superinfection is suggested. Sputum produced during influenza usually contains only moderate numbers of white cells of both mononuclear and polymorphonuclear varieties, and the gram stain reveals a mixed bacterial flora. Findings of many polymorphonuclear cells and a predominant bacterium in sputum smears suggest superinfection. Dense consolidation of the lung extending out to the chest wall, abscess formation, and pleural effusion are all characteristics unusual for influenza pneumonia and suggest a complicating bacterial infection. Cultures of sputum and blood for bacteria are indicated in every patient with influenza severe enough to require hospitalization.

Treatment   The main objectives in the treatment of the usual case of uncomplicated influenza are prevention of bacterial superinfection and relief of bothersome symptoms. Hydration, rest, gargles with warm saline or an antiseptic mouth wash, and an antipyretic-analgesic medication (eg, aspirin or acetaminophen) are the mainstays of therapy.

Significant hypoxia may occur during acute influenza, particularly in patients with chronic pulmonary and/or cardiac disease. Characteristic blood gas changes are decreased oxygen and pH and increased carbon dioxide. Such patients require hospitalization for oxygen therapy, ventilatory assistance, and help in clearing secretions.

In the patient with influenza pneumonia, superimposed bacterial pneumonia can progress to death very rapidly. Organisms may not be detected by smear or culture until it is too late. Such patients are frequently treated from the beginning with an antibiotic, such as penicillinase-resistant penicillin, which would be effective against the major bacterial pathogens but not so broad-spectrum as to strongly invite late infection with antibiotic-resistant organisms. Such therapy can be discontinued or altered in a few days as indicated by culture reports and clinical course. Patients with recognized secondary bacterial infections should be treated with antibiotics directed against the organism detected.

Prevention Resistance to influenza illness increases with increasing serum antibody titers. Inactivated virus vaccines containing antigens of current strains of influenza virus can induce the formation of serum antibody and provide demonstable protection. This protection is less than perfect and lasts only about one year.

The formulation of influenza vaccines is regularly reviewed and updated to include contemporary strains. Divalent or polyvalent vaccine containing antigens from two or more influenza strains is frequently employed. Monovalent vaccine may occasionally be necessary, as when Hong Kong influenza suddenly appeared in 1968 after that year's polyvalent vaccine supply had been prepared.

Influenza vaccines are grown in embryonated eggs, and, therefore, caution in administrating it to persons allergic to eggs is necessary. The vaccine is inactivated and is routinely administered subcutaneously. Highly purified vaccines containing reduced amounts of nonviral protein are available and cause relatively few local or systemic reactions when compared with standard vaccines. Because of the occasional occurrence of bothersome reactions and the less than perfect protection, influenza vaccines are generally reserved for highly exposed persons and for those in whom influenza carries a high mortality rate. The latter include patients with rheumatic heart disease or cardiac insufficiency of other causes, chronic bronchopulmonary disease, diabetes mellitus, Addison's disease, and those over age 65.

One hypothesis to explain the imperfect protection of influenza vaccines is that parenterally administered antigens are not very efficient at inducing secretory antibody. The latter appears to be important in protecting against respiratory infections, such as influenza. Results with intranasal vaccination using inactivated and attenuated influenza virus vaccines are being evaluated for effectiveness in inducing secretory antibody and immunity. Recombinant influenza virus strains that possess selected antigenic and/or growth properties are now being tested as possible vaccine strains. Another approach is the use of adjuvants that potentiate the immunologic response.

Amantadine was recently introduced for chemoprophylaxis of infections caused by influenza A_2 virus (Chap. 68). This drug appears to block influenza virus penetration into susceptible cells. Its usefulness is primarily in high-risk patients who have not been vaccinated at the time that an outbreak of influenza A_2 is identified. Preliminary data suggest that amantadine may also be useful therapeutically in influenza A_2 infections, presumably by inhibiting progressive infection of respiratory epithelial cells. Toxicities of amantadine include nervousness, dizziness, ataxia, depression, and feelings of detachment. These effects are usually noted at doses above the recommended 200 mg daily. The drug has been found by serendipity to be useful in the treatment of patients with Parkinson's disease, but the mechanism of action in the central nervous system is uncertain.

PARAINFLUENZA VIRUSES

Parainfluenza viruses are grouped by virtue of common morphologic, biochemical, and antigenic properties (Table 62-4).

Several strains of parainfluenza virus infect animals. The first reported strain, Sendai, was recovered in the early 1950s from lungs of infants who died with pneumonia, but mice were used in the work and were subsequently found to be naturally infected with Sendai virus. In the late 1950s parainfluenza viruses were recovered from human beings, with the use of tissue culture and hemadsorption to detect virus growth. The first three types of parainfluenza virus to be isolated from human beings were initially known as hemadsorption viruses (HA-1, now called parainfluenza 3; HA-2, now called parainfluenza 1) and as croup-associated virus (CA, now called parainfluenza 2). Parainfluenza types 4A and 4B were described in the early 1960s. Parainfluenza viruses of animals include Sendai virus of mice and pigs which cross-reacts serologically with parainfluenza 1, viruses from cattle and monkeys that cross-react with parainfluenza 3, and simian viruses SV5 and SV41, that are related to parainfluenza 2. The latter simian viruses frequently contaminate monkey kidney tissue cultures and may create confusion in virus isolation attempts.

Disease Human parainfluenza viruses are respiratory pathogens that usually produce acute upper respiratory illnesses with pharyngitis. Fever occurs in about one-half of the cases. Infection is detected most frequently in children, among whom parainfluenza viruses account for 10 to 20 percent of acute respiratory illness. About one-third of patients in the young age groups have severe illnesses, particularly laryngotracheobronchitis (croup), but also bronchitis, bronchiolotis, and pneumonia. The decreased frequency and mildness of parainfluenza illness in adults may result from partial immunity due to early contact with the viruses.

Epidemiology Parainfluenza viruses 1 and 3 can be recovered from children throughout the year, but they may also cause epidemics of illness in young age groups during the fall, winter, or spring. Type 2 infections tend to be more sporadic, occasionally with epidemics in the fall or winter. Infection appears to be by the airborne route, with an incubation period of two to four days. Most children have acquired antibody to types 1, 2, and 3 by age 6 or 7 years. Type 4 infection is rare and not of epidemiologic importance.

Reinfections with parainfluenza viruses have been clearly documented. However, the amount of virus shed is small, the illness tends to be milder, and antibody response may be difficult to demonstrate.

Diagnosis Respiratory syncytial virus and adenoviruses 1, 2, 3, and 5 all commonly produce illness in children that is clinically indistinguishable from that produced by parainfluenza viruses. Pharyngitis due to group A beta-hemolytic streptococci may also simulate parainfluenza illness and must be diagnosed for therapeutic reasons with appropriate cultures, smears, blood counts, and serologies. Definitive diagnosis of parainfluenza virus infection depends on virus isolation and demonstration of an increase in serum antibody titer in acute and convalescent sera.

Tissue culture cells that can be used for parainfluenza viral isolation include primary human embryonic kidney, human amnion, and especially primary monkey kidney cells. Low concentrations of hyperimmune antiserum can be added to monkey kidney tissue culture medium to inhibit growth of simian viruses without interfering with recovery of the parainfluenza viruses. Late cytopathic effects are seen with parainfluenza 2 but less frequently with other types. Growth of parainfluenza virus is usually detected by hemadsorption inhibition after 5 to 20 days of incubation. Identification may be accomplished by hemadsorption with specific antisera after virus has been grown in fresh tissue culture tubes.

Parainfluenza viruses hemagglutinate guinea pig and chicken red blood cells. Hemagglutination inhibition is useful for testing virus identification and for determining titers of serum antibody against known virus strains. Complement-fixation and neutralization tests can also be used for these purposes. With all of these serologic tests, antibody response to infection with one type of parainfluenza virus may actually be higher against a different parainfluenza type or against mumps virus. Such heterotypic antibody responses are common in human beings and probably reflect the hosts' previous experience with members of this virus group. Antibody response of parainfluenza virus-free animals to immunization or infection with a single parainfluenza strain is type-specific.

Attempts have been made to develop a more rapid diagnosis of parainfluenza virus infections than routine tissue culture and serologic techniques can provide. Electron microscopy on clinical specimens, direct testing of clinical specimens for hemagglutination, and immunofluorescent staining both of clinical specimens directly and of inoculated tissue cultures after 24 to 72 hours incubation have all been used successfully for rapid diagnosis. The latter techniques are not routinely available.

Treatment Treatment is symptomatic. Hydration, provision of a moist atmosphere, and attention to airway patency are particularly important in the management of parainfluenza infections of the lower respiratory tract in young children. Secondary bacterial infection may occur and requires early antibiotic therapy in the patient already critically ill with parainfluenza virus infection.

Prevention Immunity to parainfluenza virus following natural infection is only partial. Studies in adult volunteers suggest that secretory antibody is very important in resistance. These two observations suggest that parenteral inactivated parainfluenza virus vaccines might not be very effective. Nevertheless, a potent inactivated vaccine given parenterally with mineral oil adjuvant was found to be highly protective in cattle against parainfluenza virus infection. Studies of the efficacy of experimental, inactivated parainfluenza virus vaccines in human beings have been more equivocal in their results. Work toward more effective means of inducing resistance to parainfluenza virus is being pursued because of the importance of this group of agents in childhood respiratory disease.

MUMPS

Clinical Illness Mumps virus infection, an illness prevalent in childhood, was recognized in epidemic form as early as the fifth century BC by Hippocrates. The most frequently discussed and recognized symptom is parotitis, although the illness may have multiple manifestations that are indicative of the generalized nature of the infection. The portal of entry is thought to be the upper respiratory tract, as the virus gains direct access to the mucous membranes of the mouth and nose. Virus is transmitted by the saliva of infected persons or with materials recently contaminated with virus.

The time interval that elapses after exposure to virus and prior to the appearance of clinical symptoms is usually 14 to 21 days. The tissues in which primary viral multiplication occurs are not known with certainty. Viremia then occurs, and as a result one of several tissues and organs, including the salivary glands (predominantly the parotids), meninges, testes, pancreas, ovaries, thyroid, and heart, may become secondarily infected. Virus is also excret-ed in the urine and transient abnormalities in renal function have been found in adult males with mumps infection.

Figure 77-2 presents graphically the time relationships of the clinical features of mumps viral infection and correlates the time periods of virus excretion, communicability of the illness, and clinical symptoms. Salivary gland infection with pain, edema, and consequent swelling results in the characteristic parotid gland enlargement diagnosed as mumps. This infection may involve the parotid, submandibular, and, less often, the sublingual salivary glands. Salivary gland involvement usually precedes other clinical symptoms, lasts for two to seven days, and may be unilateral or bilateral. Any of the other manifestations of mumps infection, such as CNS disease, occasionally precede, coincide with, or occur in the absence of salivary gland involvement.

Involvement of the central nervous system with any infectious agent is cause for concern for both physician and patient. Fortunately, with mumps virus infection, the vast majority of such recognized illness is transient aseptic meningitis with few sequelae. The incidence of this type of CNS infection has been estimated to be as high as 65 percent on the basis of lumbar punctures on hospitalized patients with clinical mumps. The CNS involvement was manifested in such cases by a predominantly lymphocytic pleocytosis of the cerebrospinal fluid. Only one-half of these individuals evidenced clinical signs of meningitis. Signs of meningeal involvement are most often manifest 2 to 10 days after the onset of parotitis, last for 3 to 4 days, and are self-limited.

A more serious and fortunately much less common central nervous system manifestation of mumps is postinfectious encephalitis or encephalomyelitis. It is important to distinguish

FIG. 77-2. The course of mumps virus infection.

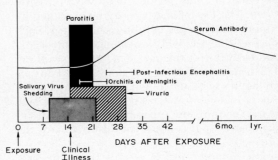

between this manifestation and the aseptic meningitis, so that the illness of the individual patient may be placed in the proper perspective for the family and for the patient. The time of onset is usually later than the transient aseptic meningitis and occurs 10 to 14 days after the clinical salivary gland involvement. The patient appears severely ill, is deeply obtunded, and may succumb to the illness. It occurs less often than the postinfectious encephalitis associated with measles or varicella and is clinically and pathologically indistinguishable from them. The typical manifestations of the preceding illness (eg, rash with measles) provide the clinical diagnosis of the underlying illness.

In hamsters experimental mumps infection may cause hydrocephalus. Sequential studies demonstrated virus replication and associated inflammatory changes during the first week after intracerebral inoculation. Virus was localized almost entirely within ependymal cells of the ventricles and choroid plexus. The animals did not show any signs of acute illness, but hydrocephalus became evident in three to six weeks after infection. These animals had aqueductal stenosis secondary to the resolving inflammation. Thus, an inapparent acute inflammation resulted in later sequelae at a time when viral antigen and infectious virus were no longer evident. Similar effects have now been described in experimental models employing influenza A_0, parainfluenza type 2, and a temperature-sensitive variant of measles virus. The clinical application of such observations remains to be established, but there are now several case reports recording mumps infection in children who subsequently developed aqueductal stenosis (although it is not certain that the infection caused the subsequent hydrocephalus).

An occasional sequel of mumps virus infection is deafness, which may occur even in the absence of other evidence of CNS involvement. The loss of hearing may be preceded by tinnitus and a sense of fullness of the ear. Such deafness is relatively uncommon, but occurs suddenly during the period of parotid swelling. It is usually unilateral, but an estimated 20 percent of those so affected may have bilateral disease. Once deafness has occurred, the damage is irreversible and apparently is caused by inflammation and subsequent destruction of the organ of Corti.

The complication of mumps infection best known to nonmedical persons is the involvement of the testes. Orchitis occurs predominantly in postpubertal males, with 20 to 30 percent of this age group manifesting testicular involvement during the course of mumps infection. Bilateral disease is present in approximately 2 to 6 percent of the total number of patients with orchitis. Inflammation of the testes is extremely painful, but the fear of this affliction stems from its association with sterility. Accurate knowledge of the incidence of sterility following mumps orchitis is not available because the occurrence is infrequent, and very large numbers of cases of mumps must be observed during the original illness to document accurately mumps viral infection as the cause of subsequent sterility. Once it has occurred, therapy of orchitis is symptomatic without any clearly demonstrated benefits from either steroid therapy or immune globulin.

Pancreatitis with typical symptoms of abdominal pain, fever, and vomiting may occur in association with mumps infection. Much less frequently, thyroiditis, mastitis, myocarditis, and oophoritis are seen.

In the normal individual, a single infection with mumps virus confers permanent immunity against clinically evident infection. It is probable that reinfection, defined as an antibody rise after exposure to the virus, may occur, but neither virus shedding nor clinical illness has been demonstrated with such reinfection. Second attacks of parotitis have been observed in the same individual, but it is wise to remember that other causes of parotitis include *Coxsackie* or lymphocytic choriomeningitis infections, starch ingestion, sarcoidosis, iodine sensitivity, and thiazide therapy. At the time of this writing, there is no documentation by culture or serology of two clinical attacks of mumps virus infection in a single individual.

The host initially responds to mumps virus infection with the production of serum IgM antibodies and subsequently antibodies predominantly of the IgG class. Neutralizing antibodies are formed within the first week of symptoms and ordinarily persist for a lifetime. Hemagglutination-inhibiting and complement-fixing antibodies may appear from the first through the third week and usually reach a peak within three to six weeks after the onset of symptoms. CF antigens have been differentiated into two distinct types. The first is the soluble (S) or nucleoprotein antigen, and the second is the virus (V) or surface antigen. CF antibodies against the S antigen are present within 2 to 3 days of onset, peak at about 10 days, and then disappear after 8 to 9 months. CF antibodies against the V antigen appear at about the tenth day of infection and persist for years. The transient nature of the S antibodies may sometimes assist in defining recent infection.

Special consideration should briefly be given to those persons commonly thought to be at increased risk from virus infections. The pregnant woman or her fetus is frequently considered at higher risk with regard to particular infections, such as varicella and rubella. At this time, conflicting reports relating to mumps infection during pregnancy have been published. There is no confirmed evidence of the occurrence of congenital anomalies in the human fetus as a result of mumps infection sustained by the pregnant mother and transmitted to her fetus in utero.

Patients who have altered immunity, either humoral (eg, the agammaglobulinemic) or cellular (eg, the natural occurring lymphopenic or the immunosuppressed patient), do not appear to be at increased risk with respect to mumps infection. Live virus vaccine is contraindicated for pregnant women and for the groups of persons with altered immunity.

The mumps intradermal skin tests has been utilized in attempts to define an individual's previous experience with mumps antigen. There is no doubt that there can be a demonstrable delayed type of hypersensitivity response which is dependent upon previous lymphocyte sensitization to the antigen, but this skin test is less reliable than such antigens as IPPD. There are a significant number of false negative and false positive tests, so that in an individual case the skin test will not be helpful.

Pathology Examination of involved tissues is unusual because of the ordinarily benign nature of the illness. There is no disruption of the general architecture of salivary glands after several days of illness. The involved salivary ducts demonstrate changes in the epithelial lining cells, ranging from swelling to complete desquamation. The ducts are dilated, and the lumen may be filled with cellular debris and polymorphonuclear cells. There is a moderate amount of periductal edema around the involved ducts, and the interstitial inflammatory cell is predominantly mononuclear.

The pathology of other involved tissues, eg, the testes, is similar, with mononuclear interstitial infiltrates, edema, and no specific hallmarks allowing the diagnosis of mumps infection to be made solely on the basis of the observed pathology.

Epidemiology Mumps virus infection is predominantly a disease of childhood, with the majority of clinically evident infections being seen between the ages of 5 and 10 years. It has been estimated that 90 percent of the population is immune by the time they reach 15 years of age. Although mumps virus infection is contagious, it is less communicable than are measles and varicella. The degree of communicability is estimated most accurately by serologic surveys of exposed individuals, since as many as one-fourth of the infections with mumps virus occur without clinical symptoms.

Isolation of the patient within the hospital setting or in homes has not effectively curtailed spread of disease. This is usually attributed to the period of virus shedding, which occurs prior to symptomatic onset of illness and thus precedes recognition of infection. As previously mentioned, one-fourth of patients have an asymptomatic infection, but they also excrete virus. Their infection is self-limited, and their immunity is comparable to those with symptomatic infection. To the best of our knowledge, there are no animal reservoirs or human carriers of mumps virus.

Diagnostic Approach The work of Johnson and Goodpasture first established that mumps is caused by a filterable virus and demonstrated that rhesus monkeys could be experimentally infected. The description of the complement-fixation test and successful propagation of virus in chick embryos preceded the now generally employed standard tissue culture techniques. These methods employ monolayers of one of several cell types, including primary monkey kidney, human amnion and human kidney cells, and cell lines, such as HeLa cells. With these techniques, virus has been isolated from such varied sources as blood, CSF, urine, saliva, salivary gland tissue, and human milk.

In many academic and large hospital settings, viral diagnostic laboratories are available, and virus isolation can be attempted from clinical materials. The responsible laboratory will provide directions for submitting materials for culture. Saliva or urine can be collected at the time of clinical CNS symptoms and submitted for culture. Mumps isolation in tissue culture is usually not necessary for either diagnosis or patient care, but techniques and facilities are available for defining the unusual or complicated situation.

For practical reasons, many diagnostic laboratories can offer more extensive serologic diagnosis than cultural facilities for virus isolation. They will evaluate sera for the presence of antibodies to mumps virus. The serum for evaluation should be obtained as early as possible in the illness, and a convalescent specimen should be obtained after an interval of two to three weeks. A pair of sera can determine whether a specific illness is mumps infection by demonstrating an increase in antibody titer. A single serum can determine whether a person has ever had mumps infection but cannot define when it occurred. As indicated previously there are several types of antibody elicited by mumps infections. As with other virus infections, understanding the time sequence of mumps antibody formation and the specificity of a given type of antibody will allow determination of the significance of a laboratory-determined antibody titer.

Treatment   No specific therapy is available for mumps infection. Symptomatic management of patients includes adequate hydration, analgesic and antipyretic therapy, and local measures, such as elevation and application of cold packs in orchitis.

Prophylaxis and Immunization   The problem repeatedly occurs of what to do after exposure to mumps infection. Usually the person concerned is an adult without previous symptomatic mumps infection. Hyperimmune globulin or pooled serum IgG has been administered after exposure, without proven decrease in the number of patients acquiring illness or lessened severity of illness. However, there has been a controlled study purporting to demonstrate that the administration of hyperimmune globulin after the appearance of parotitis can decrease the incidence and severity of orchitis. For this reason, hyperimmune globulin may be

administered to postpubertal males who have parotitis.

Live attenuated mumps virus vaccine was licensed in 1968 and is available for prophylactic use. It is recommended for administration to children more than 1 year of age and to young adults for induction of immunity parallel to that induced by natural infection. Vaccine should not be given to pregnant women because of the potential vulnerability of the fetus. Although no data exist which demonstrate transmission of attenuated virus to the fetus, placental infection has been documented after maternal immunization. There is only a single serologic strain of mumps virus, hence, a single infection with either natural or attenuated virus confers immunity. The vaccine is a live attenuated virus produced in tissue cultures of chick embryo fibroblasts and is administered parenterally. Virus is not shed by the vaccinee, and immunization does not cause any side effects. The vaccine produces 95 to 100 percent serologic conversion from the antibody negative to the positive state. The antibody levels parallel those produced by natural infection but are considerably lower. They persist for the 9 to 10 years that vaccines have been available for study. Immunized children in contact with naturally occurring mumps have been protected against clinical illness.

The vaccine will not offer protection against mumps if someone has already been exposed to natural infection and is in the incubation period of illness. On the other hand, no harmful effects have been noted after administration of vaccine to an exposed susceptible individual.

FURTHER READING

INFLUENZA

Beare AS, Hall TS, Schild GC, Kundin WD: Antigenic characteristics of swine influenza virus closely related to human Hong Kong strain and results of experimental infection in volunteers. Lancet 1:305, 1971

Dowdle WR, Coleman MT, Gregg MB: Natural history of influenza Type A in the United States, 1957-1972. Prog Med Virol 17:92, 1974

Galbraith AW, Oxford JS, Schild GC, Potter CW, Watson GI: Therapeutic effect of 1-adamantanamine hydrochloride in naturally occurring influenza A$_2$ Hong Kong infection. Lancet 2:113, 1971

Jackson GG, Muldoon RL: Viruses causing common respiratory infections in man. V. Influenza A (Asian). J. Infect Dis 131:308, 1975

Kasel JA, Rossen RD, Fulk RV, et al: Human influenza:

aspects of the immune response to vaccination. Ann Intern Med 71:369, 1969

Knight V (ed): Viral and Mycoplasmal Infections of the Respiratory Tract. Philadelphia, Lea & Febiger, 1975

Loosli CG (ed): Conference on Newer Respiratory Viruses. Am Rev Respir Dis 88 (Part 2), 1963

Louria DB, Blumenfeld HL, Ellis JT, Kilbourne ED, Rogers DE: Studies on influenza in the pandemic of 1957-1958. II. Pulmonary complications of influenza. J Clin Invest 38:213, 1959

Martin CM, Kunin CM, Gottlieb LS, et al: Asian influenza A in Boston, 1957-1958. I. Observations in thirty-two influenza-associated fatal cases. Arch Intern Med 103:515, 1959

Pereira HG: Influenza: antigenic spectrum. Prog Med Virol 11:46, 1969

Petersdorf RG, Fusco JJ, Harter DH, Albrink WS: Pulmonary infections complicating Asian influenza. Arch Intern Med 103:262, 1959

Robinson RQ: Natural history of influenza since the introduction of the A2 strain. Prog Med Virol 6:82, 1964

Schulman JL: Effects of immunity on transmission of influenza: experimental studies. Prog Med Virol 12:128, 1970

Stuart-Harris CH: Influenza and Other Virus Infections of the Respiratory Tract. Baltimore, Williams & Wilkins, 1965

Tateno I, Kitamoto O, Kawamura A Jr: Diverse immunocytologic findings of nasal smears in influenza. N Engl J Med 274:237, 1966

Ward TG: Viruses of the respiratory tract. Prog Med Virol 15:126, 1973

Webster RE, Campbell CH: Studies on the origin of pandemic flu: Selection and transmission of "new" viruses in vivo. Virology 62:404, 1974

World Health Organization, Scientific Group. Respiratory Viruses. WHO Technical Report Series, No 408. Geneva, World Health Organization, 1969

PARAINFLUENZA VIRUSES

Bisno AL, Barratt NP, Swanston WH, Spence LP: An outbreak of acute respiratory disease in Trinidad associated with parainfluenza viruses. Am J Epidemiol 91:68, 1970

Chanock RM: Parainfluenza viruses. In Lennette EH, Schmidt NJ (eds): Diagnostic Procedures for Viral and Rickettsial Infections. New York, American Public Health Association, 1969, p 434

Chanock RM, Johnson KM, Cook MI, Wong DC, Vargosko A: The hemadsorption technique, with special reference to the problem of naturally occurring simian parainfluenza virus. Am Rev Respir Dis 83:125, 1961

D'Alessio D, Williams S, Dick EC: Rapid detection and identification of respiratory viruses by direct immunofluorescence. Appl Microbiol 20:233, 1970

Doane FW, Chatiyanonda K, McLean DM, et al: Rapid laboratory diagnosis of paramyxovirus infections by electron microscopy. Lancet 2:751, 1967

Herrmann EC Jr, Hable KA: Experiences in laboratory diagnosis of parainfluenza viruses in routine medical practice. Mayo Clin Proc 45:177, 1970

Higgins PG: Epidemiology of respiratory infection in adults. J Clin Pathol [Suppl 2] 21:23, 1968

Hsiung GD: Parainfluenza-5 virus. Infection of man and animal. Prog Med Virol 14:241, 1972

Jackson GG, Muldoon RL: Viruses causing common respiratory infections in man. II. Enteroviruses and paramyxoviruses. J Infect Dis 128:387, 1973

Smith CB, Purcell RH, Bellanti JA, Chanock RM: Protective effect of antibody to parainfluenza type 1 virus. N Engl J Med 275:1145, 1966

Tyrell DAJ: Common Colds and Related Diseases. Baltimore, Williams & Wilkins, 1965

World Health Organization, Scientific Group. Respiratory Viruses. WHO Technical Report Series, No 408. Geneva, World Health Organization, 1969

MUMPS

Bang H, Bang J: Involvement of CNS in mumps. Acta Med Scand 113:487, 1943

Brunell PA, Brickman A, O'Hare D, Steinberg S: Ineffectiveness of isolation of patients as a method of preventing the spread of mumps. N Engl J Med 279:1357, 1968

Enders JF, Cohen S: Detection of antibody by complement fixation in sera of man and monkey convalescent from mumps. Proc Soc Exp Biol Med 50:180, 1942

Gellis SS, McGuiness AC, Peters M: A study of the prevention of mumps orchitis by gamma globulin. Am J Med Sci 210:661, 1945

Habel K: Cultivation of mumps virus in the developing chick embryo and its application to studies of immunity to mumps in man. Public Health Rep 60:201, 1945

Johnson CD, Goodpasture EW: An investigation of the etiology of mumps. J Exp Med 59:1, 1934

Johnson RT, Johnson KP, Edmonds CJ: Virus induced hydrocephalus: development of aqueductal stenosis in hamsters after mumps infection. Science 157:1066, 1967

Levens JH, Enders JF: The hemagglutinative properties of amniotic fluid from embryonated eggs infected with mumps virus. Science 102:117, 1945

Weibel RE, Buynak EB, Stokes J, Hilleman RR: Persistence of immunity following monovalent and combined live measles, mumps, and rubella virus vaccines. Pediatr 51:467, 1973

Weller TH, Craig JR: Isolation of mumps virus at autopsy. Am J Pathol 25:1105, 1949

Witte JJ, Karchmer AW: Surveillance of mumps in U.S. as background for use of vaccine. Public Health Rep 83:95, 1968

Yamauchi T, Wilson C, St. Geme JW Jr: Transmission of live attenuated mumps virus to the human placenta. N Engl J Med 290:710, 1974

78
Pseudomyxoviruses

MEASLES (RUBEOLA)

History Because of its distinctive clinical features, measles was recognized as a disease entity long before the demonstration of its viral etiology. Early medical writings by Hebrew and Arabic physicians include clear descriptions of the illness. In 1758, Home, a Scottish physician, first demonstrated the transmissibility of the disease by scarification of susceptible individuals with blood taken from infected patients.

Measles virus was first isolated in tissue culture in 1954 by Enders and associates. With the demonstration that the virus replicated in renal cell cultures of human or simian origin, investigations of the virus and its properties were undertaken. The use of attenuated vaccines began in 1963 and has continued to extend throughout the world. A childhood disease which was accepted as inevitable may become a rarity if the programs for control are successfully conducted. In the United States, mortality from measles has resulted consistently in 1 death per 10,000 cases. In nations with less well developed health services, the mortality rate has often exceeded 10 percent among children suffering from nutritional disorders and other debilitating conditions.

Clinical course. Measles has a regular incubation period varying from 10 to 14 days (Fig. 78-1). A prodromal stage is marked by catarrhal symptoms of cough, coryza, and conjunctivitis. Fever accompanies these symptoms and rises steadily each day, until the appearance of rash two to four days after the onset. Preceding the skin eruption, the pathognomonic Koplik spots may be found on the lateral buccal mucosa. These are pinpoint, grayish white spots surrounded by bright red inflammation. They are found over the lateral buccal mucosa as well as the inner lips and may spread to involve the entire inner anterior mouth. The exanthem begins on the head, behind the ears, on the forehead, and on the neck. Discrete macular and papular lesions progress downward to involve the trunk and upper extremities. Over a period of three days, the entire body becomes involved. When the lower extremities first show discrete lesions, those on the head and neck have begun to coalesce. With rash reaching the lower extremities, the high fever recedes dramatically. The bright red rash fades, to leave a brown discoloration which does not blanch with pressure and represents capillary leakage and hemorrhage into the skin.

The respiratory tract manifestations of measles vary in severity but include laryngitis, tracheobronchitis, bronchiolitis, and some degree of interstitial pneumonitis as manifestations of the primary viral infection that damages surface mucosal cells. With defervescence there is improvement, but secondary bacterial infections of the respiratory tract may complicate the recovery phase in 5 to 15 percent of patients. These include otitis media, sinusitis,

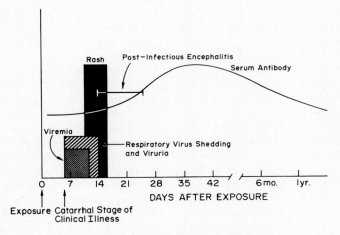

FIG. 78-1. The course of measles virus infection.

mastoiditis, and pneumonia. The most dread complication of measles is an encephalomyelitis, which occurs in approximately 0.1 percent of cases. Classically, this follows a period of three to four days' recovery from the acute illness and is marked by a sudden onset, with seizures, confusion, and coma. The mortality rate of central nervous system involvement approaches 25 percent. Additionally, nearly half of those who survive are left with some sequelae involving impaired intellectual, motor, or emotional development. More recently, the association of measles infection with a late central nervous system complication, subacute sclerosing panencephalitis (SSPE), has been established. This is discussed in greater detail in Chapter 82.

Measles is acquired as an infection of the respiratory tract, and the principal damage is to the mucosal lining cells of respiratory tract surfaces. The virus spreads via the lymphatics and through the blood to give widespread involvement, particularly in lymphoid cells. The large, multinucleated giant cells which are found in these tissues are quite similar to those produced by measles virus when grown in vitro. Patients excrete large amounts of virus during the catarrhal phase prior to the appearance of the characteristic exanthem. Virus can be recovered from the blood, particularly from the white cell fraction, for several days before rash appears but rarely therafter. The urine may remain positive for virus up to four days after the onset of rash. The pathology of central nervous system involvement includes edema, congestion, and scattered petechial hemorrhages with perivascular cuffs of round cells. There may be some perivascular demyelination in the later stages.

The exact nature of the measles rash is uncertain, but viral microtubular aggregates have been observed by electron microscopy of nuclei and cytoplasm of skin biopsies. They are also found in the oral lesions (Koplik spots). Evidence of the interaction of measles infections and cellular immune mechanisms is the loss of delayed hypersensitivity to tuberculoprotein among tuberculin-positive patients with measles. This may persist for several weeks to months following the acute infection. Closely correlated is the repeated observation of the worsening or exacerbation of underlying tuberculosis in children or adults who acquire measles infection.

Epidemiology   Measles is one of the most highly communicable of all viral infections, so that nearly all susceptible children acquire the infection. In rural settings or among isolated communities, it has been possible for a population to reach adult life without experiencing the infection. Under such circumstances, the introduction of measles virus has produced devastating epidemics. Particularly noteworthy are those that have occurred among island populations. An epidemiologic classic is Panum's description in 1846 of such an outbreak in the Faroe Islands. He showed the persistence of lifelong immunity among individuals who had acquired the infection six and seven decades previously.

In the temperate zones, measles has occurred in winter–spring epidemics at two-year or three-year cycles, apparently related to the new groups of susceptible children born during the interval since the last outbreak. Maternal antibody is transplacentally acquired by the infant, so that infection under six months of age is rare. As shown in Figure 78-1, the catarrhal stage of the illness is marked by extensive respiratory virus excretion, so that infected droplet nuclei within families, schoolrooms, or other crowded settings provide the usual mode of transmission. A single attack confers lifelong immunity.

Although measles virus is closely related to the agents of canine distemper and rinderpest of cattle, there is no evidence of natural spread from one species to another. Their biologic similarities and serologic overlapping offer an interesting area for evolutionary speculation. Except for minor variations, only one distinct serotype of measles virus has been identified. Infection sustained in any part of the world confers uniform geographic protection.

Diagnosis   Diagnosis is clinical, based on the characteristic history and findings. Examination of the urinary sediment or of nasal smears will show characteristic inclusion-bearing syncytia, and there is peripheral leukopenia. Indirect immunofluorescent microscopy has been used to show measles antigen in nasopharyngeal cells. Although virus can be isolated from blood, respiratory tract secretions, conjunctival secretions, or urine, this is not ordinarily required. In cell culture systems, the cytopathic effect is similar to that of the histology observed in vivo with measles infections.

A number of serologic tests are available,

based on the antigens of the measles virion. These include virus neutralization, hemagglutination inhibition, complement fixation, and immunofluorescence. Antibody appears very rapidly after the appearance of rash and rise to high titers in the next 30 to 60 days. A pair of sera obtained early in the course of the illness and 7 to 14 days thereafter will show a marked rise in antibody titer by any of the methods described. Because of its ease and rapidity, the hemagglutination-inhibition test is most often utilized.

Treatment and Prevention The primary disease is not presently amenable to any therapy. Supportive mesures may be employed to reduce fever, ameliorate cough, amd maintain hydration. Secondary bacterial complications are treated with antibiotics selected by culture of appropriate specimens. The use of antimicrobials prior to the appearance of secondary bacterial complications has not diminished their incidence but has altered the flora, so that more resistant organisms have survived. The treatment of encephalomyelitis is also symptomatic, with careful attention to the maintenance of an airway, control of seizures, and provision of fluid, electrolyte, and caloric requirements. The use of gammaglobulin early in the incubation period of measles may completely abort or modify the infection, depending on the amount employed. At a dose of 0.04 ml per kg body weight, gamma globulin will reliably modify measles so that a more benign course ensues, followed by lasting immunity. Using a dose of 0.2 ml per kg body weight, it is possible to abort the infection completely so that no clinical symptoms result, and the patient may remain susceptible after catabolism of the exogenous globulin.

The prevention of measles by proper use of the available attenuated active viral vaccines offers the most reliable and enduring protection against the infection. Vaccines are recommended for all healthy children shortly after 1 year of age. Several different vaccines are available, but they all originate from the Edmonston strain of virus. They are given parenterally, with successful infection in at least 95 percent of susceptibles. The infection is usually occult but may cause fever in 15 percent of recipients. Rarely there is moderate, transient rash following the fever. This attenuated infection is noncommunicable and results in antibody responses somewhat lower than those which follow the natural infection. In patients studied to date, antibodies have persisted for periods up to 15 years after immunization. When exposed to natural infection, immunized children remain solidly protected. For several years an inactivated measles vaccine was available. It has been abandoned now because of experiences that revealed a severe and unusual illness following the exposure of these children to naturally occurring measles several years after the receipt of the inactivated vaccine. They developed fever, pneumonitis, and petechiae. It seemed to represent a hypersensitivity reaction in patients whose previous immunity had waned after inactivated vaccine. These inactivated vaccines have been withdrawn from the market.

In the initial five years after the onset of vaccine use in the United States, reported cases of measles were reduced by 90 percent. Figure 78-2 graphically demonstrates the striking decline in reported cases of measles in the United States since vaccine licensure in 1963 and widespread public health immunization programs beginning in 1966. In the next two years

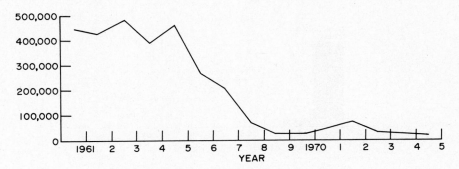

FIG. 78-2. Cases of measles reported in the United States.

there was a small upswing of cases due to a failure to immunize the new crops of susceptible infants. In those instances in which outbreaks have occurred, epidemiologic studies revealed that most of the patients were unimmunized infants and children. Continued attention to immunization of all children 1 year of age or older is needed in order to attain the goal of measles eradication.

RESPIRATORY SYNCYTIAL VIRUS

Clinical Illness   Respiratory syncytial virus (RSV) was first described in 1956 and, since that time, has become recognized as the single most important respiratory tract pathogen of infants and young children. Twenty to thirty percent of acute respiratory disease of hospitalized young children is attributable to RSV. The type and severity of the illness produced by this agent vary markedly with the age of the individual infected, although other determinants are also operative.

Infection has been produced experimentally by introducing virus into the upper respiratory tract of volunteers and chimpanzees. The communicability of the disease among children is consistent with acquisition of the virus by inhalation of contaminated secretions. Thus the virus comes into contact with the mucosal surfaces of the nasopharynx, but the nature of the cells in which it multiplies is not presently defined. Viremia has not been documented with RSV infection. Infection appears to be limited to the respiratory tract; virus has been isolated only from respiratory tissues or secretions.

The incubation period preceding clinical illness is ordinarily one to four days after exposure to virus. Virus excretion from the respiratory tract may precede clinical symptoms for one to three days and continue for four to seven days after the onset of symptoms (Fig. 78-3).

Severe disease caused by RSV is most often manifest as bronchiolitis or pneumonitis and occurs predominantly in children less than six months of age. These very young children have fever and lethargy and are severely ill. Physical examination and chest x-rays reveal changes ranging from hyperaeration to consolidation. Involvement of the lungs may be sufficiently extensive to necessitate respiratory assistance and may be fatal in a small percentage of children.

Children between the ages of 1 and 3 years usually have symptomatic disease or illness limited to the upper respiratory tract, classified as tracheobronchitis and croup. Older children and adults may have colds or asymptomatic disease with only serologic or cultural evidence of infection.

Reinfection with RSV may be either symptomatic or asymptomatic. Patients less than 2 years of age are most frequently symptomatic; virus is excreted, and an antibody rise occurs. Antigenic variation of RSV does not explain reinfection of human beings, since different isolates of virus differ only slightly antigenically.

The severity and frequency of RSV infection in infants have prompted studies to guide the development of preventive procedures. Maternal IgG class antibody against RSV crosses the placenta to the fetus, persists for the first months of life, and then gradually declines. Infants infected with the virus develop serum antibodies within 10 to 14 days after the onset

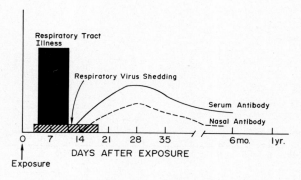

FIG. 78-3. The course of RSV infections.

of infection that persist for long periods and may show an anamnestic response upon reinfection. They do not cross-react with any other virus.

Antibodies to RSV of the IgA class appear in respiratory secretions, beginning 10 to 14 days after challenge. Their presence correlates better with protection against RSV infection than that of serum IgG class antibodies. There appears to be an inverse correlation between the titer of nasal wash antibody and the quantity of virus excreted and the antibody rise. Persons with high levels of specific IgA antibody challenged with RSV excrete little virus and may show no antibody rise in secretions or serum, whereas persons with low or absent levels of specific nasal IgA show excretion of increased amounts of virus and do develop rises in antibody.

Pathology Infants with RSV infection show severe changes in their lungs. Pulmonary tissues from children with pneumonia show marked inflammation, with mononuclear cell infiltrates in interstitial tissues, alveoli, small bronchioles, and alveolar ducts. There may be demonstrated syncytia (giant cell) formation and intracytoplasmic inclusions which are consistent with, but not pathognomonic of, RSV infection. Infants with bronchiolitis show less extensive interstitial and alveolar involvement but instead have moderate to marked changes in the bronchioles. Epithelial necrosis and plugs consisting of cell debris and fibrin are seen, as well as peribronchiolar lymphocytic infiltrates. Virus has been isolated from tissues of children with both types of illness, but preliminary information indicates that larger quantities of virus may be present in pneumonia.

Epidemiology RSV infection is worldwide in distribution and tends to cause yearly outbreaks of illness alternating from midwinter to late spring in occurrence. Attack rates of 30 to 60 percent have been estimated for exposed infants less than 1 year of age. Investigations conducted simultaneously on different populations in the same geographic setting showed that patients seen in private practice had RSV infection at an older age than did either urban or rural clinic patients. Presumably features, such as the number of siblings in the home and breast feeding, are associated with the altered epidemiologic pattern of disease in these groups.

Diagnosis Presumptive clinical diagnosis can be made in an infant with bronchiolitis or pneumonia with no demonstrable bacterial pathogens. A definite etiologic diagnosis of RSV infection can be made only by serologic tests or virus isolation. The virus can be grown in the laboratory utilizing cell cultures such as the Hep2 line.

The virus is extremely labile, and respiratory secretions, throat swab material, lung biopsy, or postmortem material must be processed immediately by a knowledgeable laboratory utilizing techniques to preserve the virus. Knowledge that the virus has been isolated may assist in management of severely ill infants, but all too frequently this information is not available until the patient has completed the natural course of illness.

Several laboratories have demonstrated RSV in throat swab material by utilizing fluorescent antibody techniques. Exfoliated cells are transferred from the swab to a glass slide, and indirect immunofluorescent methods employing rabbit anti-RSV serum and fluorescein-conjugated anti-rabbit globulin are then used to demonstrate the presence of this virus. This technique affords a rapid means for identifying RSV but is not generally available.

Serologic techniques allow the recognition of RSV antibodies by complement-fixation, neutralization, or plaque-reduction techniques. The last are the most sensitive. RSV does not possess a hemagglutination antigen as do most other myxoviruses. Acute and convalescent sera are necessary to define the significance of measured antibody. A four-fold or greater antibody rise indicates recent infection. A single value will indicate only previous experience with the virus at an undetermined time.

Therapy The therapy of RSV infection is entirely nonspecific and consists of support of the respiratory system, control of fever, adequate hydration and nutrition, and therapy of secondary bacterial infection.

Prevention The prevalence of RSV infection has resulted in attempts to develop an effective vaccine. A formalin-inactivated, alum-precipitated virus vaccine has been prepared and utilized in field trials. The vaccine produced a rise in serum antibodies in adults and children but no rise in secretory antibody. During naturally occurring outbreaks of RSV disease, the attack rate among infants immunized with inactivated vaccine was the same as that in the control (unimmunized) population. This indicated that immunization did not protect from subsequent infection. In addition, the clinical illness was more severe in vaccinees, and the age group suffering severe disease was extended to include older infants. Such unanticipated observations stopped the use of the inactivated vaccine. The reason for the exaggeration of the disease is not clear. It is of interest in this regard that the most severe illness usually occurs in individuals (infants or vaccinees) who possess serum antibodies but little or no secretory IgA. It has been postulated, therefore, that the interaction of serum IgG and virus plays a role in the pathogenesis of severe disease when no respiratory tract IgA exists to prevent infection. Alternatively, the severe disease may be a result of an anaphylactic type response to the virus that requires sensitization of the infant in the first weeks of life.

Attempts are being made to develop a live virus vaccine that will induce respiratory tract IgA formation. Temperature-sensitive RSV mutants that multiply at temperatures no higher than 33 to 35C have been isolated. It is hoped that such mutants will multiply only in the upper respiratory tract and thus reproduce the immunologic events of natural infection without causing illness.

Further Reading

MEASLES

Babbott FL Jr, Gordon JE: Modern measles. Am J Med Sci 228:334, 1954

Barkin RM: Measles mortality. Am J Dis Child 129:307, 1975

Enders JF, Katz SL, Milovanovic MJ, Holloway A: Studies on an attenuated measles virus vaccine. I. Development and preparation of the vaccine: techniques for assay of effects of vaccination. N Engl J Med 263:153, 1960

Fulton RE, Middleton PJ: Immunofluorescence in diagnosis of measles infections in children. J Pediatr 86:17, 1975

Krugman S, Ward R: Infectious Diseases of Children, 5th ed. St. Louis, Mosby, 1973

Morley DC: Measles in the developing world. Proc R Soc Med 67:112, 1974

Nader PR, Horwitz MS, Rousseau J: Atypical exanthem following exposure to natural measles: 11 cases in children previously inoculated with killed vaccine. J Pediatr 72:22, 1968

Panum PL: Observations made during the epidemic of measles on the Faroe Islands in the year 1846. New York, American Public Health Association, 1940

RESPIRATORY SYNCYTIAL VIRUS

Chanock RM, Kapikian AZ, Mills J, Kim HW, Parrott RH: Influence of immunological factors in respiratory syncytial virus disease of the lower respiratory tract. Arch Environ Health 21:347, 1970

Chanock RM, Kim HW, Vargasko AJ, et al: RSV. I. Virus recovery and other observations during 1960 outbreak of bronchiolitis, pneumonia, and minor respiratory diseases in children. JAMA 176:647, 1961

Chin J, Magoffin RL, Shearer LA, Schieble JB, Lennette EH: Field evaluation of a respiratory syncytial virus vaccine and a trivalent parainfluenza virus vaccine in a pediatric population. Am J Epidemiol 89:449, 1969

Fulginiti VA, Eller JJ, Sieber OF, et al: Respiratory virus immunization 1. A field trial of two inactivated respiratory virus vaccines; an aqueous trivalent parainfluenza virus vaccine and an alum precipitated respiratory syncytial virus vaccine. Am J. Epidemiol 89:435, 1969

Gardner PS, McQuillin J: Application of immunofluorescent antibody technique in rapid diagnosis of RSV infection. Br Med J 3:340, 1968

Gardner PS, McQuillin J, Court SDM: Speculation on pathogenesis of death from respiratory syncytial virus infection. Br Med J 1:327, 1971

Gharpure MA, Wright PF, Chanock RM: Temperature sensitive mutants of RSV. J Virol 3:414, 1969

Glezen WP, Denny FW: Epidemiology of acute lower respiratory disease in children. N Engl J Med 288:498, 1973

Glezen WP, Loda FA, Clyde WA Jr, et al: Epidemiologic patterns of acute lower respiratory disease of children in a pediatric group practice. J Pediatr 78:397, 1971

Kapikian AZ, Mitchell RH, Chanock RM, Shvedoff RA, Steward CE: An epidemiologic study of altered clinical reactivity to respiratory syncytial (RS) virus infection in children previously vaccinated with an inactivated RS virus vaccine. Am J Epidemiol 89:405, 1969

Kim HW, Arrobio JO, Brandt CD, et al: Safety and antigenicity of temperature sensitivity (TS) mutant respiratory syncytial virus (RSV) in infants and children. Pediatr 52:56, 1973

Kim HW, Canchola JG, Brandt CD, et al: Respiratory syncytial virus disease in infants despite prior administration of antigenic inactivated vaccine. Am J Epidemiol 89:422, 1969

Mills J, Van Kirk JE, Wright PF, Chanock RM: Experimental RSV infection of adults. Possible mechanism of resistance to infection and illness. J Immunol 107:123, 1971

Morris JA, Blount RE Jr, Savage RE: Recovery of cytopathogenic agent from chimpanzees with coryza. Proc Soc Exp Biol Med 92:544, 1956

Parrott RH, Vargosko AJ, Kim HW, et al: RSV II. Serologic studies over a 34 month period of children with bronchiolitis, pneumonia and minor respiratory diseases. JAMA 176:653, 1961

79
Rhabdoviruses

RABIES

History The infectious nature of rabies has been recognized since early in the nineteenth century, although it was not until the 1880s that Pasteur deduced its viral etiology and prepared the first vaccine for immunization. With recovery of the filterable agent in 1903, Negri described the now classical intracytoplasmic inclusion bodies that bear his name (Negri bodies) and remain to the present as the pathognomonic histopathologic feature of this disease. Earlier and more accurate diagnosis is now possible using a fluorescent antibody test. This has made animal inoculation practically obsolete as a laboratory test. Effective control of disease in domestic animals has been accomplished with vaccines that provide protective immunity for several years. Treatment of human cases by active and passive immunization is now feasible using hyperimmune serum and vaccines prepared in nonneural tissue.

All of these developments have contributed to the progressive decline in the incidence of rabies in the domestic animal population and a concurrent reduction in the number of recorded human cases. The problem, however, both clinically and epidemiologically, remains a serious one, since the risk of human exposure to rabid animals is omnipresent, the encephalitic illness in man is invariably fatal, and treatment remains unsatisfactory despite some recent progress.

The Disease Rabies is usually transmitted to man by the bite or scratch of a rabid animal, although bats can infect susceptible animals and, presumably, man, by aerosol transmission of the virus. The virus is not always present in the saliva of rabid animals, which accounts in part for the discrepancy between the number of bites and the incidence of the disease, even without treatment. Disease develops in about 5 to 10 percent of individuals following a peripheral superficial bite by a rabid animal and in about 40 percent of those incurring penetrating and multiple wounds about the head and neck. Other factors that contribute to these incidence figures are the amount of tissue destruction, the inoculum size, the location of the bite, and, finally, the effectiveness of the emergency cleansing and debridement of the injured area.

The incubation period is highly variable, ranging from six days to as long as a year. This seems to depend on the severity and location of the animal bite. Penetrating wounds about the face and neck are followed by an incubation period which is relatively short compared to that commonly observed following superficial injuries to the extremities. This is explained by the length of the peripheral nerve pathway along which the virus presumably spreads to enter the central nervous system and produce disease. Although the hematogenous route has been proposed as an alternative pathway for virus spread, it has not been proven in man.

The disease usually begins with vague symptoms of restlessness, irritability, and paresthesias about the wound site. This is followed in the next few days by a state of neuromuscular excitability, characterized by increased muscle tone and painful muscle contractions. As a result, pharyngeal muscles may suddenly contract when attempting to drink, or this may even occur with the mere sight or sound of liquids (hydrophobia).

The patient usually becomes acutely agitated and delirious and develops hallucinations. Convulsions may ensue at any stage of the encephalitic illness. Focal neurologic signs often referable to brainstem dysfunction frequently occur. The subsequent clinical course is usually characterized by paralysis, mental confusion, obtundation, and eventually coma. Death, often from respiratory failure, commonly occurs within one to two weeks after the onset of symptoms, although much longer survival has been recorded. Secondary infection is always a concern and may be the immediate cause of death. Although a fatal outcome has been considered inevitable in this disease, recent experience with one patient suggests that this may not always be the case (p. 1007).

Pathology The brain is the primary focus of disease, although inflammatory necrosis is sometimes seen in lacrimal glands, pancreas, and other visceral organs. Grossly, the brain is swollen and congested. The microscopic features include all those classically seen with a viral encephalitis, namely, necrosis of nerve cells and neuronophagia, perivascular cuffing with mononuclear cells, and a variable meningeal infiltration with the same cell type. Although neurons at all levels of the neuraxis may be involved, these changes are most prominent in the pyramidal cells of the hippocampus, the

Purkinje cells of the cerebellum, the nuclei of the medulla and pons, and the trigeminal ganglia. Negri bodies, intracytoplasmic acidophilic inclusions which are frequently but not invariably seen within neurons, are the most distinctive histopathologic feature of this disease. The spinal cord may also show inflammatory necrosis, accounting for the flaccid paralysis that sometimes occurs.

Epidemiology Rabies occurs in practically every species of animal, both wild and domestic. Skunks and bats appear now to be the most frequently infected animals, whereas the incidence of laboratory-confirmed rabies in dogs has fallen in recent years. In 1974 there were 1157 reported cases in skunks, 512 in bats, and only 240 in dogs.

These statistics underscore the growing concern with wildlife rabies, now that the infection in domestic animals has been effectively controlled with immunization programs. Especially is this true when one considers the problem in bats, which seem to harbor virus, often in the absence of overt disease. This presents an ongoing threat to both animals and man, since the numbers of bats are so great, their geographic distribution so unpredictable, and the possibility of aerosol spread of virus to unsuspecting hosts ever present. Despite these considerations, which continue to concern public health officials, the incidence of bat rabies has not shown any threatening increase in recent years.

Infection is transmitted to animals in the same manner that it is to man. Larger domestic animals, such as cattle, often become lethargic, weak, paralyzed, and die (dumb rabies) without ever developing the hyperactivity and neuromuscular excitability considered so classic for this disease. This poses a serious economic problem in certain areas of the world, but, quite apart from this consideration, it may present an occupational hazard to the unsuspecting individual working with these animals.

The number of proven cases of animal rabies in the United States in 1974 was 3123. However, this figure probably does not reflect the true incidence in the animal population, since there is evidence from laboratory and field studies to indicate that inapparent nonfatal infection occurs quite commonly. Studies in human beings have also shown a small but significant number of individuals with rabies-neutralizing antibodies in their sera who have had no known exposure to the virus. Reports of human disease in the United States are rare, occurring, on the average, once or twice per year. None were reported in 1974.

Diagnosis The diagnosis of rabies in an ill animal can be most rapidly and accurately made by demonstrating the antigen in the brain, using the fluorescent antibody technique. The brain can also be examined for Negri bodies by making suspension smears and staining these by the Seller's method (basic fuchsin and methylene blue). The direct isolation of virus in tissue culture can be done but is not always successful even in the presence of infection. The infection can be reliably transmitted to animals by intracerebral inoculation of infected saliva or brain suspension into suckling mice. However, since the incubation period may be as long as 21 days, during which the status of the patient's exposure remains in question, this is no longer the laboratory technique of choice. Serologic tests are available for man as well as animals, but because of the low titers of antibody usually attained and the difficulties with the assays, these are not routinely employed in diagnostic laboratories.

If the suspected animal appears well, it should be observed in quarantine for 10 days. If illness does not occur, the animal can reliably be judged not to have rabies, and all therapy can be discontinued.

Treatment and Prevention IN ANIMALS. The 1973 sixth report of the WHO Expert Committee on Rabies recommends the compulsory immunization of dogs after three months of age with MLV (nervous tissue vaccine) or 2 doses of inactivated cell culture vaccine. An annual booster is recommended if other than MLV or SMB (suckling mouse brain) types is used. Cats should be immunized at about three months of age with any of the inactivated or MLV vaccines but not with the LEP Flury strain, since it may prove pathogenic. Cattle should be immunized in areas where the disease is prevalent, notably Latin America. Other recommendations include elimination of stray dogs, quarantine requirements before international transfer of dogs or cats, and elimination by poisoning, gassing, or trapping of certain wild animal species in enzootic rabies areas.

TABLE 79-1
I. Local Treatment of Wounds Involving Possible Exposure to Rabies

A. Recommended in all exposures
 1. First-aid treatment
 Since elimination of rabies virus at the site of infection by chemical or physical means is the most effective mechanism of protection, immediate washing and flushing with soap and water, detergent, or water alone are imperative (recommended procedure in all bite wounds, including those unrelated to possible exposures to rabies). Then apply either 40 to 70% alcohol, tincture or aqueous solutions of iodine, or 0.1% quaternary ammonium compounds.*
 2. Treatment by or under direction of a physician
 (a) Treat as above (1) and then:
 (b) Apply antirabies serum by careful instillation in the depth of the wound and by infiltration around the wound
 (c) Postpone suturing of wound; if suturing is necessary, use antiserum locally as stated above
 (d) Where indicated, institute antitetanus procedures and administer antibiotics and drugs to control infections other than rabies

II. Specific Systemic Treatment

Nature of Exposure	Status of Biting Animal Irrespective of Previous Vaccination		Recommended Treatment
	At Time of Exposure	During 10 Days†	
Contact but no lesions; indirect contact; no contact	Rabid	—	None
Licks of the skin; scratches abrasions minor bites (covered areas of arms, trunk, and legs)	Suspected as rabid†	Healthy	Start vaccine. Stop treatment if animal remains healthy for 5 days†§
		Rabid	Start vaccine. Administer serum upon positive diagnosis and complete the course of vaccine
	Rabid; wild animal or animal unavailable for observation		Serum + vaccine
Licks of mucosa; major bites (multiple or on face, head, finger, or neck)	Suspect‡ or rabid domestic or wild‖ animal, or animal unavailable for observation		Serum + vaccine. Stop treatment if animal remains healthy for 5 days†§

*Where soap has been used to clean wounds, all traces of it should be removed before the application of quaternary ammonium compounds, because soap neutralizes the activity of such compounds.
†Observation period in this chart applies only to dogs and cats.
‡All unprovoked bites in endemic areas should be considered suspect unless proved negative by laboratory examination (brain FA).
§Or if its brain is found negative by FA examination.
‖In general, exposure to rodents and rabbits seldom, if ever, requires specific anti-rabies treatment.

IN MAN. Following possible exposure to rabies, immediate first-aid treatment to the wound site is essential, followed by specific systemic therapy (Table 79-1). The antirabies vaccine currently recommended is prepared in embryonic duck tissue. This preparation, which is not very immunogenic, is nevertheless associated with fewer postvaccination neurologic complications than are those produced in neural tissue. Daily subcutaneous injections should be given for a minimum of 14 days, followed by booster doses at 10, 20, and 90 days after the last daily dose. This is recommended regardless of whether hyperimmune serum is administered locally or systemically early in the treatment program.

The neuroparalytic complications following this type of immunization are rare, reportedly about 1 for every 25,000 persons treated. If encephalomyelitis develops, the vaccination program should be stopped and treatment initiated with either corticosteroids or ACTH, despite their questionable value in this type of illness.

When antirabies serum (ARS) is indicated (Table 79-1) as part of the treatment, human rabies immune globulin (HRIG) should be used. Serum sickness was a frequent complication when ARS of equine origin was used, because of the relatively large amount of foreign protein it contained. Now that HRIG is available, the risks of treatment complications have greatly diminished. It should be administered in a single dose of 20 IU/kg body weight at the same time as the first dose of vaccine is given.

The several types of vaccines and immunization programs presently available all fail to produce optimal protection or lasting immunity. For these reasons and because of postvaccination complications, the routine use of these vaccines for anyone prior to rabies exposure, other than the individual at high risk, is contraindicated at this time. Efforts to develop a tissue culture vaccine which would be safer and more immunogenic are underway, and if they are successful, mass immunization may become feasible. Progress in this direction, however, has been hampered for years because of the risks to personnel working with this virus in the laboratory.

Once the encephalitic illness begins, it is generally conceded that even with optimal care, the inevitably fatal outcome is never altered, only possibly delayed. This traditional view has recently been challenged by the complete recovery of a child who apparently had rabies encephalitis. Although this case has been contested as possibly an instance of postvaccination encephalitis mimicking rabies, its importance as a model of exemplary care remains and deserves to be emphasized. Vital functions should be continuously monitored and support provided before complications develop. Proper sedation is essential to control seizures and excessive excitation since these can lead to injury, hypoxia, or aspiration. Infection must be recognized and treated early, and gastrointestinal bleeding, which may develop in anyone with encephalitis, should be anticipated and treated promptly. If this is done effectively, those individuals who have had proper emergency attention to the wound site followed by appropriate immunization may avoid secondary complications, which quite often are the immediate causes of death. If, however, the inflammatory necrosis involves vital brainstem functions, it seems unlikely that any amount of supportive care will alter the outcome.

It may be that one of the antiviral compounds now becoming available for certain virus infections will prove effective in the treatment of rabies. Arabinosyl cytosine inhibits the replication of certain rabies virus strains in some cell culture systems, but the effectiveness of this or related compounds in the human disease is presently unknown.

THE MARBURG AGENT

History In 1967, a serious illness occurred in a group of laboratory workers, all of whom were working with either the tissues or cell cultures from African green (vervet) monkeys or were secondarily exposed to patients ill with the disease. The outbreaks occurred in Marburg and Frankfurt, Germany, and in Belgrade, Yugoslavia. Seven patients died within 8 to 17 days of the onset of symptoms; 24 patients recovered.

The Disease The incubation period varies from three to nine days. It is followed by the sudden onset of fever, headache, myalgias, epigastric pain, watery diarrhea, and uncontrollable vomiting, leading at times to severe dehydration and renal failure. A maculopapular rash typically appears on the fifth to eighth days of illness. It is seen first on the face and buttocks and subsequently progresses to involve the trunk and extremities. At about the end of the second week the rash fades and is followed by desquamation of the skin, especially on the palms and soles. A number of patients develop spontaneous bleeding from the nose, gingiva, and gastrointestinal and urinary tracts. The average duration of illness is 15 to 20 days, although occasionally relapses occur during which there is recurrence of fever and further increases in serum transaminase (SGOT,SGPT) levels. The majority of patients recover with no sequelae, although hepatic damage, testicular atrophy, and persistent changes in peripheral leukocytes have been observed.

Significant laboratory findings include markedly elevated transaminase levels, thrombocytopenia, hypoproteinemia, and leukopenia. There is frequently a relative lymphocytosis, with many atypical lymphocytes and some increase in plasma cells. The electrocardiogram may show changes suggestive of myocarditis as well as disturbances in rhythms.

Pathology Necrotic lesions are seen in most organs, although the liver and lymphatic tissues are most prominently affected. The lymphoid tissue and mucosal surfaces of the intestine are infiltrated with large atypical lymphocytes and plasma cells. Basophilic inclusion bodies have been identified in the cytoplasm of cells marginal to necrotic foci in the liver. The neuropathologic changes have included nonspecific swelling, vascular engorgement, and petechia and, in a few cases, diffuse encephalitis marked by glial nodules.

Epidemiology Since 1967, many different primate species, including numerous vervet monkeys from Africa and elsewhere, have been tested for evidence of complement-fixing or neutralizing antibodies against the Marburg agent. The survey indicated that a significant number of African primates were antibody-positive, whereas only a rare monkey from Asia had evidence of previous exposure to this virus. Human beings known to have worked with these animals in several countries were studied in a similar manner. Only 2 out of 79 African animal handlers who were tested demonstrated Marburg CF and neutralizing antibodies in their sera. No new instances of human disease have been reported in the years since 1967.

These data indicate that the virus has a restricted range of susceptible hosts, and that, although a frequent pathogen of certain African primates, it does not appear to produce overt illness in these animals. The disease in man has not recurred despite probable exposure to infected animals. It may be that the virus responsible for the 1967 outbreak was a particularly virulent strain which occurs only sporadically, but this has not been established.

The portal of entry of the virus in human cases is unknown, although two possibilities seem most likely. The virus may be inoculated directly through a defect in the skin, or it may gain entry through the gastrointestinal (GI) tract, either by aerosol dissemination or by hand-to-mouth transfer. It is known that primates can transmit infection without any physical contact. An aerosol spread, therefore, seems to occur in animals and possibly in man. The prominence of the liver and gut pathology is another factor favoring the GI tract as a route of virus entry.

Diagnosis The agent can be recovered from the blood, urine, throat washings, and seminal fluid. It grows in a number of cell systems, including primary vervet kidney cells, AH-1-GMK, BHK-21, and human amnion cells. The most common laboratory animal employed to demonstrate its infectivity has been the guinea pig, although hamsters have also been infected. The monkey is the most susceptible animal host, but its usage in laboratory diagnosis is not practical.

The agent can now be identified by neutralization with specific antiserum and visualized directly with the electron microscope. Its overall morphology resembles that of the rhabdoviruses, but the length of individual particles is highly variable, some particles being over five times as long as others (Fig. 79-1).

Treatment The most important therapeutic consideration is to minimize the incidence of human exposure to animals with clinical or serologic evidence of disease. This implies a surveillance program which properly quarantines African primates and screens their sera for antibodies against the agent before they are sacrificed and their tissues are dis-

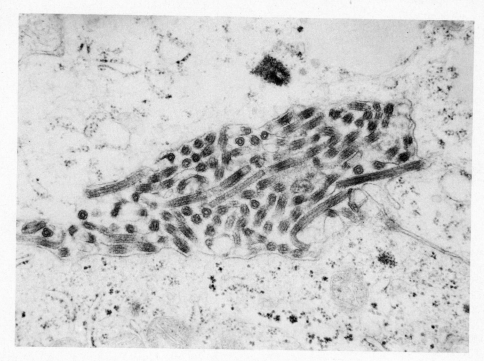

FIG. 79-1. The Marburg agent (1975 isolate from South Africa). ×75,000. (Courtesy of Dr. Erskine Palmer, Center for Disease Control, Atlanta, Ga)

persed in the laboratory. In addition, all personnel working with these animals or cell cultures derived from them should exercise the most rigid antiseptic precautions under circumstances of optimal laboratory facilities to minimize the risk of viral contamination. These same sterile precautions also apply to personnel attending a suspected or proven human case, since secondary infections do occur.

There is no specific therapy apart from the general measures designed to support blood pressure and respiration, combat hemorrhage, counteract infection, and control the complications which often attend coma and renal failure. Some of the later cases were given hyperimmune serum obtained from convalescent patients, with seemingly favorable results.

FURTHER READING

RABIES

Correa-Giron EP, Allen R, Sulkin ES, The infectivity and pathogenesis of rabies virus adminstered locally. Am J Epidemiol 91:203, 1970

Crick J, Brown F: Efficacy of rabies virus prepared from virus grown in duck embryo. Lancet 1:1106, 1970

Doege TC, Northrop RL. Evidence for inapparent rabies infection. Lancet 2:826, 1974

Rabies. Center for Disease Control. Zoonosis Surveillance US Dept of Health, Education and Welfare, 1974

WHO Expert Committee on Rabies, Sixth Report. Geneva, World Health Organization Technical Report Series, No 523. 1973

Rouche B: The incurable wound and further narratives of medical detection. New York, Berkley Publishing Co, 1964, p 33

THE MARBURG AGENT

Bowen ETW, Simpson DIH, Bright WF, Zlotnik I, Howard DMR: Vervet monkey disease: studies on some of the physical and chemical properties of the causative agent. Br J Exp Path 50:400, 1969

Gordon Smith CE, Simpson DIH, Bowen ETW, Zlotnik I: Fatal human disease contracted from green monkeys. Lancet 2:1119, 1967

Kissling RE, Murphy FA, Henderson BE: Marburg virus. Ann NY Acad Sci 174:932, 1970

Martini GA, Siegert R (eds): Marburg Virus Disease. New York, Springer Verlag, 1971

Martini GA: Marburg virus disease. Postgrad Med J 49:542, 1973

80
Hepatitis

History Classically two forms of hepatitis have been distinguished: one which may be orally or parenterally transmitted and is characterized by short incubation, the other appearing after a much longer incubation period and thought in the past to require parenteral transmission of virus. Short-incubation hepatitis has also been termed "epidemic jaundice," "catarrhal jaundice," "infectious hepatitis," "virus A," or "MS-1 hepatitis." The long-incubation disease has at various times been called "homologous serum jaundice," "serum hepatitis," "virus B," or "MS-2 hepatitis." Although the present chapter deals exclusively with these classic forms of hepatitis, it is important to remember that the clinical manifestations of liver inflammation comprise a syndrome and that nearly identical symptoms and signs may result from infections caused by *Leptospira*, treponemes, protozoa, bacteria, and a variety of viruses.

The most evident manifestation of hepatic dysfunction in hepatitis is the yellow discoloration of skin and sclerae which reflects the presence of elevated levels of circulating bilirubin and is termed "jaundice" (from the French *jaunice*) or icterus (Greek derivation). For thousands of years, observers noted that occasional clusters of jaundice were seen, suggesting the presence of a common factor—dietary, atmospheric, or a transmissible agent. During military campaigns these epidemics of jaundice were described in association with the crowding and poor sanitation prevalent in wartime. Although the more severe illnesses may have reflected the presence of yellow fever, leptospirosis, or malaria, it is certain that some of these cases were manifestations of virus hepatitis.

Sporadic cases of hepatitis were recognized early in the twentieth century, and a viral etiology had been postulated. However, attempts to transmit recognizable infection to a variety of animals were unsuccessful. Even after it became apparent that hepatitis was a transmissible disease, the existence of two epidemiologically distinct entities was not initially appreciated.

As early as 1885 an observant German doctor reported an outbreak of what was apparently long-incubation hepatitis among several hundred factory workers in Bremen. Although this physician remained uncertain about the etiology of the disease, he traced it epidemiologically to the administration two to six months previously of smallpox vaccine, which at that time was prepared with human lymph and serum. In the 1930s yellow fever vaccine virus, grown in eggs, was stabilized with pooled human serum. Subsequently, clusters of hepatitis were recognized in vaccinees, although the problem was not adequately recognized until later, when mass yellow fever immunization of military personnel was followed by thousands of cases of hepatitis.

The importance of this debilitating, transmissible disease to the military led to a major investigative effort in the United States during World War II. Hepatitis was transmitted experimentally by filtrates to man. Much of our information concerning these diseases was accumulated during volunteer studies performed upon military personnel and prisoners. These studies suggested that two distinct infectious agents existed: one (virus A) responsible for a short-incubation illness, and another (virus B) causing a disease exhibiting a long-incubation period. These early investigations defined the stability and resistance of the viruses to chemicals and temperature and, very significantly, demonstrated that many inoculated individuals exhibited chemical evidence of hepatic dysfunction although they remained in apparent good health and did not become jaundiced (anicteric hepatitis).

Clinical Course Table 80-1 summarizes many distinguishing features (clinical, virologic, and epidemiologic) of virus A and virus B hepatitis. Patients with short-incubation hepatitis remain asymptomatic after exposure for 15 to 50 days (Fig. 80-1). The onset of symptoms is abrupt, ushered in with anorexia, fever, nausea, vomiting, lassitude, and occasionally right upper quadrant abdominal pain. Smokers often lose their taste for cigarettes. Symptoms persist for several days to one week, after which jaundice, if any, becomes manifest. During the preicteric phase rashes may occur transiently. With the appearance of jaundice the fever and associated symptoms usually subside. Icterus is accompanied by the appearance of dark urine and light-colored or white stools. During the acute phase of hepatitis, functional intrahepatic obstruction of biliary flow may be as complete as with mechanical blockage of the common bile duct. With the appearance of jaundice most patients begin to recover. The feces and blood

TABLE 80-1   Long-incubation and Short-incubation Hepatitis

Property	Short Incubation	Long Incubation
Etiologic agent	Virus A	Virus B
Size of virus	Approximately 27 nm	Dane particle approximately 42 nm (HB$_s$ 20 nm) spheres and filaments
Resistance to heat	Survives 56C for 30 minutes	Survives 60C for 4 hours
Route of infection	Oral and parenteral	Parenteral, oral and sexual transmission probably also occur
Virus in blood	Late incubation and early acute illness	Incubation period and acute phase (may persist)
Virus in stools	Incubation period and acute phase	Probably present
Virus in urine	Acute phase	Uncertain, may be present
Duration of carrier state:		
blood	Probably not beyond acute illness	Protracted (indefinite) carrier state may occur
stools	Several weeks or months	Present, duration uncertain
Incubation period	15–50 days	45–160 days
Type of onset	Sudden	Insidious
Seasonal incidence	Autumn and winter	All year
Fever	Common during pre-jaundice prodome	Less common
Age group	Children and young adults	All ages
Jaundice	More common in adults	More common in adults
SGOT elevation	Transient	More prolonged
Thymol turbidity	Usually elevated	Usually normal
IGM	Usually elevated	Usually normal
HAA	Not present	Present incubation and acute phase, may persist
Gamma globulin prophylaxis	Excellent	Fair to poor

of these patients are highly infectious during late incubation and throughout the period of acute illness. During convalescence, which may be quite prolonged, patients often remain weak, anorexic, easily fatigued, and depressed (posthepatitis asthenia).

The usual course of hepatitis is benign, and recovery is generally complete. However, in some cases the disease is fulminant and fatal. The illness is liable to be more severe during pregnancy and in postmenopausal females. Persistence of symptoms or relapses over a two-

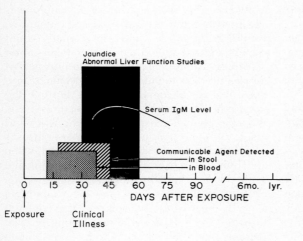

FIG. 80-1 The course of infectious hepatitis virus infection.

month period are usually designated subacute and, at an indefinite period thereafter, chronic hepatitis.

Virus B hepatitis, previously called "serum hepatitis," when it was thought to be transmitted only with blood products, is characterized by a long incubation period (45 to 160 days). The onset of clinical symptoms in virus B hepatitis is usually insidious, and patients are often afebrile (Fig. 80-2). Frequently, the initial evidence of disease is the appearance of jaundice. Although the onset is subtle, the overall course of this form of hepatitis is usually more severe than that of short-incubation disease. A significant mortality rate accompanies this infection, occasionally rising to as high as 10 to 20 percent.

Pathologic findings in virus A and virus B hepatitis are indistinguishable. Both illnesses are characterized by the development of inflammatory infiltrates in the liver parenchyma, variable degrees of distorted architecture, and bile stasis. Fatal fulminant hepatitis is accompanied by severe and widespread necrosis of parenchymal cells. The extrahepatic pathology is nonspecific, being manifest primarily as a mild lymphoid hyperplasia, accompanied, in some cases, by a moderate nephritis.

During the incubation period and prodromal phase, patients may exhibit a leukopenia with the associated presence of some atypical lymphocytes. Liver function tests (particularly serum transaminase) become abnormal during late incubation. These chemical changes may persist for a prolonged period following long-incubation hepatitis.

Epidemiology. Short-incubation hepatitis is primarily a disease of children, with maximum incidence between the ages of 5 and 14. Infection is widespread, transmitted primarily by the fecal–oral route, and apparently conveys lasting protection to the host against reinfection by the same agent. The effectiveness of pooled gamma globulin in ameliorating or preventing this infection (p. 1016) implies that most adults have had prior infection with this virus.

It is evident that since few people are aware of having had hepatitis, many infections must be anicteric and unrecognized. This supposition has been borne out by volunteer and careful epidemiologic studies in which the ratio of anicteric to icteric cases has been estimated to be as high as 10 to 1 or greater. As with many other childhood diseases, morbidity increases with the occurrence of disease in older individuals. Army studies have indicated that morbidity associated with hepatitis may be twice as high at age 40 as it is in individuals of 20. It is paradoxical that improved sanitation and the resultant postponement of contact with hepatitis may be associated with the appearance of increased overall morbidity.

Short-incubation hepatitis spreads rapidly from person-to-person. Thus, there is a high risk of infection among secondary contacts in households and within closed communities. Epidemics are frequent in homes for the retarded, army units, and childrens' homes. Common-source explosive outbreaks are usually traced to contaminated water supplies, milk, or food. Shellfish taken from sewage-contaminated estuaries may carry and transmit infec-

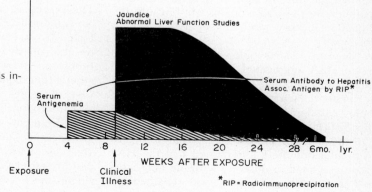

FIG. 80-2 The course of serum hepatitis infection.

tion. The incidence of short-incubation hepatitis varies inversely with population density, perhaps reflecting the existence of more crude sanitary facilities in rural communities. In general, there is a seasonal pattern to the occurrence of this disease, with a rise demonstrable in late summer, autumn, and early winter. Occasionally huge outbreaks occur. Thirty thousand cases of hepatitis were recognized in New Delhi during a six-week period in 1955 following floods which disrupted water supplies.

Characterization of the Agents of Virus A and B Hepatitis   In 1965, Blumberg and associates were seeking to define different allotypes of beta-lipoproteins in connection with genetic studies. They employed an Ouchterlony agar gel double diffusion technique and used the serum of a multiply-transfused individual (presumably carrying antibodies to a variety of circulating antigens) to screen various test serums. An antigen was recognized in the serum of an Australian Aborigine (called Australia antigen or Au) which appeared rarely in serum from North Americans (0.1 percent), though more commonly in residents of the tropics. Since the Au antigen was found frequently in association with cases of hepatitis, it was thereafter referred to as the hepatitis-associated antigen (HAA). Initial studies indicated that 41 percent of patients with transfusion-associated hepatitis possessed HAA, while 22 percent of patients with presumed infectious hepatitis were positive. Although the antigen was most consistently related to hepatitis, it was also found frequently in association with Down's syndrome, lepromatous leprosy, and certain forms of leukemia. It was uncertain whether this association related to the increased possibilities for transmission of hepatitis to these patients, to their genetic susceptibility to the infection, or to a combination of these and other factors.

Electron microscopic studies performed upon HAA aggregated by antibody revealed many spherical and filamentous particles with a mean diameter of 20 nm and some large spherical double-shelled particles, described first by Dane, with a mean diameter of 42 nm. On the basis of human inoculation studies it was then definitely ascertained that the HAA was associated exclusively with the long-incubation hepatitis (B), and it was renamed HB

antigen. The 20 nm particles probably are aggregated noninfectious surface antigen of the 42 nm Dane particles, which probably represent the complete virions of virus B hepatitis (HBV). Cores of the virus, which are present in infected liver, contain double-stranded DNA, a DNA polymerase, and core antigens termed HB_c; the surface antigens (responsible for the original immunodiffusion reactions) are designated HB_s. The presence of HB_s in clinical specimens coincides reliably with the presence of infectious HBV.

Several rapid and sensitive techniques have been developed to test for HB_s. These include complement fixation, indirect hemagglutination, high voltage crossover immunoelectrophoresis (CIE), and radioimmunoassay (RIA). HB_s RIA, which requires 24 hours, is probably more sensitive than the more rapid (2 to 4 hours) CIE technique but its use is limited to those institutions that possess the more elaborate and expensive radiation-detection equipment. About 30 to 50 percent of hepatitis carriers can be detected by these techniques.

Long-incubation hepatitis was thought for some time to be transmissible only by the parenteral route. Using the HB marker, it was demonstrated that the virus could be acquired by the oral route and that it probably exists in infectious form in feces as well as in blood. Antigen also occasionally appears in saliva, and sexual transmission has been implied by some epidemiologic observations. The dosage required for induction of infection following ingestion of virus may be 50 times as high as that necessary for parenteral transmission.

Certain individuals become permanent carriers following infection with long-incubation hepatitis, and recognition of these persons has been sought to avoid their use as blood donors. The presence of the HB antigen provides a convenient marker. The antigen is usually detected two weeks to two months prior to the onset of jaundice and persists for a mean duration of one to two months. If it remains demonstrable four months after the onset of acute disease, it seems likely to persist indefinitely. Apparently a chronic carrier state is induced more frequently. following mild cases of virus B hepatitis. Thus the persistent carrier is unlikely to be aware of his own previous illness. Mosley estimates that 5 to 10 percent of infected persons become carriers.

Anti-HB$_s$ appears and persists in most cases as the clinical symptoms resolve. Antibody to core antigen (anti-HB$_c$) is detectable soon after the onset of the icteric phase of the disease and subsides gradually after the disease resolves. In carriers anti-HB$_c$ usually persists elevated, while anti-HB$_s$ is not detectable.

With the development of sensitive detection methods for hepatitis B, persistent antigenemia was found associated with several conditions, including some cases of chronic hepatitis and some of glomerulonephritis. Persistent antigenemia occurs in a variety of individuals with depressed or altered immunologic reactivity, including some patients with chronic renal disease and others with certain malignancies. The early recognition by Blumberg of antigenemia in a proportion of individuals with Down's syndrome, certain forms of leukemia, and patients with lepromatous leprosy probably reflect the varying degrees of immunologic compromise associated with these conditions.

Hepatitis B has proven to be particularly troublesome in renal dialysis units. Dialysis patients are at high risk of acquisition of hepatitis B infection (frequently subclinical), and a persistent carrier state is frequently established. Staff workers are thus heavily exposed and are also at high risk.

Hepatitis B can be transmitted congenitally or during the perinatal period. If acute hepatitis B occurs during gestation, the virus can apparently be transmitted transplacentally. The risk of this transmission increases as gestation progresses. In contrast, maternal HBV carriers rarely transmit the virus prenatally, although a significant proportion of the babies of long-term carriers acquire hepatitis B infection during the first year of life. Many babies who acquire HBV infection in the perinatal period become chronic carriers, and it is presently presumed that perinatal infection with HBV is responsible for the existence of many (? most) asymptomatic carriers. A variable proportion of these infants manifest some degree of hepatic dysfunction. The high prevalence of HBV carriers in some parts of the world may be perpetuated by these circumstances. There is, in addition, some evidence that genetic factors are relevant to the establishment of prolonged or permanent HBV carriage.

Hepatitis B identification procedures employing immunodiffusion reveal precipitin spurs, indicating the existence of immunologically distinguishable subtypes of HB$_s$. All hepatitis B surface antigens manifest a group-specific determinant, a, as well as specific subtype determinants. The most common pairs of mutually exclusive determinants are d/y and w/r. The antigenic types HB$_{ad}$ and HB$_{ay}$ have been termed subtypes D and Y, respectively. The prominence and distribution of these subtypes has varied in different countries and social groups. The clinical significance of these variants is, as yet, uncertain.

The mortality of long-incubation hepatitis varies from 0 to 20 percent and increases with age. Approximately 6 to 8 per 1000 transfused develop this illness. Plasma, serum, fibrinogen, and thrombin may transmit the infection. Washed packed red blood cells (and frozen glycerinized blood) seem less likely to be contaminated with the virus.

Long-incubation hepatitis appears to be a sporadic disease, reflecting poor transmissibility under ordinary circumstances. This form of hepatitis is probably more frequent among adults. In contrast, short-incubation hepatitis is more often a disease of children. An attack of either disease apparently conveys permanent immunity. Since hepatitis A and B viruses are quite unrelated, no cross-immunity is conferred.

In 1973 Feinstone, Kapikian, and Purcell visualized 27 nm particles by immune electron microscopy in the stools of patients with acute virus A hepatitis. Using similar methods they were able to detect specific antibody to these particles, indicating that they were very likely the etiologic agents of virus A hepatitis. Morphologically they resemble picornaviruses or parvoviruses, and they probably contain RNA. Hepatitis A virus can be transmitted to marmosets, and complement-fixation and immune-adherence serologic tests to it have been developed.

Thus, although neither virus A nor virus B has been replicated in vitro, specific identifying tests have been developed which permit the further elucidation of hepatitis epidemiology. It appears that virus B is a DNA virus, and that virus A is a smaller RNA agent.

There remains a significant (perhaps greater than 50 percent) cluster of hepatitis cases that are for the moment best termed "non A-non B." It remains to be determined whether these cases will eventually prove to be related etiologically to additional viruses.

Diagnosis   Table 80-1 lists some distinguishing features of long-incubation and short-incubation hepatitis. Clinical differentiation of these conditions may be difficult.

In both illnesses, liver function may become abnormal during the preicteric phase. The most sensitive measures of hepatic dysfunction are provided by the levels of serum glutamic-oxaloacetic and pyruvic transaminase (SGOT and SGPT). If jaundice develops, bile appears in the urine, and the stools become acholic. There may be a leukopenia, and a few atypical lymphocytes usually appear among the peripheral circulating white blood cells.

The diagnosis of hepatitis is supported by epidemiologic data. However, it is well to remember that aside from the specific tests described for hepatitis A and B, no single feature of these diseases absolutely distinguishes them from carcinoma (primary or metastatic) affecting the liver, other infectious entities, or even obstructive jaundice due to a calculus or tumor.

Treatment   The treatment of uncomplicated hepatitis is nonspecific. In the past much attention has been paid to the control of activity and diet. It now appears quite certain that the activity of patients need not be restricted. The persistence of residual hepatic dysfunction and the development of chronic hepatitis are apparently unaffected by early ambulation. Activity should be regulated simply by the patient's state of well-being. If nausea and anorexia are prominent, intravenous fluids are indicated. Subsequently, diet may be managed without specific restrictions. However, if symptoms suggestive of hepatic coma supervene, control of diet becomes much more important. In this instance the level of blood ammonia must be controlled, and thus protein intake should be restricted and intestinal antibiosis instituted to reduce the bacterial breakdown of nitrogenous products. If the prothrombin time is prolonged, vitamin K may be administered. Exchange transfusion or hemodialysis may be employed in order to reduce the blood ammonia and other toxic products. Although of symptomatic importance, these measures probably will not alter the final outcome of the specific infection.

Steroids have been used in the management of hepatitis, but although the use of these agents may be associated with a more rapid fall in temperature, as well as of serum transaminase and bilirubin values, the ultimate time of recovery and the risk of development of chronic hepatitis are not significantly influenced. Since a variety of steroid-associated complications may occur, there does not appear to be a place for this therapy in acute hepatitis.

Prevention   It was anticipated that with the characterization of the hepatitis viruses a major effort would be made to develop a vaccine. It has been shown that inoculation of volunteers with heat-killed short-incubation hepatitis virus is followed by the development of a protective immune response.

Pooled gamma globulin protects against short-incubation hepatitis effectively when administered prior to or shortly after exposure in a dosage of 0.02 to 0.04 ml per kg of body weight. In the face of intensive and chronic exposure 0.06 ml per kg may be given. If exposure will be chronic (in an endemic area) this dose may be repeated after six months. Thereafter the development of passive-active (permanent) immunity is assumed. It is noteworthy that gamma globulin inoculation may reduce the clinical manifestations of short-incubation hepatitis without actually preventing infection. Unaware of the presence of an active process, patients who have received gamma globulin may still be infectious and are capable of spreading the virus.

The prevention of serum hepatitis is more complex. All blood to be used in clinical medicine should be screened for the presence of HB_s. Donors with a past history of hepatitis should be excluded. Blood and pooled plasma should be used sparingly. There is virtually never an indication to administer a single unit transfusion. Whenever possible washed packed red blood cells should be employed. Needles, dental equipment, and syringes should be carefully sterilized or disposable.

Large doses of pooled gamma globulin given before or simultaneously with blood transfusions probably reduce the incidence of virus B hepatitis. There is evidence that hyperimmune anti-HB_s globulin administered to exposed individuals reduces the severity or even the likelihood of HBV infection without increasing the risk of the establishment of the carrier state. The use of hyperimmune globulin in neonates born to HBV carrier mothers is presently suggested to reduce the likelihood of early infection with the associated high risk of the establishment of the carrier state.

The management of HBV carriers presents very significant medical and moral dilemmas. It has been suggested that medical personnel and food handlers (for example) be tested and, if HB_s positive, change their employment or take other drastic measures to reduce the likelihood of HBV transmission. HBV transmission has (rarely) been reported under these circumstances in association with the carrier state, and most studies to date have been reassuring in this regard. Thus, in the United States at present, there are no specific recommendations for testing other than blood donors, workers, and patients in dialysis units, other patients considered at high risk, or those under diagnostic study.

Active immunization against type B hepatitis is apparently feasible, and initial human trials of a subunit vaccine will soon be underway.

FURTHER READING

Books and Reviews

Blumberg BS, Sutnick AI, London WT, Millman I: The discovery of Australia antigen and its relation to viral hepatitis. Perspect Virol 7:223, 1971

MacCallum FO (ed): Viral hepatitis (a collection of reviews). Br Med Bull 28:103, 1972

Symposium on Viral Hepatitis, Washington, DC, National Academy of Sciences, March 17-19, 1975. Am J Med Sci (in press).

Selected Papers

Alter HJ, Chalmers TC, Freeman BM, et al: Health-care workers positive for hepatitis B surface antigen; are their contacts at risk? N Engl J Med 292:454, 1975

Feinstone SM, Kapikian AZ, Purcell RH: Hepatitis A: detection by immune electron microscopy of a viruslike antigen associated with acute illness. Science 182: 1026, 1973

Feinstone SM, Kapikian AZ, Purcell RH, Alter HJ, Holland PV: Transfusion-associated hepatitis not due to viral hepatitis type A or B. N Engl J Med 292:767, 1975

Gerety RJ, Hoofnagle JH, Markenson JA, Barker LF: Exposure to hepatitis B virus and development of the chronic HBAg carrier state in children. J Pediatr 84:661, 1974

Krugman S, Friedman H, Lattimer C: Viral hepatitis A identified by complement fixation and immune adherence. N Engl J Med 292:1141, 1975.

Krugman S, Giles JP: Viral hepatitis, type B (MS-2 strain). N Engl J Med 288:755, 1973

London WT, DiFiglia M, Sutnick AI, Blumberg BS: An epidemic of hepatitis in a chronic-hemodialysis unit. N Engl J Med 281:571, 1969

Nielsen JO, Le Bouvier GL, Copenhagen Hepatitis Acute Program: Subtypes of Australia antigen among patients and health carriers in Copenhagen. N Engl J Med 288: 1257, 1973

Stevens CE, Beasley RP, Tsui J, Lee WC: Vertical transmission of hepatitis B antigen in Taiwan. N Engl J Med 292: 771, 1975

Szmuness W, Hirsch RL, Prince AM, et al: Hepatitis B surface antigen in blood donors: further observations. J Infect Dis 131:111, 1975

Villarejos VM, Visoná KA, Gutiérrez A, Rodríguez A: Role of saliva, urine and feces in the transmission of type B hepatitis. N Engl J Med 291:1378, 1974

81
Rubella (German Measles)

History From the midnineteenth century until 1941, rubella was regarded as a benign childhood exanthem. When the Australian ophthalmologist, Sir Norman Gregg, reported the association of intrauterine rubella infection with congential cataracts, this attitude changed completely. Subsequently, congenital heart disease and other malformations were found to result from maternal rubella during the first months of pregnancy. Despite heightened interest in all aspects of this infection, it was not until 1962 that Weller in Boston and Buescher in Washington were able simultaneously to report successful laboratory techniques for the isolation, propagation, and study of rubella virus. With the adaptation and modification of these techniques by other laboratories, a number of groups were prepared to study the effects of an epidemic of rubella that swept through the United States and many other nations in 1964 and 1965. From that single major outbreak, basic data about the virologic, immunologic, and pathogenetic events were acquired. Stimulated by this new knowledge, several laboratories mounted major efforts to derive immunizing antigens which would effectively prevent rubella. By 1969, attenuated active rubella virus preparations were licensed in the United States and Western Europe. They offered the first real promise of controlling this major cause of congenital malformations.

Earlier investigators had demonstrated the viral etiology of rubella by transmission studies in monkeys and later in children, using filtered respiratory tract secretions from infected patients. The absence of any serologic tests made reliable clinical and epidemiologic studies very difficult. With the newer techniques after 1962, it became apparent that many diseases that had previously been diagnosed clinically as rubella were not. Studies of the enteroviruses and adenoviruses revealed that many mild rash diseases that were clinically indistinguishable from rubella were actually caused by members of these large virus groups. Since these are not known to be teratogenetic, the importance of laboratory differentiation became crucial.

Clinical Features Rubella is a mild rash disease which occurs principally in children but is seen at all ages. As shown in Figure 81-1, the incubation period is approximately 16 to 18 days, with minimal prodromal signs or symptoms. Most often the first awareness of illness is mild fever and respiratory signs immediately preceding the onset of rash. The exanthem is pink in color with macules and papules. They appear at first on the face and then spread to the neck, trunk, and extremities where they remain discrete and rarely coalesce. The rash is shorter-lived than that of measles and has ordinarily disappeared by the third day. Preceding and accompanying the rash there is lymphadenopathy, which may involve the postauricular, suboccipital, and cervical nodes. Rash may be observed commonly among children, but infection may be occult in as many as one-third of adult patients. Although major complications are rare (thrombocytopenic purpura and encephalitis), the incidence of arthralgia and arthritis is much greater than generally appreciat-

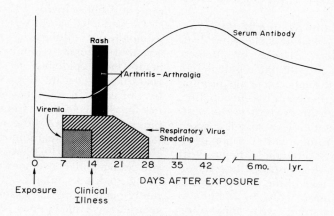

FIG. 81-1. The course of rubella virus infection.

ed. The frequency of joint involvement is directly correlated with increasing age and appears to be more common among women.

The route of infection is via the respiratory tract, with spread to lymphatic tissues and then to the blood. Both viremia and respiratory tract shedding of virus may precede the rash by one week, and the latter may follow it for another several weeks. Because the major excretion of virus occurs prior to the recognition of illness, secondary infection of intimate contacts has usually transpired before the primary patient has been diagnosed. Little is known of the actual pathology of the postnatal disease because it is not a fatal one. However, the pathogenesis of congenital infection has been well studied during and since the 1964 outbreak. Maternal viremia is followed by infection of the placenta with characteristic lesions described. Placental infection may then lead to virus invasion of the fetus. Multiple tissues and organs support the replication of virus, which continues to multiply throughout the remainder of pregnancy and in the postnatal period. A large percentage of maternal infections that occur in the first three months of pregnancy result in fetal illness. There is a diminishing number in the fourth month, and it is uncertain whether any fetal infections have resulted from maternal rubella in later pregnancy. Although the exact mechanism of the damage to fetal organs is not clear, rubella infection of human embryonic cells in vitro is associated with both chromosomal breakage and inhibition of normal mitosis. Infants with congenital rubella have a subnormal number of cells in some infected organs, which suggests that these same features may also occur in vivo.

Congenital rubella infection may result in a large variety of abnormalities, including deafness, congenital heart disease, eye defects (cataracts, glaucoma, retinitis, microphthalmia), growth retardation, thrombocytopenic purpura, osteitis, hepatitis, pneumonitis, encephalitis, and cerebral damage. In contrast to the postnatal infection, intrauterine disease is marked by a continued replication and excretion of virus, which may persist throughout the first year of life and has been demonstrated in selected tissues, such as the lens of the eye, as long as three or four years postnatally. In addition to malformations compatible with life, intrauterine rubella infection may also produce fetal death, abortion, and neonatal death. Although many of the acute neonatal manifestations resolve over the first months of life, long-term sequelae result in multiple developmental handicaps. Recent studies also indicate a significant increase in diabetes mellitus, chronic pneumonitis, and degenerative encephalitis among long-term survivors of intrauterine infection.

The immunity which follows naturally acquired postnatal rubella is similar to that observed with other common viral infections, such as measles and mumps. Only one serologic type of virus has been identified, and a single attack apparently confers lifelong immunity. The immunologic events that accompany intrauterine infection differ strikingly. The antibody response in utero is one of IgM rather than IgG. Although IgG specific for rubella is found in fetal circulation, it is mainly of maternal origin and transplacentally acquired. Despite the presence of specific IgM and IgG in the fetal circulation, chronic infection of cells continues, as already mentioned above. Postnatally, the infant infected in utero synthesizes rubella-specific IgG. A small number of congenitally infected infants have developed unusual forms of hypogammaglobulinemia in the first year of life. Another small group have lost all their detectable rubella antibody postnatally but have proven resistant to challenge with attenuated rubella viruses. The explanations for a number of these apparent immunologic paradoxes are not yet known.

Epidemiology   In most urban communities, rubella infection is acquired during early childhood, principally in the school years. Because it is not as highly communicable as measles or varicella, as many as 15 to 20 percent of women reach childbearing age without having acquired natural immunity. In the United States, large epidemics have occurred at six-year to eight-year intervals, with smaller numbers of cases in the intervening years. Usual transmission is by the respiratory route, but the prolonged viruria of the congenitally infected infant may be of great importance in spread to close contacts. In situations where adolescents and young adults have been placed in crowded living conditions, rubella outbreaks have recurrently been observed. Examples are regularly seen among Armed Forces recruits, preparatory school and college groups, and summer camps. Deliberate efforts to expose susceptibles in the hopes of their acquiring natural immunity have not been uniformly successful. The reasons for these failures include the lack of clinical reliability of the diagnosis of rubella so that many of the alleged outbreaks were due to other agents and, secondly, the apparent necessity for fairly intimate and prolonged contact to ensure transmission.

Diagnosis Until 1962, the diagnosis was entirely a clinical one and therefore sometimes unreliable. Current viral isolation techniques are reliable but not readily available. They involve the use of cell culture systems susceptible to the virus, with direct observation for cytopathic effect, or the use of an interfering agent as an indicator of viral replication. Because these are time-consuming and somewhat fastidious, serologic tests are more commonly used. The antigens of rubella virus are responsible for induction of a number of antibody types that can be assayed in serum. These include complement-fixing, virus-neutralizing, hemagglutination-inhibiting (HI), and immunofluorescent antibodies. The rapidity and reliability of the HI test have made it the most commonly employed. Paired serum specimens obtained early in the course of illness and 14 to 21 days thereafter will demonstrate a rise in the particular antibody tested. The presence in many sera of nonspecific inhibitors of hemagglutination makes the HI test susceptible to some error unless care is taken first to treat the sera with kaolin, heparin, or manganese chloride to remove inhibitors. The HI test is also valuable for screening populations to determine serosusceptibility or immunity and in the consideration of the use and efficacy of vaccines. The diagnosis of intrauterine rubella is more complicated but may be accomplished on a single serum specimen if neonatal blood is assayed for IgM antibodies specific to rubella virus. If such a technique is not available, it may be necessary to assay paired specimens obtained over a period of several months in order to determine whether there is active postnatal antibody synthesis by the infant or merely a decline of transplacentally acquired antibody.

Treatment and Prevention. There is no specific therapy for rubella virus infection. In the case of documented maternal infection during the first trimester of pregnancy, therapeutic abortion is commonly employed. Even though

rubella is confirmed virologically and/or serologically in the mother, it is not possible to be certain that fetal infection has occurred. It is estimated that maternal rubella in the first month of gestation carries a 30 to 50 percent incidence of fetal infection, in the second month of gestation a 25 percent risk, and in the third month a 10 percent incidence. After the third month there are insufficient numbers to quantitate the minimal risk of fetal involvement. Amniocentesis has been employed in a few cases to examine cells and fluid for evidence of rubella virus infection. However, there are insufficient data at present to evaluate the reliability of this method.

The use of immune serum globulin to prevent fetal rubella in an exposed pregnant woman has been the subject of long, continued controversy. With the availability of virologic and serologic testing, the lack of efficacy of ordinary gamma globulin has been repeatedly demonstrated. Studies utilizing a high-titered convalescent rubella gamma globulin preparation have led to encouraging results, but this material is investigational and not otherwise available. In most situations, it has been difficult to ascertain for how long a mother has been exposed to the virus. As depicted in Figure 81-1, it is conceivable that she may have had one week's exposure to respiratory shedding from a family member by the time she develops rash disease. With this in mind, the expectation of globulin prevention of secondary infection is not very high.

Since 1969 several attenuated active rubella virus vaccines have become available. Studies to date suggest that these vaccines confer lasting effective immunity. They have been prepared in cell cultures of duck embryo, rabbit kidney, and a human diploid line. The use of all these vaccines is followed by respiratory shedding of the vaccine virus. In contrast to the shedding which follows natural infection, this is not transmissible. A serologically detectable antibody response is produced in more than 95 percent of susceptible vaccine recipients within four to six weeks of immunization. As with acquired rubella, vaccination may be followed by joint complaints, but in a much smaller percentage of recipients than is noted after natural disease. Whether the attenuated strains of virus might also be teratogenic for the fetus or embryo is not known. Vaccine virus can cross the placenta to reach the products of conception.

The use of vaccine in pregnant women is therefore strictly contraindicated. Before administering attenuated rubella vaccine to a susceptible woman of childbearing age, it is essential to be certain that she is not pregnant and that she will follow an acceptable method of pregnancy prevention for two to three months thereafter. Reinfection with naturally acquired rubella virus has been demonstrated to occur following either naturally acquired or vaccine-induced immunity. This usually occurs in individuals whose antibody titers have fallen to low levels. The virologic events of such reinfection are markedly abbreviated, and it has not been possible to demonstrate viremia, but there is brief respiratory shedding of virus and a rapid secondary type antibody response with no overt illness. There is no evidence to date that would suggest that such a reinfection phenomenon would threaten the fetus of a woman in early pregnancy. Continued study will be required to answer fully all the questions raised by the vaccines. In seven years of utilization they have been accompanied by a striking reduction in reported cases of intrauterine rubella.

FURTHER READING

Blattner RJ, Williamson AP, Heyes FM: Role of viruses in the etiology of congenital malformations. Prog Med Virol 51:1, 1973

Cooper LA: Congenital rubella in the United States. Infections of the fetus and the newborn infant. In Krugmans, S, Gershon AA (eds): Progress in Clinical and Biological Research. New York, Alan R. Liss, 1975, vol 3

Fuccillo DA, Sever JL: Viral teratology. Bacteriol Rev 37: 19, 1973

Gregg NM: Congenital cataract following German measles in the mother. Trans Ophthalmol Soc Aust 3:35, 1942

Johnson RT: Progressive rubella encephalitis. N Engl J Med 292:1023, 1975

Krugman S, Ward R: Infectious Diseases of Children, 5th ed. St. Louis, Mosby, 1973

Modlin JF, Brandling-Bennett AD: Surveillance of the congenital rubella syndrome, 1969-1973. J Infect Dis 130:316, 1974

Modlin JF, Brandling-Bennett AD, Witte JJ, Campbell CC, Meyers JD: A review of five years' experience with rubella vaccine in the United States. Pediatrics 55:20, 1975

Ziring PR, Florman AL, Copper LA: The diagnosis of rubella. Pediatr Clin North Am 18:87, 1971

82
Slow Virus Infections

TABLE 82-1 PARALLELS BETWEEN "SLOW" AND ACUTE ("FAST") VIRAL INFECTIONS OF THE CNS

	Kuru 3–5 years	Creutzfeldt-Jakob Unknown	SSPE Months–years	Acute Viral Infections (Enteroviruses, Arboviruses, Herpesviruses, etc) 1–3 weeks
Incubation Period	3–5 years	Unknown	Months–years	1–3 weeks
Signs and symptoms	Ataxia, tremor, behavioral change	Tremor, dysarthria, behavioral change, weakness, spasticity	Behavioral change, myoclonic seizures, spasticity, coma	Behavioral change, seizures, coma
Course	6–9 months, afebrile, death	Months–years, afebrile, death	Months–years, afebrile, death	2–6 weeks average, febrile, recovery usual, death sometimes during acute illness
Laboratory	Normal blood and cerebrospinal fluid (CSF)	Normal blood and CSF	Increase in gamma globulin in CSF	Leukocytosis, CSF pleocytosis, and protein elevation
Antibody response	None demonstrable	None demonstrable	Measles antibody in serum and CSF	Specific for causative agent
Genetic susceptibility	Fore tribe (New Guinea)	Familial and sporadic cases	None	None
Diseased organ	Brain	Brain	Brain	Brain, multiple organs sometimes involved
Neuropathology	Neuronal degeneration, status spongiosus, astrocytic hypertrophy, no inflammation	Neuronal degeneration, status spongiosus, no inflammation	Neuronal degeneration, gliosis, inclusion bodies, inflammation	Necrosis, hemorrhage, edema, inflammation
Animal transmission	Chimpanzee, spider monkey	Chimpanzee	None	Often successful in suckling rodents
Agent recovery	None	None	Measles from co-cultured brain cells	By inoculating susceptible cells with brain tissue or CSF

(Clinical: Signs and symptoms, Course, Laboratory, Antibody response)

Definition

A slow virus infection refers only to the tempo of the disease as it is appreciated clinically and not to a specific type of virus or pathogenetic mechanism, although these may ultimately be proven. In clinical terms, it implies a subacute or chronic virus disease of one organ, usually the central nervous system (CNS), following a prolonged incubation period of months or years during which the patient remains well. It is this feature which best serves to differentiate this order of disease from the conventional viral encephalitides and menigitides afflicting man (Table 82-1).

Certain chronic diseases of other organ systems may eventually be explained on a similar basis, especially hepatitis (Chapter 80), infectious mononucleosis (Chap. 73), and certain renal and hematopoietic disorders. However, since most of our present knowledge of slow virus infections has resulted from the study of CNS disease, only these conditions will be discussed in this section.

History

The modern era of slow infections of the nervous system began in 1954 when Sigurdsson, a veterinarian pathologist, proposed certain criteria to define a group of chronic infectious diseases of sheep. These included: (1) a prolonged initial period of latency lasting for months or years, (2) a regular protracted course after clinical signs had appeared, ending in serious disease or death, (3) limitation of infection to a single host species, and (4) localization of anatomic lesions in a single organ or tissue system. Although these criteria were initially proposed for a group of animal diseases, it soon became apparent that certain mysterious human diseases seemed to evolve in a similar manner.

For years, rabies (Chap. 79) has been known to occur after an incubation period of weeks to months, during which the virus is thought to spread from the periphery to the CNS along nerves. In a restricted sense rabies was the first of the slow virus infections caused by a conventional agent. More recent observation, however, both in animals and man, have defined another order of slow virus diseases of the CNS

that are caused by poorly defined agents, which have indefinite incubation periods and result in progressive degeneration of the brain rather than inflammation.

KURU

The best known disorder of this type, kuru, was found in a tribe of New Guinea natives. It is characterized by cerebellar degeneration, resulting in progressive tremor and ataxia, leading inevitably to death, usually within a year. It may begin during the childhood, adolescent, or young adult years, and although the sex incidence is approximately equal for children, there is an overwhelming preference for women over men (25:1) among the adult cases. Careful study of the disease pattern indicated that it was transmitted by either inoculation of the abraded skin with infected tissue removed from relatives in the act of cannabalism or the actual ingestion of such specimens. Now that this ritual has been abolished, the disease seems to be rapidly disappearing.

The pathologic changes in the brains of patients resemble those seen in scrapie, a degenerative nervous system disorder of sheep with an incubation period of three to five years. When the scrapie agent is injected into sheep or selected other animal species, it produces a disease clinically and pathologically indistinguishable from the natural disease after an incubation period of several months. The scrapie agent, unlike viruses, is highly resistant to physicochemical inactivation, including ultraviolet irradiation. It is intimately cell-associated, and to date no virions have been visualized with the electron microscope.

These observations prompted more vigorous efforts to demonstrate an infectious etiology for kuru. This was eventually accomplished by injecting kuru brain suspensions intracerebrally into chimpanzees. After 16 months, the first of these animals developed an illness that conformed in all essential details to the human disease, and over the ensuing months, they all became ill. This observation has now been repeatedly confirmed, making kuru the first proven human chronic degenerative CNS disease with an infectious etiology. However, the causative agent is not well defined and, like scrapie, has never been seen with the electron microscope. It is very resistant to physico-chemical agents, including ultraviolet irradation.

SPONGIFORM ENCEPHALOPATHY (CREUTZFELDT-JAKOB DISEASE)

Creutzfeldt-Jakob disease is a dementing illness of midadult life that occurs sporadically in this country and elsewhere. It shares with kuru a common neuropathologic feature, namely, a vacuolar or spongiform change in the cortex. This occurs in neurons and glial cells and has become the distinguishing finding for a group of conditions with similar clinical features now collectively referred to as the "spongiform encephalopathies." These are presently being studied in the manner described for kuru.

An illness similar to the human disease, both clinically and pathologically, has now been transmitted to chimpanzees by the intracerebral inoculation of a brain suspension from a Creutzfeldt-Jakob brain. This occurred only after an incubation period of 12 to 14 months. Efforts are now underway to examine several other neurologic illnesses with progressive dementia which may share a common etiology despite minor variations in clinical presentation.

The filterable, transmissible agent recovered from the brains of these patients has not yet been defined. As in kuru, it has eluded electron microscopic detection and does not appear to be antigenic.

SUBACUTE SCLEROSING PANENCEPHALITIS (SSPE)

In the past few years, evidence has accumulated to implicate measles virus or a closely related agent in the pathogenesis of subacute sclerosing panencephalitis.

Clinical Features This condition occurs almost exclusively in children and adolescents, usually between the ages of 5 and 10 years and predominantly in males (3:1). Rarely, young infants are affected, and a few cases have been reported in the adult population. It usually presents clinically with subtle changes in personality, impaired school performance, and a gradual intellectual deterioration over several weeks or months (Table 82-2). This is characteristically followed by myoclonic seizures, focal neurologic deficits, and a gradual or sometimes precipitous diminution in conscious level. The progress of the disease may appear to be arrested for periods of years, usually when the patient is in coma, but almost invariably the patients die, often of intercurrent infection. A few older patients with well-documented disease have recovered, but this is extremely rare.

Epidemiology The true incidence of SSPE in this country is unknown, although crude estimates based on case reporting have suggested a figure of approximately 200, or about 1 per million population. The majority of patients give a history of uncomplicated natural measles at a slightly younger age than average, and all remain well during the interim of months or years until the onset of their CNS disease. Occasionally no prior history of measles is elicited, or live attenuated measles vaccine is the only known exposure to measles antigen. No immunologic defects in either cell-mediated or humoral immunity have been demonstrated in these individuals in their re-

TABLE 82-2 Subacute Sclerosing Panencephalitis (SSPE)

	Clinical
Early	Personality change; declining school performance; intellectual deterioration often manifested by impaired memory, altered judgment, and inappropriate behavior; occasionally chorioretinitis; impaired motor activity, gait difficulty, speech difficulty; myoclonic jerks progressing to repetitive, often sound-sensitive myoclonic seizures; gradual deterioration in consciousness; coma; death
	Laboratory
EEG	Paroxysmal, synchronous spike discharges with interim suppression of electrical activity
CSF	Usually acellular, sometimes modest mononuclear pleocytosis; normal total protein; increased gamma globulins (IgG); detectable measles antibody
Blood	Markedly elevated measles antibody
Brain	Specific immunofluorescence to measles antigen; SSPE virus recovered in tissue culture

sponses to either routine infections or immunizations. Their in vitro lymphocytic responses to stimulation with measles antigen are normal.

Some recent epidemiologic data have suggested that the disease may be more common in the Southeastern United States, that the primary measles infection seems to occur at a statistically younger age in such patients, and that rural rather than urban residents seem to be at greater risk.

Diagnosis The diagnosis can usually be suspected on the basis of history and the clinical findings of progressive changes in personality, myoclonus, and variable focal neurologic deficits, including impaired vision, sometimes as a result of chorioretinitis. A characteristic spike wave discharge is frequently seen on the electroencephalogram (EEG), and the cerebrospinal fluid is usually normal apart from a first zone colloidal gold sol rise and sometimes a slight lymphocyte pleocytosis. The diagnosis is confirmed by the finding of measles antibodies in the CSF. Brain biopsy is no longer necessary for diagnosis, but should tissue become available, it may show perivascular round cell infiltration, neuronal degeneration, gliosis, and type A Cowdry intranuclear inclusion bodies when stained with hematoxylin and eosin (H & E) and examined with the light microscope.

With the electron microscope, these inclusion bodies resemble microtubular filaments, corresponding in size and configuration to the nucleocapsids of measles virus (Fig. 82-1). With appropriate fluorescent antibody staining, measles antigen can be demonstrated at these sites. Finally, when brain tissue is cultivated in the laboratory, serially passaged and cocultured with either HeLa or Vero cells, complete infectious virus may be recovered. This SSPE agent is almost identical to rubeola virus but differs slightly in its behavior both in vitro and in vivo, in its affinity for the cell nucleus, and in certain of its molecular characteristics. The definition of these differences is currently the focus of intensive studies.

Treatment Numerous approaches to therapy for this condition have been attempted, but since its pathogenesis is so poorly understood, these attempts have quite predictably failed.

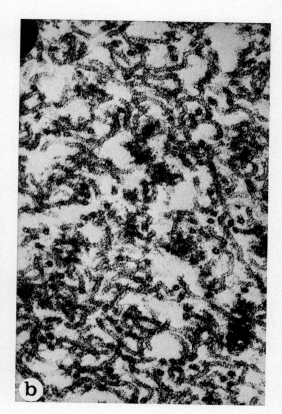

FIG. 82-1. a. Nucleus of a neuron from a patient with SSPE showing microtubular filaments. The nuclear chromatin is displaced to the periphery. ×16,000. b. Higher power view of microtubules, showing their irregular, convoluted appearance and circular contour on cross section ×50,000.

At present, one can only provide general supportive care for the patient, attempt to control seizures, and try to allay parental anxiety by early diagnosis and proper explanation.

Progressive Rubella Encephalitis A progressive rubella encephalitis has recently been described in four children as an apparent late sequel to congenital infection with this virus. The neuropathologic changes and clinical picture of spasticity, ataxia, intellectual deterioration, and seizures are remarkably similar to that seen in SSPE. It typically begins in the second decade of life in children with varying stigmata of congenital rubella, including mental retardation, cataracts, and deafness. The course is progressively downhill, with loss of motor and mental skills. Death occurred in two of the cases.

Elevated antibody titers to rubella virus were detected in the sera and CSF of patients who were tested, and rubella virus was removed from the brain tissue of one following cocultivation with CV-1 cells.

A clearer understanding of the incidence and pathogenesis of this condition must await further study of more patients with congenital rubella. It is tempting to conclude that rubella virus persists in neural tissue from the time of primary infection, rather than being acquired postnatally, but even this is uncertain.

FURTHER READING

Fuccillo DA, Kurent JE, Sever JL: Slow virus diseases. Annu Rev Microbiol 28:231, 1974

Gajdusek DC, Gibbs CJ Jr, Alpers M (eds): Slow, latent, and temperate virus infections. NINDB Monograph No. 2, PHS No. 1378. Washington, US Gov Printing Office, 1965

Gibbs CJ Jr, Gajdusek DC: Infection as the etiology of spongiform encephalopathy (Creutzfeldt-Jakob disease). Science 165:1023, 1969

Gibbs CJ Jr, Gajdusek DC: Cell-virus interactions in slow infections of the nervous system. In Schmitt FO, Worden FG (eds): Neurosciences. Boston, MIT Press, 1974, p 1025

Hamilton R, Barbosa L, Dubois M: Subacute sclerosing panencephalitis measles virus: Studies of biological markers. J Virol 12:632, 1973

Johnson RT, Gibbs CJ, Jr: Koch's postulates and slow infections of the nervous system. Arch Neurol 30:36, 1974

Payne FE, Baublis JV, Itabashi HH: Isolation of measles virus from cell cultures of brain from a patient with subacute sclerosing panencephalitis. N Engl J Med 281: 585, 1969

Peterson DA, Wolfe LG, Deinhardt F, Gajdusek DC, Gibbs CJ Jr: Transmission of kuru and Creutzfeldt-Jakob disease to marmoset monkeys. Intervirology 2:14, 1973/74

Sigurdsson B: Observations on three slow infections of sheep. Br Vet J 110:255, 307, 341, 1954

Weil ML, Itabashi HH, Cremer NE, et al: Chronic progressive panencephalitis due to rubella virus simulating subacute sclerosing panencephalitis. N Engl J Med 292: 994, 1975

Zeman W, Lennette EH: Slow Virus Diseases. Baltimore, Williams & Wilkins, 1974.

83
Progressive Multifocal Leukoencephalopathy (PML)

History
Clinical Features
Epidemiology

Progressive multifocal leukoencephalopathy (PML) is a disease of the human central nervous system which usually occurs in chronically ill, immunosuppressed patients with lymphoproliferative disorders, especially Hodgkin's disease and chronic lymphocytic leukemia. Rarely, it has occurred in otherwise normal individuals.

History The first neuropathologic description of the lesions in this condition was by Hallervorden in 1930, but it was not until 1958 that PML was recognized as a distinct clinical pathologic entity occurring in chronically ill individuals. A viral etiology was entertained but lacked proof until 1965, when the electron microscope was first used to study the lesions, and aggregates of small round particles were observed in distended ogliogodendroglial nuclei (Fig. 83-1). These resembled papovaviruses, yet all attempts to culture an agent from these brains using conventional tissue culture techniques and animal inoculation were unsuccessful. Finally, in 1971, a virus was recovered by inoculating human fetal astrocyte cultures with dispersed brain cells from a case of PML. The isolate, which was called "JC virus" after the patient from whom it was recovered, proved to be a new papovavirus, similar in size and appearance to SV40 but antigenically distinct (Chap. 67). About the same time workers recovered an SV40 virus from two separate cases of PML. This virus, called "SV40-PML," proved to be very similar to, but not identical with, SV40 (Chap. 79).

The isolation of these two papovaviruses within a short period suggested that PML might be caused by a number of different but related agents. Since that time all subsequent virus isolations have been of the JC type, with one exception (COL virus) which reacts with JC antiserum and probably is a variant of this virus. Another new human papovavirus, the BK virus, was initially recovered from the urine of an immunosuppressed patient but to date has not been implicated in either PML or any other disease.

Clinical Features Progressive multifocal leukoencephalopathy has been observed only in adults, most commonly in the fifth to seventh decades of life. The course is relentlessly progressive, usually leading to death within three to six months from the onset of symptoms. The clinical signs are variable, depending on the location and size of the lesions. The cerebral hemispheres, both gray and white matter, are most frequently involved, but any part of the neuraxis can be affected, including cerebellum, brainstem, and spinal cord. The patients usually develop visual disturbances, progressive mental deterioration, and at times focal motor weakness, cranial nerve dysfunction, ataxia, and aphasias. There is no associated fever or spinal fluid abnormality. Occasionally the course fluctuates with periods of apparent remission, but inevitably death ensues. Whether this is primarily the result of the underlying systemic disease or a sequel to the brain involvement is often difficult to determine. The disease that occurs in patients with JC virus infection differs in no appreciable way from that seen in patients from which SV40-PML was isolated.

Pathologic lesions occur in both the gray and white matter. These are classically small, discrete areas of demyelination which may become confluent. Cytologically, the outstanding features are the unusual astrocytes with bizarre chromatin patterns and the atypical oligodendroglia with enlarged, ill-defined inclusions. As a result of the altered function of these oligo-

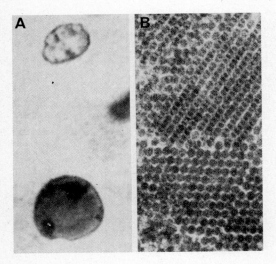

FIG. 83-1. A. Abnormal oligodendroglial nucleus (bottom) with hetrochromatic patches suggestive of inclusions. Astrocytic nucleus on top. B. Paracrystalline array of virus particles in glial nucleus. (From zuRhein: Acta Neuropathol 8:57, 1967)

dendroglia, demyelination ensues, making this the first reported instance of a virus-induced demyelinating disease in man.

Epidemiology Approximately 100 cases of PML have been reported; it is thus a very rare disorder. Infection with JC virus, however, is prevalent. One seroepidemiologic survey showed that 69 percent of adults sampled had antibody against JC virus and that this developed in most individuals before 14 years of age. Fifty percent of children in another study had antibody to the virus by the age of 3 years. It is more difficult to determine the incidence of naturally occurring infection with SV40-PML, but it seems to be of much rarer occurrence. In 80 randomly sampled sera, antibodies to SV40 were found in 1.3 percent and antibody to JC virus in 58.8 percent. Although BK virus has not been linked with human disease, it is an extremely common infection of childhood. By 10 to 11 years of age, 100 percent of children in one study had acquired antibodies to this virus, making the peak incidence of infection earlier than for JC virus.

The pathogenesis of the nervous system infection with JC virus is unknown. The leading hypotheses propose either that it is a result of the activation of virus latent in the host since early life or that it results from a recently acquired infection in an immunocompromised host not previously exposed to the virus. Nothing is known at this time of the mode of transmission of the virus to human beings, the sites of extraneural replication, or the clinical expression of primary disease. Until the PML story unfolded, the only virus of this family implicated in human disease was the common wart virus, which has no cross-reactivity with the agents recovered from the brains of patients with PML.

SV40-PML, JC, and BK viruses are antigenically distinguishable from each other and share common antigens with SV40. With the use of immune electron microscopy, the antigenic nature of the virions in suspect cases of PML can now be identified prior to virus isolation in cell culture. This is done by cross-reacting type-specific antisera prepared with PML isolates with virions extracted directly from brain. Not only has this permitted rapid identification of virus type, but it has now been shown conclusively that the SV40-PML agent was a brain isolate and did not result from recombination with latent simian agents in cell cultures, as was originally suspected.

No proven specific therapy is yet available for the treatment of PML. Cytosine arabinoside has been tried in a few patients, with encouraging results and probably warrants further study, considering the uniformly fatal course of the disease.

FURTHER READING

Astrom KE, Mancall EL, Richardson EP Jr.: Progressive multifocal leuko-encephalopathy: a hitherto unrecognized complication of chronic lymphatic leukemia and Hodgkin's disease. Brain 81:93, 1958

Dougherty RM, diStefano HS: Isolation and characterization of a papovavirus from human urine. Proc Soc Exp Biol Med 146:481, 1974

Lewandowski LJ, Leif FS, Verini MA, et al: Analysis of a viral agent isolated from multiple sclerosis brain tissue: Characterization as parainfluenzavirus type 1. J Virol 13:1036, 1974

Padgett BL, Walker DL: Prevalence of antibodies in human sera against JC virus, an isolate from a case of progressive multifocal leukoencephalopathy. J Infect Dis 127:467, 1973

Padgett BL, Walker DL, zuRhein GM, Eckroade RJ: Cultivation of papova-like virus from human brain with progressive multifocal leukoencephalopathy. Lancet 1:257, 1971

Penney JB Jr, Weiner LP, Herndon RM, Narayan O, Johnson RT: Virions from progressive multifocal leukoencephalopathy: rapid serological identification by electron microscopy. Science 178:60, 1972

Portolani M, Barbanti-Brodano G, LaPlaca M: Malignant transformation of hamster kidney cells by BK virus. J Virol 15:420, 1975

Richardson EP Jr: Our evolving understanding of progressive multifocal leukoencephalopathy. Ann NY Acad Sci 230:358, 1974

Shah KV, Daniel RW, Warszawski RM: High prevalence of antibodies to BK virus, an SV40 related papovavirus in residents of Maryland. J Infect Dis 128:784, 1973

Takemoto KK, Rabson AS, Mullarkey MF, et al: Isolation of papovavirus from brain tumor and urine of a patient with Wiskott-Aldrich syndrome. J Natl Cancer Inst 53:1205, 1974

Walker DL, Padgett BL, zuRhein GM, Albert AE: Human papovavirus (JC): Induction of brain tumors in hamsters. Science 181:674, 1973

Weiner LP, Herndon RM, Narayan O, et al: Isolation of virus related to SV40 from patient with progressive multifocal leukoencephalopathy. N Engl J Med 286:385, 1972

Weiss AF, Portmann R, Fischer H, Simon J, Zang KD: Simian virus 40-related antigens in three human meningiomas with defined chromosome loss. Proc Natl Acad Sci USA 72:609, 1975

zuRhein GM, Chou SM: Particles resembling papovaviruses in human cerebral demyelinating disease. Science 148:1477, 1965

84
Miscellaneous Viral Infections

LYMPHOCYTIC CHORIOMENINGITIS (LCM)
    VIRUS
REOVIRUSES
CORONAVIRUSES
HUMAN PAPILLOMA VIRUS

LYMPHOCYTIC CHORIOMENINGITIS

Lymphocytic choriomeningitis (LCM) has historical significance, since it was the first of the aseptic meningitides proven to have a viral etiology. When the original isolate was injected into mice or monkeys, it resulted in a lymphocytic infiltration of the meninges and choroid plexus, hence the name, lymphocytic choriomeningitis.

The human disease is usually mild, often escaping clinical detection and only exceptionally involving the central nervous system (CNS). The illness frequently begins with symptoms common to most acute viral infections, including fever, headache, malaise, generalized pain, and varying respiratory and gastrointestinal complaints. When meningitis develops, nuchal rigidity, drowsiness, severe headache, and sometimes stupor and coma usually follow within one to three days from the onset of symptoms. Occasionally encephalitis occurs, resulting in focal neurologic abnormalities. As with any inflammatory process involving the CNS, the cerebrospinal fluid (CSF) pressure may be very elevated, resulting in papilledema and signs of transtentorial herniation. The symptoms gradually subside within one to three weeks. Complete recovery is the rule, accounting for the paucity of pathologic studies of this condition.

The CSF characteristically contains a moderate lymphocytic pleocytosis (10 to 600 cells/cu mm) and an elevated protein content. A peripheral leukocytosis with atypical lymphocytes may occur, but often the blood count and differential are normal even at the height of the illness.

The incidence of this infection in humans and its pathogenesis are poorly understood. Screening studies for LCM antibody among large populations of healthy individuals and others with flulike illnesses indicate that approximately 10 percent of individuals have experienced infection with this agent. Whether chronically infected mice are important vectors for human disease has not been established with certainty but seems probable, since the virus is endemic in rodents, and LCM infections have been observed in individuals living in mouse-infested houses. Other rodents, especially hamsters, have also been implicated in the pathogenesis of human disease. Recent outbreaks of LCM in the United States and Germany have been traced to pet hamsters, and sporadic cases are well documented among laboratory personnel working with hamsters. Experimental observations and those made possible by the recent outbreak from pet hamster exposure suggest that virus is spread by the airborne or droplet route and that direct physician contact is not required. Human to human transmission is not known to occur.

The diagnosis can be suspected in any patient with a lymphocytic pleocytosis in the CSF but can only be established by the demonstration of a rise in specific antibodies in the serum or, rarely, by the isolation of the agent. The treatment is supportive only, since uneventful recovery is to be expected, providing secondary complications do not occur.

Newborn mice infected with LCM develop high titers of virus in their blood as they grow without obvious signs of illness. The reason for the persistence of virus in these animals was formerly thought to result from an inability of the immature host to produce antibody (ie, immunologic tolerance). It is now known that antibody is formed but is complexed with viral antigen which is present in excess. As a result, the antibody cannot be detected except by special techniques. Adult mice inoculated with LCM virus either become ill and die or recover with antibody production and subsequent immunity. This potentially lethal choriomeningitis can be converted by the use of cyclophosphamide into a nonfatal carrier infection, further emphasizing the role of the immune system in the pathogenesis of viral persistence.

REOVIRUSES

Reoviruses are ubiquitous viruses that have been recovered worldwide from animals as well as from man. Three serotypes are recognized that share a common complement-fixing antigen. Some strains were initially classified as ECHO virus type 10. However, as the multiple dissimilarities from picornaviruses were recognized, establishment of a new virus group was suggested in 1959, with the first two letters of the name, reoviruses, serving to emphasize an association with the respiratory and enteric tracts.

Human infection with reoviruses is common.

Reovirus has been recovered from healthy persons, as well as from persons with non-specific fever, exanthem, upper respiratory illness, pneumonia, diarrhea, steatorrhea, hepatitis, meningoencephalitis, and Burkitt lymphoma. In all cases the presence of reovirus was without certain etiologic significance. Viruses related to reoviruses have recently been shown by electron microscopy and serology to be important causes of acute nonbacterial gastroenteritis in infants and young children throughout the world, and this represents an area of currently active investigation.

Little is known about the epidemiology of these viruses. Diagnosis of infection depends upon recovery of the virus, using any of a number of tissue culture cell lines, demonstration of the virus morphologically using electron microscopy, and/or demonstration of changing antibody titers (neutralization, hemagglutination inhibition, complement fixation, immuno-fluorescence, and/or agglutination recognized by electron microscopy). Treatment of suspected reovirus illness is symptomatic. Methods for prevention of infection are unknown.

CORONAVIRUSES

A new respiratory virus was recovered in 1966 by Hamre and Procknow from the respiratory tracts of students with upper respiratory illnesses. The prototype strain, 229E, was an ether-sensitive RNA virus about 90 nm in diameter, unrelated serologically to known myxoviruses. Tyrrell and Bynoe had reported in 1965 on work with an agent, B814, found in respiratory secretions from a boy with a cold. B814 could be passed serially in human fetal tracheal epithelium organ culture, but not in tissue culture, and it produced colds in volunteers. Almeida and Tyrrell reported in 1967 that the

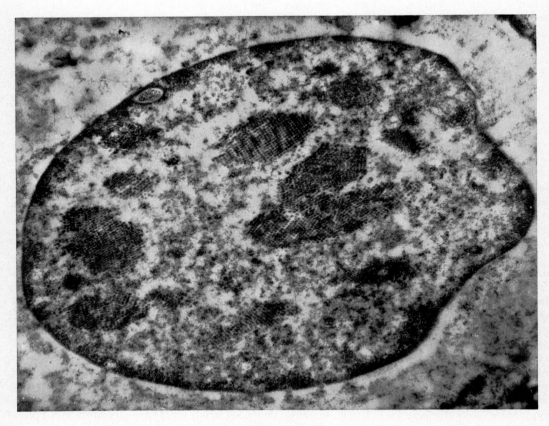

FIG. 84-1. Nucleus of   human skin cell in the upper stratum granulosum containing wart virus arranged in paracrystalline formation. ×13,000. (From Almeida, Howatson, and Williams: J Invest Dermatol 38:337, 1962)

morphology of these viruses resembled that of avian infectious bronchitis virus, and Becker et al further reported recognition of a morphologic resemblance to mouse hepatitis virus (Chap. 62).

Coronavirus infections account for 5 percent or less of common colds, but sharp outbreaks of infection have been described in winter and spring. Symptomatic reinfections and asymptomatic infections have been documented. Diagnosis can be made by demonstrating a rise in antibody titer (complement fixation, neutralization). Recovery of the virus from respiratory secretions requires the use of ciliated epithelium organ culture and tissue culture cell lines known to be sensitive to the virus group. Treatment of coronavirus illness is symptomatic. Little is known about immunity or possibilities for immunoprophylaxis.

HUMAN PAPILLOMA VIRUS (Warts, Verrucae)

The human papilloma virus is the cause of the common wart (verruca vulgaris), as well as of the plane (juvenile), filiform, plantar, and genital warts.

Warts commonly occur on exposed areas subject to abrasion, such as hands and knees, and can be spread by direct or indirect contact, as well as by autoinoculation through scratching. The incubation period varies widely, from four weeks to five to six months. Inclusions consisting of paracrystalline arrays of virus particles are commonly observed in transformed cells, especially in those in plantar warts (Fig. 84-1). Individuals carrying warts possess specific 19 S IgM antibodies directed against human papilloma virus, but the antibody response never develops further; the reason for this is not clear.

The tumors caused by the human papilloma virus are benign and generally regress after a period ranging from months to years. The reasons for regression are not clear. The only papilloma-caused human tumor that ever becomes malignant is the genital variety, condyloma acuminatum (venereal warts), which forms moist, soft, pedunculated excrescences on the external genitalia, which may turn into a form of malignant papillomatosis behaving as an erosive, destructive carcinoma. Podophyllin is said to be an effective therapeutic agent in the treatment of this condition, but it has no effect on warts of other kinds in man.

FURTHER READING

LYMPHOCYTIC CHORIOMENINGITIS (LCM) VIRUS

Armstrong C, Lillie RD: Experimental lymphocytic choriomeningitis of monkeys and mice produced by a virus encountered in studies of the 1933 St. Louis encephalitis epidemic. Public Health Rep 49:1019, 1934

Diebel R, Woodall JP, Decher WJ, Schryver GD: Lymphocytic choriomeningitis virus in man. JAMA 232:501, 1974

Gliden D, Cole GA, Monjan AA, Nathanson N: Immunopathogenesis of acute central nervous system disease produced by lymphocytic choriomeningitis virus. J Exp Med 135:860, 1972

Hotchin J, Sikora E, Kinch W, Hinman A, Woodall J: Lymphocytic choriomeningitis in a hamster colony causes infection of hospital personnel. Science 185:1173, 1974

Merritt HH: Textbook of Neurology, 3rd ed. Philadelphia, Lea & Febiger, 1963

Volkert M: Studies on immunologic tolerance to LCM virus. Perspect Virol 4:269, 1965

REOVIRUSES

Bishop RF, Davidson GP, Holmes IH, Ruck BJ: Virus particles in epithelial cells of duodenal mucosa from children with acute non-bacterial gastroenteritis. Lancet 2:1281, 1973

Bishop RF, Davidson GP, Holmes IH, Ruck BJ: Detection of a new virus by electron microscopy of fecal extracts from children with acute gastroenteritis. Lancet 1:149, 1974

Davidson GP, Bishop RF, Townley RRW, Holmes IH, Ruck BJ: Importance of a new virus in acute sporadic enteritis in children. Lancet 1:242, 1975

Flewett TH, Bryden AS, Davies H: Epidemic viral enteritis in a long-stay children's ward. Lancet 1:4, 1975

Flewett TH, Bryden AS, Davies H, et al: Relation between viruses from acute gastroenteritis of children and newborn calves. Lancet 2:61, 1974

Jackson GG, Muldoon RL: Viruses causing common respiratory infection in man. IV. Reoviruses and adenoviruses. J Infect Dis 128:811, 1973

Kapikian AZ, Cline WL, Mebus CA, et al: New complement-fixation test for the human reovirus-like agent of infantile gastroenteritis. Nebraska calf diarrhea virus used as antigen. Lancet 1:1056, 1975

Rosen L: Reovirus group. In Horsfall FL, Tamm I (eds): Viral and Rickettsial Infections of Man, 4th ed. Philadelphia, Lippincott, 1965, p 569

Stanley NF: Reoviruses Br Med Bull 23:150, 1967

CORONAVIRUSES

Bradburne AF, Tyrrell DAJ: Coronaviruses of man. Prog Med Virol 13:373, 1971

Bradburne AF, Bynoe ML, Tyrrell DAJ: Effects of a "new" human respiratory virus in volunteers. Br Med J 3:767, 1967

Cavallaro JJ, Monto AS: Community-wide outbreak of

infection with a 229E-like coronavirus in Tecumseh, Michigan, J Infect Dis 122:272, 1970

Coronaviruses. Nature 220:650, 1968

Hamre D, Procknow JJ: A new virus isolated from the human respiratory tract. Proc Soc Exp Biol Med 121:190, 1966

Hendley JO, Fishburne HG, Gwaltney MJ Jr: Coronavirus infections in working adults. Eight-year study with 229E and OC43. Am Rev Respir Dis 105:805, 1972

Jackson GG, Muldoon RL: Viruses causing common respiratory infections in man. III. Respiratory syncytial viruses and coronaviruses. J Infect Dis 128:674, 1973

Kapikian AZ, James HD Jr, Kelly SJ, et al: Isolation from man of "avian infectious bronchitis virus-like" viruses (cornonaviruses) similar to 229E virus, with some epidemiological observations. J Infect Dis 119:282, 1969

McIntosh K, Kapikian AZ, Hardison KA, Hartley JW, Chanock RM: Antigenic relationships among the coronaviruses of man and between human and animal coronaviruses. J Immunol 102:1109, 1969

Tyrrell DAJ: Hunting common cold viruses by some new methods. J Infect Dis 121:561, 1970

Wenzel RP, Hendley JO, Davies JA, Gwaltney JM Jr: Coronavirus infections in military recruits. Three-year study with coronavirus strains OC43 and 229E. Am Rev Respir Dis 109:621, 1974

HUMAN PAPILLOMA VIRUS

Almeida JD, Howatson AF, William MG: Electronmicroscopic study of human warts, sites of virus production and nature of the inclusion bodies. J Invest Dermatol 38:337, 1962

Rowson KEK, Mahy BWJ: Human papova (wart) virus. Bacteriol Rev 31:110, 1967

SECTION 6
MEDICAL MYCOLOGY

85
General Characteristics of Fungi

Mycology is the study of fungi. The term "mycology" derives from the Greek word *mykos*, meaning "mushroom." Traditionally the fungi have been considered to be members of the plant kingdom. There are approximately 100,000 species of fungi, and variation in the structure and physiologic characteristics of the different species is quite pronounced. Fortunately, less than 100 species of fungi have been implicated directly as agents of human and animal disease, and perhaps 90 percent of all fungous infections can be attributed to less than a dozen species. Nevertheless, it is necessary to know something about the characteristics of fungi in general in order to understand how they develop, how they can be recognized and diagnosed, and how some of them become pathogenic. This latter concept is especially relevant.

All fungi are eukaryotic organisms, and, as such, fungous cells possess at least one nucleus, a nuclear membrane, endoplasmic reticulum, and mitochondria. Fungous cells resemble those of higher plants and animals and are quite advanced microorganisms. As plants, however, fungi are primitive, having undefined root, stem, and leaf systems. Some fungi do exhibit cellular organization into tissue, and the more advanced groups show more than rudimentary differentiation into tissues and specialized structures. Unlike other members of the plant kingdom, fungi lack the property of photosynthesis.

The natural habitats for most fungi are water, soil, and decaying organic debris. All fungi are obligate or facultative aerobes. They are chemotrophic organisms, obtaining their nutrients from chemicals found in nature. Most fungi survive by secreting enzymes that degrade a wide variety of organic substrates into soluble nutrients, which are then passively absorbed or taken into the cell by active transport systems.

MORPHOLOGY

Fungi grow in two basic forms, as yeasts or molds. Growth in the mold form refers to the production of multicellular, filamentous colonies. These colonies consist basically of branching cylindrical tubules varying in diameter from 2 to 10 μm and termed "hyphae" (sing, hypha). Hyphal growth occurs by apical elongation, ie, extension in length from the tip of a filament. The hyphal diameter of a given species remains relatively constant during growth. The mass of intertwined hyphae that accumulate during active growth in the mold form is called a "mycelium" (pl, mycelia). Some hyphae are divided into cells by septa (sing, septum), or crosswalls, that are typically formed at regular intervals during filamentous growth. Other molds are composed of nonseptate hyphae. Since fungous septa are perforated, cytoplasmic continuity is maintained in septate as well as nonseptate mycelia.

Molds perferentially grow on the surface of natural substrates or of laboratory media. Under these conditions, hyphae which penetrate the supporting medium and absorb nutrients are called "vegetative" hyphae or mycelium. Other hyphal filaments project above the surface of the mycelium into the air, and such "aerial" mycelium usually bears the reproductive structures of the fungus. Identification of most filamentous fungi can be made by observation of their morphology. Macroscopic examination of a mold isolate should include notation of such characteristics as the rate of growth, topography (eg, glabrous, verrucose), surface texture (eg, pasty, cottony, powdery), and any pigmentation (surface, reverse, or diffusible into the medium). Microscopically, the type of reproductive spores produced (pigment, size, shape, mode of attachment) are characteristic for each species.

The other basic form of fungous growth occurs as single cells called "yeasts," which are usually spherical to ellipsoidal in shape and vary in diameter from 3 to 15 μm. Yeasts generally reproduce by budding. The budding process is initiated when the yeast cell develops a swelling at a specific point. This swollen portion enlarges and evaginates, and, following nuclear division, a daughter nucleus migrates into the newly formed bud. The bud may then continue to enlarge. The cell wall grows together at the constricted point of attachment. Eventually the bud breaks off from the parent cell, and the cycle is complete and ready to be repeated. Some yeasts retain a characteristic scar on their cell walls where a bud was once attached. Other species typically produce multiple buds before detachment occurs. If single buds are formed which fail to separate, chains of spherical yeast cells are formed. Other species of yeasts produce buds that characteristically fail to detach and become elongated; the continuation of the budding process then produces a chain of elongated yeast cells that resemble hyphae and are called "pseudohyphae."

In addition to growth as a yeast or mold, some species of fungi are dimorphic, capable of growing in more than one form under different environmental conditions. For example, some of the systemic pathogenic fungi grow as yeasts at 37C and in the mold form at 25C.

The fine structure of fungi consists of a unique cell wall, cell membrane, and cytoplasm containing an endoplasmic reticulum, nuclei, nucleoli, storage vacuoles, mitochondria, and other organelles.

Some fungi elaborate a gelatinous, largely polysaccharide capsule. The capsular material may be very slimy and produced in great quantity. Encapsulated yeasts typically produce mucoid or wet colonies. Cryptococci are yeasts that produce polysaccharide capsules of definite thickness and antigenic specificity.

The cell walls of fungi are thick, rigid structures that often appear highly refractile under the light microscope. The microscopic appearance of fungous cell walls as well as their resistance to mild alkaline digestion and special staining properties all help to differentiate and identify fungous pathogens in clinical specimens. With electron microscopy, fungous cell walls often display a fibrillar structure composed of polysaccharides and polysaccharide–protein complexes. The most commonly occurring cell wall polysaccharide is chitin, which is found in varying amounts in most of the fungi. Chitin is a β-1, 4-linked polysaccharide of N-acetylglucosamine; this particular linkage of the glycosidic bonds resembles that found in cellulose of plant and some fungous walls. Two other polysaccharides frequently occurring in fungal cell walls are glucan and mannan, polymers of glucose and mannose, respectively. These polysaccharides apparently occur in the compact cell wall as branching chains of various lengths. Cross-linkages with oligopeptides involve cystine residues and disulfide bonds. One theory of morphogenesis, advanced by Nickerson, suggests that during growth in the yeast form reduction of the disulfide bridges in the cell wall permits cell division and budding and that elongation and hyphal formation result from continuous growth without budding. With certain dimorphic species studied by Nickerson and

others, the addition of -SH groups to the medium maintains the yeast form of growth. With other species, morphogenesis appears to be controlled by other factor(s), such as the amino acids or carbon dioxide in the environment.

All fungous cell walls probably stain grampositive. However, this stain is rarely applied to fungi because it often masks other structures, and the biochemical cell wall differences detected by the gram reaction in bacteria do not pertain to fungi.

The fungous cell membrane appears to have the same bilayer structure found in many other organisms. Enzymes required for active transport are associated with the cell membrane. Fungous membranes contain lipid, primarily as sterols in their cell membranes; the most common sterol in fungous membranes is ergosterol. This sterol component is highly significant because it permits the polyene antibiotics that chemically bind sterols, to be effective antifungous chemotherapeutic agents. Bacteria, with the exception of the mycoplasmas, lack sterols and consequently are not affected by the polyene group of antibiotics (eg, amphotericin B and nystatin). Since certain mammalian cell membranes contain sterols, polyene antibiotics do have major side effects. However, human cells contain cholesterol rather than ergosterol, for which the heptane amphotericin B is more selective. Other polyenes with less specific binding properties cannot be used parentally in the treatment of fungous infections.

Fungi, both yeasts and molds, often contain several nuclei. Indeed, all hyphae can be considered to be multicellular, since cytoplasmic continuity is maintained. Hyphal filaments with septa or crosswalls have pores which permit streaming of cytoplasmic contents and migration of organelles, including nuclei, through the hyphae.

ASEXUAL REPRODUCTION

Fungi reproduce via asexual, sexual, and/or parasexual processes. Asexual reproduction can occur simply as growth and expansion of a mold or yeast colony. When a few yeast cells or fragments of hyphae are transferred to a fresh substrate, such as is routinely performed in the laboratory when fungi are transplanted

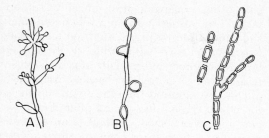

FIG. 85-1. Various types of asexual spores (thallospores). A. Blastospores and pseudohyphae. B. Chlamydospores. C. Arthrospores. (From Conant et al: Manual of Clinical Mycology, 3rd ed, 1971. Courtesy of W.B. Saunders Co)

from one culture to another, the transferred portion grows to produce a new colony. Asexual reproduction, however, usually refers to the production of spores which are generally more resistant to adverse growth conditions. The properties of spores that facilitate their dispersion are often essential for the dissemination and propagation of the fungus in nature. For example, they are usually dry and easily airborne. Some spores are equipped with rough surfaces for adherence to fomites. Asexual spores are of two general types: "thallospores", derived from cells of the thallus or body of the fungus, ie. via transformation of the yeasts or hyphal cells per se, and "conidia" (sing., conidium), asexual spores borne on specialized spore-producing structures.

Buds formed on yeast cells or pseudohyphae are often called "blastospores". Technically, blastospores are a type of thallospore, since they derive from the thallus, which is the yeast cell in this case (Fig. 85-1A). Another thallospore is the "chlamydospore", a large, round, thickwalled, unicellular structure formed by enlargement of a hyphal cell. Chlamydospores may be produced in a position lateral, intercalary, or terminal to a hypha (Fig. 85-1B). An "arthrospore" is a unicellular, asexual spore produced by condensation of the cytoplasm and thickening of the wall of a hyphal cell. Usually adjacent cells, or alternate cells, as in the case of *Coccidioides immitis*, undergo this transformation into small, dense spores to produce a chain of rectangular arthrospores from a hypha. With maturation the arthrospores become desiccant, and the hyphal strand fragments to form an easily aerosolized batch of spores, quite uniform in size (Fig. 85-1C). Arthrospores, chlamydospores, and blastospores are not specific for any single species; a given fungus may produce none, one, or more of these thallospores.

A conidium is a specialized, resistant asexual spore easily carried by air currents and capable of maintaining viability for years. Conidia that are not normally dislodged from the mycelium upon maturation are called "aleuriospores." Unicellular conidia are termed "microconidia," multicellular ones "macroconidia." A fungous

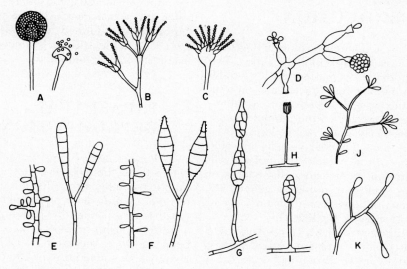

FIG. 85-2. Various types of asexual spores (conidia). A. Sporangia and sporangiospores. B. *Penicillium* type. C. *Aspergillus* type. D. *Phialophora* type. E,F. Microconidia and macroconidia. G, I. Macroconidia. H, J, K. Other types of conidia and conidiophores. (From Conant et al: Manual of Clinical Mycology, 3rd ed, 1971. Courtesy of W.B. Saunders Co)

species may characteristically produce either or both macroconidia and microconidia (Fig. 85-2). The specialized conidium-bearing hypha is called the "conidiophore," which may be a simple and undistinguished stem to which the conidium is attached. Other conidiophores are branched, complexly modified, or uniquely shaped. For example, *Aspergillus* species produce a swollen knob at the end of the conidiophore from which short "sterigmata" project, and these in turn produce spherical, unicellular, often pigmented microconidia in radiating chains (Fig. 85-2C). This type of conidial formation is "basipetal," since the conidia are extruded from the attached end of the chain. The newest and youngest conidium is the one nearest the point of attachment of the chain to the sterigmata. "Acropetal" sporulation occurs with other fungi (eg, *Cladosporium*), whereby chains of spores are produced by a budding process from the youngest spore at the distal end.

Asexual spores in many of the lower fungi are produced in a saclike structure termed a "sporangium" (pl, sporangia) (Fig. 85-2A). The sporangium develops at the tip of a "sporangiophore", and the spores formed within it are called "sporangiospores." Upon maturation, the sporangial wall ruptures to release its spores.

SEXUAL REPRODUCTION

Sexual reproduction in fungi follows the same pattern as in other biologic forms. The process is initiated by plasmogamy, whereby two compatible, haploid nuclei are brought together in the same cell. Karyogamy is the fusion of these two nuclei to form a diploid nucleus. Karyogamy may immediately follow plasmogamy, or it may be delayed, as in some higher fungi, with the development of a mycelium consisting of binucleate cells. Sooner or later meiosis occurs, resulting in genetic exchange, reduction, and then division to yield four haploid progeny nuclei. This sequence occurs in all the fungi for which a sexual cycle has been discovered, but many variations exist among the different kinds of fungi. Some fungi produce distinct sex organs and gametes. In others, the somatic nuclei perform the sexual function. In some species, nuclei within a single thallus are capable of fusion, and in others, sexual compatibility is genetically determined, and compatible thalli are required for mating. Nuclei from two compatible thalli may be brought together by specialized gametangia or by anastomosis of their hyphae and exchange of nuclei by migration from the hypha of one to the other. Hyphal fusion and migration of nuclei and cytoplasmic contents from one filament to another are a common phenomenon among the same species of fungi.

Since for many fungi the sequence of plasmogamy, karyogamy, and meiosis is not a single continuous event, it is helpful to describe the life cycle of a fungus as consisting of (1) a haplophase, during which the uninuclear or multinuclear thallus contains only haploid nuclei, (2) a dikaryophase, in which two genetically distinct haploid nuclei occupy each cell of the thallus, and (3) a diplophase, referring to the diploid nucleus formed as a result of karyogamy. Most of the lower fungi lack a distinct dikaryophase, and the haplophase is the predominant state. In the more complex higher fungi the dikaryophase assumes greater significance. For example, with mushrooms, the binucleate mycelium of the dikaryophase constitutes most of the structures and pertains most of the time. In some species both the haplophase and dikaryophase occupy significant portions of the life cycle, and asexual sporulation may serve to propagate both phases.

Following meiosis, the progeny nuclei develop into sexual spores. The basic type of sexual spore that is formed, as well as the supporting tissue, if any, that is produced, define the major taxonomic groups of fungi.

PARASEXUAL REPRODUCTION

Parasexuality refers to a sequence of events that culminates in genetic exchange via mitotic recombination. First described by Pontecorvo, parasexual reproduction has become a new laboratory tool for the genetic analysis of many imperfect fungi. It has also been shown to occur in, several species of ascomycetes and basidiomycetes (see following classification scheme).

Parasexuality is initiated by the formation of a heterokaryon, a thallus containing haploid nuclei of two different genotypes. Heterokaryons are most commonly formed by hyphal anastomosis and nuclear exchange between genetically different strains of the same species. Rarely, nuclear fusion will occur with the formation of a stable diploid heterozygote that multiplies along with the two haploid nuclei. It is during mitosis of the diploid nuclei that homologous chromosomes may pair up and permit somatic recombination to occur. The cycle is completed when the diploid undergoes haploidization to the original chromosome number, and the haploid recombinant is isolated.

The parasexual process, or mitotic recombination, provides a natural mechanism for genetic exchange among imperfect fungi. It also provides a model for genetic manipulation in other somatic systems, such as mammalian tissue cultures.

CLASSIFICATION

Mycologic taxonomy is constantly being revised. The following is an abridged and oversimplified list of taxonomic groups of special interest in medical mycology. The classification of fungi depends primarily on the type of spore formation that follows sexual reproduction.

Class Myxomycetes The myxomycetes, or slime molds, are those fungi whose vegetative form is an aseptate mass of protoplasm called a "plasmodium," containing many diploid nuclei.

Class Zygomycetes The zygomycetes and several smaller classes of fungi are commonly referred to as "phycomycetes," a term that is no longer taxonomically legitimate. These fungi include water molds, arthropod parasites, and various types of motile, flagellated fungi. In most cases the thallus of these fungi lacks crosswalls. The class Zygomycetes contains molds that reproduce sexually by the fusion of two compatible gametes to form a zygospore and asexually with the production of conidia or sporangiospores.

ORDER MUCORALES. Asexual reproduction occurs by the production of sporangia. It includes the genera *Rhizopus*, *Absidia*, *Mucor*, *Phycomyces*, *Pilobolus*, *Mortierella*.

ORDER ENTOMOPHTHORALES. Asexual reproduction occurs by conidia that are forcibly discharged, such as *Basidiobolus*, *Entomophthora*, and *Conidiobolus*.

Ascomycotina Sexual reproduction involves a saclike structure, an "ascus" (pl, asci), that contains the spores produced following karyogamy and meiosis.

ORDER EUROTIALES. Asci are produced with a cleistothecium (pl, cleistothecia), a closed structure composed of compact specialized hyphae. Many of the medically important, imperfect fungi, for which sexual phases have been discovered, have now been reclassified in this order.

Family Gymnoascaceae. This family produces spherical cleistothecia with unorganized peridial hyphae. Genera include *Arthroderma*, *Nannizzia*, *Emmonsiella*, and *Ajellomyces*, which are the perfect genera for *Trichophyton* species, *Microsporum* species, *Histoplasma*, and *Blastomyces*, respectively.

Family Eurotiaceae. With these molds the peridial hyphae around the cleistothecium is more compact and tissuelike. This group contains many of the perfect forms of *Aspergillus* species (eg, *Eurotium*, *Sartorya*, *Emericella*) and of *Penicillium* species (eg, *Talaromyces*, *Carpenteles*).

Basidiomycotina Sexual reproduction results in progeny spores supported on the surface of a special structure called a "basidium." This is a large and complex class of fungi, some members of which show a high degree of differentiation. The basidiomycetes include many plant and insect pathogens, the smuts and rusts, puffballs, bracket fungi, toadstools, and mushrooms.

Deuteromycotina (Fungi Imperfect) This group contains all the fungi for which a sexual reproductive cycle has not been discovered.

Family Cryptococcaceae. This group contains the imperfect (asexual) yeasts, some of which produce hyphae. The genera include

Cryptococcus, Candida, Torulopsis, Trichosporon, Pityrosporum, and *Rhodotorula*.

ORDER MONILIALES.   Asexual reproduction occurs by budding or by conidia which are not borne on a highly specialized tissue stroma.

Family Moniliaceae.   This family includes all the imperfect molds which produce conidia on unorganized, hyaline or brightly colored conidiophores. Most of the pathogenic fungi are placed in this group. Some of the genera are *Aspergillus, Penicillium, Trichophyton, Microsporum, Epidermophyton, Blastomyces, Histoplasma, Geotrichum, Sporothrix, Paracoccidioides*.

Family Dematiaceae.   The hyphae and/or conidia of these molds are typically darkly pigmented. Some examples: *Hormodenum, Cladosporium, Alternaria*, and *Phialofora*.

FURTHER READING

Ainsworth GC, Susman AS: The Fungi. New York, Academic Press, 1966-1974

Alexopoulos CJ: Introductory Mycology, 2nd ed. London, Wiley, 1962

Barron GL: The Genera of Hyphomycetes from Soil. Baltimore, Williams & Wilkins, 1968

Bessey EA: Morphology and Taxonomy of Fungi. New York, Hafner, 1961

Burnett JH: Fundamentals of Mycology. New York, St. Martin's Press, 1968

Nickerson WJ: Symposium on the biochemical basis of morphogenesis in fungi. IV. Molecular basis of form in yeast. Bacteriol Rev 27:305, 1963

Pontecorvo G: The parasexual cycle in fungi. Annu Rev Microbiol 10:393, 1956

86
Fungous Diseases Involving Internal Organs

FUNGOUS DISEASES

Fungi, like bacteria, are ubiquitous. Many of the saprophytic forms play indispensable roles in the cyclic transformation of organic matter, not only in the decomposition of substances, such as hemicelluloses and lignins, but also in the synthesis of complex organic compounds. Their economic importance can be illustrated by the large volumes that have been written on the industrial uses of yeasts and molds.

Fungi are frequent causes of diseases in plants, but of the thousands of known species, less than 100 are capable of invading man or animals, and less than a dozen of them produce fatal infections. It is fortunate, moreover, that only a few of the fungi, the *dermatophytes*, can spread from man to man or animal to man and initiate epidemics.

A few fungi, eg, *Candida albicans*, can be considered as endogenous because they can be carried by the normal individual apparently in the same manner as staphylococci, pneumococci, and meningococci. Males are attacked more frequently than females but never in a ratio greater than 3 to 1, in contrast to infections caused by exogenous fungi, where males are infected 7 to 20 times as frequently as females.

The habitat of exogenous fungi is the soil, and males because of their occupations are exposed to the infectious materials more intimately and frequently than are females. The exogenous group also contains many of the more pathogenic fungi. Where there are concentrated sources of infection in environments, such as *Coccidioides immitis* in certain areas of the southwest and *Histoplasma capsulatum* in the Mississippi Valley, as many as 50 to 80 percent of the adult population can be demonstrated, by positive skin tests, to have been infected at some time during their residency in the area. Where fungi, such as *H. capsulatum* and *Sporotrichum schenckii*, have been found to contaminate heavily restricted areas, epidemics of active infection have occurred.

There is a general feeling the prolonged use of broad-spectrum antibiotics, antileukemic drugs, corticosteroids, and immunodepressants predisposes to activation of latent or subclinical fungous infections. In our clinics the occurrence of systemic cryptococcosis following a kidney transplant and the therapy necessary to maintain the new organ is a frequent finding. Also, increased susceptibility to cryptococcosis and histoplasmosis occurs in malignant diseases of the reticuloendothelial system, while phycomycosis (mucormycosis) frequently has been associated with uncontrolled diabetes mellitus.

The diseases produced by pathogenic fungi resemble those caused by *Mycobacterium tuberculosis* in that they evolve slowly and develop characteristic chronic infections which persist for weeks, months, and even years. The organisms grow slowly in the tissues, produce neither endotoxins nor exotoxins, and induce slowly developing granulomatous reactions. In most mycoses a state of hypersensitivity analogous to that found in tuberculosis develops. Lesions, such as tissue necrosis and abscess formation, often are produced as direct results of this hypersensitivity. Sensitizing antibodies, measured as agglutinins, precipitins, and complement-fixing antibodies, develop as a result of mycotic infections.

The pathogenic fungi are much larger than bacteria, and it is not surprising that a fungus was the first microorganism to be proved as an etiologic agent of a disease. Schöenlein, in 1839, reported that favus was caused by a fungus that later was named *Achorion schoenleinii* by Remak in 1845. In 1839 Langenbeck demonstrated yeastlike fungi in thrush. The ringworm fungi were described by Gruby (1843) and Malmsten (1845) as *Microsporum audouinii* and *Trichophyton tonsurans*, respectively. In 1871 Harz described the fungous nature of eczema marginatum caused by the organism now known as *Epidermophyton floccosum*.

Most of the fungi that cause disease in man and animals had been isolated and identified before 1900. The slow development of medical mycology, in contrast to that of medical bacteriology, can be attributed in part to the complexity of their morphologic forms but primarily to the fact that the fungi do not produce epidemic diseases as do some of the bacteria, viruses, and rickettsiae. Since the major bacterial, spirochetal, rickettsial, and viral diseases now have been identified, the microbiologist belatedly is taking up the study of the pathogenic fungi.

Methods of Studying Fungi

The general methods of bacteriology are applicable to the study of the fungi in so far as cultural techniques are concerned. All of the fungi can be cultivated on routine bacteriologic media under aerobic conditions both at room temperature and at incubator temperature. Since most of the fungi are slow-growing, cultures must be maintained for a week and should be protected against drying during this period.

The microscopic examination of cultures differs somewhat from the usual bacteriologic methods of examination. Identification of fungi is based on the types of spores produced and the arrangement of the spores on the hyphae. Smears are quite useless when prepared in the manner in which bacterial films are spread on slides, since the cell walls are crushed and the arrangement of diagnostic structures is displaced. Preparations must be made with the least possible disorganization of the fungus or by careful dissection of parts of the culture. Cultures may be examined undisturbed by placing the culture tube on the stage of the microscope and examining the growth at the top of the slant with the low-power objective. Also, numerous types of culture preparations may be made for microscopic examinations, cell cultures, and slide cultures. Microscopic preparations may be made by placing a portion of the colony in a drop of mounting medium on a slide, carefully teasing it with needles, and covering the preparation with a coverglass. Lactophenol-cotton blue may be used for this purpose. Yeast and yeastlike colonies are best examined microscopically by emulsifying a bit of the culture in a drop of water on a slide and covering the preparation with a coverglass.

Clinical materials, such as skin, hair, and nails, should be placed on a slide with a drop of 10 percent potassium hydroxide and covered with a coverglass. Such preparations may be heated over a low flame of a Bunsen burner and immediately examined. Sputum, pus, or other exudates should be examined as fresh preparations, ie, placed on a slide, coverglass added, and examined, untreated and unstained, with reduced light under the low-power and high-power objectives of the microscope.

CRYPTOCOCCOSIS

Cryptococcosis, caused by *Cryptococcus neoformans,* usually is referred to as "European blastomycosis" in the European literature and "torulosis" in the older American and European literature. The disease, however, occurs sporadically throughout the world, and a defining geographic term, such as "European

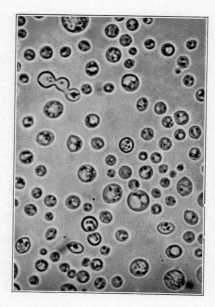

FIG. 86-1. *Cryptococcus neoformans.* Small round yeast-like cells from Sabouraud's glucose agar. ×736. (From Conant et al: Manual of Clinical Mycology, 3rd ed, 1971. Courtesy of W.B. Saunders Co)

blastomycosis," is misleading, and "torulosis" would imply a different etiologic agent.

The first case of meningitis was described by von Hansemann in Germany, but interest in the United States dates from the monograph published by Stoddard and Cutler.

MORPHOLOGY. Although hyphal strains have been described, *C. neoformans* appears in tissue and culture as a thin-walled, oval to spherical, budding cell, 5 to 15 μm in diameter (Fig. 86-1). The cells are surrounded by a wide gelatinous capsule that may equal or exceed the diameter of the cell itself. Identification is facilitated by emulsifying a portion of the colony, pus from abscesses, sputum, or the sediment from spinal fluid in a drop of India ink under a coverglass (Fig. 86-2). The presence of the large, gelatinous capsule, clearly seen in such preparations, differentiates this fungus from all other yeastlike organisms. In culture and in tissue this yeastlike organism reproduces by budding, except in those instances noted above where hyphal forms were seen in some strains. Micromorphology, as seen in ultrathin sections, has been described.

CULTURAL CHARACTERISTICS. *C. neoformans* grows readily on all the usual laboratory

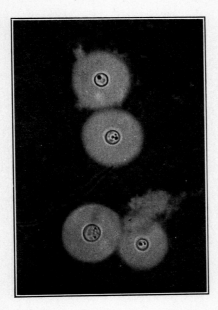

FIG. 86-2. *Cryptococcus neoformans.* India ink preparation of spinal fluid. ×736.

media at room temperature and at 37C. In primary cultures from spinal fluid, blood, or tissues the colonies usually appear in 2 to 4 days, but in some isolations the growth is delayed, and definite colonies cannot be detected until after 10 to 14 days' incubation. Cultured on Sabouraud's glucose agar at room temperature, white, mucoid, glistening colonies appear, which gradually develop a cream to light tan pigmentation (Fig. 86-3). In a liquid medium, growth is confined to the bottom of the tube except in old cultures, in which a ring may be

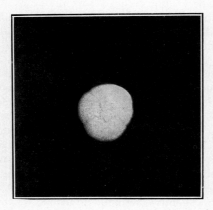

FIG. 86-3. *Cryptococcus neoformans.* Colony on Sabouraud's glucose agar at room temperature for 15 days.

formed at the surface. In a synthetic medium, *C. neoformans* synthesizes all of its growth requirement substances with the exception of thiamine.

C. neoformans does not ferment sugars, assimilate potassium nitrate (KNO_3), or reduce nitrates to nitrites. In carbon assimilation tests with various carbohydrates, however, positive tests are obtained with glucose, maltose, sucrose, and galactose, while lactose is negative. A positive urease test is obtained on Christensen's urea agar.

C. neoformans can be isolated from heavily contaminated materials (pigeon nests, and so on) on a selective medium containing creatinine as a nitrogen source, chloramphenicol and diphenyl to control contaminants, and *Guizotia abyssinica* for a marker. Colonies of *C. neoformans* will have a brownish color on this medium, while other yeastlike colonies remain white.

FUNGOUS METABOLITES. A polysaccharide has been obtained from the capsular material, and the extracellular starch is usually produced in liquid and solid media. Many investigators have been concerned with the capsular material, and the consensus lists xylose, mannose, and uronic acid and the polysaccharide to inhibit phagocytosis. A skin test antigen has been obtained from *C. neoformans*, and the presence of a positive skin test would indicate a subclinical infection in an otherwise healthy person.

ANTIGENIC STRUCTURE. Antibodies are produced as a result of infection with *C. neoformans*. The demonstration of antibody and a decreasing antigen titer in serum or CSF by various tests provides diagnostic and prognostic information about the patient's disease.

CLINICAL TYPES OF INFECTION IN MAN. *C. neoformans* may infect any part of the body but has a predilection for the brain and meninges, where it produces a disease closely simulating tuberculous meningitis, brain abscess, or brain tumor.

Cutaneous lesions appear as acneform pustules, punched-out granulomatous ulcers, subcutaneous tumors, or tumorlike masses, which have been mistaken for myxomatous tumors. Such lesions usually result from metastases to the subcutaneous tissues from an established systemic infection. Primary infections of the lungs may simulate tuberculosis or neoplasm. From this primary focus the organism disseminates to the rest of the body, invading the skin, bones, viscera, and eventually the brain and meninges.

The terminal meningitis is frequently diagnosed as tuberculous meningitis. Lymphadenopathy associated with cryptococcosis may be diagnosed correctly as coexistent lymphoblastoma or sarcoidosis. Also, coexistent myelogenous leukemia, lymphatic leukemia, and monocytic leukemia have been reported. In fact, the debilitated patient, from whatever cause, is a good candidate for cryptococcosis.

TRANSMISSION. Crytococcosis is a sporadic infection with a worldwide distribution. Although spontaneous infections in animals have been reported, there are no known instances of transmission from animal to man. Furthermore, there have been no reports of man-to-man transmission. Emmons and Ajello have isolated this fungus from the soil, and it has been isolated from pigeon habitats in Washington, DC, Maryland, Cincinnati, New York City, and Milwaukee. This natural habitat for *C. neoformans* would indicate its exogenous source, from which both man and animals become infected.

TREATMENT. Since proven cases have been known to have remissions for more than eight years, the value of any specific therapy can be judged accurately only after long periods of time. Intravenous use of amphotericin B, however, is being used with reasonable success for the treatment of cryptococcosis, and the oral use of 5-fluorocytosine shows great promise.

BLASTOMYCOSIS

Blastomycosis, caused by *Blastomyces dermatitidis*, manifests itself as a slowly evolving, chronic infection of the skin, as a subacute suppurative infection of the lungs, or as a generalized systemic infection which may involve any or all organs of the body with the exception of the intestinal tract.

The organism was seen first by Gilchrist in sections of a skin lesion which resembled tuberculosis. From a second case Gilchrist and

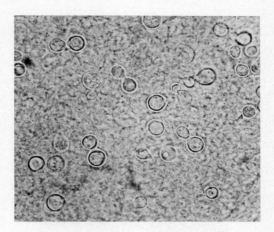

FIG. 86-4. *Blastomyces dermatitidis.* Budding yeastlike cells in pus. ×762. (From Conant et al: Manual of Clinical Mycology, 3rd ed, 1971. Courtesy of W.B. Saunders Co)

Stokes cultured the fungus and named it *Blastomyces dermatitidis*. Other isolates from blastomycosis were given a variety of different names, but comparative studies of cultures of these fungi have shown them to be identical with *B. dermatitidis*.

Ajellomyces dermatitidis, the perfect state, is obtained by pairing cultures on a suitable medium.

MORPHOLOGY. In sputum, pus, exudates, and tissues, *B. dermatitidis* appears as large, round, thick-walled cells, 5 to 15 μm in diameter, which reproduce by budding from a broad base. In sections of various tissues small forms measuring 2 to 5 μm in diameter have been described. Such small forms might be mistaken for *Histoplasma capsulatum* in tissue. However, the small forms can be distinguished by their nuclei: *B. dermatitidis* is multinucleate, whereas *H. capsulatum* has a single nucleus (Fig. 86-4).

CULTURAL CHARACTERISTICS. On blood agar or brain-heart infusion glucose agar incubated at 37C, the fungus develops soft, waxy, wrinkled colonies not unlike those of *Mycobacterium tuberculosis*. Microscopic examination reveals round, budding forms, identical in appearance to those found in tissues or in discharges from lesions. Temperature alone is responsible for the yeast growth at 37C, and when it is grown on a chemically defined medium, no accessory growth factors were found to be essential for its growth (Figs. 86-5 and 86-6).

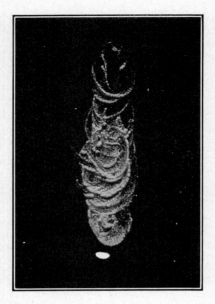

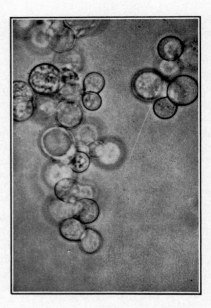

FIG. 86-5. *Blastomyces dermatitidis.* Culture on blood agar at 37C for seven days.

FIG. 86-6. *Blastomyces dermatitidis.* Budding yeastlike cells from culture on blood agar at 37C. ×700. (From Conant et al: Manual of Clinical Mycology, 3rd ed, 1971. Courtesy of W.B. Saunders Co)

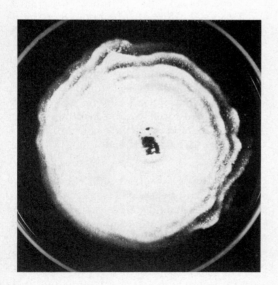

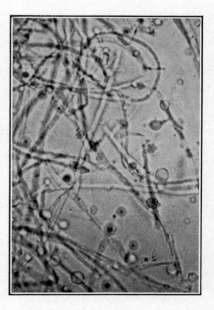

FIG. 86-7. *Blastomyces dermatitidis.* Colony on Sabouraud's glucose agar for 14 days.

FIG. 86-8. *Blastomyces dermatitidis.* Mycelium and conidia from culture on Sabouraud's glucose agar at room temperature. ×736.

On Sabouraud's glucose agar at room temperature, the fungus develops a white to light brown filamentous colony. Microscopic examination reveals branching septate hyphae with lateral, spherical to pyriform conidia, 5 to 8 μm in diameter. If this filamentous growth is transferred to fresh media and incubated at 37C, the fungus will revert to the tissue or yeast phase (Figs. 86-7 and 86-8).

A. dermatitidis, the perfect state of *B. dermatitidis,* develops if cultures are grown on yeast extract agar with ethylene oxide sterilized bone meal. Mature cleistothecia, 200 to 300 μm in diameter and tan in color, are seen in two and one-half to five weeks. Asci contain eight smooth, spherical, hyaline or very light tan, uninucleate ascospores, 1.5 to 2.0 μm in diameter. Cultures are said to be heterothallic.

Antibiotics (chloramphenicol 0.05 mg and cycloheximide 0.5 mg per ml) are used in the medium to isolate *B. dermatitidis* from contaminated clinical materials. However, cycloheximide and chloramphenicol should not be used in cultures to be incubated at 37C, since these two antibiotics are inhibitory for the yeast phase at this temperature.

FUNGOUS METABOLITES. Neither endotoxins nor exotoxins have been demonstrated. A hemolysin against guinea pig erythrocyte occurs in the supernate of disintegrated yeast cells. It is destroyed by autoclaving at 15 pounds pressure for 15 minutes but not at 60C for 30 minutes.

Lipids have been extracted from *B. dermatitidis,* and the soaps of their fatty acids have been shown to inhibit tissue enzymes. Carbohydrates and proteins also have been isolated.

ANTIGENIC STRUCTURE. The yeast phase may be used as an antigen in the complement-fixation test with animal sera and with human sera. Blastomycin, a filtrate of a filamentous culture, also has been used as an antigen in the complement-fixation test and as an antigen for collodion particle sensitization for an agglutination test. Soluble antigens from whole yeast cells and sonic-treated cells have been used in the complement-fixation test with animal and human sera. A carbohydrate obtained from the supernatant fluid of yeast cell suspensions was shown to sensitize sheep cells, which could then be used in a hemagglutination test with patients' sera. Precipitins in the serum of patients with blastomycosis have been reported. A summary of serologic methods is given by Kaufman.

Heat-killed (60C for one hour) saline suspensions of a 1:1,000 dilution of the yeast phase and blastomycin elicit a positive skin test in 24 to 48 hours if animals or human beings have been sensitized to the fungus or its products. Unfortunately, however, only about 50 percent of those infected give positive skin tests to the above materials. These materials also will react on *Histoplasma*-infected animals or human beings. Positive skin tests have been elicited in patients by the carbohydrate and protein fractions obtained from *B. dermatitidis.* Dyson and Evans have reported a specific skin test antigen obtained from yeast culture supernates by alcohol precipitation. A soluble extract from sonic-treated cells, a cell-free extract from ground cells, and various carbohydrate fractions have been obtained from *B. dermatitidis* for dermal sensitivity studies and for serologic investigations. Kaufman and Kaplan reported fluorescent antibody techniques to distinguish common and distinct antigens of *B. dermatitidis* and *H. capsulatum.*

EXPERIMENTAL INFECTION IN LABORATORY ANIMALS. Rabbits, guinea pigs, and mice can be infected experimentally, but mice are the most susceptible and, after an intraperitoneal injection of 1 ml of a 1:200 suspension of the yeast phase, usually develop extensive infection within three weeks. Intravenous injection of the yeast phase into mice produces a rapidly fatal infection. This animal, therefore, has been used extensively to test drugs for in vivo activity against *B. dermatitidis* and for possible use as chemotherapeutic agents for blastomycosis. Guinea pigs inoculated intrathoracically develop systemic infections with early serologic findings which correlate with the extent of infection. Experimentally infected guinea pigs held at 35 to 37C have minimum infection, whereas those held at 10 to 20C demonstrate maximum infection.

CLINICAL TYPES OF INFECTION IN MAN. It is convenient to classify blastomycosis into three clinical forms: cutaneous, pulmonary, and systemic. In primary cutaneous blastomycosis, the lesions usually occur on the exposed parts of the body. The lesion, following trauma and introduction of the organism, begins as a papule or papulopustule which slowly increases in size. The regional lymphatics become involved, with resulting lymphadenopathy which is characteristic of primary cutaneous infection. On further extension the lesion becomes raised above the surrounding skin, and irregular, smooth, glistening, reddish or dark-colored, wartlike papilliform elevations appear. The lesion is defined sharply from the surrounding skin by an abrupt, elevated, dark red or purple, verrucous border which contains minute dermal abscesses. The diagnosis can be made by microscopic examination and culture of the small amount of pus expressed from these abscesses.

Multiple subcutaneous abscesses may occur anywhere on the body and may rupture to evolve into cutaneous lesions as described. The lack of lymphadenopathy distinguishes these lesions from the primary cutaneous type. They are the result of metastases to the subcutaneous tissues from an established systemic infection.

Pulmonary blastomycosis usually begins as isolated pneumonic lesions in any part of the lung, as a result of inhalation of the organism. The lesions most often are diagnosed incorrectly as either tuberculosis or neoplasm. Many patients have been sent to sanatoriums for tuberculosis, and we know of several patients who underwent pneumonectomy because of the incorrect diagnosis of neoplasm. Occasionally the organisms invade the chest wall and produce multiple-draining sinuses. The sputum may or may not contain blood but usually contains numerous yeastlike budding *Blastomyces*. Two instances of a self-limited, untreated, pulmonary infection have been reported. No calcium is found in healed pulmonary blastomycosis.

Systemic blastomycosis results from a dissemination of the fungus from a pulmonary lesion. In some cases, however, no focus can be detected either in the lungs or on the skin, and the patient presents himself with involvement of the subcutaneous tissues, vertebrae, ribs, brain, or other internal organs.

TRANSMISSION.   North American blastomycosis occurs within the borders of the United States and Canada. The rare patient with this disease reported elsewhere — for example in Mexico or in Europe — invariably has a history of previous residence in the United States. However, several autochthonous cases have been reported from Africa within the past few years. The chronicity of blastomycosis allows for several years to intervene between infection and demonstrable signs and symptoms of active disease. Several epidemiologic studies of blastomycosis have been reported. Spontaneous infections have been reported in dogs, but there are no proven cases of animal-to-man transmission.

Since *B. dermatitidis* has been isolated from the soil, both the dog and man become infected from this source. The infection does not spread from man to man, although a few cases have occurred as a result of wound at the necropsy table, and a case of conjugal blastomycosis has been reported.

TREATMENT.   In localized cutaneous blastomycosis, dihydroxystilbamidine has been used successfully in many patients. Relapses have occurred, however, following therapy, probably as a result of the poor immunologic status of the patient. Amphotericin B is a very effective antibiotic in the treatment of systemic blastomycosis and is considered to be the drug of choice.

LOBOMYCOSIS

Lobomycosis, caused by *Loboa loboi*, is a chronic disease of the skin and subcutaneous tissues of the body, causing fibrous tumors or keloids. Most of the cases have been described in natives from the Amazon valley of Brazil, but the disease is also found in Venezuela, Colombia, and French Guiana in South America and from cases in Costa Rica, Honduras, and Panama in Central America. With one exception, the disease occurs in adult males, all of whom have been agricultural workers. The description of the disease in a dolphin is the sole reference to its occurrence in an animal.

MORPHOLOGY.   *Loboa loboi* occurs in the keloidean tissues in great masses as large, thick-walled cells, 10 to 60 μm in diameter, appearing singularly or in chains held together by narrow tubes (Fig. 86-9). In spite of the abundance of the organism, it has never been

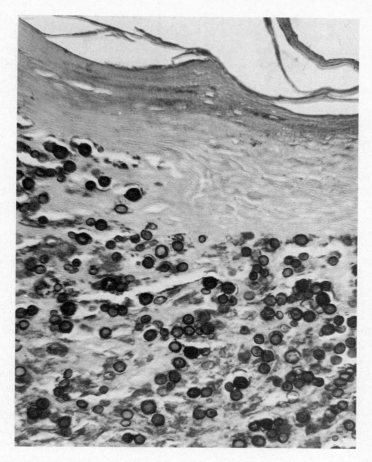

FIG. 86-9. Lobomycosis. Section of skin. Numerous organisms are seen just below the skin surface. Grocott-Gomori methenamine silver stain. ×400. (From Villegas: Mycopathal Mycol Appl 25:376, 1965)

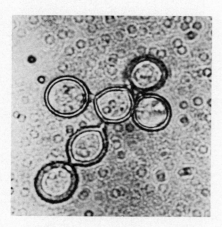

FIG. 86-10. Lobomycosis. KOH preparation of macerated skin showing the large, thick-walled, catenulate organisms. ×1,500. (From Villegas: Mycopathal Mycol Appl 25:376, 1965)

cultured nor have experimental animals been infected.

Diagnosis is made by curettage or biopsy of the lesion. Simple KOH preparations of the macerated material will reveal the typical organism (Fig. 86-10). Histologic sections of the nodules show the multitude of cells characteristic of this disease.

CULTURAL CHARACTERISTICS AND ANTIGENIC STRUCTURE. Many attempts to culture the organisms have failed. The few cultures reported appeared to be identical with *Paracoccidioides brasiliensis*, which is quite a different organism.

The failure to cultivate the agent has hindered any attempt to obtain materials for immunologic studies. The patient has no systemic reaction to this skin disease, so no detectable antibodies have been described.

TREATMENT.   The only effective treatment is surgery of very young or limited lesions. No drug therapy has been found to be successful.

HISTOPLASMOSIS

Histoplasmosis, caused by *Histoplasma capsulatum*, is an infection primarily of the reticuloendothelial system. It occurs chiefly as a primary, benign, subclinical infection. Occasionally, however, dissemination may take place, resulting in enlargement of the liver, spleen, and lymph nodes.

The organism was seen first by Darling in sections of livers and spleens removed from natives of the Canal Zone who had died of a disease resembling visceral leishmaniasis. He named the organism *Histoplasma capsulatum* and thought it was a protozoan closely related to *Leishmania donovani*. Final proof of the mycotic nature of the infection was furnished by Hansmann and Schenken and De Monbreun, who were the first to culture *H. capsulatum*.

MORPHOLOGY.   *H. capsulatum* is a small (2 to 4 μm), budding, oval, yeastlike organism which, in the body, appears to grow exclusively in the cytoplasm of endothelial and mononuclear cells. The organisms are about the size and shape of *L. donovani* but lack the central nuclear material and blepharoplast seen in stained preparations of this protozoan. They can be demonstrated in tissue sections by the gram stain or, more clearly, by Giemsa's stain and the methenamine silver stain. Smears of peripheral blood, bone marrow, sputum, and exudates should be made on coverglasses and stained by the Giemsa method (Fig. 86-11).

CULTURAL CHARACTERISTICS.   The tissue stage of *H. capsulatum* can be grown on blood agar slants at 37C if the tubes are sealed after inoculation (Fig. 86-12). The colonies, which are yeastlike, smooth, and white to cream in color, closely resemble the colonies of *Staphylococcus aureus*. Microscopically the growth is composed of small, oval, single budding cells, 2 by 5 μm in size (Fig. 86-13).

A filamentous growth occurs on Sabouraud's glucose agar at room temperature. The growth at first is cottony and white but gradually becomes buff to brown with age (Fig. 86-14). In young cultures the branching, septate hyphae

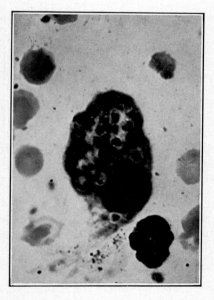

FIG. 86-11. *Histoplasma capsulatum.* Parasitized mononuclear cell in peripheral blood smear. ×1,540.

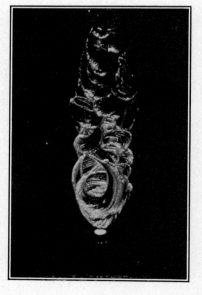

FIG. 86-12. *Histoplasma capsulatum.* Yeastlike growth on blood agar at 37C for five days.

bear small, 2.5 to 5 μm, smooth, round to pyriform microconidia on short lateral branches. In older cultures there are numerous round to pyriform, thick-walled macroconidia (8 to 20 μm), which are covered with fingerlike projections. These tuberculate spores are characteristic and diagnostic for *H. capsulatum* (Fig. 86-15).

By pairing cultures, the perfect stage of *H. capsulatum* has been obtained. This sexual stage has been named *Emmonsiella capsulata* and is classified among the Gymnoascaceae.

FUNGOUS METABOLITES. The filtrates of broth cultures of the mycelial phase of *H. capsulatum* contain substances which may be used to detect hypersensitivity to the organism. This material, known as "histoplasmin," is prepared by growing the filamentous culture for two to four months in a synthetic medium. A polysaccharide and a protein have been obtained from the mycelial phase and from histoplasmin. The serology may become positive in response to a skin test with histoplasmin in a previously histoplasmin-positive individual. However, if blood is drawn no later than two days after the skin test, the serology by a variety of tests will be negative. A single positive skin test or repeated tests in a skin test-negative individual have no effect on antibody titer. Edwards and Palmer have reported on the geographic variation and prevalence of histoplasmin sensitivity and *Histoplasma* infection in the United States, while Edwards and Klaer have reported the incidence of infection and histoplasmin sensitivity throughout the world. A polysaccharide extract of culture filtrates of *H. capsulatum* has

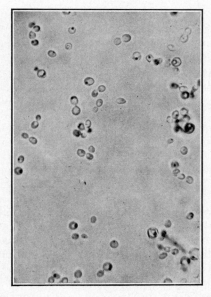

FIG. 86-13. *Histoplasma capsulatum.* Yeastlike cells from blood agar culture at 37C. ×700.

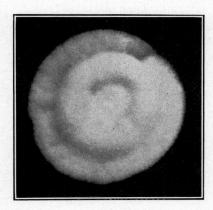

FIG. 86-14. *Histoplasma capsulatum.* Colony on Sabouraud's glucose agar at room temperature for 22 days. (From Conant et al: Manual of Clinical Mycology, 3rd ed, 1971. Courtesy of W.B. Saunders Co)

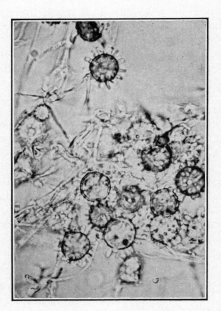

FIG. 86-15. *Histoplasma capsulatum.* Typical tuberculate macroconidia from Sabouraud's glucose agar culture. ×658. (From Smith: Am J Med 2:594, 1947)

been shown to be comparable to histoplasmin in skin test surveys.

ANTIGENIC STRUCTURE.

Yeast cells and histoplasmin have been used as antigens in a complement-fixation test with sera from human beings and infected and immunized animals. Campbell and Binkley reported frequent cross-reactions of histoplasma antigens with sera from patients with blastomycosis and a few cross-reactions with sera from patients with coccidioidomycosis. Sorensen and Evans precipitated an antigen by zinc and alcohol from the supernates of yeast phase cultures. This antigen proved to be specific in complement-fixation tests with sera from infected rabbits. Collodion particles sensitized with histoplasmin have been used in an agglutination test to demonstrate antihistoplasma antibodies in animal and human sera. A hemagglutination test also has been reported. Precipitins to histoplasmin and four fractions isolated from it have been demonstrated in sera from infected rabbits. Salvin and Furcolow used histoplasmin in a precipitin test with human sera. Precipitins could be demonstrated in the sera of patients with mild and severe acute histoplasmosis.

A histoplasmin-latex agglutination test, whole cell agglutination test, capillary tube agglutination test, and an agar gel precipitin test have been used to demonstrate antibody in animal and human sera.

Mice and guinea pigs acquire resistance to histoplasmosis after inoculation with acetone-dried dead yeast cells and a cell wall fraction of the yeast cells obtained by disruption in a Mickle tissue disintegrator followed by differential centrifugation. Also, mice show some resistance to infection after immunization with polysaccharide.

A specific fluorescent antibody for yeast phase *H. capsulatum* has been described. Yeast phase growth can be standardized for serologic testing by obtaining the organisms in the exponential phase of growth and testing their viability with Janus Green B.

EXPERIMENTAL INFECTION IN LABORATORY ANIMALS.

The pathogenesis of experimental histoplasmosis has been investigated in mice, hamsters, guinea pigs, and dogs. Intranasal, intracerebral, intraperitoneal, and intravenous routes of inoculation have been used.

CLINICAL TYPES OF INFECTION IN MAN.

Histoplasmosis is primarily a subclinical pulmonary disease of man resulting from inhalation of the fungus from contaminated areas of his environment. This benign type of self-limiting, pulmonary histoplasmosis is the most common type of infection, as evidenced by positive skin tests to histoplasmin in tens of thousands of individuals residing in the central Mississippi Valley.

Such patients are asymptomatic, but x-ray shadows of the lung taken during the first few months of the disease show numerous small, soft areas of infiltration 2 to 3 mm in size. After three or four years these areas become calcified and simulate the calcification seen in primary pulmonary infections. In many instances the hilar lymph nodes are enlarged and calcified. Such patients give a markedly positive skin test to a 1:1,000 dilution of a standard histoplasmin. In endemic areas studies of a number of individuals with multiple calcified foci in their lungs have shown that the negative tuberculin, positive histoplasmin reactors far outnumber those with positive tuberculin and negative histoplasmin tests.

This primary complex is essentially identical with that of tuberculosis in that there is a primary pulmonary focus with affected corresponding lymph nodes. Also, splenic calcification has been reported to be a part of the primary infection with *H. capsulatum*.

Chronic progressive (cavitary) histoplasmosis closely resembles the reinfection type of tuberculosis. The disease is characterized by exacerbations, with cough, profuse sometimes blood-tinged sputum, elevation of temperature and sedimentation rate, and moderate weight loss. Apical pneumonia or cavitary lesions, occasionally bilateral, are found. Progressive disease, with dissemination of the fungus throughout the body, occurs after varying periods of time. This results in ulceration of the lymphoid tissue, enlargement of the mesenteric nodes, hepatosplenomegaly, and generalized lymphadenopathy suggestive of Hodgkin's disease or visceral leishmaniasis or lymphoblastoma. Lesions on the mucosa of the nose, lips, mouth, pharynx, or larynx usually are secondary manifestations of widespread infection. These lesions may simulate carcinoma or tuberculosis. A granulomatous ocular infection poses a problem in differential diagnosis, which should include histoplasmosis. Such a diagnosis is based on clinical evidence of chorioretinitis, calcified pulmonary lesions, and a negative tuberculin and positive histoplasmin skin test.

TRANSMISSION. *H. capsulatum* has been isolated from animals, from soil, and from keratinaceous materials, such as feathers, in the soil. Several epidemics have been described, which have resulted from groups having contact with a common exposure and not by direct transmission from person to person. The isolation of *H. capsulatum* from bird and bat guano in caves has allowed histoplasmosis to be considered a spelunker's risk. Infections acquired in such areas result in a pneumonitis, with eventual development of miliary calcification in the lungs. Also, the isolation of *H. capsulatum* from bat tissues and feces has led investigators to speculate about this animal as the source of the infective agent. However, there is no known transmission from animal to animal or from animal to man. Young children frequently are infected with *Histoplasma*, the youngest reported patient being only one month of age, but 10 other cases have been reported in which the disease occurred during the first 12 months of life. Before the age of 10 years both sexes are affected equally, but in the older age groups males contract clinical infec-

tion seven times as frequently as do females. Such a sex distribution suggests that the reservoir of infection is in the fields or woods, where males would naturally be more exposed, but it indicates also that the organism can be brought into the home, where infants of both sexes would be exposed equally.

Histoplasmosis in its generalized form is a highly fatal disease, although a few spontaneous recoveries have been reported.

TREATMENT. Successful surgical removal of pulmonary cavities and segmental resection of coin lesions have been reported. The use of amphotericin B combined with the surgical removal of localized cavitary lesions offers the best management for chronic pulmonary histoplasmosis.

COCCIDIOIDOMYCOSIS

Coccidioidomycosis is an exogenous, dustborne infection caused by *Coccidioides immitis*. Two forms of the disease are known: primary coccidioidomycosis, which usually is an acute, benign, self-limiting, respiratory infection, and progressive coccidioidomycosis, which is a chronic, malignant, disseminated

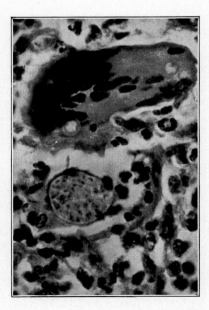

FIG. 86-16. *Coccidioides immitis.* Section of lung showing mature spherule and giant cell containing immature cells. ×736.

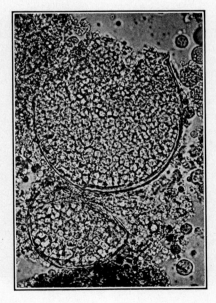

FIG. 86-17. *Coccidioides immitis.* Large spherules with endospores in pus. ×315. (From Smith: Am J Med 2:594, 1947)

disease that involves cutaneous, subcutaneous, visceral, and osseous tissues.

The disease was described first in the Argentine as a case of mycosis fungoides caused by a protozoan. Later cases were reported from California, and the etiologic agent was named *Coccidioides immitis* under the impression it also was a protozoan. The mycotic nature of the infection, however, was subsequently proven by Ophüls and Moffitt, who isolated a fungus from the infection and reproduced the disease in animals.

MORPHOLOGY.   *C. immitis* in the tissues develops into spherical, thick-walled structures, 15 to 80 μm in diameter, which are filled with numerous small endospores 2 to 5 μm in diameter (Figs. 86-16 and 86-17). When the spherules rupture, the endospores are freed and become distributed throughout the tissues, where they increase gradually in size and develop into mature spherules which become filled with endospores. Immature cells may contain no endospores and in size and appearance resemble the nonbudding forms of *B. dermatitidis*. Occasional reports have described mycelium as well as spherules in the tissues and sputum of patients with coccidioidal cavities of the lungs.

CULTURAL CHARACTERISTICS.   *C. immitis* grows readily on Sabouraud's glucose agar at room temperature. After four to six days' incubation, a flat membranous type colony appears, which during the course of the next week becomes covered with an abundance of cottony, aerial mycelium that at first is snow-white but gradually becomes tan to brown (Fig. 86-18). Microscopic examination of young cultures shows branching septate hyphae and many socalled racquet hyphae. In older cultures the hyphae broaden and break up into numerous, thick-walled, rectangular, ellipsoidal, or barrel-shaped arthrospores about 2.5 to 4.5 by 3.5 to 8 μm in size which alternate with empty spaces in the hyphae (Fig. 86-19). Nutritional requirements for growth and arthrospore formation have allowed abundant sporulation of this type. These small arthrospores are detached easily by jarring or shaking the culture, and numerous laboratory infections have resulted from the inhalation of these detached spores. Atypical cultures are identified by mouse inoculation and the subsequent demonstration of endosporulating spherules. When clinical materials are heavily contaminated with bacteria or sapro-

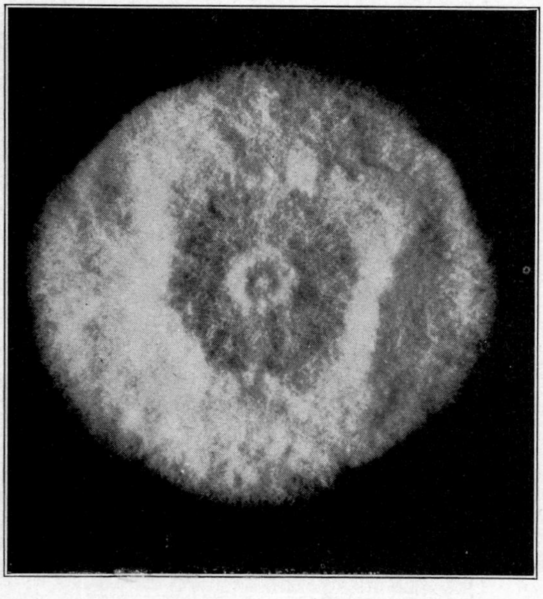

FIG. 86-18. *Coccidioides immitis.* Colony on Sabouraud's glucose agar at room temperature for 19 days. (From Conant et al: Manual of Clinical Mycology, 3rd ed, 1971, Courtesy of W. B. Saunders Co)

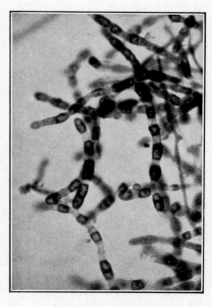

FIG. 86-19. Typical arthrospore formation in hyphae. From Sabouraud's glucose agar at room temperature. ×736.

phytic fungi, *C. immitis* may be cultured on antibiotic agar.

The spherules, or tissue phase, have been cultivated on artificial media. Physiologic studies of spherule production reveal certain amino acids and amino acid derivatives to be important for conversion from the mycelium.

The fungus is identified by its characteristic arthrospore formation in culture and its spherule production when inoculated intraperitoneally into mice.

FUNGOUS METABOLITES. No endotoxins or exotoxins are produced by *C. immitis*. A skin test material, coccidioidin, is prepared by growing for a period of three to six months a single or several strains of the fungus in Long's synthetic medium with the addition of 1 percent glucose. Such cultures are Seitz-filtered, and Merthiolate (1:10,000 final concentration) is added. The filtrate is used as a skin test material for the detection of dermal sensitivity and is comparable to tuberculin hypersensitivity. Coccidioidin also may be used as an antigen in the complement-fixation test, tube precipitin test, and immunodiffusion test. However, only certain samples of coccidioidin can be used for the complement-fixation test, since many preparations are anticomplementary.

Coccidioidin is heat stable. It resists 80C for 30 minutes and autoclaving. A position coccidioidin test in a healed patient does not induce serologic response in complement-fixation, tube precipitin, and immunodiffusion tests.

ANTIGENIC STRUCTURE. Probably there is only one antigenic type of *C. immitis*, since coccidioidins prepared from different strains have been found to give identical skin reactions when tested on sensitive individuals. In the complement-fixation reaction, sera from infected patients from Texas, Arizona, and California all may fix complement with a single antigen.

Immunogenic substances reside in the cell wall of the spherule.

EXPERIMENTAL INFECTION IN LABORATORY ANIMALS. Mice, rats, rabbits, guinea pigs, dogs, and monkeys are infected readily with *C. immitis*. Many of these animals have been used for investigations concerning the pathogenesis of

coccidioidomycosis and for immunologic studies relative to the possible production of a vaccine suitable for active immunization against coccidioidomycosis. A cytolytic factor for monuclear leukocytes has been described in the plasma and serum of guinea pigs infected with *C. immitis*.

CLINICAL TYPES OF INFECTION IN MAN. In certain areas in the southwestern part of the United States, from 50 to 80 percent of the population react to coccidioidin skin tests, suggesting that most cases of primary coccidioidomycosis, 60 percent, either are completely asymptomatic or cannot be differentiated from mild, nonspecific, respiratory infections. Goldstein and McDonald studied 75 soldiers who developed the primary form of coccidioidomycosis while on maneuvers in the desert during World War II. The incubation periods ranged from 8 to 21 days, and the symptoms were those of bronchitis or flu. About 19 percent of the soldiers developed skin lesions of the erythema nodosum type, and 28 percent had arthralgia. This hypersensitivity to the disease has been known for years as the "bumps" or "desert rheumatism."

Hypersensitivity to coccidioidin develops between the second and third weeks of the infection. The standard dose of coccidioidin is 0.1 ml of a 1:1,000 dilution of a standardized product, and the material is injected intracutaneously. A 1:100 dilution is necessary to elicit reactions in many patients, but those who have had previous skin lesions often give severe reactions even with a 1:10,000 dilution. Precipitins and complement-fixing antibodies are absent in mild cases but appear in the more severe infections, only to disappear with recovery.

Reports by Smith et al and Smith and Saito describe the use of serology in coccidioidomycosis and the pattern of reactions in 39,500 serologic tests.

Progressive coccidioidomycosis or coccidioidal granuloma usually develops from the more severe cases of the primary disease. One should suspect the progressive form of the disease if the temperature remains elevated after the third or fourth week, if the precipitin and complement-fixation titers increase, and if new shadows appear in the parenchyma of the lungs. As the disease progresses, metastatic lesions appear in the bones, subcutaneous tissues, and internal organs. Many patients die in coma from a terminal meningitis.

Generalized delayed hypersensitivity to coccidioidin can be transferred in man with leukocyte extracts from sensitive donors. Repeated intradermal testing with coccidioidin does not create sensitivity in previously nonsensitized individuals.

Transmission. Coccidioidomycosis is a dustborne, respiratory infection occurring in endemic areas in the arid regions of the southwestern United States, particularly in Southern California, the San Joaquin Valley in California, the area around Phoenix and Tucson in Arizona, New Mexico, and the contiguous southeastern and southwestern corners of Denver and Utah, respectively, and in central west Texas. Cases have been reported in Honduras and Guatemala in Central America, the northern states of Mexico, and Venezuela, Colombia, Bolivia, Paraguay, and Argentina in South America. The Chaco region of Argentina may prove to be a major endemic area in South America. A few cases have been reported from Italy, southeastern Europe, the Hawaiian Islands, and France. There is no known man-to-man or animal-to-man transmission of the disease. There has been one report, however, of transmission from an adult monkey to its offspring. Animals living in the endemic areas probably are infected, as is man, by the inhalation of contaminated dust, and infected rodents may serve to indicate the extent of endemic areas.

Travel through or within an endemic area is not without hazard. Also, infection from fomites outside known endemic areas has been documented.

Treatment. No particular treatment is necessary for the cases of primary coccidioidomycosis other than assigning the patient to bed until the sedimentation rate is normal, the lungs are clear when examined by x-ray, and the complement-fixation reaction becomes negative. Most patients with the progressive form of the disease (coccidioidal granuloma) will need specific therapy, although an occasional patient recovers after a prolonged illness. At the present time amphotericin B would seem to be the drug of choice for specific treatment of coccidioidomycosis. The chronicity of

the disseminated form of the disease, however, demands withholding judgment of the final efficacy of chemotherapy.

Surgery has been successful for pulmonary cavities which cause distressing symptoms.

Vaccination of large nonimmune population groups (troops) moving into endemic areas would minimize the danger of dissemination following primary pulmonary infections.

PARACOCCIDIOIDO-MYCOSIS

Paracoccidioidomycosis, caused by *Paracoccidioides brasiliensis,* is a chronic granulomatous infection of the mucous membranes of the mouth, skin, lymph nodes, and internal organs. The disease has been described in several countries in South America and in Costa Rica, Guatemala, Honduras, and Mexico. The cases described in the United States had a history of previous residence in Latin America. The greatest number of cases, however, has been reported from Brazil.

Lutz in Brazil described the first case of this disease, and he reported it as a case of paracoccidioidal granuloma because he thought the invading fungus was similar to *C. immitis.* Almeida obtained authentic cultures of *C. immitis* and compared them with the South American isolates and showed them to be quite different. On the basis of these comparative studies, he renamed the South American fungus *Paracoccidioides brasiliensis.*

Morphology.   *P. brasiliensis* occurs in tissue, exudates, and sputum as large, round, thick-walled, multiple budding cells, 10 to 60 μm in diameter. The entire surface of the parent cell may be covered with small buds, 1 to 5 μm in diameter, or it may show only a few larger buds, 10 to 30 μm in diameter. Single budding cells occasionally resemble the yeastlike tissue form of *B. dermatitidis.* The transformation of the yeast forms from the mycelium has been studied by Carbonell and Rodriguez.

Cultural Characteristics.   Smooth, waxy, yeastlike colonies develop on blood agar or beef infusion glucose agar at 37C (Fig. 86-20). Microscopically such cultures are composed

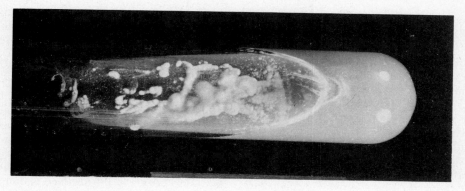

FIG. 86-20. *Paracoccidioides brasiliensis.* Growth on beef infusion glucose agar at 37C for 12 days.

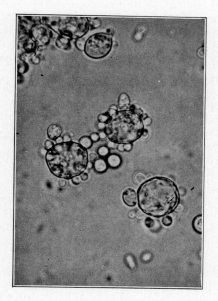

FIG. 86-21. *Paracoccidioides brasiliensis.* Multiple budding yeastlike cells from beef infusion glucose agar at 37C. ×790. (From Conant: Am Rev Tuberc 61:690, 1950)

of multiple budding cells, 6 to 30 μm in diameter, with surface buds, 1 to 5 μm in diameter (Fig. 86-21).

On Sabouraud's glucose agar at room temperature, the colonies develop slowly, reaching a diameter of 1 to 2 cm after two or three weeks' incubation. Such colonies may be covered with a short, white, aerial mycelium which later becomes light brown in color (Fig. 86-22), or it may become heaped, folded, and cerebriform. Microscopically, the mycelium consists of hyphae with numerous chlamydospores, noncharacteristic hyphal swellings, and short, broad, thick-walled cells. A subculture of this filamentous phase will revert to the yeast phase if incubated at 37 C.

FUNGOUS METABOLITES. No exotoxins or endotoxins have been described. Filtrates of broth cultures contain the substance, paracoccidioidin, which has been used as a skin testing antigen and as an antigen in the complement-fixation test.

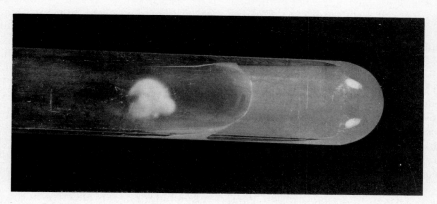

FIG. 86-22. *Paracoccidioides brasiliensis.* Colony on Sabouraud's glucose agar at room temperature for 25 days.

ANTIGENIC STRUCTURE. A filtrate of Sabouraud's broth, paracoccidioidin, in which 19 different strains of *P. brasiliensis* have been grown for several months, elicits a positive skin reaction in 48 hours upon intracutaneous inoculation into sensitive patients. Such patients do not react to coccidioidin, but may give a positive test to blastomycin. Paracoccidioidin can be used as the antigen in complement-fixation tests with the serum and spinal fluid of patients with systemic infections. Skin testing antigens also can be prepared by making saline suspensions of the yeast phase grown on chocolate agar and heating at 80C for one-half hour on three successive days or diluting infected pus 1:10 in saline and heating at 70C for one-half hour on three successive days. Also, the yeast phase growth has been used as antigen in the complement-fixation test. Cross-reactions occur, however, with serum from patients with blastomycosis. A filtrate of the yeast phase culture grown at 37C has been used successfully as a skin testing antigen. A polysaccharide obtained from an autoclaved yeast cell suspension also served as an antigen in a precipitin test and in the complement-fixation test and as a skin testing antigen.

An agar gel immunodiffusion test with patients' sera and filtrates from the mycelial and yeast phases was found to be simple to perform and specific.

Flourescent antibody could be made specific with sera from rabbits immunized with formalin-killed cells, but cross-reactions with several other fungi occurred with sera from infected rabbits.

EXPERIMENTAL INFECTION. Intratesticular injection of guinea pigs and intraperitoneal injection of mice, using the cultural yeast phase or clinical materials containing the budding forms, result in lesions similar to those produced by *B. dermatitidis*. Dissemination of infection is readily produced in mice when inoculated by the bronchopulmonary route and by intravenous injection. Guinea pigs and rabbits also develop systemic infections after intracardiac inoculation. Repeated passage of inoculum by intratesticular inoculation of guinea pigs was reported to increase the virulence of *P. brasiliensis*.

CLINICAL TYPES OF INFECTION IN MAN. Paracoccidioidomycosis usually is classified clinically into mucocutaneous, lymphatic, visceral, and mixed types. In the mucocutaneous infection the fungus enters the mouth and produces ulcerative lesions on the tonsils, tongue, cheek, gums, and palate. The skin lesions about the mouth and nose usually are secondary to the spreading, vegetative, papillomatous lesions of the buccal mucosa. Such lesions are similar to yaws and mucocutaneous leishmaniasis.

The lymphatic type most commonly involves the glands of the neck, which may become infected by an extension of the buccal lesions, but it also occurs in the absence of demonstrable lesions in the mouth. Lymphatic spread results in hard, painful glands which adhere to the skin, soften, and finally ulcerate. Massive lymphadenopathy of the mesenteric glands may be mistaken for Hodgkin's disease or a tumor, particularly when located in the ileocecal region.

Visceral infections are widespread, with involvement of the spleen, liver, pancreas, kidneys, and intestines. With hematogenous dissemination, the lungs and brain also are invaded.

Mixed infections include various combinations of the types just described.

TRANSMISSION. The hundreds of cases reported from Brazil would indicate that the disease is endemic in certain regions and that the fungus exists in the soil or on vegetation of some kind.

P. brasiliensis has been isolated from the soil and from the intestinal tracts of bats, *Artibus lituratus*, in Recife and Colombia, South America, respectively.

TREATMENT. Paracoccidioidomycosis, more than any other fungous infection, responds to sulfonamide therapy. Oliveira Ribeiro described the first cases which were treated successfully with sulfanilamide, sulfathiazole, and sulfadiazine, and Decourt et al in Brazil and Negroni and Nino in Argentina have reported cures using sulfadiazine, sulfamerazine, and sulfathiazole. The drug must be given in large doses (4 g daily) over a period of months. Sulfamethoxpyridazine and sulfadimethoxine in doses of 1 g daily for the first week and maintenance doses of 0.5 g daily until apparent cure is an effective treatment regimen.

Amphotericin B is effective in the treatment of paracoccidioidomycosis and should be considered for those patients showing sensitivity to sulfonamides. However, the organism can remain quiescent for prolonged periods of time in spite of the treatment used.

CLADOSPORIOSIS

Cladosporiosis is an infection of the brain caused by species of dematiaceous fungi, particularly by *Cladosporium bantianum.*

Binford et al in 1952 described what was considered to be the first case of brain abscess caused by *Cladosporium trichoides.* Previously, however, Banti in 1911 had described a cerebral lesion due to a dematiaceous fungus. The strain from Banti's case was named *Torula bantiana* by Saccardo in 1912. *T. bantiana* and *C. trichoides* were said to be identical by Borelli in 1960, and the new combination *Cladosporium bantianum* (Sacc.) Borelli has replaced *C. trichoides.*

Since the original report of this disease, many infections throughout the world have been described.

Fonsecaea pedrosoi was found to cause brain abscess in Japan and in the Congo, while *Phialophora dermatitidis* was isolated from a brain abscess in a Japanese.

MORPHOLOGY. Regardless of the species causing the brain abscesses, they all appear as branching, septate, brown hyphae in the pus and tissue. Individual cells in the hyphae may assume a dumbbell shape and become swollen and rounded, or the hyphae may appear moniliform. Such hyphae are seen readily in the pus when a drop of the exudate is mounted on a slide under a coverglass (Fig. 86-23). No special staining is necessary for tissue sections, since the brown-pigmented hyphae are easily detected. Cultures are necessary for species identification of the fungus responsible for the infection.

CULTURAL CHARACTERISTICS. *C. bantianum* develops an olive gray to olive brown colony on Sabouraud's glucose agar. The surface is velvety and develops radial folds in old cultures. The slow spreading growth of the colony (4 cm in two weeks) is typical of that for cultures of *Hormodendrum pedrosoi* and not of that for the rapidly growing, large, powdery colonies of saprophytic *Cladosporium* species (Fig. 86-24).

Sporulation is of the *Cladosporium* type, with septate conidiophores bearing long-branched chains of conidia (Fig. 86-25). The conidia are elliptical, 2 to 2.5 μm by 4 to 7 μm, brown, smooth-walled, and separated in the chain by the typical disjunctors seen in *Cladosporium* species.

The biochemical activity of cultures of *C. bantianum* differentiates this species from saprophytic strains. *C. bantianum* does not liquefy gelatin or Löffler's coagulated serum, coagulate milk, digest starch, or utilize tributyrin and

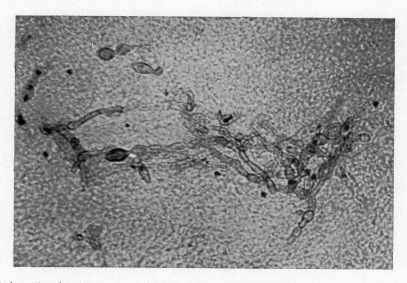

FIG. 86-23. *Cladosporium bantianum.* Brown hyphae seen in pus from brain abscess. ×750.

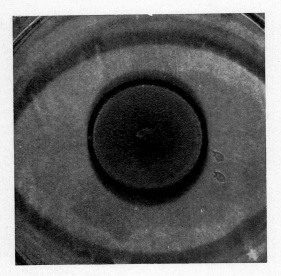

FIG. 86-24. *Cladosporium bantianum.* Colony on potato dextrose agar at room temperature for 14 days. (Courtesy of C.W. Emmons. National Institutes of Health, Bethesda, Maryland)

cellulose. Saprophytic species are positive in these tests, with the exception of tributyrin and cellulose. Although its optimum temperature for growth is 37 to 38C, its maximum temperature for growth is 42 to 43C.

EXPERIMENTAL INFECTION IN LABORATORY ANIMALS. *C. bantianum* is pathogenic for the mouse and rabbit. Intravenous inoculation of a saline suspension produced brain abscesses in these animals. Duque also reported dissemination to the brain when mice were inoculated intraperitoneally with *C. bantianum.* Shimazono et al found their isolate of *B. dermatitidis* to produce brain abscesses in mice following intravenous inoculation. Iwata and Wada inoculated mice and guinea pigs intraperitoneally with their isolate of *F. pedrosoi.** They describe fatal systemic infections in these animals with abscesses "in the liver, spleen, mesentery and other internal organs, the kidney, however, being not so much affected." No mention was made of lesions in the brains of these animals.

CLINICAL TYPES OF INFECTION IN MAN. The signs and symptoms are those produced by any space-occupying lesion in the brain or may be those of a chronic meningitis. In a review of 23 cases Shimazono et al found headache, drowsiness, hemiplegia, and meningeal signs to be the most prominent. In 17 of these cases the patients showed loss of mobility, with 12 demonstrating hemiplegia. In addition, 14 complained of headache, 9 had fever, 8 were disoriented, 7 had meningeal signs, and 3 each had disturbance of vision, convulsive seizures, and ataxia.

C. bantianum probably occurs in nature.

*Iwata K, Wada J: Mycological studies on the strains isolated from a case of chromoblastomycosis in central nervous system. Jap J Microbiol 1:355, 1957

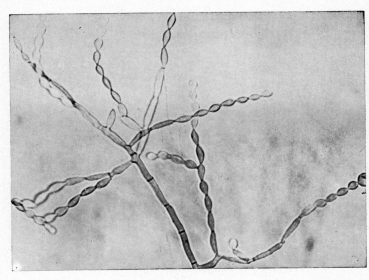

FIG. 86-25. *Cladosporium bantianum.* Conidiophore showing branching chains of conidia. ×690. (From Emmons et al: Medical Mycology, 2nd ed, 1970. Courtesy of Lea & Febiger)

Infection by pulmonary inhalation of spores with eventual dissemination to the brain by the bloodstream is the most likely route to cerebral infection. Experimental infection of mice by intravenous inoculation of *C. bantianum* would seem to prove the above assumption. Also, an abscess in the lung has been noted in one instance of human infection from which *C. bantianum* was isolated from both the lung and the brain.

TREATMENT. There has been no report of successful therapy for this infection. Many drugs have been used without effect for the several patients whose infection had not been diagnosed until autopsy or surgical removal of the abscess. In the first case reported by Binford et al the patient remained well following surgery.

FURTHER READING

CRYPTOCOCCOSIS

Bennett JE, Hasenclever HF, Baum LG: Evaluation of a skin test for cryptococcosis. Am Rev Resp Dis 91:616, 1965

Bindschadler DD, Bennett JE: Serology of human cryptococcosis. Ann Intern Med 69:45, 1968

Gordon MA, Vedder DK: Serologic tests in diagnosis and prognosis of cryptococcosis. JAMA 197:961, 1966

Hamilton JD, Elliott DM: Combined activity of amphotericin B and 5-fluorocytosine against *Cryptococcus neoformans* in vitro and in vivo in mice. J Infect Dis 131:129, 1975

Jennings A, Bennett JR, Young V: Identification of *Cryptococcus neoformans* in a clinical laboratory. Mycopathologia 35:256, 1968

Kaufman L, Blumer S: Latex-cryptococcal antigen test. Am J Clin Pathol 60:285, 1973

Kaufman L, Cowart G, Blumer S, Stine A, Wood R: Evaluation of a commercial latex agglutination test kit for cryptococcal antigen. Appl Microbiol 27:620, 1974

Newberry WM Jr, Walter JE, Chandler JW Jr, Tosh FE: Epidemiological study of *Cryptococcus neoformans*. Am Inst Med 67:724, 1967

Sarosi GA, Parker JD, Doto IL, Tosh FE: Amphotericin B in cryptococcal meningitis. Am Med 71:1079, 1969

Shields AB, Ajello L: Medium for selective isolation of *Cryptococcus neoformans*. Science 151:208, 1966

Steer PL, Marks MI, Klite PD, Eickhoff TC: 5-fluorocytosine: An oral antifungal compound. A report on clinical and laboratory experience. Ann Intern Med 76:15, 1972

Utz JP, Tynes BS, Shadomy HJ, et al: 5-fluorocytosine in human cryptococcosis. Antimicrob Agents Chemother 8:344, 1968

BLASTOMYCOSIS

Abernathy RS: Clinical manifestations of pulmonary blastomycosis. Ann Intern Med 51:707, 1959

Abernathy RS, Jansen GT: Therapy with amphotericin B in North American blastomycosis. Am J Intern Med 53:1196, 1960

Baum GL, Schwartz J: North American blastomycosis. Am J Med Sci 238:661, 1959

Campas Magalhoes MJ, Droulet E, Destombes P: Premier cas de blastomycose à *Blastomyces dermatitidis* observé au Mozambique. Guériscon par l'amphotéricin B. Bull Soc Pathol Exot 61:210, 1968

Craig MW, Davey WN, Green RA: Conjugal blastomycosis. Am Rev Respir Dis 102:86, 1970

Denton JF, DiSalvo AF: Isolation of *Blastomyces dermatitidis* from natural sites at Augusta, Georgia. Am J Trop Med Hyg 13:716, 1964

Duttera MJ, Osterhout S: North American blastomycosis: a survey of 63 cases. South Med J 62:295, 1969

Furcolow ML, Smith CD: A new interpretation of the epidemiology, pathology and ecology of *Blastomyces dermatitidis* with some additional data. Trans NY Acad Sci 35:421, 1973

Gilchrist TC, Stokes WR: A case of pseudo-lupus vulgaris caused by a *Blastomyces*. J Exp Med 3:53, 1898

Johnson WW, Mantiulli J: The role of cytology in the primary diagnosis of North American blastomycosis. Acta Cytol 17:200, 1970

Kepron MW, Schaenperlen CB, Hershfield ES, Zylak CJ, Cherniack RM: North American blastomycosis in Central Canada. Can Med Assoc J 106:243, 1972

McDonough ES: Blastomycosis—Epidemiology and biology of its ecologic agent *Ajellomyces dermatitidis*. Mycopathologia 41:195, 1970

McDonough ES, Lewis AL: The ascigenous stage of *Blastomyces dermatitidis*. Mycologia 40:76, 1968

Menges RW: Blastomycosis in animals. Vet Med 55:45, 1960

Parker JD, Doto IJ, Tosh FE: A decade of experience with blastomycosis and its treatment with amphotericin B. Am Rev Respir Dis 99:895, 1969

Sarosi GK, Hammerman KJ, Tosh FE, Kronenberg RS: Clinical features of acute pulmonary blastomycosis. N Engl J Med 290:540, 1974

Sudman MS, Kaplan W: Antigenic relationship between American and African isolates of *Blastomyces dermatitidis* as determined by immunofluorescence. Appl Microbiol 27:496, 1970

LOBOMYCOSIS

Boreli D: Lobomicosis: Nomenclatura de su agente. Med Cutanea 3:151, 1968

Ciferri R, Azevedo PC, Campos S, Carneiro LS: Taxonomy of Jorge Lobo's disease fungus. Inst Micol Recife Pernambuco Brasil 53:121, 1956

Fouseca Filho O, Avea Leao AE: Cantribucao para conhecimento dos gramumatoes blastomicoides O agente etiologico da doenca Jorge Lobo. Med Cir Brazil 48:147, 1940

Lobo J: Um caso de blastomycose produzida por uma especie nova, encontrada em Recife. Rev Med Pernambuco 1:763, 1931

Migaki G, Valerio MG: Lobo's disease in an Atlantic bottle-nosed dolphin. J Am Vet Med Assoc 159:578, 1970

Silva ME, Kaplan W, Miranda JL: Antigenic relationships between *Paracoccidioides loboi* and other pathogenic fungi determined by immunofluorescence. Mycopathol Mycol Appl 36:98, 1968

Wiersema JP, Niemel PLA: Lobo's disease in Surinam patients. Trop Geogr Med 17:89, 1965

HISTOPLASMOSIS

Ajello L: Geographic distribution of *Histoplasma capsulatum*. Mukosen 1:147, 1958

Campbell DD: Serology in the respiratory mycoses. Sabouraudia 5:240, 1967

Darling STA: A protozan general infection producing pseudotubercles in the lungs, and focal necrosis in the liver, spleen, and lymph nodes. JAMA 46:1283, 1906

De Monbreun WA: The cultivation and cultural characteristics of Darling's *Histoplasma capsulatum*. Am J Trop Med 14:93, 1934

Emmons CW: Isolation of *Histoplasma capsulatum* from soil. Public Health Rep 64:892, 1949

Furcolow ML: Opportunism in histoplasmosis. Lab Invest 11:1134, 1962

Furcolow ML: Recent studies on the epidemiology of histoplasmosis. Ann NY Acad Sci 72:127, 1958

Howard DH, Otto V: Lymphocyte mediated cellular immunity in histoplasmosis. Infect Immun 4:605, 1971

Kwon-Chung KJ: Sexual stage of *Histoplasma capsulatum*. Science 175:326, 1972

Kwon-Chung KJ: Studies on *Emmonsiella capsulata*. I. Heterothallism and development of the ascocarp. Mycologia 65:109, 1973

Larsh HW, Bartels PA: Serology of histoplasmosis. Mycopathologia 41:115, 1970

COCCIDIOIDOMYCOSIS

Ajello L, Maddy K, Crecelius G, Hugenholtz PG, Hall LB: Recovery of *Coccidioides immitis* from the air. Sabouraudia 4:92, 1965

Albert BL, Sekevs TE Jr: Coccidioidomycosis from formites. Arch Intern Med 112:151, 1963

Culwell JA, Tillman SP: Early recognition and therapy of disseminated coccidioidomycosis. Am J Med 31:676, 1961

Dickson EL: "Valley fever" of the San Joaquin Valley and fungus *Coccidioides*. Calif West Med 47:151, 1937

Emmons CW: Isolation of *Coccidioides* from soil and rodents. Public Health Rep 57:109, 1942

Fiese MJ: Coccidioidomycosis. Springfield, Ill, Thomas, 1958

Gehlbach, SH, Hamilton HD, Conant NF: Coccidioidomycosis. An occupational disease in cotton mill workers. Arch Intern Med 131:254, 1973

Huppert M: Serology of coccidioidomycosis. Mycopathologia 41:107, 1970

Kruse RH: Potential aerogenic laboratory hazards of *Coccidioides immitis*. Am J Clin Pathol 37:150, 1962

Kruse RH, Green TD, Leeder WD: Infection of control monkeys with *Coccidioides immitis* by caging with inoculated monkey. Proceedings of Second Coccidioidomycosis Symposium. Tucson, Univ of Arizona Press, 1967, pp 387-395

Levine HB: Development of vaccines for coccidioidomycosis. Mycopathologia 41:177, 1970

Levine HB, Couzalez Ochoa, A, Ten Eyck DR: Dermal sensitivity to *Coccidioides immitis*: A comparison of response elicited by spherulin and coccidioides immitis: A comparison of response elicited by spherulin and coccidioidin. Am Rev Resp Dis 107:379, 1973

Ophüls W, Moffitt HC: A new pathogenic mold (formerly described as a protozoan: *Coccidioides immitis*). Preliminary report. Phila Med J 5:1471, 1900

Smith CE, Saito MT, Simons SA: Pattern of 39,500 serologic tests in coccidioidomycosis. JAMA 160:546, 1956

Smith CE, Beard RR, Rosenberger HG, Whiting EG: Effect of season and dust control on coccidioidomycosis. JAMA 132:833, 1946

Smith CE, Whiting EG, Baker EE, et al: The use of coccidioidin. Am Rev Tuberc 57:300, 1948

PARACOCCIDIOIDOMYCOSIS

Albornoz MB: Isolation of paracoccidioidomycosis from rural soil in Venezuela. Sabouraudia 9:248, 1971

Almeida RP: Estados comparativos do granuloma coccidioidica nos Estados Unidos e no Brasil. Novo genero para a parasita brasiliero. An Fac Med Univ Sao Paulo 5:3, 1931

Groose E., Tausitt JR: *Paracoccidioides brasiliensis* recovered from intestinal tract of three bats *(Artibeus literatus)* in Columbia, S.A. Sabouraudia 4:121, 1971

Londero AT: The lung in paracoccidioidomycosis. In proceedings of the First Pan American Symposium. PAHO, WHO. Scientific Publ 254:109, 1972

Lutz A: Uma mycose peudoscoccidica localizada na boca e observada no Brazil. Contribuição ao conhecimenta das hytoblastomycoses americanas. Brazil-Med 22: 121, 1908

Murray HW, Littman ML, Roberts RB: Disseminated paracoccidioidomycosis (South American blastomycosis) in the United States. Am J Med 56:209, 1974

Negroni P: Prolonged therapy for paracoccidioidomycosis—approaches, complications and risks. In proceedings of the First Pan American Symposium, PAHO, WHO, Scientific Publ 254:147, 1972

Oliveira Ribeiro D: Mora terapeutica para blastomycose. Publ Med Sao Paulo 12:35, 1940

Restrepo MA: La prueba de immuno diffusion en el diagnostico de la paracoccidioidomycosis. Sabouraudia 4: 223, 1966

Restrepo MA, Correa I: Comparison of two culture media for primary isolation of *Paracoccidioidomycosis brasiliensis* from sputum. Sabouraudia 10:260, 1973

Sampaio SAP: Tratamento da blastomicose sul-americana com Anfotericina B. Tese de professovado. Sao Paulo, 1960

CLADOSPORIOSIS

Binford CH, Thompson RK, Gordon ME, Emmons CW: Mycotic brain abscess due to *Cladosporium trichoides*, a new species. Am J Clin Path 22:535, 1952

Borelli D: *Torula bantianum*, agent di un granuloma cerebrale. Rev Anat Pat Oncol 17:615, 1960

Crichlow DK, Enrile FT: Cerebral abscess due to *Cladosporium trichoides* (bantianum). Am J Clin Pathol 60: 416, 1973

Duque O: Meningo-encephalitis and brain abscess caused by *Cladosporium* and *Fonsecaea*. Am. J Clin Pathol 36:505, 1961

Fuentes CA, Bosch ZE: Biochemical differentiation of the etiologic agents of chromoblastomycosis from the nonpathogenic *Cladosporium* species. J Invest Dermatol 34:419, 1960

Shimazono Y, Isaki K, Torii H, Otsuka R: Brain abscess due to *Hormodendrum dermatitidis* (Kano) Conant, 1953. Report of a case and review of the literature. Folia Psychiat Neurol Jap 17:80, 1963

FURTHER READING

Books

Baker RD: The Pathogenic Anatomy of Mycoses. Berlin-Heidelberg-New York, Springer Verlag, 1971

Beneke ES: Human Mycoses. Kalamazoo, The Upjohn CO, 1972

Conant NF, Smith DT, Baker RD, Callaway JL: Manual of Clinical Mycology, 3rd ed. Philadelphia, Saunders, 1971

Emmons CW, Binford CH, Utz JP: Medical Mycology, 2nd ed. Philadelphia, Lea & Febiger, 1970

Fetter BF, Klintworth GK, Hendry WS: Mycoses of the Central Nervous System. Baltimore, Williams & Wilkins, 1967

Hazen EL, Gordon MA, Reed FC: Laboratory Identification of Pathogenic Fungi Simplified, 3rd ed. Springfield, Ill, Thomas, 1970

Lodder L, Kreger-Van Rij NJW: The Yeasts, a Taxonomic Study. Amsterdam, North-Holland Publishing Co, 1970

Rippon JW: Medical Mycology. The Pathogenic Fungi and the Pathogenic Actinomycetes. Philadelphia, Saunders, 1974

Vanbreuseghem R, Wilkinson J: Mycoses of Man and Animals. Springfield, Ill, Thomas, 1958

Wilson JW: Clinical and Immunological Aspects of Fungus Diseases. Springfield, Ill, Thomas, 1957

Winner HI, Hurley R: *Candida albicans*. Boston, Little, Brown, 1964

Manuals

Ajello L, Georg LK, Kaplan W, Kaufman L: Laboratory Manual for Medical Mycology. PHSP No. 994. Superintendent of Documents, Washington, DC, US Government Printing Office, 1963

Beneke ES, Rogers A: Medical Mycology Laboratory Manual, 3rd ed. Minneapolis, Burgess Publishing Co, 1971

Rebell G, Taplin D: Dermatophytes, Their Recognition and Identification, 2nd ed. Coral Gables, Univ of Miami Press, 1970

Selected Papers

Ajello L: The medical mycological iceberg. Proceedings — International Symposium on Mycoses Sci Pub PAHO No. 205:3, 1970

Ajello L: A comparative study of the pulmonary mycoses of Canada and the United States. Public Health Rep 84: 869, 1969

Buechner HA, Seabury JH, Campbell CC, et al: The current status of serologic, immunologic and skin tests in the diagnosis of pulmonary mycoses. Chest 63:259, 1973

DuToit CJ: Sporotrichosis on the Witwatersrand. Proc. Mine Med Oft Assoc 22:111, 1942

Hutter RVP: Phycomycetous infection (mucormycosis) in cancer patients; a complication of therapy. Cancer 12: 330, 1959

Kaplan W: Epidemiology of the principal systemic mycoses of man and lower animals and the ecology of their etiologic agents. Am Vet Med Assoc 163:1043, 1973

McGinnis MR, Padhye AA, Ajello L: Storage of stock cultures of filamentous fungi, yeasts and some aerobic actinomycetes in sterile distilled water. Appl Microbiol 28: 218, 1974

Palmer CE: Nontuberculous pulmonary calcification and sensitivity to histoplasmin. Public Health Rep 60:513, 1945

Smith CE, Beard RR, Rosenberger HG, Whiting EG: Effect of season and dust control on coccidioidomycosis JAMA 132:833, 1946

Sudman MS: Protothecosis. A critical review. Am J Clin Pathol 61:10, 1974

Utz JP: The treatment of systemic mycoses. Mod Treat 7: 509, 1970

87

Fungous Diseases of the Skin and Subcutaneous Tissues

SPOROTRICHOSIS

Sporotrichosis, caused by *Sporotrichum schenckii*, is a chronic progressive infection of the skin and subcutaneous tissue characterized by a sporotrichotic chancre at the site of inoculation, followed by the development and the formation of subcutaneous nodules along the lymphatics draining the primary lesion. Extracutaneous lesions (pulmonary, osseous, and mucosal) are being recognized more frequently.

Schenck in Baltimore isolated a fungus, *Sporotrichum* species, from a patient with refractory subcutaneous abscesses on his arm. A second case in the United States was reported by Hektoen and Perkins, who named the fungus *Sporothrix schenckii*. Several other species of *Sporotrichum* have been described from infections of man and animals, but they have been reduced to synonymy with *S. schenckii* by many investigators.

MORPHOLOGY. *S. schenckii* is rarely seen in human tissues or exudates unless stained by the Schiff-McManus technique. This periodic acid-Schiff stain for fungus in tissue stains the organisms red and allows them to be seen easily. Also, the methenamine silver stain makes them more noticeable. The organisms appear as fusiform bodies or round budding cells, 3 to 5 μm in diameter. Occasionally, asteroid bodies are seen. These are round, single-budding cells, 5 to 10 μm in diameter, surrounded by a homogeneous eosinophil-staining material. Infrequently, hyphal elements may be seen. Cultures must be obtained, however, for a definitive diagnosis.

CULTURAL CHARACTERISTICS. *S. schenckii* grows readily on Sabouraud's glucose agar at room temperature or on blood agar at 37C. On Sabouraud's glucose agar, growth appears in four to five days as small, white to cream-colored colonies, which rapidly enlarge, becoming smooth, leathery, and folded. Some strains remain cream-colored, while other strains develop a brownish to black pigmentation (Fig. 87-1). Such colonies are very characteristic and diagnostic. Microscopically, the mycelium is seen to be 1.5 to 2 μm in diameter with lateral branches of various lengths which support clusters (2 to 15) of pyriform conidia 2 to 4 by 2 to 6

μm in size (Fig. 87-2). Such spores also may be borne directly from the sides of hyphae as well as at the tips of conidiophores.

When cultures are grown on blood agar at 37C, they become soft and yeastlike (Fig. 87-3) and are composed of fusiform, round, oval, and budding cells similar to those seen in lesions of infected animals (Fig. 87-4).

Sugar fermentations are of no value in the differentiation of species. In metabolic studies, eight strains did not differ in their nitrogen metabolism; nitrogen of various amino acids, urea, and ammonium nitrate were utilized, and no single amino acid was essential for growth. However, Mariat and others reported pyrimidine to be essential for growth, whereas previously thiamine has been shown to be a requirement.

ANTIGENIC STRUCTURE. Agglutinins can be demonstrated in the sera of cases of human and experimental sporotrichosis. It has also been shown that different isolates of *Sporotrichum* are antigenically similar by agglutinin and agglutinin-absorption tests.

Kaden has demonstrated precipitins to a carbohydrate extracted from yeast cells by an agar gel diffusion technique.

Serologic studies in 11 human cases showed the precipitin test with autoclaved antigen to be positive in 8, the complement-fixation test to be positive in 2, and the agglutination test to be positive in 4.

Intracutaneous injections of saline suspensions of killed cultures and carbohydrate ob-

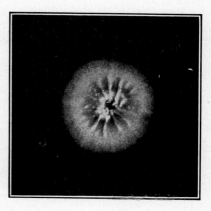

FIG. 87-1. *Sporotrichum schenckii.* Colony on Sabouraud's glucose agar at room temperature for 12 days.

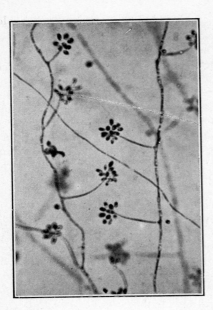

FIG. 87-2. *Sporotrichum schenckii.* Clusters of pyriform conidia from the ends of conidiophores. ×650. (From Conant et al: Manual of Clinical Mycology, 3rd ed, Courtesy of W.B. Saunders Co)

chosis follows immunization with formalin-killed antigen or preinfection with S. *schenckii.* The direct fluorescent antibody technique has been used for detecting S. *schenckii* in smears of exudates from animal and human lesions and in smears made from cultures.

EXPERIMENTAL INFECTION IN LABORATORY ANI-MALS.   Mice, rats, cats, and dogs may be infected experimentally by several routes of inoculation. The mouse and the rat show a marked orchitis in which the fungus may be seen in smears or may be cultured. The temperature at which infected rats are held, 10 to 20C or 31C, determines the extent of the infection. At 10 to 20C metastatic lesions are seen, while at 31C the infection is minimal.

Howard and Orr found that several strains isolated from nature were not pathogenic for laboratory animals, although they were morphologically identical and antigenically related to human pathogenic isolates. MacKinnon et al, however, found seven isolates from nature to be pathogenic for mice.

tained from cultures elicit positive skin tests in 24 to 48 hours. Sporotrichin elicited positive reactions in 32.3 percent of nursery workers and 11.2 percent of all persons tested at Charity Hospital and Angola Penitentiary in Louisiana. This would indicate subclinical infection among plant nursery employees.

In experimental sporotrichosis in mice, soluble antigens from the peritoneal fluid and various tissues were found to precipitate in anti-*Sporotrichum* rabbit serum. Also, capsules could be demonstrated on the fungous cells recovered from infected mice.

Slight protection of mice against sporotri-

CLINICAL TYPES OF INFECTION IN MAN.   In the monograph by de Beurmann and Gougerot, sporotrichosis was divided into six clinical types: lymphatic, disseminated, epidermal, mucosal, skeletal, and visceral. To these should be added the pseudoneoplastic form described by Smith. The localized lymphatic type of infection is seen most frequently in the United States. The primary lesion occurs on the hand or arm, where the fungus is introduced by trauma. The lesion begins as a hard, inelastic nodule, which at first is pink but slowly changes to a purplish color and finally develops into a black necrotic ulcer. The lymphatics draining the area become cordlike, and chains of subcu-

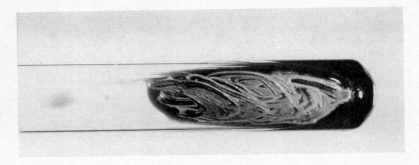

FIG. 87-3. *Sporotrichum schenckii.* Yeast culture on brain-heart infusion blood agar for seven days at 37C. (From Conant et al: Manual of Clinical Mycology, 3rd ed, 1971. Courtesy of W.B. Saunders Co)

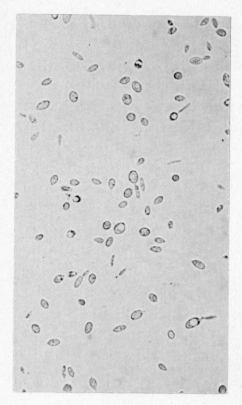

FIG. 87-4. *Sporotrichum schenckii.* Fusiform, round, oval cells from culture on blood agar at 37C. ×790. (From Conant et al: Manual of Clinical Mycology, 3rd ed, 1971. Courtesy of W.B. Saunders Co)

taneous nodules develop along the lymphatic vessels. Such secondary nodules also may soften and ulcerate to become chronic ulcerating lesions. In contrast to tularemia, the patients with sporotrichosis have little if any fever and do not appear ill. The regional lymph nodes usually are not involved, with the possible exception of the epitrochlear node.

The disseminated and visceral forms of the disease have been reported more frequently outside the United States. However, sporotrichosis of the viscera, bones, and joints should be considered in the differential diagnosis of infection of unknown etiology. Not infrequently, synovitis of the knee has been caused by S. *schenckii.*

Primary pulmonary sporotrichosis, caused by inhalation of infectious particles, must be more frequent than realized. Occasional reports of pulmonary infection do not indicate the possible extent of self-limited infections. A suitable

skin test antigen and its use in epidemiologic surveys, as for histoplasmosis and coccidioidomycosis, might provide the answer to the existence of benign infections.

TRANSMISSION. S. *schenckii* occurs as a saprophyte in nature, where it can infect both man and animals. Man may become infected by wounds from plant materials, such as thorns and barbs, or by the handling of infected animals or contaminated dressings. Recently a number of infections acquired in the laboratory have come to our attention. Sporotrichosis occasionally assumes importance as an occupational disease. The most remarkable epidemic of sporotrichosis, however, occurred in the gold mines of South Africa, where a total of 2,825 cases were reported. Males are infected more frequently than females, especially farmers, laborers, and horticulturists.

BIOLOGIC PRODUCTS. Vaccines may be prepared from the tissue phase of S. *schenckii* from cystine agar cultures at 37C. Heat-killed saline suspensions may be used for skin testing, agglutination reactions, and desensitization. Also, polysaccharides obtained from cultures have been used and found effective as skin testing antigens.

TREATMENT. Potassium iodide has a specific curative action in sporotrichosis. Large doses should be employed and continued for four to six weeks after apparent recovery. An occasional case may require supplementary vaccine therapy if a marked degree of hypersensitivity has developed during the infection. Successful treatment with stilbamidine, dihydroxystilbamidine, and amphotericin B has been reported.

PHAEOSPORO-TRICHOSIS

Phaeosporotrichosis, caused by a variety of deeply brown pigmented fungi, occurs in the debilitated patient as a disease of the subcutaneous tissue in which a single lesion occurs in the skin as a subcutaneous abscess, a dermal cyst, or a foreign body granuloma. In such lesions, the fungus appears as brown budding cells, fragmented hyphae, or chains of monili-

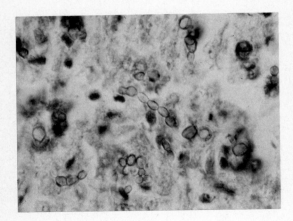

FIG. 87-5. *Phialophora gougerotii.* Moniliform hyphae and yeast cells in wall of subcutaneous abscess. ×828. (From Nielsen: Manual of Clinical Microbiology, 2nd ed., 1974 Courtesy of American Society for Microbiology)

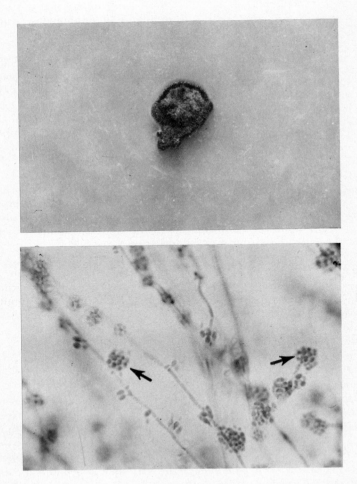

FIG. 87-6. *Phialophora gougerotii.* Top. Culture on Sabouraud's glucose agar at room temperature for 14 days. Bottom. Spores produced along hyphae and from conidiophores. ×687. (From Conant et al: Manual of Clinical Mycology, 3rd ed, 1971. Courtesy of W.B. Saunders Co)

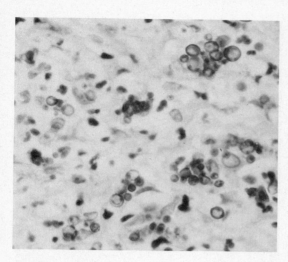

FIG. 87-7. *Phialophora spinifera.* Pigmented yeastlike cells in tissue. (From Nielsen and Conant: Sabouraudia 6: 228, 1968)

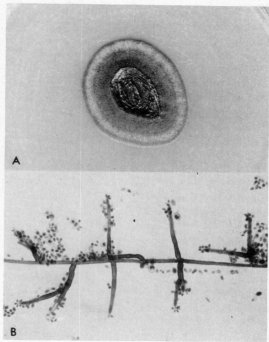

FIG. 87-8. *Phialophora spinifera.* A. Culture on corn meal agar at room temperature. B. Deeply pigmented, rigid conidiophores on corn meal agar. ×450. (From Conant et al: Manual of Clinical Mycology, 3rd ed, 1971. Courtesy of W.B. Saunders Co)

form cells in the necrotic center of the lesion. The organisms isolated from such lesions have been identified as *Phialophora gougerotii,* *Phialophora spinifera,* and *Phialophora richardsiae.*

MORPHOLOGY. *P. gougerotii* occurs in abscesses of the skin as brown budding cells, short fragments of moniliform cells, or bits of hyphae. The pigmentation of these fungous cells separates this disease from sporotrichosis, with which it was formerly confused. Also, a single lesion rather than multiple lesions along the regional lymphatics would tend to separate these two diseases (Fig. 87-5).

When material is obtained from a lesion and cultured on Sabouraud's agar, the colony is at first soft, yeastlike, and black. This colony type and the black yeastlike budding cells are similar to those of a *Pullularia* species (Fig. 87-6A).

A gradual change in the morphology of the culture takes place, with time, when the colonies become overgrown with a grayish mycelium. Many spores are produced in clusters from small protuberances along this mycelium and from the ends of conidiophores of the phialophora type. These species are 2 to 3 μm by 2.5 to 4 μm in size (Fig. 87-6B).

P. spinifera occurred in a granulomatous mass on the nose of a patient as clusters of brown, ovoid, budding cells 2 to 10 μm in diameter (Fig. 87-7).

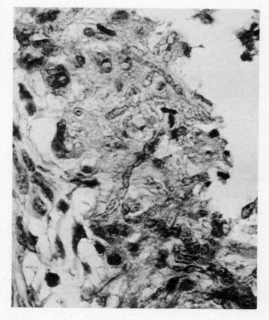

FIG. 87-9. *Phialophora richardsiae.* Pigmented hyphae seen in wall of abscess.

When this material was cultured on Sabouraud's agar, the colonies were dark, moist, soft, and yeastlike. This growth consists of unicellular, budding yeast cells 2.5 to 3.0 μm by 3 to 6 μm, and segments of toruloid hyphae (Fig. 87-8a).

Eventually, a short naplike mycelium is produced. Deeply pigmented, spinelike conidiophores, single or branched, come off the hyphae at right angles and terminate in clusters of spores 2.5 by 3.5 μm in size (Fig. 87-8B).

P. richardsiae, a contaminant of wood pulp, has been isolated from a dermal cyst in which it appeared in the necrotic material as dark hyphal strands (Fig. 87-9).

When the necrotic material was cultured on Sabouraud's agar, a brownish short wool-like mycelial mat was produced (Fig. 87-10). Simple, long, tapering conidiophores are produced at right angles to the hyphae, which produce dark spores, 4 μm in size, from the base of a conspicuous saucer-shaped tip (Fig. 87-11).

These miscellaneous pigmented (dematiaceous) fungi have occurred infrequently as the cause of wound infections. They occur in nature and are introduced into the tissues at the time of injury where they slowly develop lesions in the subcutaneous tissues of the debilitated patient.

The surgical removal of the single lesion produced by these fungi is adequate treatment.

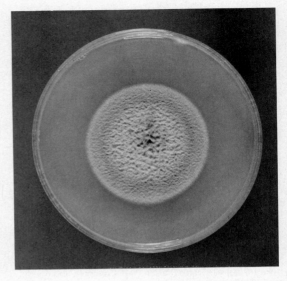

FIG. 87-10. *Phialophora richardsiae.* Culture on Sabouraud's glucose agar at room temperature for two weeks. (From Conant et al: Manual of Clinical Mycology, 3rd ed, 1971. Courtesy of W.B. Saunders Co)

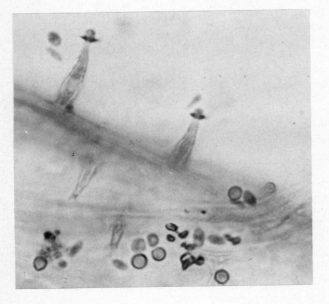

FIG. 87-11. *Phialophora richardsiae.* Conidiophores with terminal saucer-shaped cup. ×1387. (From Conant et al: Manual of Clinical Mycology, 3rd ed, 1971. Courtesy of W.B. Saunders Co)

MADUROMYCOSIS

Mauduromycosis, caused by a variety of filamentous fungi, is a slowly progressive, unilateral infection of the subcutaneous tissues, characterized by chronicity, tumefactions, and multiple sinus formation from which granules are extracted.

Colebrook, of the Madura Dispensary in India, used the term "Madura foot" for an infection of the feet commonly seen in India and previously described by Gill. Vandyke-Carter established the fungous nature of the infection and suggested the name "mycetoma" (fungous tumor). It became evident that species of *Nocardia* (Actinomycetes) as well as species of typically filamentous fungi could be the etiologic agents of the disease. Pinoy suggested that the infection be designated "actinomycosis" when the causative fungus was an Actinomycete and "true mycetoma" when the infection was caused by the higher fungi. Following this, Chalmers and Archibald proposed the two divisions: actinomycotic mycetoma, and maduromycosis. This latter classification is now in general use.

The fungi appear in the tissues as large lobulated granules composed of fungous hyphae. The character of the granule varies with the etiologic agent (color, size, shape, architecture) and often provides a clue to its identity.

In the United States the following fungi have been isolated from cases of maduromycosis: *Monosporium apiospermum (Allescheria boydii)*, *Madurella grisea*, and *Phialophora jeanselmei*, which in other parts of the world *Madurella mycetomii*, *Cephalosporium falciforme*, *Leptosphaeria senegalensis*, *Leptosphaeria tompkinsii*, and *Pyrenochaeta romerai* have been isolated from cases of maduromycosis.

Monosporium apiospermum, which has been isolated from several cases of maduromycosis in the continental United States, will be described as one of the etiologic agents of the disease.

MORPHOLOGY. *M. apiospermum* occurs in the tissues or serosanguineous exudates from draining sinuses as a lobulated, yellowish white granule, 0.5 to 2 mm in diameter. Micro-

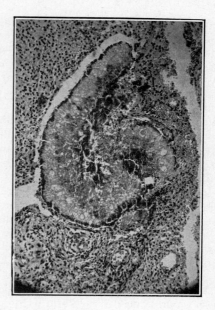

FIG. 87-12. Maduromycosis. Section of tissue from foot showing granule. ×112. (From Fineberg: Am J Clin Pathol 14:239, 1944)

scopically, the granule is composed of broad, septate hyphae, 2 to 4 μm in diameter, with numerous swollen cells, 15 μm in diameter, particularly around the periphery of the granule (Fig. 87-12).

CULTURAL CHARACTERISTICS. On Sabouraud's glucose agar at room temperature the colony at first is white and cottony, but later the aerial mycelium becomes grayish in color

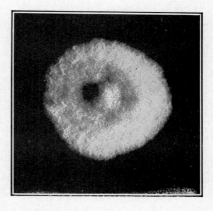

FIG. 87-13. *Monosporium apiospermum*. Colony on Sabouraud's glucose agar at room temperature for 15 days.

(Fig. 87-13). Microscopically, the conidia appear singly on the ends of conidiophores, occasionally from the sides of the hyphae or in small two to three clusters (Fig. 87-14). The spores are ovoid to clavate, with a truncate base at the point of attachment to the conidiophores, and are 5 to 7 by 8 to 10 μm in size.

Emmons has shown that a Canadian strain of *M. apiospermum* not only produces the imperfect spore form just described but also produces cleistothecia and asci, allowing the strain to be identified as *Allescheria boydii*, which was isolated from maduromycosis by Boyd and Crutchfield and described by Shear. According to the rules of botanical nomenclature, therefore, the name *M. apiospermum* should be discarded, since it represents merely the conidial stage of an ascomycetous fungus.

ANTIGENIC STRUCTURES. Reifferscheid and Seeliger reported positive agglutinins, precipitins, and complement-fixing antibodies in the serum of a patient with chronic maduromycosis due to *M. apiospermum*. Skin tests with culture filtrate and a polysaccharide extract gave positive, delayed, 48-hour reactions.

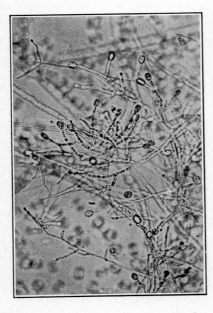

FIG. 87-14. *Monosporium apiospermum.* Single conidia on ends of conidiophores. ×305. (From Conant et al: Manual of Clinical Mycology, 3rd ed, 1971. Courtesy of W.B. Saunders Co)

Seeliger reported several strains of *M. apiospermum*, two strains of *A. boydii*, and one strain each of *Acremoniella lutzi* and *Madurella americana* to be antigenically identical.

SPONTANEOUS INFECTIONS IN ANIMALS. Infections have been reported in the horse, dog, and cat.

EXPERIMENTAL INFECTION IN LABORATORY ANIMALS. Rabbits, mice, and guinea pigs have been inoculated intravenously, subcutaneously, and intraperitoneally with little or no reaction to the fungus. Gammel and Moritz reported infection in rabbits by intraarticular inoculation of saline suspensions.

CLINICAL TYPES OF INFECTION IN MAN. Infection follows the introduction of the fungus into the tissues by injury. A slowly progressing, painless infection, taking weeks or months, evolves, with abscess formation, swelling, and the development of multiple draining fistulas from which granules are discharged in a serosanguineous fluid. If the foot is infected, it becomes deformed or club-shaped, and the small bones often show proliferative changes and punched-out areas of destruction. The infection remains localized, with extensions by direct invasion of tissue. There is no systemic reaction unless secondary bacterial infection takes place.

TRANSMISSION. Maduromycosis is a disease of the exposed parts of the body, particularly the feet and occasionally the leg and the hand. The source of the infection is exogenous, since more than half of the patients give a history of injury, such as a minor scratch, bruise, or introduction of foreign material into the skin. Strains of *A. boydii* have been isolated from soil.

A. boydii (*M. apiospermum*) also has been isolated from the sputum of a patient with a chronic, suppurative lung disease, from the blood of a patient with septicemia, from the spinal fluid of a patient with meningitis, and from patients with chronic otomycosis.

TREATMENT. Maduromycosis does not respond to the sulfonamides or known antibiotics. An occasional patient with true maduromycosis may be benefited temporarily by sulfonamides because of the elimination of superimposed bacterial infections. Seeliger reported successful treatment of a patient by intramuscular and peroral therapy with 2'2-dioxy-5'5-dichlordiphenysulfide. Neuhauser reported favorable response to DDS when a patient with infection by *M. grisea* was treated for an extended period of time. Strains of *M. apiospermum* have different sensitivity levels to amphotericin B. Most, however, are sensitive to 100 mg per ml, and the drug may be used locally. Surgical intervention for removal of diseased tissue and for adequate drainage must accompany any form of drug therapy.

CHROMOBLASTO-MYCOSIS

Chromoblastomycosis is an infection of the skin characterized by the development of warty or verrucous cutaneous lesions. The disease is caused by a variety of dematiaceous fungi: *Fonsecaea pedrosoi, Fonsecaea compactum, Cladosporium carrionii,* and *Phialophora verrucosa.*

Pedroso, in Brazil, was the first to observe the disease; he noted characteristic, dark brown bodies in a biopsy section. Although he isolated a darkly pigmented fungus and was aware of the fungous nature of the disease, he failed to report his observations. Lane and Medlar in Boston reported a new fungus, *Phialophora verrucosa,* which they isolated from lesions on the buttocks of an Italian patient in whose tissues they found spherical, dark brown bodies. Pedroso and Gomes then reported four Brazilian cases of "verrucous dermatitis" caused by *P. verrucosa.* Brumpt, however, renamed their fungus *Hormodendrum pedrosoi,* and Terra and others named the disease "chromoblastomycosis." One of the fungi isolated from the four Brazilian cases, however, was found later to be *P. verrucosa.* The third etiologic agent to be identified with this disease was described from Puerto Rico as *Fonsecaea compactum* by Carrión, and the fourth was described from Venzuela, South Africa, and Australia as *Cladosporium carrionii.*

MORPHOLOGY.   In spite of the variety of different fungi which have been isolated from

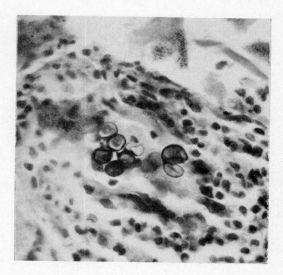

FIG. 87-15. *Fonsecaea pedrosoi.* Section of skin showing giant cell containing brown bodies. × 736.

chromoblastomycosis, they appear identical in clinical materials. They all appear in the pus, crusts, and in sections as thick-walled, dark brown, spherical bodies, 6 to 12 µm in diameter, which divide by septation rather than by budding (Fig. 87-15). The different genera and species can be identified only in culture where typical spore formation occurs. Only three of the fungi which cause chromoblastomycosis will be discussed below; a full discussion of the known agents of this disease has been published by Carrión and Silva.

CULTURAL CHARACTERISTICS.   *F. pedrosoi,* on Sabouraud's glucose agar at room tempera-

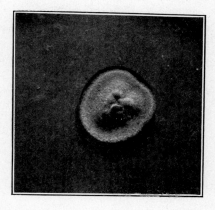

FIG. 87-16. *Fonsecaea pedrosoi.* Colony on Sabouraud's glucose agar at room temperature for 20 days.

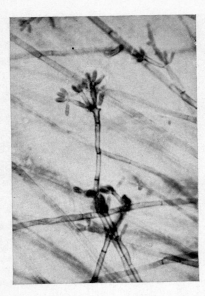

FIG. 87-17. *Fonsecaea pedrosoi.* Hormodendrum type of conidiophore. ×400. (From Conant et al: Manual of Clinical Mycology, 3rd ed, 1971. Courtesy of W.B. Saunders Co)

ceous conidia from conidiophores of varying length, *Hormodendrum* type (Fig. 87-17), (2) single ovoid conidia borne on the sides of swollen club-shaped ends of the conidiophores, *Acrotheca* type (Fig. 87-18), and (3) small conidia borne from the cuplike tip of flask-shaped conidiophores, *Phialophora* type. The prominence of each spore type varies with individual strains.

The three types of spore production exhibited by *F. pedrosoi* in culture have caused confusion in the classification of this fungus, and several attempts have been made to place *F. pedrosoi* in the single genus that would be acceptable.

F. compactum, on Sabouraud's glucose agar at room temperature, is a slow-growing, heaped, brittle colony covered with a coarse aerial mycelium, olive black in color (Fig. 87-19). Microscopically, subspherical conidia are borne in tight, compact, chain formation on the ends of conidiophores (Fig. 87-20). A *Phialophora* type of conidiophore also is developed by this fungus.

C. carrionii, on Sabouraud's glucose agar at room temperature, is a slow-growing, heaped, black colony usually only 2 to 4 cm in diameter in three to four weeks (Fig. 87-21).

Microscopically, this fungus produces loose, long, branching chains of elliptical spores not unlike the typical saprophytic species (Fig. 87-22). A *Phialophora* type of conidiophore is not found in this species.

P. verrucosa, on Sabouraud's glucose agar at room temperature, is a slow-growing, dark

ture, is a slow-growing, flat colony covered with a feltlike, short, aerial mycelium, dark green to brown or black in color (Fig. 87-16). Microscopically three types of spore formation are seen: (1) branching chains of ovoid oliva-

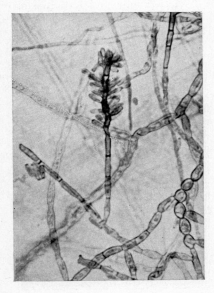

FIG 87-18. *Fonsecaea pedrosoi.* Acrotheca type of conidiophore. ×400 (From Conant et al: Manual of Clinical Mycology, 3rd ed, 1971. Courtesy of W.B. Saunders Co)

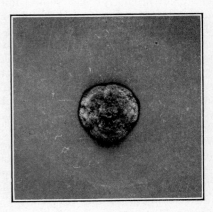

FIG. 87-19. *Fonsecaea compactum.* Colony on Sabouraud's glucose agar at room temperature for 14 days. (From Conant et al: Manual of Clinical Mycology, 3rd ed, 1971. Courtesy of W.B. Saunders Co)

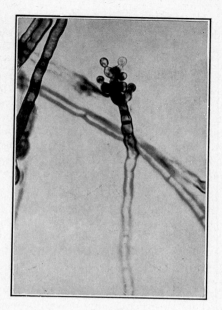

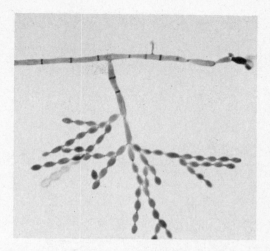

FIG. 87-22. *Cladosporium carrionii.* Conidiophore showing loose, branching chains of elliptical spores. ×825. (From Conant et al: Manual of Clinical Mycology, 3rd ed, 1971. Courtesy of W.B. Saunders Co)

FIG. 87-20. *Fonsecaea compactum.* Conidiophore with compact spore head. ×816. (From Conant et al: Manual of Clinical Mycology, 3rd ed, 1971. Courtesy of W.B. Saunders Co)

brown to black colony, with olivaceous to gray aerial mycelium (Fig. 87-23). Microscopically, the characteristic structures on the end of flask-shaped conidiophores is diagnostic for this species (Fig. 87-24). Abortive perithecia also have been reported in one strain.

The biochemical activity of these fungi is of little help in their identification. Fuentes and Bosch were able to show, however, that pathogenic strains differed in their biochemical activities from nonpathogenic, saprophytic species of *Cladosporium*. The pathogenic strains did not liquefy gelatin or Löffler's medium, coagulate milk, digest starch, or utilize tributyrin and cellulose. The nonpathogenic strains were positive in all of these tests, except that they did not attack tributyrin or cellulose.

ANTIGENIC STRUCTURE. Positive complement-fixation tests have been described by Martin et al. They found that several different

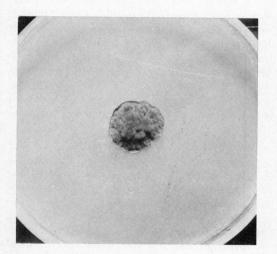

FIG. 87-21. *Cladosporium carrionii.* Colony on Sabouraud's glucose agar at room temperature for four weeks.

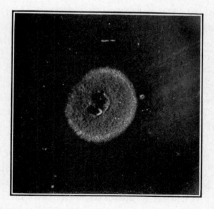

FIG. 87-23. *Phialophora verrucosa.* Colony on Sabouraud's glucose agar at room temperature for 20 days.

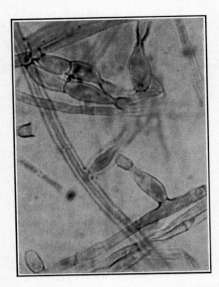

FIG. 87-24. *Phialophora verrucosa.* Typical conidiophore. ×1,500.

fungous antigens and several sera from noninfected human beings gave negative results in control tests and also that a close antigenic relationship exists between two morphologically different fungi, *F. pedrosoi* and *P. verrucosa,* in that a high-titered serum from a patient with chromoblastomycosis caused by' *F. pedrosoi* had complement-fixing antibodies for both fungi. Rabbits immunized with *F. pedrosoi, F. compactum,* and *P. verrucosa* produced complement-fixing antibodies for *F. compactum* and *P. verrucosa,* but anti-*P. verrucosa* rabbit serum contained complement-fixing antibodies only for the homologous antigen.

Seeliger and co-workers used agglutination, agglutinin-absorption, and precipitin tests for antigenic analyses of this group of fungi. Al-Doory and Gordon used fluorescent antibody techniques to distinguish *C. carrionii* from *Cladosporium bantianum.* Inaki reported precipitin, precipitin-absorption, and agar gel diffusion tests to give cross-reactions with antigens from 14 strains of these dematiaceous fungi.

EXPERIMENTAL INFECTION IN LABORATORY ANIMALS.   A chronic, progressive disease similar to that seen clinically in human beings has not been produced in animals, but local and systemic infections of a granulomatous type have resulted from experimental inoculations.

Duque reported that *Cladosporium trich-*

oides, F. pedrosoi, and *F. compactum* produced extensive lesions in the brains of young mice following intracerebral inoculation. Only *C. trichoides,* however, produced brain lesions following intraperitoneal injection. Saprophytic strains were not pathogenic. Feliger and Friedman reported similar results in experimental infections, with the exception that intraperitoneal inoculation resulted in dissemination to the brain. Experimental infections in man have been reported. These infections produce typical cutaneous chromoblastomycosis.

CLINICAL TYPES OF INFECTION IN MAN. Chromoblastomycosis is a unilateral infection, usually of the foot and leg, caused by the introduction of the fungus by trauma. The lesion begins on the skin as a papule, which evolves slowly over months or years and gradually develops into a verrucous, cauliflowerlike growth with the development of numerous satellite lesions. Metastases have been reported in only two cases. Early lesions that fail to show a typical verrucous appearance or lesions that occur on the hand, arm, neck, or face may not be suspected to be of fungous origin until the typical brownish bodies are seen in biopsy sections. A very benign, pigmented, superficial infection of the skin on the palmar aspect of the hand, tinea nigra palmaris, is caused by *Cladosporium werneckii.*

TRANSMISSION.   *P. verrucosa* exists in nature as one of several fungi that cause staining of logs, lumber, and wood pulp, from which it has been isolated and identified under the name *Cadophora americana.* The fungi isolated from chromoblastomycosis and those from nature have been shown to be both morphologically and antigenically identical. *F. pedrosoi* and *C. carrionii* also have been isolated from nature.

TREATMENT.   Small discrete lesions may be excised. Extensive lesions are treated best with sodium iodide administered intravenously, potassium iodide by mouth, and x-ray therapy to the local lesions. Iontophoresis, using copper sulfate, has been used with some benefit. Sulfonamides and antibiotics may be used to combat secondary bacterial infections.

The use of 5-fluorocytosine has proved successful in the treatment of twelve patients.

RHINOSPORIDIOSIS

Rhinosporidiosis, caused by *Rhinosporidium seeberi*, is an infection of man and domestic animals characterized by the formation of friable, sessile, or pedunculated polyps on the mucous membranes of the nose, nasopharynx, soft palate, and conjunctivas of the eyes, and rarely, in the ear, in the vagina, on the penis, or on the skin.

Seeber, in Buenos Aires, reported two cases of protozoan infection of the nose with polyp formation. The organism was named *Coccidium seeberi* by Wernicke in 1903. O'Kinealy, in India, reported the third case, and the organism was named *Rhinosporidium kinealyi* by Minchin and Fantham. Later, Seeber reported the identity of these two organisms, and the name *R. seeberi* was established. Until Ashworth's classic study of material from nasal polyps, the organism had been considered a protozoan. Although he was unable to obtain cultures, he demonstrated a morphologic similarity between the organism and rudimentary plants, such as those of the Chytridales. Until proved by culture, however, the position of *R. seeberi* must remain doubtful.

Of the many cases that have been reported in the United States, all have been infections of the conjunctivas.

MORPHOLOGY. *R. seeberi* occurs in the polypoid masses as round, thick-walled sporangia, 40 to 300 μ in diameter. The mature sporangia are filled with hundreds or thousands of spores, 6 to 8 μm in diameter (Fig. 87-25).

SPONTANEOUS INFECTIONS IN ANIMALS. Spontaneous infections have been reported in domestic animals, such as cattle, horses, and mules.

EXPERIMENTAL INFECTION IN LABORATORY ANIMALS. There have been no reports of successful animal inoculations.

CLINICAL TYPES OF INFECTION IN MAN. The most prevalent infection in man occurs on the mucosa of the nose, with initial symptoms of painless itching, accompanied by a mucoid discharge. Sessile lesions develop into polypoid masses, which bleed easily when traumatized. Such masses are pedunculate and may hang down from the nose or fall back into the posterior pharynx to cause obstruction. The polypoid masses are soft, nodular, and pale pink to purplish red in color, with minute, whitish, opaque areas (sporangia) scattered beneath the surface.

Infection of the conjunctivas may be minimal and not be detected by the patient, or the growths may be large enough to cause symptoms similar to those of foreign bodies. Granular, reddish, irregular masses may be seen on either the bulbar or palpebral conjunctiva.

TRANSMISSION. It is not known exactly how or where infection by *R. seeberi* is con-

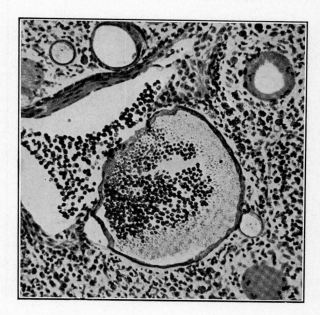

FIG. 87-25. Rhinosporidiosis. Section of nasal polyp showing mature and immature sporangia. ×175. (From Conant et al: Manual of Clinical Mycology, 3rd ed, 1971. Courtesy of W.B. Saunders Co)

tracted. Epidemiologic studies of large numbers of cases in India suggest infection during contact with stagnant water. However, an examination of water, silt, soil, and fish from stagnant waters did not reveal the organism. Inoculation of fish and snails with materials from human lesions was unsuccessful. Implantation of tissues on animals, cultures on a variety of media, serologic studies, and skin tests to demonstrate dermal sensitivity gave negative results. So far as is known, there is no transmission from man to man or from animal to man.

Tʀᴇᴀᴛᴍᴇɴᴛ. Removal of the masses by dissection and cauterization usually is effective, but recurrences are frequent when the masses are removed by snares. As an adjunct to surgical removal, Neostibosan may prove helpful.

FURTHER READING

SPOROTRICHOSIS

Du Toit CJ: Sporotrichosis on the Witwatersand. Proc Transval Mine Med Off Assoc 2nd ed, III, 1942

Fetter BF, Tindall JP: Cutaneous sporotrichosis. Clinical study of nine cases utilizing an improved technique for demonstration of organisms. Arch Pathol 781:613, 1964

Hektoeu L, Perkins CF: Refractory subcutaneous abscesses caused by *Sporothrix schenckii,* a new pathogenic fungus. J Exp Med 5:77, 1900

Ishizaki H: Some antigenic substances from culture filtrate of *Sporotrichum schenckii.* Jap J Dermatol 80:16, 1970

Karlan JV, Nielsen HS Jr: Serologic aspects of sporotrichosis. J Inf Dis 121:316, 1970

Mackinnon JE, Conti-Diaz IA, Geznde E, Civila E, Luz S da: Isolation of *Sporothrix schenckii* from nature and considerations of its pathogenicity and ecology. Sabouraudia 7:38, 1969

Mohr JA, Patterson CD, Eaton BG, Rhodes ER, Nichols NB: Primary pulmonary sporotrichosis. Am Rev Respir Dis 106:260, 1972

Norden A: Sporotrichosis. Clinical and laboratory features and a serological study in experimental animals and humans. Acta Path Microbiol Scand [Suppl] 89:13, 1951

Schenck BR: On refractory subcutaneous abscess caused by a fungus possibly related to *sporotricha.* Bull Johns Hopkins Hosp 9:286, 1898

Welsh MS, Dolan CT: Sporothorix whole yeast agglutination test. Am Clin Pathol 39:82, 1973

Wilson DE, Mann JJ, Bennett JE, Utz JP: Clinical features of extracutaneous sporotrichosis. Medicine 46:265, 1967

PHAEOSPOROTRICHOSIS

Kempson RH, Steinberg WH: Chronic subcutaneous abscesses caused by pigmented fungi. A lesion distinguishable from cutaneous chromoblastomycosis. Am J Clin Pathol 39:598, 1963

Mariat F, Segretain G, Destombes P, Darrasse H: Kyste souscutane mycosique (Pheo-sporotrichose) a *Phialophora gougerotii* (Martruchot 1910) Borelli 1955, observe au Senegal. Sabouraudia 5:209, 1967

Nielsen HS, Conant NF: A new pathogenic *Phialophora.* Sabouraudia 6:228, 1968

Schwartz IS, Emmons CW: Subcutaneous cystic granuloma caused by a fungus of wood pulp *(Phialophora richardsiae).* Am J Clin Pathol 49:500, 1968

Young JM, Ulrich E: Sporotrichosis produced by *Sporotrichum gougeroti.* Arch Dermatol 67:44, 1953

MADUROMYCOSIS

Emmons CW: *Allescheria boydii* and *Monosporium apiospermum.* Mycologia 36:188, 1944

Feiger JW: Mycetoma: review of the literature. Milit Med 128:762, 1963

Green WO Jr, Adams TE: Mycetoma in the United States. A review and report of seven additional cases. Am J Clin Pathol 42:75, 1964

Murray IG, Maligoub ES: Further studies in the diagnosis of mycetoma by double diffusion in agar. Sabouraudia 6:106, 1968

Nielsen HS Jr: Effects of amphotericin B in vitro on perfect and imperfect strains of *Allescheria boydii.* Appl Microbiol 15:86, 1967

Seeliger H: A serologic study of hyphomycetes causing mycetoma in man. J Invest Dermatol 26:81, 1958

CHROMOBLASTOMYCOSIS

Al-Doory Y: Chromomycosis. Missoula, Montana, Mountain Press Publishing Co, 1972

Callaway JL, Layman JD, Conant NF: Chromoblastomycosis. Laboratory infection with *Cladosporium carrionii.* Cutis 6:60, 1970

Carrion AL, Silva-Hunter M: Taxonomic criteria for fungi of chromoblastomycosis with reference to *Fonsecaea pedrosoi.* Int J Dermatol 10:35, 1971

Costello MJ, DeFeo CP, Littman ML: Chromoblastomycosis treated with local infiltration of amphotericin B solution. Arch Dermatol 79:184, 1959

Duque O: Meningo-encephalitis and brain abscess caused by *Cladosporium* and *Fonsecaea.* J Clin Pathol 36:505, 1961

Fuentes CA, Bosch ZE: Biochemical differentiation of the etiologic agents of chromoblastomycosis from nonpathogenic *Cladosporium* species. J Invest Dermatol 34:419, 1960

Gordon MA, Al-Doory Y: Application of fluorescent-antibody procedures to the study of pathogenic dematiaceous fungi. II. Serologic relationships of the genus *Fonsecaea.* J Bacteriol 89:551, 1965

Lopes CF, Cisalpino EO: Treatment of chromomycosis with 5-fluorocytosine. Int J Dermatol 10:182, 1971

Trejos A: *Cladosporium carrionii* n. sp. and the problem of Cladosporia isolated from chromoblastomycosis. Rev Biol Trop 2:75, 1954

Whiting DA: Treatment of chromoblastomycosis with high local concentrations of amphotericin B. Br J Dermatol 29:345, 1967

RHINOSPORIDIOSIS

Grover S: *Rhinosporidium seeberi* with a preliminary study of the morphology and life cycle. Sabouraudia 7:249, 1970

Karpova, MF: On the morphology of the rhinosporidiosis. Mycopathologia 23:281, 1964

Kameswaran S: Surgery in rhinosporidiosis. Experience with 293 cases. Int Surg 46:602, 1966

Cameron HM, Gatei D, Brenner AD: The deep mycoses in Kenya: a histopathological study. 4. Rhinosporidiosis. East Afr Med J 50:413, 1973

Vanbreuseghem R: Ultrastructure of *Rhinosporidium seeberi*. Int J Dermatol 12:20, 1973

88
The Dermatomycoses

THE DERMATOPHYTES

The dermatophytes are parasites of man and animals that live in the superficial keratinized areas of the body: the skin, hair, and nails. The fungi responsible for such infections have been placed in three genera: *Microsporum*, *Trichophyton*, and *Epidermophyton*. Species of these genera are considered to be keratinophilic fungi because of their specialized attack on the keratin of the body.

Such infections are known to the layman as "athlete's foot," "jockey itch" and "ringworm," and although they do not kill, they are unsightly and often disabling and present a serious problem both to the private practitioner and the public health authorities. *Microsporum audouinii* has caused extensive epidemics of ringworm of the scalp among schoolchildren in certain areas of this country, while *Trichophyton tonsurans* has been reported as the cause of epidemics in the adult and adolescent.

After a technique for culturing keratinophilic fungi from soil was described, many species of *Microsporum* and *Trichophyton* have been isolated from soil samples collected in various parts of the world. A natural grouping of the dermatophytes has resulted in the following divisions: anthropophilic, zoophilic, and geophilic. The anthropophilic organisms are found to infect man only, the zoophilic organisms to infect animals and man, and the geophilic organisms to be widespread in nature where they are found in the soil. The geophilic organisms may infect man or animals, but a considerable number of them are considered to be saprophytic species. Thus, there are saprophytic soil isolates that do not produce lesions on the hair, skin, or nails of man or animals but whose morphology would place them among the dermatophytes, where they are called "related species."

Using a hair-baiting technique, it has been possible to grow the perfect state (sexual stage) of some of the dermatophytes. These perfect states produce sexual spores (ascospores), allowing the fungi to be placed in the class Ascomycetes of the family Gymnoascaceae, where the genera *Nannizzia* and *Arthroderma* have been created.

Morphology The dermatophytes present only rudimentary structures in their parasitic habitats of hair, skin, and nails. As seen in potassium hydroxide preparations, the fungi appear as mycelial fragments in the skin and nails (Fig. 88-1) or as arthrospores arranged inside or outside the hair (Figs. 88-2, 88-3, and 88-4). To establish an identification of the fungus, however, it is necessary to culture the organisms on artificial media in order to observe the type and arrangement of spore forms.

Cultural Characteristics The dermatophytes grow on a variety of simple media, but they usually are cultivated on Sabouraud's glucose agar at room temperature. Both the appearance of the colonies and the microscopic morphology are necessary for generic and specific classification. The nutritional investigations of some of the dermatophytes have provided more satisfactory differential media upon which colony formation, pigmentation, and spore production are more consistent.

The isolation of dermatophytes from contaminated clinical materials is greatly facilitated by the use of Sabouraud's glucose agar to which has been added chloramphenicol (0.05 mg per ml) and cycloheximide (Acti dione) in a concentration of 0.5 mg per ml.

A brief description of the important genera and species as they appear in culture follows.

GENUS EPIDERMOPHYTON. This genus contains a single species that invades the skin and nails but does not invade the hair. The fungus

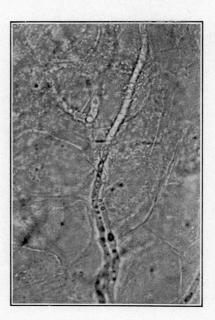

FIG. 88-1. Branching hypha seen in potassium hydroxide preparation of the skin. ×275.

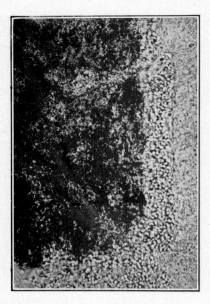

FIG. 88-2. Microsporum spore sheath around hair. ×350.

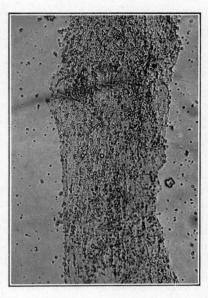

FIG. 88-4. Trichophyton hair of favus type with numerous hyphae and bubbles. ×305.

is seen in these clinical materials as broken fragments of hyphae and cannot be distinguished from species of *Microsporum* or *Trichophyton* without a culture. This genus is characterized by numerous oval to broadly cla-

vate (club-shaped), smooth-walled macroconidia produced in clusters or directly from the sides of hyphae. No microconidia are produced.

Epidermophyton floccosum. Perfect state: unknown. On Sabouraud's glucose agar the colony is powdery and greenish yellow and quickly develops a white, cottony, aerial myce-

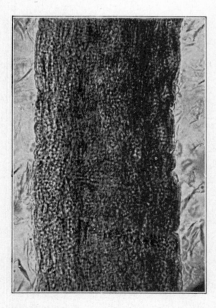

FIG. 88-3. Trichophyton hyphae and spores inside hair of endothrix type. ×170. (From Conant et al: Manual of Clinical Mycology, 3rd ed, 1971. Courtesy of W.B. Saunders Co)

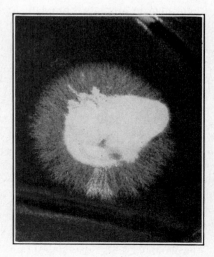

FIG. 88-5. *Epidermophyton floccosum.* Colony on Sabouraud's glucose agar at room temperature for 12 days.

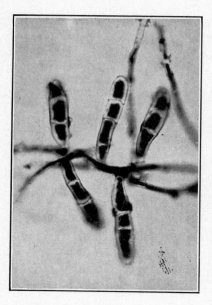

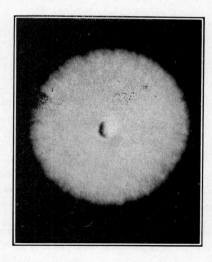

FIG. 88-7. *Microsporum audouinii.* Colony on Sabouraud's agar at room temperature for 12 days.

FIG. 88-6. *Epidermophyton floccosum.* Typical macroconidia borne laterally on hyphae. ×736.

lium which spreads eventually to cover the surface (Fig. 88-5). Numerous clavate, two- to six-celled, smooth-walled macroconidia, 7 to 12 by 20 to 40 μm in size, are produced from the sides of hyphae or in clusters (Figs. 88-6). Chlamydospores are numerous throughout the culture. This species is considered to be anthropophilic in that it affects only humans.

Genus Microsporum. This genus contains species that invade the hair and skin but rarely the nails. In the hair, the genus is characterized by a mosaic sheath of small spores which surrounds the hair shaft and as mycelium fragments in the skin. Some species give infected hair a greenish fluorescence under the Wood's light.

This genus is characterized by numerous echinulate, multiseptate, fusiform to obovate, thin- to thick-walled macroconidia and by few clavate microconidia.

Microsporum audouinii. Perfect state: unknown. On Sabouraud's glucose agar the colony is slow-growing, matted, and velvety, later developing radial grooves and producing an orange pigmentation in the agar (Fig. 88-7). Macroconidia are scarce and, when found, usually are immature and appear as expanded ends of hyphae which have failed to develop fully.

Rarely a few bizarre forms may be found (Figs. 88-8, 88-9). Microconidia may appear in primary cultures, but they become more numerous in subsequent transfers. Pectinate hyphae and raquette hyphae may be numerous. This species is considered anthropophilic in that it infects only humans. It is the cause of epidemic tinea capitis in children. Infected hairs exhibit a

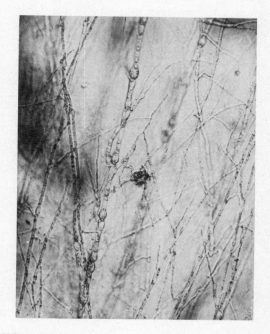

FIG. 88-8. *Microsporum audouinii.* Showing raquette hyphae and a nodular body. ×1,000.

bright yellow-green fluorescence in Wood's light.

Microsporum canis. Perfect state: unknown. On Sabouraud's glucose agar the colony is fast-growing, with a loose, white, aerial mycelium that becomes tan to brown in color and develops an orange pigmentation in the agar. Macroconidia are abundant and appear as thick-walled, echinulate, fusiform 6- to 14-celled spores, 8 to 15 by 40 to 150 μm in size (Fig. 88-10). Microconidia become numerous on transfer. Raquette hyphae and chlamydospores are numerous. This species is considered zoophilic in that it is primarily an animal parasite which causes sporadic infections in humans. When isolated from man, it generally was called *Microsporum lanosum*, but if cultured from an animal, it generally was named after the animal, hence, such designations as *Microsporum canis, Microsporum felineum,* and *Microsporum equinum.* Infected hairs exhibit bright yellow-green fluorescence in the Wood's light.

Microsporum gypseum. Perfect state: *Nannizzia gypsea* and *Nannizzia incurvata.* On Sabouraud's glucose agar the colony is fast-growing, powdery, and cinnamon brown in color, with an orange pigmentation in the agar

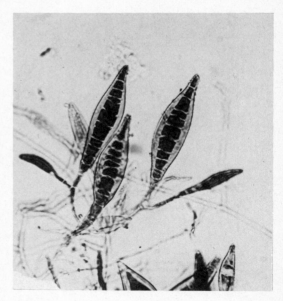

FIG. 88-10. *Microsporum canis.* Typical fusiform macroconidia. ×736.

(Fig. 88-11). Echinulate macroconidia are abundant and appear as thin-walled, elipsoid, four- to six-celled spores, 8 to 12 by 30 to 50 μm in size (Fig. 88-12). Microconidia become numerous on transfer. Raquette hyphae and chlamydospores are produced.

This species has been cultured from soil throughout the world and is said to be "geophilic." It is primarily an animal parasite which

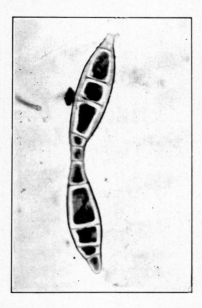

FIG. 88-9. *Microsporum audouinii.* Bizarre type of macroconidium. ×736.

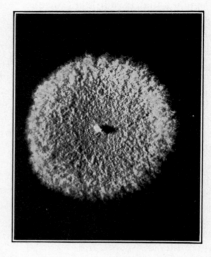

FIG. 88-11. *Microsporum gypseum.* Colony on Sabouraud's glucose agar at room temperature for seven days.

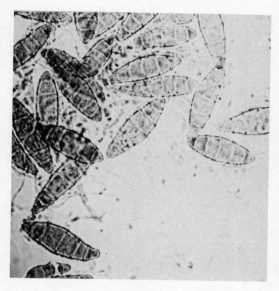

FIG. 88-12. *Microsporum gypseum.* Typical thin-walled macroconidia. ×1,000.

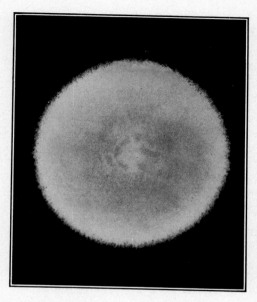

FIG. 88-13. *Trichophyton mentagrophytes.* Colony on Sabouraud's glucose agar (gypseum type) at room temperature for 10 days.

causes sporadic infection in humans. Infected hairs have no or poor fluorescence under the Wood's light.

Of the other species of *Microsporum* which have been described, some have been isolated from soil, while others have been reported as an infrequent cause of infection in man and animals.

GENUS TRICHOPHYTON. This genus contains seveal species that invade the hair, skin, and nails. The genus is more difficult to characterize because spores are lacking in some species, and it is necessary to resort to an artificial grouping of species by colony characteristics rather than by microscopic morphology. The nutritional studies mentioned previously have aided greatly in the identification of certain species. When grown on suitable media containing accessory growth substances, better growth and sporulation are induced. When macroconidia are produced, they are few in number, smooth-walled, elongated, thin-walled, clavate, smooth spores. The numerous microconidia, which are subspherical, pyriform, or clavate, develop from the sides of hyphae, en thyrses, or in grapelike clusters, en grappe.

Trichophyton mentagrophytes. Perfect state: *Arthroderma benhamiae.* On Sabouraud's glucose agar the colonies may be pow-

dery and tan to buff in color—gypseum type—or the aerial hyphae may be compact, white and cottony—interdigitale type (Figs. 88-13, 88-14). Typical for this species is the development of numerous subspherical microconidia in grapelike clusters (Figs. 88-15) or along the sides of

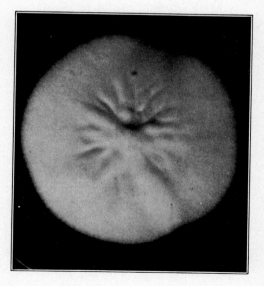

FIG. 88-14. *Trichophyton mentagrophytes.* Colony on Sabouraud's glucose agar (interdigitale type) at room temperature for eight days.

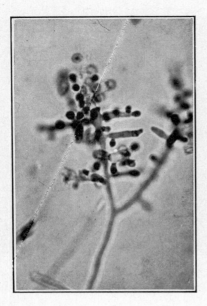

FIG. 88-15. *Trichophyton mentagrophytes.* Conidiophores from which clusters of microconidia (en grappe) develop. ×375. (From Conant et al: Manual of Clinical Mycology, 3rd ed, 1971. Courtesy of W.B. Saunders Co)

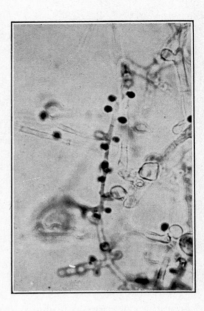

FIG. 88-16. *Trichophyton mentagorphytes.* Microconidia borne laterally on hypha (en thyrses) ×375. (From Conant et al: Manual of Clinical Mycology, 3rd ed, 1971. Courtesy of W.B. Saunders Co)

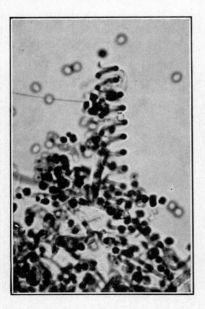

FIG. 88-17. *Trichophyton mentagrophytes.* Coiled hypha. ×375. (From Conant et al: Manual of Clinical Mycology, 3rd ed, 1971. Courtesy of W.B. Saunders Co)

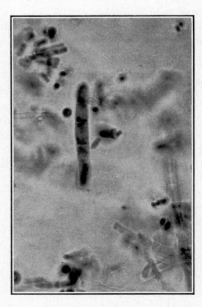

FIG. 88-18. *Trichophyton mentagrophytes.* Typical clavate macroconidium. ×736.

the hyphae (Fig. 88-16) and the coils of hyphae (Fig. 88-17). Macroconidia, when produced, are elongated, clavate, thin-walled spores, 4 to 6 by 10 to 50 μm in size (Fig. 88-18). This species is found in ectothrix infections of the hair and in infections of the beard. This species can be differentiated from *Trichophyton rubrum* by giving a positive urease test within a week and by producing perforations in hair when grown in vitro.

Trichophyton rubrum. Perfect state: unknown. On Sabouraud's glucose agar the colony at first is white, but it quickly develops a reddish to purplish pigmentation both in the aerial mycelium and in the agar (Fig. 88-19). Different strains will vary greatly in the amount of pigment produced and may remain cottony white, with the pigment confined to the reverse side of the colony in the agar. Consistent pigment formation is developed on corn meal dextrose agar, and characteristic macroconidia are developed on heart infusion agar plus tryptose and blood agar base. Macroconidia are smooth, long, slender, and pencil-shaped; microconidia are more numerous, elongated, clavate, and single-celled. The appearance of these conidia helps distinguish this species from *T. mentagrophytes*. This species, which often is referred to as *T. purpureum*, causes recalcitrant lesions of the skin and nails.

Trichophyton equinum. Perfect state: unknown. This species is very similar to *T. mentagrophytes* and has been placed in synonymy with it by several investigators. However, Georg et al have shown this species to differ in morphologic characteristics and in nutritional requirements for growth. *T. equinum* has an absolute requirement for nicotinic acid. *T. equinum* has caused epizootic equine ringworm in the United States and in other parts of the world, and man becomes infected by contact with these animals. This species causes ectothrix infection of the hair.

Trichophyton tonsurans. Perfect state: unknown. On Sabouraud's glucose agar the slow-growing, velvety colony becomes heaped, folded, and cream to yellowish in color (Fig. 88-20). Some strains have a central crater (crateriform). Macroconidia are rare or lacking, but the microconidia are elongated, with clavate spores attached to the sides of the hyphae. Characteristic macroscopic morphology of typical strains of this species is developed on Sabouraud's glucose agar. Microscopic morphology and spore production develop better on wort agar. Suspected atypical cultures can be identified by the requirement of this species for thiamine. There are many synonyms for this species because of the great variations in the gross colony characteristics of different strains. This species is found in endothrix infections of the hair and, like other endothrix fungi, is difficult to eradicate.

Whereas *M. audouinii* causes epidemic ringworm of the scalp only in children, epidemics caused by *T. tonsurans* are carried over into adult life, or the fungus can directly infect the adult scalp.

Trichophyton violaceum. Perfect state: unknown. On Sabouraud's glucose agar, the slow-

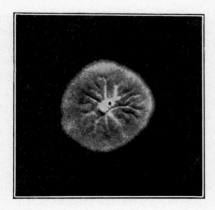

FIG. 88-19. *Trichophyton rubrum.* Colony on Sabouraud's glucose agar at room temperature for 12 days.

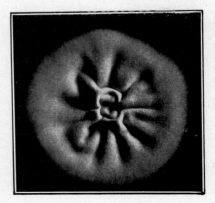

FIG. 88-20. *Trichophyton tonsurans.* Colony on Sabouraud's glucose agar at room temperature for 35 days.

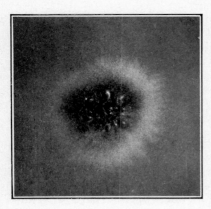

FIG. 88-21. *Trichophyton violaceum.* Colony on Sabouraud's glucose agar at room temperature for 27 days.

growing colony is folded, heaped, smooth, and waxy and develops a deep violet pigmentation (Fig. 88-21). On subsequent transfers a white aerial overgrowth may develop. Better colony formation is obtained by the addition of thiamine or pyrimidine to the medium. Microscopically, spore forms are lacking, and only swollen hyphae and chlamydospores are seen. This fungus is found in endothrix infections of the hair and causes lesions which are difficult to cure. This species infects the adult scalp, on which are found black dots characterized by the hair having broken off at the follicle.

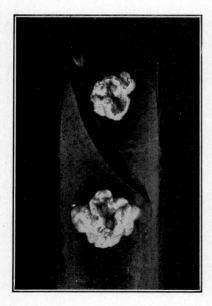

FIG. 88-22. *Trichophyton schoenleinii.* Colony on Sabouraud's glucose agar at room temperature for 28 days.

Trichophyton schoenleinii. Perfect state: unknown. On Sabouraud's glucose agar the slow-growing colony becomes smooth, waxy, and folded (Fig. 88-22). A short aerial mycelium may develop in subsequent transfers. Except in special media, spore forms are lacking or scarce, but when present they are typical of the genus *Trichophyton.* Morphologically, the fungus is composed of short-celled, swollen hyphae with numerous chlamydospores and favic chandeliers, so called because they appear as antlerlike processes on the ends of hyphae in the agar. The generic name *Achorion,* however, has been discarded because the fungus clearly belongs to the genus *Trichophyton,* species of which cause a variety of lesions. This fungus is isolated from typical favus lesions and causes a particular type of endothrix infection of the hair. It infects the adult scalp.

Trichophyton verrucosum. Perfect state: unknown. On Sabouraud's glucose agar the colony is slow-growing, heaped, and deeply folded, with a smooth, waxy surface or with a fine, white surface down. Better growth is obtained on Sabouraud's glucose agar with added thiamine. On enriched thiamine medium both macroconidia and microconidia are produced.

This species produces ringworm in cattle and other domestic animals, from which man becomes infected. It causes large-spored ectothrix infection of the hair.

Other species of *Trichophyton* that have been described occur in other parts of the world and are not encountered in ringworm infections in the United States.

Fungous Metabolites   Neither endotoxins nor exotoxins are produced by the dermatophytes. Saline extracts of dried and powdered cultures, filtrates of a two- to three-months' culture mat ground up with its own liquid medium, and other such preparations have been shown to contain allergens which elicit positive skin tests in sensitized individuals. Such skin testing material has been called "tricophytin." Protein and carbohydrate fractions have been isolated from synthetic media in which *T. mentagrophytes* and *T. rubrum* were grown. Since many of the dermatophytes produce pigments in culture, the nature of these substances has been the subject of numerous investigations.

Antigenic Structure The dermatophytes contain group-specific antigens, which can be demonstrated by the Schultz-Dale technique in guinea pigs or by the Prausnitz-Küstner technique in humans. A protein fraction obtained from broth filtrates of *T. mentagrophytes* and *T. rubrum* gave positive precipitin reactions in sera of rabbits immunized by the homologous fungus. No cross-reactions occur with these antigens in heterologous sera. Kitamura reported polysaccharide and protein fractions of *T. mentagrophytes* to give positive precipitin tests in the serum of rabbits inoculated intravenously with a suspension of live fungus.

Antigens common to *T. rubrum, T. metagrophytes, Hormodendrum* species, and *Penicillium* species have been demonstrated by agar gel diffusion, hemagglutination, and hemagglutination-inhibition tests.

The production of cutaneous infection in animals results in the development of a cellular antibody which can be demonstrated by the reaction to the intracutaneous injecton of trichophytin. Such reactions become positive in 24 to 48 hours and may last for seven days. Animals infected and subsequently sensitized with one of the dermatophytes usually react to injections of products from other dermatophytes, indicating the presence of group antigens. Keeney and Huppert induced hypersensitivity and increased resistance to infection by topical applications of a specially prepared antigen of *T. mentagrophytes*. A positive skin test in human beings signifies past or present infection and cannot be used as a means of diagnosis.

Spontaneous Infection in Animals Spontaneous dermatophytoses have been observed in the cat, dog, horse, calf, cow, sheep, squirrel, monkey, and rat. Many of these animal strains also are pathogenic for man.

Experimental Infection in Laboratory Animals Experimental cutaneous infections can be established in a variety of laboratory animals. *M. audouinii*, however, seems to be primarily a parasite of man, since infections in animals do not occur spontaneously or after experimental inoculations. Although guinea pigs infected experimentally with dermatophytes occasionally have positive blood cultures, they never show lesions of their internal organs. Dermatophytes are apparently adapted exclusively for growth in ectodermal structures. If the skin of a guinea pig is traumatized and spores are injected intravenously, no lesions of the internal organs occur, but characteristic cutaneous infections develop in the areas of trauma.

Occasional reports imply that some species can exist in and invade internal organs of experimentally infected animals.

Clinical Types of Infection in Man The most prevalent type of dermatophytosis in man is that which occurs on the feet, particularly on the webs between the toes. This type of infection is known popularly as "athlete's foot" and usually is caused by species of *Trichophyton* or *E. floccosum*. Crops of small itching vesicles appear between the toes and, after being ruptured by trauma, discharge a thin serous fluid which causes maceration and peeling of the superficial layers of the skin, accompanied by the appearance of cracks and fissures. Even in the absence of secondary bacterial infection, the lesions persist as indolent infections for months or years, with occasional acute exacerbations. A secondary infection with bacteria often results in an acute inflammatory reaction, with lymphangitis and lymphadenitis. Many patients infected with species of *Trichophyton* become highly allergic to the fungi, which not only increases the intensity of the local reaction but often results in the appearance of vesicular lesions, indistinguishable from the primary infections, in other parts of the body. Such lesions, which are particularly common on the palms of the hands, do not contain fungi and are referred to as dermatophytids.

Ringworm of the scalp, known as tinea capitis, occurs in childhood and usually heals spontaneously at puberty. However, a few of the dermatophytes, such as *T. schoenleinii, T. violaceum,* and *T. tonsurans*, produce lesions which persist into adult life. Infections with *M. canis* are acquired by contact with infected cats and dogs and usually are sporadic. In contrast, infections with *M. audouinii* and *T. tonsurans,* which are acquired by contact with other infected children, can occur in epidemic form.

Transmission The dermatophytes cause infection of man and animals, and this group contains the only known pathogenic fungi for which there is a known transmission from man to man or animal to man. Hairs infected with *M.*

audouinii cause epidemics of tinea capitis in children by direct contact, by the use of contaminated clippers in barber shops, and by contact with contaminated theater seats. Tinea pedis, or athlete's foot, is thought to be transmitted from man to man by the common use of shower bath facilities in clubs, schools, and colleges. Epidemics, such as the one due to *E. floccosum* which involved a ship's crew, occasionally occur when extraordinary conditions favor the spread of a particular type of organism. Infections can be transmitted from cats, dogs, cows, and other animals to persons coming in contact with infected animals. The infections usually are sporadic and can be traced to the animal with little difficulty.

Biologic Products   Skin testing material trichophytin, can be made in the laboratory or purchased from biologic supply companies. Occasionally the material can be used for desensitization as an adjunct to other forms of therapy.

Treatment   Since the discovery of Gentles that griseofulvin given by mouth cures experimental ringworm infections in guinea pigs, this antibiotic has been used extensively for the treatment of infection in human beings.

FURTHER READING

Ajello L: Present day concepts of the dermatophytes. Mycopathologia 17:315, 1962

Ajello L: A taxonomic review of the dermatophytes and related species. Sabouraudia 6:147, 1968

Ajello L, Georg LK: In vitro hair cultures for differentiation between atypical isolates of *Trichophyton mentagrophytes* and *T. rubrum*. Mycopathol Mycol Appl 8:1, 1957

English MP: Tinea pedis as a public health problem. Br J Dermatol 81:705, 1969

English MP: Some unusual dermatophyte infections. Sabouraudia 7:265, 1970

Friedman L, Derbes VJ: The question of immunity in ringworm infections. Ann NY Acad Sci 89:178, 1960

Gentles JC: The treatment of ringworm with griseofulvin. Br J Dermatol 71:427, 1959

Georg LK, Camp LB: Routine nutritional tests for the identification of dermatophytes. J Bacteriol 74:113, 1957

Georg LK: Animal ringworm in public health. Diagnosis and nature. US Department of Health, Education, and Welfare. PHS, Bureau of States Services, CDC, 1959

Grappel SF, Fethiere A, Blank F: Macroconidia of *Trichophyton schoenleinii*. Sabouraudia 9:144, 1971

Griseofulvin and Dermatomycoses. An International Symposium. Arch Dermatol 81:5, 1960

Lepper AWD: Immunological aspects of dermatomycosis in animals and man. Rev Med Vet Mycol 6:435, 1969

Padhye AA, Blank F, Koblenzes PJ, Spatz S, Ajello L: *Microsporum persicolor* infection in the United States. Arch Dermatol 108:561, 1973

Rippon JW, Malkinso, FD: *Trichophyton simii* infection in the United States. Arch Dermatol 102:552, 1970

Taplin D, Zaias N, Rebell G, Blank H: Isolation and recognition of dermatophytes on a new medium (DTM). Arch Dermatol 99:203, 1969

Vanbreuseghem R: Technique biologique pour l'isolement des dermatophytes du sol. Ann Soc Belg Med Trop 32: 173, 1952

Vanbreuseghem R, DeVroey C, Takashio M: Production of macroconidia by *Microsporum ferrugineum* Ota 1922. Sabouraudia 7:252, 1970

89
Opportunistic Fungous Infections

CANDIDIASIS

Lagenbeck was the first to demonstrate a yeastlike fungus in the lesions of thrush. The fungus was named *Oidium albicans* by Robin and *Monilia albicans* by Zopf. Berkhout proposed the generic name *Candida* to include these fungi, which developed a pseudomycelium and reproduced by budding, but before 1930 many generic names and over 100 species had been recorded in the literature. The single genus *Candida* has been accepted generally, and the recognized human pathogenic species, to be included in this genus have been reduced. Of these species only *Candida albicans* is considered to be pathogenic, but other species are encountered in pathologic conditions. The review of the yeastlike fungi by Skinner and Fletcher is an excellent summary of the information available concerning these organisms, while Winner and Hurley's book, *Candida albicans*, gives a definitive account of that species.

C. *albicans*, which had been isolated heretofore only from human or animal sources, has been isolated from soil and vegetable sources in nature.

MORPHOLOGY. *C. albicans* is a small, oval, budding yeastlike fungus, 2.5 by 4 by 6 μm. It develops a pseudomycelium by elongation of cells which fail to detach. In sputum, tissue, and exudates both the budding cells and fragments of pseudomycelium may be seen (Fig. 89-1). Typical chlamydospores serve to distinguish *C. albicans* from other species of *Candida* (Fig. 89-2). Hasenclever, however, has discussed other species that can produce this structure (*Candida stellatoidea* and *Candida tropicalis*). Also, *C. albicans* can be identified by pseudomycelial formation on selected media and by pigment production in the colony.

CULTURAL CHARACTERISTICS. *C. albicans* grows readily (24 to 48 hours) at both room and incubator temperatures on Sabouraud's glucose agar. The colonies are of moderate size, smooth, and pasty, and have a characteristic yeasty odor. Older colonies (giant colonies) may be honeycombed in the center and develop radial furrows (Fig. 89-3). There is no surface growth in broth (48 hours). Glucose and

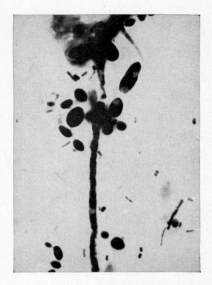

FIG. 89-1. *Candida albicans.* Gram stain of sputum smear showing budding cells and pseudohyphae. ×1,175.

maltose are fermented with acid and gas, sucrose with acid only, and lactose is not fermented. The fermentations are apt to be irregular unless conditions are carefully controlled.

C. *albicans* produces a distinctive filamentous colony in two days on a streaked plate of Levine eosin-methylene blue agar at 37C in 10

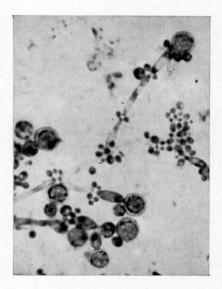

FIG) 89-2. *Candida albicans.* Characteristic chlamydospores from corn meal agar. ×790. (From Conant: Am Rev Tuberc 61:696, 1950)

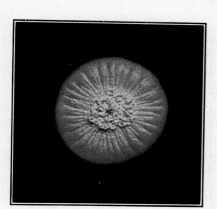

FIG. 89-3. *Candida albicans.* Giant colony on Sabouraud's glucose agar at room temperature for 20 days.

percent CO_2. Different species of *Candida* may be identified rather accurately by (1) the type of colony developed on blood agar plates at 37C (10 days), (2) the type of growth in Sabouraud's glucose broth at 37C (48 hours), (3) development and morphology of blastospores, chlamydospores, and pseudomycelium on corn meal agar at room temperature, and (4) the fermentation reaction after 10 days at 37C in glucose, maltose, sucrose, and lactose.

FUNGOUS METABOLITES. Salvin reported toxemia in mice inoculated intraperitoneally with a suspension of killed *C. albicans* and tubercle bacilli. Mourad and Friedman also produced a toxemia in mice by intravenous injection of soluble substances obtained by sonic oscillation of *C. albicans, Candida robusta,* and *Candida reukaufi.* However, Ekmen could not demonstrate toxins from sonic extraction, mechanical disruption, or acetone-treated cells of *C. albicans.* *C. albicans* has been shown to have a capsular polysaccharide. Neytcheff reported polysaccharides of *C. albicans* extracted with phenol to have a minimum pyrogenic activity at 0.9 mg per kilogram and to be 55 to 580 times as potent as polysaccharides obtained from *C. tropicalis, Candida krusei,* and *Candida pseudotropicalis.* Mannans have been extracted from *Candida* cell walls.

ANTIGENIC STRUCTURE. Serologic studies have shown recognized species of *Candida* to be closely related antigenically. Some of the species could be differentiated specifically by absorbed serums, but *C. albicans* and *C. tropi-*

calis seemed to be antigenically identical. Vogel and Collins reported a specific hemagglutination test to detect antibodies in anti-*C. albicans* rabbit serum. Tsuchiya and others have proposed an antigenic structure for seven species of *Candida* and have reported heat-stable and heat-labile antigens based on antigenic analyses. Their type-specific sera have allowed accurate and rapid identification of species within the genus. Gordon reported anti-*C. albicans* fluorescent conjugate to be specific and to differentiate *C. albicans* from *C. stellatoidea,* particularly if absorbed with *Candida parakrusei.* Kaplan and Kaufman reported two distinct serologic groups of *C. albicans* based on fluorescent antibody techniques. Hasenclever and Mitchell demonstrated two antigenic groups for *C. albicans* by agglutination and agglutinin-absorption studies. These groups (A and B) were shown to be antigenically similar to *C. tropicalis* and *C. stellatoidea,* respectively. Mannans extracted from these species have been used as agglutinin-inhibiting antigens with conflicting results. Organisms of groups A and B differed little in their pathogenicity for rabbits and mice, and a study of isolates from patients did not reveal one group to be more pathogenic than the other. Gordon et al also used immunofluorescence to separate *C. albicans* groups A and B, *C. stellatoidea, C. tropicalis,* and *Torulopsis glabrata.*

Since *C. albicans* may be found in the mouth, intestinal tract, and vagina of many normal individuals, little diagnostic significance can be attached to the findings of a positive skin test or agglutinins. Drake reported that a high percentage of sera from normal individuals contained agglutinins for *C. albicans.* Chew and Theus found group A *C. albicans* mannan precipitins in concentrated globulin fractions of sera from healthy individuals in Peer immunodiffusion tubes.

EXPERIMENTAL INFECTION IN LABORATORY ANIMALS. The rabbit is particularly susceptible to infection with *C. albicans* but relatively, if not absolutely, resistant to the other species of *Candida.* Rabbits injected intravenously with 1 ml of a 1 percent saline suspension of *C. albicans* die in four to five days with typical abscesses in the kidneys. Rabbits having a high agglutinin titer because of previous immunization are not protected against a subsequent injection of lethal dose of the organism.

A number of reports have shown enhancement of infection in mice with *C. albicans* when they have also received gastric mucin, alloxan, tetracyclines, and/or cortisone. However, mice are uniformly susceptible to *C. albicans* by intravenous inoculation. Therefore, these animals have been used extensively for studies on the pathogenesis of *C. albicans* infections. They have also been used to demonstrate active immunity to *C. albicans* infection after injection of living cells, sonically ruptured cells, and cell wall preparations.

The ability of *C. albicans* to produce pseudomycelium quickly upon injection into animals is said to interfere with phagocytosis and thus enhance its virulence. Balish and Svilha showed the mycelial form of *C. albicans* to differ in cell wall structure, storage of an essential amino acid, methionine, in the form of S-adenosylmethionine, and structure of the cytoplasmic membranes, each of which was thought to enhance virulence.

CLINICAL TYPES OF INFECTION IN MAN.

It is difficult to evaluate the presence of *C. albicans* in cultures obtained from clinical materials. In infections of the lungs, for example, the fungus is found often as a secondary invader superimposed upon tuberculosis or a malignancy. In sprue and pernicious anemia the fungus is isolated frequently from stool specimens, but these findings merely indicate the presence in greater quantity of an organism that can be isolated from the normal intestinal tract. The fungus also may be cultured from mouth lesions which were initiated by dietary deficiencies.

The extensive use of antibiotics, particularly the tetracyclines, has resulted in candidiasis' complicating the primary disease. Infection of the mucous membranes, the mucocutaneous areas (thrush, perleche, vaginitis, and vulvovaginitis) and generalized candidiasis have been reported following the use of these antibiotics.

In disseminated candidiasis in the adult, other predisposing factors include treatment with adrenal glucocorticoids, surgery of the vascular system, cardiac surgery, and organ transplantation which might necessitate prolonged use of plastic intravenous catheters.

C. albicans, however, can produce infections of various types in which the fungus can be recognized as the primary etiologic agent. Candidiasis (thrush) of the oral mucous membranes occurs in infants and eldery people with wasting diseases. Vaginitis, vulvovaginitis, and infection of the vaginal mucosa are not uncommon in diabetes and during pregnancy.

Candidiasis of the skin may follow maceration of tissue resulting from constant exposure to water (housewives or bartenders) or from friction of adjacent parts in obese patients (axillas, inframammary areas, and inguinal region). The presence of *C. albicans* in the intestinal tract may serve to infect such areas.

Generalized candidiasis is rare, but *C. albicans* has been the primary cause of meningitis. Endocarditis following cardiac surgery has been reported.

TRANSMISSION.

Since *C. albicans* is found in the mouth and intestinal tract of a high percentage of human beings, the fungus may spread from such locations to cause skin and nail infections. Aspiration of material may lead to bronchopulmonary infections, which eventually, though rarely, may initiate generalized infection. Such types of infection can be assumed to be endogenous in origin. Infections due to *C. albicans* can be transmitted, however. Balanoposthitis has been observed in the husbands of women with vaginitis, and cutaneous candidiasis about the nipples of nursing mothers has been caused by infants with oral thrush. Thrush frequently occurs in infants who became infected by passage through the birth canal of a mother with vaginitis.

TREATMENT.

Nystatin has proved to be useful in the treatment of candidiasis. Amphotericin B and 5-fluorocytosine, however, are potent antifungous agents and have been used successfully in the treatment of *Candida* infections.

ASPERGILLOSIS

Aspergillosis, caused by *Aspergillus fumigatus* most frequently but by other species of *Aspergillus* as well, is an acute or chronic inflammatory granulomatous infection of the sinuses, bronchi, lungs, and occasionally other parts of the body.

Since species of *Aspergillus* are ubiquitous, it is difficult to ascribe pathogenicity to an isolate from any orifice in the body or from the sputa of patients with undiagnosed pulmonary infections. *A. fumigatus*, however, is a recognized pathogen of birds, both wild and domestic, as well as of animals and man. As early as 1856 Virchow reported autopsy findings in human pulmonary aspergillosis, and Renon in 1897 discussed aspergillosis in both human and animal infections. Aspergillosis has been recognized as an occupational disease occurring among those who handle and feed squabs and among the handlers of furs and hair.

MORPHOLOGY *A. fumigatus,* in the sputum of patients with pulmonary aspergillosis, appears as broken fragments of hyphae, and occasionally conidia may be seen. When hyphal fragments or conidia are seen, cultures must be obtained for identification. Only repeated cultures from such materials are indicative of etiologic significance.

Aspergillus may appear as a hyphal mass or ball in a cyst or closed cavity in the lungs. This is referred to as an "aspergilloma." Mycelium and spore heads may be seen lining the wall of an open cavity or in bronchial casts seen in sputum in bronchitis. In tissues, septate, twisted, dichotomously branching hyphae may be seen in gram-stained sections but are better stained with the PAS technique (periodic acid – Schiff stain) (Fig. 89-4). Frequently the hyphae invade the walls of blood vessels, eventually their lumens, and cause infarction.

CULTURAL CHARACTERISTICS. *A. fumigatus* grows rapidly on Sabouraud's glucose agar to form a white, cottony colony which becomes velvety (Fig. 89-5). As spores are produced, it attains a dark green powdery appearance. Microscopically the typical *Aspergillus* conidiophore is seen (Fig. 89-6). The vesicle is covered on the upper half with phialides, which produce chains of dark green, spherical conidia.

RESISTANCE. The discovery by Fourneau and others that sulfanilamide was the active ingredient of Prontosil was based on the fungistatic activity of this material during in vitro studies on the growth of *Aspergillus niger, Aspergillus fumigatus, Aspergillus jeanselmei,* and *Lichtheimia italica.* It is interesting to note, therefore, that the first in vitro demonstration of the drug, from which so many important derivatives have been made, was based on fungistatic rather than on bacteriostatic experiments.

A. niger is inhibited for 24 hours by 1 : 10,000, for 8 to 10 days by 1 : 1,000, and for two months by 1 : 100 concentrations of sulfanilamide. Senturia and Wolf showed that 20 to 30 mg of sulfanilamide powdered over the surface of the culture inhibited *A. niger, A. fumigatus, A. glaucus,* and *A. sydowi,* while sulfathiazole, sulfadiazine, sulfaguanidine, and sulfamerazine

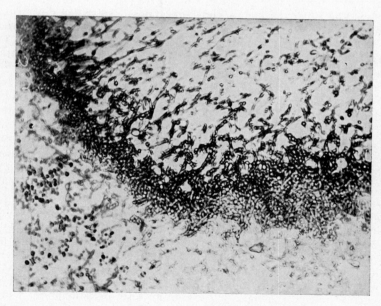

FIG. 89-4. Aspergillosis. Hyphae forming dense mass in section of lung. ×245. (From Weed et al: Mayo Clin Proc 24:463, 1949)

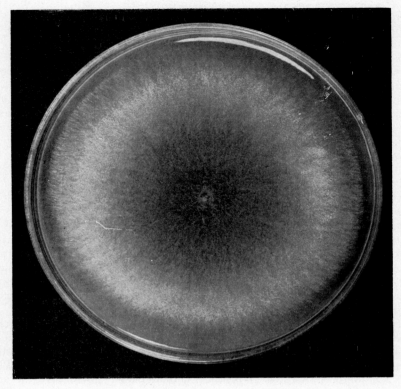

FIG. 89-5. *Aspergillus fumigatus.* Colony on Sabouraud's glucose agar at room temperature for six days. (Conant et al: Manual of Clinical Mycology, 3rd ed, 1971. Courtesy of W.B. Saunders Co)

were ineffective. Strains isolated from broncho-pulmonary aspergillosis by Hinson, et al were insensitive to penicillin, streptomycin, chloramphenicol, and aureomycin. Amphotericin B, however, has inhibited some strains of *Aspergillus* in concentrations of 0.1 to 40 μg per ml of medium.

Endotoxins have been demonstrated in *A. fumigatus* and in *A. flavus.* A polysaccharide of low toxicity for the rabbit and a lipoid which causes monocytosis and tubercle formation and which shows adjuvant properties have been reported. From another pathogenic species, *Aspergillus nidulans,* extracted cell sap was found to be nontoxic for rabbits and guinea pigs but produced a delayed reaction on intracutaneous injection for previously infected rabbits. On the other hand, Bodin and Gauthier found a toxic substance in filtrates of cultures of *A. fumigatus* which was lethal for rabbits but harmless for pigeons and guinea pigs. These various extracts from *A. fumigatus* may produce dermatonecrotic, hemolytic, or nephrotoxic

reactions. A substance designated aspergillin O has been extracted from filtrates of culture media of *Aspergillus oryzae.* This extract has proteolytic, fibrinolytic, and anticoagulant properties.

ANTIGENIC STRUCTURE.   Henrici's cell sap toxin on injections into rabbits results in the production of precipitins and antihemolysins. The polysaccharide isolated from *A. fumigatus* by Stanley and the cell sap isolated from *A. nidulans* by Drake were found to be antigenic in that precipitins could be demonstrated in the sera of previously inoculated rabbits. Immune serum from rabbits has been shown to prevent effects of toxins in experimental animals. Henrici was able to immunize rabbits actively against toxins of *A. fumigatus.*

Pepys and others reported positive immediate wheal reactions and direct bronchial sensitivity tests in asthmatics. A peculiar delayed skin reaction, reaching its maximum in 24 hours, was considered to be an Arthus type of

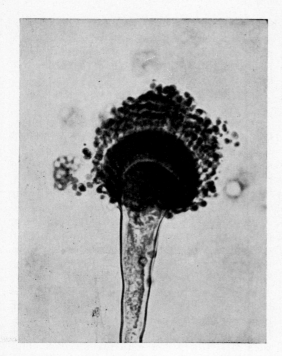

FIG. 89-6. *Aspergillus fumigatus.* Typical conidiophore. ×824. (From Conant et al: Manual of Clinical Mycology, 3rd ed, 1971. Courtesy of W.B. Saunders Co)

reaction because of its eosinophilic nature. This reaction was said to be due to precipitating antibody in patients' sera. Complement-fixing antibodies to *Aspergillus* antigens have been reported by Junke and Theone and by Seeliger. Precipitation, hemagglutination, collodion, and latex particle agglutination tests have been described with a variety of antigens from species of *Aspergillus* and *Penicillium.* The agar-gel diffusion technique also has been used. This test has shown common antigens to be shared by *Aspergillus* species and other saprophytic and pathogenic fungi.

Species of *Aspergillus* cause a variety of diseases in many different animals: pulmonary infection in lambs, mycotic abortion in cattle, and aspergillosis in chickens and a variety of wild and captive birds. The presence of aspergilli in moldy substrates makes billions of spores readily available for inhalation infections.

EXPERIMENTAL INFECTION IN LABORATORY ANIMALS. Cattle, chickens, pigeons, rabbits, and guinea pigs may be infected by inoculating spores intravenously or intraperitoneally or by introducing them into the respiratory passages.

Ford and Friedman compared the relative virulence of several species of *Aspergillus* for mice. They could find no physiologic or morphologic differences that would explain degrees of virulence.

CLINICAL TYPES OF INFECTION IN MAN. Otomycosis probably is secondary to bacterial infections of the ear, with the fungus existing saprophytically on the macerated tissue or earwax. Hearing may be impaired by obstruction of the canal with a mycelial mass and epithelial debris. The symptoms are those of intense itching and edema, and not infrequently the pain may become unbearable.

Involvement of the sinuses simulates infection by pyogenic bacteria.

Infection of the subcutaneous tissues of the foot produces the typical picture of maduromycosis.

Infection of the nails simulates infection by dermatophytes.

Bronchial infections simulate bronchitis caused by bacteria and may be associated with asthma.

Bronchiectasis complicated by infection with an *Aspergillus* may result in a so-called aspergilloma in which the mass of fungus distends and occupies a large area of cavitation. The fungus does not invade the bronchial wall. Repeated hemoptysis is the only symptom. The x-ray is characteristic and diagnostic.

Bronchopulmonary aspergillosis may be characterized by frequent pyrexial attacks associated with severe cough, purulent, occasionally blood-tinged sputum with flecks of white or brownish material containing mycelium, and a high eosinophilia. Serial roentgenograms show sifting shadows appearing with pyrexial attacks.

Systemic aspergillosis results from predisposing factors which, in the debilitated patient, interfere with humoral and tissue defense mechanisms. Patients with preexisting leukemia, Hodgkin's disease, collagen diseases, malignancies, and so on, are frequently infected with *A. fumigatus.* The therapy, antibiotics and antimetabolites, available for the primary diseases may also predispose to secondary mycotic infections.

Transmission.   Species of *Aspergillus* are ubiquitous. They are found in the soil, water, and air, on foodstuffs and animal products, and may be cultured from almost any body orifice. Members of the genus are constant contaminants of clinical materials, such as sputum, pus, feces, wax from the ear, and exudates from open lesions. They may be cultured from the gastric contents, and at autopsy they frequently are seen and cultured from necrotic lesions of the lungs resulting from neoplasma or tuberculosis.

Conditions creating moisture and prolonged dampness are conducive to the growth of molds, and a moldy environment predisposes to infection by *A. fumigatus*.

Treatment.   Surgery has been effective in certain types of pulmonary aspergillosis. Demonstrated sensitivity in aspergillosis has been treated by desensitization with autogenous vaccines. Sodium iodide intravenously and potassium iodide by mouth may prove effective. Amphotericin B is perhaps the only antibiotic useful in drug therapy of aspergillosis.

PHYCOMYCOSIS

Phycomycosis, caused by species of *Mucor*, *Absidia*, and *Rhizopus*, is a rapidly fatal disease of man, in whom primarily the brain but occasionally the lungs and other organs are invaded. The disease has been reported most often in patients with uncontrolled diabetes mellitus and is characterized by intraorbital cellulitis and a meningoencephalitis, with invasion of the wall and lumen of blood vessels resulting in acute inflammation and vascular thrombosis.

A subcutaneous infection caused by *Basidiobolus meristosporus* is seen in India, southeast Asia, and central Africa. This is a chronic infection of the subcutaneous tissues of the thorax and upper arm which occurs in children and many adults, with a tendency to spontaneous healing after various periods of time.

Many cases of phycomycosis in man and animals have been described in the literature. With few exceptions, cultures were not obtained, and the diagnosis was based on postmortem studies of tissues. Bauer and others and McCall and Strobos have cultured *Rhizopus oryzae*, while Harris cultured *Rhizopus arrhizus* from diabetic patients with cerebral infections. A culture of *Rhizopus rhizopodiformis* has been obtained from a cutaneous lesion of a diabetic by Baker et al.

Morphology.   Large, broad, nonseptate, branching hyphae, 7 to 15 μm in diameter and 100 to 200 μm in length, are seen in the affected tissues, particularly in the wall and lumen of blood vessels which contain thrombi infiltrated with hyphae. The fungus can be readily demonstrated in hematoxylin and eosin-stained sections (Fig. 89-7). In fresh preparations or potassium hydroxide mounts of scrapings from sinuses, the fungus appears as extremely wide, nonseptate, hyaline, branching hyphae (Fig. 89-8).

The mycelium of the Phycomycetes differs from that of all other fungi in that it is broad, nonseptate, and coenocytic. These characteristics allowed the hyphal fragments seen in tissues to be identified with the Phycomycetes rather than with other possible groups of fungi, and the term "mucormycosis" was given to infections in which such hyphae were seen. Since fungi belonging to different genera of the Phycomycetes have been cultured from tissues in which nonseptate hyphae have been seen, the term "phycomycosis" has been adopted for diseases caused by these fungi.

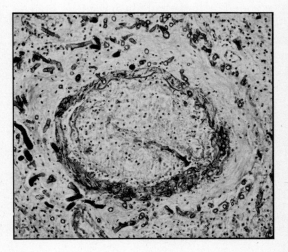

FIG. 89-7. Phycomycosis. Hyphae in wall and lumen of blood vessel and in pulmonary alveoli. ×150. (From Conant et al: Manual of Clinical Mycology, 3rd ed, 1971. Courtesy of W. B. Saunders Co)

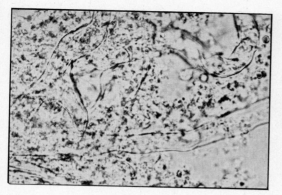

FIG. 89-8. *Rhizopus arrhizus.* Wide, nonseptate hyphae seen in potassium hydroxide preparation in scraping from lesion on palate.

CULTURAL CHARACTERISTICS. *Absidia co-rymbifera* has been isolated from bovine phycomycosis, while *R. oryzae* and *R. arrhizus* have been isolated from human cases. Species of these two genera of the Mucorales grow quickly and fill the test tube or petri dish with loose, grayish mycelium in three to four days (Fig. 89-

9). *Absidia* and *Rhizopus* produce runners, stolons, which attach themselves to the walls of the test tube or to the cover of the petri dish with holdfasts, rhizoids. The rhizoids may be seen microscopically by focusing through the test tube wall or petri dish cover with the low-power objective (Fig. 89-10).

In *Absidia* the sporangiophores arise in fascicles from the arching internodes of the stolons between the rhizoid-bearing nodes. The sporangia are terminal and pyriform, the columella hemispheric with papillate apical prolongation, and the sporangiospores small.

In *Rhizopus* the sporangiophores arise in fascicles from the node of the stolon directly opposite the tuft of rhizoids. The sporangia are terminal and globose, the columella hemispheric, and the sporangiospores oval or angular, smooth, or with longitudinal striations.

In *Mucor* stolons are not produced, and the sporangiophores arise directly from the mycelium. They are simple or branched and terminate in a sporangium. The sporangia are large, globose, and have an evanescent wall; the columella is continuous with the sporangiophore

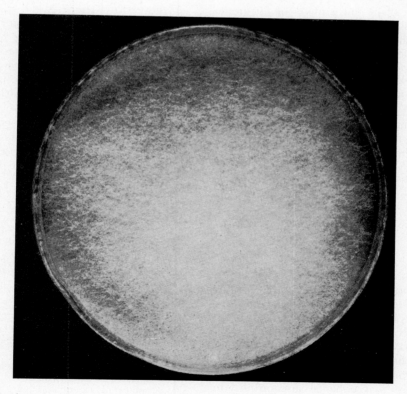

FIG. 89-9. *Rhizopus arrhizus.* Culture on Sabouraud's glucose agar at room temperature for seven days.

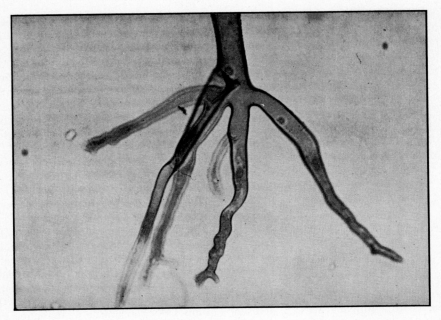

FIG. 89-10. *Rhizopus oryzae.* Rhizoids typical of the genus *Rhizopus.* ×450. (From Baur et al: Am J Med 18:822, 1955)

and varies in shape but is never hemispheric, and sporangiospores are globose to elliptical, with a smooth thin wall.

Genera and species in the *Phycomycetes (Mucorales)* can be differentiated only by their methods of sporulation, sexual and asexual, which occur in culture on suitable media. The three species belonging in two genera of the *Mucorales* mentioned previously, therefore, appeared identical in tissue and were identified by isolation and a study of their cultural characteristics.

Since the species mentioned above have been, and others may yet be, isolated from cases of phycomycosis, identification of cultures from this disease can be obtained only by reference to monographs on this group of fungi.

EXPERIMENTAL INFECTION IN LABORATORY ANIMALS.   Cerebral and pulmonary phycomycosis has been produced with *R. oryzae* and *R. arrhizus* in rabbits made diabetic with alloxan. Pulmonary infection could be established only in the acute toxic diabetic rabbit. The reaction of the chronic diabetic rabbit did not differ greatly, and the prolonged use of broad-spectrum antibiotics also may enhance susceptibility to the disease.

TREATMENT.   There is no specific treatment for phycomycosis. The majority of cases have been diagnosed at necropsy. In one instance the disease was diagnosed by biopsy and culture, and the patient recovered with control of her diabetes, desensitization with autogenous vaccine, and potassium iodide therapy. The surgical removal of a localized, intracerebral, septic formation, caused by a phycomycete, resulted in complete recovery.

In the absence of a known specific treatment, amphotericin B should be used in proven cases of phycomycosis.

FURTHER READING

CANDIDIASIS

Hasenclever HF: The consistent formation of chlamydospores by *Candida tropicalis.* Sabouraudia 9:164, 1971

Herrell WE: The antifungal activity of 5-fluorocytosine. Clin Med 78:11, 1971

Kozinn PJ, Taschdjian CL, Seelig MS, Cardine L, Teitler A: Diagnosis and therapy of systemic candidiasis. Sabouraudia 7:98, 1969

Louria DB, Stiff DP, Bennett B: Disseminated moniliasis in the adult. Medicine 41:307, 1962

Schöneback J, Steen L, Tarnvik A: 5-fluorocytosine treatment of *Candida* infections of the urinary tract and other sites. Scand J Urol Nephrol 6:37, 1972

Schöneback J, Polak A, Fernex M, Scholer HJ: Pharmacokinetic studies on the oral antimycotic agent 5-fluorocytosine in individuals with normal and impaired kidney function. Chemotherapy 18:321, 1973

Schönebeck J, Åuséhn S: The occurrence of yeast-like fungi in the urine under normal conditions and in various types of urinary tract pathology. Scand J Urol Nephrol 6:123, 1972

Stickle D, Kaufman L, Blumer O, McLaughlin DW: Comparison of a newly developed latex agglutination test and an immunodiffusion test in the diagnosis of systemic candidiasis. Appl Microbiol 23:490, 1972

Taschdjian CL: Routine identification of *Candida albicans*, current methods and a new medium. Mycologia 49:332, 1957

Taschdjian CL, Kozinn PJ: Opportunistic yeast infections with special reference to candidiasis. Ann NY Acad Sci 174:431, 1970

Vandevelde AG, Mauceri AA, Johnson JE: 5-flourocytosine in the treatment of mycotic infections. Ann Intern Med 77:43, 1972

Weld JT: *Candida albicans*. Rapid identification in culture with carbon dioxide and modified eosin-methylene blue medium. Arch Dermatol Syph 66:691, 1952

Winner HL, Hurley R: *Candida albicans*. Boston, Little, Brown 1964

ASPERGILLOSIS

Austwick PKC: In Raper KB, Fennell DI (eds): The Genus *Aspergillus*. Baltimore, Williams & Wilkins, 1965, Chap 7

Bardana EJ, McClatchy JK, Farr RS, Minden P: The primary interaction of antibody to components of aspergilli. I. Immunological chemical characterization of nonprecipitating antigen. J Allergy Clin Immunol 50:208, 1972

British Thoracic and Tuberculosis Report. Aspergilloma and residual tuberculous cavities—The results of a resurvey. Tubercle 51:227, 1970

Coleman RM, Kaufman L: Use of immunodiffusion test in the serodiagnosis of aspergillosis. Appl Microbiol 23:301, 1972

Ikenoto H, Watanbe K, and Mori T: Pulmonary aspergilloma. Sabouraudia 9:30, 1971

Kwon-Chung KJ, Fennell DI: A new pathogenic species of *Aspergillus*. Mycologia 63:478, 1971

Meyer RD, Rosen P. et al Aspergillosis complicating neoplastic disease. Am J Med 54:6, 1973

Stevens EAM, Russchen CJ, Hilvering C, Orie NGM: Steroid effect on *Aspergillus* antibodies. Scand J Respir Dis 51:55, 1970

Young RC, Bennett JE: Invasive aspergillosis. Absence of detectable antibody response. Am Rev Respir Dis 104:710, 1971

Young RC, Jennings A, Bennett JE: Species identification of invasive aspergillosis in man. Am J Clin Pathol 58:554, 1972

PHYCOMYCOSIS

Addleston RD, Baylin GJ: Rhinocerebral mucormycosis. Radiology 115:113, 1975

Baker RD, Seabury JH Schneidau JD Jr: Subcutaneous and cutaneous mucormycosis and subcutaneous phycomycosis. Lab Invest 11:1091, 1962

Bauer H, Ajello L, Adams E, Hernandez DU: Cerebral mucormycosis: pathogenesis of the disease, description of the fungus, *Rhizopus oryzae* isolated from a fatal case. Am J Med 18:822, 1955

Burkitt DP, Wilson AMM, Jelliffe DB: Subcutaneous phycomycosis: a review of thirty-one cases seen in Uganda. Br Med J 1:1669, 1964

Emmons CW: Phycomycosis in man and animals. Rev Patol Vegetale 4:329, 1964

Haim S, Better OS, Lichtig C, Erlik D, Barzilai A: Rhinocerebral mucormycosis following kidney transplantation. Isr J Med Sci 6:646, 1970

Harris JS: Mucormycosis. Report of a case. Pediatrics 16:857, 1955

Hutter RVP: Phycomycosis infection (mucormycosis) in cancer patients, a complication of therapy. Cancer 12:330, 1959

Klokke AH, Job CK, Warlow PFM: Subcutaneous phycomycosis in India. Report of four cases with review of the disease. Trop Geogr Med 18:20, 1966

Landau JW, Newcomer VD: Acute cerebral phycomycosis (mucormycosis). J Pediatr 61:363, 1962

Langston C, Roberts DA, Porter GA, Bennett WM: Renal phycomycosis. J Urol 109:941, 1973

Lowe JT, Hudson WR: Rhinocerebral phycomycosis and internal carotid-artery thrombosis. Arch Otolarngol 101:100, 1975

McCall W, Strobos RRJ: Survival of a patient with cerebral nervous system mucormycosis. Neurology 7:290, 1957

Medoff G, Kobayashi GJ: Pulmonary mucormycosis. N Engl J Med 286:86, 1972

Meyer RD, Kaplan MH, Marin O, Armstrong D: Cutaneous lesions in disseminated mucormycosis. JAMA 225:737, 1973

Meyer RD, Rosen P, Armstrong D: Phycomycosis complicating leukemia and lymphoma. Ann Intern Med, 77:871, 1972

Reinhardt DJ, Kaplan W, Ajello L: Experimental cerebral zygomycosis in alloxan diabetic rabbits. Infect Immun 2:404, 1970

Smith JMB: Mycoses of the elimentary tract. Gut 10:1035, 1969

Straatsma BR, Zimmerman LE, Gass JDM: Phycomycosis. A clinicopathologic study of fifty-one cases. Lab Invest 11:963, 1963

90
Miscellaneous Mycoses

MYCOTIC KERATITIS

Fungous infection of the cornea by a large variety of fungi follows trauma and bacterial infection. Of recent concern, however, is the increasing incidence of mycotic infection of the diseased eye following antibiotic and topical cortisone treatment.

Leber in 1879 described the first case of keratomycosis, proved its fungous etiology, and reproduced the disease in laboratory animals. For a number of years, *Aspergillus fumigatus* has been responsible for the majority of cases proven by culture. Since the advent of antibiotics and corticosteroids, the list of fungi known to infect the cornea has increased to include many saprophytic as well as a few pathogenic fungi.

MORPHOLOGY. In corneal scrapings the filamentous fungi appear as septate, branching mycelial fragments (Fig. 90-1). Such a finding does not allow identification of the fungus. Cultures must be made and identified by their characteristic sporulating structures. Occasionally, budding yeast cell with pseudomycelium may be seen in microscopic preparations from the diseased eye. A tentative identification of *Candida* species may be made under these circumstances.

The fungi may not be visible in hematoxylin-eosin-stained sections of the eye. Sections should be stained by the Gridley, the PAS, or the Gomori methenamine silver stain. In the Gridley- and PAS-stained sections the fungous elements will appear red, and in the Gomori methenamine silver-stained sections they will appear black.

CULTURAL CHARACTERISTICS. The fungi are situated deep in the corneal stroma. Scrapings deep in the ulcer or at its edge must be made to obtain material for examination and culture. Sabouraud's glucose agar with chloramphenicol (0.05 mg per ml) should be used to avoid bacterial contamination. Pieces of the curetted materials are placed on the agar slant, and the cultures are held at room temperature. Many different fungi have been isolated from the ulcerated cornea. The diversity ranges from yeastlike species of *Candida* to any filamentous fungus that occurs as a saprophyte in nature. Cultures made from corneal scrapings may be identified as *Aspergillus* species, *Fusarium* species, *Penicillium* species, *Scopulariopsis* species, *Cephalosporium* species, *Monosporium* species, *Curvularia* species, and others.

FUNGOUS METABOLITES. Little is known about the metabolites that would allow saprophytic fungi to invade the corneal tissue. Injury seems to be necessary for invasion, but the continued growth and destructive abilities of the various fungi are probably dependent on products elaborated during growth. Burda and Fisher reported that a crude mycelial extract of *Cephalosporium serrae* produced corneal destruction in the rabbit eye, and further purification of this material allowed them to believe it to be a constitutive proteinase. Dudley and Chick found a mycelial extract of *Fusarium moniliforme* to produce intracorneal necrosis in the rabbit eye.

EXPERIMENTAL INFECTION IN LABORATORY ANIMALS. Many investigators have produced experimental corneal ulceration in laboratory animals. Primary pathogenicity can be demonstrated by inoculation following trauma. Ley produced corneal infections in rabbits by the use of cortisone and oxytetracycline.

CLINICAL TYPES OF INFECTIONS IN MAN. Infection is initiated by trauma due to vegetable substances (twigs, corn stalks, and so on) or by wounds caused by foreign bodies which lodge in the cornea. The fungous spores carried into the wound germinate to produce a mycelial growth.

A white plaque develops at the site of trauma. The cornea usually is not vascularized, and ulceration develops in the corneal tissue surrounding these opacities.

TREATMENT. Nystatin and amphotericin B drops have proved effective in some cases. The drugs can reach the fungus only after removal of as much necrotic tissue as possible. All corticosteroids should be withdrawn from treatment.

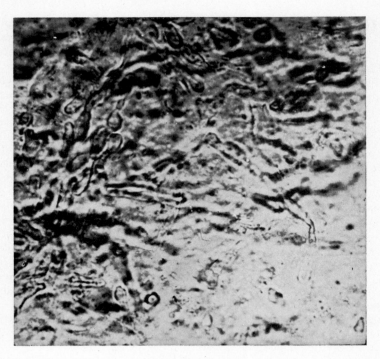

FIG. 90-1. Corneal scraping showing hyphae of invading fungus. (Courtesy of E. W. Chick, Veterans Administration Hospital, Durham, North Carolina)

TINEA VERSICOLOR

Tinea versicolor is an infection of the skin caused by *Malassezia furfur*. The lesions usually appear on the trunk, but they may also occur on the neck, face, and arms. They appear as irregular, circumscribed, brownish red, furfuraceous patches which fluoresce under the Wood's light. Cultures are not made, since the clinical diagnosis can be confirmed by microscopic examination of the furfuraceous scales.

MORPHOLOGY. In potassium hydroxide preparations or stained preparations of the scales, the fungus appears as clusters of round, budding cells, 3 to 8 μm in diameter, intermixed with short fragments of hyphae (Fig. 90-2). Newer techniques for obtaining scales for staining and microscopic examination have been described. Keddie and others have used cellulose tapes applied to the skin to remove the horny layer with its flora of yeast cells and hyphae characteristic for tinea versicolor. These tapes may be stained in a variety of ways

or placed on suitable media for direct culture of the fungus. A particular tape, Eastman No. 910 Monomer, removes the layer of horny cells and hairs. Such preparations show the localization of *M. furfur* within follicles as well as in the surrounding stratum corneum.

CULTURAL CHARACTERISTICS. For a number of years it was not known with certainty if *M. furfur* had been or could be cultured from scales. In spite of the abundance of fungous elements seen in microscopic preparations of scraping taken from the lesions, numerous negative reports attested to the variety of media. Gordon in 1951, however, was able to grow a yeastlike fungus from the scales of normal skin and from tinea versicolor scales on Sabouraud's glucose slants overlaid with olive oil. Antibiotics, penicillin (20 units per ml) and streptomycin (40 units per ml), were added to the medium to prevent growth of contaminating bacteria. The culture obtained, *Pityrosporum obiculare*, was a white to cream colored, yeastlike growth on incubation at 30 to 37C. The

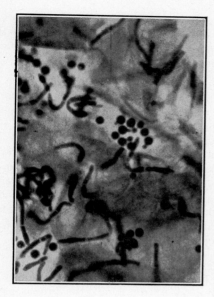

FIG. 90-2. *Malassezia furfur.* Clusters of round cells and short hyphal segments ×736.

yeast cells are spherical with buds attached by a narrow isthmus, 2.8 to 3.8 μ in diameter. *P. obiculare* does not grow at 25C or at higher temperatures without oils or other fatty substances and is considered to be lipophilic.

TRANSMISSION. Tinea versicolor is rarely, if ever, transmitted from person to person. The rare report of conjugal infection and repeated failures to infect healthy skin with scales or cultures of *P. obiculare* have prevented epidemiologic investigations or studies concerning the pathogenesis of this disease. Burke in 1961, however, was able to infect a patient who had Cushing's syndrome, a patient on steroid therapy, and a patient with nutritional deficiency. These results would indicate biochemical or physiologic changes in the skin to be necessary predisposing factors for tinea versicolor. In a later study, an analysis of lipid level, fatty acid, and amino acid content of normal skin and skin of patients with tinea versicolor did not reveal significant differences. It is felt, however, that predisposition by one or many factors is necessary for infection.

ANTIGENIC STRUCTURE. Sternberg and Keddie and Keddie and Shadomy have shown by immunofluorescent techniques that *P. obiculare* and the fungus in scales are antigenical-

ly similar. These investigators also showed that a patient's serum would agglutinate cells of *P. obiculare* and, by the indirect immunofluorescent technique and by absorption tests, that antigenic similarity exists.

SPONTANEOUS INFECTION IN ANIMALS. Tinea versicolor is a human disease, and all attempts to infect animals have failed.

CLINICAL TYPES OF INFECTION IN MAN. The infection often is asymptomatic, with only an occasional complaint of pruritis. The lesions are superficial, furfuraceous, irregular, or circumscribed brownish red patches. Of diagnostic value is the ease with which the scales are scraped from the lesion, either by curette or the edge of a glass slide, or even by the fingernail.

The lesions fluoresce under the Wood's light. This characteristic aids in the management of the disease by locating and outlining areas for treatment.

TREATMENT A weak, keratolytic agent removes the fungus-laden scales.

PIEDRA

Piedra is a term applied to two types of fungous infection of the hair. Black piedra, caused by *Piedraia hortai*, is characterized by hard, black nodules which are adherent to the hair. White piedra, caused by *Trichosporon beigelii*, is distinguished by the soft and light-colored nodules which are detached easily from the hair.

MORPHOLOGY. *P. hortai* appears on hair as a discrete, hard, adherent, black, nodular, mycelial mass composed of broad (4 to 12 μm), closely septate, dichotomously branched hyphae (Fig. 90-3). Scattered throughout the mycelial mass are numerous oval asci, 30 by 50 μm, which contain eight curved or fusiform ascospores, 10 by 30 μm, each with a single terminal, cilium-like appendage.

T. beigelii appears on hair as soft, gelatinous, easily detached, elongate sheaths of transparent mycelial masses composed of round, oval, and rectangular cells, from 2 to 4 μm to 10 μm in diameter (Fig. 90-4). The fungus reproduces both by arthrospore formation and by budding,

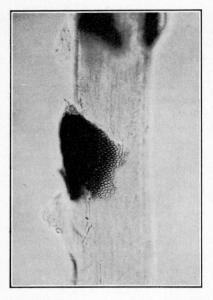

FIG. 90-3. *Piedraia hortai.* Hard black nodule on hair shaft. ×147.

and the elements are held together in a gelatinous substance.

CULTURAL CHARACTERISTICS.   *P. hortai* develops slowly on Sabouraud's glucose agar as an adherent, black to greenish black, glabrous, wrinkled colony. *T. beigelii* develops somewhat faster on Sabouraud's glucose agar as a soft, cream-colored yeastlike, wrinkled colony.

For clinical purposes a diagnosis is based on the microscopic appearance of the fungous nodules on the hair in KOH preparations.

SPONTANEOUS INFECTIONS IN ANIMALS. Black piedra has been reported on the pelts of chimpanzees. These museum pelts had been obtained from animals killed in the Cameroons. Kaplan, in a study of pelts from a wide variety of primates, reported black piedra in 195 of 438 specimens. These pelts had been obtained from primates of Asia, Africa, and the New World. Also, Kaplan reported white piedra from a live monkey, and Miguens has reported this type of infection on a horse.

TRANSMISSION.   *P. hortai* infections are common in Brazil, where the fungus causes epidemics more often among men than among women, probably because the latter take better care of their hair. It is not known where in nature the fungus may be located or how epidemics are established. Greasy hair preparations may have some significance, since their use is wisespread in those areas where the infection is common.

In the United States, infection may be found on recent arrivals, but autochthonous cases have been reported.

T. beigelii, which causes sporadic infections of the hair, is much less contagious, and the fungus is found more frequently on the hairs of the mustache and beard than on the scalp.

TREATMENT.   Infected hairs should be cut or shaved off, and, after their removal, the area should be treated by applications of a solution of bichloride of mercury (1:2,000) or ammoniated mercury ointment (3 percent).

PROTOTHECOSIS

Protothecosis, caused by species of *Prototheca,* is a cutaneous disease in man and a systemic disease in lower animals caused by an achlorophyllous alga. In man the cutaneous lesions have been described as papular and ulcerating papula pustular. Such lesions have finally been characterized by hyperkeratosis

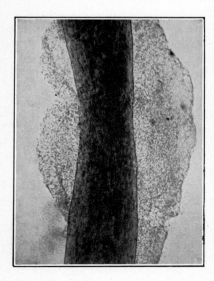

FIG. 90-4. *Trichosporon beigelii.* Soft nodule on hair shaft. ×147.

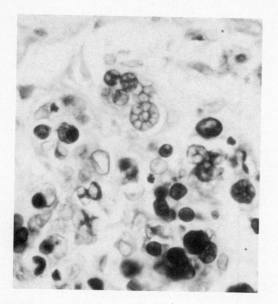

FIG. 90-5. *Prototheca wickerhamii* in wall of ulcer on the skin. ×1,000. (From Klintworth et al: J Med Microbiol 1: 211, 1968)

and pseudoepitheliomatous hyperplasia. In animals (cow, deer, dog) various internal organs and lymph nodes, as well as skin, have been involved.

Prototheca are ubiquitous in nature and enter the skin of man through abrasions of various kinds. The patient usually has an underlying disease which lowers his resistance to attack by these organisms.

MORPHOLOGY.   In the skin the algae are seen in stained preparations (PAS) as single, ovoid to spherical, nonbudding bodies 2 to 18 μm in diameter. There is little reaction to these bodies (Fig. 90-5).

Multiplication takes place by the formation of autospores (4 to 5 μm in diameter) within the oval bodies. This takes place by cleavage of the cytoplasm within the parent cell until approximately 50 spores are produced. These spores are freed by rupture of the parent cell membrane.

CULTURAL CHARACTERISTICS.   Biopsy material can be cultured at room temperature on a variety of bacteriologic media. When grown on Sabouraud's glucose medium the culture develops quickly (four to five days) as a smooth, white, yeastlike, soft growth composed of single, nonbudding, oval cells 8 to 20 μm in size (Figs. 90-6 and 90-7). The alga reproduces itself by producing spores (up to 50) within the cell.

Species of *Prototheca* can be characterized by assimilation tests on various sugars and al-

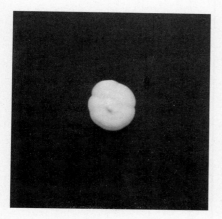

FIG. 90-6. *Prototheca wickerhamii.* Yeastlike colony on Sabouraud's glucose agar at room temperature for two weeks. (From Tindall and Fetter: Arch Dermatol 104:490, 1971)

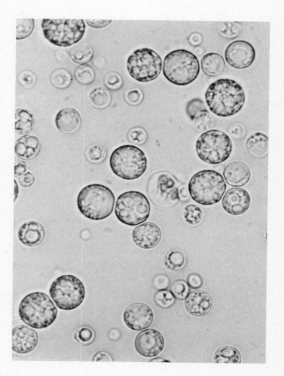

FIG. 90-7. *Prototheca wickerhamii.* Cells from yeastlike culture. ×100.

cohols and by specific immunofluorescence tests on cultures and tissues.

FURTHER READING

MYCOTIC KERATITIS

Anderson B Jr, Chick EW: Mycokeratitis: Treatment of fungal corneal ulcers with amphotericin B and mechanical debridement. South Med J 56:270, 1963

Bakerspigel A: Fungi isolated from keratomycosis in Ontario, Canada. I. *Monosporium apiospermum (Allescheria boydii)*. Sabouraudia 9:109, 1971

Chick EW, Conant NE: Mycotic ulcerative keratitis, a review of 148 cases from the literature (abstact). Invest Ophthalmol 1:419 1962

Laverde S, Moncada LH, Restrepo A, Vera CB: Mycotic keratitis; 5 cases caused by unusual fungi. Sabouradia 11:119, 1973

Rippon JW: Mycotic infections of the eye. Diagnosis and treatment. Ophthalmol Digest 34:18, 1972

Zimmerman LE: Mycotic keratitis. Lab Invest 11 [part 2]: 1151, 1962

TINEA VERSICOLOR

Gordon MA: Lipophilic yeast-like organisms associated with tinea versicolor. J Invest Dermatol 17:267, 1951

Gordon MA: The lipophilic mycoflora of the skin. Mycologia 43:524, 1951

Keddie F, Shadomy S: Etiologic significance of *Pityrosporum obiculare* in tinea versicolor. Sabouraudia 3:21, 1963

Keddie, F, Shadomy J, Shadomy S, Barfatani M: Intrafollicular tinea versicolor demonstrated on monomer plastic strips. J Invest Dermatol 41:103, 1963

Roberts SOB: Pityriasis: A clinical and mycological investigation. Br J Dermatol 81:315, 1969

Roberts SOB: *Pityrosporon obiculare*. Incidence and distribution on clinically normal skin. Br J Dermatol 81:264, 1969

Sternberg, TH, Keddie EM: Immunofluorescence studies in tinea versicolor. Arch Dermatol 84:999, 1961

PIEDRA

Kaplan W: Piedra in lower animals. J Am Vet Med Assoc 134:113, 1959

Kaplan W: The occurrence of black piedra in primate pelts. Trop Geogr Med 11:115, 1959

Mackinnon JE, Schouten GB: Investigaciones sobre las en denominadas "piedra." Arch Soc Biol Montevideo 10:227, 1942

Takashio M, Vanbreuseghem R: Production of ascospores by *Piedraia hortai* in vitro. Mycologia 63:612, 1971

PROTOTHECOSIS

Sudman MS: Prototheosis. A critical review. Am J Clin Pathol 61:10, 1974

SECTION 7
MEDICAL PARASITOLOGY

Parasitology is the science or study of parasitism—that is, the relations between parasites and the organisms (hosts) that harbor them. In the fields of medicine and public health, the subject matter of parasitology is limited to parasitism in man. In a broad sense, this would involve the study of all organisms parasitic on or within the human body. However, this broad approach, including both plant and animal parasites, is not usually feasible for teaching purposes, since there are many specialized fields involved. Thus, it is customary to study parasites of the plant kingdom in medical bacteriology, virology, and mycology, and those of the animal kingdom in medical parasitology. The most important species of animal parasites of man belong to four groups of animals: the Protozoa, or single-celled animals, the Nematoda, or true roundworms, the Platyhelminthes, or flatworms, and the Arthropoda, which includes not only the true insects but ticks, mites, and others. Although arthropods affect the health of man in many ways, space does not permit a consideration of them in the present discussion.

In presenting the material, an attempt will be made to coordinate the medical and biologic approaches to the subject—that is, to give proper attention to both the host and the parasite. The life cycle of the parasite will be given, followed by a brief consideration of the principal damage produced in the host and the striking signs and symptoms resulting therefrom. After these discussions of each infection, the laboratory diagnosis and treatment will be given. By relating the important host-parasite relations, rather than emphasizing certain factors concerned only with the host or the parasite, it has been my experience that the student gains a better appreciation and understanding of these infections. In following this approach, however, it will be necessary to limit the space customarily given to details of classification, morphology of the parasite, pathology, and so forth. For those interested in more complete information, there are many excellent references available, including those listed below.

It has not been practical, for reasons of space, to cite bibliographic references, but the writer wishes to acknowledge the fact that this material is based on the published studies of others.

There are many sources of information dealing with all phases of medical parasitology. The few references listed below are among the best as sources of information to supplement the material in these chapters.

FURTHER READING

Belding DL: Textbook of Parasitology, 3rd ed. New York, Appleton-Century-Crofts, 1965

Brown HW: Basic Clinical Parasitology, 4th ed. New York, Appleton-Century-Crofts, 1975

Faust EC, Beaver PC, Jung RC: Animal Agents and Vectors of Human Disease, 4th ed. Philadelphia, Lea & Febiger, 1975

Faust EC, Russell PF, Jung RC: Craig and Faust's Clinical Parasitology, 8th ed. Philadelphia, Lea & Febiger, 1970

Hunter GW, III, Frye WW, Swartzwelder JC: Manual of Tropical Medicine, 4th ed. Philadelphia, Saunders, 1966

Kenny M: In Thomas BA (ed): Scope Monograph on Pathoparasitology. A Color Atlas of Parasites in Tissue Sections, Kalamazoo, Mich, Upjohn Company, 1973

Larsh JE, Jr: Parasitology. In Race GJ (ed): Laboratory Medicine. Hagerstown, Md, Harper and Row, 1973

Markell EK, Voge M: Medical Parasitology, 3rd ed. Philadelphia, Saunders, 1971

91

Protozoa and Protozoan Infections

Protozoa are unicellular animals composed of a nucleus, or nuclei, and cytoplasm. The nucleus is concerned with reproduction. The cytoplasm is differentiated into an inner portion, the endoplasm, and an outer layer, the ectoplasm. The endoplasm is concerned mainly with nutrition, whereas the ectoplasm performs the functions of protection, ingestion of food, and so forth. Locomotion, if accomplished, is carried out by special ectoplasmic organelles. Four groups of Protozoa contain important parasites of man: (1) Rhizopodea (amebae), (2) Ciliatea (ciliates), (3) Mastigophora (flagellates), and (4) Sporozoa. The amebae locomote by means of pseudopodia, the ciliates by cilia, and the flagellates by flagella, whereas the sporozoans lack definite organelles for locomotion.

In the presentation of the material of this chapter, the protozoa will be grouped according to their usual location within the body of man. By so doing, there are two main groups to be considered: the intestinal, oral, and genital protozoa, and the blood and tissue protozoa.

INTESTINAL, ORAL, AND GENITAL PROTOZOA

This group will include six amebae (Rhizopodea), one organism in the class Ciliatea (*Balantidium coli*), and five flagellates (Mastigophora). Most of these reside in the intestinal tract, but two occur in the mouth (an ameba and a flagellate), and one occurs in the genital organs (another flagellate). Emphasis will be placed on the agents of clinical importance, but it will be necessary to include information on the common so-called nonpathogenic agents, especially in relation to microscopic differentiation.

The Amebae

Of the six amebae commonly found in man, only one *(Entamoeba gingivalis)* occurs in the mouth; the remaining five species (*Entamoeba histolytica, Entamoeba coli, Endolimax nana, Iodamoeba bütschlii,* and *Dientamoeba fragilis)* are located in the large intestine. Since *E. histolytica,* the cause of amebiasis, is the most important of the amebae, it will be given

special attention. There is evidence that heavy infections with one or more of the other four amebae living in the large intestine may produce irritation resulting in certain cases of diarrhea. Furthermore, there is some evidence that at least one of these so-called nonpathogenic amebae *(D. fragilis)* may exhibit pathogenicity in some individuals. Nevertheless, until more information becomes available, our main concern with these four amebae lies in the fact that one or more may coexist with *E. histolytica,* making differentiation necessary. For this reason, they will be mentioned only in connection with the laboratory diagnosis of *E. histolytica.* The remaining ameba, *E. gingivalis,* may be dismissed, since it is now considered a commensal organism. It is common in those with carious teeth and diseased gums and tonsils.

MORPHOLOGY AND LIFE CYCLE OF ENTAMOEBA HISTOLYTICA. There are three distinct stages in the life cycle that are recovered from stool specimens: the trophozoite, the precyst, and the cyst (Fig. 91-1). The trophozoites vary considerably in size (8 to 60 μm). In warm smears prepared from fresh material, they are active and exhibit progressive and directional motility by the action of ectoplasmic pseudopodia. These are glasslike and are formed in explosive fashion. After extrusion of a pseudopodium, the remaining material of the cell is drawn toward it, tending to give a degree of polarity to the organism. The nucleus usually is not visible, so that the only inclusions noted are within the food vacuoles, where digestion takes place. If red blood cells are present in the material being examined, they often will be seen as well within the food vacuoles, but it should be emphasized that trophozoites from cases of chronic amebiasis usually do not contain these cells. The usual inclusions are indistinct, being presumably debris of tissue cells in various stages of digestion. When undergoing degeneration, the trophozoites become sluggish, and bacteria as well as large vacuoles can be seen within them.

In stained preparations the structure of the nucleus is distinctive. The nuclear membrane is delicate and has on its inner surface a single layer of minute chromatin beads, and the karyosome is small and usually located centrally. Again, when undergoing degeneration, changes

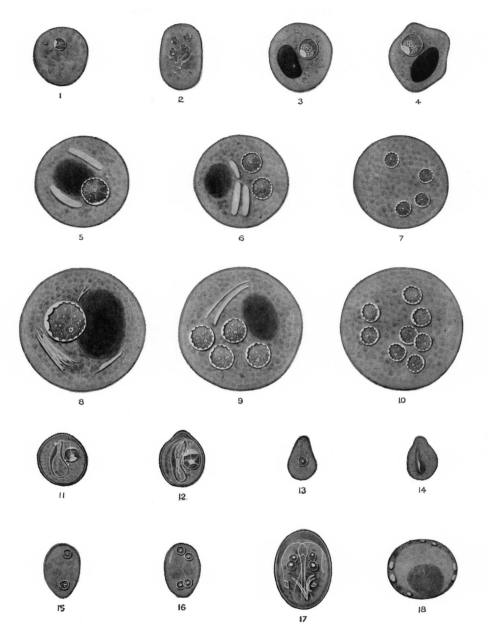

Plate 91-I.   Cysts of intestinal protozoa treated with iodine. × 2000. 1 and 2, *Endo-limax nana*; 3 and 4, *Iodamoeba bütschlii*; 5, 6, and 7, *Entamoeba histolytica*; 8, 9, and 10, *Entamoeba coli*; 11 and 12, *Chilomastix mesnili*; 13 and 14, *Embadomonas intestinalis*; 15 and 16, *Enteromonas hominis*; 17, *Giardia lamblia*; 18, *Blastocystis hominis*, a yeast resembling a protozoan cyst. (From Belding: Textbook of Clinical Parasitology, 2nd ed, Appleton-Century-Crofts.)

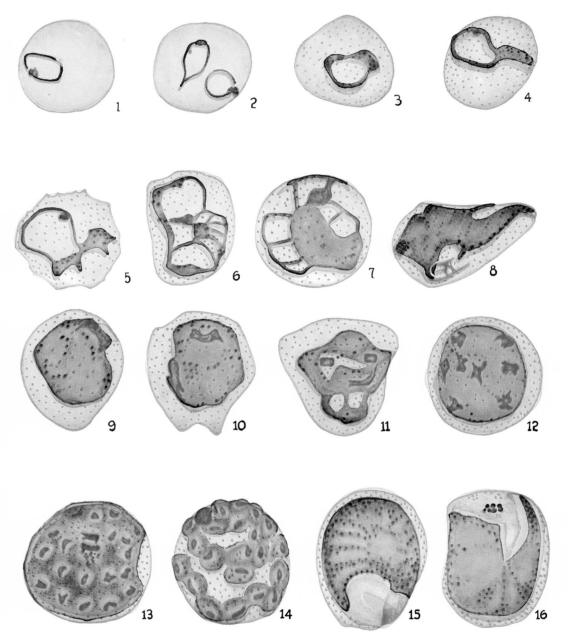

Plate 91-II. *Plasmodium vivax.* Sexual and asexual developmental forms of the parasite within the red cells of man from a case of benign tertian malaria, as seen in dried blood films stained with Romanovsky stain. Approx. × 3200. 1 and 2, ring forms; 3-9, growth of trophozoite, enlargement and change in red cell, formation of Schüffner's dots, and deposition of pigment in cytoplasm of parasite; 10-14, growth of schizont; 15, female gametocyte (macrogametocyte); 16, male gametocyte (microgametocyte). (From Belding: Textbook of Clinical Parasitology, 2nd ed, Appleton-Century-Crofts.)

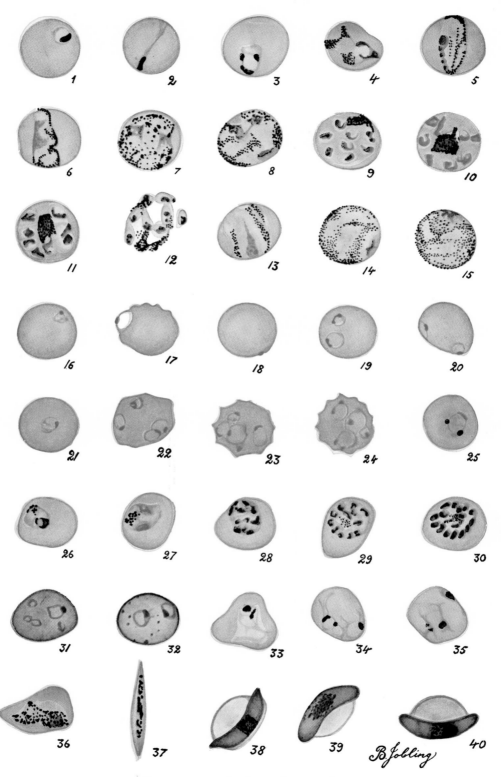

[See reverse side for explanation.]

Plate 91-III. *Plasmodium malariae* (1–15) and *Plasmodium falciparum* (16–40) as seen in dried blood films stained with Leishman stain. × 2,000. *Plasmodium malariae:* 1, young ring form; 2, young band form; 3, slightly older parasite with granule of pigment; 4–6, growth of trophozoite; 7–12, development of schizont; 13, older band form of nearly mature gametocyte; 14, female gametocyte (macrogametocyte); 15, male gametocyte (microgametocyte). *Plasmodium falciparum;* 16–24, ring forms; 25 and 26, growth of trophozoite and development of pigment; these forms usually occur in the internal organs, but are occasionally seen in the peripheral blood; 27–30, development of schizont; these forms occur rarely in the peripheral blood; 31 and 32, deeply stained cells containing ring forms and showing Stephens' and Christopher's or Maurer's dots on the surface of the cell; 33–35, irregular or ameboid young forms, showing tendency to fusion of one or more parasites (*"Plasmodium tenue"* of Stephens); 36 and 37, developing gametocytes; 38 and 40, female gametocytes (macrogametocytes) showing remains of host cell; 39, male gametocyte (microgametocyte). (From Wenyon: Protozoology, London, Baillière, Tindall and Cox, 1926. This plate was made from the original drawing now in the Museum of Medical Science, Wellcome Research Institution, obtained through the courtesy of Professor Wenyon and the Publishers. From Belding. Textbook of Clinical Parasitology, 2nd ed, Appleton-Century-Crofts.)

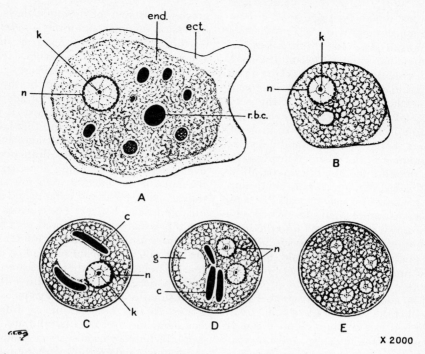

FIG. 91-1. Schematic representation of *Entamoeba histolytica*. A, trophozoite containing red blood cells undergoing digestion; B, precystic ameba devoid of cytoplasmic inclusions; C, young uninucleate cyst; D, binucleate cyst; E, mature quadrinucleate cyst; c, chromatoid bodies; ect., ectoplasm; end., endoplasm; g, glycogen vacuole; k, karysome; n, nucleus; r.b.c., red blood cells. (From Belding: Textbook of Clinical Parasitology, 2nd ed, 1952. Courtesy of Appleton-Century-Crofts)

occur in the nucleus that cause it to lose its characteristic appearance.

The precystic stage is intermediate between the trophozoite and cyst stages. Due especially to reorganization of the nuclear material, this stage is not diagnostic. The trophozoites become sluggish in action, and, after extrusion of food particles, there is a rounding of the cytoplasm. This results in a reduction in size compared with that of the motile amebae. Motility ceases, and a cyst wall is secreted.

The cyst stage is more resistant than the other stages and is, under most conditions, the infective stage. Cysts range in size from 5 to 20 μm, are usually spherical, and contain one, two, or four nuclei with the same structure noted in the trophozoites. Also present in some are paired chromatoid bars (bodies) with rounded ends and a glycogen vacuole. The chromatoid bars and the vacuole disappear gradually as the cyst reaches maturity by division of the nucleus to the quadrinucleate stage.

The life cycle of *E. histolytica* is comparatively simple. The parasite is passed in the stools of infected individuals. If the specimen is dysenteric or diarrheic or has been obtained following purgation, trophozoites will predominate. Few cysts are observed in such specimens because, presumably, evacuation is too rapid for encystment. Cysts, therefore, usually are found only in normally passed stools that are formed, at least in part. Cysts will remain viable only if kept moist and if other favorable conditions exist, as they are readily destroyed by desiccation, sunlight, heat, and other factors. Reinfection of the same individual or infection of a new host(s) may occur directly, via contaminated fingers (hand-to-mouth infection), or indirectly, chiefly via contaminated food and/or fluids. The ingested cysts pass through the stomach and excyst in the small intestine. A metacystic ameba containing the four cystic nuclei emerges from each cyst. Cytoplasmic division takes place to form four small metacystic trophozoites, which feed and soon grow to full size. Hence, cysts provide for reproduction as well as transmission. The trophozoites pass along the intestinal canal until conditions are favorable for colonization, which occurs as the result of rapid and repeated transverse binary fission. This usually occurs first at the cecal area but may take place at a lower level of the large intestine. Tissue invasion is probably accomplished both by lytic and physical means. After entering the tissue, lytic digestion of host cells provides food for the ameba, allowing it to advance. Under certain conditions, some of the trophozoites may metastasize to the liver and other extraintestinal sites. When some of the trophozoites are extruded into the intestinal lumen, they begin their passage from the body. If this passage is not too rapid, they pass through the precystic stage and occur in the stool as cysts.

It should be added that many workers are of the opinion that the small strain of *E. histolytica* (12 μm or less) is a commensal organism living in the lumen of the intestine, and a separate species, *Entamoeba hartmanni*, has been established for it. However, it is known that geographic strains vary in pathogenicity, that the bacterial flora of the intestine, the resistance, and the nutritional status of the host all are factors in determining whether demonstrable pathology results from a given infection. Thus, it would seem wise, until final proof has been established, to consider all strains capable of damaging the host.

PATHOLOGY AND SYMPTOMATOLOGY OF AMEBIASIS. The intestinal pathology of amebiasis is most commonly observed in the cecal area, followed by the sigmoidorectal area, but lesions may occur at any point from the lower ileum downward. The process begins with a small lesion produced at the site of entry into the tissue. A minute cavity is formed from lytic necrosis. As viewed from the surface, these small lesions are surrounded by a raised yellowish ring and are separated by mucosa that appears normal. Usually showing no evidence of inflammatory reaction, these lesions fail to suggest the degree of subsurface damage, which may be considerable. As the colony of amebae increases, a narrow channel often is formed to the base of the mucosa. There, due probably to the greater resistance of the muscularis mucosae, the lesion enlarges and forms an early, characteristic, flask-shaped or teardrop ulcer. This appears to be a critical stage, determining whether or not extensive damage will be produced, and it may, therefore, be thought of as an expression of the degree of adaptation between the parasite and the host. If the organisms are unable to penetrate this layer, repair may keep pace with the damage, and in some cases the amebae may be eliminated. If, however, the organisms erode a passage through the muscularis mucosae into the submucosa, they usually spread out radially and produce an enlarged ragged ulcer. The mucosa surrounding this usually is rolled and elevated due to the undermining. Secondary infections usually are not observed in these lesions, despite extensive necrosis, and there is essentially no tissue reaction present. Later the surface of the ulcer sloughs off, exposing shaggy overhanging edges. At this time secondary infections are common, and the ulcer is infiltrated with neutrophilic leukocytes and other wandering cells, tending to thicken the overhanging edges. In severe cases the organisms may spread from the submucosa through the muscular coats into the serosa, where they are likely to cause perforation. Also, from the intestinal wall, the amebae may enter the portal venules or, less commonly, the lymphatics and be carried to the liver and other organs. Liver involvement is most common, followed by involvement of the lungs, which usually is by direct extension from the liver abscess. Lesions outside of the intestinal tract are always secondary to those in the intestine.

In intestinal amebiasis there often is no definite pattern of symptoms; in fact, the disease may manifest itself clinically in a deceptive fashion. In acute amebiasis (amebic dysentery), the individual usually is acutely ill, complains of general abdominal discomfort and tenderness, and passes numerous stools, which in most cases are dysenteric. The symptoms usually are referable to the cecal area and may resemble appendicitis and various other conditions. In subacute infections, the picture is similar but less striking. Considering the number of cases involved and the difficulty of diagnosis, the major problem is chronic amebiasis. The symptomatology in this case exhibits even greater latitude. Some patients may have periodic bouts of diarrhea or, less commonly, dysentery, but longer periods of constipation are characteristic. Others are without distinctive signs or symptoms and complain of a low fatigue threshold, moderate loss of weight, mental dullness, and the like. In many such cases, tenderness can be demonstrated in the right lower quadrant. Still others found to be infected are entirely asymptomatic.

The pathology of amebic liver abscess results from the establishment and multiplication of trophozoites in that organ. The early abscess is small, with a grayish brown matrix of necrosed hepatic cells. Connective tissue does not appear to be destroyed by the lytic property. As the abscess increases in size, the center liquefies, the wall thickens, and in most cases the contents become a viscid (creamy), chocolate-colored mass. At all stages of abscess formation, the amebae are seen invading the marginal tissue. Abscesses occur more frequently in the right lobe than in the left and tend to be solitary rather than multiple. The latter are usually seen in individuals with active dysentery, and these abscesses usually develop in a relatively brief period after the intestinal phase becomes acute. It is important to emphasize that liver abscess may be a sequela of chronic intestinal amebiasis as well as of the acute type (amebic dysentery). In fact, liver abscess without evidence of intestinal involvement and without organisms in the stool is not unusual.

The symptomatology of amebic liver abscess is characterized by hepatomegaly, tenderness over the liver, and referred pain around the right or left scapula, bulging and fixation of the right or left leaf of the diaphragm, moderate leukocytosis, and a low-grade, inconstant fever.

LABORATORY DIAGNOSIS OF E. HISTOLYTICA. In the diagnosis of intestinal amebiasis, various methods are used, depending upon the type of specimen and other factors. If the fecal specimen is dysenteric or diarrheic or has been obtained following purgation, it is likely to contain only trophozoites. If possible, it should be examined while still warm, because the trophozoites may soon lose their characteristic features. Two fecal smears should be prepared side by side, and about 1 cm apart, on a microscope slide. One smear is made by emulsifying a bit of the specimen in a drop of tepid physiologic salt solution, and the other by emulsification in a drop of tepid Quensel's supravital stain. To avoid overstaining, the latter may require the addition of a small drop of tepid salt solution. Coverglasses are added to both preparations, and careful examinations are made under the low power and high dry power of a compound microscope. The salt solution smear is examined first and is most useful in permitting the observation of the characteristic locomotion of the trophozoites, and the Quensel-stained smear, viewed about five minutes after preparation, will permit the observation of the characteristic stained nucleus. Other supravital staining methods are available. If, in suspected cases of amebiases, such direct examinations fail to reveal the organism, and especially if Charcot-Leyden crystals or other microscopic materials suggestive of amebiasis have been noted, it is worthwhile to culture some of the stool.

If the fecal specimen is formed, or at least semiformed, it is likely to contain mostly cysts (Fig. 91-1). Again, direct examinations should be made of dual preparations. In this case, one smear is made in the salt solution, especially to observe the refractive chromatoid bars, and the other is made in D'Antoni's iodine solution. The latter stains the cyst, making visible the internal diagnostic characteristics. If direct examinations fail to reveal cysts, a concentration method should be employed (eg, the simplified zinc sulfate method).

Differentiation of *E. histolytica* from the other four intestinal amebae must be made. Since all of these except *D. fragilis* have a cyst stage, differentiation involves both stages, with this one exception. The single character that is most diagnostic is the structure of the nucleus (Fig. 91-2). Two of the five intestinal amebae, *E. histolytica* and *E. coli*, have conspicuous peripheral chromatin on the inner surface of the nuclear membrane, whereas such material is lacking or is not conspicuous in the other three. In *E. histolytica*, the nuclear membrane is delicate, and the chromatin on the inner surface appears as fine beads; the karyosome is small and usually central. In *E. coli*, the membrane is thicker, and the chromatin on the inner surface is in the form of coarse plaques; the

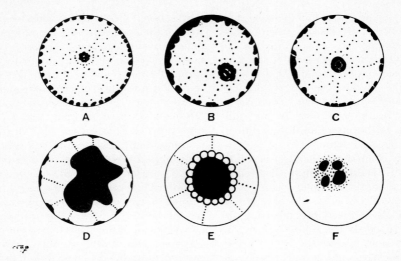

FIG. 91-2. Diagrammatic representation of the various types of nuclei in the amebae of man. A. *Entamoeba histolytica;* B, *Entamoeba coli;* C, *Entamoeba gingivalis;* D, *Endolimax nana;* E, *Iodamoeba bütschlii,* F, *Dientamoeba fragilis.* (From Belding: Textbook of Clinical Parasitology, 2nd ed, 1952. Courtesy of Appleton-Century-Crofts)

karyosome is much larger than that of *E. histolytica* and is located eccentrically. The striking feature of the nucleus of *E. nana* is the large karyosome located in the center or slightly off center. In the case of *I. bütschlii*, the karyosome is also large but is surrounded by a ring of achromatic granules, giving a halo effect around the karyosome. *D. fragilis* usually has two nuclei, but organisms with a single nucleus are not rare. In all cases, the nucleus is composed of a central mass with four to six chromatin granules, one of which usually is larger and stains more deeply than the others. The characteristics of the cysts of the amebae after staining with iodine are shown in Color Plate 91-I.

In addition to stool specimens, proctoscopic aspirates are sometimes submitted for direct examination. These should be examined immediately after being obtained in unstained preparations and in preparations stained with one of the supravital stains. Usually a variety of host tissue cells is present, so it is important to observe the typical motility of the trophozoites before deciding definitely on the diagnosis.

In the diagnosis of amebic liver abscess, the aspirated specimen should be treated with streptococcal DNAase to free the trophozoites from the coagulum. After this the material should be examined in unstained and supravital-stained smears, and some of the material

should be placed in culture. It should be added that many have come to rely upon the indirect hemagglutination test as one of the means of diagnosis, and liver scans have been widely used.

It is important to emphasize that the laboratory diagnosis of chronic amebiasis, especially in children, often is difficult. Best results will be obtained following the use of a battery of tests for examinations of a series of suitable specimens (eg, one or more normally passed specimens, one following purgation, and one following administration of an enema).

TREATMENT OF AMEBIASIS.   For the treatment of intestinal amebiasis, a large number of effective antiamebic drugs is at hand. Excellent results have been obtained following the use of Terramycin alone, but many recommend combining the use of this antibiotic with Diodoquin (63.9 percent iodine), using the full schedules and dosages recommended for each. For the treatment of liver abscess, chloroquine diphosphate is the recommended drug. It should be added that many now recommend the use of metronidazole (Flagyl), which is effective against both the intestinal and the extraintestinal (liver abscess and so on) phases of infection.

The Ciliated Protozoan

Balantidium coli (Fig. 91-3) is the only ciliate parasitic in man and is by far the largest of the protozoa found in the human body. The trophozoite varies considerably in size (50 to 100 μm by 40 to 70 μm, or even larger), is ovoidal in shape, and is covered entirely with short, constantly moving cilia. A funnel-shaped peristome (mouth) leads into the cytostome (gullet), and a minute cytopyge is located at the posterior end. One or two contractile vacuoles may be seen within the cytoplasm, as well as two nuclei, a large, kidney-shaped macronucleus, and, usually within the concavity, a small micronucleus. The cyst, observed less frequently than the trophozoite, is smaller (45 to 65 μm in diameter), is almost spherical in shape, and is covered with a double transparent wall. Stained cysts reveal clearly the nuclear components.

This organism occurs usually in the cecal area but may be found at both higher and lower levels. The trophozoites feed upon bacteria and other substances in the lumen but take in host cells after they enter the tissues. They reproduce by transverse binary fission, and in certain hosts they may become numerous. The mucosal layer appears to be penetrated mainly by boring action, and because of the size of the organism, the opening is much larger than that produced by *E. histolytica*. Having gained entrance into the mucosa, the organism appears to have little difficulty in passing through the muscularis mucosae into the submucosa, where it spreads out radially and may produce considerable destruction. Unlike *E. histolytica*, it apparently invades the muscular layers only on rare occasions, and although observed in lymphatics, it has not been found in extraintestinal sites. The ulcers produced may occur at all levels of the large intestine but are most common in the cecal and sigmoidorectal areas. They often resemble those produced by *E. histolytica*, especially after bacteria invade them. When this occurs, extensive inflammatory reactions are noted around the organisms as well as a diffuse infiltrate throughout the tissue.

Many harboring *B. coli* are asymptomatic, but others show symptoms ranging from mild to profuse diarrhea and even fulminating, fatal dysentery.

Laboratory diagnosis usually is made by finding the characteristic trophozoites in the stool. Because of their great size, they are easily detected. However, free-living ciliates may occur as contaminants of the stool or saline solution used in making the smear, resulting in a mistak-

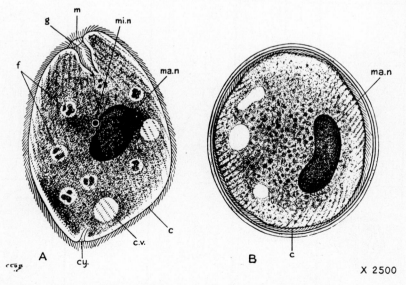

X 2500

FIG. 91-3. Schematic representation of *Balantidium coli*. A, trophozoite; B, cyst; c, cilia; cy., cytopyge; c.v., contractile vacuole; f, food vacuole; g. "gullet"; m, "mouth"; ma.n, macronucleus; mi.n, micronucleus. (From Belding: Textbook of Clinical Parasitology, 2nd ed, 1952. Courtesy of Appleton-Century-Crofts)

en diagnosis. Cysts also may be found, depending somewhat upon the condition of the stool specimen.

Balantidiasis can be treated effectively with Diodoquin or Terramycin given orally.

The Flagellated Protozoa

MORPHOLOGY AND LIFE CYCLES. *Giardia lamblia* is found in the small intestine, and it has trophozoite and cyst stages. The trophozoite (10 to 18 μm by 6 to 11 μm) is bilaterally symmetrical, with two nuclei and four pairs of flagella (Fig. 91-4). It has no oral opening, but on the ventral surface near the anterior end there is a characteristic adhesive disk. Two axostyles extend through the center portion to the posterior end, which is tapered and from which a pair of flagella emerges. Other structures, such as the blepharoplasts, may be seen, but no food particles are evident. Since there is no cytostome, the food substances must be absorbed through the surface of the cell. The cyst (8 to 14 μm by 6 to 10 μm) is ovoid, and the wall is relatively thickened (Fig. 91-4, Color Plate 91-I). When stained, two, four, or occasionally more nuclei can be seen, as well as curved fibrils.

The trophozoites usually are found in the intestinal crypts at the duodenal level, where they are firmly attached to the epithelial surface. At times they are also found at lower levels of the intestine and in the common bile duct and gallbladder. As revealed in electron micrographs, they also may occur within epithelial cells. Multiplication is by longitudinal binary fission, which may result in myriads of organisms. Because of their location, trophozoites are not seen in the stool unless the individual has been given a saline cathartic or is extremely diarrheic. Therefore, only cysts usually are found in stool specimens. These occur intermittently and may be very numerous. Under moist conditions, the cysts may remain viable for long periods. They presumably reach the mouth of the same person or others by the avenues of transmission listed above for *E. histolytica*. They pass unharmed through the stomach and excyst in the upper intestine. Two trophozoites, or sometimes more, result from

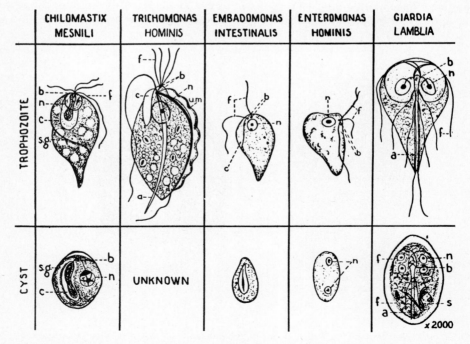

FIG. 91-4. Intestinal flagellates of man. a, axostyle; b, blepharoplasts; c, cytostome; f, flagella; n, nucleus; s, shields; s.g., spiral groove; u.m. undulating membrane. (From Belding: Textbook of Clinical Parasitology, 2nd ed., 1952. Courtesy of Appleton-Century-Crofts)

each cyst, hence this stage provides for reproduction as well as for transmission.

Chilomastix mesnili in the trophozoite stage (Fig. 91-4) is pear-shaped and ranges usually from 10 to 15 μm in length and from 3 to 4 μm in width. There are three anterior flagella and a fourth situated within the cytostome. A large spherical nucleus with one or more blocks of chromatin is located near the anterior end of the cell. Numerous food vacuoles, filled mainly with bacteria, are crowded in the cytoplasm. The most characteristic features of this organism are the peripheral spiral groove and the caudostyle, a spinelike projection at the posterior end. The lemon-shaped cysts usually range from 7 to 9 μm in length and from 4 to 6 μm in width, have a thickened portion at the anterior end, and in stained smears show the nucleus and cytostomal structures (Fig. 91-4, Color Plate 91-I).

The trophozoites live in the lumen of the large intestine and multiply by longitudinal binary fission. They may occur in large numbers in unformed stools, but usually only cysts are seen in formed stools. These are more resistant than most protozoan cysts, as they have a thermal death point of 72C and may survive in clean water for longer than 200 days. Infection is acquired from swallowing viable cysts in feces-contaminated food and/or drink or from viable cysts introduced into the mouth from feces-contaminated fingers.

Three species of trichomonads are common in man and all are known only in the trophozoite stage (*Trichomonas tenax, Trichomonas hominis, Trichomonas vaginalis*). They have the following common characteristics: a pear-shaped appearance as a result of the rounded anterior end and somewhat pointed posterior end, a slender rodlike axostyle that extrudes through the posterior tip, a small cytostome, a large spherical nucleus near the anterior end, and the most characteristic structural feature, an undulating membrane (Fig. 91-5). Multiplication is by longitudinal binary fission.

T. tenax, 6 to 12 μm in length, has four anterior flagella, and the undulating membrane extends posteriorly about two-thirds the length of the cell. The flagellum on its outer edge does not extend beyond the end of the membrane (Fig. 91-5). The normal habitat is the mouth, and the rate of infection is considerably higher in those with diseased gums and carious teeth than in those with normal mouths. Transmis-

sion, no doubt, usually occurs by the transfer of trophozoites during kissing, but contaminated dishes, glasses, and the like may be involved.

T. hominis lives in the lumen of the large intestine and is usually from 7 to 15 μm long and from 4 to 7 μm wide. There are usually four anterior flagella, but organisms with three or five are seen at times. In addition to these, there is a flagellum, attached to the outer edge of the undulating membrane, which becomes free at the posterior end of the cell (Figs. 91-4, 91-5). The membrane, in this case, extends the full length of the cell. Transmission occurs by the ingestion of trophozoites in contaminated food and/or drink. The organism can survive for many days in undiluted feces stored at temperatures ranging from 5 to 31C, and there is evidence that houseflies may play a role in transmission.

T. vaginalis (Fig. 91-5) is an inhabitant of the human vagina and of the male genital tract and is often found in the urine of infected subjects. It usually is much larger than the other two trichomonads, reaching 25 μm or more in length and 18 μm in width. It has four anterior flagella and one on the margin of the undulating membrane. The membrane in this case is very short, usually not extending below the upper half of the cell, and the flagellum on its margin does not extend beyond the side of the cell. Transmission in most cases is accomplished through sexual intercourse, but many infections cannot be explained on this basis. Some of these may have resulted from a transfer of organisms from female to female through the use of a common vaginal douche or a contaminated toilet seat or from grossly contaminated clothing.

PATHOLOGY AND SYMPTOMATOLOGY. Three of these organisms are not important clinically, except in unusual cases. *T. tenax*, like *E. gingivalis*, is now considered a harmless organism that grows best in those who fail to practice good dental and oral hygiene. Also, *C. mesnili* and *T. hominis* are considered to be nonpathogenic. However, there is some evidence that these organisms, when present alone or together in large numbers, may irritate the intestine and play a role in diarrhea, since the condition often subsides upon eradication of the parasite(s). The remaining two flagellates, *G. lamblia* and *T. vaginalis*, are important clinically whether or not they are classified as pathogen-

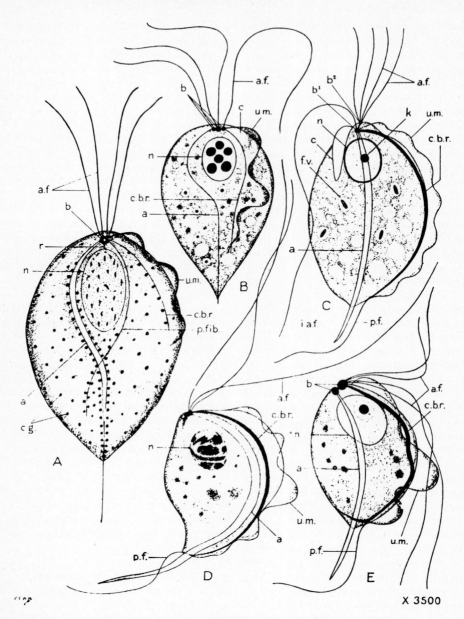

FIG. 91-5. Trichomonads of man. A, *Trichomonas vaginalis;* B, *Trichomonas tenax;* C, *Pentatrichomonas ardin delteili;* D, *Tritrichomonas fecalis;* E, *Trichomonas hominis,* a, axostyle: a.f., anterior flagella; b, b¹, b², blepharoplasts; c, cyto-stome; c.b.r., chromatoid basal rod; c.g., chromatin granules; f.v., food vacuole; i.a.f., inferior anterior flagellum; k, karyosome; n, nucleus; p.f., posterior flagellum; p.fib., parabasal fiber; r. rhizoplast; u.m., undulating membrane. (From Belding: Textbook of Clinical Parasitology, 2nd ed, 1952. Courtesy of Appleton-Century-Crofts)

ic. Although many persons found to be infected with *G. lamblia* are entirely asymptomatic, others complain of periodic epigastric or abdominal pain and show a history of recurrent or persistent diarrhea (with much mucus), whereas others, mostly adults, may have symptoms referable to the duodenum and gallbladder. In

some of the latter cases, the symptoms may approximate the typical syndrome of chronic cholecystitis. Many patients with a giardial infection, after a period when anorexia and diarrhea are pronounced, lose weight and may become dehydrated. *T. vaginalis* infection is not limited to females, as a large number of males with nongonorrheal urethral discharges are found to be infected. In the latter, the symptoms usually are slight until the infection is aggravated by secondary bacterial invasion, after which the condition becomes a purulent urethritis and prostatovesiculitis. In the female, many infections do not result in a complaint of symptoms, but the vaginal secretions are altered invariably. In typical cases of *T. vaginalis* vaginitis, the normal pH of the vagina (3.8 to 4.4 during sexual maturity) becomes more alkaline, and the glycogen stores of the vaginal mucosa, especially in the superficial layers, are reduced greatly. The normal processes of cellular destruction make the glycogen available to the Döderlein bacillus, an inhabitant of the normal vagina, which metabolizes glycogen and excretes lactic acid. This maintains the normal acid state of the vagina. In the absence of normal stores of glycogen, the numbers of this organism are reduced, and in severe cases it may be eliminated. When these events occur, the physiologic protection offered by the normal vaginal acidity is altered, and the growth of *T. vaginalis* and other organisms is encouraged. Those with *T. vaginalis* have a profuse, watery leukorrheic discharge that produces a chafing of the vagina, vulva, and perineum, and pruritus vaginae and vulvae are distressing.

LABORATORY DIAGNOSIS. Fecal smears made from fresh material will reveal *G. lamblia*, *C. mesnili*, and *T. hominis*. If the specimen is formed, the cysts of *G. lamblia* and *C. mesnili* may be expected, but if it is liquid or semiformed, the trophozoites of all three forms may be seen. If cysts are difficult to find, indicating that few are present, they may be concentrated. Aside from the structural differences listed above, the trophozoites of each species exhibit characteristic movements. *G. lamblia* has a fluttery, falling-leaf movement, *C. mesnili* a graceful, progressive spiral movement, and *T. hominis* a nervous, jerky movement. *G. lamblia* trophozoites may also be obtained by duodenal aspiration and, if the gallbladder is involved, from bile aspirate.

T. tenax sometimes is difficult to demonstrate in smears, but may be demonstrated by cultures.

T. vaginalis may be recovered in the urine, prostatic, or urethral discharges of the male and in the urine and vaginal discharges of the female.

TREATMENT. Atabrine by mouth is recommended for the removal of *G. lamblia*, Carbarsone or Diodoquin for *C. mesnili* and *T. hominis*. Treatment for *T. tenax* is not necessary. Metronidazole (Flagyl), an oral drug, is considered the drug of choice for treating both males and females infected with *T. vaginalis*.

BLOOD AND TISSUE PROTOZOA

Flagellated Protozoa

These flagellates differ greatly from those discussed above. Besides having an entirely different structure, the blood and tissue flagellates are found in different tissues in man and require a bloodsucking arthropod to complete their life cycles. Six species are involved, three in the genus *Trypanosoma* (*Trypansoma gambiense*, *Trypanosoma rhodesiense*, and *Trypanosoma cruzi*), and three in the genus *Leishmania* (*Leishmania donovani*, *Leishmania tropica*, and *Leishmania brasiliensis*).

The Trypanosomal Parasites MORPHOLOGY AND LIFE CYCLES. *T. gambiense* and *T. rhodesiense*, agents of the African trypanosomiases, cannot be separated by morphologic characteristics. Both circulate primarily in the bloodstream as the trypanosomal (trypomastigote) stage. The most diagnostic feature of this stage is the long undulating membrane that originates near the posterior end of the cell and extends along the margin of the cell to the tip of the anterior end, where the free flagellum may be seen (Fig. 91-6). These parasites are polymorphic in their appearance in the blood. Short and broad forms, long and slender forms, and intermediate forms ranging in length from 15 to 30 μm may be seen in the same stained preparation. When blood containing *T. rhodesiense* is injected into mice or other laboratory animals, forms with a nucleus located posteriorly may occur, permitting differentiation from *T. gambiense*. The trypanosomal stage in the blood of man is taken with a blood meal by the vector, one of the tsetse flies. *Glossina palpalis* is the most common vector for *T. gambiense*, whereas *Glossina morsitans* is the principal vector of *T. rhodesiense*. In the vector, the trypanosomal

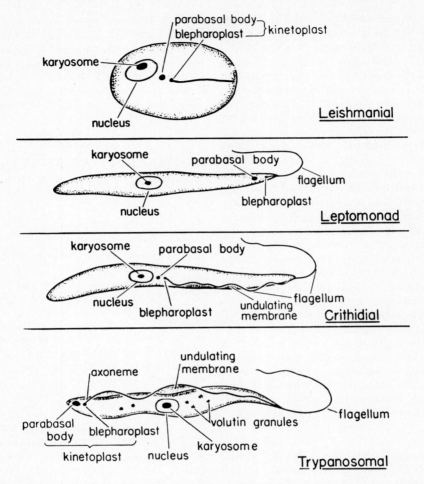

FIG. 91-6. Schematic representation of morphologic forms in the *Trypanosoma* and *Leishmania* genera. (From Mackie, Hunter, and Worth: A Manual of Tropical Medicine, 2nd ed., 1954. Courtesy of W. B. Saunders Co)

forms pass through the proventriculus into the midgut, where multiplication by longitudinal binary fission results in the production of slender trypanosomes. These finally make their way into the salivary glands, where multiplication results in the production of crithidial (epimastigote) forms (Fig. 91-6). These resemble the trypanosomal stage, but the undulating membrane is shorter, originating anterior to the nucleus. Later, these transform into infective-stage trypanosomes (metacyclic forms), which accumulate in the ducts of the salivary glands. The entire development within the fly requires about two weeks *(T. rhodesiense)* or three weeks *(T. gambiense).* Infection of man occurs when the fly, containing infective-stage trypanosomes, takes a blood meal.

T. cruzi, agent of Chagas' disease or American trypanosomiasis, differs from the other two trypanosomes in that it has an intracellular phase involving not only cells of the lymphoid-macrophage system but also those of the myocardium, endocrine glands, and the glial cells of the brain. In this phase, the parasite is a typical leishmanial (amastigote) form (Fig. 91-6), being ovoid in shape, 1.5 to 5 μm in the longer diameter, and having a large nucleus and a deeply staining kinetoplast composed of a parabasal body and a blepharoplast. A delicate axoneme may sometimes be seen arising from the blepharoplast. No true flagellum or undulating membrane is present. When freed from the host cell, this stage enters the bloodstream, where it transforms into a typical, or C-shaped, trypanosomal (trypomastigote) stage, about 20 μm long, which is the stage taken by the vector. The vector, in this case, is a triatomid (cone-nosed) bug. Many species of these bugs have been found infected naturally with *T. cruzi*, but *Panstrongylus megistus*, *Triatoma infestans*, and *Rhodnius prolixus* appear to be the most important vectors. When taken into the bug, the trypanosomal stage of the parasite is carried into the midgut, where it transforms into the crithidial stage (preceding). Later, following multiplication in the hindgut, the infective-stage trypanosomes are formed, which pass out in the liquid feces of the bug when it is taking a blood meal or immediately thereafter. This usually occurs at night, and the pruritus produced by the bite often results in an infection caused by rubbing into the wound, or nearby skin or mucous membrane, the excrement containing the infective parasites. The entire cycle in the bug requires about two weeks.

PATHOLOGY AND SYMPTOMATOLOGY. *T. rhodesiense* is much more likely than *T. gambiense* to run a rapid, fulminating course with a fatal outcome. In *T. gambiense* infections, there usually are three progressive stages of tissue relation: parasitemia, when the parasites are numerous in the blood, lymphadenitis, when they are concentrated in the lymph nodes, and central nervous system involvement, when the parasites are numerous in the brain substance and arachnoid spaces. Lymphadenitis is most pronounced in the posterior cervical triangle (Winterbottom's sign). Physical weakness and mental lethargy follow invasion of the central nervous system. Sleepiness develops and becomes progressively pronounced until, in the advanced stage, the patient sleeps continuously.

An early, almost constant sign of acute *T. cruzi* infection, especially in infants, is edema of the face and eyelids (Romaña's sign). The acute form predominates in younger age groups, is usually of short duration, and has a high case fatality rate in untreated young children. The chronic disease follows the development of the parasite in several visceral organs. Here they multiply as leishmanial type organisms, destroying the host cells and bringing about inflammatory reactions in the involved tissues. The principal pathologic changes are noted grossly in the heart and brain, and the predominant symptoms are those of cardiac failure. The

spleen and liver are enlarged and congested in relation to the degree of cardiac failure. The brain is congested and edematous and often contains scattered petechial hemorrhages. Collections of organisms may be associated with glial nodules.

LABORATORY DIAGNOSIS. *T. gambiense* and *T. rhodesiense* occur in the circulating blood during febrile episodes and sometimes can be demonstrated in thick smear preparations. However, lymph node aspirates reveal more infections. After involvement of the central nervous system, examination of spinal fluid may yield positive results. For the reason explained above, this method applies only to *T. gambiense* infections. If these various methods fail to establish the diagnosis, susceptible laboratory animals (guinea pigs, white rats, and others) may be inoculated intraperitoneally with some of the patient's blood and later examined at intervals for the parasites.

T. cruzi also may be found in the circulating blood during febrile periods, but they are never numerous and therefore are difficult to demonstrate even in thick film preparations. Laboratory animals may be inoculated with blood from suspected cases, and a widely used xenodiagnostic test is available. The latter involves the use of parasite-free, laboratory-raised triatomids, which are allowed to take blood from the patient. Examination of the feces or intestinal contents of the bugs after 8 to 10 days usually will reveal trypanosomes if they were present in the blood of the patient. The organisms also may be cultivated easily on various media [Nicolle, Novy, MacNeal (NNN), Chang's, and others] and in tissue cultures, all of which reveal the crithidial and trypanosomal forms. Finally, a complement-fixation test is available in attempts to diagnose latent and chronic cases of the disease.

TREATMENT. For treating early cases (blood and lymph stages) of both *T. gambiense* and *T. rhodesiense*, suramin sodium (Bayer 205) is the drug of choice. In the late stages (after invasion of the central nervous system), Mel B is the drug of choice. These two drugs can be obtained from the Center for Disease Control (see page 1138).

T. cruzi infections can be treated with Bayer 7602. This drug causes the disappearance of trypansomes from the blood and improves the clinical condition. However, it does not destroy leishmanial stages in the tissues, hence relapses occur.

The Leishmanial Parasites Morphology and Life Cycles.   The size and other morphologic characters of *L. donovani*, *L. tropica*, and *L. brasiliensis* are indistinguishable. In man, they occur as typical leishmanial (amastigote) forms (2 to 3 μm long and 1 to 1.5 μm wide), often referred to as "Leishman-Donovan bodies," with structures similar to those noted in this form during the tissue stage of *T. cruzi* (Fig. 91-6). *L. donovani* causes visceral leishmaniasis, or kala-azar, and the organisms are usually numerous in the endothelial cells of the blood and lymph capillaries and in circulating macrophages. They have been described from almost all organs but occur especially in the spleen, liver, bone marrow, and lymph nodes. The organisms probably are distributed throughout the body by the bloodstream after reaching this site upon rupture of the host cells. They multiply, as do all members of the Mastigophora, by longitudinal binary fission. *L. tropica* causes cutaneous leishmaniasis, or oriental sore, and so on. There is no general dissemination of the parasites, and only exposed skin areas are affected. The parasites often can be demonstrated within endothelial macrophages. *L. brasiliensis* causes mucocutaneous leishmaniasis, or uta, and so on. The primary location of the organisms is in the skin, but in most cases they migrate to develop in secondary sites in mucous membranes near cutaneous junctions. The nose and/or mouth usually are involved, but extension into the pharynx may occur.

In the case of all three organisms, several species of small biting flies belonging to the genus *Phlebotomus* are mainly responsible for their transmission to man and reservoirs. The flies ingest the leishmanial form by direct ingestion from the infected skin or by ingestion of blood or tissue juices. After being ingested, the parasites develop into the leptomonad (promastigote) stage in the midgut (Fig. 91-6). This stage is characterized by having a free flagellum at the anterior end without having an undulating membrane. They multiply rapidly, and within three to five days many have migrated into the proboscis. In this location they are ready to be injected into the skin of the next individual when the fly takes another blood meal.

Pathology and Symptomatology.   *L. donovani* infections cause hyperplasia of the cells of the lymphoid-macrophage system, especially of the spleen, liver, and bone marrow. Both the liver and spleen become enlarged. The usual signs and symptoms include an undulant type fever, loss of weight (which may be masked by edema), abdominal protuberance, visible pulsation of the carotid arteries, bleeding of the gums, lips, and nares, and hemorrhage from the intestinal mucosa. The case fatality rate in some areas may be as high as 90 percent in untreated cases. *L. tropica* and *L. brasiliensis* infections produce local lesions that appear first as a macule, then as a papule with a slightly raised center. Later the lesion opens at the center to discharge necrotic material. The *L. tropica* ulceration usually occurs late, after which rapid healing is the rule, always with the formation of a scar. However, secondary infections may occur, slowing healing and causing more extensive scarring. The lesion produced by *L. brasiliensis* develops more rapidly, and ulceration and secondary infection usually occur early in the disease. After extension to the mucous membranes, destruction of tissue usually is considerable, and even if healing occurs, the scars are disfiguring to the extent of causing deformity of the face.

Laboratory Diagnosis.   *L. donovani* may be demonstrated sometimes in stained blood smears, but cultivation of the organisms by inoculating the blood into special media (NNN, Chang's, and others) and incubating at 20 to 25C is more likely to be successful. The leptomonad stage occurs in cultures (Fig. 91-6). Many workers perfer to prepare stained tissue smears following removal of a specimen by biopsy. In the past, spleen and liver specimens were most often used, but today most workers favor the use of a bone marrow specimen from the iliac crest obtained by the van den Bergh technique. A portion of each sample should also be handled aseptically and cultured. If these various methods fail to reveal the parasites in suspect cases, hamsters may be inoculated. A complement-fixation test of great diagnostic value is available.

L. tropica and *L. brasiliensis* may be demonstrated in stained smears made from the crater of an early lesion or, less often, from material obtained from the indurated margin of older lesions. The material can also be cultured, but care must be taken to cleanse the area before taking a sample, as the organisms seldom will grow in the presence of bacteria. A complement-fixation test and a skin test are available for diagnosis of both *L. tropica* and *L. brasiliensis*, but the skin test has been more widely used in clinics and in the field to diagnose *L. brasiliensis*.

TREATMENT. Pentostam, a pentavalent organic antimonial, is the drug of choice for treating infections with *L. donovani*, except in the Egyptian Sudan and parts of East Africa, where the aromatic diamidine, stilbamidine (or the less toxic hydroxystilbamidine) is the choice. In other areas the latter, due to greater toxicity, is reserved for antimony-resistant cases. The drug of choice for treating *L. tropica* and *L. brasiliensis* is Pentostam. After secondary bacterial infections of ulcers, sulfa drugs or antibiotics are used to destroy these agents before giving Pentostam. This drug can be obtained from the Center for Disease Control (see page 1138).

The Malarial Parasites

The malarial parasites belong to the subphylum Sporozoa, subclass Haemosporina, and genus *Plasmodium*, and their life cycle involves both an asexual phase (schizogony in man as the intermediate host) and a sexual phase (sporogony in certain female anopheline mosquitoes as the definitive host). There are three common species of human malarial parasites: (1) *Plasmodium vivax*, agent of benign, tertian malaria, is the most widely distributed and, on a worldwide basis, is the most prevalent species, (2) *Plasmodium falciparum*, agent of malignant, subtertian malaria, is as prevalent as *P. vivax* in subtropical and tropical regions but fails to establish in areas where there are long cold seasons, and (3) *Plasmodium malariae*, agent of quartan malaria, is limited almost entirely to tropical and subtropical areas, where it is considerably less prevalent than are *P. vivax* and *P. falciparum*. A fourth valid species, *Plasmodium ovale*, will not be included in this discussion. It has been reported sporadically from widely separated tropical and subtropical regions, but it is not the dominant type even in parts of Africa where it is well established. The parasite resembles *P. vivax* in certain characters and *P. malariae* in others.

In addition to the human species, various malarial parasites of monkeys can develop in man. The demonstration of the natural transmission of one of these to man poses a serious problem for those working toward worldwide eradication of malaria.

GENERAL ASEXUAL CYCLE IN MAN. Although there are striking morphologic differences among the three parasites selected for study, the general features of the cycles are the same. Specific differences will be considered on page 1132 (Color Plates 91-II and 91-III). The cycle in man begins with the inoculation of infective sporozoites by a female anopheline mosquito. Within 30 minutes, the sporozoites disappear from the circulating blood, and no parasites can be demonstrated in red blood cells for many days. It is now known that during this negative phase the parasite is residing in fixed tissue cells (parenchymal cells of the liver and perhaps others). Although the various stages of the parasite observed in exoerythrocytic foci resemble those seen later within the red blood cells, the characteristic malarial pigment (hemozoin), derived from the breakdown of hemoglobin, is, of course, not seen. After development in exoerythrocytic foci for many days, the density of the parasites increases, and certain of the progeny enter the bloodstream and initiate erythrocytic infection. It should be added that the exoerythrocytic forms of *P. vivax*, and those of *P. malariae* as well, may persist long after the eradication of the erythrocytic forms and thus are believed to be the cause of later episodes of parasitemia and clinical relapses. Following the use of Giemsa or other blood stains, all of the red blood cell stages are seen with the nucleus or chromatin red, the cytoplasm blue, and the malarial pigment a light brown to dense black, depending upon the species. The first stage observed within the red blood cells is the trophozoite. The youngest trophozoite is referred to as a "ring," which has a central vacuole and a ring of cytoplasm containing a chromatin dot. The growth of the parasite proceeds gradually, the vacuole disappears, and the cytoplasm increases in size. With the increase in volume of the cytoplasm, pigment may be observed within it. The pigment increases in amount with increasing age of the parasite, since it is a waste product of hemoglobin me-

tabolism. When the single nucleus of the trophozoite stage divides to form two nuclei, the
schizont stage is formed. The chromatin continues to divide until the number characteristic for
the species is reached. At this point the preseg-
menter has been produced. The segmenter or
mature schizont is observed soon thereafter,
when each chromatin mass has been provided,
after division of the cytoplasm, with an envelope of cytoplasm to form the merozoites. By
this time the pigment, scattered previously, has
become clumped, usually near the center of the
parasite. The red blood cell ruptures, and some
of the merozoites enter new cells to begin again
the asexual cycle. The length of this cycle, from
entry of merozoite to the rupture of the host
cell, varies with the species of parasite, being
48 hours for *P. vivax* (although a 44-hour strain
has been demonstrated), 72 hours for *P. malariae*, and 36 to 48 hours for *P. falciparum*. The
last cycle, however, has considerably less
synchronization than that of the other two species. In addition to trophozoites and schizonts,
a third stage, gametocyte, is seen within the red
blood cells. The gametocytes, male and female
sex cells, nearly fill the red blood cell and have
only a single chromatin mass. It is this stage
that initiates the sporogenous cycle in the female anopheline. In summary, there are only
three distinct stages within the red blood cells
of man: the trophozoite, the schizont, and the
gametocyte.

GENERAL SEXUAL CYCLE IN ANOPHELINE MOS-
QUITO.   After a susceptible female anopheline
ingests a blood meal containing ripe gametocytes of both sexes, the sexual cycle begins. In
the lumen of the midgut, the gametocytes escape from the host cells and soon undergo
changes preparatory to fertilization. The female
gametocyte (macrogametocyte) extrudes polar-
like bodies, which is indicative that the haploid
condition is being assumed. The male gametocyte (microgametocyte), through a process
known as "exflagellation" forms a number of
spermlike bodies. Because these changes in
both cells are noted within about 20 minutes
under favorable conditions, it is suggestive that
the lining up process within the nucleus of
each actually begins in the human bloodstream.
In any event, fertilization occurs when a micro-
gamete enters a macrogamete and a zygote is
formed. Being motile, this form is referred to as
the "ookinete." The ookinete penetrates be-

neath the peritrophic membrane lining the
midgut and, after about 24 hours, penetrates
through the cells and becomes encysted under
the hemocoelic membrane on the outside wall
of the midgut. Here the oocyst is formed, which
when mature, contains large numbers of sporozoites. The oocyst ruptures into the body cavity
(hemocoel) after about two weeks, and many of
the sporozoites eventually find their way into
the trilobed salivary glands. After a few days
under optimum conditions, the sporozoites
become infective and are capable of initiating
an infection in a susceptible individual after
being inoculated when the mosquito punctures
the skin to take a blood meal.

PATHOLOGY AND SYMPTOMATOLOGY. The
most characteristic features of the pathology of
malaria are anemia, pigmentation of certain
organs, and hypertrophy of the liver and, especially, the spleen. The anemia, a microcytic,
hypochromic type, may be produced not only
by the direct loss of red blood cells as a result of
their destruction by the parasite but also from
interference with hematopoiesis, by increased
phagocytosis of red blood cells, and as the result of capillary hemorrhages. In acute cases, *P.
falciparum* produces the greatest degree of
anemia, especially because of the marked loss
of red blood cells by the growth of the parasite
within them. In chronic cases, and especially
during malarial cachexia, the anemia is particularly outstanding. During the latter cases, leukopenia, with a 20 percent or more monocytosis, is considered diagnostic of malaria. The
pigmentation noted in the tissues of malaria
victims is due to the phagocytosis of hemozoin,
the true malarial pigment, released into the
blood upon rupture of the host cells at the termination of each asexual cycle. It is taken up in
large amounts by cells of the lymphoid-macrophage system, especially by the macrophages
in the spleen and bone marrow and the Kupffer
cells in the liver. The pigmentation constantly
increases with the age of the infection, so that it
may be observed grossly in autopsied cases of
chronic malaria. As would be expected from the
massive blood destruction, there is also deposition of hemosiderin in the tissues. The liver is
enlarged because of congestion during acute
malaria, and it increases considerably in size
during chronic infections. The spleen, the organ affected most seriously in malaria, is also
enlarged, first as a result of congestion, follow-

ing cavernous dilatation of the sinusoids, and later as a result of a great increase in macrophage elements, especially in Billroth's cords. With repeated attacks, the enlargement becomes progressively greater, and the organ may reach considerable size, especially in width, in chronic malaria. Fibrosis of the cords of Billroth is outstanding here. Splenomegaly in malaria is so characteristic that palpation of this organ has been used for a long time as a rapid and effective means of appraising the malaria problem in communities. Changes in the bone marrow, although much less striking, are similar in character to those in the spleen.

In addition to these changes that may be expected, to a degree, from any malarial infection, especially those of long standing, another important change, capillary occlusions, should be mentioned. These are most characteristic in *P. falciparum* infections and are most dangerous in the brain. The parasitized red blood cells become sticky, some believe as a result of a specific antibody-antigen reaction, and agglutinate. Such cells marginate at the periphery of the vessel lumen, probably as a result of centrifugal force, and later the capillary becomes occluded. Following this, hemorrhages occur about such vessels, exclusively in the subcortical and paraventricular white matter, producing a ring effect. The tissue immediately surrounding the vessel is necrotic, and the ring hemorrhage is somewhat removed from the vessel. Usually associated with ring hemorrhages are the so-called malarial granulomas, consisting essentially of a rosette of one or several layers of glial cells arranged around the necrotic zone. Anoxia with necrosis of tissue in the immediate vicinity must be the logical consequence of occluded vessels.

Blackwater fever should be mentioned, as it is associated with malarial infections, especially *P. falciparum* infections. The etiology is unknown. The disease is characterized by intravascular hemolysis with hemoglobinemia and hemoglobinuria. Hemoglobinuric casts occur in the distal convoluted tubules in the kidney. Degeneration—and some regeneration—of the tubular epithelium is also seen.

The symptomatology of malaria differs between *P. vivax* and *P. malariae* infections and that caused by *P. falciparum*. The typical paroxysm caused by the former two parasites involves, usually after a brief prodromal period, a cold stage (shaking chill), followed by a fever stage (a characteristic remittent type fever reaching suddenly a level of 104 to 105F (40C) and, after many hours, returning suddenly to near normal), and a marked terminal sweating stage resulting from the sudden fall in body temperature. *P. falciparum* paroxysms differ in many ways: the chill stage is less pronounced (there may be only a chilly sensation), the fever stage is more prolonged and intensified (fever tends to be a continuous type), and because the fever fails to remit sharply, the sweating stage is usually absent. *P. falciparum* infection is more dangerous than those of the other two species, since it often is accompanied by pernicious manifestations, such as coma, convulsions, and/or cardiac failure. *P. falciparum* parasites may localize in any organ, and those bearing the brunt of the attack will give rise to the most striking signs and symptoms. Therefore, the symptomatology of *P. falciparum* malaria may resemble that of many other diseases.

LABORATORY DIAGNOSIS. Stained blood smears are examined, under the oil immersion objective, for the presence of malarial parasites. Comparative information on the three malarial parasites of man, including the most important differential diagnostic characters, is given in Table 91-1 (see also Color Plates 91-II 91-III).

TREATMENT. Therapeutic (and suppressive) activity is directed primarily against the stages within the red blood cells. Many effective drugs are available: Atabrine among the old antimalarials, and Aralen (chloroquine), Paludrine (chlorguanide), Daraprim (pyrimethamine), and others among the newer ones. The drugs in this group will terminate clinical attacks promptly. Also, when taken in suppressive amounts, they will usually prevent clinical attacks and, if continued long enough, will cure *P. falciparum* malaria. Of the drugs exerting this type of activity, chloroquine, a 4-aminoquinoline, is the most efficient and effective drug. However, drug-resistant strains of *P. falciparum* malaria, in Southeast Asia and elsewhere pose a serious problem that must be solved with other drugs. Curative activity is directed against the persisting tissue stages, especially of *P. vivax* malaria. Primaquine, an 8-aminoquinoline, is a very effective curative agent. It is recommended that the acute attack

TABLE 91-1 DIFFERENTIAL DIAGNOSIS OF MALARIAL PARASITES IN STAINED THIN BLOOD SMEARS

Most Striking Differences	Plasmodium vivax	Plasmodium malariae	Plasmodium falciparum
Abundance of parasites	More abundant than P. malariae	Least abundant	Most abundant
Stages of parasite usually observed	Trophozoites, schizonts, gametocytes	As for P. vivax	Young trophozoites, gametocytes
Changes in infected red blood cells	Enlarged, mal-shaped, blanched Schüffner's dots*	Changes not common	Changes not common
Trophozoites ring stage	Small and large (1/3 diameter of r.b.c.) with vacuole and usually one chromatin dot	Much like P. vivax	Very small (1/6 diameter of r.b.c. with vacuole often with 2 chromatin dots, peripheral forms (accolé) common, multiple-infected cells very common*
half-grown	Ameboid, irregular with vacuoles, pigment yellow-brown rods	Oval, band forms (25%), compact, pigment coarse black granules*	Not usually seen
Schizonts (mature)	12 – 24 merozoites* (usually 16 – 18)	8 – 12 merozoites (usually 8 – 10)* arranged in rosette	Not usually seen
Gametocytes	Spherical or oval (9 – 15μ)	As for P. vivax (smaller)	Kidney-bean shape, round or pointed ends*

Most diagnostic

be treated immediately with chloroquine, and concomitantly, or soon thereafter, primaquine treatment should be instituted.

The Toxoplasma Organism

Toxoplasma gondii, an obligate intracellular organism, is now known to be a cosmopolitan parasite of man, producing an infection known as "toxoplasmosis." It has an amazing lack of host specificity, being found in various primates, carnivores, rodents, and birds.

MORPHOLOGY OF THE STAGES IN MAN. The individual cells (trophozoites), 4 to 7 by 2 to 4 μm, usually are crescentic in shape with one end pointed and the other rounded. The cell of the organism is made up of distinct cytoplasm and nuclear chromatin, but there are no flagella or other visible structures. The absence of inclusions, other than the nucleus, differentiates this organism from the leishmanial stage of *Leishmania* species and *Trypanosoma cruzi*, but its morphologic similarity to other organisms (*Histoplasma*, and so on) may confuse the diagnosis. *Toxoplasma* organisms may oc-

cur singly or during acute infections in clusters (pseudocysts within fixed host cells. They may be found at times within wandering macrophages in exudates (peritoneal, pleural, or cerebral), and in circulating blood and technical preparations some may be extracellular. The cells of the lymphoid-macrophage system are most often involved, but the parenchymal cells of the liver, lungs, brain, and other tissues may be parasitized. A peculiar cyst, 5 to 100 μm, may be observed under certain conditions. It is formed by aggregates of *Toxoplasma* merozoites and has a delicate, delimiting argyrophilic membrane produced by the parasite. Tissue reaction seldom is associated with cysts (which are usually in the lungs, heart, or brain). Hence, they are believed to be the basis for the persistence of the organisms during chronic and latent infections. The release of merozoites from cysts must be responsible for the fulminating *Toxoplasma* infections reported in immunosuppressed patients. Such reports raise the question of whether suppression similarly affects other previously established protozoan infections.

LIFE CYCLE. Recent evidence indicates that *T. gondii* is a coccidial parasite, hence it belongs along with the malarial parasites in the subphylum Sporozoa. In the definitive (final) host (the domestic cat and other Filidae), an asexual cycle (similar to the malarial one in human RBCs) as well as a sexual cycle (similar to the malarial one in the infected anopheline mosquito) occurs in the epithelial cells of the small intestine. The end result is the production of oocysts, which are passed in the feces. After a few days, these sporulate so that each oocyst contains two sporocysts, each with four sporozoites. If these mature oocysts are ingested by an intermediate host (animals other than the Filidae, including man), infection results and trophozoites may be produced in many tissues. Therefore, it is now assumed that human infection can occur not only by ingestion of cysts in undercooked meat, as has been known for years, but by ingestion of mature oocysts as well.

PATHOLOGY AND SYMPTOMATOLOGY. These organisms may give rise to at least five types of infections: (1) a congenital infection with onset in utero, (2) an acquired encephalitic infection in older children, (3) an acute febrile illness, usually in adults, resembling typhus or spotted fevers and often producing pulmonary involvement (a typical diffuse interstitial pneumonitis), myocarditis, and so on, (4) an infection resembling infectious mononucleosis with lymphadenopathy, fever, marked weakness, and so on, and (5) a latent infection, in children or adults, which usually can be recognized only by the presence of specific antibodies in the serum. In addition, there is evidence of an association between *Toxoplasma* organisms and granulomatous uveitis and chorioretinitis in adults. The congenital infection has been reported most frequently. With its onset in utero, it occurs as a fetal or neonatal encephalomyelitis, which often is fatal soon after birth but which may remain asymptomatic until much later. Marked lesions and necrosis usually occur in the central nervous system, associated with calcification there and in the eyes. Bilateral chorioretinitis is very common. At times hydrocephaly or microcephaly and psychomotor disturbances are evident. In other types of infections, lesions in the viscera are more common than those in the central nervous system. In summary, it may be stated that during toxoplasmic infections the sites most commonly attacked are the lymph nodes, brain, eyes, and lungs.

LABORATORY DIAGNOSIS. Three approaches are available: direct examination, isolation of organisms, and examinations for a presumptive diagnosis. For direct examination under the oil-immersion objective, impression films of suspected tissues or fluids should be air-dried and stained with Giemsa's stain. The preparations usually examined are tissues taken by biopsy, sputum, vaginal exudates, and the sediment of spinal, pleural, or peritoneal fluids. In an attempt to isolate the organisms, white mice should be inoculated intraperitoneally with fresh, untreated tissue or fluids most likely to contain the organisms. If present, a generalized infection will be produced in 5 to 10 days, at which time the organisms usually can be demonstrated easily in the extensive peritoneal exudate. It should be added that this is an excellent source of organisms to prepare antigens for serologic tests. The animals that die may be examined for *Toxoplasma* organisms by preparing films and/or sections of the peritoneal fluid, lungs, brain, and other tissues. A presumptive diagnosis can be made by a positive delayed skin reaction or by serologic means. Several serologic tests are available (complement fixation, and so on) to assist in the diagnosis, but the dye test is most widely used. This test is dependent on the fact that in the presence of specific antibodies the cytoplasm of the organism loses its affinity for methylene blue. Newer tests, such as the indirect hemagglutination test, have been reported, and of all tests available the indirect fluorescent antibody test appears to be the best.

TREATMENT. Triple sulfonamides (equal part of sulfadiazine, sulfamerazine, and sulfamethazine) and pyrimethamine (Daraprim), acting synergistically, are effective and should be used as the treatment of choice for toxoplasmosis (plus the addition of a steroid in treating eye involvement).

TREATMENT OF PROTOZOAN INFECTIONS

The following references are recommended to those who wish to check the doses and pertinent details about the administration of the various drugs mentioned in the text above.

FURTHER READING

Brown HW: Basic Clinical Parasitology, 4th ed. New York, Appleton-Century-Crofts, 1975

Faust EC, Beaver PC, Jung RC: Animal Agents and Vectors of Human Disease, 4th ed. Philadelphia, Lea & Febiger, 1975

Hunter GW III, Frye WW, Swartzwelder JC: Manual of Tropical Medicine, 4th ed. Philadelphia, Saunders, 1966

Markell EK, Voge M: Medical Parasitology, 3rd ed. Philadelphia, Saunders, 1971

NOTE: In addition to the drugs listed in the text, there are other effective ones not yet released on the market in this country (eg, dehydroemetine for severe intestinal amebiasis and extraintestinal amebiasis). These are available to physicians *on an investigational basis* and can be obtained from Dr. M.G. Schultz, Center for Disease Control, Atlanta, Georgia 30333.

92

Helminths and Helminthic Infections

In addition to the Protozoa, or one-celled animals, there are large numbers of many-celled animals, often referred to as Metazoa, that parasitize man. As stated above, the present discussion will deal with those that belong to two phyla of the animal kingdom, the Nematoda (the nematodes or roundworms) and Platyhelminthes (flatworms). The species of medical and public health importance in the phylum Platyhelminthes belong to two groups: the Cestoda or tapeworms, and the Trematoda or flukes. Collectively, the parasitic worms are termed "helminths." The most important members of the three separate groups will be discussed in the order listed: the nematodes, cestodes, and trematodes.

NEMATODES

The adult nematodes, or roundworms, are characterized by having an elongate, cylindrical body, which is round in cross-section. They are covered with a cuticle and have a complete digestive tract, with mouth and anus, as well as excretory, nervous, and reproductive systems. As in all parasitic worms the latter is the most conspicuous. The sexes are separate, and the males are almost invariably smaller than the females. Nematodes vary considerably in size, from forms difficult to see readily by the unaided eye to others many centimeters in length. They pass through a series of molts, or ecdyses, which are accomplished by shedding the cuticle. A complete series of stages in the life cycle includes the ovum (unfertilized egg), egg, rhabditiform larva (larva of intestinal nematodes having an open mouth and conspicuous esophageal bulb), filariform larva (larva with a closed mouth and slender esophagus), and adult.

In presenting the material of this section, nematodes will be grouped according to the usual location of the adult worms in man. This results in two main groups to be considered: the intestinal nematodes and the tissue nematodes. As an aid to the student, the intestinal nematodes will be divided into two groups: those infective for man in the egg stage and those infective for man in a larval stage. Also, under each grouping, they will be presented in increasing order of the complexity of the life cycle.

Intestinal Nematodes Infective for Man in the Egg Stage

Enterobius vermicularis (the Pinworm of Man, Causing Enterobiasis)   LIFE CYCLE.   These worms live usually in the cecum but many extend into other areas of the large intestine. They attach insecurely to the mucosa. The females, 8 to 13 mm long, are considerably larger than the males, 2 to 5 mm (Fig. 92-1). Both have a characteristic cephalic (head) swelling. The males apparently disappear soon after copulation. The gravid females begin to migrate from the body after the uterus fills with eggs. This migration usually occurs at night. They cling temporarily to the rectal mucosa but soon pass out of the anus onto the perianal and perineal skin (in female subjects, especially young girls, they may reach the vulva and enter the vagina and may at times even reach the inner ends of the fallopian tubes). The female worms oviposit as they crawl about on the skin, and often the body wall ruptures, spilling all of the eggs (about 11,000 per female). These are fully developed, each containing a coiled, first-stage larva (Fig. 92-2). The outer membrane of the eggs is albuminous, causing them to adhere to one another and to the skin and hairs. The intense pruritus produced by the crawling females and/or the eggs results in scratching of the affected part(s). In this way, eggs are transferred to the fingertips and may become lodged beneath the nails. Reinfection follows when the fingers, or food contaminated by the fingers, are placed in the mouth. Aside from this common type of direct transfer of eggs, often referred to as a hand-to-mouth transfer, the eggs may reach the mouth of the infected individual and/or others via one or more indirect routes. The eggs adhere to clothing and bed linen, and some get in air currents to settle later on objects. Thus, the household becomes contaminated, and all members sooner or later swallow some of the eggs. After the infective eggs are swallowed, they hatch in the duodenum, freeing the contained first-stage larvae. These pass slowly toward the cecal area, undergoing the usual number of molts. Upon reaching the cecum, the worms attach, and mating occurs to begin the cycle again. The complete life cycle may be as brief as 15 to 28 days. However, it is known that some of the eggs deposited on the perineum may hatch, and the larvae may

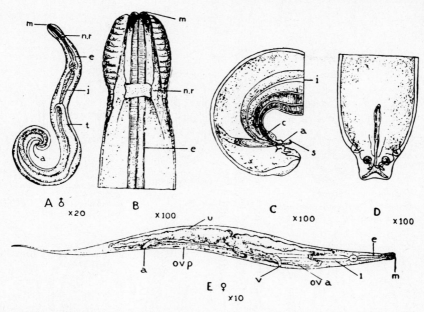

FIG. 92-1. *Enterobius vermicularis.* A, male; B, anterior end of worm; C, posterior end of male, lateral view; D, posterior end of male, ventral view; E, female; a, anus; c, cloaca; e, esophagus; i, intestine; m, mouth; n.r., nerve ring; ov.a., anterior ovary; ov.p., posterior ovary; s, spicule; t, testis; u, uterus; v, vulva. (From Belding: Textbook of Clinical Parasitology, 2nd ed, 1952. Courtesy of Appleton-Century-Crofts)

enter the anus, producing retrofection. When this occurs the cycle may be lengthened considerably.

PATHOLOGY AND SYMPTOMATOLOGY. Inflammation, of an acute or chronic nature, often is produced in the areas of worm attachment. Sometimes necrosis of the mucosa occurs, and sympathetic nerve endings are exposed. This, and probably absorbed metabolites of the worms, is thought to be responsible for the commonly observed reflex nervous symptoms. In some cases the worms probably play a role in appendicitis. Anal pruritus is outstanding, and the scratching that follows may produce scarification, which is subject to invasion by bacteria and other infectious agents. In addition, especially in children, insomnia or restless sleep, low fatigue threshold, and especially nervous symptoms are common.

LABORATORY DIAGNOSIS. The characteristic eggs usually are not found in the stool but may be recovered easily from the perianal area by use of a simple Scotch-tape or other swab. These eggs are asymmetrical, being flattened on the ventral side, and ranging in size from 50 to 60 by 20 to 30 μm (Fig. 92-2). They are composed of two layers and contain the first-stage, infective larva, which usually is active within the shell. Sometimes the diagnosis is made by finding the female worms on the perianal area or, less commonly, in a stool specimen, especially following an enema.

TREATMENT. The drug of choice is oral piperazine citrate, or as a single-dose treatment, oral pyruvinium pamoate.

Trichuris trichiura (Human Whipworm, Causing Trichuriasis). LIFE CYCLE. The anterior three-fifths of the adult whipworms are attenuated, whereas the posterior portion is more fleshy (Fig. 92-3). The male measures 35 to 45 mm in length, the female 35 to 50 mm. The anterior end of the worm is sewed into the mucosa of the large intestine, typically of the cecum and appendix, and the posterior end swings freely in the lumen. After copulation, the females begin to oviposit, the daily egg production probably being 2,000 to 4,000. The characteristic barrel-shaped eggs occur in the stool

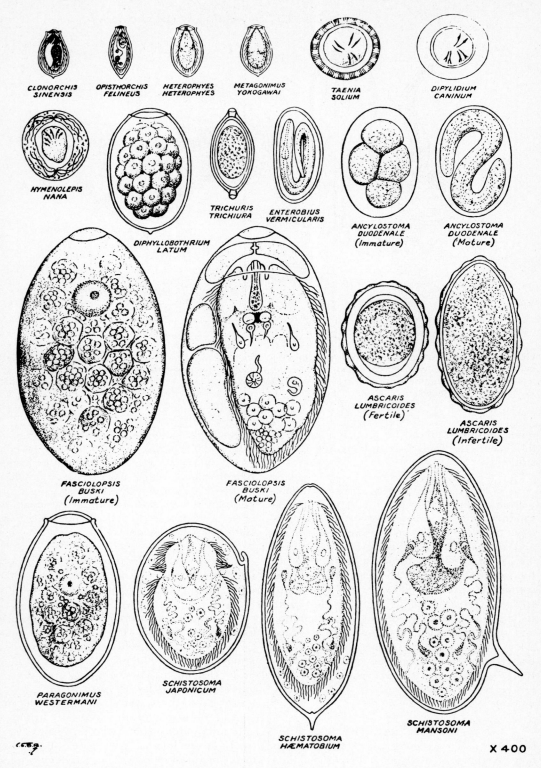

CLONORCHIS
SINENSIS

OPISTHORCHIS
FELINEUS

HETEROPHYES
HETEROPHYES

METAGONIMUS
YOKOGAWAI

TAENIA
SOLIUM

DIPYLIDIUM
CANINUM

HYMENOLEPIS
NANA

DIPHYLLOBOTHRIUM
LATUM

TRICHURIS
TRICHIURA

ENTEROBIUS
VERMICULARIS

ANCYLOSTOMA
DUODENALE
(Immature)

ANCYLOSTOMA
DUODENALE
(Mature)

FASCIOLOPSIS
BUSKI
(Immature)

FASCIOLOPSIS
BUSKI
(Mature)

ASCARIS
LUMBRICOIDES
(Fertile)

ASCARIS
LUMBRICOIDES
(Infertile)

PARAGONIMUS
WESTERMANI

SCHISTOSOMA
JAPONICUM

SCHISTOSOMA
HÆMATOBIUM

SCHISTOSOMA
MANSONI

X 400

FIG. 92-2. Eggs of the common helminths of man. The size of this illustration has been increased by 1/5. (From Belding: Textbook of Clinical Parasitology, 2nd ed, 1952. Courtesy of Appleton-Century-Crofts)

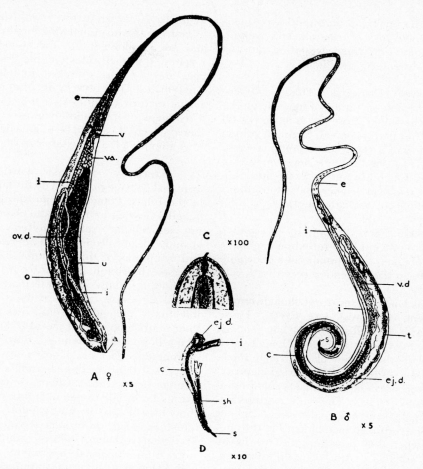

FIG. 92-3. *Trichuris trichiura.* A, female; B, male; C, anterior end showing spear; D, cloaca and copulatory organs of male; a, anus; c, cloaca; e, esophagus; ej.d., ejaculatory duct; i, intestine; o, ovary; ov.d., oviduct; s, spicule, sh., sheath of spicule; t, testis; u, uterus; v, vulva; va, vagina; v.d., vas deferens. (From Belding: Textbook of Clinical Parasitology, 2nd ed, 1952. Courtesy of Appleton-Century-Crofts)

while still in the one-cell stage (Fig. 92-2). Under favorable conditions (warm temperature, shade, moisture, sandy humus soil) the eggs embryonate and become infective (after the contained larvae molt into the second stage) within three to five weeks. They lack the great resistance of *Ascaris* eggs, and their survival is considered to be relatively brief. When infective eggs are ingested, they hatch in the duodenum. The freed larvae enter nearby intestinal crypts and penetrate into the glands and stroma. They leave these sites after about 10 days and are found in the large intestine. The worms are sexually mature after approximately 90 days, and they may live for several years.

PATHOLOGY AND SYMPTOMATOLOGY. These bloodsucking worms damage the tissues penetrated and may carry into these sites bacteria and other infectious agents. If the heads of the worms penetrate into blood capillaries, petechial hemorrhages are produced. The degree of damage corresponds to the number of worms involved. In light infections relatively little damage results, but in heavy infections the mucosa is hyperemic and eroded superficially and may be inflamed extensively. Extreme irritation in the wall of the lower colon and rectum may provoke prolapse of the rectum. Depending upon the degree of infection and reaction of the individual, the signs and symptoms vary from mild (discomfort in the right lower quadrant, flatulence, loss of appetite and weight, and so on) to severe (nausea, vomiting, mucous diarrhea or dysentery, and anemia).

LABORATORY DIAGNOSIS.   This is dependent upon the demonstration of the characteristic eggs in the stool. These are about 20 by 50 μm in size and barrel-shaped, having a golden brown color and a transparent prominence at each pole (Fig. 92-2). They may be few in number and difficult to find in fecal smears, in which cases it is of assistance to use the simplified zinc sulfate concentration method.

TREATMENT.   Hexylresorcinol (crystoids), given as a 0.3 percent high-retention enema(s), is used. Mebendazole (Vermox) in a chewable tablet has been recommended recently.

Ascaris lumbricoides (Large Roundworm of Man, Causing Ascariasis) LIFE CYCLE. These large nematodes (males 15 to 31 cm, females 20 to 35 cm or more in length) usually live unattached in the lumen of the small intestine (Fig. 92-4). After reaching sexual maturity, copulation occurs, and the females soon thereafter begin to oviposit. The daily egg production per female is phenomenal, averaging about 200,000. The fertilized eggs are still in the one-cell stage when they pass from the host in the feces (Fig. 92-2). In rtile eggs, differing considerably in morph gic detail from the fertilized eggs, are some imes seen (Fig. 92-2). If the stool containing the fertilized eggs is deposited in a warm, shady, moist area, the eggs will develop. They have considerable resistance to cold and desiccation but lie dormant under these conditions. At temperatures between 22 and 33C, the eggs develop to the infective stage within two to three weeks. By this time the first-stage rhabditiform larva within each egg has molted into the second-stage rhabditiform larva. These infective eggs may remain viable on the soil for many months, even years in some cases. Accidental ingestion of infective eggs results in infection. The eggs hatch in the duodenum, and the emerging larvae penetrate the intestinal wall, enter the circulatory system, and are carried to the right heart and thence to the lungs. They are filtered out of the lung capillaries and later penetrate into the alveoli (Fig. 92-4). After about two weeks in the lungs and after two additional

molts have occurred, the fourth-stage larvae migrate up the respiratory tract to the epiglottis and are swallowed into the stomach. Upon reaching the small intestine, the final molt occurs, and the worms develop into adult males and females. The entire cycle, from infection to sexual maturity, requires from 8 to 12 weeks. The longevity of the adult worms is rarely more than one year. It should be emphasized that the lung migration is a necessary part of the cycle.

PATHOLOGY AND SYMPTOMATOLOGY.   The principal damage produced by the larvae occurs in the lungs. Petechial hemorrhages are produced following entry into the alveoli. A striking serocellular exudate collects, in which eosinophils are prominent. The cardinal signs and symptoms of this pneumonitis consist of dyspnea, dry cough, fever, and eosinophilia. X-ray findings show scattered mottling of the lungs suggestive of tuberculosis and other infections. The adult worms derive most of their nourishment from the semidigested food of the host, and if abundant, they may have a detrimental effect on the host's nutrition. However, most light infections produce little or no change in the host. Effects from the adult worms are usually noted in children, who often show loss of appetite and weight, intermittent intestinal colic, and various nervous symptoms. The greatest danger from the adult worms results from abnormal migrations within the body. They may enter the ampulla of Vater and block the common bile duct or penetrate into the liver parenchyma or the pancreas. They also have been found on rare occasions in other abnormal sites in the body. Sometimes they perforate the intestinal wall, but much more often, especially in young children, a mass of tangled worms causes an acute obstruction of the small intestine. There is evidence that absorption of the toxic and allergenic metabolites of the adult worms accounts for various referred symptoms, especially those of a neurologic nature.

VISCERAL LARVA MIGRANS.   This clinical condition is observed in young children. It usually results from the larvae of *Toxocara canis* (the dog ascarid) that hatch from eggs in the small intestine and migrate into the liver, lungs, or other organs. These larvae, not adapted to man, remain immature and eventually perish within a granulomatous host capsule.

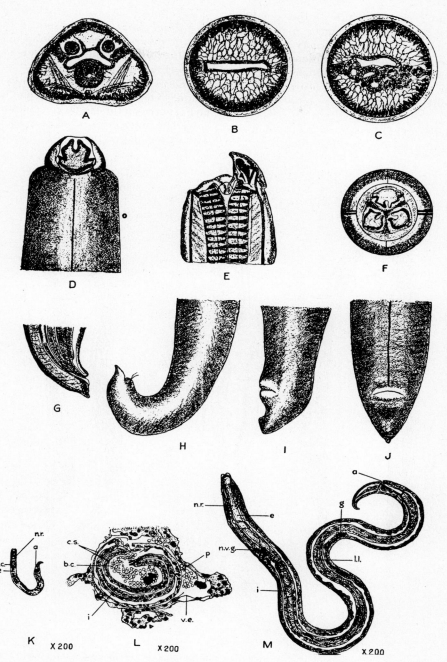

FIG. 92-4. *Ascaris lumbricoides*. A, cross-section through posterior portion of male showing intestine, ejaculatory ducts, and spicules; B and C, cross-sections showing longitudinal lines, musculature, and intestine; D, anterior end showing lips, dorsal view; E, longitudinal section of anterior end; F, papillated lips, front view; G, longitudinal section of posterior end of male, showing cloaca, ejaculatory duct, and spicular sheath; H, posterior end of male with extended spicules, lateral view; I, posterior end of female, lateral view; J. posterior end of female, ventral view; K, larva from liver of mouse; L, section of lung of rat showing larva in air vesicle; M, fully developed larva from lung of rat; a, anus; b.c., red blood cells; c.c., circum-esophageal collar; c.s., cuticular surface; e., esophagus; g, gonads; i, intestine; l.l., lateral line; n.r., nerve ring; n.v.g., nucleus ventral gland; p, pigment; v.e., epithelium of air vesicle. (From Belding: Basic Clinical Parasitology. 1st ed., 1958. Courtesy of Appleton-Century-Crofts)

Outstanding characteristics of this condition are persistent eosinophilia, or hypereosinophilia, enlarged liver, pulmonary infiltration, fever, cough, and hyperglobulinemia. There is no specific treatment, but evidence indicates that oral thiabendazole may prove to be the drug of choice.

LABORATORY DIAGNOSIS.   Except when only male worms are present (less than 5 percent of infections), the characteristic fertilized eggs of *A. lumbricoides* are present in the stool in large numbers and can be found in smears by examination under the low power of the microscope (Fig. 92-2). Concentration methods are not necessary. This egg is bluntly ovoid in shape, 45 to 70 by 35 to 50 μm, and has several layers between the single egg cell and the outside. The outer layer is coarsely mammillated. The various layers account for the thick shell,

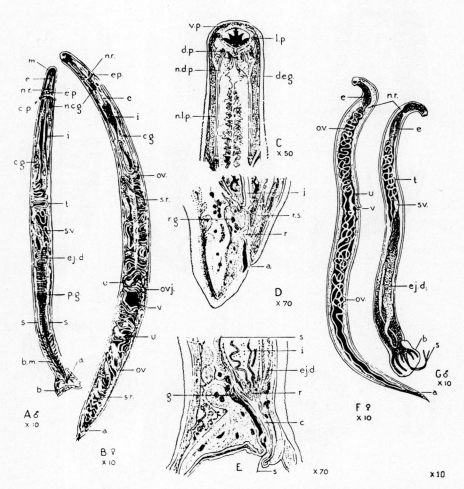

FIG. 92-5. Important hookworms of man. A, adult male *Ancylostoma duodenale* from ventral side; B, young adult female *A. duodenale* from right side; C, anterior end of *A. duodenale* from dorsal side; D, longitudinal section through end of female *A. duodenale*, somewhat diagrammatic; E, longitudinal section through end of male *A. duodenale*, not quite median; F, female *Necator americanus*; G, male *N. americanus*; a, anus; b, bursa; b.m., bursal muscles; c, cloaca; c.g., cervical gland; c.p., cervical papilla; d.e.g., dorsal esophageal gland; d.p., dorsal papilla; e, esophagus; e.p., excretory pore; ej.d., ejaculatory duct; g, gubernaculum; i, intestine; l.p., lateral papilla; m, mouth; n.c.g., nucleus of cephalic gland; n.d.p., nerve of dorsal papilla; n.l.p., nerve of lateral papilla; n.r., nerve ring; ov., ovary; ovj., ovejector; p.g., prostatic glands; r, rectum; r.g., rectal ganglion; r.s., rectal sphincter; s, spicules; s.r., seminal receptacle; s.v., seminal vesicle; t, testis; u, uterus; v, vulva; v.p., ventral papilla. (From Belding: Textbook of Clinical Parasitology, 2nd ed, 1952. Courtesy of Appleton-Century-Crofts)

which is characteristic. The eggs usually are bile-stained by the time they are passed from the body and usually appear brown in color.

TREATMENT.   The drug of choice for eliminating the adult worms is piperazine citrate given by mouth in a syrup.

Intestinal Nematodes Infective for Man in a Larval Stage

Hookworms   Four species are involved in human infections: two (*Necator americanus* and *Ancylostoma duodenale*) are true human parasites, and two (*Ancylostoma braziliense* and *Ancylostoma caninum*) are parasites of cats and dogs. The latter, especially *A. braziliense*, produce a dermatitis (cutaneous larva migrans or creeping eruption) in man following penetration of the skin by the filariform larvae (p. 1148). All hookworms have certain common morphologic characteristics, the most striking being the umbrellalike copulatory bursa of the males, the twinned ovaries, oviducts, and uteri of the females, and the thin-shelled eggs (Figs. 92-2, 92-5, 92-6). *A. duodenale* males (8 to 11

mm long) and females (10 to 13 mm long) are somewhat larger than those of *N. americanus* (7 to 9 mm; 9 to 11 mm long), and the structures for attachment to the intestinal mucosa differ in the two species. In *A. duodenale*, the buccal capsule is provided with paired toothlike processes, whereas semilunar cutting plates are present in *N. americanus* (Fig. 92-6). The females of *A. duodenale* produce more eggs per day (10,000 to 20,000) than those of *N. americanus* (5,000 to 10,000), and the *A. duodenale* infections usually are more severe and less amenable to treatment. *N. americanus*, the American killer, is the only human species of importance throughout the hookworm belt of the southern United States. It will be necessary, however, to be on the alert for *A. duodenale*, as it is known that some military personnel have returned from other parts of the world with this species. The life cycles of these various hookworms are similar.

LIFE CYCLE.   The adult worms are usually attached to the upper levels of the small intestine. The head is anchored securely to the intestine, the tip of a villus usually being drawn into the mouth of the worm, and blood is

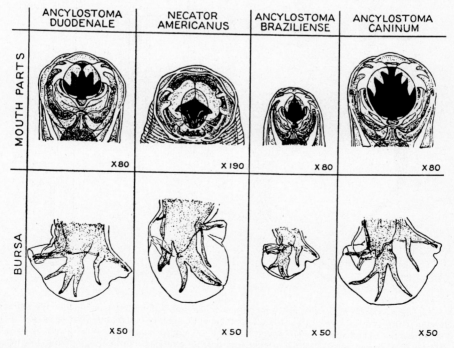

FIG. 92-6. Mouth parts and bursae of hookworms. (From Belding: Textbook of Clinical Parasitology, 2nd ed, 1952. Courtesy of Appleton-Century-Crofts)

sucked from the capillaries. After copulation, the females oviposit, and the eggs occur in the stool (Fig. 92-2). These usually are in the four- to eight-cell stage, but much further development is noted within eggs passed from constipated individuals. Under favorable conditions (especially warm temperature, shade, and moist sandy-loam soil) the eggs will embryonate and hatch in the deposited feces within 24 to 48 hours. The first-stage larvae, freed from the eggs, are typically rhabditiform and have a long buccal chamber (Fig. 92-7). They feed actively, especially on bacteria in the feces, and molt into the second stage after two or three days. This stage, also rhabditiform, continues to feed and grow for two or three days, when it molts into the third stage. The third-stage filariform larvae remain within the old cuticles (of the second molt) and thus cannot feed (Fig. 92-7). These larvae have sharply pointed tails and

are the infective stage. Except under optimum conditions, most of the filariform larvae probably die within a few weeks in the absence of a suitable host. The usual means of human infection is penetration by these larvae, after they escape from the old cuticles, into the tender skin between the toes of barefooted individuals. After many hours, the larvae enter the cutaneous blood vessels and are carried through the right heart to the lungs. After a few days, they have succeeded in penetrating from the pulmonary capillaries into the alveoli, have ascended the respiratory tract to the epiglottis, and, after having been swallowed, have descended to the upper small intestine. During this time they undergo a third molt and acquire a temporary buccal capsule. After attaching to the villi, the young worms undergo a fourth molt and in about six weeks grow into sexually mature males and females. Although some of

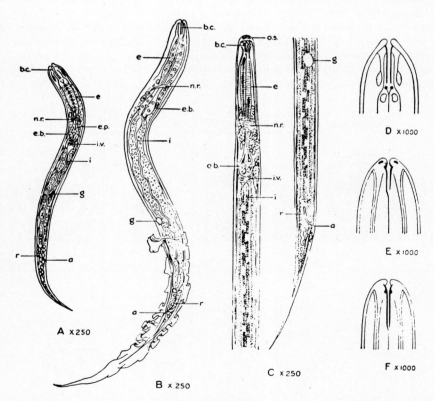

FIG. 92-7. Larvae of *Ancylostoma duodenale*. A, recently hatched rhabditiform larva, lateral view; B, rhabditiform larva during late stage of first ecdysis; C, filariform larva, lateral view; D, anterior end rhabditiform larva (schematic); E, anterior end filariform larva (schematic); F, anterior end filariform larva of *N. americanus* (schematic); a, anus; b.c., buccal cavity; e, esophagus; e.b., esophageal bulb; e.p., excretory pore; g, genital primordium; i, intestine; i.v., intestinal valve; n.r., nerve ring; o.s., old sheath; r, rectum. (From Belding: Textbook of Clinical Parasitology, 2nd ed, 1952. Courtesy of Appleton-Century-Crofts)

the worms in man live for 10 years, most of them will have been lost from the host after 1 to 2 years.

PATHOLOGY AND SYMPTOMATOLOGY. At the site of entry of the filariform larvae into the skin, most individuals experience intense itching and burning, followed by edema and erythema. A papule may appear, which transforms into a vesicle. This condition, known as ground itch, is more serious in those sensitized by previous infections and in those developing secondary infections. The larvae reaching the lungs produce small focal hemorrhages as they penetrate from the capillaries into the alveoli, but usually only a subclinical pneumonitis is produced. The greatest damage results from the adult worms attached to the small intestine. The superficial mucosa within the buccal cavity of the worm becomes denuded, and the surrounding mucosa usually shows a mild inflammatory infiltrate. More important is the blood loss. Blood is sucked from the capillaries of the villi, and it passes through the digestive tract of the worms. Apparently only highly refined products (amino acids, vitamins, and so on) are removed, the remainder being extruded through the anus in a wasteful fashion. Adding to this blood loss, which may average more than 0.2 ml per worm daily, is that occurring after a change(s) in site of attachment. The former wound continues to ooze blood for a time after the worm has released the tissue. Blood loss from the intestinal wall constitutes the greatest damage in hookworm infection. This loss, unless compensated adequately, will give rise to a microcytic, hypochromic anemia. Whether an individual with hookworm infection develops hookworm disease is dependent, in general, upon the number of worms harbored and his nutritional status. Even moderately heavy infections may fail to produce a significant anemia if the individual has been on an adequate, well-balanced diet rich in animal proteins, iron and other minerals, and vitamins. However, in heavy infections, even with a highly fortified diet, the hematopoietic mechanism is unable to keep pace with the great loss of red blood cells.

In many endemic areas of hookworm, the natives are infected repeatedly from early childhood. Thus, chronic hookworm disease is most characteristic. Common signs and symptoms are anemia, epigastric burning, flatulence,

sallow skin, tender abdomen, irritability, alternating diarrhea and constipation, dry skin, blurred vision, and so on. When the condition finally produces marked physical weakness, the individual is not fit for any type of manual labor. This accounts for the early term "lazy disease." Cardiac symptoms are evident in many, and, especially in severe cases, death may result from cardiac failure. Physical (including sexual) stunting is characteristic in children, and many are also retarded mentally.

CUTANEOUS LARVA MIGRANS OR CREEPING ERUPTION. The filariform larvae of the dog and cat hookworms (*A. caninum* and, especially, *A. braziliense*) are the agents of this clinical condition, which is most often observed in children. The condition is common along the sandy coastal areas from New Jersey to the Florida Keys and elsewhere. At each point of entry into the skin there is produced an itching, reddish papule. After a few days, the larvae have developed a serpiginous tunnel in the skin as they proceed (usually at the rate of several millimeters a day). Over a period of weeks or months this results in extensive skin involvement (Fig. 92-8). At times, severe systemic illness may result. These movements, limited to the skin of man, and the resulting irritation, produce an intense pruritus. This leads to scratching and often opens the lesions to pyogenic organisms. Oral or topical thiabendazole is the drug of choice.

LABORATORY DIAGNOSIS. To diagnose human hookworm infection, the characteristic eggs are demonstrated in the stool. These are bluntly ovoid in shape, 40 by 60 μm, have a thin, transparent shell, and usually are in the four-cell stage (Fig. 92–2). Simple fecal smears are sufficient in detecting most infections, but a concentration method (zinc sulfate, and so on) may be necessary to detect light infections. An estimate of the worm burden may be obtained by use of the Stoll or Beaver technique.

TREATMENT. Evidence obtained from numerous worldwide studies indicates that bephenium hydroxynaphthoate (Alcopar) should now be considered the drug of choice. In addition to its striking effectiveness against hookworms, it removes a high percentage of the adult worms of *Ascaris* and certain other intestinal helminths in combined infections.

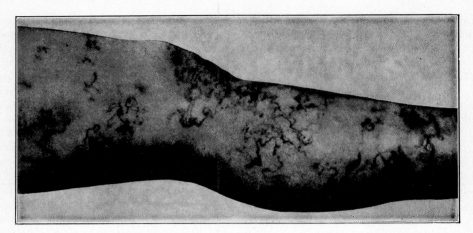

FIG. 92-8. Creeping eruption of *Ancylostoma braziliense*. Multiple, rapidly developing lesions of about 2 weeks' duration. (From Belding: Textbook of Clinical Parasitology, 2nd ed, 1952. Courtesy of Appleton-Century-Crofts)

Moreover, no serious side effects have been reported even in anemic persons with greatly reduced hemoglobin levels, and purgatives are not necessary. However, it should be added that Mebendazole (Vermox) is considered by many to be more effective against *N. Americanus*.

Strongyloides stercoralis (Human Threadworm, Causing Strongyloidiasis) LIFE CYCLE. Four different cycles may be involved. The direct cycle is the most common. The parasitic females are slender filiform worms about 2 mm in length. They usually reside among the epithelial and gland cells or in the tunica propria in the upper levels of the small intestine. Here, apparently in the absence of males, they lay several dozens of eggs daily (Fig. 92-9), at least during the first few months of infection. As the eggs filter through the mucosa toward the lumen they develop and hatch, freeing the first-stage rhabditiform larvae (Fig. 92-9). These make their way to the lumen and are passed in the stool. Under favorable conditions, as mentioned above for hookworm larvae, the filariform larvae (Fig. 92-9) make their appearance within a few days and enter exposed human skin to initiate a new infection. Their migration to the lungs and thence to the small intestine is similar to that described above for the hookworm larvae, but it should be noted that *S. stercoralis* larvae molt twice in the lungs. After reaching the tissue of the small intestine, the larvae develop into mature females in about 25 days, and these worms may live for several

years. They probably are parthenogenetic. This type of cycle is similar to that of the hookworm cycle, except that part of the early *S. stercoralis* cycle (embryonation and hatching of the eggs, and growth of the first-stage rhabditiform larvae) occurs in man. A second type of cycle, common only in the tropics, involves the interpolation of one or more free-living generations. This is the indirect cycle. In this case, the rhabditiform larvae in the stool retain the rhabditiform type of esophagus and develop into free-living males and females. Eventually some of the rhabditiform larvae produced develop into filariform larvae to begin the parasitic cycle. The intrahuman cycle is the same as that of the direct cycle. The indirect cycle was no doubt the original cycle from which the parasitic cycle evolved. Being able to live a free or a parasitic existence suggests that *S. stercoralis* has become a parasite of man in comparatively recent times.

The third, and perhaps least common, type of cycle is that known as internal autoinfection, or hyperinfection. In this case, the rhabditiform larvae, before leaving the inside of the body, metamorphose into the filariform larvae, which, after entering the intestinal wall, migrate through the tissues of the body. Some reach the lungs, as in other cycles, and return to the small intestine, but many find their way into various other tissues, where considerable damage may result. This is most common in those with low tissue resistance, and it may produce a fatal outcome.

It should be noted that immunosuppression

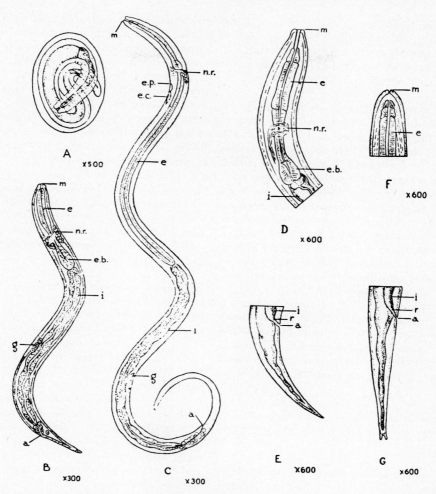

FIG. 92-9. Larvae of *Strongyloides stercoralis*. A, egg containing mature larva of *S. simiae;* B, rhabditiform larva; C, filariform larva; D, anterior end of rhabditiform larva; E, posterior end of rhabditiform larva; F, anterior end of filariform larva; G, posterior end of filariform larva; a, anus; e, esophagus; e.b., esophageal bulb; e.c., excretory cell; e.p., excretory pore; g, genital rudiment; i, intestine; m, mouth; n.r., nerve ring; r, rectum. (From Belding: Textbook of Clinical Parasitology, 2nd ed, 1952. Courtesy of Appleton-Century-Crofts)

has been reported to cause this type of cycle in those harboring *S. stercoralis*. Therefore, it is necessary to consider the presence of this and possibly other helminthic infections (as well as mycotic and other infections) in patients selected for such suppression.

The fourth type of cycle results from external autoinfection when precociously developed filariform larvae on fecal contaminated areas penetrate the skin, usually in the perianal area.

PATHOLOGY AND SYMPTOMATOLOGY. A severe pneumonitis may be produced by the larvae in the lungs, but the main damage is produced in the wall of the small intestine by the females, eggs, and rhabditiform larvae. Mechanical, and perhaps lytic, damage is produced, especially by the females, which move about considerably. Cellular infiltration, often striking, consists chiefly of eosinophils, lymphocytes, and epithelioid cells. This may be general throughout large areas of the mucosa and not limited to areas adjacent to the worms. The affected tissue becomes increasingly nonfunctional, and at times sloughing of the tissue occurs. There is evidence of systemic damage consisting of sensitization and probably toxic reactions. As stated above, autoinfection may produce severe damage in various tissues, with striking signs and symptoms. The most characteristic symptoms of the usual type of infection are midepigastric pain, a watery-mucous diarrhea, and eosinophilia.

Laboratory Diagnosis.　This usually is made by finding the characteristic rhabditiform larvae in the stool (Fig. 92-9). These are about 200 by 15 μm in size. There usually is no confusion with hookworms, but it might be added that the structure of these larvae differs from that of hookworms. The difference in the buccal chamber alone is sufficient to differentiate the two. As mentioned above, the rhabditiform larvae of hookworms have a long buccal chamber, whereas those of S. stercoralis have a short inconspicuous chamber. The filariform larvae likewise may be differentiated by a single difference. Those of hookworms have a sharply pointed tail, those of S. stercoralis have a notched tail (Figs. 92-7, 92-9). Many times duodenal aspirates will reveal larvae when stools are negative, but at times the reverse is true. Sometimes the larvae can be recovered from urine, sputum, or aspirates from body cavities.

Treatment.　Thiabendazole by mouth has been shown to be an effective drug against this parasite.

Trichinella spiralis (Cause of Trichinellosis or Trichinosis) Life Cycle.　Man is infected by ingesting infective larvae (Fig. 92-10) encysted in striated muscles of a reservoir host, swine being the most important. Gastric digestion frees most of the larvae. They soon enter the small intestine and penetrate into the mucosa. Within two days they have undergone the necessary molts to reach the adult stage (Fig. 92-10). The males measure 1.4 to 1.6 mm in length and have a pair of characteristic conical papillae (bursae) guarding the terminal cloaca. The females, more than twice the length of the males, have the vulvar opening at about one-fifth the body length from the anterior end. Copulation occurs, and the females, after burrowing more deeply into the mucosa or even to lower levels, begin to larvaposit. This is thought to begin about 5 days after infection and is completed for the most part by 14 days. The total number of larvae released by each female is about 500. The larvae released from

the females are small, about 100 by 6 μm. They enter the circulation and are distributed throughout the body. However, only those entering striated muscles are capable of further development. Here, within three weeks after infection, encapsulation begins. This host reaction, initiated by infiltration mainly by round cells and eosinophils, results in the formation of a double-walled, adventitious capsule (Fig. 92-10). The larvae within grow to about 0.8 mm in length and become coiled tightly. The larvae are infective for a new host a few days after encapsulation has begun. Some remain viable within cysts for many years, despite the fact that calcification of the cyst is usually observed after six months. As noted, this parasite is completely parasitic, as there is no free existence in its cycle.

Pathology and Symptomatology.　Trichinosis has been confused with many other diseases, because the parasite may damage various tissues of the body. For a clear understanding of the disease, it is necessary to consider in turn the various stages involved. During the first stage, the adult worms are becoming established in the mucosa of the small intestine. Due to extensive burrowing, tissue is destroyed, and an intense inflammatory reaction results. Nausea, vomiting, diarrhea, and fever may be experienced. These and other signs and symptoms resemble salmonellosis and other enteric infections. This stage usually lasts for about 10 days; thus it overlaps the second stage. The second stage, set arbitrarily between 7 and 14 days after infection, involves most of the larvae in the circulation. The fever usually reaches a peak (41C), and there is characteristic edema (especially of the face) and eosinophilia. In addition, dyspnea, difficulty in mastication and speech, and petechial hemorrhages, especially in the conjunctivas and retinal vessels, may be noted. Cardiac and neurologic signs and symptoms often are noted, and it should be remembered that any organ may be damaged by the migrating larvae. The features of this stage are most pronounced during the second week but continue throughout the period of larvaposition. The third stage, after 14 days, is a culmination of the traumatic, allergenic and toxic effects of the infection. Also myositis is outstanding, so that muscular pains are usually the chief complaint. Larvae entering muscle fibers cause a severe reaction. The infiltrate

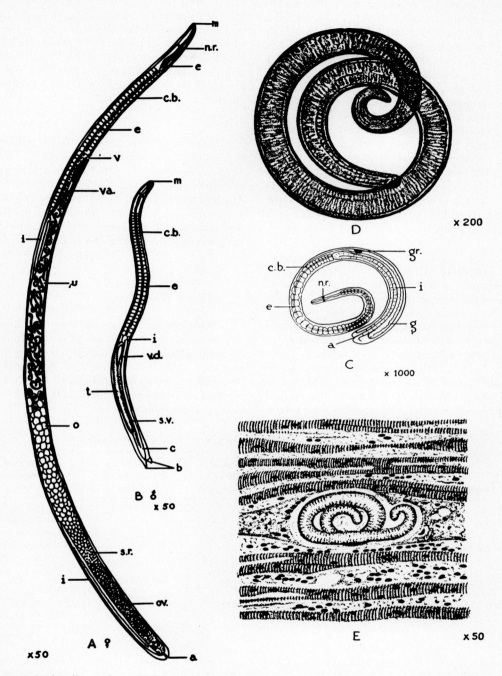

FIG. 92-10. *Trichinella spiralis.* A, adult female; B, adult male; C, young larva; D, mature larva from digested muscle; E, early encysted larva in muscle; a, anus; b, "bursa"; c, cloaca; c.b., cell bodies; e, esophagus; g, gonads (anlage); gr., granules; i, intestine; m, mouth; n.r., nerve ring; o, eggs; ov., ovary; s.r., seminal receptacle; s.v., seminal vesicle; t, testis; u, uterus; v, vulva; va., vagina; v.d., vas deferens. (From Brown and Belding: Basic Clinical Parasitology, 2nd ed, 1964. Courtesy of Appleton-Century-Crofts)

consists chiefly of plasma cells, lymphocytes, and especially, eosinophils. This host response results in the formation of the characteristic cyst. The edema, especially around the eyes, persists, as does the hypereosinophilia, which reaches a peak about 21 days after infection. Cachexia may be profound. Many fatal cases show congestive heart failure due to myocardial lesions, respiratory paralysis, and anaphylaxis. Those surviving usually are cured symptomatically five to eight weeks after infection, but a much longer period is required in some cases. Except during epidemics, most cases are relatively asymptomatic, due presumably to the consumption of small numbers of larvae. However, it should be kept in mind that death will result inevitably if large numbers are ingested.

LABORATORY DIAGNOSIS. A specific means of diagnosis is provided by biopsy of a small piece of the deltoid or other muscle. The larvae may be demonstrated by pressing the tissue firmly between two microscope slides prior to microscopic examination or by recovering the larvae following digestion in artifical gastric juice. To relate the presence of larvae to the present illness, it is important to consider the stage of cyst formation. For example, the finding of calcified cysts only could not be related

to an illness of recent origin. Various serologic tests are available, but the bentonite flocculation test is considered the best to detect acute infections. An intradermal test is available. Finally, the degree of and changes in the eosinophilic response, although not specific and not always striking, are of assistance and should be charted.

TREATMENT. In general, only palliative and supportive measures are of value. However, cortisone and related drugs are of great assistance during the larval encystment period. Allergic reactions to, or toxic effects from, the metabolites of the worms often show amelioration after use of cortisone, and on occasion this drug has appeared to be lifesaving.

Tissue Nematodes

This group includes six species of filariae (Filarioidea) and *Dracunculus medinensis* (Dracunculoidea). Information regarding these parasites is given in Table 92-1. Among those listed, *Wuchereria bancrofti* is of the greatest interest and importance, hence it will be discussed in more detail.

TABLE 92-1   FILARIAE AND DRACUNCULUS MEDINENSIS

Parasite	Disease	Location of Adults in Man	Location of Microfilariae in Man	Arthropod Intermediate Hosts
Wuchereria bancrofti	Bancroft's filariasis	Lymphatics	Blood	Mosquitoes; especially *Anopheles, Culex, Aëdes* spp.
Brugia malayi	Malayan filariasis	Lymphatics	Blood	Mosquitoes: *Mansonia, Anopheles* spp.
Onchocerca volvulus	Onchocerciasis	Subcutaneous nodules	Skin tissues	*Simulium* spp., black flies
Loa loa	Loasis	Subcutaneous tissues	Blood	*Chrysops* spp., deer flies
Acanthocheilonema perstans	Acanthocheilonemiasis	Body cavities, especially perirenal tissues	Blood	*Culicoides* spp., biting midges
Mansonella ozzardi	Ozzard's filariasis	Body cavities, especially mesentery fat	Blood	*Culicoides* spp., biting midges
Dracunculus medinensis	Dracontiasis	Visceral connective tissues, in subcutaneous tissues	No microfilarial stage; female discharges rhabditform larvae	*Cyclops* spp., small crustaceans

Wuchereria bancrofti (Cause of Bancroft's Filariasis) Life Cycle. The adults, usually coiled together, live within the lymphatic system of man. The males are about 40 mm in length, and the females about 90 mm. Both sexes are threadlike, being no more than 0.3 mm in diameter. Following copulation, the females give off living embryos, termed microfilariae. These ultimately find their way into the bloodstream. In most strains, they circulate in the blood in largest numbers at night and are said to have nocturnal periodicity. In certain other strains either no particular periodicity is noted, or there is a tendency for the occurrence of the largest numbers at dusk. The circulating microfilariae, 125 to 320 μm in length by 7 to 10 μm in cross-section, are active within a sheath, the retained transparent egg membrane that was stretched about the embryos during development in utero. These forms will develop only in certain mosquitoes. Hence, pathology will not result if blood containing them is transfused into a recipient. Female mosquitoes of various genera (especially *Culex, Aedes,* and *Anopheles*) serve as necessary intermediate hosts for this parasite. When feeding upon an infected individual, they ingest the microfilariae from the peripheral bloodstream. These pass into the midgut, and after escaping from their sheaths, many invade the intestinal wall. Within 24 hours, most of these find their way to the thoracic muscles. Under favorable conditions of temperature and humidity, they undergo metamorphosis to third-stage infective larvae in one to three weeks. This stage is active and migrates to the tip of the proboscis sheath, from which it penetrates onto the skin of the human host at the time of the next blood meal. It probably enters the wound made by the mosquito. After entering the skin, these larvae pass to the lymphatic system and grow to maturity; in most cases this probably requires at least one year. The adult worms may live for many years in certain individuals.

Pathology and Symptomatology. In endemic areas, most of the natives are more or less asymptomatic. In these, there appears to be an excellent host-parasite adjustment. The host experiences little or no disturbance, and the parasite is able to develop normally, which results in the release of large numbers of microfilariae. These individuals, therefore, are the main source of infection for the mosquito host,

as man is the only known definitive host. In those showing clinical evidence of the infection, two distinct stages are evident. In the acute stage there is a characteristic, and often profound, lymphatic inflammation in response to trapped worms and/or their metabolites. Tissue changes tend eventually to constrict the wall of the lymphatic vessel or other affected parts of the system. This partial obstruction results in lymph stasis and edema. The cardinal manifestation is a recurrent lymphangitis, usually with an associated lymphadenitis. Some experience a low-grade fever, usually of short duration. The location of the obstruction determines the part of the body affected, the external genitalia of both sexes being the most common. In the absence of reinfections, there usually is steady improvement in the individual, each relapse being milder than the former. Thus, even without specific therapy this condition is self-limiting and presumably will not become chronic in those acquiring the infection during a brief sojourn in an endemic area. It is of interest to note that microfilariae are difficult to demonstrate during the acute phase, indicating a pronounced disturbance in the host-parasite equilibrium. Lymph node biopsy (p. 1156) has been used in special cases to demonstrate adult worms. Sectioning the tissues reveals the worms; the females are readily recognized by the microfilariae in utero. The characteristic reaction here consists of a necrotic zone around the worms and a palisaded area of foreign body giant cells, epithelioid cells, and eosinophils.

There is good evidence that the advanced chronic type of filariasis, known as elephantiasis, develops only in a small percentage of highly reactive individuals infected repeatedly for many years. Following lymphatic obstruction, striking proliferative changes occur, and the worms die and are absorbed or become calcified. The edema, soft at first, becomes fibrotic following the growth of connective tissue in the area. The redundant skin, being nourished poorly, cracks and becomes fissured and often is secondarily infected with pyogenic or mycotic organisms. This resemblance to elephant skin accounts for the term "elephantiasis" applied to this chronic, disfiguring condition. Although microfilariae may appear in the blood of chronic cases, due to new active infections superimposed upon the older ones, they are not often demonstrated. Thus, it appears that the more reactive the host, the less likely is the development of the worms and the release of embryos.

From this account, it is obvious that undue emphasis has been placed on the advanced chronic type of filariasis, which involves a relatively few individuals even in highly endemic areas.

LABORATORY DIAGNOSIS.   A final diagnosis is made by demonstrating the microfilariae, usually in thick blood smears. In most areas of the world, they are present in appreciable numbers only at night, usually with greatest frequency between 10 PM and 2AM. It should be remembered that microfilariae cannot be demonstrated during the incubation period and, usually, not during the acute phase of the infection. In the absence of microfilariae, a presumptive diagnosis can be made on the basis of the history of exposure, clinical evidence of the disease, and positive serologic tests and/or a positive intradermal test. It may be added that lymph node biopsy, during clinical quiescence only, often will reveal adult or immature worms. This, however, is a research tool and should not be used except in unusual circumstances and then only by adhering to strict surgical techniques.

TREATMENT.   Patients with acute infections resulting from recent primary exposure should be removed from the endemic area, if possible. Bed rest and supportive measures, such as hot and cold compresses, are of assistance in reducing the edema. Psychotherapy often is necessary, especially for young males with scrotal involvement.

The anthelmintic of choice is Hetrazan, an antimonial taken orally.

CESTODES

The adult cestodes, or tapeworms, are strobilate, ie, they consist of a chain of units made up of the scolex (head), the neck, and a series of proglottids (segments). The scolex is adapted for attachment to the intestinal mucosa. It is provided with cupped suckers or sucking grooves according to the species. In some cases hooklets are also present. The delicate, unsegmented neck region, immediately behind the scolex, is a budding zone that gives rise to all of the more distal parts of the worm. Sexually im-

mature proglottids arise directly from the neck, then mature units containing fully developed male and female reproductive organs, and distalmost the gravid units. The number of proglottids varies considerably among the different species. In contrast to the prominent male and female genital systems, tapeworms have simple nervous and excretory systems, and a digestive system is lacking.

In presenting the material of this section, the cestodes will be grouped according to their common habitat in the body, the intestinal tract and various tissues. The intestinal cestodes live as adults in man, whereas the tissue cestodes occur in a larval stage.

Intestinal Cestodes

This discussion will be limited to the four most common intestinal cestodes of man: *Diphyllobothrium latum* (fish or broad tapeworm), *Taenia saginata* (beef tapeworm), *Taenia solium* (pork tapeworm), and *Hymenolepis nana* (dwarf tapeworm). The first three are very large, ranging in length from 3 to 10 meters or more, whereas the fourth is, by comparison, a dwarf, being 45 mm or less in length. To conserve space, the four species will be considered together under each topic.

LIFE CYCLES.   *D. latum*, being a more primitive form, differs from the other species in many ways, both in structure and complexity of the life cycle. The scolex is spatulate and is provided with a median ventral and dorsal grooved sucker (Fig. 92-11). The proglottids are broad, and the centrally located uterus has a characteristic rosette arrangement. Eggs within the fully developed uterus are discharged continuously in large numbers from the uterine pore (Figs. 92-2, 92-11). These are undeveloped when passed in the stool and will embryonate only upon reaching cool fresh water. Embryonation is completed after two weeks or more, and hatching occurs. A ciliated embryo (coracidium) escapes from the shell and swims about actively (Fig. 92-12). If this stage is ingested by one of the first intermediate hosts (copepods of the genus *Diaptomus* or *Cyclops*), the embryo, after losing the ciliated covering, burrows into the body cavity (hemocoel) and transforms, within two or three weeks, into a

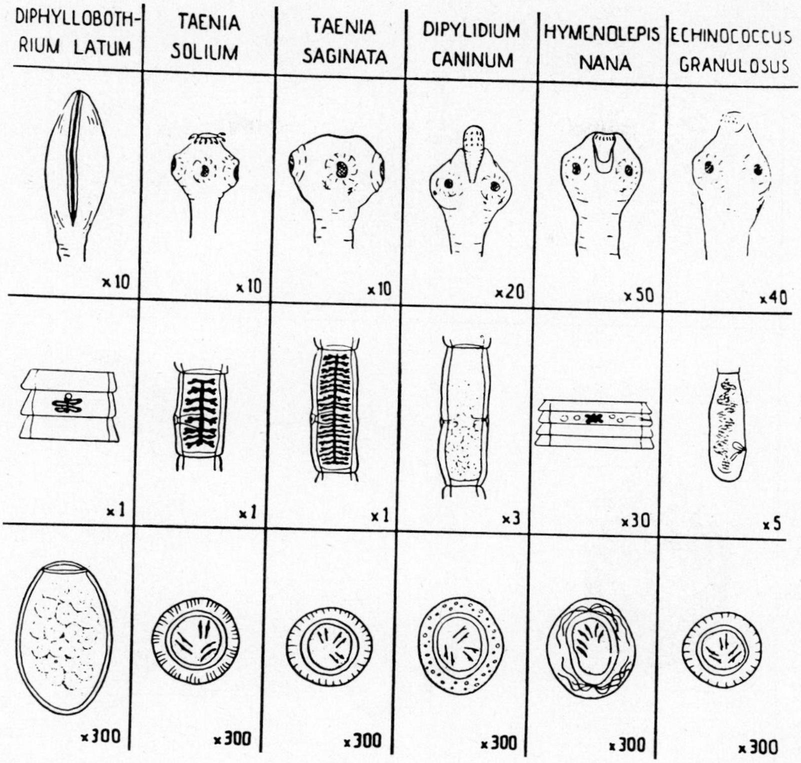

FIG. 92-11. Differential characteristics of common tapeworms of man. (Modified from Belding: Textbook of Clinical Parasitology, 2nd ed, 1952. Courtesy of Appleton-Century-Crofts)

mature first larval stage (procercoid, Fig. 92-12). Ingestion of the first intermediate host with these mature larvae by the second intermediate host (many different fresh-water fishes) continues the cycle. The larvae migrate into the flesh (often between the muscle fibers) of the fish and metamorphose, within several weeks, into a second larval stage (plerocercoid, Fig. 92-12). Larger (edible) fishes acquire the infection from eating their infected young or infected smaller species. Consumption by man or other definitive hosts (dogs, bear, and so on) of fish flesh containing mature plerocercoid larvae completes the cycle. The worm, usually only one, develops to maturity in the small intestine in three to five weeks, and egg production begins. The worm may live for many years.

The scolex of *T. saginata* is rhomboidal and has cup-shaped suckers (Fig. 92-11). These are the sole means of attachment, since the rostellum is devoid of hooklets. The distalmost gravid proglottids (Fig. 92-11), each containing about 80,000 mature eggs, become separated from the strobila and actively migrate out of the anus or are evacuated in the stool. If grazing cattle, the only intermediate host, ingest the proglottids, or more commonly, the eggs freed after disintegration of the proglottids on moist earth or in sewage, the cycle proceeds. The six-hooked embryos (onchospheres) escape from the eggs, following hatching in the duodenum, and penetrate into the intestinal tissue to reach, ultimately, the circulation. They are carried about, and most of them reach skeletal muscles or the heart. In these sites, they transform in 60 to 75 days into a typical cysticercus stage. (*Cysticercus bovis*), which contains a scolex, similar to that of the adult worm, invaginated into the fluid-filled bladder (Fig. 92-13). Man is infected by ingesting these larvae in beef, either raw or processed inadequately. The head of the larva attaches to the wall of the ileum, and the adult worm, usually only one, develops to maturity in 8 to 10 weeks and may live for several years.

The scolex of *T. solium* bears, in addition to

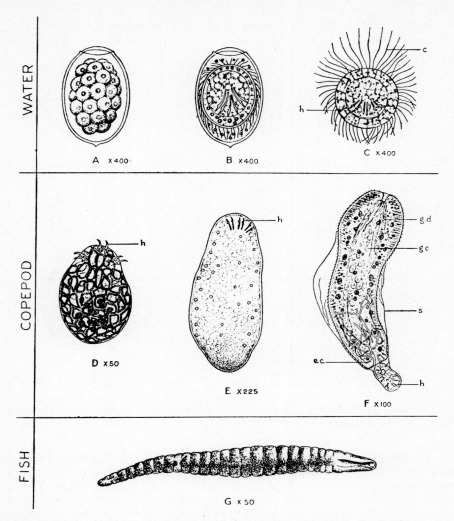

FIG. 92-12. Eggs and larvae forms of *Diphyllobothrium latum*. A, undeveloped egg; B, hexacanth embryo in eggshell; C, ciliated coracidium; D, larva, seven days after infection of copepod; E, larva, 20 days; F, procercoid larva; G, plerocercoid larva; c, cilia; e.c., excretory cell; g.c., gland cells; g.d., ducts of glands; h, hooklets; s, old membrane of onchosphere. (From Belding: Textbook of Clinical Parasitology, 2nd ed, 1952. Courtesy of Appleton-Century-Crofts)

the four cup-shaped suckers, 22 to 32 small hooklets on the rostellum (Fig. 92-11). The length of the worm is shorter than that of *T. saginata*, and the structure of the proglottids differs in the two species (Fig. 92-11). The life cycles of the two species are similar, except that the hog is the usual intermediate host for *T. solium*. The scolex of this larval stage (*Cysticercus cellulosae*) is provided with four suckers and a crown of hooklets. This stage may also occur in man and cause serious injury (p. 1160). For this reason, *T. solium* has greater medical and public health importance than *T. saginata*.

The scolex of *H. nana* has four cup-shaped suckers and a rostellar circle of 20 to 30 hooklets (Fig. 92-11). Unlike the three large species that usually occur singly, the adults of *H. nana* may be numerous. The terminal gravid proglottids usually disintegrate before separation from the strobila, so that the mature eggs are passed in the stool (Figs. 92-2, 92-11). In the direct cycle, these eggs initiate infection upon ingestion. Such infections may be of a direct hand-to-mouth type or of an indirect type via contaminated food and/or drink. The eggs hatch in the duodenum, and the liberated six-hooked em-

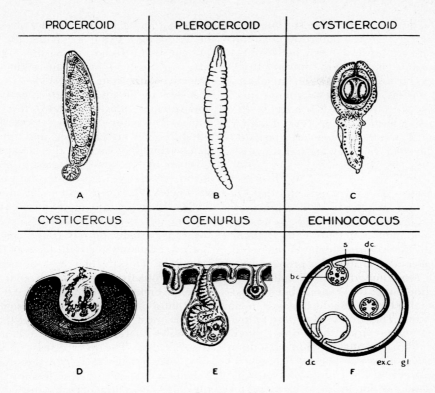

FIG. 92-13. Larval forms of tapeworms, b.c., brood capsule; d.c., daughter cyst; ex.c., external laminated cuticla; g.l., germinal or inner nucleated layer; s, scolex. (From Belding: Textbook of Clinical Parasitology, 2nd ed, 1952. Courtesy of Appleton-Century-Crofts)

bryos penetrate into nearby villi. The resulting larval stage (cysticercoid), mature in about four days, penetrates into the intestinal lumen, attaches to the mucosa, and develops in about two weeks into the adult worm. This cycle, with both the larval and adult stages in the same host, is unique for a cestode. In the indirect cycle, insects, especially certain beetles, serve as the intermediate host. Accidental ingestion of those containing the mature cysticercoids (Figs. 92-13) results in infection.

PATHOLOGY AND SYMPTOMATOLOGY. The adult stage of the three large cestodes usually causes little damage and gives rise only to vague signs and symptoms, such as epigastric distress, false hunger pains, and nervous manifestations, but there are important exceptions to this rule. The most important of these is the so-called bothriocephalus anemia exhibited by certain individuals infected with *D. latum*. This disease is a true symptomatic pernicious anemia. It appears that the living worm and the

host compete for vitamin B_{12}. If the worm is in the proximal part of the small intestine, a deficiency in this substance may result, causing pernicious anemia. After a period of time, a poor supply of extrinsic factor and/or reduced production of intrinsic factor contributes to the development of this condition.

Heavy infections with *H. nana*, particularly in children, usually give rise to serious conditions, such as striking abdominal pain, bloody-mucous stools, and exaggerated nervous disorders.

LABORATORY DIAGNOSIS. This is based on the recovery of the species-characteristic eggs of *D. latum* and *H. nana* and gravid proglottids of *T. saginata* and *T. solium*. The eggs of *D. latum* are unembryonated, about 70 by 45 μm in size, have an operculum at one end and a thickened shell, often with a knob, at the opposite end (Fig. 92-2). Those of *H. nana* are nearly spherical, measure about 50 μm in diameter, and have polar filaments arising from the inner membranous shell that surrounds the embryo (Fig. 92-2). When the fresh proglottids of *T. saginata* are pressed gently between two microscope slides and held in front of a bright light, it is easy to see 15 to 20 main lateral arms of the uterus (Figs. 92-11). *T. solium* has only 7 to 13 of these arms (Figs. 92-11), making differentiation a simple procedure. Eggs of both *T. saginata* and *T. solium* are recovered occasionally from the stool, but they are indistinguishable (Figs. 92-2, 92-11).

TREATMENT.   Evidence indicates that Atabrine is the drug of choice in all four infections, although hexylresorcinol (crystoids) is used by some to treat light infections with *H. nana.* Success with the Atabrine treatment depends, in large measure, upon adequate preparation of the patient. Most important is the administration of a saline purge the evening before treatment, since effective treatment depends on an empty intestine. The drug is given the following morning on an empty stomach as a single dose along with an equal amount of sodium bicarbonate or other substance to counteract nausea and vomiting. Two hours later a second saline purgation is employed to evacuate the worm(s), which usually is passed intact and stained a deep yellow.

Tissue Cestodes

As noted above, two of the intestinal cestodes may have a tissue stage in man, *T. solium* and *H. nana.* In addition, there are two species of small cestodes in the genus *Echinococcus* that are dangerous tissue parasites of man, *Echinococcus granulosus* and *Echinococcus multilocularis.* Until 1951 there was general agreement that the various types of *Echinococcus* larval development in man were of the single species, *E. granulosus.* It is now clear that this species produces a larval cyst known as the unilocular hydatid cyst (p. 1161), whereas the other species, *E. multilocularis,* is responsible for a peculiar, branching type, larval cyst, the alveolar hydatid cyst. Since space permits discussion of only one of these parasites, *E. multilocularis* will be omitted. However, to compare it with the more common and widespread *E. granulosus,* a few comments should be made.

LIFE CYCLE.   *E. multilocularis* adults (smaller and morphologically differentiated from *E. granulosus*) occur in the small intestine of wild canines, the fox being the most important definitive host (domestic dogs and cats may be involved in certain endemic areas). Infective eggs occur in the stool, and if they are ingested by an intermediate host (wild mice and voles are most important), the cycle continues. The embryos migrate to the liver (less often to other visceral sites) and grow by exogenous budding to form the larval stage, the alveolar hydatid cyst. Infected viscera with a mature cyst(s), if ingested by the canine host, completes the cycle when contained protoscolices develop into adult worms. Man serves accidentally as an intermediate host by ingesting eggs, usually on raw fruit, such as strawberries, contaminated with feces of the definitive host. The alveolar cyst in man lacks a strong protective layer, which appears to encourage branching formations of cavities with little fluid and few, if any, protoscolices. The liver is most often involved, and the damage resembles that produced by a large amebic liver abscess. The liver disease is almost always fatal. Skin and serologic tests can be used to make a diagnosis, and biotherapy (p. 1161) is the only known form of treatment.

The most important of the various larval cestodes in man are *C. cellulosae* (larval stage of *T. solium,* p. 1156) and *E. granulosus.* They will be considered together for this discussion.

THE INVOLVEMENT OF MAN IN THE LIFE CYCLE. The egg is the stage that infects man in both cases. In the case of *C. cellulosae,* three means of infection are known. A patient harboring the adult worm may become infected by transferring mature eggs from the anus to the mouth on unclean fingertips (external autoinfection), or these eggs may be transferred indirectly to another person (heteroinfection). The third type, internal autoinfection, is thought to occur when detached gravid proglottids are regurgitated into the stomach and return to the intestine, where some of the eggs become liberated. In the case of *E. granulosus,* the situation is entirely different, in that man does not harbor the adult worms. These occur, usually in large numbers in dogs and other definitive hosts. Many animals may serve as intermediate hosts, but the most important are sheep and hogs. Man serves in this capacity, but, as in trichinosis, he is a blind alley for the parasite. Human infection usually occurs by the accidental transfer of the mature eggs from the fur of the dog to the human mouth. The eggs hatch in the small intestine, and the embryos penetrate into the circulatory system. They are filtrated out in various tissues. Any organ or tissue may be involved, but the liver and lungs are the most common sites. By a remarkable process of asexual reproduction, the embryos metamorphose into hydatid cysts. These vacuolated larval cestodes are called "unilocular hydatid cysts." Cysts in soft tissues (liver, lungs, and so on) are somewhat similar, but the type in bone (osseous) tends to elongate as it flows into, and erodes, the bony canal. The unilocular hydatid cyst of the liver is the most common in man. It consists typically of a central fluid-filled cavity lined with a germinative (protoplasmic) layer, surrounded by a cuticular (protective) layer that tends to become laminated. It usually requires many years for the cyst to reach a large size. In time it becomes covered with a fibrous, host tissue capsule. Arising from the germinative layer, internal buds (brood capsules) are produced (Fig. 92-13). When full size, each forms vesicles along its inner margin. Typically, each vesicle (10 to 20 or more) develops into a small protoscolex (usually invaginated, which serves to protect the 20 to 30 rostellar hooklets) and a short neck region. Thus, a large mature cyst containing thousands of these protoscolices produces a heavy infection of adult worms when eaten by a definitive host. The optimum conditions for perpetuation of the parasite are provided in the dog-sheep cycle.

PATHOLOGY AND SYMPTOMATOLOGY. *C. cellulosae* may occur in various tissues of man, but of greatest concern is the common involvement of the eyes and the brain. Ocular cysticercosis may result in uveitis, dislocation of the retina, and other conditions. Pain, flashes of light, and grotesque figures in the field of vision and other complaints have been noted. Cerebral cysticercosis usually follows involvement of the meninges, with Jacksonian epilepsy as the most characteristic consequence, and the fourth ventricle, with hydrocephalus, headache, and diplopia being noteworthy.

The hydatid cysts of *E. granulosus* are usually single, but they may be multiple. Their size and contour depend upon the site of implantation and the age of the cysts. Because of the slow growth of cysts, vital processes usually are not disturbed sufficiently to be of concern to the patient until many years after infection. Ultimately, however, there may be great tissue de-

struction and striking signs and symptoms. The type and degree of this damage and the resulting clinical manifestations correspond to the exact location and size of the cyst(s). It should be added that systemic intoxication or sensitization often occurs in those with a unilocular hydatid cyst having a vascularized wall permitting leakage of sensitizing fluids. Sensitized individuals exhibit marked eosinophilia, and in some urticaria or angioneurotic edema is evident. Anaphylaxis may be precipitated by the sudden release of hydatid fluid, as in the case of spontaneous rupture of a large intraabdominal cyst or rupture following a severe blow to the area.

LABORATORY DIAGNOSIS. Both infections usually are diagnosed by indirect means, such as x-ray and intradermal and serologic tests.

TREATMENT. Surgery, in most instances, is the only therapeutic procedure of value in both infections. In ocular cysticercosis removal of the parasite while it is still alive usually prevents total loss of sight. In cerebral cysticercosis, procedures are well developed for extirpation of solitary cysts, and a majority of patients recover completely. However, operative techniques are not recommended in cases with generalized cerebral infections. In the case of hydatid cysts, surgical intervention is limited to those with unilocular cysts in operable sites. Meticulous care must be taken to prevent spilling the cyst contents into the operative cavity for the reason mentioned above. For the treatment of cysts in inoperable sites or for treatment of multiple cysts in several anatomic locations, biologic therapy has been employed widely. This involves the use of sterile hydatid fluid, or only the protein component, to desensitize the host, which usually is followed in time by death and gradual absorption of the cysts.

TREMATODES

The exact form of adult digenetic trematodes is dependent upon the state of contraction, but they usually are flat, elongated, and leaf-shaped. They vary considerably in size, from less than 1 mm to several centimeters. Characteristic external features include an oral and, in most species, a ventral sucker, the acetabulum, an excretory pore at the posterior extremity, and a genital pore near the anterior border of the ventral sucker. The principal internal organs include a blind, bifurcate intestinal tract, an excretory system, prominent male and/or female reproductive organs, and a primitive nervous system. The arrangement, shape, and size of these various structures are characteristic for different species.

Endoparasitic trematodes have complicated life cycles involving alternation of generations and hosts.

Information concerning the most important trematodes of man and the infections they cause is listed in Table 92-2 (see also Fig. 92-2). The schistosomes, or bloodflukes, being of the greatest medical and public health importance, deserve further consideration.

The Schistosomes

Schistosomes differ in many ways from the other digenetic trematodes. The important differences include the presence in schistosomes of separate sexes, nonoperculated eggs with spines, forktailed cercariae, and the absence of a true metacercarial stage in the life cycle. As noted in Table 92-2 there are three species that occur commonly in man: *Schistosoma japonicum*, *Schistosoma mansoni*, and *Schistosoma haematobium*. Although the other two species lack important natural reservoirs, *S. japonicum* has many mammalian reservoirs (cats, dogs, cattle, water buffaloes, and so on). However, it may be stated that man usually is the most important source of eggs of all three species. The adult worms occur characteristically in pairs in mesenteric veins *(S. japonicum* and *S. mansoni)* and vesical veins *(S. haematobium)*. The male attaches to the wall of the blood vessel, holding the female in a ventrad groove, the gynecophoral canal. The female is able to extend its anterior end into the smaller calibered venules where the eggs are discharged. As would be judged from the last two statements, the males are stouter (0.5 to 1.1 mm being the range in width among the species) than the females (0.16 to 0.30 mm). The females, on the other hand, are longer (14 to 20 mm being the range among the species) than the males (10 to 15 mm).

LIFE CYCLES.   The adults of *S. japonicum* and *S. mansoni* are found normally in the tribu-

taries of the superior and inferior mesenteric veins, respectively, whereas those of *S. haematobium* find the vesical plexus the optimum location. Although these are the usual locations, it should be remembered that the worms may be found in other sites. Perhaps most important in this connection is the well-known fact that following infection with *S. haematobium* a small percentage of the worms fail to reach the normal site and remain in the rectal vessels. Thus, some of the eggs released may occur in the stools rather than in the urine as expected in this infection. After copulation, the females give off a considerable number of eggs over a long period of time. These are undeveloped when laid but usually contain a fully developed ciliated larva (miracidium) after they have succeeded in passing through the wall of the intestine or bladder to occur in the stools or urine (Fig. 92-2). Upon reaching fresh water, hatching occurs through a tear in the shell, and the miracidium swims about in the water. If appropriate intermediate hosts are present in the immediate vicinity, the miracidium will penetrate into the soft tissues. These hosts are certain snails (eg, *Oncomelania quadrasi* for *S. japonicum* in the Philippines, *Biomphalaria glabrata* for *S. mansoni* in the Americas, and *Bulinus contortus* for *S. haematobium* in Egypt). The intrasnail cycle lasts for several weeks and involves three distinct stages, the first (mother) and second (daughter) generation sporocysts and cercariae. The latter, with characteristic forked tails, escape from the snail at intervals and swim about in the water. In contact with the skin of man, or other susceptible definitive hosts, they discard their tails and digest their way into the skin. These schistosomules reach the bloodstream and are carried through the right heart to the lungs. Here they pass the capillary filter and are carried to the left heart and thence into the large arterial vessels. From the mesenteric artery, where most of them are carried, they pass through the capillaries into the intrahepatic portal blood. They feed and grow in this site, and when sexual maturity approaches (after about 16 days of residence) they migrate against the portal blood flow to the areas where oviposition is to occur. *S. haematobium* is thought to pass from the rectal veins through hemorrhoidal anastomoses into the pudendal vein to reach ultimately the vesical venous plexus. Several weeks are required for the maturation of the adult worms (4

TABLE 92-2 IMPORTANT TREMATODES OF MAN

Parasite	Disease	Location of Adults Where Eggs are Laid	Stage Passed From Man	Second Intermediate Host (Certain Snails are the First Intermediate Host)	Means of Human Infection	Laboratory Diagnosis
Fasciolopis buski	Fasciolopsiasis	Small intestine	Undeveloped eggs in stool	Water caltrop, certain other freshwater plants	Ingestion of metacercariae	Eggs in stool (140 × 80 μm)
Clonorchis sinensis	Clonorchiasis	Distal bile ducts of liver	Developed eggs in stool	Certain freshwater fishes	Ingestion of metacercariae	Eggs in stool (30 × 16 μm)
Paragonimus westermani	Paragonimiasis	In lung capsules	Undeveloped eggs in stool and sputum	Certain freshwater crabs and crayfishes	Ingestion of metacercariae	Eggs in stool and sputum (85 × 50 μm)
Schistosoma japonicum	Schistosomiasis japonica	Venules of superior and inferior mesenteric veins	Developed eggs in stool	None	Penetration of skin by cercariae	Eggs in stool (89 × 66 μm with rudimentary lateral spine)
Schistosoma mansoni	Schistosomiasis mansoni	Venules of inferior (and, at times, superior) mesenteric vein	Developed eggs in stool, rarely in urine	None	Penetration of skin by cercariae	Eggs in stool or urine (150 × 60 μm), with large lateral spine)
Schistosoma haematobium	Schistosomiasis haematobia	Venules of vesical and pelvic plexuses	Developed eggs in urine, rarely in stool	None	Penetration of skin by cercariae	Eggs in urine or stool (150 × 60 μm, with large terminal spine)

to 5 for *S. japonicum,* 6 to 7 for *S. mansoni,* and 10 to 12 weeks after skin penetration in the case of *S. haematobium*), and they may live for many years. Thus, it can be seen that there is justification for the common statement that the life cycle of the schistosomes is a marvel of biology.

PATHOLOGY AND SYMPTOMATOLOGY.   In the case of all three species, penetration of the skin by the cercariae produces small hemorrhages, and after the schistosomules break out of the capillaries in the lungs they cause an acute inflammatory reaction predominated by eosinophils. Upon arrival in the intrahepatic portal blood, an acute hepatitis may follow as well as systemic intoxication and sensitization, all due presumably to the toxic and/or allergenic metabolites released. Many patients exhibit toxic manifestations, such as fever and sweats, epigastric distress, and pain in the back, groin, or legs. Some develop giant urticaria, and toxic diarrhea is common. These reactions may continue long after the worms have migrated to the area of oviposition. Although the penetration of the cercariae and the migrations of the schistosomules and later the movements of the developing worms usually produce detrimental effects, the main agents of pathology in schistosomiasis are the eggs released from the females.

The period of egg deposition and extrusion from the body usually is referred to as the acute stage. In the case of the two intestinal forms, *S. japonicum* and *S. mansoni,* the events of this stage are, in general, similar. However, it is important to add that the females of *S. japonicum* release considerably more eggs, hence the damage is proportionately greater. In both species the intestinal tissue is first to be damaged, usually the small intestine in the case of *S. japonicum* and the colon in the case of *S. mansoni.* Considerable trauma and hemorrhage are produced by the eggs as they are filtered through the perivascular tissues into the lumen. Eggs trapped in these sites are walled off, usually individually, by an eosinophilic abscess, which later transforms into a characteristic pseudotubercle (granuloma). The egg, or its shell only, is usually surrounded by foreign body giant cells and epithelioid cells. The entire lesion often is surrounded by a peripheral ring of connective tissue, eosinophils, plasma cells, and lymphocytes. The acute stage is ush-

ered in with diarrhea or dysentery and the appearance of eggs in the stools. Daily fever, anorexia, loss of weight, severe abdominal pain, and anemia are common. Many of the eggs are swept into the intrahepatic portal vessels, where they provoke pseudotubercle formation. Liver involvement is more rapid and severe in *S. japonicum* infections. The liver becomes tender and enlarged. Coarse bands of dense connective tissue, chiefly about the large radicals of the portal vein, have been responsible for the term, "Symmer's clay pipestem fibrosis," associated with schistosomiasis japonica and mansoni. It should be added that nests of *S. japonicum* eggs often occur also in ectopic sites, such as the brain and heart.

The chronic stage of schistosomiasis is one of tissue proliferation and repair. The intestinal wall becomes thickened by fibrosis, and the lumen may be reduced considerably. Anal polyps are common, as are papillomas and fistulas. Hemorrhoids may be the first indication of the infection, due to portal obstruction. The liver may become increasingly damaged due to extensive periportal fibrosis, and there may be a compensatory congestive enlargement of the spleen, especially in *S. japonicum* infections. Thus in many there is a rapidly developing dysfunction of the intestinal wall and periportal tissues. In the late stages of the disease in those with heavy infections, emaciation is severe, and many victims die of exhaustion or a concurrent infection.

In the case of *S. haematobium,* the acute stage involves mainly the wall of the urinary bladder, but the lungs also may be involved. The latter involvement is due to eggs, and at times worms, which are probably carried via the common iliac vein, the inferior vena cava, and the right heart to reach the pulmonary arterioles. Here pseudotubercles are produced as described above, and in time pulmonary heart disease (cor pulmonale) may develop. The damage produced in the wall of the urinary bladder is similar to that described above for the wall of the intestine. Hematuria usually is the first evidence of infection. As time passes, the bladder wall becomes thickened by dense fibrosis of the muscular and submucous coats, and multiple urinary polyps, papillomas, and fistulas are common. The superficial mucosa of the bladder may show metaplasia, an intense inflammatory infiltrate, and eggs (many calcified). Fever, suprapubic tenderness, and difficulty in urination are common. Bladder colic is a cardinal symptom. In addition to the bladder, other parts of the genitourinary system often become involved. Finally, it is worth noting that in some areas there is a close association between chronic schistosomiasis of the bladder and carcinoma, since eggs .in capillaries are seen in the midst of an infiltrating carcinoma. In fact, the term "Egyptian irritation cancer" is well known.

LABORATORY DIAGNOSIS. In a majority of cases, *S. haematobium* eggs can be demonstrated in the sediment that settles out of urine. In some instances, a small bladder biopsy specimen will reveal the eggs when they cannot be demonstrated in urine. If these measures fail in suspected cases, stool examinations and/or rectal biopsies should be considered, since these worms may involve the rectum as well. The mature eggs contain a miracidium, are rounded at the anterior pole, and have a terminal spine (Fig. 92-2). They range from 112 to 170 μm in length by 40 to 70 μm in width (average 150 by 60 μm). Intradermal and serologic tests, although available, usually are not needed to provide evidence of infection.

The eggs of *S. japonicum* and *S. mansoni* usually can be recovered from the stools of patients during the acute stage, but they tend to be released in clutches, making it necessary to perform repeated examinations at intervals for a period of one month before ruling out the infection. *S. japonicum* eggs are rotund, measure 70 to 100 μm by 50 to 70μm (average, 89 by 66 μm), and have a rudimentary lateral spine within a hook cavity (Fig. 92-2). Those of *S. mansoni* are rounded at both ends, measure 114 to 175 μm by 45 to 70 μm (average, 150 by 60 μm), and have a conspicuous lateral spine near one pole (Fig. 92-2). The eggs of *S. japonicum* are more numerous and tend to be mixed with the feces. For this reason, a cross-section of the bolus should be used for examination. On the other hand, eggs of *S. mansoni* tend to be concentrated in the outer layer, especially in mucus. In both infections, but especially in those with *S. mansoni*, simple fecal smears may fail to reveal the eggs, making it necessary to use a concentration technique. Sedimentation alone is helpful, but best results are obtained following the use of the acid-ether-detergent method or the acid-sodium sulfate-ether-detergent method. In chronic cases, rectal biopsy often will reveal eggs when they have not been found in many different stool specimens. Intradermal and complement-fixation tests with schistosome antigen are available.

TREATMENT. Potassium antimony tartrate, given intravenously, is the only effective drug against *S. japonicum*. For treating cases of *S. mansoni* and *S. haematobium*, Fuadin (intramuscular) or Miracil D (oral) is recommended. The latter is preferred by most clinicians treating cases in the United States, since it appears to be as effective as Fuadin, is less toxic, and is easier to administer, especially to children.

TREATMENT OF HELMINTHIC INFECTIONS

The following references are recommended to those who wish to check the doses and pertinent details about the administration of the various drugs listed in the text above.

Brown HW: Basic Clinical Parasitology, 4th ed. New York, Appleton-Century-Crofts, 1975

Faust EC, Beaver PC, Jung RC: Animal Agents and Vectors of Human Disease, 4th ed. Philadelphia, Lea & Febiger, 1975

Hunter GW III, Frye WW, Swartzwelder JC: Manual of Tropical Medicine, 4th ed. Philadelphia, Saunders, 1966

Markell EK, Voge M: Medical Parasitology, 3rd ed. Philadelphia, Saunders, 1971

NOTE: In addition to the drugs listed in the text, there are other effective ones not yet released on the market in this country (eg, Ambilhar for the treatment of schistosomiasis). These are available to physicians *on an investigational basis* and can be obtained from Dr. M.G. Schultz, Center for Disease Control, Atlanta, Georgia 30333.

Index

A particles, 890
A protein, 923
a subunits, 898
A-type particles, 901–2
A₂ antibodies, 364
AAV, 785, 807
ABO blood group system, 363
Abortive infection, 853
Absidia, 1043, 1102, 1103
  corymbifera, 1103
Acanthocheilonema perstans, 1154
Accelerated reaction, 939–40
Acetoin, 56
Acetylcholine, 318
  anaphylaxis and, 318–19
N-Acetylmuramul-ʟ-alanyl-ᴅ-*iso*-glutamine, 100
N-Acetylneuraminic acid, 459, 801
Acholeplasmataceae, 756
Achondroplasia, 351–52
Achorion schoenleinii, 1046
Acidaminococcus, 655
  identification of, 639
Acid-fast
  bacilli, 510
  bacteria
    envelope components of, 90
    integument of, 97–98
  stain, 25
Acids as sterilizing agents, 232
Acinetobacter, 457
  differential properties of, 458
Acremoniella lutzi, 1076
Acridine orange, 127, 145
Acrotheca type of conidiophore, 1078
ACTH, 1007
Actinobacillus, 622
  actinomycetemcomitans, 477, 622
Actinomadura, 549, 551
  pelletierii, 553
Actinomyces, 654
  bovis, 544
    differential characteristics of, 548
  dental caries and, 716
  identification of, 639
  israelii, 544, 545, 546
    differential characteristics of, 538
  naeslundii, 544, 547
    differential characteristics of, 548
  as normal flora in humans, 641

Actinomyces (cont.)
  Propionibacterium and, 654
Actinomycetaceae, 544
Actinomycetes, 503, 543–54
  aerobic, 549–54
    comparison of pathogenic, 550
  anaerobic, 544–49
    antigenic structure, 547
    clinical infection, 547–49
    cultural characteristics, 545–46
    epidemiology, 547
    laboratory identification, 546–47
    morphology, 544–45
    pathogenesis, 547–49
    treatment, 549
  maduromycosis and, 1075
Actinomycin, 206
  inhibiting protein synthesis, 207
Actinomycosis, 549, 1075
  abdominal, 549
  cervicofacial, 549
  thoracic, 549
Actinomycotic mycetoma, 554, 1075
Activated C3, receptors for, 324
Activation, metabolite, 190
Acute poststreptococcal glomerulonephritis (AGN), 439–40
Acute rheumatic fever (ARF), 438–39
α-Adamantanamine, 869, 871
Adaptation of viruses, 770
Addison's disease, idiopathic, 337
Adeno-associated satellite virus, 798
Adeno-associated viruses, 785, 807
  adenoviruses and, 864
Adenoidal tissues, 271
Adeno-satellite viruses, 960–61
Adenosine 3′, 5′-cyclic monophosphate (AMP), 182
  cyclic, 63, 176
Adenosine deaminase, 351
Adenosine triphosphatase, 72
Adenosine triphosphate (ATP), 49
  key position of, 50–51
S-Adenosylmethionine, 164
Adenoviridae, 805–6
Adenovirus-associated viruses, 960–61
  selected readings on, 961
Adenovirus(es), 783, 785, 792, 793, 959–60
  adeno-associated viruses and, 864
  base composition of, 798, 799

1169